MW01196233

Will Maclean
Jane Lyttleton

Clinical
Handbook
of Internal
Medicine

The Treatment of Disease with Traditional Chinese Medicine

Volume 3
Qi, blood, fluid and channel disorders

Pangolin Press

National Library of Australia Cataloguing–in–Publication data:
Maclean, Will and Lyttleton, Jane
Clinical Handbook of Internal Medicine, Volume 3

Bibliography
Includes Index
ISBN: 978–0–9579720–1–8

1. Internal diseases 2. Medicine, Chinese

Published and distributed by Pangolin Press (www.pangolinpress.com.au)

Cover Design: Yolande Gray Design
Illustrations: Karen Vance

ABOUT THE AUTHORS

Will Maclean studied Chinese medicine in Australia and China, and has been in practice since 1987. He is the author, with Jane Lyttleton, of the Clinical Handbook series, and with Kathryn Taylor of the Clinical Manual of Chinese Herbal Patent Medicines. He has lectured in Australia and New Zealand, the United States, Europe and South Africa, and continues to be actively involved in the development and practice of Chinese medicine.

Jane Lyttleton began her studies in science in New Zealand and then London with doctoral studies in genetics before succumbing to the siren song of Chinese medicine. She is the author of Treatment of Infertility with Chinese Medicine (Elsevier) and is in great demand world wide as a lecturer. She has always had a keen interest in the way Chinese medicine can be applied to gynecological disorders in a modern western context, and has run Chinese medicine clinics in women's health centres and general medical centres since the early 1980s. In addition to her own busy practice she has established a number of clinics which work closely with IVF clinics and the University of Western Sydney, and which are providing the platform for data collection and clinical research.

ACKNOWLEDGEMENTS

Thanks to all who contributed to this work in some way, in particular my coauthor and editor Jane Lyttleton, my wonderful and patient wife Kathryn who's forbearance and editing skills went beyond the call of duty, and daughter Molly for keeping me entertained. Special thanks to Bill Maclean, and Christine Flynn for her feedback. Thanks also to the good people of Darjeeling where much of this book took shape, especially Subash and Hera Temang, Norbu and Lhamu Deveka and Mahommed Latif. All care has been taken to ensure accuracy and efficacy of the material presented. Any omissions or errors are wholly my own. WM.

All the people Will has mentioned above I would like to thank too, even the ones I don't know personally, because they all have played a part in the making of this final tome in the Handbook series. It has taken us a long time to finish this volume, partly because its contents cover topics that are more complex and more inaccessible than some of the other material we have presented. It is thanks to Will's creative and persistent determination that it all finally came together. My colleagues in the various clinics I work with continue to be a constant support and source of inspiration (especially the new generation of Chinese medical doctors coming up behind us). My family have put up with an awful lot of my back view as I am hunched over the computer, and I hope they know how much their patience is appreciated. JL.

TERMINOLOGY

We have tried, to the best of our ability, to present this work in plain English, which we feel is perfectly adequate for expressing the essential clinical concepts of Chinese medicine. In general, we follow the Eastland press terminology, with a few variations.

Supplement is used instead of tonify (*bǔ* 补), as it is slightly better at suggesting the replacement of something missing; activate replaces invigorate (*huó* 活) when applied to blood; pungent (*xīn* 辛) replaces acrid when describing that attribute of herbs; network vessels (*luò* 络) replaces collaterals.

Capitalized organs are the internal organs (*zàng fǔ* 脏腑) of Chinese medicine. Lower case organs are the physical organs of anatomical medicine.

Contents

THE TEXT

The introduction to each pattern attempts to give an overview of the pattern and the mechanisms behind it.

Prescriptions

The prescriptions in this text have been modified to suit the specific conditions being treated, and to remove endangered animal and plant species (those listed in Appendix 1 of the Convention on International Trade in Endangered Species [CITES], in which all trade is banned). Items legally traded with permits (CITES Appendix 2), remain viable, but may be difficult to obtain. Alternatives for endangered species are recommended in Appendix 6, p.935. Herbs in italics are modifications to the original prescription. Prescriptions are also described as modified when doses of specific ingredients are altered from the standard to address particular conditions.

Prepared medicines

The prepared medicines recommended in this text are all available from reputable manufacturers who adhere to Good Manufacturing Practice (GMP) standards. The majority (those available for sale in Australia) are registered with the Australian Therapeutic Goods Administration (TGA). Although some prepared medicines retain the name of an endangered species (for example Mu Xiang Shun Qi Wan), the endangered herb has been replaced with substitutes of similar activity.

Acupuncture

The acupuncture points recommended are derived from standard acupuncture texts, and more points than should be used in an individual treatment are listed to allow for variations. The points listed for any pattern are not meant to be exhaustive or definitive.

Key to the symbols following acupuncture points

absence of a symbol denotes an even method (*ping bu ping xie* 平补平泻)

+ apply a supplementing method (*bu fa* 补法)

− apply a reducing method (*xie fa* 泻法)

▲ use moxa; stick, warm needle, rice grain, moxa box or equivalent

Ω apply cups

↓ bleed with a surgical lancet

Clinical notes

Information regarding prognosis, probable treatment lengths and other auxiliary aspects of treatment are based on the authors combined forty years of clinical experience.

ABDOMINAL MASSES

In Chinese medicine abdominal masses are known as *zhēng jiǎ jī jù*[1] 癥瘕积聚. Zheng jia ji ju is a collective term for both physical masses and transitory swellings in the abdominal cavity.

Zheng and ji are solid masses associated with structural pathology of affected tissues. Tumors, cysts, fibroids, abscesses and inflammatory lesions are examples of zheng and ji type masses. Jia and ju masses are transitory swellings resulting from functional disorder of the affected tissues. They are associated with spasm, congestion, edema and constipation, and are not associated with structural change. Ji ju masses and swellings are found in the upper abdomen. Zheng jia are found in the lower abdomen and are associated with reproductive structures.

This chapter focuses on masses associated with structural pathology. The transitory swellings, the ju and jia types, will typically present with symptoms such as abdominal pain, distension or constipation, rather than a palpable mass or swelling. Analysis of these conditions can be found in Volume 2 of the Clinical Handbook series.

There are four types of abdominal mass, blood, phlegm, heat and cold. In practice, mixtures of pathology are common. Most masses are due to blood stasis or phlegm, or a combination of both, with or without heat or cold. Some masses are due to focal accumulation of heat or cold, with blood stasis or phlegm as secondary complications. Blood stasis or phlegm accumulation may be the result of, or a contributing factor to, pathology such as toxic heat or damp heat, cold, qi constraint, organ system weakness and deficiencies of qi, blood, yin and yang.

Traditionally, abdominal masses were detected by palpation. The advent of mod-

BOX 1.1 PATTERNS OF ABDOMINAL MASSES

Blood
Liver
Epigastrium
Spleen
Intestines
Low abdomen, hypogastrium
  – with cold
  – mild stasis

Phlegm
Liver
Abdomen, non specific
Spleen
Epigastrium
Hypogastrium

Heat
Liver
  – toxic heat
  – damp heat
  – chronic damp heat with
    qi and yin deficiency
  – yin deficiency
Epigastrium
Intestines
Hypogastrium

Cold, yang qi deficiency
Liver, Gallbladder
Liver yang deficiency
Epigastrium
Lower abdomen
Hypogastrium
  – Kidney deficiency
  – qi and blood deficiency

---

1 Practical Dictionary of Chinese Medicine (1998) – 'concretions, conglomerations, accumulations and gatherings'

ern imaging techniques has increased our ability to examine the abdominal cavity and detect masses that may be undetectable by palpation. Imaging enables precise determination of the structures or organs affected. If an impalpable mass is detected by ultrasound or CT scanning in the course of investigation, it can be treated as a mass in Chinese medical terms, even though traditionally it would not be diagnosed according to the Chinese medical disease category of abdominal mass. Knowledge of the presence of a mass, before it becomes palpable, simply enhances our ability to treat it at a more responsive phase.

ETIOLOGY

Emotional factors

Any emotional factor that leads to stagnation of qi can lead to blood stasis, as qi leads the blood. The emotions most likely to contribute to abdominal masses are those that influence the Liver and Spleen, Intestines and Uterus. Unexpressed frustration, chronic stress, anger and resentment disrupt free flow of Liver qi. Sexual frustration can also be a contributing factor to qi and blood stagnation in the lower abdomen, especially in women. Masses related to Liver dysfunction appear in the regions dominated by the Liver system, the hypochondriac region and the liver organ itself, the lower abdomen and the reproductive system. Chronic Liver qi constraint can cause further complication. Repeated invasion of the Spleen by pent up Liver qi weakens digestion and leads to dampness and phlegm. Qi constraint can generate heat, which can combine with damp to generate damp heat or be congealed further into phlegm. Heat can also damage yin and congeal blood.

Worry, obsessive thinking and prolonged concentration in combination with a sedentary lifestyle and poor diet, can weaken Spleen qi and disrupt the qi dynamic. Once the qi dynamic is blocked, the movement of qi and blood through the abdomen is compromised, blood slows and stagnates, the Spleen and Stomach are weakened, and damp and phlegm are produced.

Diet

The type of food consumed, and the way it is consumed, can contribute to the formation of abdominal masses. An excess of cold, raw or greasy foods, and/or irregular eating times weaken Spleen qi, resulting in poor circulation of qi and blood and the generation of dampness and phlegm. Any dietary habit that re-

BOX 1.2 BIOMEDICAL CAUSES OF ABDOMINAL MASS

hepatic cirrhosis
hepatosplenomegaly
  – lymphoma
  – leukemia
  – malaria
tumors of the stomach, intestines, liver, uterus, ovaries, pancreas, lymph nodes, bladder
mesenteric lymphadenopathy
aortic aneurysm (pulsatile swelling)
diverticular disease
appendiceal abscess
Crohn's disease
fibroids
ovarian cyst
polycystic or enlarged kidney
pancreatic pseudocyst
pancreatic abscess
cholecystitis
pregnancy
ectopic pregnancy
distended urinary bladder

Table 1.1 Characteristics of abdominal masses

Type	General features	Pain and location
Blood	Mass may be well defined with clear but rough or irregular edges, or be an area of increased tissue density and hard texture within otherwise normal feeling tissue. Mass is firm or hard and immobile. No change with prolonged pressure. May appear quite dense and irregularly shaped with ultrasound.	Often (but not always) painful when pressed; the pain stays the same or is made worse with continued pressure; fixed, always found in the same spot. Blood stasis masses tend to grow within organ or muscle tissue.
Phlegm	Mass is well defined, smooth, soft or rubbery and rounded. Fixed in position, but may be able to be moved slightly over basement tissues. Appears solid and round on ultrasound. If visualized by laparoscopy, the surface of the mass may appear shiny and pearl-like or opaque.	The mass itself is usually not painful or tender with palpation, but it may impinge on other pain producing structures. These masses may be pedunculated, growing on the surface of organs or in between tissue layers.
Heat	Mass feels warmer than the surrounding tissue and usually soft and squishy. May appear regular in shape with imaging.	Can be quite tender to palpation, with muscle guarding over the lesion, and rebound tenderness.
Cold	Soft mass under tissue that feels cooler than that surrounding it; abdominal wall usually cool, pale and lax.	Generally non tender or only mildly tender with palpation, depending on degree of complicating blood stasis and/or yang qi deficiency.

peatedly introduces heat or damp heat into the body can lead to accumulation of damp heat and mass formation. An example of this is seen in the nodules formed in the cirrhotic liver of one who drinks to excess. The damp heat introduced by an excessive intake of alcohol blocks the circulation of qi and blood through the Liver, causing the gradual development of blood stasis and fibrotic nodules.

Overeating leads to food stagnation, disruption of the qi dynamic and the generation of heat, damp heat and phlegm. Chronic heat or damp heat from overeating may injure Intestinal yin, congeal blood and disrupt the integrity of the intestinal lining. Phlegm accumulation will block the free movement of qi and eventually evolve into blood stasis.

External pathogens

The external pathogens with the greatest potential to create abdominal masses are damp heat and cold. Damp heat can invade through the mouth or genitals, or be introduced in the diet. Once damp heat has lodged in the body, most commonly in the reproductive system, Liver and Large Intestine, it can be difficult to dislodge and will often become chronic. The effects of chronic damp heat may be subclinical, but its presence still obstructs qi and blood, and blood stasis may complicate it over time. This is seen in the liver tumors that may complicate chronic

Figure 1.1 Regional guide to mass pathology. Page reference in bold.

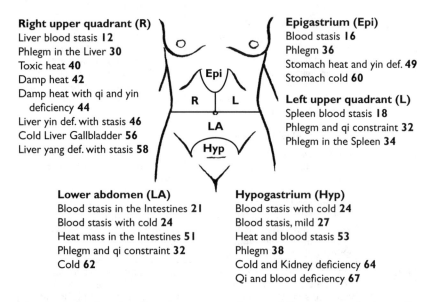

Right upper quadrant (R)
Liver blood stasis **12**
Phlegm in the Liver **30**
Toxic heat **40**
Damp heat **42**
Damp heat with qi and yin
  deficiency **44**
Liver yin def. with stasis **46**
Cold Liver Gallbladder **56**
Liver yang def. with stasis **58**

Epigastrium (Epi)
Blood stasis **16**
Phlegm **36**
Stomach heat and yin def. **49**
Stomach cold **60**

Left upper quadrant (L)
Spleen blood stasis **18**
Phlegm and qi constraint **32**
Phlegm in the Spleen **34**

Lower abdomen (LA)
Blood stasis in the Intestines **21**
Blood stasis with cold **24**
Heat mass in the Intestines **51**
Phlegm and qi constraint **32**
Cold **62**

Hypogastrium (Hyp)
Blood stasis with cold **24**
Blood stasis, mild **27**
Heat and blood stasis **53**
Phlegm **38**
Cold and Kidney deficiency **64**
Qi and blood deficiency **67**

hepatitis, the chronic inflammatory masses that can follow an unresolved sexually transmitted disease (for example a tubal infection) or chronic dysentery (causing a liver abscess or diverticular abscess).

External cold can easily penetrate the female reproductive system, especially during menstruation and after childbirth. Once cold is present, it constricts qi and blood movement through the local area, and over time contributes to blood stasis and mass formation.

Deficiency

Weakness of qi and yang can lead to slowing of blood circulation and pooling of blood. The lower burner is where blood tends to pool, being the lowest point of the abdominal cavity. Sluggish circulation may be due to Heart and Lung qi deficiency and weakness of qi and blood movement in general, or to weak Kidney qi that specifically affects lower burner qi movement. Deficient yang adds the constriction of cold to the poor circulation, and so is even more likely to produce blood stasis. Weak qi also contributes to the development of phlegm by causing poor fluid metabolism and Spleen weakness. Physiological fluids congeal into phlegm when sluggish, and the damp created by Spleen deficiency can thicken into phlegm simply by languishing, or by being cooked by heat.

Deficiency of yin and blood can also lead to blood stasis; yin deficiency because of the combined effect of the thickening of yin fluids characteristic of yin depletion, and the evaporating effect of the heat derived from yin deficiency, and blood deficiency by allowing the blood to congregate in pools, in the same way as stagnant pools form in the bed of a diminishing river.

BOX 1.3 CAUTIONS

- An impacted stool can be mistaken for a mass, especially in the elderly, when they may experience spurious diarrhea
- A pulsatile mass in the midline around the umbilicus is an aortic aneurysm
- Lesions of the abdominal wall (scars, adhesions) can be mistaken for masses
- A biomedical investigation is essential when a mass is detected
- A mass that changes quickly is malignant until proven otherwise

Inheritance

A predisposition to some types of mass runs through families. For example, a tendency to qi and blood stasis and phlegm accumulation can be inherited. This is observed in the increased incidence of gynecological masses like fibroids and cysts, and bowel polyps and tumors within family groups.

ABDOMINAL PALPATION

When a mass is palpable, it should be assessed according to the criteria in Table 1.1, p.3. When a mass is not able to be palpated, the abdomen can still provide valuable diagnostic clues. Even though a mass is by definition an excess pathology, the constitution of the patient and the etiology giving rise to the mass may be deficient. The tone of the abdominal wall, temperature variations, and pain and the response of pain to palpation are assessed. A thorough discussion of this valuable diagnostic technique is beyond the scope of this book, but see Abbate (2001) and Matsumoto and Birch (1988) for a full review.

Abdominal tone

A firm or resistant abdominal wall suggests an excess condition. A soft or flaccid abdominal wall suggests a deficient condition. An increase or decrease in tone can be regional, with some areas firm and others weak and flaccid. This is commonly seen in mixed patterns. Muscle resistance along the margin of the ribs with a toneless epigastric region suggests Liver qi constraint and Spleen deficiency. A patient with blood stasis in the lower abdomen plus a weakness of Spleen yang may exhibit a cool epigastrium with weak tone but a firm lower abdomen.

Temperature

Regional variation in temperature can provide clues about the underlying state of qi and blood circulation, and the yang qi and yin. A cool lower abdomen below the navel is often seen in Kidney yang deficiency, while a cool epigastrium is seen in Spleen yang deficiency. A tender mass that feels warmer than the surrounding tissue suggests heat or damp heat, while a firm mass that feels cooler than the surrounding tissue suggests qi and blood stasis from cold or yang deficiency.

Pain

Masses may be tender or non tender with palpation. Masses with blood stasis or heat are more likely to be tender than those with phlegm or cold. A mass that is painful when pressed and stays worse with continued pressure is of an excess type, regardless of the deficient or otherwise weak state of the patient. Pain that is

Figure 1.2 Anatomy and landmarks (female)

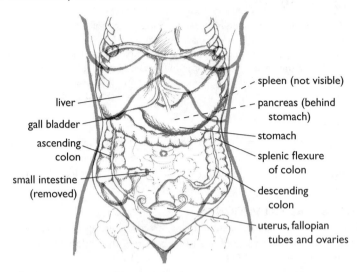

relieved by, or at least no worse with pressure, can be associated with either excess or deficiency, depending on the firmness of the mass. A hard and irregular but non tender mass is still an excess type, requiring an attacking strategy, regardless of the weak or deficient appearance of the patient. A soft non tender mass is most likely associated with deficiency of yang qi, phlegm or cold.

When a pattern appears contradictory, the abdominal palpation findings can help discrimination. For example, a thin pale patient with obvious signs of qi deficiency might complain of right lower abdominal pain which is definitely worse with palpation. Even though the patient is weak, the therapy should be aimed at clearing the excess in the lower abdomen, with secondary support for zheng qi.

TREATMENT

The aim of treatment is to resolve the mass. In general, this requires an attacking strategy that uses strong dispersing and mass resolving herbs or acupuncture techniques. Strong attacking and dispersing treatments can disperse both the pathogen and the patient's zheng qi, and thus have the potential for iatrogenic depletion of qi and blood. Even when a patient appears deficient and weak however, a strong treatment is usually required, as attacking and eliminating the stasis will result in enhanced creation and distribution of new qi and blood.

Elderly and feeble patients with a mass of an excess type should be treated 'cautiously but courageously', and monitored closely for signs of increasing deficiency. Strong attacking treatment can be moderated with appropriate supplements to offset their potential negative effects if necessary. If such a patient is going to react badly to a strong treatment they usually do so quite quickly, before too much damage is done.

Having said this, there are however some masses, specifically those in the lower abdomen, that are the result of pooling of blood from yang deficiency and that respond to treatment of the deficiency rather than direct attack upon the mass. Experience has demonstrated supplementation and yang activation to be effective in resolving masses of this type. Similarly, when treating masses due to the drying and contracting effects of yin deficiency, the main aim is to replenish the yin, with gentle dispersal of the stasis in support. Salty herbs that draw liquid back into the damaged tissues while gently softening hardness are ideal (Table 1.2, p.8).

Masses associated with heat require heat clearing as the primary strategy, in combination with blood activation. Blood activation plays a secondary but important role here, by enabling the heat clearing herbs, as well as healing qi and blood to access the lesion. The heat is usually in the form of damp heat or toxic heat.

Cold masses are warmed and dispersed with phlegm transformation, blood activation or supplementation as appropriate.

Successful treatment depends on selecting the correct course of action, and the type of biomedical disease state. Chinese medicine is an appropriate treatment choice for some types of abdominal mass, such as those associated with chronic inflammation, benign gynecological tumors and cysts. The prognosis for other types of mass, such as malignant tumors, scarring and stricture, is poorer, and treatment requires a combined Western and Chinese medical approach.

Figure 1.3 Regions and pathology of abdominal masses

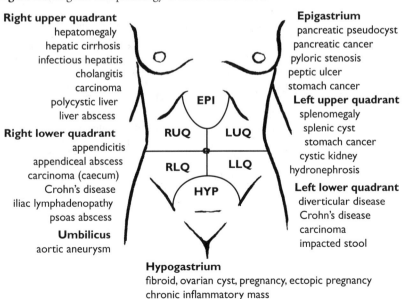

Right upper quadrant
hepatomegaly
hepatic cirrhosis
infectious hepatitis
cholangitis
carcinoma
polycystic liver
liver abscess
Right lower quadrant
appendicitis
appendiceal abscess
carcinoma (caecum)
Crohn's disease
iliac lymphadenopathy
psoas abscess
Umbilicus
aortic aneurysm

EPI

RUQ   LUQ

RLQ   LLQ

HYP

Epigastrium
pancreatic pseudocyst
pancreatic cancer
pyloric stenosis
peptic ulcer
stomach cancer
Left upper quadrant
splenomegaly
splenic cyst
stomach cancer
cystic kidney
hydronephrosis
Left lower quadrant
diverticular disease
Crohn's disease
carcinoma
impacted stool

Hypogastrium
fibroid, ovarian cyst, pregnancy, ectopic pregnancy
chronic inflammatory mass
ovarian, endometrial, bladder and prostate cancer
endometriosis

Table 1.2 Herbs that soften hardness, transform phlegm and dissipate masses

Zhe Bei Mu Fritillaria thunbergii Bulbus 浙贝母	Xiao Luo Wan 消瘰丸	Zhejiang fritillaria tuber; bitter, cold; Heart, Lung. Dissipates nodules. For phlegm masses anywhere in the body, usually in combination with **mu li** and **xuan shen**. 9-12 grams in decoction.
Mu Li Ostreae Concha 牡蛎		Oyster shell; salty, astringent, cool; Liver, Kidney. Softens hardness and dissipates masses and nodules. For a variety of masses and swellings from phlegm and blood stasis, including hepatospleno-megaly, benign gynecological tumors, goitre and thyroid nodules. 15-30 grams in decoction.
Xuan Shen Scrophularia Radix 玄参		Scrophularia root; salty, sweet, bitter, cool; Kidney, Lung. Softens hardness, dissipates masses and nodules, cools the blood and nourishes yin. For phlegm masses and inflammatory masses anywhere, but especially those in the neck and gynecological systems, and those associated with yin deficiency. 12-24 grams in decoction.
Wa Leng Zi Arcae Concha 瓦楞子		Ark shell; sweet, salty, neutral; Lung, Stomach, Spleen, Liver. Activates blood, disperses phlegm, softens hardness and dissipates masses. Used for phlegm and blood stasis masses, especially gynecological tumors such as fibroids and endometriosis. Also used for masses in the neck. 15-30 grams in decoction.
Hai Zao Sargassum 海藻 **Kun Bu** Eckloniae Thallus 昆布		Hai Zao (sargassum seaweed) – bitter, salty, cold; Kun Bu (kelp) – salty, cold; both enter the Liver, Stomach and Kidney. Used together to disperses phlegm and dissipate nodules. For phlegm masses and nodules anywhere, but especially those in the gynecological system, neck and testicles. 15-30 grams of each in decoction.
Wei Ling Xian Clematidis Radix 威灵仙		Chinese clematis root; pungent, salty, warm; enters all organs and channels. Dispels wind damp, dissipates phlegm and blood stasis, and stops pain. Primarily used for painful masses from either phlegm and/or blood stasis. Contraindicated in very deficient patients. 6-12 grams in decoction.
Zao Jiao Gleditsiae Fructus 皂角		Chinese honeylocust fruit; pungent, salty, warm, slightly toxic; Lung, Large Intestine. Zao jiao is used for phlegm masses, especially those in the Stomach and Intestines. It is also laxative and can expel roundworms. 3-6 grams in decoction, or better, 0.8-1.5 grams in pills or powder.

Table 1.3 Herbs that activate blood and dissipate masses

E Zhu Curcumae Rhizoma 莪术 **San Leng** Sparganii Rhizoma 三棱	E zhu (curcuma); bitter, pungent, warm. **San leng** (sparganium); bitter, pungent, neutral; both enter the Liver and Spleen, break up blood stasis and disperse masses. These herbs are the most important and widely used pair for blood stasis masses. Used together for both benign and malignant tumors. 6-12 grams of each in decoction. When processed with vinegar, their analgesic effect is enhanced; when processed with wine the ability of **san leng** to break up blood stasis and dissipate masses is enhanced.
Bie Jia Trionycis Carapax 鳖甲	Soft shelled turtle shell; salty, cold; Liver, Spleen. Activates blood, softens hardness, dissipates nodules and nourishes yin. For blood stasis abdominal masses, especially those associated with swelling of the Liver and Spleen, and masses in the reproductive system. Most suitable when there is yin deficiency. 15-30 grams in decoction.
Hu Po Succinum 琥珀	Amber; sweet, neutral; Liver, Heart, Urinary Bladder. Activates blood and dissipates masses. For a variety of abdominal masses from blood stasis. Best for painful masses in the lower burner and Uterus. 1.5-3 grams in powder or pills.
Wang Bu Liu Xing Vaccariae Semen 王不留行	Vaccaria seed; bitter, neutral; Liver, Stomach. Activates blood and reduces swelling. For abdominal masses from blood stasis and chronic inflammation, especially in the lower burner and prostate. Substitutes for the scales of the endangered pangolin, chuan shan jia 穿山甲. 3-9 grams in decoction.
Jiu Da Huang Rhei Radix et Rhizoma 酒大黄	Rhubarb root; bitter, cold; Heart, Liver, Stomach, Large Intestine. An important herb for all acute and chronic blood stasis masses, including those from trauma. Prepared in alcohol and cooked for at least 20 minutes to enhance its blood activating properties. 3-15 grams in decoction.
Ling Xiao Hua Campsis Flos 凌霄花	Trumpet creeper flower; sweet, sour, cool; Liver, Pericardium. Activates blood and dissipates masses. For abdominal masses from blood stasis and heat. 6-9 grams, decocted.
Shui Hong Hua Zi Polygoni orientale Semen 水红花子	Polygonum orientale seed; salty, cool; Liver. Activates blood, softens hardness, dissipates masses and stops pain. For a variety of abdominal blood stasis masses, especially of the Liver, Spleen and lymphatic systems. Best when there is pain. 15-30 grams in decoction.
Ma Bian Cao Verbenae Herba 马鞭草	Verbena; bitter, cool; Liver, Spleen. Activates blood, dissipates masses and kills parasites. For blood stasis with heat in the Liver and lower burner. For Liver abscess, chronic malaria, chronic inflammatory masses and gynecological masses. 15-30 grams in decoction.
Di Bie Chong Eupolyphaga/ Steleophaga 地鳖虫	Field cockroach; salty, cold, toxic; Liver. For blood stasis abdominal masses, including hepatosplenomegaly, benign gynecological tumors and ectopic pregnancy. The mildest of the insect products. 5-10 grams in decoction, or 1-2 grams in pills or powder.

Table 1.4 Herbs that treat inflammatory masses

Xia Ku Cao Prunellae Spica 夏枯草	Selfheal spike; bitter, pungent, cold; Liver, Gallbladder. Cools the Liver and dissipates masses and nodules. An important herb for all masses with heat. Used for both acute and chronic inflammatory masses. 12–18 grams in decoction.
Bai Jiang Cao Patriniae Herba 败酱草	Patrinia; pungent, bitter, cool; Liver, Stomach, Large Intestine. Clears toxic heat, activates blood and reduces abscesses. For a variety of acute and chronic inflammatory masses, especially in the gastrointestinal and reproductive systems. Usually combined with **hong teng**. 10–30 grams in decoction.
Hong Teng Sargentodoxae Caulis 红藤	Sargentodoxa vine; bitter, neutral; Stomach, Large Intestine. Clears toxic heat, activates blood, reduces abscesses and stops pain. For a variety of inflammatory masses, especially with pain. Usually combined with **bai jiang cao**. 10–30 grams in decoction.
Yi Ren Coicis Semen 苡仁	Job's tears; sweet, bland, cool; Spleen, Stomach, Lungs, Kidney. Clears damp heat, promotes urination and aids in discharge of pus. An important herb for inflammatory masses from persistent damp heat, such as Intestinal abscess (chronic appendicitis or diverticulitis). 15–30 grams in decoction. Excellent for long term use.
Zao Jiao Ci Gleditsiae Spina 皂角刺	Chinese honeylocust thorn; pungent, warm; Liver, Stomach. Zao jiao ci reduces swelling and aids in the discharge of pus. Used for abscesses, sores and inflammatory masses to encourage suppuration and rupture. Has the ability to penetrate and open up congested areas and enable other herbs to gain better access. 3–9 grams in decoction.

See also Xuan Shen (Table 1.2), Ma Bian Cao (Table 1.3), Ling Xiao Hua (Table 1.3), Wang Bu Liu Xing (Table 1.3) and Bai Hua She She Cao (Table 1.5)

Table 1.5 Herbs with anti–cancer properties

Bai Hua She She Cao Hedyotidis Herba 白花蛇舌草	Hedyotidis or oldenlandia; sweet, bitter, cool; Liver, Spleen, Kidney. Clears toxic heat, dispels blood stasis and reduces abscesses. An important herb for all tumors and suppurative sores. Usually combined with **ban zhi lian**. For cancer the dose is up to 60-120 grams in decoction.
Ban Zhi Lian Scutellaria barbatae Herba 半枝莲	Scutellaria barbata; bitter, cool; Liver, Lung, Stomach, Kidney. Clears toxic heat. For a wide variety of tumors, particularly early stage liver and gastrointestinal tumors. Usually in combination with **bai hua she she cao**. 15-60 grams in decoction.
Ban Bian Lian Lobeliae chinensis Herba 半边莲	Lobelia; sweet, bland, cool; Lung, Liver, Kidney. Clears toxic heat. For stomach, intestinal and lymphatic cancer, and cancer with ascites. 15-30 grams in decoction.
Long Kui Solanum nigrum Herba 龙葵	Black nightshade; bitter, slightly sweet, cold, slightly toxic; Liver, Spleen, Lung, Urinary Bladder. Clears toxic heat, disperses blood stasis and reduces swelling. Used for a variety of cancers in particular cervical, liver and breast. 10-15 grams in decoction.
Huang Yao Zi Dioscoreae bulbiferae Rhizoma 黄药子	Dioscorea bulbifera rhizome; bitter, cold, toxic; Liver, Stomach, Heart, Lung. Dissipates nodules and goitre. Treats Liver heat and phlegm heat patterns. Used for a variety of cancers, including stomach, intestine and thyroid. Can cause liver damage. Toxicity precludes its use in those with hepatic dysfunction (chronic hepatitis, cirrhosis). 3-15 grams in decoction.
Teng Li Gen Actinidia arguta Radix 藤梨根	Actinidia; sour, astringent, cool; Liver, Stomach, Urinary Bladder. Clears toxic heat, activates blood and reduces swelling. For cancer of the stomach and esophagus. 60-120 grams in decoction.
Shu Yang Quan Solanum lyratum Herba 蜀羊泉	Solanum; slightly bitter, cold; Liver, Gallbladder. Clears toxic heat. For cancer of the liver, cervix, stomach and esophagus. Also used for early cirrhosis and schistosomiasis. 15-30 grams in decoction.
She Mei Duchesnea indica Herba 蛇莓	Duchesnea; sweet, bitter, cold; Liver, Spleen, Large Intestine. Clears toxic heat, disperses blood stasis and accumulations. For cancer of the stomach, intestine and cervix. 10-30 grams in decoction.
Zi Bei Tian Kui Semiaquilegia adoxoides Herba 紫背天葵	Semiaquilegia; sweet, slightly bitter, cold; Liver, Spleen, Kidney. Clears toxic heat, disperses accumulations and reduces swelling. For liver and breast cancer and lymphoma. 10-15 grams in decoction.
Gui Zhen Cao Bidens bipinnata Herba 鬼针草	Bidens; bitter, cool; Liver, Spleen. Stomach, Large Intestine. Clears toxic heat, activates blood and disperses blood stasis. For cancer of the digestive system. 15-60 grams in decoction.
Mao Zhua Cao Ranunculi ternati Radix 猫爪草	Ranunculus; sweet, pungent, warm; Liver. Clears toxin and dissipates nodules. For cancer of the lymphatic system. 10-30 grams in decoction.

1.1 BLOOD MASSES

1. Liver
2. Stomach
3. Spleen
4. Intestines
5. Lower burner
6. Lower burner, mild

肝
臟
血
瘀

1.1.1 BLOOD MASS IN THE LIVER

A blood stasis mass in the liver can be the product of prolonged Liver qi constraint or the prolonged presence of a pathogen such as damp heat. Masses and swellings of this type are chronic, and there will usually be a long history of Liver pathology. In some cases, a mass can develop silently, with few symptoms and little or no pain, until it is discovered upon routine examination.

Chronic Liver blood stasis is frequently complicated by other pathology, in particular qi and yin deficiency.

Clinical features
- Swollen liver with a hard irregular edge, or with a hard, nodular or irregular mass or masses. The liver and masses are likely to be tender with palpation, but may not be. In some cases there may be a palpable mass in the upper left quadrant as well (hepatosplenomegaly).
- hypochondriac pain, if present, is fixed and nagging, or intermittently sharp and intense
- dark or purplish spider nevi or distended vessels over the abdomen and ribs, on the face and around the inner ankle and knee
- dull, sallow or darkish complexion, dark rings under the eyes, dark or purplish lips and conjunctiva
- hectic or irregularly spiking fever, worse at night
- may be easy bruising, purpura, vomiting blood, melena or bleeding from the nose and gums
- marked left iliac fossa pressure pain (p.925–926)
- fatigue, listlessness, weakness
- abdominal distension, loss of appetite, weight loss
- may be dull yellow or dark yellow jaundice

T dark or purple, or with brown or purple stagnation spots; dark congested sublingual veins
P wiry, choppy

Treatment principle
Activate qi and blood and disperse blood stasis
Soften hardness and dissipate masses
Support qi and yin as necessary

Prescription

GE XIA ZHU YU TANG 膈下逐瘀汤
Drive Out Blood Stasis Below the Diaphragm Decoction

dang gui (Angelicae sinensis Radix) 当归 9–12g
chi shao (Paeoniae Radix rubra) 赤芍 9–12g
chuan xiong (Chuanxiong Rhizoma) 川芎 6–9g
tao ren (Persicae Semen) 桃仁 9–12g
hong hua (Carthami Flos) 红花 9–12g
xiang fu (Rhizoma Cyperi) 香附 9–12g
wu yao (Linderae Radix) 乌药 9–12g
zhi ke (Aurantii Fructus) 枳壳 6–9g
gan cao (Glycyrrhizae Radix) 甘草 6–9g
mu dan pi (Moutan Cortex) 牡丹皮 6–9g
chao wu ling zhi (stir fried Trogopterori Faeces) 炒五灵脂 9–12g
cu yan hu suo (vinegar fried Corydalis Rhizoma) 醋延胡索 6–12g
Method: Decoction. **Dang gui**, **chi shao** and **chuan xiong** nourish and activate the blood; **tao ren**, **hong hua** and **chao wu ling zhi** transform and dispel static blood, free the network vessels and stop pain; **mu dan pi** activates and cools the blood; **xiang fu**, **wu yao**, **cu yan hu suo** and **zhi ke** move qi, dredge the Liver and stop pain; **gan cao** protects and harmonizes the Stomach. (Source: *Shi Yong Zhong Yi Nei Ke Xue* [*Yi Lin Gai Cuo*])

Modifications

- With very hard, nodular masses, add **cu e zhu** (vinegar fried Curcumae Rhizoma) 醋莪术 9–12g, **cu san leng** (vinegar fried Sparganii Rhizoma) 醋三棱 9–12g and **bie jia** (Trionycis Carapax) 鳖甲 12–15g. See also Table 1.3, p.9.
- With nodules from hepatic cirrhosis, add **dan shen** (Salviae miltiorrhizae Radix) 丹参 12–15g.
- With round, regular, phlegm type nodules, combine with XIAO LUO WAN (Reduce Scrophula Pill 消瘰丸, pp.8 and 921).
- With stabbing pain, add **shui hong hua zi** (Polygoni orientale Semen) 水红花子 15–30g and **wei ling xian** (Clematidis Radix) 威灵仙 9–12g, or **zhi mo yao** (Myrrha preparata) 炙没药 6–9g and **zhi ru xiang** (Olibanum preparata) 炙乳香 6–9g.
- With diffuse pain and distension, add **yu jin** (Curcumae Radix) 郁金 9–12g and **chuan lian zi** (Toosendan Fructus) 川楝子 9–12g.
- With jaundice, a greasy yellow tongue coat and slippery pulse, add **yin chen** (Artemisiae scopariae Herba) 茵陈 12–18g, **jin qian cao** (Lysimachiae/Desmodii Herba) 金钱草 30–60g, **shan zhi zi** (Gardeniae Fructus) 山栀子 9–12g and **yu jin** (Curcumae Radix) 郁金 9–12g.
- With fever, add **zhi mu** (Anemarrhenae Rhizoma) 知母 9–12g and **shui niu jiao** (Bubali Cornu) 水牛角 15–30g [cooked first].
- With constipation, add **da huang** (Rhei Radix et Rhizoma) 大黄 6–9g.
- With food stagnation, add **shen qu** (Massa medicata fermentata) 神曲 12–15g, and **jiao shan zha** (scorched Crataegi Fructus) 焦山楂 9–12g.
- With fluid in the peritoneal cavity (ascites) and scanty urination, add **hou po** (Magnoliae officinalis Cortex) 厚朴 12–15g, **che qian zi** (Plantaginis

Semen) 车前子 12–15g and **da fu pi** (Arecae Pericarpium) 大复皮 12–15g or combine with **Wu Ling San** (Five Ingredient Powder with Poria 五苓散, p.219–220).

- With bleeding from the digestive tract, or purpura, add **xian he cao** (Agrimoniae Herba) 仙鹤草 12–15g, **san qi fen** (powdered Notoginseng Radix) 三七粉 3–9g [added to the strained decoction], and **qian cao gen** (Rubiae Radix) 茜草根 9–15g, or combine with the prepared medicine **Yun Nan Bai Yao** (Yunnan White Powder 云南白药).
- With Liver yin deficiency, combine with **Yi Guan Jian** (Linking Decoction 一贯煎, p.816).
- With Liver yin deficiency and marked deficient heat, night sweats and fever, combine with **Qing Gu San** (Cool the Bones Powder 清骨散, p.391).
- With Spleen qi deficiency, anorexia, abdominal bloating, loose stools, weakness and fatigue, combine with **Xiang Sha Liu Jun Zi Tang** (Six Gentlemen Decoction with Aucklandia and Amomum 香砂六君子汤, p.618).
- With qi and blood deficiency, fatigue, anxiety, spontaneous sweating and purpura, combine with **Gui Pi Tang** (Restore the Spleen Decoction 归脾汤, p.387).
- With cancer or tumors, add herbs from Table 1.5, p.11, in particular **bai hua she she cao** (Hedyotidis Herba) 白花蛇舌草, **ban zhi lian** (Scutellariae barbatae Herba) 半枝莲, **zi bei tian kui** (Begonia fimbristipulata Herba) 紫背天葵 or **shu yang quan** (Solanum Lyratum Herba) 蜀羊泉.

Prepared medicines
Concentrated powder
Ge Xia Zhu Yu Tang (Tangkuei & Corydalis Combination)
Xue Fu Zhu Yu Tang (Persica & Carthamus Combination)
Xiao Luo Wan (Scrophularia & Fritillaria Combination)
  – combine with one of the above when there is phlegm

Pills
Ge Xia Zhu Yu Wan (Stasis in the Lower Chamber Teapills)
Xue Fu Zhu Yu Wan (Stasis in the Mansion of Blood Teapills)
Nei Xiao Luo Li Wan (Nei Xiao Luo Li Teapills)
Ji Sheng Ju He Wan (Citrus Aurantium Compound Pills, Citrus Seed Pills)
  – the latter two are salty formulae to soften hardness and disperse phlegm;
    combine with a suitable blood activating formula
Yun Nan Bai Yao (Yunnan Paiyao)
Sheng Tian Qi Pian (Raw Tian Qi Ginseng Tablets)
  – either of the latter two can be added when there is bleeding

Topical therapies
Poultice
- A poultice can be prepared by boiling 50 grams of **shui hong hua zi** (Polygoni orientale Semen) 水红花子 in 2–3 cups of water until reduced by half. Strain off the dregs and soak a cloth in the warm liquid, apply to the right hypochon-

drium and leave for as long as possible. Keep the poultice warm.

Acupuncture (select from)

Liv.14 (qimen –) ....alarm point of the Liver, activates Liver qi and blood, dispels static blood

Liv.13 (zhangmen –) ....alarm point of the Spleen and meeting point of the internal yin organs, strengthens the Spleen, promotes Liver function, harmonizes the Liver and Spleen

Sp.21 (dabao –) ....local point, use if tender

ahshi points ....over the right hypochondrium

Bl.17 (geshu –) ....transport point for the diaphragm, meeting point for blood, dispels static blood

Bl.18 (ganshu –) ....transport point of the Liver, dredges the Liver and activates qi and blood

SJ.6 (zhigou –) ....these points together are effective for pain

GB.34 (yanglingquan –)   in the lateral part of the trunk and hypochondrium

GB.40 (qiuxu –)

Liv.3 (taichong –) ....source point of the Liver, activates blood, nourishes yin and stops pain

• with severe pain, add LI.4 (hegu –) and Liv.6 (zhongdu –)
• with nausea and vomiting, add PC.6 (neiguan)
• with Spleen deficiency, add Ren.12 (zhongwan) and St.36 (zusanli)
• with heat in the Liver, add Liv.2 (xingjian –)
• with spasms or cramping pain, add Du.8 (jinsuo –)
• with depression, apply rice grain moxa to Liv.1 (dadun)
• with jaundice, add Du.9 (zhiyang –) and Bl.19 (danshu –)
• Ear points: abdomen, liver, gallbladder, zero point, shenmen, sympathetic, subcortex

Clinical notes

• Blood stasis masses in the liver may be diagnosed as liver cancer, hepatomegaly from chronic malaria or lymphoma, hepatic cirrhosis, hepatic hemangioma or focal nodular hyperplasia. When cancer is the diagnosis a combination of Western and Chinese medicine is required. In cases of cirrhosis, as long as it is not too far advanced, results can be surprisingly good.
• For dietary recommendations see Clinical Handbook, Vol. 2, p.878 and 886.

胃
脘
血
瘀

1.1.2 BLOOD MASS IN THE EPIGASTRIUM

This is a firm, usually palpable, mass in the epigastrium associated with chronic pathology of the stomach or pancreas. This type of mass is most commonly the result of chronic Liver and Spleen Stomach disharmony, or chronic heat and yin deficiency. In both cases, there will be a long history of indigestion, heartburn, pain and upper digestive tract symptoms.

Clinical features

- A firm or hard mass in the epigastrium accompanied by distension and/or pain when palpated. The pain is worse with palpation.
- may be difficulty swallowing with vomiting or regurgitation; vomit may resemble coffee grounds
- may be black or tarry stools, or occult blood in the stools
- poor appetite, weight loss, emaciation
- weakness, fatigue
- left iliac fossa pressure pain (p.925–926)

T mauve or purple body, with brown or purple spots, and dark, congested sublingual veins; with yin deficiency, dry with no coat; with qi and blood deficiency pale mauve and swollen

P wiry, choppy

Treatment principle

Activate blood and rectify qi
Soften hardness, dispel static blood and disperse accumulation

Prescription

SAN LENG TANG 三棱汤
Sparganium Decoction

---

jiu san leng (wine fried Sparganii Rhizoma) 酒三棱 9–12g
e zhu (Curcumae Rhizoma) 莪术 9–12g
dang gui (Angelicae sinensis Radix) 当归 9–12g
bai zhu (Atractylodis macrocephalae Rhizoma) 白术............................ 12–15g
bing lang (Arecae Semen) 槟榔.. 9–12g
mu xiang (Aucklandiae Radix) 木香... 9–12g

Method: Decoction. **Jiu san leng** and **e zhu** activate blood, break up static blood and dissipate masses; **bing lang** and **mu xiang** regulate qi and direct qi downwards; **bai zhu** strengthens the Spleen and supplements qi; **dang gui** nourishes and protects blood. (Source: *Shi Yong Zhong Yi Nei Ke Xue* [*Xuan Ming Fang Lun*])

Modifications

- With sharp or stabbing pain, add **pu huang** (Typhae Pollen) 蒲黄 9–12g and **wu ling zhi** (Trogopterori Faeces) 五灵脂 9–12g.
- With qi stagnation, epigastric focal distension and distending pain, add **chuan lian zi** (Toosendan Fructus) 川楝子 9–12g and **yan hu suo** (Corydalis Rhizoma) 延胡索 9–15g.
- With lack of appetite or indigestion, add **shan zha** (Crataegi Fructus) 山楂

12–15g and **shen qu** (Massa medicata fermentata) 神曲 12–15g.

- With difficulty swallowing or dysphagia, add **dan shen** (Salviae miltiorrhizae Radix) 丹参 9–12g, **xuan fu hua** (Inulae Flos) 旋覆花 12–15g and **dai zhe shi** (Haematitum) 代赭石 12–15g [the last two cooked in a cloth bag].
- With black tarry stools (melena) or occult blood in the stools, add **san qi fen** (powdered Notoginseng Radix) 三七粉 3–9g [added to the strained decoction], **di yu** (Sanguisorbae Radix) 地榆 9–12g, **huai hua mi** (Sophorae Flos immaturus) 槐花米 9–12g and **xian he cao** (Agrimoniae Herba) 仙鹤草 12–15g.
- With phlegm, morning nausea, a thick greasy central tongue coat and slippery pulse, add **zhi ban xia** (Pinelliae Rhizoma preparatum) 制半夏 9–12g, **chen pi** (Citri reticulatae Pericarpium) 陈皮 9–12g, **yi ren** (Coicis Semen) 苡仁 18–30g and **fu ling** (Poria) 茯苓 12–15g.
- With qi and blood deficiency, combine with Ba Zhen Tang (Eight Treasure Decoction 八珍汤, p.275).
- With Stomach yin deficiency, combine with a formula such as Yi Guan Jian (Linking Decoction 一贯煎, p.816) or Sha Shen Mai Men Dong Tang (Glehnia and Ophiopogonis Decoction 沙参麦门冬汤, p.918).
- With cancer or tumors, add herbs from Table 1.5, p.11, in particular **gui zhen cao** (Bidens bipinnata Herba) 鬼针草, **teng li gen** (Actinidia arguta Radix) 藤梨根, **shu yang quan** (Solanum lyratum Herba) 蜀羊泉, **ban zhi lian** (Scutellariae Barbatae Herba) 半枝莲 and **bai hua she she cao** (Hedyotis diffusae Herba) 白花蛇舌草.

Prepared medicines
Concentrated powder
Xue Fu Zhu Yu Tang (Persica & Carthamus Combination)

Pills
Xue Fu Zhu Yu Wan (Stasis in the Mansion of Blood Teapills)
Dan Shen Pian (Dan Shen Pills)
Yun Nan Bai Yao (Yunnan Paiyao)
Sheng Tian Qi Pian (Raw Tian Qi Ginseng Tablets)
   – add one of the last two when there is bleeding
Fu Ke Wu Jin Wan (Woo Garm Yuen Medical Pills)
   – with blood stasis, qi deficiency and cold

Topical therapies
Poultice
See p.14.

Acupuncture (select from)
ahshi points ....over the site of the mass, to disperse local accumulation of qi and blood in the epigastrium and Stomach
Ren.12 (zhongwan –) ....alarm point of the Stomach, reducing method disperses blood stasis
Ren.13 (shangwan –) ....local point for excess patterns of the Stomach
St.21 (liangmen –) ....alleviates epigastric pain

St.34 (liangqiu –) ....cleft point of the Stomach, activates circulation of qi, activates blood in the Stomach and stops pain

St.36 (zusanli –) ....sea point of the Stomach, activates qi and blood and regulates the Stomach

Sp.10 (xuehai –) ....regulates and activates blood

Sp.4 (gongsun) ....connecting point of the Spleen, regulates the Spleen and Stomach, stops epigastric pain

Bl.17 (geshu –)...................meeting point for blood, disperses blood stasis

Bl.18 (ganshu –).................transport point of the Liver, dredges the Liver and activates Liver blood

Bl.21 (weishu –).................transport point of the Stomach, disperses blood stasis from the Stomach

- with nausea and vomiting, add PC.6 (neiguan)
- with irritability or depression, add Liv.3 (taichong) or Liv.1 (dadun ↓)
- with anxiety, add yintang (M–HN–3) and Du. 24 (shenting)
- with difficulty swallowing, add Ren.22 (tiantu) and Ren.17 (shanzhong)
- with cold, add moxa
- Ear points: abdomen, stomach, zero point, shenmen, sympathetic, subcortex

Clinical notes
- A blood stasis mass in the epigastrium may be diagnosed as stomach or pancreatic cancer, pyloric stenosis, esophageal varices, perforated peptic ulcer or bleeding peptic ulcer.
- This type of mass can respond to focused and prolonged treatment. When the diagnosis is stomach cancer, a perforated peptic ulcer or a mechanical stricture, a combination of Chinese and Western medicine is required.
- For dietary recommendations, see Clinical Handbook, Vol. 2, p.878 and 886.

1.1.3 BLOOD MASS IN THE SPLEEN
脾臟症積

This type of mass is associated with swelling of the spleen due to chronic malaria, leukemia or lymphoma. This is a chronic pattern and often complicated by yin and/or qi and blood deficiency.

Clinical features
- A firm mass, sometimes large, in the left upper quadrant. The mass may or may not be tender with palpation.
- distension, fullness, discomfort and pain under the ribs
- low grade, hectic or irregularly spiking fever, worse at night
- tiredness, malaise
- loss of appetite, nausea, weight loss
- bleeding, purpura, melena
- dull, sallow or darkish complexion, dark ring under the eyes, dark or purplish lips and conjunctiva
- spider nevi and distended vessels over the ribs, upper abdomen and lower legs, around the inner knee and ankle
- left iliac fossa pressure pain (p.925–926)

T dark or purple, or with brown or purple stasis spots; dark congested sublingual veins; with yin deficiency, dry with no coat; with qi and blood deficiency pale mauve and swollen
P wiry, choppy

Treatment principle
Activate blood and dispel blood stasis
Soften hardness and dissipate masses

Prescription

BIE JIA WAN 鳖甲丸
Turtle Shell Pills

This prescription is used for swelling of the spleen in a patient with reasonably robust qi.

zhi bie jia (honey fried Trionycis Carapax) 炙鳖甲 120g
duan wa leng zi (calcined Arcae Concha) 煅瓦楞子 120g
chao mai ya (stir fried Hordei Fructus germinantus) 炒麦芽 60g
jiu san leng (wine fried Sparganii Rhizoma) 酒三棱 60g
e zhu (Curcumae Rhizoma) 莪术 60g
di bie chong (Eupolyphaga/Steleophaga) 地鳖虫 60g
xiang fu (Cyperi Rhizoma) 香附 30g
qing pi (Citri reticulatae viride Pericarpium) 青皮 30g
Method: Pills. Grind ingredients to a powder and form into 9 gram pills with honey. The dose is one pill 2–3 times daily. Can also be decocted with a 80–90% reduction in dosage, and **zhi bie jia** and **duan wa leng zi** cooked first for 30 minutes. **Zhi bie jia** and **duan wa leng zi** soften hardness, activate blood and dissipate masses; **chao mai ya** protects the Stomach and assists in dispersing phlegm; **jiu san leng**, **e zhu** and **di bie chong** break up blood stasis and dissipate masses; **xiang fu** and **qing pi** break up qi stagnation and regulate qi. (Source: *Shi Yong Zhong Yao Xue* [*Gu Shi Yi Jing*])

Modifications
- With yin deficiency and heat, add **sheng di** (Rehmanniae Radix) 生地 60g, **xuan shen** (Scrophulariae Radix) 玄参 90g, **mu dan pi** (Moutan Cortex) 牡丹皮 60g and **zhi mu** (Anemarrhenae Rhizoma) 知母 60g.
- With bleeding or purpura in a patient with heat or yin deficiency, add **han lian cao** (Ecliptae Herba) 旱莲草 60g and **nu zhen zi** (Ligustri lucidi Fructus) 女贞子 60g.
- With bleeding or purpura accompanied by signs of qi deficiency and the Spleen not holding the blood in the vessels, combine with GUI PI TANG (Restore the Spleen Decoction 归脾汤, p.387), and **san qi fen** (powdered Notoginseng Radix) 三七粉 30g.
- With severe qi and blood deficiency, combine with REN SHEN YANG YING TANG (Ginseng Decoction to Nourish the Nutritive Qi 人参养营汤, p.384).
- With cancer or tumors, add herbs from Table 1.5, p.11., especially **gui zhen cao** (Bidens bipinnata Herba) 鬼针草, **zi bei tian kui** (Begonia fimbristipulata Herba) 紫背天葵, **ban zhi lian** (Scutellariae Barbatae Herba) 半枝莲 and **bai hua she she cao** (Hedyotis diffusae Herba) 白花蛇舌草.

Prepared medicines
Concentrated powder
Ge Xia Zhu Yu Tang (Tangkuei & Corydalis Combination)
Xue Fu Zhu Yu Tang (Persica & Carthamus Combination)
  – qi and blood stasis

Pills
Ge Xia Zhu Yu Wan (Stasis in the Lower Chamber Teapills)
Xue Fu Zhu Yu Wan (Stasis in the Mansion of Blood Teapills)
Nei Xiao Luo Li Wan (Nei Xiao Luo Li Teapills)
  – can be added to enhance the mass dispersing action of the primary formula
Yun Nan Bai Yao (Yunnan Paiyao)
Sheng Tian Qi Pian (Raw Tian Qi Ginseng Tablets)
  – add one of the last two when there is bleeding

Acupuncture (select from)
Liv.13 (zhangmen –) ....alarm point of the Spleen and meeting point of the yin organs, strengthens the Spleen and improves digestion, harmonizes the Liver and Spleen
Sp.21 (dabao) ....use if tender
ahshi points ....over the left hypochondrium
SJ.6 (zhigou –) ....these points together alleviate pain in the lateral
GB.34 (yanglingquan –)   trunk and hypochondrium
GB.40 (qiuxu –)
Bl.17 (geshu –)..................meeting point for blood, dispels blood stasis
Bl.18 (ganshu –)................transport point of the Liver, moves qi and blood
Sp.4 (gongsun) ....connecting point of the Spleen, regulates the Spleen and Stomach, stops pain
Sp.8 (diji –) ....cleft point of the Spleen, activates blood
• with severe pain, add LI.4 (hegu –) and Liv.6 (zhongdu –)
• with nausea and vomiting, add PC.6 (neiguan)
• with Spleen deficiency, add Ren.12 (zhongwan) and St.36 (zusanli)
• with phlegm, add St.40 (fenglong –) and Sp.3 (taibai)
• with spasms or cramping pain, add Du.8 (jinsuo –)
• Ear points: abdomen, spleen, zero point, shenmen, sympathetic, subcortex

Clinical notes
• Blood masses in the spleen may be diagnosed as chronic malaria, chronic lymphoma, splenomegaly from leukemia, splenic cysts, or tumors of the splenic flexure.
• When the diagnosis is cancer, a combination of Chinese and Western medicine is required.
• For dietary recommendations, see Clinical Handbook, Vol. 2, p.878 and 886.

肠
腹
血
瘀

1.1.4 BLOOD MASS IN THE INTESTINES

Blood masses in the intestines often have a familial component, and may also be associated with chronic Liver Spleen disharmony, damp heat in the Intestines or pooling of blood from yang deficiency. Regardless of the cause, the stasis is usually complicated by qi and blood deficiency.

Clinical features
- Mass, usually palpable, in the abdomen (commonly in lateral lower right or left quadrant); the mass is hard and usually painful with palpation
- distension, fullness and/or pain in the abdomen that is worse for pressure
- loose stools, diarrhea or alternating constipation and diarrhea
- may be melena or rectal bleeding; may be mucus in the stools and tenesmus
- loss of appetite, weight loss, emaciation
- distended or spider veins and nevi over the abdomen and lower legs
- dark rings around the eyes

T mauve, dark or purple, or with brown or purple stagnation spots; dark congested sublingual veins; with qi and blood deficiency the tongue is pale mauve and swollen

P wiry, choppy

Treatment principle
Activate blood and rectify qi
Soften hardness and dissipate masses
Support qi and blood as necessary

Prescription

GE XIA ZHU YU TANG 膈下逐瘀汤
Drive Out Blood Stasis Below the Diaphragm Decoction, modified

tao ren (Persicae Semen) 桃仁	9–12g
hong hua (Carthami Flos) 红花	9–12g
dang gui wei (rootlets of Angelicae sinensis Radix) 当归尾	9–12g
chi shao (Paeoniae Radix rubra) 赤芍	9–12g
chuan xiong (Chuanxiong Rhizoma) 川芎	6–9g
chao wu ling zhi (stir fried Trogopterori Faeces) 炒五灵脂	9–12g
xiang fu (Rhizoma Cyperi) 香附	9–12g
cu yan hu suo (vinegar fried Corydalis Rhizoma) 醋延胡索	12–15g
e zhu (Curcumae Rhizoma) 莪术	12–15g
jiu san leng (wine fried Sparganii Rhizoma) 酒三棱	9–12g
wa leng zi (Arcae Concha) 瓦楞子	15–30g

Method: Decoction. **Wa leng zi** is cooked for 30 minutes prior to the other herbs. **Tao ren, hong hua** and **chao wu ling zhi** activate and dispel static blood, free the network vessels and stop pain; **dang gui, chi shao** and **chuan xiong** nourish and activate the blood; **xiang fu** and **cu yan hu suo** move qi and blood, dredge the Liver and stop pain; **e zhu, jiu san leng** and **wa leng zi** break up blood stasis, soften hardness and dissipate masses. (Source: *Zhong Yi Zhi Liao Yi Nan Za Bing Mi Yao [Yi Lin Gai Cuo]*)

Modifications

- With pain, add **shui hong hua zi** (Polygoni orientale Semen) 水红花子 15–30g, **zhi mo yao** (Myrrha preparata) 炙没药 6–9g and **zhi ru xiang** (Olibanum preparata) 炙乳香 6–9g.
- With Spleen qi deficiency, add **dang shen** (Codonopsis Radix) 党参 12–15g, **bai zhu** (Atractylodis macrocephalae Rhizoma) 白术 9–12g, **fu ling** (Poria) 茯苓 12–18g, **yi ren** (Coicis Semen) 苡仁 18–30g and **shan yao** (Dioscoreae Rhizoma) 山药 12–18g, or combine with SHEN LING BAI ZHU SAN (Ginseng, Poria and White Atractylodes Powder 参苓白术散, p.270).
- With Spleen yang deficiency and watery early morning diarrhea, add **bu gu zhi** (Psoraleae Fructus) 补骨脂 9–12g, **wu wei zi** (Schizandrae Fructus) 五味子 3–6g, **rou dou kou** (Myristicae Semen) 肉豆蔻 3–6g and **wu zhu yu** (Evodiae Fructus) 吴茱萸 1–3g.
- With Liver and Spleen disharmony, abdominal pain and diarrhea, add **bai shao** (Paeoniae Radix alba) 白芍 12–18g, **bai zhu** (Atractylodis macrocephalae Rhizoma) 白术 12–15g, **fang feng** (Saposhnikovae Radix) 防风 9–12g and **chen pi** (Citri reticulatae Pericarpium) 陈皮 6–9g.
- With qi and blood deficiency, combine with REN SHEN YANG YING TANG (Ginseng Decoction to Nourish the Nutritive Qi 人参养营汤, p.384).
- With cancer or tumors, add several herbs from Table 1.5, p.11, especially **gui zhen cao** (Bidens bipinnata Herba) 鬼针草, **huang yao zi** (Dioscoreaea bulbiferae Rhizoma) 黄药子, **ban zhi lian** (Scutellariae Barbatae Herba) 半枝莲 and **bai hua she she cao** (Hedyotis diffusae Herba) 白花蛇舌草.

Topical therapies

Poultice

1. Powder **da huang** (Rhei Radix et Rhizoma) 大黄 and **mang xiao** (Natrii Sulfas) 大黄 and mix with a suitable carrier paste, such as sorbolene or lanolin. Apply on a cloth to the affected area. This poultice is best when there is heat.
2. A poultice can be prepared by boiling 50 grams of **shui hong hua zi** (Polygoni orientale Semen) 水红花子 in 2–3 cups of water until reduced by half. Strain off the dregs and soak a cloth in the warm liquid, apply to the abdomen and leave for as long as possible. Keep the poultice warm. This poultice is best when blood stasis is primary.
3. A poultice prepared with castor oil can be effective. Warm the castor oil to body temperature, soak a thick cloth the size of the area to be treated in the oil and place on the skin. The cloth can be held in place with cling film or a bandage. Place a hot water bottle over the oil soaked cloth for 20 minutes to one hour.

Retention enema

This prescription is suitable for blood stasis masses in the intestines or lower burner. The herbs are decocted in the normal fashion, strained and cooled to body temperature before 60–150 milliliters are inserted into the rectum with a commercial enema device. The enema is given once daily for 7–14 days, and can be retained with the patient lying down for 30 minutes to 2 hours with the hips elevated.

e zhu (Curcumae Rhizoma) 莪术 9g

san leng (Sparganii Rhizoma) 三棱 9g
chi shao (Paeoniae Radix rubra) 赤芍... 12g
zao jiao ci (Gleditsiae Spina) 皂角刺 12g
Method: Decoction and retention enema. **E zhu**, **san leng** and **chi shao** break up blood stasis and dissipate masses; **zao jiao ci** opens up congested areas and enables the other herbs to gain better access. (Source: *Zhong Yi Fu Chan Ke Xue*)

Prepared medicines
Concentrated powder
Ge Xia Zhu Yu Tang (Tangkuei & Corydalis Combination)
Shao Fu Zhu Yu Tang (Fennel Seed & Corydalis Combination)
   – with cold
Xue Fu Zhu Yu Tang (Persica & Carthamus Combination)
   – qi and blood stasis

Pills
Ge Xia Zhu Yu Wan (Stasis in the Lower Chamber Teapills)
Shao Fu Zhu Yu Wan (Stasis in the Lower Palace Teapills)
Xue Fu Zhu Yu Wan (Stasis in the Mansion of Blood Teapills)
Yun Nan Bai Yao (Yunnan Paiyao)
   – add when there is bleeding

Acupuncture (select from)
ahshi points ....over the site of the lesion plus distal points on the corresponding channel: the Stomach channel between St.36 (zusanli) and St.41 (jiexi), Spleen between Sp.6 (sanyinjiao) and Sp.8 (diji), or Kidney between Kid.7 (fuliu) and Kid.10 (yingu)
St.25 (tianshu –).................alarm point of the Large Intestine, regulates Intestinal function and eliminates stagnation
Bl.17 (geshu –)...................these points activate blood and disperse blood stasis
Sp.10 (xuehai –)
Sp.8 (diji –)
Sp.6 (sanyinjiao)................strengthens the Spleen and Kidneys, dredges the Liver, activates qi and blood, and removes obstruction from the channels and network vessels
LI.4 (hegu –) ....the 'four gates', both source points, move qi and
Liv.3 (taichong)   activate blood, ease muscle spasm and stop pain
• with focal pain, add Sp.4 (gongsun –) and St.34 (liangqiu –)
• Ear points: abdomen, large intestine, zero point, shenmen, sympathetic

Clinical notes
• Blood stasis masses in the intestines may be diagnosed as appendiceal abscess, stricture of the ileocaecal valve, tumors of the large intestine, Crohn's disease, lymphoma or mesenteric adenitis. When the diagnosis is cancer or stricture, a combination of Chinese and Western medicine is required.
• For dietary recommendations, see Clinical Handbook, Vol. 2, p.878 and 886.

寒
凝
血
瘀

1.1.5 BLOOD MASS IN THE LOWER ABDOMEN AND HYPOGASTRIUM, WITH COLD

Blood masses with cold often produce more severe pain due to the combined effects of the stasis and the vessel constricting effects of the cold. The cold may be from the exterior or be generated by yang deficiency. The most common site for masses of this type in the lower burner is the uterus, but other structures, such as the prostate, bladder and pelvic portion of the intestines, may be affected.

Clinical features

• Firm or hard mass in the lower burner, which is usually painful with pressure (but not always). When there is pain with palpation, it is relatively sharp or stabbing, fixed in location, worse with increasing pressure, but alleviated by warmth
• dark or purplish spider nevi or broken vessels on the trunk and around the inner ankle and knee
• dark, ashen, sallow or purplish complexion, dark or purplish lips and conjunctiva, dark ring around the eyes
• in women, the menses may be painful, irregular, purple and clotted, and there may be pelvic pain during intercourse; in men there may be urinary difficulty, urinary bleeding with clots or occult blood
• the lower abdomen feels firm and cold to the touch
• cold intolerance, cold extremities

T mauve, purple or blue, or with brown or purple stasis spots; sublingual veins dark and congested; with qi or yang deficiency, pale mauve and swollen
P wiry, choppy, fine

Treatment principle

Warm the lower burner and dispel cold, activate and dispel static blood
Soften hardness and dissipate masses, stop pain

Prescription

SHAO FU ZHU YU TANG 少腹逐瘀汤
Drive Out Blood Stasis in the Lower Abdomen Decoction, modified

dang gui (Angelicae sinensis Radix) 当归	9–12g
chi shao (Paeoniae Radix rubra) 赤芍	9–12g
pu huang (Typhae Pollen) 蒲黄	9–12g
chao wu ling zhi (stir fried Trogopterori Faeces) 炒五灵脂	9–12g
yan hu suo (Corydalis Rhizoma) 延胡索	9–12g
chuan xiong (Chuanxiong Rhizoma) 川芎	6–9g
xiao hui xiang (Foeniculi Fructus) 小茴香	9–12g
mo yao (Myrrha) 没药	6–9g
rou gui (Cinnamomi Cortex) 肉桂	3–6g
pao jiang (Zingiberis Rhizoma preparatum) 炮姜	3–6g
tao ren (Persicae Semen) 桃仁	9–12g
e zhu (Curcumae Rhizoma) 莪术	9–12g

jiu san leng (wine fried Sparganii Rhizoma) 酒三棱 9–12g
Method: Decoction. **Dang gui, chi shao, pu huang, chao wu ling zhi, chuan xiong, tao ren**
and **mo yao** activate blood and dispel blood stasis; **chuan xiong, xiao hui xiang** and **yan hu suo**
regulate qi, activate blood and stop pain; **rou gui** and **pao jiang** warm yang and stimulate the
circulation of qi and blood; **rou gui** warms cold and promotes generation of new blood; **e zhu** and
jiu san leng break up blood stasis, dissipate masses and stop pain. (Source: *Shi Yong Zhong Yi Nei
Ke Xue* [*Yi Lin Gai Cuo*])

Modifications

- To augment the mass softening action of the formula, add **bie jia** (Trionycis
  Carapax) 鳖甲 12–15g and **hu po** (Succinum) 琥珀 1.5–3g [taken separately
  as powder]. See also Table 1.3, p.9.
- With a chronic inflammatory mass, add **huang qi** (Astragali Radix) 黄芪
  15–30g and **zao jiao ci** (Gleditsiae Spina) 皂角刺 6–9g.
- If a mass follows a traumatic injury or surgical procedure, add **wang bu liu
  xing** (Vaccariae Semen) 王不留行 9–12g and **san qi fen** (powdered Notogin-
  seng Radix) 三七粉 3–9g [added to the strained decoction].
- With post surgical adhesions, add **hong hua** (Carthami Flos) 红花 6–9g and
  ze lan (Lycopi Herba) 泽兰 9–12g.
- With lower back ache or aching legs before or after menstruation, add **du zhong**
  (Eucommiae Cortex) 杜仲 9–12g and **xu duan** (Dipsaci Radix) 续断 9–12g.
- With qi stagnation, add **mu xiang** (Aucklandiae Radix) 木香 9–12g, **hou po**
  (Magnoliae officinalis Cortex) 厚朴 9–12g and **bing lang** (Arecae Semen) 槟
  榔 9–12g.
- With qi deficiency, add **huang qi** (Astragali Radix) 黄芪 15–30g, **dang shen**
  (Codonopsis Radix) 党参 15–30g and **chao bai zhu** (stir fried Atractylodis
  macrocephalae Rhizoma) 炒白术 12–15g.
- With yang deficiency, add **bu gu zhi** (Psoraleae Fructus) 补骨脂 9–12g, **xian
  ling pi** (Epimedii Herba) 仙灵脾 12–15g and **rou dou kou** (Myristicae Semen) 肉豆蔻 3–6g.
- With blood deficiency, add **huang qi** (Astragali Radix) 黄芪 15–30g and **shu
  di** (Rehmanniae Radix preparata) 熟地 18–24g.
- With phlegm damp and a thick greasy tongue coat, add **cang zhu** (Atractylodis Rhizoma) 苍术 9–12g, **yi ren** (Coicis Semen) 苡仁 15–30g and **fu ling**
  (Poria) 茯苓 12–18g.
- With cancer, add herbs from Table 1.5, p.11, especially **shu yang quan** (Solanum lyratum Herba) 蜀羊泉, **ban zhi lian** (Scutellariae Barbatae Herba) 半
  枝莲 and **bai hua she she cao** (Hedyotis diffusae Herba) 白花蛇舌草.

Prepared medicines

Concentrated powder
Shao Fu Zhu Yu Tang (Fennel Seed & Corydalis Combination)

Pills
Shao Fu Zhu Yu Wan (Stasis in the Lower Palace Teapills)
Fu Ke Wu Jin Wan 妇科乌金丸 (Woo Garm Yuen Medical Pills)
    – for blood stasis, fibroids and other benign masses with yang deficiency
Tao Hong Si Wu Wan (Tao Hong Si Wu Tang Teapills)

– for mild cases with blood deficiency
Qian Lie Xian Wan (Prostate Gland Pills)
– blood stasis swelling in the prostate
Yun Nan Bai Yao (Yunnan Paiyao)
– add when there is bleeding

Acupuncture (select from)

ahshi points ....over the site of pain in the abdomen, treated with a reducing method

St.29 (guilai –) ....these points regulate the movement of qi and blood
zigong – (M–CA–18 ▲)   in the lower burner and reproductive system, and
Ren.6 (qihai –▲)   with Sp.8 (diji) and Sp.6 (sanyinjiao), disperse blood stasis

Sp.8 (diji –) ....cleft point of the Spleen, activates qi and blood
Sp.6 (sanyinjiao –)..............these points activate blood and disperse stagnant
Sp.10 (xuehai –)   blood from the lower burner
LI.4 (hegu –)
Liv.3 (taichong –)...............source point of the Liver, regulates qi and activates blood, supplements Liver yin and blood, frees the channels and network vessels and stops pain

Bl.17 (geshu –)...................meeting point for blood, disperses stagnant blood

• Non–scarring moxa cones burnt over the renmai points of the lower abdomen and zigong (M–CA–18) are helpful in activating local blood circulation.
• Bleeding ahshi points or congested veins over the sacral foramina followed by strong cupping, can activate blood in the reproductive system. This treatment is good for fibroids, but only in robust patients.
• Ear points: uterus, liver, kidney, endocrine, shenmen, sympathetic, subcortex

Topical therapies
Poultice and retention enema
The same poultices and retention enema used for blood stasis in the Intestines is suitable. See pp.22–23.

Clinical notes
• Blood stasis with cold in the lower burner may be diagnosed as chronic pelvic inflammatory disease, fibroids, endometriosis, ovarian cysts or cancer, inflammatory masses, chronic appendicitis, placental retention, diverticular disease, prostatitis, prostatic cancer, bladder cancer, intestinal obstruction and adhesions.
• Depending on the biomedical pathology, relatively good results can be attained. When the diagnosis is cancer or stricture, a combination of Chinese and Western medicine is required.
• For dietary recommendations, see Clinical Handbook, Vol. 2, p.878 and 886.

瘀
血
留
结

1.1.6 MILD BLOOD STASIS IN THE HYPOGASTRIUM

A small blood mass or masses in the hypogastrium, with few clear systemic signs and symptoms, is a common finding in clinical practice. These masses are typically found in the uterus and associated structures, and are usually benign masses such small as fibroids or cysts, but may represent endometriosis, adenomyosis and chronic inflammatory masses. They are usually discovered during investigation for some other problem such as infertility.

Clinical features
- Small, well defined mass or masses in the lower burner, usually non palpable. If a mass is palpable, it is relatively soft and may be moveable, with mild to moderate tenderness.
- in many cases menstruation is normal and obvious blood stasis signs are absent or mild, but when present may include: dysmenorrhea (or urinary disruption and a sense of fullness or discomfort in the perineum in men), menorrhagia or persistent uterine bleeding of dark or clotted blood, a long menstrual cycle and infertility
- spider veins on the medial knee and ankle

T unremarkable, pale or slightly mauve, may be with brown or purple stasis spots; sublingual veins dark and congested

P deep, wiry, choppy, fine

Treatment principle
Activate blood and gradually transform and disperse blood stasis
Soften hardness and dissipate masses

Prescription

GUI ZHI FU LING WAN 桂枝茯苓丸
Cinnamon Twig and Poria Pill

gui zhi (Cinnamomi Ramulus) 桂枝 9–12g
fu ling (Poria) 茯苓 9–12g
chi shao (Paeoniae Radix rubra) 赤芍.. 9–12g
tao ren (Persicae Semen) 桃仁 9–12g
mu dan pi (Moutan Cortex) 牡丹皮 9–12g

Method: Grind the herbs to a fine powder and form into 3 gram pills with honey. The dose is two pills 2–3 times daily on an empty stomach. May also be decocted with the doses as shown. **Gui zhi** frees the channels and network vessels and invigorates the circulation of yang qi; **fu ling** strengthens the Spleen, leaches out damp and calms the shen; **tao ren** activates blood and dispels blood stasis; **chi shao** and **mu dan pi** cool the blood and dispel blood stasis. (Source: *Shang Han Lun*)

Modifications
- For tender or quite firm masses, with fixed pain and dark clotted bleeding, add **cu e zhu** (vinegar fried Curcumae Rhizoma) 醋莪术 6–9g and **bie jia** (Trionycis Carapax) 鳖甲 9–12g.
- For ovarian cysts, leukorrhea and signs of phlegm damp, add **zao jiao ci** (Gleditsiae Spina) 皂角刺 6–9g, **xuan shen** (Scrophulariae Radix) 玄参 9–12g, **zhe bei mu** (Fritillariae thunbergii Bulbus) 浙贝母 9–12g and **mu li** (Ostreae

Concha) 牡蛎 12–15g.
- For a chronic inflammatory mass, add **dan shen** (Salviae miltiorrhizae Radix) 丹参 30g, **huang qi** (Astragali Radix) 黄芪 12–15g, **xia ku cao** (Prunellae Spica) 夏枯草 12–15g and **bai jiang cao** (Patriniae Herba) 败酱草 12–15g.
- With colicky or spasmodic pain, add **bai shao** (Paeoniae Radix alba) 白芍 9–12g and **gan cao** (Glycyrrhizae Radix) 甘草 3–6g.
- With cold, add **xiao hui xiang** (Foeniculi Fructus) 小茴香 6–9g and **pao jiang** (Zingiberis Rhizoma preparatum) 炮姜 3–6g.
- For damp accumulation, edema or fluid filled masses (like hydrosalpinx), double the dose of **fu ling** and add **yi mu cao** (Leonurus Herba) 益母草 12–15g and **lu lu tong** (Liquidambaris Fructus) 路路通 15–30g.
- With heat, a warm lower abdomen and yellow leukorrhea, decrease the dose of **gui zhi** by 20% and increase the dose of **mu dan pi** by 20%.
- With qi constraint, distending pain and premenstrual symptoms, add **xiang fu** (Cyperi Rhizoma) 香附 9–12g and **qing pi** (Aurantii Fructus immaturus) 青皮 9–12g, or combine with Xiao Yao San (Rambling Powder 逍遥散, p.435).
- With blood deficiency, combine with Dang Gui Shao Yao San (Tangkuei and Peony Powder 当归芍药散, p.234).

Prepared medicines
Concentrated powder
Gui Zhi Fu Ling Wan (Cinnamon & Poria Formula)
Xiao Luo Wan (Scrophularia & Fritillaria Combination)
– add with phlegm masses

Pills
Gui Zhi Fu Ling Wan (Cinnamon and Poria Teapills)
Ji Sheng Ju He Wan (Citrus Aurantium Compound Pills, Citrus Seed Pills)
– add with phlegm masses
Qian Lie Xian Wan (Prostate Gland Pills)
– add with swollen prostate

Acupuncture (select from)
St.29 (guilai –) ....these points regulate the movement of qi and blood
zigong – (M–CA–18)   in the lower abdomen and reproductive system, and
Ren.6 (qihai –)   with Sp.8 (diji) and Sp.6 (sanyinjiao), disperse blood stasis
Bl.31–34 (baliao) ....regulate the circulation of qi and blood in the lower burner; the most tender points are selected
Sp.8 (diji –) ....cleft point of the Spleen, rectifies qi and activates blood
Sp.6 (sanyinjiao –)..............these points activate blood and disperse stagnant
Sp.10 (xuehai –)   blood from the lower burner
LI.4 (hegu –)
Liv.5 (ligou –)...................connecting point of the Liver, regulates qi and blood in the lower abdomen

Bl.17 (geshu –).................meeting point for blood, disperses stagnant blood
- with Kidney deficiency, add Bl.23 (shenshu +)
- with edema, add Sp.9 (yinlingquan –)
- with heat, add Liv.2 (xingjian –)
- with qi stagnation, add PC.6 (neiguan) and Liv.3 (taichong)
- Ear points: uterus, liver, kidney, endocrine, shenmen, sympathetic

Topical therapies
Poultice and retention enema
See p.22–23.

Clinical notes
- This pattern is chronic and will usually take some time to resolve. It is erroneous to try and increase the intensity of the treatment to resolve the mass quickly, as this will usually deplete qi and blood and ultimately aggravate the condition. Several months to a year or more may be required to gently and gradually disperse the mass. Herbs are preferred due to convenience and efficacy. A small but regular dose over a long period of time keeps the qi and blood activated and chips away at the stasis.
- The masses in this pattern are usually silent. They may not cause any specific complaints and are often unrecognized until investigations are undertaken for some other condition such as infertility.
- Masses in this category include small fibroids, functional or other small cysts, silent endometriosis, polycystic ovaries and adenomyosis. Masses of this type can also be induced iatrogenically, such as ovarian hyper stimulation syndrome, as part of IVF treatment.
- A reasonable level of activity is essential to keep qi and blood moving. Activities that focus on the pelvic region, such as walking and rowing, are especially helpful.
- For dietary recommendations, see Clinical Handbook, Vol. 2, p.878 and 886.

1.2 PHLEGM

1. Liver
2. Abdomen
3. Spleen
4. Epigastrium
5. Lower burner

肝
脏
痰
结

1.2.1 PHLEGM MASS IN THE LIVER

This pattern is associated with cysts or adenomas in the liver. There is usually a constitutional component and the patient may exhibit systemic signs of phlegm.

Clinical features
• Round, regular single or multiple masses in the liver; usually not palpable but able to be detected with imaging. In many cases patients with cysts in the liver are asymptomatic, but when the cysts are large, there may be signs of phlegm or blood stasis such as distension or discomfort of the upper abdomen and under the right ribs.
• may be other signs of constitutional phlegm, such as a tendency to be over-weight, heaviness and poor energy, cystic swellings in other locations (ovaries, kidneys, breasts, lipomata etc.)
• spider nevi over the ribs
T swollen; stasis spots or swollen dark sublingual veins
P slippery, soft or soggy

Treatment principle
Soften hardness and transform phlegm damp to dissipate masses
Strengthen the Spleen and supplement qi

Prescription

HUA JIAN ER CHEN TANG 化坚二陈丸
Two Aged [Herb] Pill to Soften Hardness

zhi ban xia (Pinelliae Rhizoma preparatum) 制半夏	9–15g
chen pi (Citri reticulatae Pericarpium) 陈皮	9–15g
fu ling (Poria) 茯苓	9–12g
zhi gan cao (Glycyrrhizae Radix preparata) 炙甘草	3–6g
huang lian (Coptidis Rhizoma) 黄连	3–6g
dan nan xing (Arisaema cum Bile) 胆南星	6–9g
quan gua lou (Trichosanthis Fructus) 全栝楼	18–24g
hou po (Magnoliae officinalis Cortex) 厚朴	9–12g
bai zhu (Atractylodis macrocephalae Rhizoma) 白术	9–12g
bai jie zi (Sinapsis Semen) 白芥子	6–9g
shan zha (Crataegi Fructus) 山楂	12–15g
shen qu (Massa medicata fermentata) 神曲	12–15g

Method: Pills or powder. **Zhi ban xia** dries damp and transforms phlegm; **chen pi** dries damp, transforms phlegm and rectifies the qi dynamic; **fu ling** strengthens the Spleen and leaches damp out through the urine; **zhi gan cao** supplements qi and harmonizes the formula; **huang lian** clears heat generated by phlegm accumulation; **dan nan xing** and **quan gua lou** transform phlegm and open up qi flow through the upper abdomen; **hou po** directs qi downward and transforms phlegm; **bai zhu** strengthens the Spleen, supplements qi and dries damp; **bai jie zi** expels phlegm and dissipates masses; **shan zha** and **shen qu** assist digestion. (Source: *Xian Zai Zhong Yi Gan Zang Bing Xue*)

Modifications

- With liver pain, add **yu jin** (Curcumae Radix) 郁金 9–12g and **ze lan** (Lycopi Herba) 泽兰 9–12g.
- With resistent or large nodules, add **xuan shen** (Scrophulariae Radix) 玄参 12–15g, **mu li** (Ostreae Concha) 牡蛎 15–30g [cooked first] and **zhe bei mu** (Fritillariae thunbergii Bulbus) 浙贝母 9–12g. This is **Xiao Luo Wan**, p.8, 921.
- With blood stasis, add **bie jia** (Trionycis Carapax) 鳖甲 12–15g and **dan shen** (Salviae miltiorrhizae Radix) 丹参 12–15g.
- With a greasy yellow tongue coat and heat intolerance, add **yin chen** (Artemisiae scopariae Herba) 茵陈 12–15g and **hu zhang** (Polygoni cuspidati Rhizoma) 虎杖 9–12g.
- With qi deficiency, add **huang qi** (Astragali Radix) 黄芪 12–15g.
- With sluggish stools or constipation, add **da huang** (Rhei Radix et Rhizoma) 大黄 6–9g and **zhi shi** (Aurantii Fructus immaturus) 枳实 6–9g.
- With loose stools or diarrhea, add **su geng** (Perillae Caulis) 苏梗 6–9g and **huo xiang geng** (Pogostemonis/Agastaches Caulis) 藿香梗 9–12g.

Prepared medicines

Concentrated powder

Ju He Wan (Citrus Seed Formula)
Shi Liu Wei Liu Qi Yin (Tangkuei Sixteen Herbs Combination)
Xiao Luo Wan (Scrophularia & Fritillaria Combination)

Pills

Ji Sheng Ju He Wan (Citrus Aurantium Compound Pills, Citrus Seed Pills)

Acupuncture (select from)

Liv.14 (qimen –) ....alarm point of the Liver, activates Liver qi and blood
Sp.21 (dabao) ....use if tender
ahshi points ....over the right hypochondrium
St.40 (fenglong –) ....connecting and source points of the Spleen and
Sp.3 (taibai –)   Stomach, strengthen the Spleen and transform phlegm
PC.5 (jianshi –).................river point of the Pericardium, transforms phlegm and clears heat
Bl.17 (geshu –)..................meeting point for blood, dispels blood stasis
Bl.18 (ganshu –)................transport point of the Liver, moves qi and blood
Bl.20 (pishu) ....transport point of the Spleen, strengthens the Spleen to transform phlegm
- with pain, add SJ.6 (zhigou –) and GB.34 (yanglingquan –)
- with foggy head, add Du.20 (baihui)

- Ear points: abdomen, liver, zero point, shenmen, endocrine, sympathetic

Clinical notes

- Small liver cysts are usually asymptomatic and are discovered in the course of a general examination. Most small cysts do not need treatment, but larger cysts may cause symptoms, and thus require attention. The conventional medical treatment to drain the fluid from the cyst or cysts does not cause any more than temporary improvement and the cysts tend to recur.
- Phlegm cysts in the liver can be variable in response; small cysts are more amenable to treatment than large or multiple cysts. Even when the cysts are unresponsive to treatment, however, constitutional treatment is worth while to prevent further phlegm complications.
- For dietary recommendations, see Clinical Handbook, Vol. 2, p.880.

1.2.2 ABDOMEN – PHLEGM AND QI CONSTRAINT

腹中痰凝

The phlegm in this pattern is the product of Liver and Spleen disharmony, qi constraint, Spleen weakness and accumulation of damp that gradually coalesces into phlegm. The phlegm congeals along the pathway of the Liver and Spleen channels in the abdomen, inguinal region and neck. The masses are found in the left upper abdomen and may be distributed through the abdomen (especially in the spleen and lymphatic system).

Clinical features

- Rubbery, non–tender mass palpable under the margin of the left rib cage (and occasionally the right), and at various non–specific locations in the abdomen
- muscle tightness beneath the ribs
- fullness and distension in the abdomen; chest oppression
- puffy face; may be peripheral edema
- sluggish bowels or alternating constipation and diarrhea
- loss of appetite, weight loss
- may be occasional low grade fever
- non tender lymphadenopathy

T mauve or pale and swollen with a greasy white coat
P wiry and slippery, or fine and wiry

Treatment principle

Soften hardness, transform phlegm and dissipate masses
Harmonize the Liver and Spleen, mobilize qi and alleviate qi constraint
Strengthen the Spleen and supplement qi as necessary

Prescription

CHAI HU SHU GAN SAN 柴胡疏肝散
Bupleurum Powder to Dredge the Liver, modified

chai hu (Bupleuri Radix) 柴胡	9–12g
bai shao (Paeoniae Radix alba) 白芍	12–18g
zhi ke (Aurantii Fructus) 枳壳	9–12g

xiang fu (Cyperi Rhizoma) 香附 9–12g
chuan xiong (Chuanxiong Rhizoma) 川芎 6–9g
qing pi (Aurantii Fructus immaturus) 青皮 6–9g
zhi gan cao (Glycyrrhizae Radix preparata) 炙甘草 3–6g
dan shen (Salviae miltiorrhizae Radix) 丹参 12–15g
bai hua she she cao (Hedyotis diffusae Herba) 白花蛇舌草 30–45g
mu li (Ostreae Concha) 牡蛎 15–30g
zhe bei mu (Fritillariae thunbergii Bulbus) 浙贝母 9–12g

Method: Decoction. **Mu li** is cooked for 30 minutes prior to the other herbs. **Chai hu** dredges the Liver and regulates qi, **bai shao** softens the Liver, nourishes yin and blood and assists **chai hu** in regulating qi; **zhi ke**, **qing pi** and **xiang fu** mobilize and break up qi constraint; **chuan xiong** moves qi and activates blood; **zhi gan cao** strengthens the Spleen and, with **bai shao**, alleviates any cramping and spasmodic pain; **dan shen** activates blood; the saltiness of **mu li** softens hardness and dissipates knotted phlegm; **zhe bei mu** assists **mu li** in softening hardness; **bai hua she she cao** clears toxic heat and dissipates masses. (Source: *Zhong Yi Zhi Liao Yi Nan Za Bing Mi Yao / Zheng Zhi Zhun Sheng*)

Modifications

- With Spleen qi deficiency, add **bai zhu** (Atractylodis macrocephalae Rhizoma) 白术 9–12g and **huang qi** (Astragali Radix) 黄芪 12–15g.
- With heat, low grade fever and a yellow tongue coat, add **xia ku cao** (Prunellae Spica) 夏枯草 15–24g, **da qing ye** (Isatidis Folium) 大青叶 15–18g and **xuan shen** (Scrophulariae Radix) 玄参 12–18g.
- With constipation or sluggish stools, substitute **zhi shi** (Aurantii Fructus immaturus) 枳实 9–12g for **zhi ke**.
- With cancer, add herbs from Table 1.5, p.11, especially **mao zhua cao** (Ranunculi ternati Radix) 猫爪草 12–15g and **ban bian lian** (Lobelia Herba) 半边莲 12–15g.

Prepared medicines

Concentrated powder

Chai Hu Shu Gan San (Bupleurum & Cyperus Combination) plus Ju He Wan (Citrus Seed Formula)
Shi Liu Wei Liu Qi Yin (Tangkuei Sixteen Herbs Combination)
San Zhong Kui Jian Tang (Forsythia & Laminaria Combination)
    – with heat

Pills

Chai Hu Shu Gan Wan (Bupleurum Soothe Liver Teapills) plus Ji Sheng Ju He Wan (Citrus Aurantium Compound Pills, Citrus Seed Pills)

Acupuncture (select from)

Liv.13 (zhangmen –) ....alarm point of the Spleen and meeting point of the yin organs, strengthens the Spleen and improves digestion, harmonizes the Liver and Spleen
Sp.21 (dabao) ....use if tender
ahshi points ....over the left hypochondrium
Bl.20 (pishu) ....transport points of the Spleen and Stomach,
Bl.21 (weishu –)   strengthen the middle burner to transform phlegm

St.36 (zusanli –) ....sea point of the Stomach, strengthens the Spleen to transform phlegm

St.40 (fenglong –) ....connecting and source points of the Spleen and
Sp.3 (taibai –)   Stomach, strengthen the Spleen and transform phlegm

Liv.3 (taichong –) ....source point of the Liver, regulates and activates qi and blood

- with sluggish bowels, add St.25 (tianshu –) and SJ.6 (zhigou –)
- with edema, add Sp.9 (yinlingquan –)
- with nausea and vomiting, add PC.6 (neiguan)
- Ear points: abdomen, spleen, zero point, shenmen, sympathetic, subcortex

Clinical notes
- A phlegm and qi constraint mass may be diagnosed as splenomegaly and abdominal lymphadenopathy from chronic infection, glandular fever, leukemia or lymphoma. When the diagnosis is cancer, a combination of Chinese and Western medicine is required.
- For dietary recommendations, see Clinical Handbook, Vol. 2, p.880.

脾
脏
痰
结

1.2.3 PHLEGM KNOTTING IN THE SPLEEN
Phlegm knotting in the spleen is a type of cyst that can be associated with trauma or parasites.

Clinical features
- Round, nodular, well defined mass in the spleen. The mass is usually not palpable unless quite large, and is discovered when investigating the pain it causes. A palpable mass may be seen to move with inspiration.
- dull left hypochondria and lateral rib pain; the pain may sporadically be sharp and piercing
- shortness of breath
- fatigue, weakness

T pale or mauve and swollen with brown or purple spots and a greasy coat
P fine, wiry, slippery

Treatment principle
Soften hardness, transform phlegm and dissipate masses
Strengthen the Spleen and supplement qi
Activate blood and stop pain

Prescription
HUA TAN RUAN JIAN FANG 化痰软坚方
Transform Phlegm and Soften Hardness Formula

huang qi (Astragali Radix) 黄芪 18–30g
chao bai zhu (stir fried Atractylodis macrocephalae Rhizoma) 炒白术 12–15g
shan yao (Dioscoreae Rhizoma) 山药 12–15g
yi ren (Coicis Semen) 苡仁 18–30g

zhi tian nan xing (Arisaematis Rhizoma preparatum) 制天南星 9–12g
zhi ban xia (Pinelliae Rhizoma preparatum) 制半夏 9–12g
chen pi (Citri reticulatae Pericarpium) 陈皮 9–12g
xia ku cao (Prunellae Spica) 夏枯草 15–18g
gan cao (Glycyrrhizae Radix) 甘草 6–9g
di bie chong (Eupolyphaga/Steleophaga) 地鳖虫 9–12g
shu yang quan (Solanum lyratum Herba) 蜀羊泉 15–30g
xu chang qing (Cynanchi paniculati Radix) 徐长卿 15–30g
Method: Decoction. **Huang qi, chao bai zhu, shan yao** and **yi ren** strengthen the Spleen and supplement qi; **zhi tian nan xing, zhi ban xia, chen pi** and **xia ku cao** transform phlegm; **di bie chong, xu chang qing** and **shu yang quan** break up stagnant qi and blood, free the channels and network vessels and stop pain. (Source: *Zhong Yi Zhi Liao Yi Nan Za Bing Mi Yao* [*Jing Yan Fang*])

Modifications
• With severe pain, add **yan hu suo** (Corydalis Rhizoma) 延胡索 9–12g and **chuan lian zi** (Toosendan Fructus) 川楝子 9–12g, or **zhi mo yao** (Myrrha preparata) 炙没药 6–9g and **zhi ru xiang** (Olibanum preparata) 炙乳香 6–9g.

Prepared medicines
Concentrated powder
Ju He Wan (Citrus Seed Formula)
Shi Liu Wei Liu Qi Yin (Tangkuei Sixteen Herbs Combination)
Xiao Luo Wan (Scrophularia & Fritillaria Combination)
Tuo Li Xiao Du Yin (Gleditsia Combination)

Pills
Ji Sheng Ju He Wan (Citrus Aurantium Compound Pills, Citrus Seed Pills)
Nei Xiao Luo Li Wan (Nei Xiao Luo Li Teapills)

Acupuncture (select from)
Liv.13 (zhangmen –) ....alarm point of the Spleen and meeting point of the yin organs, strengthens the Spleen and harmonizes the Liver and Spleen
Sp.21 (dabao) ....use if tender
ahshi points ....over the left hypochondrium
GB.39 (xuanzhong –).........these points are for pain over the lateral ribs
SJ.5 (waiguan –)
PC.5 (jianshi –).................river and metal point of the Pericardium, transforms phlegm
St.40 (fenglong –) ....connecting and source points of the Stomach,
Sp.3 (taibai –)   strengthen the Spleen and transform phlegm
• with stabbing pain, add LI.4 (hegu –) and Liv.6 (zhongdu –)
• with spasm or cramping pain, add Du.8 (jinsuo –) and GB.34 (yanglingquan –)
• with nausea and vomiting, add PC.6 (neiguan)
• with Spleen deficiency, add Ren.12 (zhongwan) and St.36 (zusanli +)
• Ear points: spleen, zero point, shenmen, sympathetic, subcortex

Clinical notes
- Phlegm cysts in the spleen or left upper quadrant are unusual, but can respond to treatment when relatively small. If large, surgery is usually required.
- For dietary recommendations, see Clinical Handbook, Vol. 2, p.880.

胃
胰
痰
结

1.2.4 PHLEGM MASS IN THE EPIGASTRIUM

A phlegm mass in the epigastrium may be the result of Liver and Spleen/Stomach disharmony, disruption to the qi dynamic or long term damp that gradually congeals into phlegm. There may be a constitutional component in some patients. The mass may affect the stomach, pancreas or lymphatics.

Clinical features
- Firm, rounded, well defined mass in the epigastrium; the mass may be moderately tender with palpation
- epigastric distension and discomfort
- loss of appetite, weight loss
- nausea and vomiting of a watery or frothy mucus like material
- heartburn, acid reflux, dysphagia
- constipation alternating with diarrhea

T swollen with a thick greasy white or yellow coat
P wiry or slippery

Treatment principle
Soften and transform phlegm and dissipate masses
Downbear counterflow Stomach qi

Prescription

HAI ZAO YU HU TANG 海藻玉壶汤
Sargassum Decoction for the Jade Flask, modified

hai zao (Sargassum) 海藻	30g
kun bu (Eckloniae Thallus) 昆布	30g
zhe bei mu (Fritillariae thunbergii Bulbus) 浙贝母	9–12g
zhi ban xia (Pinelliae Rhizoma preparatum) 制半夏	9–12g
dan nan xing (Arisaema cum Bile) 胆南星	6–9g
xia ku cao (Prunellae Spica) 夏枯草	15–30g
zao jiao ci (Gleditsiae Spina) 皂角刺	9–12g
ting li zi (Lepidii/Descurainiae Semen) 葶苈子	9–12g
gua lou ren (Trichosanthis Semen) 栝楼仁	9–12g
mu li (Ostreae Concha) 牡蛎	15–30g
wa leng zi (Arcae Concha) 瓦楞子	12–15g

Method: Decoction. **Mu li** and **wa leng zi** are cooked for 30 minutes prior to the other herbs. **Hai zao, kun bu** and **zhe bei mu** soften hardness, resolves phlegm and dissipate nodules; **zhi ban xia** and **dan nan xing** dry damp and dispel phlegm; **xia ku cao** clears phlegm heat and dissipates nodules; **zao jiao ci** dissipates masses and enables other herbs to gain better access to the mass; **ting li zi** and **gua lou ren** transform phlegm and direct qi downwards; **mu li** and **wa leng zi** soften hardness, activate blood, transform phlegm and neutralize gastric acid. (Source: *Zhong Yi Zhi Liao Yi Nan Za Bing Mi Yao* [*Wai Ke Zheng Zong*])

Modifications
- With severe vomiting, reflux or dysphagia, add **xuan fu hua** (Inulae Flos) 旋覆花 9–12g and **hou po** (Magnoliae officinalis Cortex) 厚朴 6–9g.
- With cancer, add herbs from Table 1.5, p.11, especially **mao zhua cao** (Ranunculi ternati Radix) 猫爪草 12–15g, **ban bian lian** (Lobelia Herba) 半边莲 12–15g and **huang yao zi** (Dioscoreaea bulbiferae Rhizoma) 黄药子 6–15g.
- With Spleen deficiency, combine with Liu Jun Zi Tang (Six Gentlemen Decoction 六君子汤, p.916).

Prepared medicines
Concentrated powder
Ju He Wan (Citrus Seed Formula)
Shi Liu Wei Liu Qi Yin (Tangkuei Sixteen Herbs Combination)
San Zhong Kui Jian Tang (Forsythia & Laminaria Combination)
Xiao Luo Wan (Scrophularia & Fritillaria Combination)
Ban Xia Xie Xin Tang (Pinellia Combination)
  – can be combined with one of the above when reflux is severe

Pills
Ji Sheng Ju He Wan (Citrus Aurantium Compound Pills, Citrus Seed Pills)
Nei Xiao Luo Li Wan (Nei Xiao Luo Li Teapills)

Acupuncture (select from)
Ren.12 (zhongwan –).........alarm point of the Stomach, downbears counterflow Stomach qi and dissipates stagnation
Ren.13 (shangwan –)..........local point for excess patterns of the Stomach
ahshi points ....over the site of the mass, to disperse local accumulation of qi and phlegm
Bl.20 (pishu) ....transport points of the Spleen and Stomach,
Bl.21 (weishu –)   strengthen the middle burner to transform phlegm
St.40 (fenglong –) ....connecting and source points of the Spleen and
Sp.3 (taibai –)   Stomach, strengthen the Spleen to transform phlegm
PC.5 (jianshi –).................river and metal point of the Pericardium, resolves phlegm and clears heat
- with pain, add St.34 (liangqiu –)
- with reflux, nausea and vomiting, add PC.6 (neiguan)
- with dysphagia, as Ren.17 (shanzhong –) and Ren.22 (tiantu)
- with Spleen deficiency, add St.36 (zusanli)
- with spasms or cramping pain, add Du.8 (jinsuo –)
- Ear points: spleen, zero point, shenmen, sympathetic, subcortex

Clinical notes
- A phlegm mass in the epigastrium may be diagnosed as a cyst in the stomach, lymphoma, pancreatic pseudocyst or chronic abscess.
- For dietary recommendations, see Clinical Handbook, Vol. 2, p.880.

少
腹
痰
凝

1.2.5 PHLEGM MASS IN THE HYPOGASTRIUM

This type of mass, (often multiple masses), is often seen in patients with a constitutional tendency to phlegm, but can also be the result of chronic qi constraint
and Spleen qi deficiency. These masses are often complicated by blood stasis.

Clinical features
- Soft or firm and rubbery mass or masses in the hypogastrium which can be
  quite large and easily palpable. The mass may be relatively mobile and is not
  tender with palpation.
- lower abdominal distension; may be intermittent lower abdominal pain
- irregular menstruation, scanty menstruation or amenorrhea
- profuse sticky white vaginal discharge
- lethargy and heaviness
- foggy head, poor concentration, dizziness
- patients may be overweight
- there may be phlegm type masses in other locations, like the breasts and neck

T thick greasy white coat
P deep and slippery or wiry and slippery

Treatment principle
Transform and soften phlegm to dissipate masses
Regulate qi and activate blood

Prescription

CANG FU DAO TAN WAN 苍附导痰丸
Guide Out Phlegm Pill with Atractylodes and Cyperus, modified

cang zhu (Atractylodis Rhizoma) 苍术 9–12g
xiang fu (Cyperi Rhizoma) 香附 6–9g
zhi ban xia (Pinelliae Rhizoma preparatum) 制半夏 9–12g
fu ling (Poria) 茯苓 9–15g
chen pi (Citri reticulatae Pericarpium) 陈皮 6–9g
gan cao (Glycyrrhizae Radix) 甘草 3–6g
dan nan xing (Arisaema cum Bile) 胆南星 6–9g
zhi ke (Aurantii Fructus) 枳壳 6–9g
sheng jiang (Zingiberis Rhizoma recens) 生姜 6–9g
shen qu (Massa medicata fermentata) 神曲 12–15g

Method: Pills. Grind the herbs to a fine powder and form into 6 gram pills with water. The dose
is one pill 2–3 times daily. **Zhi ban xia**, **cang zhu**, **fu ling**, **chen pi** and **gan cao** strengthen the
Spleen, dry damp and transform phlegm; **xiang fu** and **zhi ke** regulate qi and alleviate qi constraint;
dan nan xing dries dampness and phlegm; **sheng jiang** and **shen qu** harmonize and protect the
Stomach. (Source: *Zhong Yi Fu Chan Ke Xue* [*Ye Tian Shi Nu Ke Zhi Liao Mi Fang*])

Modifications
- With a solid mass or masses, combine with **XIAO LUO WAN** (Reduce Scrophula
  Pill 消瘰丸, p.921).
- With Spleen qi deficiency, add **huang qi** (Astragali Radix) 黄芪 12–18g and
  dang shen (Codonopsis Radix) 党参 12–15g, or combine with **LIU JUN ZI**

Tang (Six Gentlemen Decoction 六君子汤, p.916).
- With blood stasis, add **lu lu tong** (Liquidambaris Fructus) 路路通 9–12g and **yi mu cao** (Leonurus Herba) 益母草 12–15g.
- With amenorrhea, add **chuan xiong** (Chuanxiong Rhizoma) 川芎 6–9g, **dang gui** (Angelicae sinensis Radix) 当归 6–9g and **ji xue teng** (Spatholobi Caulis) 鸡血藤 15–30g.
- With cold, add **gui zhi** (Cinnamomi Ramulus) 桂枝 6–9g.
- With heat, add **huang qin** (Scutellariae Radix) 黄芩 6–9g.
- With Liver qi constraint, add **qing pi** (Aurantii Fructus immaturus) 青皮 6–9g and **mu xiang** (Aucklandiae Radix) 木香 6–9g.

Prepared medicines
Concentrated powder
Ping Wei San (Magnolia & Ginger Formula) and Er Chen Tang (Citrus & Pinellia Combination) plus Xiao Luo Wan (Scrophularia & Fritillaria Combination) or Qing Qi Hua Tang Wan (Pinellia & Scute Formula)
Wei Ling Tang (Magnolia & Poria Combination)
Ju He Wan (Citrus Seed Formula)

Pills
Ji Sheng Ju He Wan (Citrus Aurantium Compound Pills, Citrus Seed Pills) plus Ping Wei San (Calm Stomach Teapills, Tabellae Pingwei)

Acupuncture (select from)
ahshi points ....over the site of the mass, treated with a reducing method
St.29 (guilai –) ....these points regulate the movement of qi and blood
St.28 (shuidao –)   in the lower abdomen and reproductive system
zigong (M–CA–18 –)
Bl.18 (ganshu –).................transport point of the Liver, activates qi and blood
Bl.20 (pishu) ....transport point of the Spleen, strengthens the Spleen to transform phlegm
St.40 (fenglong –) ....connecting and source points of the Spleen and
Sp.3 (taibai –)   Stomach, strengthen the Spleen to transform phlegm
PC.5 (jianshi –).................river and metal point of the Pericardium, resolves phlegm and clears heat
- with pain, add Sp.4 (gongsun –) and Liv.5 (ligou –)
- Ear points: uterus, ovaries, spleen, zero point, shenmen

Topical therapies
Poultice
- A poultice prepared with castor oil, p.22, can be helpful.

Clinical notes
- Phlegm masses in the hypogastrium may be diagnosed as ovarian cysts, adenomas, polycystic ovaries, fibroids, ovarian hyperstimulation syndrome, ovarian cancer or benign prostatic hypertrophy.
- For dietary recommendations, see Clinical Handbook, Vol. 2, p.880.

1.3 HEAT MASSES

1. Liver / Gallbladder – toxic heat
2. Liver – damp heat
3. Liver – damp heat with qi and yin deficiency
4. Liver – yin deficiency
5. Epigastrium
6. Intestines
7. Uterus, adnexa

热
毒
雍
聚

1.3.1 LIVER / GALLBLADDER – TOXIC HEAT MASS

A toxic heat mass in the Liver or Gallbladder is associated with an abscess or empyema. It may be seen after episodes of dysenteric disorder or Intestinal abscess.

Clinical features
- Soft tender swelling in the upper right quadrant, pain worsens with palpation; the liver may be enlarged and smooth but not hard; pain may refer to the right shoulder; there may be muscle guarding over the liver.
- high fever with rigors or alternating fever and chills
- profuse sweating
- malaise, anorexia, nausea and vomiting
- sallow or ashen complexion; red, sore eyes
- thirst, dry mouth, bitter taste in the mouth
- concentrated urine
- maybe disturbances of consciousness

T red with a dry or greasy yellow coat
P surging and rapid

Treatment principle
Clear toxic heat from the Liver and Gallbladder
Cool and activate blood and dispel stasis

Prescription

HUANG LIAN JIE DU TANG 黄连解毒汤
Coptis Decoction to Resolve Toxicity, plus
DA CHAI HU TANG 大柴胡汤
Major Bupleurum Decoction, modified

---

huang qin (Scutellariae Radix) 黄芩 9–12g
huang lian (Coptidis Rhizoma) 黄连 6–9g
huang bai (Phellodendri Cortex) 黄柏 9–12g
da huang (Rhei Radix et Rhizoma) 大黄 6–9g
shan zhi zi (Gardeniae Fructus) 山栀子 9–12g
chai hu (Bupleuri Radix) 柴胡 9–12g
zhi shi (Aurantii Fructus immaturus) 枳实 9–12g
chi shao (Paeoniae Radix rubra) 赤芍 9–12g
jin yin hua (Lonicera Flos) 金银花 18–30g

zi hua di ding (Violae Herba) 紫花地丁 9–12g
ban bian lian (Lobeliae chinensis Herba) 半边莲 15–30g
lian qiao (Forsythiae Fructus) 连翘 9–12g
yi ren (Coicis Semen) 苡仁 18–30g
bai jiang cao (Patriniae Herba) 败酱草 18–30g
zao jiao ci (Gleditsiae Spina) 皂角刺 9–12g

Method: Decoction. **Huang qin, huang lian, huang bai** and **shan zhi zi** clear damp heat and toxic heat; **da huang** breaks up stagnant blood and clears heat through the Intestines; **chai hu** and **huang qin** harmonize shaoyang; **zhi shi** regulates and directs qi downwards; **chi shao** cools and activates blood; **jin yin hua, zi hua di ding, ban bian lian** and **bai jiang cao** clear toxic heat; **lian qiao** clears toxic heat and dissipates nodules; **bai jiang cao, yi ren** and **zao jiao ci** aid in discharge of pus and relieve swelling. (Source: *Shi Yong Zhong Yi Wai Ke Xue* [*Wai Tai Yi Bao* / *Shang Han Lun*])

Modifications

- With severe pain, add **ma bian cao** (Verbenae Herba) 马鞭草 15–30g, **zhi mo yao** (Myrrha preparata) 炙没药 6–9g and **zhi ru xiang** (Olibanum preparata) 炙乳香 6–9g.
- With severe or persistent fever, add **shui niu jiao** (Bubali Cornu) 水牛角 30–60g [cooked first].
- With severe nausea or vomiting, a decoction of **zhi ban xia** (Pinelliae Rhizoma preparatum) 制半夏 9–12g and **zhu ru** (Bambusae Caulis in taeniam) 竹茹 6–9g can be sipped through a straw before the main decoction is ingested.

Topical therapies
Poultice
See p.14.

Prepared medicines
Concentrated powder
Da Chai Hu Tang (Major Bupleurum Combination) or Long Dan Xie Gan Tang (Gentiana Combination) plus Huang Lian Jie Du Tang (Coptis & Scute Combination)
Pu Ji Xiao Du Yin (Scute & Cimicifuga Combination)
Xian Fang Huo Ming Yin (Angelica & Mastic Combination)

Pills
Pu Ji Xiao Du Wan (Universal Benefit Teapills)
Huang Lian Jie Du Wan (Huang Lian Jie Du Teapills) plus Wu Wei Xiao Du Wan (Five Flavor Teapills)

Acupuncture (select from)
LI.4 (hegu –) ....source point of the Large Intestine, clears heat, stops pain, activates qi and blood
LI.11 (quchi –) ....sea point of the Large Intestine, clears heat
Du.10 (lingtai –) ....these points clear heat and treat suppurative lesions
Du.12 (shenzhu –)
Liv.2 (xingjian –) ....fire point of the Liver, clears heat and fire
Bl.40 (weizhong –↓) ....lower sea point of the Urinary Bladder, clears heat, cools the blood and treats toxic lesions

- with severe pain, add GB.41 (zulinqi –) and SJ.5 (waiguan –)
- with nausea and vomiting, add PC.6 (neiguan)
- with disturbances of consciousness, bleed the tips of the fingers
- Ear points: liver, shenmen, subcortex, endocrine

Clinical notes
- A toxic heat mass in the Liver/Gallbladder may be diagnosed as a bacterial or amebic abscess, or empyema and suppuration in the gall bladder.
- This is potentially a dangerous condition and should be managed in hospital.
- Acupuncture is used to alleviate the heat, fever and pain of this condition. Herbs are essential to clear toxic heat from within the Liver.

湿 热 瘀 毒 1.3.2 LIVER – DAMP HEAT MASS
This pattern is associated with damp heat toxin and blood stasis, and represents an inflammatory presentation of liver cancer or cirrhosis, or inflammation of the liver from infection or poisoning.

Clinical features
- Large, firm, tender swelling or mass palpable beneath the right ribs; when palpated the mass feels firm and spongy like a fluid filled bag
- severe abdominal pain and distension
- sallow or dark complexion; may be jaundice
- low grade or afternoon fever, or alternating fever and chills
- night sweats
- nausea, vomiting, bitter taste in the mouth
- irritability and anger
- concentrated urine
- constipation

T red or red purple with a greasy yellow coat and stasis spots; swollen dark sublingual veins
P slippery, wiry and rapid

Treatment principle
Clear damp heat from the Liver
Activate blood, dispel blood stasis and dissipate masses
Opens the bowels to clear heat and move stagnation

Prescription

DANG GUI LONG HUI WAN 当归龙会丸
Tangkuei, Gentian and Aloe Pill, modified

dang gui (Angelicae sinensis Radix) 当归 12–15g
long dan cao (Gentianae Radix) 龙胆草 12–15g
lu hui (Aloe) 芦荟 12–15g
shan zhi zi (Gardeniae Fructus) 山栀子 12–15g
huang qin (Scutellariae Radix) 黄芩 12–15g
huang lian (Coptidis Rhizoma) 黄连 6–9g

huang bai (Phellodendri Cortex) 黄柏 9–12g
da huang (Rhei Radix et Rhizoma) 大黄 6–9g
qing dai (Indigo Naturalis) 青黛 9–12g
mu xiang (Aucklandiae Radix) 木香 6–9g
chai hu (Bupleuri Radix) 柴胡 9–12g
chuan xiong (Chuanxiong Rhizoma) 川芎 12–15g
shui hong hua zi (Polygoni orientale Semen) 水红花子 15–20g
Method: Decoction. **Qing dai** is added to the strained decoction. **Huang lian, huang qin, huang bai** and **shan zhi zi** clear damp heat and fire from all three burners; **long dan cao, qing dai** and **lu hui** purge fire from the Liver and Gallbladder; **da huang** purges fire through the bowels and provides an outlet for the heat; **mu xiang** and **dang gui** regulate qi and blood and protect them from the harsh bitter cold of the other herbs; **da huang** and **dang gui** activate blood; **chai hu** dredges the Liver, clears heat and regulates qi; **chuan xiong** activates qi and blood; **shui hong hua zi** softens hardness and dissipates masses. (Source: *Zhong Liu Ke Zhuan Bing*)

Modifications

- With Liver pain, add **yu jin** (Curcumae Radix) 郁金 12–15g and **qing pi** (Aurantii Fructus immaturus) 青皮 12–15g.
- With jaundice, add **yin chen** (Artemisiae scopariae Herba) 茵陈 30g.
- For skin rashes or purpura, add **mu dan pi** (Moutan Cortex) 牡丹皮 12–15g and **chi shao** (Paeoniae Radix rubra) 赤芍 12–15g.
- With high fever, add **zhi mu** (Anemarrhenae Rhizoma) 知母 9–12g and **shui niu jiao** (Bubali Cornu) 水牛角 15–30g [cooked first].
- With cancer or tumors, add herbs from Table 1.5, p.11, especially **bai hua she she cao** (Hedyotidis Herba) 白花蛇舌草, **ban zhi lian** (Scutellariae barbatae Herba) 半枝莲, **zi bei tian kui** (Begonia fimbristipulata Herba) 紫背天葵 or **shu yang quan** (Solanum Lyratum Herba) 蜀羊泉.

Topical therapies
Poultice
See p.14.

Prepared medicines
Concentrated powder
Dang Gui Long Hui Wan (Tangkuei, Gentiana & Aloe Formula)

Acupuncture (select from)
Liv.14 (qimen –) ....alarm point of the Liver, clears damp heat, dredges
                              the Liver, activates qi and blood and transforms
                              blood stasis
GB.24 (riyue –) ....alarm point of the Gallbladder, clears damp heat
Bl.18 (ganshu –)................transporting point of the Liver, dredges the Liver
                              and clears damp heat
Du.9 (zhiyang –) ....promotes Gallbladder function, clears damp heat
                              and alleviates jaundice
SJ.6 (zhigou –) ....these points clear heat and promote qi movement
GB.34 (yanglingquan –)   through the bowels and the Liver and Gallbladder
Liv.5 (ligou –).....................connecting point of the Liver, clears damp heat

Liv.2 (xingjian –) ....fire point of the Liver, clears heat
Sp.9 (yinlingquan –)...........sea point of the Spleen, promotes urination and
            drains damp
- with high fever, add Du.14 (dazhui)–) and LI.11 (quchi –)
- with alternating fever and chills, add SJ.5 (waiguan –) and GB.39 (xuanzhong –)
- with abdominal distension, add Ren.12 (zhongwan –) and St.25 (tianshu –)
- with nausea, add PC.6 (neiguan –)
- Ear points: liver, zero point, sympathetic, shenmen

Clinical notes
- A mass or swelling associated with damp heat and blood stasis may be diagnosed as an inflammatory phase of liver cancer, hepatitis or cirrhosis.
- With cancer a combination of Western and Chinese medicine is required. For hepatitis or cirrhosis, Chinese medicine treatment can alleviate inflammation and pain, and improve liver function.
- For dietary recommendations, see Clinical Handbook, Vol. 2, p.882.

正
虚
邪
恋

1.3.3 LIVER – CHRONIC DAMP HEAT MASS WITH QI AND YIN DEFICIENCY

This is a chronic liver abscess, and usually follows an unresolved or poorly managed acute toxic heat abscess. The presence of the toxic heat consumes qi and damages yin, and the body is unable to throw off the remaining pathogen. There is usually some degree of blood stasis as well.

In many cases there will be a history of dysenteric disorder or an intestinal abscess in the months before. The lesion may also form gradually with vague or non–specific symptoms for a period of time before imaging or physical examination reveals the mass.

Clinical features
- Enlarged, smooth, or nodular liver, that is moderately tender with palpation
- persistent low grade, undulant or recurrent fever
- night sweats
- abdominal discomfort
- loss of appetite, nausea, weight loss
- fatigue, lethargy
- pale complexion, or pale with flushed cheeks
- spider nevi over the ribs

T normal or slightly red with a greasy yellow coat; may be stasis spots
P soggy, soft and weak

Treatment principle
Support, strengthen and nourish qi and yin
Expel the remaining pathogen
Gently activate blood as necessary

Prescription

HUANG QI BIE JIA TANG 黄芪鳖甲汤
Astragalus and Turtle Shell Decoction, modified

huang qi (Astragali Radix) 黄芪 15–30g
bie jia (Trionycis Carapax) 鳖甲 12–15g
chai hu (Bupleuri Radix) 柴胡 9–12g
tian hua fen (Trichosanthes Radix) 天花粉 9–12g
qin jiao (Gentianae macrophyllae Radix) 秦艽 9–12g
bai shao (Paeoniae Radix alba) 白芍 9–12g
zhi mu (Anemarrhenae Rhizoma) 知母 9–12g
jie geng (Platycodi Radix) 桔梗 6–9g
zhi gan cao (Glycyrrhizae Radix preparata) 炙甘草 3–6g
xian he cao (Agrimoniae Herba) 仙鹤草 12–15g
ma bian cao (Verbenae Herba) 马鞭草 12–15g

Method: Decoction. **Huang qi** supplements qi and aids in discharge of pus; **bie jia** deeply nourishes yin and softens hardness to dissipate masses; **chai hu** clears heat from the Liver; **tian hua fen** clears heat and generates fluids; **qin jiao** clears deficiency heat from the Liver, activates blood and alleviates pain; **bai shao** protects yin and blood and softens the Liver; **zhi mu** clears heat from deficiency; **jie geng** aids in discharge of pus; **zhi gan cao** supports **huang qi** in supplementing qi; **xian he cao** kills parasites; **ma bian cao** clears heat and dissipates masses. (Source: *Xian Zai Zhong Yi Gan Zang Bing Xue* [*Wei Sheng Bao Jian*])

Modifications

• With persistent fever, add **qing hao** (Artemisiae annuae Herba) 青蒿 15–30g and **mu dan pi** (Moutan Cortex) 牡丹皮 9–12g.
• For amebic abscess, add **qing hao** (Artemisiae annuae Herba) 青蒿 15–30g.
• To enhance the ability of the herbs to access the mass, add **zao jiao ci** (Gleditsiae Spina) 皂角刺 9–12g and **xuan shen** (Scrophulariae Radix) 玄参 12–15g.
• With night sweats, add **duan mu li** (calcined Ostreae Concha) 煅牡蛎 15–30g and **qing hao** (Artemisiae annuae Herba) 青蒿 9–15g.
• With blood stasis, add **tao ren** (Persicae Semen) 桃仁 9–12g, **hong hua** (Carthami Flos) 红花 6–9g and **wang bu liu xing** (Vaccariae Semen) 王不留行 6–9g.
• If tending to more qi deficiency, add **bai zhu** (Atractylodis macrocephalae Rhizoma) 白术 9–12g and **fu ling** (Poria) 茯苓 12–15g.
• If tending to more yin deficiency, add **tian dong** (Asparagi Radix) 天冬 9–12g and **sheng di** (Rehmanniae Radix) 生地 9–12g.

Topical therapies
Poultice
See p.14.

Prepared medicines
Concentrated powder
Tuo Li Xiao Du Yin (Gleditsia Combination)
– for a chronic mass with qi deficiency
Qing Hao Bie Jia Tang (Artemesia & Turtle Shell Combination)
– for a chronic mass with yin deficiency

Pills
Nei Xiao Luo Li Wan (Nei Xiao Luo Li Teapills)

Acupuncture (select from)

Liv.13 (zhangmen –) ....alarm point of the Spleen and meeting point of the
yin organs, strengthens the Spleen and improves
digestion, harmonizes the Liver and Spleen

Liv.14 (qimen –) ....alarm point of the Liver, activates qi and blood and
clears damp heat

ahshi points ....over the right hypochondrium

Bl.17 (geshu –)..................meeting point for blood, dispels blood stasis

Bl.18 (ganshu –)................transport point of the Liver, activates qi and blood

Bl.20 (pishu) ....transport point of the Spleen, strengthens the Spleen
to transform phlegm

Liv.3 (taichong –)..............source and earth point of the Liver, activates Liver qi
and blood, stops pain

Sp.6 (sanyinjiao)................regulates and activates Liver qi and blood and
strengthens the Spleen, supplements qi and yin

• with pain, add SJ.6 (zhigou –) and GB.34 (yanglingquan –)
• Ear points: abdomen, liver, zero point, shenmen

Clinical notes

• A chronic mass in the liver with qi and yin deficiency may be diagnosed as a liver abscess or subphrenic abscess. Chronic inflammatory masses in the liver can form a thick wall which can prevent access to the lesion. They can be difficult to treat and may require aspiration. At least six weeks of herbs and acupuncture should be given before deciding whether the treatment is working or not.
• For dietary recommendations, see Clinical Handbook, Vol. 2, p.870 and 876.

1.3.4 LIVER – YIN DEFICIENCY MASS WITH BLOOD STASIS

肝
阴
不
足，
血
燥
瘀
结

A mass in the Liver with concurrent yin deficiency is usually the result of a chronic heat or stasis pathology that gradually damages and depletes yin. Years of alcohol abuse which introduce damp heat, or a chronic pattern of Liver heat may be seen. The mass still needs to be addressed, but the deficiency has come to the fore. Too vigorous an attacking strategy will further damage yin and weaken the patient.

Clinical features

• Firm or nodular palpable mass or masses in the liver, generally non tender or only mildly tender
• dull ache in the right upper quadrant
• firm distended abdomen with prominent distended veins
• spider veins and nevi on the face, chest and lower legs
• low grade fever, irregularly spiking fever at night; night sweats
• weight loss, emaciation
• dark, grey or ashen complexion
• dry mouth and purple, dry, cracked, lips

- dry scaly skin
- nose bleeds, bleeding gums, melena, purpura
- concentrated urine

T red or scarlet and dry, with little or no coat; may be dark swollen sublingual veins

P wiry, choppy, fine, rapid

Treatment principle

Nourish and supplement Liver yin
Cool and activate blood and dispel blood stasis

Prescription

YI GUAN JIAN 一贯煎
Linking Decoction, modified

sheng di (Rehmanniae Radix) 生地	25–50g
gou qi zi (Lycii Fructus) 枸杞子	20–30g
sha shen (Glehniae/Adenophorae Radix) 沙参	12–15g
mai dong (Ophiopogonis Radix) 麦冬	12–15g
dang gui (Angelicae sinensis Radix) 当归	12–15g
chuan lian zi (Toosendan Fructus) 川楝子	12–10g
bie jia (Trionycis Carapax) 鳖甲	12–15g
gui ban (Testudinis Plastrum) 龟板	9–12g
mu dan pi (Moutan Cortex) 牡丹皮	9–12g
shui hong hua zi (Polygoni orientale Semen) 水红花子	12–15g

Method: Decoction. **Sheng di**, **sha shen**, **mai dong** and **gou qi zi** nourish and protect yin and blood; **dang gui** nourishes and harmonizes blood; **chuan lian zi** dredges the Liver and regulates qi; **bie jia** and **gui ban** deeply enrich yin, soften hardness and dissipate masses; **mu dan pi** activates and cools the blood and dispels blood stasis; **shui hong hua zi** softens hardness and dissipates masses. (Source: *Zhong Liu Ke Zhuan Bing* [*Xu Ming Yi Lei An*])

Modifications

- With constipation, add **gua lou ren** (Trichosanthis Semen) 栝楼仁 12–15g and **xuan shen** (Scrophulariae Radix) 玄参 12–15g.
- With fever and night sweats, add **yin chai hu** (Stellariae Radix) 银柴胡 9–12g, **di gu pi** (Lycii Cortex) 地骨皮 12–15g, **chao shan zhi zi** (stir fried Gardeniae Fructus) 炒山栀子 9–12g and **ye jiao teng** (Polygoni multiflori Caulis) 夜胶藤 15–30g.
- With scanty urination, dysuria and hematuria, add **bai mao gen** (Imperatae Rhizoma) 白茅根 15–18g.
- With bleeding or purpura, add **bai mao gen** (Imperatae Rhizoma) 白茅根 15–18g, **ce bai ye** (Platycladi Cacumen) 侧柏叶 12–15g and **san qi fen** (powdered Notoginseng Radix) 三七粉 3–9g [taken separately].
- With ascendant yang, headaches and dizziness, add **mu li** (Ostreae Concha) 牡蛎 15–30g [cooked first].
- With sharp pain, add **yu jin** (Curcumae Radix) 郁金 9–12g and **dan shen** (Salviae miltiorrhizae Radix) 丹参 9–12g.

- With cancer or tumors, add herbs from Table 1.5, p.11, especially **bai hua she she cao** (Hedyotidis Herba) 白花蛇舌草, **ban zhi lian** (Scutellariae barbatae Herba) 半枝莲, **zi bei tian kui** (Begonia fimbristipulata Herba) 紫背天葵 or **shu yang quan** (Solanum Lyratum Herba) 蜀羊泉.

Topical therapies
Poultice
See p.14.

Prepared medicines
Concentrated powder
Yi Guan Jian (Linking Combination)
Liu Wei Di Huang Wan (Rehmannia Six Formula)
Ge Xia Zhu Yu Tang (Tangkuei & Corydalis Combination)
  – add a small proportion, 15–30%, of this formula to one of those above

Pills
Yi Guan Jian Wan (Linking Decoction Teapills)
Liu Wei Di Huang Wan (Six Flavor Teapills)
Ge Xia Zhu Yu Wan (Stasis in the Lower Chamber Teapills)

Acupuncture (select from)
Bl.23 (shenshu +) ....these points supplement Liver and Kidney yin
Bl.18 (ganshu +)
Liv.14 (qimen) ....alarm point of the Liver, activates Liver qi and blood
SJ.6 (zhigou –) ....these points clear heat and promote qi movement
GB.34 (yanglingquan –)   through the bowels and the Liver and Gallbladder
Liv.3 (taichong +) ....source point of the Liver, supplements Liver yin and
                               blood, activates qi and blood, stops pain, pacifies
                               hyperactive Liver yang
Sp.6 (sanyinjiao +) ....strengthens the Spleen, dredges the Liver and
                               regulates qi, benefits the Kidneys and supplements
                               qi and yin
Liv.8 (ququan –) ....sea point of the Liver, supplements Liver yin and
                               clears damp heat
Ear points: liver, kidney, gallbladder, spleen, shenmen

Clinical notes
- Liver yin deficiency with blood stasis may be diagnosed as hepatic cirrhosis or primary liver cancer.
- When the diagnosis is cancer, a combination of Western and Chinese medicine should be used.
- For dietary recommendations see Clinical Handbook, Vol. 2, p.878 and 886.

胃
热
伤
阴

1.3.5 EPIGASTRIC MASS – STOMACH HEAT AND YIN DEFICIENCY

This pattern is usually the result of long term Liver and Stomach disharmony. The qi constraint generates heat which damages yin and congeals blood.

Clinical features

- Small, firm epigastric mass that is tender with palpation. The epigastrium feels warm and dry to the touch. There is a burning or acidic sensation in the epigastrium.
- vomiting, acid reflux, heartburn
- may be vomiting blood or melena
- abdominal and epigastric distension
- dry mouth, tongue and lips, thirst
- sense of heat in the chest, palms and soles
- low grade afternoon or evening fever
- loss of appetite, weight loss constipation
- concentrated urine
- flushed complexion or red cheeks

T red, dry and cracked with little or no coat or a centrally peeled coat
P fine and rapid

Treatment principle

Nourish Stomach yin and clear heat
Soften hardness, gently activate qi and blood and dissipate masses

Prescription

SHA SHEN MAI MEN DONG TANG 沙参麦门冬汤
Glehnia and Ophiopogonis Decoction, modified

sha shen (Glehniae/Adenophorae Radix) 沙参 15–20g
mai dong (Ophiopogonis Radix) 麦冬 15–20g
yu zhu (Polygonati odorati Rhizoma) 玉竹 15–20g
gan cao (Glycyrrhizae Radix) 甘草 3–6g
sheng di (Rehmanniae Radix) 生地 15–20g
zhi mu (Anemarrhenae Rhizoma) 知母 9–12g
shan yao (Dioscoreae Rhizoma) 山药 18–30g
xi yang shen (Panacis quinquefolii Radix) 西洋参 9–12g
bai hua she she cao (Hedyotis diffusae Herba) 白花蛇舌草 15–30g
chong lou (Paridis Rhizoma) 重楼 12–15g
Method: Decoction. **Sha shen, mai dong, yu zhu, sheng di** and **zhi mu** nourish yin and clear heat; **bai hua she she cao** and **chong lou** clear heat and toxins and treat tumors; **shan yao, xi yang shen** and **gan cao** support Stomach qi and yin. (Source: *Zhong Liu Ke Zhuan Bing* [*Jing Yue Quan Shu*])

Modifications

- With nausea, add **zhu ru** (Bambusae Caulis in taeniam) 竹茹 12–15g.
- With fever, add **yin chai hu** (Stellariae Radix) 银柴胡 9–12g.
- With severe reflux, add **xuan fu hua** (Inulae Flos) 旋覆花 9–12g, **dai zhe shi**

(Haematitum) 代赭石 9–12g and **wa leng zi** (Arcae Concha) 瓦楞子 12–15g [separately as powder].
- One or two herbs from Table 1.5, p.11 can be added to augment the anti–cancer property of the formula. Relatively small doses should be used initially as the bitterness that characterizes these herbs can further damage yin.

Topical therapies
Poultice
See p.14.

Prepared medicines
Concentrated powder
Sha Shen Mai Men Dong Tang (Glehnia & Ophiopogon Combination)
Yu Nu Jian (Rehmannia & Gypsum Combination)
Pills
Qing Wei San Wan (Qing Wei San Teapills) plus Yu Quan Wan (Jade Spring Teapills) or Sheng Mai Wan (Great Pulse Teapills)

Acupuncture (select from)
Ren.12 (zhongwan –) ....these points harmonize the Liver and Stomach,
St.21 (liangmen –)   regulate qi and stop pain
Ren.4 (guanyuan +)............supplements yin systemically
ahshi points ....locally, and along the course of the Stomach
                              channel, between St.36 (zusanli) and St.41 (jiexi)
Bl.21 (weishu +) ....transport points of the Stomach and Kidneys,
Bl.23 (shenshu +)   supplement Stomach yin
St.44 (neiting –) ....these points clear heat from the Stomach
LI.4 (hegu –)
Sp.6 (sanyinjiao +)..............supplement Spleen, Stomach, Kidney and Liver yin
St.36 (zusanli –) ....sea point of the Stomach, strengthens the Spleen and
                              Stomach and clears heat
PC.7 (daling) ....source and stream point of the Pericardium, harmonizes the Stomach and clears Heat
- with severe pain, add St.34 (liangqiu –) and Sp.4 (gongsun –)
- with reflux and heartburn, add PC.6 (neiguan –) and Sp.4 (gongsun –)
- with hematemesis, add PC.4 (ximen –)
- with fever, add LI.11 (quchi –)
- Ear points: stomach, zero point, abdomen, kidney, shenmen, sympathetic

Clinical notes
- An epigastric mass associated with Stomach heat and yin deficiency type may be diagnosed as stomach cancer, cancer associated with chronic gastritis or peptic ulcer disease.
- When the diagnosis is cancer, a combination of Western and Chinese medicine should be used.
- For dietary recommendations, see Clinical Handbook, Vol. 2, p.884 and 876.

瘀
毒
阻
滞

1.3.6 HEAT MASS IN THE INTESTINES

This is an acute accumulation of toxic heat or damp heat in the Intestines.

Clinical features

- Tender mass in the lower burner, usually left or right iliac fossa, with muscle guarding in the overlying tissues. The pain is intermittent, colicky or spasmodic, and worse with pressure. There may be rebound tenderness on palpation, and the patient may flex their hip to provide some degree of relief.
- intermittent low grade fever, or fever and chills
- abdominal distension, loss of appetite, nausea, maybe vomiting
- constipation or diarrhea; may be mucus or blood in the stools

T thin, greasy white or yellow coat
P slippery and rapid

Treatment principle

Open the bowels to purge the accumulating pathogen
Move qi and activate blood, clear heat

Prescription

DA HUANG MU DAN TANG 大黄牡丹汤
Rhubarb and Moutan Decoction, modified

da huang (Rhei Radix et Rhizoma) 大黄 9–18g
dong gua ren (Benincasae Semen) 冬瓜仁 18–30g
tao ren (Persicae Semen) 桃仁 12–15g
mu dan pi (Moutan Cortex) 牡丹皮 9–12g
mang xiao (Natrii Sulfas) 芒硝 6–9g
san leng (wine fried Sparganii Rhizoma) 三棱 9–12g
e zhu (Curcumae Rhizoma) 莪术 9–12g
Method: Decoction. **Da huang** is added a few minutes before the end of cooking, **mang xiao** is dissolved in the strained decoction. **Da huang** opens the bowels to clear heat and purges accumulation; **tao ren** activates blood and disperses blood stasis; **dong gua ren** aids in discharge of pus and clears heat; **mang xiao** softens hardness to support the purging and heat clearing action of the **da huang**; **mu dan pi** cools the blood and disperses static blood; **san leng** and **e zhu** break up blood stasis and dissipate masses. (Source: *Shi Yong Zhong Yi Nei Ke Xue* [*Jin Gui Yao Lüe*])

Modifications

- The dose of **da huang** can vary depending on the degree of heat and constipation, and the robustness of the patient. It is usually best to begin at the low end of the dosage range, then increase it on the second dose if necessary. Without constipation, processed **da huang** (**zhi da huang** 制大黄) may be used. Remember that it usually takes about six hours for **da huang** to move the bowels.
- With more intense heat, add two or three of the following herbs: **hong teng** (Sargentodoxae Caulis) 红藤 30g and **bai jiang cao** (Patriniae Herba) 败酱草 30g, **pu gong ying** (Taraxici Herba) 蒲公英 15–30g, **lian qiao** (Forsythia Fructus) 连翘 9–12g and **jin yin hua** (Lonicera Flos) 金银花 15–30g.
- With marked abdominal distension, add **zhi shi** (Aurantii Fructus immaturus) 枳实 9–12g and **gua lou ren** (Trichosanthis Semen) 栝楼仁 9–12g.

- With severe pain, add **yan hu suo** (Corydalis Rhizoma) 延胡索 9–12g, **chuan lian zi** (Toosendan Fructus) 川楝子 9–12g and **mu xiang** (Aucklandiae Radix) 木香 6–9g.
- With nausea, add **zhu ru** (Bambusae Caulis in taeniam) 竹茹 12–15g.

Topical therapies
Poultice
A poultice over the lesion may assist to soften the mass directly and accelerate resolution. Poultice No. 1 or 3 is recommended, p.22.

Retention enema
See p.55.

Prepared medicines
Concentrated powder
Da Huang Mu Dan Pi Tang (Rhubarb & Moutan Combination)
Pills
Ge Xia Zhu Yu Wan (Stasis in the Lower Chamber Teapills)

Acupuncture (select from)
ahshi points ....If the appendix is affected, lanweixue (M–LE–13), about one cun below St.36 (zusanli), will be exquisitely tender; if the focus is in another part of the intestine (usually the left iliac fossa), points on the Stomach channel between St.36 (zusanli) and St.37 (shangjuxu) will be tender.

St.25 (tianshu –)..................alarm point of the Large Intestine, regulates Intestinal function and eliminates stagnation

St.37 (shangjuxu –) ....lower sea point of the Large Intestine, eliminates stagnation and accumulation from the Stomach and Intestines and clears damp heat

Sp.8 (diji –) ....cleft point of the Spleen, regulates and activates blood

- with fever, add LI.11 (quchi –), LI.4 (hegu –) and St.44 (neiting –)
- with severe pain, add St.34 (liangqiu –), St.43 (xianggu –) and Sp.4 (gongsun)
- with nausea and vomiting, add PC.6 (neiguan) and Ren.13 (shangwan)
- with abdominal distension, add Ren.6 (qihai) and St.41 (jiexi –)
- with constipation, add SJ.6 (zhigou), Sp.14 (fujie) and GB.34 (yanglingquan)
- Ear points: appendix, large intestine, abdomen, zero point, sympathetic

Clinical notes
- A mass of this type may be diagnosed as an inflammatory lesion such as appendicitis, diverticulitis, salpingitis or an abscess in the iliac fossa.
- When treated early enough, masses of this type respond quickly to treatment.
- The development of toxic heat (fever, increasing pain, malaise, pallor) is ominous and may indicate a rupture and peritonitis, and should be managed in hospital.

热
郁
血
瘀

1.3.7 HEAT MASS IN THE HYPOGASTRIUM, WITH BLOOD STASIS

The heat and blood stasis masses in this pattern affect the uterus and associated structures. The heat can manifest in the form of constrained heat or damp heat.

Clinical features

- Soft tender mass in the central lower burner, that may or may not be palpable. The lower abdomen is firm and warm to the touch and painful with palpation.
- lower abdominal distension, warmth and focal pain or burning pain
- short menstrual cycle, menorrhagia or persistent uterine bleeding; dark, clotted, sticky menstrual flow
- yellow vaginal discharge; may be offensive
- persistent low grade or intermittent fever, or fever and chills
- night sweats
- insomnia, fitful sleep
- concentrated urine
- constipation

T red with a dry yellow or greasy yellow coat
P wiry, slippery and rapid or wiry and fine

Treatment principle

Clear heat, activate blood, dispel blood stasis and dissipate masses

Prescription

XIAO CHAI HU TANG 小柴胡汤
Minor Bupleurum Decoction, plus
TAO HE CHENG QI TANG 桃核承气汤
Peach Pit Decoction to Order the Qi, modified

chai hu (Bupleuri Radix) 柴胡	6–12g
huang qin (Scutellariae Radix) 黄芩	6–9g
zhi ban xia (Pinelliae Rhizoma preparatum) 制半夏	6–9g
ren shen (Ginseng Radix) 人参	6–9g
zhi gan cao (Glycyrrhizae Radix preparata) 炙甘草	3–6g
sheng jiang (Zingiberis Rhizoma recens) 生姜	6–9g
da zao (Jujubae Fructus) 大枣	4 fruit
tao ren (Semen Persicae) 桃仁	9–12g
da huang (Rhei Radix et Rhizoma) 大黄	6–9g
mang xiao (Natrii Sulfas) 芒硝	6–9g
gui zhi (Cinnamomi Ramulus) 桂枝	6–9g
hong teng (Sargentodoxae Caulis) 红藤	15–30g
bai jiang cao (Patriniae Herba) 败酱草	15–30g
mu dan pi (Moutan Cortex) 牡丹皮	9–12g

Method: Decoction. **Mang xiao** is dissolved in the strained decoction. **Chai hu** and **huang qin** clear heat and harmonize shaoyang to assist in expulsion of the pathogen; **tao ren** and **da huang** activate blood and disperse static blood; **da huang** and **mang xiao** open the bowels to provide an outlet for the heat and stasis; **hong teng**, **bai jiang cao** and **mu dan pi** clear heat, cool and activate the blood and disperse blood stasis; **ren shen**, **zhi gan cao**, **sheng jiang** and **da zao** support zheng qi and assist the expulsion of the pathogen; **gui zhi** opens up the flow of yang qi through the lower burner. (Source: *Zhong Yi Fu Chan Ke Xue* [*Shang Han Lun*])

Modifications

- With damp heat and profuse vaginal discharge, add **huang bai** (Phellodendri Cortex) 黄柏 9–12g, **cang zhu** (Atractylodis Rhizoma) 苍术 6–9g and **tu fu ling** (Smilacis glabrae Rhizoma) 土茯苓 15–30g.
- With severe pain, add **yan hu suo** (Corydalis Rhizoma) 延胡索 9–12g and **chuan lian zi** (Toosendan Fructus) 川楝子 9–12g.
- With lower back or thigh pain, add **qin jiao** (Gentianae macrophyllae Radix) 秦艽 9–12g and **du huo** (Angelicae Pubescentis Radix) 独活 6–9g.
- With menorrhagia, add **yi mu cao** (Leonurus Herba) 益母草 12–15g, **di yu** (Sanguisorbae Radix) 地榆 9–12g and **qian cao gen** (Rubiae Radix) 茜草根 9–12g.
- With a large or persistent mass, add **xia ku cao** (Prunellae Spica) 夏枯草 15–18g, **pu huang** (Typhae Pollen) 蒲黄 9–12g [decocted in a cloth bag] and **zao jiao ci** (Gleditsiae Spina) 皂角刺 6–9g.

Prepared medicines

Concentrated powder

Xiao Chai Hu Tang (Minor Bupleurum Combination) plus Tao He Cheng Qi Tang (Persica & Rhubarb Combination)

San Miao San (Atractylodes & Phellodendron Formula)
 – add with damp heat

Da Huang Mu Dan Pi Tang (Rhubarb & Moutan Combination)

Pills

Qian Jin Zhi Dai Wan (Chien Chin Chih Tai Wan)

Huang Lian Jie Du Wan (Huang Lian Jie Du Teapills) plus Tao Hong Si Wu Wan (Tao Hong Si Wu Tang Teapills)

Acupuncture (select from)

St.29 (guilai –) ....these points regulate the movement of qi and blood
St.28 (shuidao –)   in the lower abdomen and clear heat
Ren.3 (zhongji –)
GB.26 (daimai –) ....regulates the daimai and clears damp heat
Liv.5 (ligou –)......................connecting point of the Liver, regulates qi and blood in the lower abdomen and clears heat
Liv.8 (ququan)....................sea point of the Liver, clears heat from the lower burner
Sp.8 (diji –) ....cleft point of the Spleen, regulates and activates blood
Sp.10 (xuehai –) ....activates blood and cools the blood
- with fever, add LI.11 (quchi –) and LI.4 (hegu –)
- with severe pain, add Sp.4 (gongsun) and PC.6 (neiguan –)
- with nausea and vomiting, add PC.6 (neiguan) and Ren.12 (zhongwan)

- with abdominal distension, add St.40 (fenglong –) and SJ.6 (zhigou –)
- with constipation, add SJ.6 (zhigou) and GB.34 (yanglingquan)
- Ear points: uterus, liver, kidney, endocrine, sympathetic, subcortex

Topical therapies

Poultice

A poultice over the lesion may assist to soften the mass directly and accelerate resolution. Poultice No. 1 or 3 is recommended, p.22.

Retention enema

This prescription is suitable for masses with blood stasis and heat. The herbs are decocted in the normal fashion, strained and cooled to body temperature before 60–150 milliliters are inserted into the rectum with a commercial enema device. The enema is given once daily for 7–14 days, and can be retained with the patient lying down for 30 minutes to 2 hours with the hips elevated.

hong teng (Sargentodoxae Caulis) 红藤 30g
bai jiang cao (Patriniae Herba) 败酱草 30g
zao jiao ci (Gleditsiae Spina) 皂角刺 30g
pu gong ying (Taraxici Herba) 蒲公英 30g
xu chang qing (Cynanchi paniculati Radix) 徐长青 30g
dan shen (Salviae miltiorrhizae Radix) 丹参 15g

Method: Decoction and retention enema. **Hong teng**, **bai jiang cao** and **zao jiao ci** dissipate inflammatory masses and aid in the discharge of pus; **pu gong ying** and **xu chang qing** clear toxic heat; **dan shen** activates blood and dispels blood stasis. (Source: *Zhong Yi Zhi Liao Yi Nan Za Bing Mi Yao*)

Clinical notes

- A heat mass with blood stasis in the hypogastrium may be diagnosed as chronic pelvic inflammatory disease, inflammatory masses, endometritis, salpingitis, adnexitis or endometriosis.
- Classically, this pattern can follow pregnancy, a termination or even menstruation, when the blood is weak and it is thought the 'blood chamber' is vulnerable to invasion from the exterior.
- For dietary recommendations, see Clinical Handbook, Vol. 2, p.882.

1.4 COLD and/or DEFICIENCY

1. Liver and Gallbladder – cold and blood stasis
2. Liver yang deficiency with blood stasis
3. Stomach
4. Lower burner
5. Lower burner – Kidney deficiency
6. Uterus – qi and blood deficiency

寒
凝
血
瘀

1.4.1 COLD MASS IN THE LIVER AND GALLBLADDER

This pattern describes masses caused by cold and blood stasis which affect the liver and gall bladder and the passage of bile.

Clinical features

- Firm palpable mass in the upper right quadrant, generally non tender
- dull jaundice with a dark tinge
- anorexia, nausea, weight loss
- loose stools, or sticky pale clay like stools
- abdominal and epigastric distension, discomfort or pain
- cold intolerance, cold or purplish extremities
- spider nevi over the ribs and on the face

T mauve with a greasy white coat; stasis spots and dark swollen sublingual veins
P soggy, soft and weak

Treatment principle

Warm and dispel cold damp
Activate blood and dispel blood stasis
Support the Spleen and harmonize the Stomach

Prescription

YIN CHEN ZHU FU TANG 茵陈术附汤
Virgate Wormwood, Atractylodes and Prepared Aconite Decoction, plus
FU YUAN HUO XUE TANG 复元活血汤
Revive Health by Activating the Blood Decoction, modified

yin chen (Artemisiae scopariae Herba) 茵陈 12–15g
chao bai zhu (stir fried Atractylodes macrocephalae Rhizoma) 炒白术 ... 9–12g
zhi fu zi (Aconiti Radix lateralis preparata) 制附子 6–12g
gan jiang (Zingiberis Rhizoma) 干姜 6–9g
chai hu (Bupleuri Radix) 柴胡 9–12g
wang bu liu xing (Vaccariae Semen) 王不留行 9–12g
tao ren (Persicae Semen) 桃仁 9–12g
hou po (Magnoliae officinalis Cortex) 厚朴 9–12g
fu ling (Poria) 茯苓 12–15g
di bie chong (Eupolyphaga/Steleophaga) 地鳖虫 6–9g

Method: Decoction. **Yin chen** promotes Gallbladder function and alleviates jaundice; **chao bai zhu** dries damp and strengthens the Spleen; **zhi fu zi** and **gan jiang** warm yang and dispel cold; **chai hu** regulates qi flow in the Liver and Gallbladder; **wang bu liu xing** (substitute for **chuan** shan jia 穿山甲), activates blood and opens the network vessels; **tao ren** and **di bie chong** break up blood stasis and dissipate masses; **hou po** directs qi downward and alleviates distension; **fu ling** strengthens the Spleen and leaches out damp. (Source: *Zhong Yi Zhi Liao Yi Nan Za Bing Mi Yao* [*Yi Xue Xin Wu* / *Yi Xue Fa Ming*])

Modifications

- With a hard, nodular mass, add **e zhu** (Curcumae Rhizoma) 莪术 9–12g, **jiu san leng** (wine fried Sparganii Rhizoma) 酒三棱 9–12g and **bie jia** (Trionycis Carapax) 鳖甲 12–15g.
- With a round, rubbery, solid or cystic mass, combine with **Xiao Luo Wan** (Reduce Scrophula Pill 消瘰丸, pp.8, 921).
- With pain, add **yu jin** (Curcumae Radix) 郁金 9–12g, **chuan lian zi** (Toosendan Fructus) 川楝子 9–12g and **yan hu suo** (Corydalis Rhizoma) 延胡索 9–15g, or **zhi mo yao** (Myrrha preparata) 炙没药 6–9g and **zhi ru xiang** (Olibanum preparata) 炙乳香 6–9g.
- With Spleen qi deficiency, combine with **Xiang Sha Liu Jun Zi Tang** (Six Gentlemen Decoction with Aucklandia and Amomum 香砂六君子汤, p.618).
- With qi and blood deficiency, combine with **Gui Pi Tang** (Restore the Spleen Decoction 归脾汤, p.387).
- With cancer or tumors, add herbs from Table 1.5, p.11, in particular **bai hua she she cao** (Hedyotidis Herba) 白花蛇舌草, **ban zhi lian** (Scutellariae barbatae Herba) 半枝莲, **ban bian lian** (Lobeliae chinensis Herba) 半边莲 or **shu yang quan** (Solanum Lyratum Herba) 蜀羊泉.

Prepared medicines

Concentrated powder

Yin Chen Wu Ling San (Capillaris & Poria Five Formula) plus Fu Yuan Huo Xue Tang (Tangkuei & Persica Combination)

Shao Fu Zhu Yu Tang (Fennel Seed & Corydalis Combination)

Ge Xia Zhu Yu Tang (Tangkuei & Corydalis Combination)

Pills

Ge Xia Zhu Yu Wan (Stasis in the Lower Chamber Teapills)

Shao Fu Zhu Yu Wan (Stasis in the Lower Palace Teapills)

Acupuncture (select from)

Liv.14 (qimen –▲)..............alarm point of the Liver, activates qi and blood

GB.24 (riyue –)...................alarm point of the Gallbladder, activates Gallbladder qi

ah shi points ....over the right hypochondrium

Bl.17 (geshu –)...................meeting point for blood, dispels blood stasis

Bl.18 (ganshu –▲)..............transport point of the Liver, moves qi and blood

Bl.19 (danshu –▲)..............transport point of the Gallbladder, regulates Gallbladder qi

SJ.6 (zhigou –) ....these points activate qi and blood through the Liver

GB.34 (yanglingquan –)   and Gallbladder organ systems, and stop pain

dannangxue (M–LE–23) ....extra point for the Gallbladder disorders; good for colicky pain, use if tender

Liv.1 (dadun –) ....well point of the Liver, for masses in the hypochon-drium with Liv.14 (qimen)
- Ear points: gallbladder, liver, zero point, sympathetic, shenmen

Clinical notes
- A cold mass with blood stasis affecting the Liver and Gallbladder may be diagnosed as a tumor of the gall bladder, the biliary tree or head of the pancreas.
- This is a difficult condition to treat and should be managed by a combination of Western and Chinese medicine.
- For dietary recommendations, see Clinical Handbook, Vol. 2, p.886.

肝阳虚弱，血瘀湿滞

1.4.2 LIVER YANG DEFICIENCY WITH BLOOD STASIS AND DAMP ACCUMULATION

This is chronic mass or masses with edema or ascites.

Clinical features
- Firm or nodular palpable mass or masses in the liver, generally non tender; the region over the right hypochondrium feels cool.
- dull ache in the right hypochondriac region
- sallow, withered or ashen complexion
- abdominal distension; fluid in the abdominal cavity
- generalized edema
- frequent scanty urination, nocturia
- loose stools or watery early morning diarrhea with undigested food
- fatigue, exhaustion
- lower back aching, weak and cold
- cold intolerance, cold or blue extremities
- spider veins on the abdomen and lower legs, the inner knees and ankles

T swollen, pale or mauve and scalloped with a thin white coat; may be stasis spots and dark swollen sublingual veins

P deep, weak, fine or imperceptible

Treatment principle
Warm yang and dispel cold
Stimulate fluid metabolism and promote urination to drain damp
Activate blood and dispel blood stasis

Prescription

JI SHENG SHEN QI WAN 济生肾气丸
Kidney Qi Pill from Formulas to Aid the Living, modified

ze xie (Alismatis Rhizoma) 泽泻	9–12g
fu ling (Poria) 茯苓	9–12g
che qian zi (Plantaginis Semen) 车前子	9–12g
shan yao (Dioscoreae Rhizoma) 山药	9–12g
mu dan pi (Moutan Cortex) 牡丹皮	9–12g
zhi fu zi (Aconiti Radix lateralis preparata) 制附子	3–6g

gui zhi (Cinnamomi Ramulus) 桂枝 3–6g
shu di (Rehmanniae Radix preparata) 熟地 3–6g
huai niu xi (Achyranthis bidentatae Radix) 怀牛膝 3–6g
huang qi (Astragali Radix) 黄芪 6–9g
chao bai zhu (stir fried Atractylodes macrocephalae Rhizoma) 炒白术 6–9g
chao bai shao (stir fried Paeoniae Radix alba) 炒白芍 6–9g
ze lan (Lycopi Herba) 泽兰 6–9g
dan shen (Salviae miltiorrhizae Radix) 丹参 6–9g
e zhu (Curcumae Rhizoma) 莪术 6–9g
Method: Powder or pills. Can be decocted at the beginning of treatment with the doses as shown until fluids are moving, after which powders or pills can be used. **Ze xie**, **fu ling** and **che qian zi** promote urination and drain damp; **gui zhi** works with **ze xie** and **fu ling** to enhance the transformation of qi and stimulate the excretion of accumulated fluids; **zhi fu zi** and **gui zhi** warm Kidney yang, dispel cold, promote the transformation of qi and promote fluid metabolism; **shu di** supports Liver and Kidney yin and blood; **shan yao** strengthens the Spleen and Kidneys and supplements qi; **mu dan pi** activates blood; **huai niu xi** supplements the Liver and Kidneys and activates blood; **huang qi** supplements qi and mobilizes fluids; **chao bai zhu** dries damp and supplements qi; **chao bai shao** softens the Liver and protects yin and blood; **ze lan** activates blood and promotes urination; **dan shen** and **e zhu** activate blood and dissipate masses. (Source: *Xian Zai Zhong Yi Gan Zang Bing Xue* [*Ji Sheng Fang*])

Prepared medicines
Concentrated powder
Ji Sheng Shen Qi Wan (Cyathula & Plantago Formula)

Pills
Jin Kui Shen Qi Wan (Fu Gui Ba Wei Wan, Golden Book Teapills)
Zhen Wu Tang Wan (True Warrior Teapills)

Acupuncture (select from)
Liv.14 (qimen +▲)............alarm point of the Liver, warms the Liver and
                                              activates qi and blood
Bl.23 (shenshu +▲) ....these points warm yang, promote Liver and Kidney
Bl.18 (ganshu +▲)   function and activate qi and blood
Bl.19 (danshu ▲)
Ren.12 (zhongwan +▲) .....local points to warm, strengthen and regulate middle
Ren.13 (shangwan +▲)   burner qi and dispel cold
SJ.6 (zhigou) ....these points promote qi movement through the
GB.34 (yanglingquan)   lateral aspect of the body
St.36 (zusanli +▲) ....sea point of the Stomach, warms and strengthens the
                                              Spleen and Stomach and supplements yang qi
• Ear points: liver, kidney, spleen, zero point, shenmen, adrenal

Clinical notes
• Liver, Spleen and Kidney yang deficiency with stasis may be diagnosed as hepatic cirrhosis or liver cancer with ascites.
• A yang warming diet is recommended. See Clinical Handbook, Vol. 2, p.873 and 886.

寒
凝
血
结

1.4.3 COLD MASS IN THE EPIGASTRIUM

A cold epigastric mass is most often in the stomach, but the pancreas may be involved. The mass is commonly the product of chronic yang deficiency of the middle burner, however it may also develop as the result of qi constraint or dysfunction of the qi dynamic, with gradual complication by yang deficiency. A mass of this type is invariably complicated by blood stasis.

Clinical features

- Epigastric mass with colicky or spasmodic pain. The pain is alleviated somewhat with heat and is worse when the patient has not eaten.
- vomiting, acid reflux, heartburn
- poor appetite, weight loss
- abdominal and epigastric distension
- pale complexion
- may be melena

T moist and pale, with a thick white coat
P weak and soft, or tight (with pain)

Treatment principle

Warm and dispel cold and dissipate masses

Prescription

AN ZHONG SAN 安中散
Calm the Middle Powder, modified

gui zhi (Cinnamomi Ramulus) 桂枝 9–12g
yan hu suo (Corydalis Rhizoma) 延胡索 9–12g
duan mu li (calcined Ostreae Concha) 煅牡蛎 15–30g
xiao hui xiang (Foeniculi Fructus) 小茴香 9–12g
sha ren (Amomi Fructus) 砂仁 3–6g
gao liang jiang (Alpiniae officinarum Rhizoma) 高良姜 3–6g
gan cao (Glycyrrhizae Radix) 甘草 3–6g
jiu san leng (wind fried Sparganii Rhizoma) 酒三棱 9–12g
cu e zhu (vinegar fried Curcumae Rhizoma) 醋莪术 9–12g

Method: Decoction. **Duan mu li** is cooked first for 30 minutes. **Gui zhi** warms the Stomach, dispels cold and assists qi transformation; **yan hu suo** activates blood and stops pain; **duan mu li** softens hardness and alleviates heartburn; **xiao hui xiang**, **sha ren** and **gao liang jiang** warm the Stomach and dispel cold; **gan cao** harmonizes and protects the Stomach; **jiu san leng** and **cu e zhu** break up blood stasis and dissipate masses. (Source: *He Ji Ju Fang*)

Modifications

- With nausea and vomiting, add **zhi ban xia** (Pinelliae Rhizoma preparatum) 制半夏 9–12g, **wu zhu yu** (Evodiae Fructus) 吴茱萸 2–3g and **sheng jiang** (Zingiberis Rhizoma recens) 生姜 6–9g.
- With severe reflux, add **xuan fu hua** (Inulae Flos) 旋覆花 9–12g and **dai zhe shi** (Haematitum) 代赭石 9–12g, or **wa leng zi** (Arcae Concha) 瓦楞子 9–12g.
- With marked pain, increase the dose of **gao liang jiang** to 9g, and add **bi ba** (Piperis Longi Fructus) 荜茇 3–6g.

- With bleeding from the digestive tract, add **san qi fen** (powdered Notoginseng Radix) 三七粉 3–9g [added to the strained decoction] and **qian cao gen** (Rubiae Radix) 茜草根 9–15g, or combine with the prepared medicine YUN NAN BAI YAO (Yunnan White Powder 云南白药).
- With cancer or a tumor, one or two herbs from Table 1.5, p.11 can be added to augment the anti–cancer property of the formula. Suitable herbs include **bai hua she she cao** (Hedyotis diffusae Herba) 白花蛇舌草, **mao zhua cao** (Ranunculi ternati Radix) 猫爪草 and **ban bian lian** (Lobelia Herba) 半边莲. Relatively small doses should be used initially as the cold bitterness that characterizes these herbs can aggravate the cold and worsen the condition.

Prepared medicines
Concentrated powder
An Zhong San (Fennel & Galanga Formula)
Fu Zi Li Zhong Tang (Aconite, Ginseng and Ginger Combination)

Pills
Fu Zi Li Zhong Wan (Fu Tzu Li Chung Wan, Li Chung Yuen Medical Pills)
Wei Tong Ding (Calm Stomach Pain)

Acupuncture (select from)
Ren.12 (zhongwan –▲) .....alarm point of the Stomach, dispels cold, regulates qi and stops pain
St.21 (liangmen –▲).........warms the Stomach and dispels cold
St.36 (zusanli +▲) ....sea point of the Stomach, warms and strengthens the Spleen and Stomach and supplements qi
St.34 (liangqiu –) ....cleft point of the Stomach, stops pain
Sp.4 (gongsun) ....connecting point of the Spleen, master point of chongmai, regulates the Spleen and Stomach and stops pain
Bl.20 (weishu +▲) ....transport point of the Stomach, warms the Stomach and disperses cold
- a moxa box over the epigastrium is helpful
- with abdominal distension, add Sp.3 (taibai) and Sp.15 (daheng)
- with severe pain, add LI.4 (hegu –) and Liv.6 (zhongdu –)
- with spasms or cramping pain, add Du.8 (jinsuo –)
- with nausea and vomiting, add PC.6 (neiguan)
- with Spleen deficiency, add Ren.12 (zhongwan) and St.36 (zusanli)
- with phlegm, add St.40 (fenglong –) and Sp.3 (taibai)
- Ear points: abdomen, spleen, large intestine, shenmen, sympathetic, subcortex

Clinical notes
- A mass associated with cold and blood stasis in the stomach may be diagnosed as lymphoma, stomach cancer or a pancreatic pseudocyst.
- When the diagnosis is cancer, a combination of Western and Chinese medicine should be used.
- For dietary recommendations, see Clinical Handbook, Vol. 2, p.873.

正虚邪陷 1.4.4 COLD MASS WITH DEFICIENCY IN THE LOWER ABDOMEN

A cold mass with deficiency reflects the residue of an incompletely resolved or badly managed acute episode of toxic heat or damp heat. Repeated courses of antibiotics can damage the Spleen and contribute to the persistence of the pathogen and weakness of yang qi. This pattern describes a chronic yin type inflammatory mass from which the heat has dissipated. Masses such as this tend to be thickly encapsulated and can be difficult to access.

Depending on the etiology and the constitution of the patient, a mass of this type is usually complicated by damp, blood stasis, qi and blood deficiency, or a mixture of all three.

Clinical features
- Soft, rubbery, well defined mass in the lower burner, that may be non–tender or mildly tender.
- The abdomen may feel taut initially, but with deeper palpation and increasing pressure, the tone is lost and the abdomen feels cool, and soft or boggy/cottony. The skin of the abdomen may be dry and coarse.
- cold intolerance, cold extremities and lower abdomen
- no fever or chills or thirst
- bowel movements may be normal, loose or sluggish
- may be melena
- copious vaginal discharge

T pale with a white coat, thicker on the root
P fine and weak, or tight

Treatment principle
Warm yang and invigorate flow of yang qi through the lower burner
Reduce swelling and dissipate the mass

Prescription

YI YI FU ZI BAI JIANG SAN 薏苡附子败酱散
Coix, Prepared Aconite and Patrinia Powder, modified

chao yi ren (stir fried Coicis Semen) 炒苡仁 20–30g
zhi fu zi (Aconiti Radix lateralis preparata) 制附子 3–6g
bai jiang cao (Patriniae Herba) 败酱草 12–15g
ren shen (Ginseng Radix) 人参 9–12g
Method: Decoction. **Zhi fu zi** is decocted for 30 minutes prior to the other herbs. **Chao yi ren** and **bai jiang cao** aid in the discharge of pus; **chao yi ren** promotes urination to clear damp; **bai jiang cao** clears any residual toxic heat, activates blood and dissipates masses; **zhi fu zi** warms and balances the cooling herbs, disperses cold and opens up the channels to facilitate the circulation of qi and blood; ren shen supplements yuan qi and assists anti–pathogenic qi in dispelling the remains of the pathogen. (Source: *Zhong Yi Fu Chan Ke Xue* [*Jin Gui Yao Lüe*])

Modifications
- With damp or phlegm, add **cang zhu** (Atractylodis Rhizoma) 苍术 9–12g and **zao jiao ci** (Gleditsiae Spina) 皂角刺 9–12g.

- With marked qi deficiency, add **huang qi** (Astragali Radix) 黄芪 18–30g, **zao jiao ci** (Gleditsiae Spina) 皂角刺 9–12g and **chao bai zhu** (stir fried Atractylodes macrocephalae Rhizoma) 炒白术 12–15g, or combine with **Xiang Sha Liu Jun Zi Tang** (Six Gentlemen Decoction with Aucklandia and Amomum 香砂六君子汤, p.618).
- With qi deficiency and melena, combine with **Gui Pi Tang** (Restore the Spleen Decoction 归脾汤, p.387).
- With diarrhea, add **pao jiang** (Zingiberis Rhizoma preparatum) 炮姜 3–6g and **chao bai zhu** (stir fried Atractylodes macrocephalae Rhizoma) 炒白术 9–12g.
- With blood stasis, add **dang gui wei** (rootlets of Angelicae sinensis Radix) 当归尾 6–9g, **chuan xiong** (Chuanxiong Rhizoma) 川芎 6–9g and **tao ren** (Persicae Semen) 桃仁 6–9g.

Variations and additional prescriptions
Cold and blood stasis
Cold and blood stasis often occur together and the relative proportions can vary, requiring different strategies. When the blood stasis becomes prominent, physical signs of stasis are more obvious. The features include left iliac fossa pressure pain, vascular congestion on the lower limbs and a mauve tongue. The treatment is primarily to active blood while warming and dispelling cold, with a formula such as **Shao Fu Zhu Yu Tang** (Drive Out Blood Stasis in the Lower Abdomen Decoction 少腹逐瘀汤, p.24) or **Gui Zhi Fu Ling Wan** (Cinnamon Twig and Poria Pill 桂枝茯苓丸, p.27).

Prepared medicines
Concentrated powders
Tuo Li Xiao Du Yin (Gleditsia Combination)
Shao Fu Zhu Yu Tang (Fennel Seed & Corydalis Combination)
Gui Zhi Fu Ling Wan (Cinnamon & Poria Formula)

Pills
Fu Ke Wu Jin Wan (Woo Garm Yuen Medical Pills)
Shao Fu Zhu Yu Wan (Stasis in the Lower Palace Teapills)
Gui Zhi Fu Ling Wan (Cinnamon and Poria Teapills)
Shi Quan Da Bu Wan (Ten Flavour Teapills)
    – combine with one of the above for qi and blood deficiency

Acupuncture (select from)

ahshi points	over the site of the lesion plus distal points on the corresponding channel: the Stomach channel between St.36 (zusanli) and St.39 (xiajuxu), Spleen between Sp.6 (sanyinjiao) and Sp.8 (diji), or Kidney between Kid.7 (fuliu) and Kid.10 (yingu)
Ren.4 (guanyuan ▲) Ren.6 (qihai ▲)	these points warm yang and promote yang movement in the lower burner
St.29 (guilai) zigong (M–CA–18 ▲)	these points regulate the movement of qi and blood in the lower abdomen and reproductive system

St.25 (tianshu –).................alarm point of the Large Intestine, regulates Intestinal function and eliminates stagnation from the Intestines

Ren.6 (qihai ▲) ....regulates qi in the lower abdomen and dispels cold damp

St.36 (zusanli +▲) ....sea point of the Stomach, strengthens the Spleen and Stomach, supplements qi and activates movement of qi and blood

Sp.6 (sanyinjiao).................strengthens the Spleen and Kidneys, regulates the Liver and activates qi and blood

Bl.17 (geshu –)...................these points activate blood and disperse blood stasis
Sp.8 (diji –)

• Ear points: large intestine, uterus, abdomen, appendix, adrenal, shenmen

Topical therapies
Poultice
A poultice prepared with castor oil can be effective. See No.3, p.22.

Retention enema
See p.22–23.

Clinical notes
• Lower burner masses of a chronic cold type may be diagnosed as chronic appendicitis, chronic pelvic inflammatory disease, chronic salpingitis, endometriosis, diverticular disease, chronic colitis or lymphoma.
• Chronic masses of this type can respond well to prolonged treatment. Cancer requires a combination of Western and Chinese medicine.
• A warm diet is recommended. See Clinical Handbook, Vol. 2, p.873 and 886.

1.4.5 COLD MASS IN THE HYPOGASTRIUM – KIDNEY DEFICIENCY WITH BLOOD STASIS

肾
虚
血
瘀

A chronic mass in the lower burner, in this case the reproductive system, will gradually deplete Kidney yang qi and yin. In practice, the pattern may tend towards either yin or yang deficiency depending on the constitution and habits of the patient. Even though Kidney deficiency is the primary feature, the mass is most commonly seen in women of reproductive age.

Clinical features
• Mass in the lower abdomen. If palpable, the mass is usually felt in the midline, and may be either soft or firm and mild to moderately tender. The abdominal wall is toneless and flaccid and may feel cool to the touch. When soft, the mass may feel like a fluid filled cyst.
• irregular menstruation, with variable quantity of menstrual flow; may be some clotting with menstruation
• abdominal pain and lower back ache during menstruation
• premenstrual edema

- infertility, loss of libido
- fatigue, weakness, exhaustion
- may be night sweats, heat in the hands and feet, and facial flushing
- dizziness, tinnitus
- loose stools or diarrhea
- urinary frequency, nocturia
- left iliac fossa pressure pain; vascular congestion on the lower legs

T pale, pink or mauve with a white coat
P deep, weak and fine

Treatment principle

Supplement the Kidneys to invigorate movement of qi and blood
Gently activate blood and disperse blood stasis

Prescription

BU SHEN QU YU FANG 补肾祛瘀方
Supplement the Kidney and Dispel Blood Stasis Formula

xian ling pi (Epimedii Herba) 仙灵脾 12–15g
xian mao (Curculiginis Rhizoma) 仙茅 9–12g
huai niu xi (Achyranthis bidentatae Radix) 怀牛膝 9–12g
shu di (Rehmanniae Radix preparata) 熟地 12–15g
shan yao (Dioscoreae Rhizoma) 山药 15–24g
xiang fu (Cyperi Rhizoma) 香附 9–12g
e zhu (Curcumae Rhizoma) 莪术 3–6g
san leng (Sparganii Rhizoma) 三棱 3–6g
ji xue teng (Spatholobi Caulis) 鸡血藤 15–30g
dan shen (Salviae miltiorrhizae Radix) 丹参 12–15g

Method: Decoction. **Xian ling pi** and **xian mao** warm Kidney yang and dispel cold; **shu di** supplements yin and blood and supports the Kidneys; **huai niu xi** activates blood and supplemenst the Kidneys; **shan yao** nourishes Spleen and Kidney qi and yin; **xiang fu** regulates qi; **e zhu** and **san leng** break up blood stasis and dissipate masses; **ji xue teng** supplements blood and stimulates the flow of qi and blood through the network vessels; **dan shen** activates blood and disperse blood stasis. (Source: *Zhong Yi Fu Chan Ke Xue [Shanghai Zhong Yi Yao Za Zhi]*)

Modifications

- With predominant yang deficiency, add **zhi fu zi** (Aconiti Radix lateralis preparata) 制附子 6–9g and **rou gui** (Cinnamomi Cortex) 肉桂 3–6g.
- With yin deficiency, night sweats and flushing, add **nu zhen zi** (Ligustri Fructus) 女贞子 9–12g and **di gu pi** (Lycii Cortex) 地骨皮 12–15g.
- With qi deficiency, add **huang qi** (Astragali Radix) 黄芪 12–15g.
- With blood deficiency, add **dang gui** (Angelicae sinensis Radix) 当归 6–9g and **he shou wu** (Polygoni multiflori Radix) 何首乌 9–12g.
- With menorrhagia, add **e jiao** (Asini Corii Colla) 阿胶 6–9g [melted in the strained decoction] and **xian he cao** (Agrimoniae Herba) 仙鹤草 12–15g.
- With lower back and leg ache, add **sang ji sheng** (Taxilli Herba) 桑寄生 12–18g and **du zhong** (Eucommiae Cortex) 杜仲 12–15g.
- With a persistent mass, add **zao jiao ci** (Gleditsiae Spina) 皂角刺 6–9g.

Prepared medicines
Concentrated powder
Ba Wei Di Huang Wan (Rehmannia Eight Formula) plus Xiao Luo Wan
  (Scrophularia & Fritillaria Combination)
  – tending to yang deficiency
Liu Wei Di Huang Wan (Rehmannia Six Formula) plus Xiao Luo Wan (Scroph-
  ularia & Fritillaria Combination)
  – tending to yin deficiency
Er Xian Tang (Curculigo & Epimedium Combination) plus Xiao Luo Wan
  (Scrophularia & Fritillaria Combination)
  – with yin and yang deficiency
Wen Jing Tang (Tangkuei & Evodia Combination)
Pills
Jin Kui Shen Qi Wan (Fu Gui Ba Wei Wan, Golden Book Teapills) plus Nei
  Xiao Luo Li Wan (Nei Xiao Luo Li Teapills)

Acupuncture (select from)
Ren.4 (guanyuan +) ....these points warm Kidney yang to promote
Ren.6 (qihai +)   yang movement in the lower burner
zigong (M–CA–18)............activates qi and blood in the Uterus and lower
                             burner
Ren.9 (shuifen) ....these points promote transformation and movement
St.28 (shuidao)   of fluids; use with soft or waterlogged masses
Bl.23 (shenshu +) ....transport point of the Kidneys
Kid.3 (taixi +)....................source point of the Kidneys, supplements Kidney
                             yin and yang
Kid.7 (fuliu) ....river point of the Kidneys, strengthens Kidney qi
Sp.6 (sanyinjiao)................supplements and strengthens the Kidneys, Liver and
                             Spleen
• with yang deficiency, add moxa
• Ear points: kidney, uterus, shenmen, adrenal, subcortex, endocrine

Topical therapies
Poultice
A poultice prepared with castor oil can be effective. See No.3, p.22.

Retention enema
See p.22–23.

Clinical notes
• A mass associated with Kidney deficiency and blood stasis may be diagnosed as
  endometriosis, fibroid, cysts or advanced ovarian cancer.
• For dietary recommendations, see Clinical Handbook, Vol. 2, p.873.

气
血
两
虚

1.4.6 COLD MASS IN THE HYPOGASTRIUM – QI AND BLOOD DEFICIENCY

This type of mass occurs in women and affects the reproductive system.

Clinical features

- Mass in the midline of the lower burner, generally soft and non tender. The abdominal wall is flaccid and toneless.
- menorrhagia, abnormal uterine bleeding of watery or pale blood
- mild dysmenorrhea or a dragging or distending sensation in the lower abdomen, that may be more noticeable after the period, at the end of the day and when tired
- pale complexion
- postural dizziness; visual weakness, blurring vision
- palpitations, tachycardia
- insomnia, dream disturbed sleep
- fatigue and weakness

T pale with a thin white coat
P fine or big, hollow and empty

Treatment principle

Supplement qi and strengthen the Spleen to hold blood
Activate circulation of qi in the lower burner to lead the blood
Nourish and replenish blood and dissipate masses

Prescription

SHI QUAN DA BU TANG 十全大补汤
All Inclusive Great Supplementing Decoction, modified

shu di (Rehmanniae Radix preparata) 熟地 9–12g
dang gui (Angelicae sinensis Radix) 当归 9–12g
bai shao (Paeoniae Radix alba) 白芍 9–12g
chuan xiong (Chuanxiong Rhizoma) 川芎 3–6g
chao bai zhu (stir fried Atractylodes macrocephalae Rhizoma) 炒白术 ... 9–12g
ren shen (Ginseng Radix) 人参 6–9g
fu ling (Poria) 茯苓 9–12g
zhi gan cao (Glycyrrhizae Radix preparata) 炙甘草 3–6g
huang qi (Astragali Radix) 黄芪 18–30g
pu huang (Typhae Pollen) 蒲黄 6–9g
ai ye (Artemisiae argyi Folium) 艾叶 9–12g
e jiao (Asini Corii Colla) 阿胶 9–12g

Method: Decoction. **Pu huang** is decocted in a cloth bag; **e jiao** is melted into the strained decoction. **Shu di** nourishes yin and blood and supplements the Kidneys; **dang gui** and **bai shao** supplement blood and soften the Liver; **dang gui** and **chuan xiong** activate blood and move qi; **dang gui** and **huang qi** work together to build blood, and **huang qi** works synergistically with **chuan xiong** to activate qi and blood; **ren shen** and **huang qi** supplement yuan qi and strengthen the Spleen; **bai zhu** strengthens the Spleen and dries damp; **fu ling** strengthens the Spleen, leaches out damp and calms the shen; **zhi gan cao** supplements qi, harmonizes the action of the other herbs, and with **bai shao** alleviates spasmodic pain; **pu huang**, **ai ye** and **e jiao** regulate blood and stop bleeding.

(Source: *Zhong Yi Zhi Liao Yi Nan Za Bing Mi Yao* [*He Ji Ju Fang*])

Modifications
- With a sinking or dragging sensation in the lower abdomen, add **sheng ma** (Cimicifugae Rhizoma) 升麻 3–6g and **chai hu** (Bupleuri Radix) 柴胡 3–6g.

Prepared medicines
Concentrated powder
Shi Quan Da Bu Tang (Ginseng & Dang Gui Ten Combination)

Pills
Ba Zhen Yi Mu Wan (Eight Treasure Pill plus Motherwort)
Gui Pi Wan (Kwei Be Wan, Gui Pi Teapills)

Acupuncture (select from)
Du.20 (baihui ▲) ....assists is elevating sinking qi and blood
Ren.4 (guanyuan +) ....these points warm Kidney yang to promote yang
Ren.6 (qihai +)   movement in the lower burner
zigong (M–CA–18) ....activates qi and blood in the Uterus
St.36 (zusanli +) ....strengthens the Spleen and supplements qi and blood
Sp.10 (xuehai) ....nourishes and activates blood
Sp.6 (sanyinjiao).................supplements and strengthens the Kidneys, Liver and Spleen, and qi and blood
- Ear points: spleen, kidney, uterus, shenmen, subcortex, endocrine

Topical therapies
Poultice
A poultice prepared with castor oil can be effective. See No.3, p.22.

Clinical notes
- A mass associated with qi and blood deficiency may be diagnosed as a fibroid.
- Fibroids of this type, if not too large, can respond reasonably well to prolonged treatment, and may shrink. Even if the mass does not change, bleeding and other symptoms of qi and blood deficiency can be improved. Treatment should continue for a least several months.
- Treatment with blood activating herbs and strategies will make this condition worse.
- For dietary recommendations, see Clinical Handbook, Vol. 2, p.870 and 874.

Table 1.6 Summary of abdominal mass patterns

Location	Pattern	Features	Biomedical disease	Prescription
Blood masses	Liver	Swollen firm liver or hard nodular mass, pain worse for pressure, spider nevi, purple tongue with stasis spots and dark sublingual veins, wiry choppy pulse	liver cirrhosis, cancer, nodular hyperplasia, hepatomegaly from malaria, hemangioma	Ge Xia Zhu Yu Tang
	Epigastrium	Hard painful mass; melena, 'coffee ground' vomitus, weight loss, mauve or purple tongue with stasis spots and dark sublingual veins, wiry, choppy pulse	stomach cancer, pyloric stenosis, esophageal varices, ulceration	San Leng Tang
	Spleen	Firm mass under left ribs; low grade fever, weight loss, bleeding, spider nevi, purple tongue with stasis spots and dark sublingual veins, wiry, choppy pulse	splenomegaly from chronic malaria, lymphoma, leukemia, tumor of the splenic flexure	Bie Jia Wan
	Intestines	Hard, tender mass in the left or right lower quadrant; distension, constipation or diarrhea, rectal bleeding, weight loss, spider nevi, mauve or purple tongue with stasis spots and dark sublingual veins, wiry, choppy pulse	appendiceal abscess, bowel cancer, lymphoma or mesenteric adenitis, Crohn's disease, scarring and adhesions	Ge Xia Zhu Yu Tang
	Lower burner, with cold	Hard mass, may be tender when palpated; spider naevi, broken vessels on the legs, dysmenorrhea, cold abdomen, mauve or purple tongue with dark sublingual veins, choppy pulse	fibroids, endometriosis, uterine, bladder and prostate cancer	Shao Fu Zhu Yu Tang
	Lower burner, mild stasis	Small mass or masses usually discovered with routine investigation; menstrual irregularities	fibroid, cyst, endometriosis, ovarian hyper stimulation, early ovarian cancer	Gui Zhi Fu Ling Wan

Table 1.6 Summary of abdominal mass patterns (cont.)

Location	Pattern	Features	Biomedical disease	Prescription
Phlegm masses	Liver	Rubbery, rounded, well defined single or multiple masses; other cystic lesions (breast etc.)	non parasitic liver cysts	Hua Jian Er Chen Tang
	Abdomen	Swollen spleen or a firm, rubbery, non-tender mass; abdominal distension, lymphadenopathy; pale or mauve tongue, wiry slippery pulse	splenomegaly from chronic infection, lymphoma, leukemia	Chai Hu Shu Gan Wan
	Spleen	Round mass in the spleen associated with dull or sharp pain; pale or mauve tongue with a greasy coat, fine, wiry, slippery pulse	splenic cyst	Hua Tang Ruan Jian Fang
	Epigastrium	Firm, rounded, well defined, moderately tender mass; epigastric distension, nausea and vomiting, swollen tongue with a thick coat, wiry slippery pulse	cysts, pancreatic pseudocyst, lymphoma	Hai Zao Yu Hu Tang
	Hypogastrium	Soft or firm rubbery, non-tender mass or masses; leukorrhea, amenorrhea, lethargy, dizziness, thick greasy tongue coat, slippery, wiry pulse	ovarian cyst, adenoma, polycystic ovarian syndrome, fibroid, benign prostatic hypertrophy	Cang Fu Dao Tan Wan
Heat masses	Liver Gallbladder – toxic heat	Focal soft swelling under right ribs with pain; high fever, malaise, red dry tongue with a dry or greasy yellow coat, surging rapid pulse	liver abscess, empyema of the gall bladder	Huang Lian Jie Du Tang + Da Chai Hu Tang
	Liver – damp heat	Acute large, firm, tender swelling or mass beneath the right rib margin; low grade fever, night sweats, nausea, red with greasy yellow tongue coat, slippery rapid pulse	alcoholic or toxic hepatitis, inflammation from liver cancer	Dang Gui Long Hui Wan
	Liver – damp heat with qi and yin deficiency	Enlarged, smooth or nodular liver that is moderately tender to palpation; low grade fever, night sweats, lethargy, pallor, pale or slightly red tongue, weak pulse	chronic encapsulated liver abscess	Huang Qi Bie Jie Tang

Table 1.6 Summary of abdominal mass patterns (cont.)

ABDOMINAL MASSES 71

Location	Pattern	Features	Biomedical disease	Prescription
Heat masses	Liver – yin deficiency	Firm or nodular non-tender mass under right ribs; spider veins, weight loss, low grade fever, red dry tongue with no coat, fine, wiry, rapid pulse	hepatic cirrhosis, liver cancer	Yi Guan Jian
	Epigastrium – with yin deficiency	Small firm tender mass; burning epigastric pain, dry mouth, heat in the palms and soles, low grade fever, red dry cracked tongue, fine rapid pulse	stomach or pancreatic cancer	Sha Shen Mai Men Dong Tang
	Intestines	Soft tender mass in either lower quadrant with rebound tenderness; low grade fever, nausea, vomiting, constipation, greasy tongue coat, slippery rapid pulse	acute appendicitis, diverticulitis, salpingitis, oophoritis	Da Huang Mu Dan Pi Tang
	Hypogastrium	Soft tender mass; abdomen feels warm, menorrhagia, short menstrual cycle, offensive leukorrhea, fever, might sweats, red tongue with greasy yellow coat, slippery rapid pulse	acute pelvic inflammatory disease, endometriosis	Xiao Chai Hu Tang + Tao He Cheng Qi Tang
Cold and/or deficiency	Liver, Gallbladder	Firm, non-tender mass; jaundice, anorexia, loose or clay like stools, cold intolerance, mauve tongue with a greasy coat and dark sublingual veins, soggy, weak pulse	cancer of the liver, gallbladder, pancreas or biliary tree	Yin Chen Zhu Fu Tang + Fu Yuan Huo Xue Tang
	Liver yang deficiency	Firm non-tender nodular mass in the liver; dull hypochondriac pain, ascites, cold intolerance, nocturia, swollen pale tongue, deep weak pulse	hepatic cirrhosis with ascites	Ji Sheng Shen Qi Wan
	Epigastrium	Mass with colicky or spasmodic pain, alleviated by heat; vomiting, distension, pallor, pale tongue, weak or tight pulse	lymphoma, cancer, pancreatic pseudocyst	An Zhong San

Table 1.6 Summary of abdominal mass patterns (cont.)

Location	Pattern	Features	Biomedical disease	Prescription
Cold and/or deficiency	Lower abdomen	Soft non tender mass; abdomen feels flaccid and cool, pallor, fatigue, loose stools or melena, leukorrhea, pale tongue, fine pulse	chronic pelvic inflammatory disease, diverticulosis, chronic intestinal abscess or colitis, lymphoma	Yi Yi Fu Zi Bai Jiang Tang
	Hypogastrium – Kidney deficiency with blood stasis	Soft or firm, non tender mass; toneless cool abdomen, abdominal pain, infertility, fatigue, irregular menses, pale, pink or mauve tongue, deep fine pulse	endometriosis, fibroid or cysts, advanced ovarian cancer	Bu Shen Qu Yu Tang
	Hypogastrium – qi and blood deficiency	Soft non tender mass; toneless abdomen, dragging sensation in low abdomen, pallor, postural dizziness, fatigue, insomnia, pale tongue, fine pulse	fibroid	Shi Quan Da Bu Tang

COLDS AND FLU, PERSISTENT

Persistent colds, flu and other acute superficial infections are defined as those that persist for longer than they normally would, or that keep on recurring. This common situation presents in clinic with patients who have a cold they 'just can't shake'. In Chinese medicine terms these patterns are associated with a lingering pathogen. The pathogen can, in certain circumstances, get locked away in various parts of the body, reaching a state of equilibrium with the body's anti–pathogenic qi.

As a general rule, acute surface invasions run a fairly predictable course. For the most part they are self limiting, re-solving in a few days to a week. Wind cold and wind heat patterns usually respond reliably to timely treatment. However, if the patient is not robust, continues to 'soldier on' through the acute phase or receives inappropriate treatment (see below) recovery may not be so rapid. Wind damp, damp heat and summerheat patterns, with the stickiness of damp, tend to be more protracted and have a greater tendency to persist when poorly managed.

> **BOX 2.1 PERSISTENT COLD AND FLU PATTERNS**
>
> Lingering pathogen in the surface
> – ying wei disharmony
> – qi deficiency with wind cold
> Lingering pathogen in the qi level
> – with qi and yin deficiency
> – damp heat
> – dampness
> – phlegm heat
> Lingering pathogen in the shaoyang
> – taiyang / shaoyang
> – shaoyang / yangming
> – damp heat

In most cases, when a patient presents with a cold that won't go away, or that keeps on reappearing as soon as the patients energy expenditure increases, or goes back to work, a residual pathogen in the qi level or shaoyang level is to blame. The symptoms can be quite diverse, but typically feature fatigue, swollen lymph nodes, persistent cough and sore throat, and sleep and digestive disturbances. Fever may occur, but is not a consistent feature.

The persistent colds and flu described in this chapter are all types of lingering pathogen, and are always directly related to a specific superficial infection, from which the patient does not fully recover. The patterns in this chapter reflect the experience of the authors, working in a mild temperate climate at sea level. Because the nature and expression of pathogenic illness is so dependent on the environment, we would expect practitioners in different climactic regions to observe some variation from the patterns we encounter.

ETIOLOGY

Wrong treatment or poor management of an acute episode

Wrong treatment or counterproductive behavior during the acute phase of an external pathogenic invasion can weaken qi, lower resistance, cut off the escape routes

Figure 2.1 Patterns of persistent colds and flu

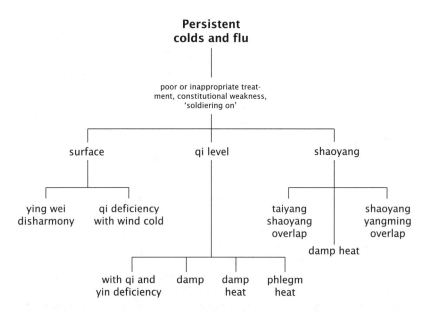

and trap a pathogen, and encourage it to move deeper into the body. Wrong treat ment includes inducing excessive sweating or purgation, and inappropriate use of astringent, supplementing or bitter cold herbs. Excessive sweating, as a re-sult of strong or inappropriate diaphoretic medications, attempts to 'sweat it out' in a sauna or vigorous exercise, depletes qi and yin. Purgation with bitter, cold herbs, enemas, antibiotics or large doses of vitamin C sufficient to cause diarrhea, weaken the Spleen and diminish anti–pathogenic qi and the ability to expel the pathogen. The diarrhea that results from purgation also helps to drag a surface pathogen deeper into the body. The use of astringent and supplementing herbs can prevent the venting and dispersal of the pathogen through the surface, and en-courage inward movement of the pathogen. The qi strengthening and pore closing action of **huang qi** (Astragali Radix) 黄芪 is a particular problem in this regard.

Attempting to ignore the acute illness is a common factor that contributes to persistent pathogens. Taking cold and flu 'over the counter' medications mask the symptoms and enable patients to 'soldier on'. Continuing to work and thus diverting qi away from the fight, dilutes the anti–pathogenic response and enables a pathogen to get a deeper foothold.

Constitutional factors

A pre–existing constitutional or acquired weakness of qi can lead to a failure to effectively combat a surface pathogen. Such weakness also allows the pathogen to quickly move deeper into the body.

Strong pathogen

A strong pathogen can overwhelm even robust defenses and gain a foothold.

TREATMENT

Persistent colds and flu are generally easy to treat and most respond swiftly to correct treatment. The herbal and acupuncture prescriptions recommended are for use during the illness and are not suitable for use in between episodes as preventative. When patients present in between colds requesting assistance in fortifying their immune response, a strategy aimed at strengthening the underlying weakness should be adopted, rather than the expelling strategies described herein. Strategies aimed at strengthening the various organ systems associated with defense against pathogenic invasion can be found in Chapter 18, Tiredness.

2.1 LINGERING PATHOGENS ON THE SURFACE

1. Ying wei disharmony
2. Qi deficiency with wind cold

营
卫
失
调

2.1.1 YING WEI DISHARMONY

A ying wei disharmony occurs when the balance of yin and yang on the surface of the body, (here represented by the yin ying and the yang wei) is disrupted. Ying qi fails to support wei qi resulting in a local deficiency. The localized deficiency at the surface allows external wind to penetrate and get a foothold in the superficial tissues. Once wind is established in the surface, it can persist for long periods, reappearing sporadically in response to changes of the weather or season.

This pattern is a type of wei qi deficiency, but differs from the next pattern, 2.1.2 Qi deficiency with wind cold, by the fact that in the ying wei disharmony pattern, the deficiency is isolated to the surface and does not necessarily affect the internal organs.

Clinical features

- Persistent sweating and clamminess in the aftermath of a cold or flu; even though there is sweating, the skin texture is generally dry; the skin may be itchy or numb in patches, and worse during cold dry weather
- aversion to wind and sudden changes of temperature
- mild, sporadic fever and chills, unrelieved by sweating
- joint and muscle stiffness and aching; joints may creak
- mild headache
- nasal congestion
- fatigue
- no thirst

T thin, white tongue coat
P floating, moderate or weak

Treatment principle

Dispel wind from the exterior
Balance the relationship between nutritive qi (ying qi) and defensive qi (wei qi)
Harmonize and support the Spleen and Stomach

Prescription

GUI ZHI TANG 桂枝汤
Cinnamon Twig Decoction

---

gui zhi (Cinnamomi Ramulus) 桂枝 6–9g
bai shao (Paeoniae Radix alba) 白芍 9–12g
sheng jiang (Zingiberis Rhizoma recens) 生姜 6–9g
zhi gan cao (Glycyrrhizae Radix preparata) 炙甘草 3–6g
da zao (Jujubae Fructus) 大枣 .... 4 fruit
Method: Decoction. Simmer the herbs in sufficient water to cover for 15–20 minutes, strain off the dregs and divide into two doses. **Gui zhi** promotes circulation of yang qi through the surface and dispels wind; **bai shao** protects yin and prevents excessive dispersal by **gui zhi**. **Bai shao** and

zhi gan cao combine sweet and sour flavours to create and protect yin. **Gui zhi** and **zhi gan cao** combine pungent and sweet flavours to create yang and promote movement and dispersal. The combined effect of these herbs is to gently dispel wind while protecting the patient's qi and yin. **Sheng jiang**, **da zao** and **zhi gan cao** support the Spleen and Stomach and harmonize the formula. (Source: *Shang Han Lun*)

Modifications

- For persistent colds and flu in postpartum women, add **dang gui** (Angelicae sinensis Radix) 当归 6–9g and **chuan xiong** (Chuanxiong Rhizoma) 川芎 3–6g.
- For frequent colds and stomach pains in pale or run down children, add **zhi huang qi** (honey fried Astragali Radix) 炙黄芪 12–18g and **yi tang** (Maltosum) 饴糖 9–15g.

Variations and additional prescriptions

Post wind attack residual cough

A persistent cough following resolution of a wind invasion is common, and there are a number of approaches depending on the accompanying symptoms. In some cases, there may be few, if any, symptoms other than the irritating cough, in which case a simple antitussive formula such as ZHI SOU SAN (Stop Coughing Powder 止嗽散) can be helpful.

bai bu (Stemonae Radix) 百部 9–12g
bai qian (Cynanchi stauntonii Rhizoma) 白前 9–12g
zi wan (Asteris Radix) 紫菀 9–12g
jie geng (Platycodi Radix) 桔梗 6–9g
chen pi (Citri reticulatae Pericarpium) 陈皮 6–9g
jing jie (Schizonepetae Herba) 荆芥 6–9g
gan cao (Glycyrrhizae Radix) 甘草 3–6g

Method: Decoction. **Jie geng** transforms phlegm, stops cough and alleviates sore throat; **zi wan**, **bai bu** and **bai qian** stop cough; **jing jie** assists in dispelling any residual pathogen; **chen pi** transforms phlegm; **gan cao** stops cough and benefits the throat. (Source: *Yi Xue Xin Wu*)

Prepared medicines

Concentrated powders

Gui Zhi Tang (Cinnamon Combination)
Zhi Sou San (Citrus & Aster Formula)

Pills

Gui Zhi Tang Wan (Gui Zhi Tang Teapills)

Acupuncture (select from)

Du.14 (dazhui −▲) .... meeting point of the yang channels, vents pathogens and secures the exterior; can be treated first with a reducing technique or cupped, then with moxa
LI.4 (hegu +) .... source point of the Large Intestine, dispels wind and diffuses the Lungs
Kid.7 (fuliu +) .... regulates sweating
GB.20 (fengchi −) .... releases wind and associated pathogens from the surface, clears the nose and alleviates headache

Bl.12 (fengmen – Ω) ....releases wind and associated pathogens from the surface

Bl.13 (feishu – Ω) ....transporting point of the Lungs, activates the Lungs dispersing and descending function to dispel wind

St.36 (zusanli +▲) ....sea point of the Stomach, strengthens the Spleen and Stomach and supplements qi; fortifies wei qi

Ren.6 (qihai +▲) ....supplements yuan qi

- with cough, add Lu.9 (taiyuan –)
- with wheezing, use dingchuan (M–BW–1)
- with copious sputum, add St.40 (fenglong –)
- with nasal congestion, add Du.23 (shangxing –) and LI.20 (yingxiang –)
- Ear points: lung, spleen, stomach, large intestine

Clinical notes
- Simple measures help to prevent colds, such as a scarf to cover the vulnerable neck area can be helpful.
- Following resolution of the wind, a strategy of supplementing anti–pathogenic qi should be adopted. Suitable Lung and Spleen qi supplementing formulae can be found in Tiredness, p.870–875.

2.1.2 LUNG AND SPLEEN QI DEFICIENCY WITH LINGERING WIND COLD

气
虚
感
冒

The deficiency in this pattern exists both at the surface and in the Lungs and Spleen. Because anti–pathogenic qi is reduced, the body's defensive response to the pathogen is weak and so the symptoms, which reflect the intensity of the struggle, are mild, but can persist for long periods of time. Concurrent qi deficiency and external wind invasion is commonly seen in children, and in those who are run down, convalescing or otherwise weak. The illness can be intermittent, with mild cold symptoms recurring each time the patient is overtired or run down.

Clinical features
- mild sporadic chills and fever; aversion to cold, cold intolerance
- persistent nasal congestion or runny nose
- pale complexion
- tiredness, listlessness, lack of vitality
- cough with white or clear sputum
- spontaneous sweating
- low voice, reluctance to speak
- shortness of breath with exertion
- persistent mild sore throat and swollen cervical lymph nodes

T pale, with a thin, white coat
P floating and weak

Treatment principle
Supplement qi and vent lingering pathogen from the exterior

Prescription

SHEN SU YIN 参苏饮
Ginseng and Perilla Leaf Decoction

ren shen (Ginseng Radix) 人参 6–9g
fu ling (Poria) 茯苓 12–15g
gan cao (Glycyrrhizae Radix) 甘草 3–6g
zi su ye (Perillae Folium) 紫苏叶 9–12g
ge gen (Puerariae Radix) 葛根 12–15g
qian hu (Peucedani Radix) 前胡 9–12g
jie geng (Platycodi Radix) 桔梗 6–9g
zhi ban xia (Pinelliae Rhizoma preparatum) 制半夏 9–12g
chen pi (Citri reticulatae Pericarpium) 陈皮 6–9g
zhi ke (Aurantii Fructus) 人参 6–9g
mu xiang (Aucklandiae Radix) 木香 6–9g
sheng jiang (Zingiberis Rhizoma recens) 生姜 .... 5 slices
da zao (Jujubae Fructus) 大枣 .... 3 fruit

Method: Decoction. The herbs should be gently simmered for no longer than 20 minutes. **Ren shen, fu ling** and **gan cao** strengthen the Spleen and supplement qi; **zi su ye** and **ge gen** dispel wind from the surface; **qian hu, jie geng, zhi ban xia** and **chen pi** assist diffusion and descent of Lung qi, transform phlegm and stop cough; **zhi ke** and **mu xiang** rectify qi; **sheng jiang, gan cao** and **da zao** harmonize the Stomach. (Source: *He Ji Ju Fang*)

Modifications

* With headache, add **chuan xiong** (Chuanxiong Rhizoma) 川芎 6–9g and **bai zhi** (Angelicae dahuricae Radix) 白芷 6–9g.
* With sweating, add **gui zhi** (Cinnamomi Ramulus) 桂枝 6–9g and **bai shao** (Paeoniae Radix alba) 白芍 6–9g.
* With cold, add **fang feng** (Saposhnikovae Radix) 防风 6–9g and **qiang huo** (Notopterygii Rhizoma seu Radix) 羌活 9–12g.
* With nasal congestion, add **cang er zi** (Xanthii Fructus) 苍耳子 6–9g and **bai zhi** (Angelicae dahuricae Radix) 白芷 6–9g.
* With damp, add **sha ren** (Amomi Fructus) 砂仁 6g and **pei lan** (Eupatorii Herba) 佩兰 9–12g.

Variations and additional prescriptions

In between episodes to strengthen wei qi

In patients who are frequently ill with colds and flu, and those who find it difficult to throw off colds or who experience mild exterior symptoms when fatigued or with exertion, the treatment is to fortify wei qi and strengthen the Spleen with **YU PING FENG SAN** (Jade Windscreen Powder 玉屏风散). This prescription is used in between episodes when the patient is symptom free to strengthen immunity. It should not be used for common cold patterns without deficiency, as **huang qi** can lock a pathogen in the body and aggravate the condition.

huang qi (Astragali Radix) 黄芪 30–120g
bai zhu (Atractylodis macrocephalae Rhizoma) 白术 60g
fang feng (Saposhnikovae Radix) 防风 60g

Method: Grind the herbs to a powder and take 6–9 grams twice daily with warm water. **Huang qi** fortifies and secures wei qi and Lung qi; **bai zhu** strengthens the Spleen and supplements qi; **fang feng** dispels wind from the surface. (Source: *Dan Xi Xin Fa*)

Prepared medicines
Concentrated powders
Shen Su Yin (Ginseng and Perilla Combination)
Ren Shen Bai Du San (Ginseng & Mint Formula)
Yu Ping Feng San (Astragalus & Siler Formula)

Pills
Ren Shen Bai Du Wan (Resilient Warrior Teapills)
Yu Ping Feng Wan (Jade Screen Teapills)

Acupuncture (select from)
GB.20 (fengchi –) ....releases wind from the surface, clears the nose and alleviates headache

Bl.12 (fengmen – Ω) ....releases wind from the surface

LI.4 (hegu –) ....source point of Large Intestine, dispels wind and diffuses the Lungs (with Lu.7 [lieque])

Lu.7 (lieque –) ....connecting point of the Lungs; diffuses the Lungs and directs Lung qi downwards, dispels wind and cold from the surface (with LI.4 [hegu])

St.36 (zusanli +▲) ....sea point of the Stomach, strengthens the Spleen and Stomach and supplements qi; fortifies and secures wei qi

Ren.6 (qihai +▲) ....supplements yuan qi

• In between episodes, Du.14 (dazhui ▲) and ST.36 (zusanli ▲) are useful to fortify wei qi
• Ear points: lungs, spleen, kidney, adrenal, shenmen

Clinical notes
• Wind invasion with underlying qi deficiency may be diagnosed as recurrent common cold, chronic fatigue syndrome and general poor immunity.
• A qi supplementing diet is recommended. See Clinical Handbook, Vol. 2, pp.870–871.

2.2 RESIDUAL HEAT IN THE QI LEVEL

1. Heat in the qi level with qi and yin deficiency
2. Damp heat
3. Phlegm heat

2.2.1 HEAT IN THE QI LEVEL WITH QI AND YIN DEFICIENCY

热
在
气
分,
气
阴
两
虚

Residual heat in the qi level is a common pattern following an unresolved upper respiratory tract or gastrointestinal infection associated with a wind heat pathogen or warm disease. If the pathogen is not cleared or is trapped, it will remain in the qi level and damage fluids, qi and yin. The more qi damage that results the less able the body is to expel the pathogen. Lingering heat in the qi level is encouraged when inappropriate purging, emesis or antibiotics for a viral illness are employed, or if the patient persists in working and does not get adequate rest during the acute phase. This pattern can persist for weeks after the initial illness.

Clinical features

- Persistent loud hacking, dry, irritating cough; the cough is worse at night and disrupts sleep. If the pattern follows a gastrointestinal infection, nausea or vomiting may be the main features.
- low grade fever
- spontaneous sweating, night sweats
- insomnia or restlessness fitful sleep broken by coughing or sweats
- thirst, dry mucous membranes
- sore throat, loss of voice, easily hoarse voice
- irritability and restlessness
- increasing fatigue
- mouth ulcers
- swollen lymph nodes and/or tonsils

T red and dry with little coat
P weak, fine, rapid

Treatment principle

Clear and vent residual heat from the qi level
Generate fluids and supplement qi

Prescription

ZHU YE SHI GAO TANG 竹叶石膏汤
Lophatherus and Gypsum Decoction

dan zhu ye (Lophateri Herba) 淡竹叶	9–15g
shi gao (Gypsum fibrosum) 石膏	15–30g
zhi ban xia (Pinelliae Rhizoma preparatum) 制半夏	6–9g
mai dong (Ophiopogonis Radix) 麦冬	6–15g
ren shen (Ginseng Radix) 人参	3–9g
zhi gan cao (Glycyrrhizae Radix preparata) 炙甘草	3–9g
jing mi (Oryzae Semen) 粳米	9–15g

Method: Decoction. **Shi gao** is decocted for 30 minutes prior to the other herbs. **Dan zhu ye** and **shi gao** vent heat from the qi level; **ren shen** supplements qi and supports the Spleen, and with **mai dong**, generates fluids and protects yin; **mai dong** assists in clearing heat; **zhi ban xia** downbears counterflow Stomach qi to stop nausea and vomiting; **zhi gan cao** and **jing mi** protect the Stomach and assist in strengthening the Spleen. (Source: *Shang Han Lun*)

Modifications
- With significant fluid damage and a peeled, mirror or geographic tongue, add **yu zhu** (Polygonati odorati Rhizoma) 玉竹 12–15g and **tian hua fen** (Trichosanthes Radix) 天花粉 12–15g.
- With marked residual heat, red tongue, rapid pulse and oral ulceration, add **zhi mu** (Anemarrhenae Rhizoma) 知母 9–12g and **tian hua fen** (Trichosanthes Radix) 天花粉 12–15g.

Variations and additional prescriptions
Lingering heat in the chest
A common variant of the above pattern involves lingering heat in the chest, affecting the Heart and shen, with little damage to qi or yin. This pattern follows an upper respiratory tract infection. The heat disturbs the shen, causing restlessness, irritability and depression, fitful sleep, low grade fever, fatigue and a burning sensation in the chest. The tongue is not especially red, reflecting the mild nature of the heat, and the pulse is often strong and floating in the distal position, reflecting the upper burner. The treatment is to clear and vent heat from the qi level and alleviate irritability with ZHI ZI CHI TANG (Gardenia and Prepared Soybean Decoction 栀子豉汤).

shan zhi zi (Gardeniae Fructus) 山栀子 6–9g
dan dou chi (Sojae Semen preparatum) 淡豆豉 9–12g
Method: Decoction. **Shan zhi zi** clears heat from all three burners and alleviates irritability; **dan dou chi** vents constrained heat from the chest. (Source: *Shang Han Lun*)

Prepared medicines
Concentrated powders
Zhu Ye Shi Gao Tang (Bamboo Leaves & Gypsum Combination)
Zhi Zi Chi Tang (Gardenia & Soja Combination)

Acupuncture (select from)
Du.14 (dazhui – Ω) ....meeting point of the yang channels, an important
point for clearing lingering pathogens
Lu.7 (lieque –)....................vents pathogens from the qi level
Du.12 (shenzhu –) ....these points diffuse the Lungs, and clear residual
Du.13 (taodao –)   heat from the chest and Lungs
Ren.17 (shanzhong) ....opens and promotes correct movement of qi in the
chest, clears heat and directs Lung qi downwards to
stop cough
LI.11 (quchi –)....................these point clear heat from the qi level
St.44 (neiting –)
- with cough, add Lu.5 (chize –)
- with nausea, add PC.6 (neiguan –)

- Ear points: lung, stomach, zero point, shenmen

Clinical notes

- Residual heat in the qi level may be diagnosed as the convalescent phase of an upper respiratory tract or gastrointestinal infection.
- Qi level residual heat is a common cause of persistent dry cough or nausea, fatigue and night–time fever in the aftermath of an acute upper respiratory tract infection or gastrointestinal infection. It may persist for weeks following the initial event.
- When correctly identified, residual pathogenic influence in the qi level can be dispelled quite reliably, and the qi and fluids replenished quite quickly. Usually only a few days to a week or two of treatment is necessary.

2.2.2 DAMP HEAT

湿
热

Damp heat is a common cause of lingering illness in the aftermath of an acute in-fection. It is more common in hot humid climates, and tends to occur in clusters, most frequently during the last humid days of late summer.

The nature of damp heat is sticky and viscous, so once in the body can linger for relatively long periods of time. It may appear to resolve only to reappear during humid weather or following periods of overwork, poor diet or stress. The damp heat can affect the whole body, muscles, or a specific organ system. The pattern described here is general in nature, with the damp heat lodged predominantly in the muscles and qi level. When the damp heat is concentrated in a particular or-gan system, other disease diagnoses may be more appropriate (see Hypochondriac pain Vol.1, Painful Urination Vol.1, Nausea and Vomiting, Vol.1, Sinusitis Vol.1).

Depending on the nature of the initial pathogen and the constitution of the patient, the balance of dampness and heat can vary. When damp is predominant, the heat signs are muted and the damp signs prominent – muscle aches, lethargy, heaviness and so on. When heat is predominant, afternoon fever and night sweats are the main features.

Clinical features

- Persistent tiredness, lethargy, heaviness in the head and limbs, foggy head, worse mid afternoon.
- low grade fever which rises or reaches a peak mid afternoon
- night sweats
- muscle aches
- chest oppression, abdominal distension
- loss of appetite
- loose stools, or sticky or difficult to pass stools
- nausea and vomiting
- no thirst
- swollen lymph nodes and/or tonsils

T thick, greasy, white or yellow coat, depending on the degree of heat

P slippery, wiry or soft; may be rapid

Treatment Principle

Clear damp heat from the muscles and qi level
Rectify the qi dynamic
Promote urination to provide an outlet for the damp heat

Prescription

SAN REN TANG 三仁汤
Three Nut Decoction

xing ren (Pruni Semen) 杏仁	12–15g
yi ren (Coicis Semen) 苡仁	18–30g
bai dou kou (Amomi Fructus rotundus) 白豆蔻	6–9g
zhi ban xia (Pinelliae Rhizoma preparata) 制半夏	9–12g
hou po (Magnoliae officinalis Cortex) 厚朴	6–9g
dan zhu ye (Lophatheri Herba) 淡竹叶	6–9g
hua shi (Talcum) 滑石	18g

Method: Decoction. **Bai dou kou** is added towards the end of cooking. **Xing ren** diffuses the Lungs and directs Lung qi downward; **bai dou kou** transforms damp and stimulates the qi dynamic; **yi ren** leaches damp heat from the lower burner and promotes urination; **zhi ban xia** and **hou po** dry damp and assist **xing ren** and **bai dou kou** in moving qi and freeing up the qi dynamic; **dan zhu ye** and **hua shi** promote urination to clear damp heat. (Source: *Wen Bing Tiao Bian*)

Modifications

- With nausea and vomiting, add **chen pi** (Citri reticulatae Pericarpium) 陈皮 6–9g, **sheng jiang** (Zingiberis Rhizoma recens) 生姜 6–9g and **zhu ru** (Bambusae Caulis in taeniam) 竹茹 9–12g.
- With relatively severe damp, a very thick tongue coat, heaviness in the body and muscle aches, add **huo xiang** (Pogostemonis/Agastaches Herba) 藿香 12–15g and **shi chang pu** (Acori tatarowii Rhizoma) 石菖蒲 6–9g.
- With sluggish or difficult stools, add **chao bai zhu** (stir fried Atractylodes macrocephalae Rhizoma) 炒白术 6–9g and **zhi shi** (Aurantii Fructus immaturus) 枳实 6–9g or **bing lang** (Arecae Semen) 槟榔 6–9g and **lai fu zi** (Raphani Semen) 莱菔子 6–9g.
- With epigastric distension and discomfort, add **chao shan zha** (stir fried Crataegi Fructus) 炒山楂 12–15g, **e zhu** (Curcumae Rhizoma) 莪术 9–12g and **chao bai zhu** (stir fried Atractylodes macrocephalae Rhizoma) 炒白术 6–9g.
- With headache or heaviness in the head, add **bai zhi** (Angelicae dahuricae Radix) 白芷 6–9g, **qiang huo** (Notopterygii Rhizoma seu Radix) 羌活 6–9g and **chuan xiong** (Chuanxiong Rhizoma) 川芎 6–9g.

Variations and additional prescriptions
With predominant damp myalgia and fatigue

Damp with little or no heat is more likely to occur when a patient with a pre-existing or constitutional tendency to yang deficiency is afflicted by an external pathogen or an immunization. Improper use or overuse of bitter cold antibiotics, which weaken the Spleen, can also contribute. The treatment is to vent and dispel damp from the muscles with **HUO PO XIA LING TANG** (Agastache, Magnolia Bark,

Pinellia and Poria Decoction 藿朴夏苓汤).
huo xiang (Pogostemonis/Agastaches Herba) 藿香 9–12g
zhi ban xia (Pinelliae Rhizoma preparata) 制半夏 9–12g
fu ling (Poria) 茯苓 9–12g
xing ren (Pruni Semen) 杏仁.. 9–12g
dan dou chi (Sojae Semen praeparatum) 淡豆豉 9–12g
yi ren (Coicis Semen) 苡仁.. 12–15g
ze xie (Alismatis Rhizoma) 泽泻 6–9g
zhu ling (Polyporus) 猪苓 6–9g
bai dou kou (Amomi Fructus rotundus) 白豆蔻............................ 3–6g
hou po (Magnoliae officinalis Cortex) 厚朴.................................. 3–6g

Method: Decoction. **Huo xiang** and **bai dou kou** transform and disperse damp from the muscles and qi level; **fu ling**, **ze xie** and **zhu ling** promote urination to leach out damp; **yi ren** leaches damp from the lower burner and promotes urination; **zhi ban xia** and **hou po** downbear counterflow Stomach qi and alleviate nausea and distension; **xing ren** directs Lung qi down; **dan dou chi** vents pathogens from the qi level. (Source: *Yi Yuan*)

Damp heat, with heat dominant, concentrated in the gastrointestinal system
When heat is predominant, the main features are persistent afternoon fever that is unrelieved by sweating, accompanied by nausea, vomiting and diarrhea, fullness in the chest and epigastrium, irritability and restlessness, concentrated urine, a greasy, yellow tongue coat and slippery rapid pulse. The treatment is to clear damp heat, move qi and transform turbidity with LIAN PO YIN (Coptis and Magnolia Bark Drink 连朴饮).

huang lian (Coptidis Rhizoma) 黄连 3–6g
hou po (Magnoliae officinalis Cortex) 厚朴.................................. 6–9g
shan zhi zi (Gardeniae Fructus) 山栀子 9–12g
dan dou chi (Sojae Semen praeparatum) 淡豆豉 9–12g
shi chang pu (Acori tatarinowii Rhizoma) 石菖蒲 6–9g
zhi ban xia (Pinelliae Rhizoma preparatum) 制半夏 6–9g
lu gen (Phragmitis Rhizoma) 芦根 30–60g

Method: Decoction. **Huang lian** and **shan zhi zi** clear damp heat; **zhi ban xia** transforms damp, downbears counterflow Stomach qi and stops vomiting; **hou po** directs qi downwards and alleviates distension; **dan dou chi** and **shan zhi zi** clear heat from the qi level and alleviate irritability; **shi chang pu** rouses the Spleen and transforms damp; **lu gen** clears heat from the Stomach, stops vomiting and promotes urination. (Source: *Huo Luan Lun*)

Prepared medicines
Concentrated powders
San Ren Tang (Triple Nut Combination)
Gan Lu Xiao Du Dan (Forsythia & Acorus Formula)
   – heat greater than damp
Xing Jun San 行军散 (Marching Powder, Five Pagodas Brand [Thailand])
   – for damp with little or no heat

Pills
Bi Xie Sheng Shi Wan (Subdue the Dampness Teapills)
   – damp greater than heat

Huo Xiang Zheng Qi Pian (Huo Hsiang Cheng Chi Pien)
 – damp predominant

Acupuncture (select from)

Lu.7 (lieque –)....................diffuses the Lungs and vents pathogens from the qi
 level
Sp.9 (yinlingquan –)...........these points promote urination and clear damp heat
Sp.5 (shangqiu –)
LI.11 (quchi –)...................these points clear damp heat from the qi level
St.44 (neiting –)
SI.4 (wangu –) ....source point of the Small Intestine, clears damp heat
Ren.5 (shimen –).................alarm point of the triple burner, clears damp heat
Ren.12 (zhongwan –).........alarm point of the Stomach, activates the qi dynamic
- with relatively high fever, add Du.14 (dazhui –)
- with nausea, add PC.6 (neiguan)
- with diarrhea, add zhixie (N–CA–3), Bl.25 (tianshu)
- with muscle aches, add Sp.21 (dabao)
- with headache, add GB.20 (fengchi)
- Ear points: spleen, lung, zero point, subcortex, sympathetic, shenmen

Clinical notes

- Damp heat type persistent illness following an acute episode may be diagnosed
  as a chronic infection such as cytomegalovirus, glandular fever, fibromyalgia,
  cholangitis, enteric fever, pyelonephritis, hepatic or pelvis abscess or undulant
  fever.
- A damp heat clearing diet can be helpful. See Clinical Handbook, Vol. 2,
  p.884.

痰
热

2.2.3 PHLEGM HEAT

Phlegm heat has both the cloying nature of phlegm and the shen agitating quality
of heat. A substantial fever is required to provide the heat to congeal fluids into
phlegm heat.

Clinical features

- Persistent fatigue following resolution of the acute symptoms of an external
  invasion. In spite of the tiredness, there is insomnia or fitful sleep with much
  dreaming, or waking in the early hours of the morning (typically around
  4am), inability to fall back to sleep.
- palpitations with anxiety and nervousness
- dizziness and vertigo; heavy or foggy head
- fullness and discomfort in the chest and abdomen
- residual phlegm congestion in the sinuses or lungs
- poor appetite, belching, acid reflux, bitter taste in the mouth
- nausea, vomiting or indeterminate gnawing hunger
- night sweats or spontaneous sweating
- swollen, rubbery lymph nodes; swollen tonsils

T thick, greasy, yellow coat
P wiry or slippery and rapid

Treatment principle
Clear heat and transform phlegm
Harmonize the Stomach and calm the shen

Prescription

WEN DAN TANG 温胆汤
Warm Gallbladder Decoction

zhu ru (Bambusae Caulis in taeniam) 竹茹 12–15g
zhi shi (Citri Fructus immaturus) 枳实 9–12g
zhi ban xia (Pinelliae Rhizoma preparata) 制半夏 9–12g
fu ling (Poria) 茯苓 12–15g
chen pi (Citri reticulatae Pericarpium) 陈皮 9–12g
sheng jiang (Zingiberis Rhizoma recens) 生姜 3–6g
gan cao (Glycyrrhizae Radix) 甘草 3–6g
Method: Decoction. **Zhu ru** clears phlegm heat and downbears counterflow Stomach qi; **zhi shi** breaks up stagnant qi, directs qi downwards and alleviates distension; **zhi ban xia** transforms phlegm damp and downbears counterflow Stomach qi; **chen pi** transforms phlegm, regulates middle burner qi and corrects the qi dynamic; **fu ling** strengthens the Spleen and leaches out damp; **gan cao** strengthens the Spleen and harmonizes the Stomach; **sheng jiang** assists the other herbs in transforming the phlegm. (Source: *San Yin Ji Yi Bing Zheng Fang Lun*)

Modifications
• With marked dizziness and mucus congestion, add **tian zhu huang** (Bambusae Concretio silicea) 天竺黄 9–12g, **zhu li** (Bambusae Succus) 竹沥 12–15g and **dan nan xing** (Arisaemae cum Bile) 胆南星 6–9g.
• With irritability, acid reflux, and a deep yellow tongue coat, add **huang lian** (Coptidis Rhizoma) 黄连 3–6g.
• With palpitations, anxiety and panic attacks, add **zhen zhu mu** (Margaritiferae Concha usta) 珍珠母 30g, **long gu** (Fossilia Ossis Mastodi) 龙骨 15–30g and **mu li** (Ostreae Concha) 牡蛎 15–30g.
• With constipation, add **da huang** (Rhei Radix et Rhizoma) 大黄 6–9g and **gua lou ren** (Trichosanthis Semen) 栝楼仁 12–18g.

Prepared medicines
Concentrated powder
Wen Dan Tang (Poria & Bamboo Combination)

Pills
Wen Dan Wan (Rising Courage Teapills)

Acupuncture (select from)
Ren.12 (zhongwan –) ....alarm point of the Stomach, harmonizes the Stomach and stimulates the qi dynamic
PC.5 (jianshi) ....river point of the Pericardium, transforms phlegm and clears heat

PC.6 (neiguan –)................connecting point of the Pericardium, downbears counterflow Stomach qi and stops vomiting, calms the shen, dredges the Liver and rectifies qi

St.36 (zusanli) ....sea point of the Stomach, strengthens the Spleen and Stomach and activates the qi dynamic

St.40 (fenglong –) ....connecting point of the Stomach, transforms phlegm and clears heat

St.43 (xianggu –)................wood point of the Stomach, clears heat

- with foggy head, add Du.20 (baihui)
- with marked heat, add PC.8 (laogong –) and St.45 (lidui ↓)
- with Stomach discomfort, add St.34 (liangqiu –)
- with dizziness, add GB.43 (xiaxi –)
- with anxiety, add Du.19 (houding) and Du.24 (shenting)
- Ear points: stomach, gallbladder, zero point, subcortex, sympathetic, shenmen

Clinical notes

- Persistent illness of a phlegm heat type responds well to treatment. Treatment needs to continue until all signs of phlegm are cleared. This can take some time. Herbs are more efficient at clearing entrenched phlegm although acupuncture often starts to improve energy levels quite quickly.
- For dietary recommendations, see Clinical Handbook, Vol. 2, p.885.

少
阳
证

2.3 SHAOYANG SYNDROME

- taiyang shaoyang overlap
- yangming shaoyang overlap
- damp heat

Shaoyang syndrome is a very common pattern that typically occurs several days after the acute phase of an upper respiratory tract infection. The progress of a pathogen into the shaoyang level is facilitated by a strong pathogen, a weakened host, inappropriate or wrong treatment during the surface phase (purgation, emesis), or by simply ignoring the illness and 'soldiering on'. The shaoyang level represents a transitional zone between the surface and the interior of the body, where pathogens can hide and get trapped, sometimes for prolonged periods. A type of equilibrium is created whereby the anti–pathogenic qi is unable to eject the pathogen, and the pathogen is locked up and unable to penetrate further. Qi is consumed in containing the pathogen, and the longer the pattern persists, the greater the degree of qi deficiency. Shaoyang patterns typically follow an unresolved wind (wei or taiyang level) invasion.

The principle of treatment described in the Shang Han Lun is to harmonize the shaoyang, which essentially means closing the space available to the pathogen, thus evicting it. Harmonizing also refers to the fact that because the disorder is no longer external and not yet internal, diaphoresis and purging are inappropriate. The author of the Shang Han Lun, Zhang Zhong–Jing, noted that only one or two clinical features need be present for the tentative diagnosis of shaoyang syndrome to be made. If diagnosed correctly a positive response will usually be swift.

Clinical features

- Some days or a week or two following an acute wind cold or wind heat pattern, the fever pattern changes from simultaneous fever and chills to periods of alternating fever and chills, in which the fever and chill episodes are quite distinct.
- increasing fatigue
- loss of appetite or anorexia
- nausea, particularly first thing in the morning
- hypochondriac pain, distension or tenderness
- fullness in the chest; chest oppression
- dizziness
- irritability
- bitter taste in the mouth

T often unremarkable, or coated only on the left side, or slightly red on the edges

P wiry

Treatment principle

Harmonize shaoyang

Prescription

XIAO CHAI HU TANG 小柴胡汤
Minor Bupleurum Decoction

chai hu (Bupleuri Radix) 柴胡 9–15g
huang qin (Scutellariae Radix) 黄芩 9–12g
zhi ban xia (Pinelliae Rhizoma preparata) 制半夏 9–12g
sheng jiang (Zingiberis Rhizoma recens) 生姜 6–9g
ren shen (Ginseng Radix) 人参 6–9g
zhi gan cao (Glycyrrhizae Radix preparata) 炙甘草 3–6g
da zao (Jujubae Fructus) 大枣 .... 4 fruit

Method: Decoction. **Chai hu** vents pathogens from shaoyang, and rectifiyies qi; **huang qin** clears heat; **zhi ban xia** and **sheng jiang** harmonize the Stomach, downbear counterflow Stomach qi and stop nausea; **ren shen** and **zhi gan cao** strenhthen anti–pathogenic qi and prevent the pathogen from penetrating further; **sheng jiang** and **da zao** support **zhi ban xia** in harmonizing the Stomach and stopping nausea and vomiting. (Source: *Shang Han Lun*)

Modifications

• With fullness in the chest, chest oppression and difficulty getting a deep breath, add **quan gua lou** (Trichosanthis Fructus) 全栝楼 18–24g.
• For postpartum colds and flu of a shaoyang type combine with SI WU TANG (Four Substance Decoction 四物汤, p.920).
• For otitis or recurrent glue ear, add **zao jiao ci** (Gleditsiae Spina) 皂角刺6–9g.
• With lingering dampness in shaoyang, causing relatively severe anorexia, muscle aches, chills greater than fever and heaviness in the body in addition to the shaoyang symptoms, add **cang zhu** (Atractylodis Rhizoma) 苍术 12–15g, **hou po** (Magnoliae officinalis Cortex) 厚朴 9–12g and **chen pi** (Citri reticulatae Pericarpium) 陈皮 9–12g.

Variations and additional prescriptions

Taiyang shaoyang overlap syndrome

Concurrent taiyang and shaoyang syndrome occurs when an external pathogen on the surface has begun to move internally and is entering the shaoyang. The features reflect the presence of a pathogen at both levels. The taiyang exterior aspects are seen in the fever and sensitivity to wind and temperature changes, joint stiffness and aching and floating pulse. The shaoyang aspects are the nausea, epigastric discomfort, bitter or odd taste in the mouth and loss of appetite. There may also be colicky abdominal pain. Depending on the proportions of pathogen inhabiting each level, the features can change, and in fact this pattern is usually dynamic and unstable, changing between taiyang and shaoyang dominance in relatively quick succession. The fever pattern is instructive. The more prominent the alternating fever and chill pattern, the more shaoyang involvement. The more taiyang involvement the chillier or cold intolerant the patient tends to be. The treatment is to harmonize shaoyang and dispel pathogens from the shaoyang and taiyang levels with CHAI HU GUI ZHI TANG (Bupleurum and Cinnamon Twig Decoction 柴胡桂枝汤).

chai hu (Bupleuri Radix) 柴胡 6–12g

huang qin (Scutellariae Radix) 黄芩.. 6–9g
zhi ban xia (Pinelliae Rhizoma preparatum) 制半夏 6–9g
ren shen (Ginseng Radix) 人参 6–9g
gui zhi (Cinnamomi Ramulus) 桂枝 6–9g
bai shao (Paeoniae Radix alba) 白芍.. 6–9g
zhi gan cao (Glycyrrhizae Radix preparata) 炙甘草.............................. 3–6g
sheng jiang (Zingiberis Rhizoma recens) 大枣 6–9g
da zao (Jujubae Fructus) 柴胡 .... 4 fruit

Method: Decoction. **Chai hu** vents pathogens from shaoyang and rectifies qi; **huang qin** clears heat; **gui zhi** dispels pathogens from the surface; **bai shao** protects yin and prevents excessive dispersal by **gui zhi**. **Bai shao** and **gan cao** combine sweet and sour flavours to create and protect yin. **Gui zhi** and **gan cao** combine pungent and sweet flavours to create yang and promote movement and dispersal. **Zhi ban xia** and **sheng jiang** harmonize the Stomach, downbear counterflow Stomach qi and stop nausea; **ren shen** and **gan cao** strengthen anti–pathogenic qi and prevent the pathogen from penetrating further; **sheng jiang** and **da zao** support **zhi ban xia** in harmonizing the Stomach and stopping nausea and vomiting; **Sheng jiang**, **da zao** and **gan cao** support the Spleen and Stomach and harmonize the formula. (Source: *Shang Han Lun*)

Shaoyang yangming overlap syndrome

Concurrent shaoyang and yangming syndrome is an acute pattern, characterized by relatively severe and increasing fever and gastrointestinal symptoms which follow some days after an unresolved external wind heat or wind cold pattern. The main features are alternating fever and chills, nausea and vomiting, abdominal and epigastric pain and constipation or urgent diarrhea. There may be jaundice. This is usually associated with the progress of a strong pathogen into the body, and may be facilitated by improper treatment, usually purgation of some sort, during the initial illness when the pathogen is on the surface. The treatment is to harmonize and dispel pathogens from the shaoyang level, and purge heat and stagnation from yangming through the bowels with DA CHAI HU TANG (Major Bupleurum Decoction 大柴胡汤).

chai hu (Bupleuri Radix) 柴胡 6–12g
huang qin (Scutellariae Radix) 黄芩.. 6–9g
bai shao (Paeoniae Radix alba) 白芍.. 6–9g
zhi ban xia (Pinelliae Rhizoma preparatum) 制半夏 6–9g
zhi shi (Aurantii Fructus immaturus) 枳实 6–9g
da huang (Rhei Radix et Rhizoma) 大黄 6–9g
sheng jiang (Zingiberis Rhizoma recens) 生姜 6–9g
da zao (Jujubae Fructus) 大枣 .... 4 fruit

Method: Decoction. **Chai hu** and **huang qin** dispel pathogens from shaoyang; **da huang** and **zhi shi** purge heat and constipation from yangming, and open the 'big exit' to provide another escape route out of the body; **bai shao** cools and softens the Liver, assisting **chai hu** and **huang qin** in clearing Liver and Gallbladder heat, and at the same time alleviating spasmodic pain; **zhi ban xia**, **sheng jiang** and **da zao** downbear counterflow Stomach qi and stop vomiting. (Source: *Shang Han Lun*)

Damp heat lodged in the shaoyang level

Depending on locality and climate, different pathogens can lodge in the shaoyang. The primary prescription above, was developed in the north of China where the prevailing pathogenic influence is wind and cold. In tropical or warm, humid climates, the prevailing pathogen is often damp heat, which produces a somewhat different clinical picture. In addition to the characteristic alternating fever and chill pattern with fever predominant, there may be night sweats, nausea and vomiting, aching and heaviness in the muscles, heavy and foggy head, thick, greasy, yellow tongue coat and a wiry, rapid and slippery pulse. The treatment is to clear damp heat from shaoyang and harmonize the Stomach with **HAO QIN QING DAN TANG** (Sweet Wormwood and Scutellaria Decoction to Clear the Gallbladder 蒿芩清胆汤).

qing hao (Artemisiae annuae Herba) 青蒿 12–15g
huang qin (Scutellariae Radix) 黄芩 6–9g
zhu ru (Bambusae Caulis in taeniam) 竹茹 9–12g
zhi ban xia (Pinelliae Rhizoma preparatum) 制半夏 9–12g
chi fu ling (Poria Rubra) 赤茯苓 9–12g
chen pi (Citri reticulatae Pericarpium) 陈皮 3–6g
zhi ke (Aurantii Fructus) 枳壳 6–9g
qing dai (Indigo naturalis) 青黛 3–6g
hua shi (Talcum) 滑石 12–18g
gan cao (Glycyrrhizae Radix) 甘草 3–6g

Method: Decoction. **Qing hao** and **huang qin** clear damp heat from shaoyang and cool the Liver and Gallbladder; **zhu ru** clears heat and stops vomiting, and with **zhi ban xia** transforms phlegm and downbears counterflow Stomach qi; **chen pi** and **zhi ke** harmonize the Stomach, transform damp and rectify the qi dynamic; **chi fu ling**, **qing dai** and **hua shi** promote urination to provide an outlet for damp heat; **gan cao** harmonizes the formula. Source: (*Chong Ding Tong Su Shang Han Lun*)

Prepared medicines
Concentrated powders
Xiao Chai Hu Tang (Minor Bupleurum Combination)
Chai Hu Gui Zhi Tang (Bupleurum & Cinnamon Combination)
Da Chai Hu Tang (Major Bupleurum Combination)

Pills
Xiao Chai Hu Wan (Minor Bupleurum Teapills)

Acupuncture (select from)
SJ.5 (waiguan –) .... these points harmonize and vent pathogens from
GB.41 (zulinqi –)   shaoyang
Bl.19 (danshu –) .... transporting point of the Gallbladder, regulates
                                 Gallbladder qi
Bl.21 (weishu) .... transporting point of the Stomach, strengthens the
                                 Stomach and harmonizes Stomach qi
Bl.22 (sanjiaoshu –)........... promotes movement, metabolism and transforma-
                                 tion of qi through the triple burner, promotes
                                 urination
- with damp heat, add Sp.9 (yinlingquan –) and Kid.7 (fuliu –)
- with night sweats, add SI.3 (houxi –)
- with Spleen qi deficiency, add St.36 (zusanli +) and Liv.13 (zhangmen +)

- with nausea, add PC.6 (neiguan –)
- with hypochondriac pain, add Liv.14 (qimen –)
- with dizziness, add GB.20 (fengchi) and GB.43 (xiaxi –)
- Ear points: liver, gall bladder, zero point, subcortex, sympathetic, shenmen

Clinical notes

- Shaoyang syndrome may be diagnosed as post viral or chronic fatigue syndrome, influenza, the convalescent phase of an upper respiratory tract infection, postpartum fever or cholecystitis.
- Shaoyang syndrome is a common cause of continuing illness in the aftermath of an acute cold or flu. Typically patients will have had an acute exterior wind cold, wind heat or damp heat pattern that was for some reason unresolved. The initial symptoms of the acute exterior disorder give way to feelings of heat and cold, fatigue and loss of appetite. Patients may harbor lurking pathogens in the shaoyang for weeks, months or even years.
- When correctly identified, shaoyang patterns respond well to treatment, indeed, patterns that have persisted for months can often be resolved within a week or two.

Table 2.1 Summary of persistent common cold and flu patterns

	Pattern	Features	Prescription
Lingering pathogens on the surface	Wind invasion with ying wei disharmony	Mild fever and chills, aversion to wind and sudden change of temperature, nasal congestion, sweating, dry itchy skin, joint and muscle pain, floating, weak pulse, thin white tongue coat	Gui Zhi Tang
	Qi deficiency with external wind	Lingering or recurrent colds, aversion to wind, nasal congestion, tiredness, cough with white or clear sputum, swollen cervical lymph nodes, weak voice, breathlessness, pale tongue with a thin, white coat, floating, weak pulse	Shen Su Yin
Lingering pathogens in the qi level	With qi and yin deficiency	Hacking dry cough, thirst, sweating, night sweats, low grade fever, irritability, insomnia, fatigue, nausea, swollen lymph nodes, mouth ulcers, red dry tongue with little or no coat, fine rapid pulse	Zhu Ye Shi Gao Tang
	Heat in the chest	Insomnia with restlessness and irritability, low grade fever, fatigue and a burning or stifling sensation in the chest, swollen lymph nodes	Zhi Zi Chi Tang
	Damp heat	Tiredness, foggy head, low grade fever, night sweats, muscle aches, loose stools, nausea, swollen lymph nodes, thick greasy tongue coat, slippery rapid pulse	San Ren Tang / Huo Po Xia Ling Tang / Lian Po Yin
	Phlegm heat	Fatigue, insomnia, palpitations and anxiety, dizziness, foggy head, mucus congestion, nausea, swollen lymph nodes, thick greasy yellow tongue coat, slippery rapid pulse	Wen Dan Tang
Lingering pathogens in the shaoyang	Uncomplicated shaoyang	Alternating fever and chills, fatigue, anorexia, nausea, bitter taste, irritability, dizziness, hypochondriac ache, swollen lymph nodes, wiry pulse	Xiao Chai Hu Tang
	Taiyang shaoyang	Fever, sensitive to wind and temperature change, stiff achy joints, nausea, epigastric discomfort, bitter taste and loss of appetite, swollen lymph nodes, floating or wiry pulse	Chai Hu Gui Zhi Tang
	Shaoyang yangming	Alternating fever and chills with fever predominant, nausea and vomiting, abdominal and epigastric pain, constipation or urgent diarrhea, swollen lymph nodes, wiry rapid strong pulse, yellow tongue coat	Da Chai Hu Tang
	Damp heat in shaoyang	Alternating fever and chills with fever predominant, night sweats, nausea and vomiting, muscle aches, foggy head, swollen lymph nodes, thick greasy yellow tongue coat, wiry rapid slippery pulse	Hao Qin Qing Dan Tang

DEPRESSION

Depression describes a group of disorders characterized by sadness, despondency, rumination, inability to experience pleasure, and feelings of hopelessness and inadequacy that are severe or persistent enough to interfere with normal function, interest in life and family and social interaction. Depressed patients experience a range of symptoms in addition to the mood component, and it is helpful to think of depression as a disorder that interferes with the basic aspects of life: the energy for activity, appetite, sex drive and sleep.

Typical symptoms of depression include reduced sex drive, decreased appetite and weight loss (although increased appetite and weight gain can occur), constant fatigue, poor concentration, withdrawal from social situations and activities, and thoughts of death or suicide. Sleep disturbance, insomnia, waking in the early hours of the morning, or somnolence are common. Patients may report headaches, vague aches and pains and digestive problems. Symptoms can vary during the day but are usually worse upon waking in the morning.

BOX 3.1 PATTERNS OF DEPRESSION

Liver qi constraint
Qi constraint with heat
Heart and Liver fire
Qi and phlegm constraint
Heart and Lung qi constraint
Spleen and Stomach qi constraint
Qi and blood stasis
Phlegm
  – phlegm damp
  – phlegm heat
Qi and blood deficiency
  – Heart and Spleen deficiency
  – Lung and Spleen qi deficiency
Yin deficiency
  – Liver yin deficiency
  – Heart and Kidney yin deficiency
Spleen and Kidney yang deficiency

True depression should be distinguished from the low mood that results from disappointment or loss, which may be better described as demoralization[1]. The negative feelings of demoralization, unlike those of depression, usually abate when circumstances improve; the duration of the low mood lasts days rather than weeks or months, and suicidal ideation and loss of function are less likely.

Patients with depressed mood can be classified into two groups: those with low mood as a response to specific circumstances, and those in which no specific trigger can be identified. These distinctions are clinically important, because if a cause can be identified, the probability of a satisfactory outcome is increased. Demoralization as a result of distressing or stressful stimuli can be a normal and appropriate response to the circumstances and will abate with time. In some cases, the response to the distressing event may be exaggerated, pathological, and indistinguishable from major depression (below). In both cases, Chinese medicine, in conjunction with counselling, lifestyle modification, and other appropriate interventions, can be of significant benefit, helping the patient to move through the process, while supporting healthy organ system function and maintaining qi and blood flow.

---

1 From the Merck Manual 18th Ed.

Depression without an identifiable cause is a more complex condition. It will usually be diagnosed as major depression, with the pathology a mix of constitutional factors, life habits and diet, and an exaggerated response to chronic stress, routine difficulties and setbacks. This type of depression can be difficult to manage effectively with a single therapeutic strategy, and may require a multifactorial approach, especially when suicide is a possibility. Practitioners should not be reluctant to harness the relatively fast acting pharmacotherapeutic approach of psychiatry, with the awareness building of cognitive behavioral therapy, and the supportive, strengthening and qi and blood mobilizing effects of Chinese medicine.

> **BOX 3.2 DSM–IV DIAGNOSTIC CRITERIA FOR DEPRESSION**
>
> Five of the following, with number 1 or 2 essential, are necessary for the diagnosis of major depression.
>
> 1. Pervasive depressed mood
> 2. Marked loss of interest or pleasure
> 3. Appetite changes (poor appetite most common); weight loss or weight gain
> 4. Insomnia or somnolence
> 5. Fatigue, lack of energy every day
> 6. Feelings of worthlessness or excessive guilt
> 7. Impaired thinking or concentration, indecisiveness
> 8. Suicidal thoughts

From a psychiatric point of view, there are three groups of depression; minor, major and masked. The Diagnostic and Statistical Manual, 4th edition (DSM–IV) lays out the standard diagnostic criteria (Box 3.2).

Minor depression

Minor depression is a mood disturbance of at least 2 weeks' duration, with two to four of the DSM–IV criteria (Box 3.2), including number 1 or 2. There are no delusions, and suicidal thoughts, if present, are fleeting and not seriously entertained. Minor depression is usually a form of demoralization (p.95).

Major depression

Major depression is a disabling condition which adversely affects all aspects of the patients life, and is characterized by the presence of a severely depressed state that persists for at least two weeks. The diagnostic criteria for major depression are shown in Box 3.2. Episodes may be isolated or recurrent, and occur without identifiable trigger events. Patients with major depression may contemplate and attempt suicide, and occasionally suffer delusions or hallucinations.

Masked depression

Masked depression is a depressed state characterized by the prominence of physical symptoms. Patients may not complain of depression, or may deny it. They usually present with multiple minor physical complaints. The mood component is hidden beneath tiredness, menstrual disorders, unusual sensations in the head and body, breathing difficulties and sleep problems. Masked depression is relatively common, and is influenced by cultural factors and perceptions of depression as a sign of weakness and social stigma.

> **BOX 3.3 CONSTRAINT AND STAGNATION**
>
> *yù* 郁 – Constraint. Refers specifically to qi stagnation with an emotional cause.
> Most commonly associated with the Liver, but the Heart and Lungs, and Spleen
> and Stomach can also be affected.
>
> *zhì* 滞 – Stagnation. Refers to local or systemic accumulation of qi associated
> with factors other than emotion. Also includes accumulation of food, damp
> and phlegm from a variety of causes.
>
> *yū* 瘀 – Stasis. Refers specifically to sluggish or obstructed blood. This may be
> the result of chronic Liver constraint, but can be due to a variety of other
> factors, such as heat, cold and deficiency.

DEPRESSION IN CHINESE MEDICINE

Mental and physical health is a product of the quality, volume and uninhibited movement of qi and blood. All mental disorders are due to disruption of one or more of the internal organ systems and their mental components, the shen, hun, po, yi and zhi (henceforth collectively known as the anima[2]), by insufficient or constrained qi and blood.

In Chinese, depression is *yù zhèng* 郁证. In the context of medicine, the word *yù* 郁 conveys the meaning of a restraining action on the flow of qi, which we render as constraint. Qi flow through the surface layers can be constrained by the 'freezing and constricting' nature of cold. Qi flow can also be constrained in various organ systems by repression of emotion. The term constraint is used to distinguish it from other forms of stagnation due to factors not related to emotion (Box 3.3). In the context of depression, constraint is most commonly applied to the effect of emotional repression on the Liver, but can also apply to the Heart and Lungs, and Spleen and Stomach. Different emotions cause constraint in different organs, with different expressions of the depressed mood.

Constraint of qi, however, is not the only cause of a depressed mood. Even though the term *yù* 郁 implies that constraint of some type is at work in depression, this is not always the case. Both deficiency and excess factors can influence the anima and produce depression. Constraint interferes with the expression and activity of the anima by restricting their movement, which in turn produces a particular shade of mood disorder. The anima can also be destabilized and scattered by a deficiency of qi, blood, yin and yang, with a different tone to the depressed state.

Characteristics and pathology of the anima
SHÉN 神

The shen resides in the Heart and is anchored by Heart yin and blood. It is responsible for all mental activity, perception, conscious awareness and the ability to feel. All perceptions and emotions are recognized and felt in the Heart. The shen perceives, but does not direct perception to action or reflection. The shen relies on input from the other anima to turn perception into action; the hun for insight,

---

2 From the latin meaning mind or soul

direction and intuition, the po for sense perception, the zhi for the drive to act upon perception and the yi to learn from experience.

Qi constraint, blood stasis and phlegm restrict the shen and prevent its expression. Blood and yin deficiency leave the shen unanchored and destabilized. Heat can irritate the shen, prevent it from resting and cause sleep disturbances. A constrained shen results in depression, lack of clarity in thinking, diminished insight and poor judgement. An unanchored shen is unstable, easily flustered and prone to anxiety, panic attacks and confusion. The shen is active while awake, but may be disturbed during sleep, causing vivid dreams and insomnia.

HÚN 魂

The hun is the mental aspect of the Liver and is anchored by Liver yin and blood. The hun is associated with creativity, artistic endeavor, intuition, the unconscious, the making of plans and the courage to follow them through. A healthy, well grounded hun enables forward planning with creativity, vision and insight. The hun is active in dreams, and is the creative impulse drawn upon when a problem is solved after 'sleeping on it'. When the hun and shen are balanced, wisdom is the result; when unbalanced the person may have many dreams but never accomplish anything.

A constrained hun leads to depression with a lack of inspiration and direction, diminished creativity and loss of insight. Patients feel themselves hemmed in by insurmountable barriers. A heated or overly stimulated hun results in manic or irrational behavior. A destabilized hun, ungrounded by deficiency of blood or yin, leads to aimlessness, lack of courage and resolve, indecisiveness and sleep walking.

PÒ 魄

The po is the mental aspect of the Lungs and is grounded by Lung qi. The po is concerned with awareness of sensation on the skin and perception through the five senses. It is the point of contact between the body and the external environment, and helps create a sense of self. A healthy po enables strong contact and engagement with the world, and establishes clear boundaries between self and others.

Weak Lung qi destabilizes and scatters the po, leading to depression and withdrawal, to a sense of raw exposure and vulnerability, extreme sensitivity to the emotions, thoughts and presence of others and a sense of disconnection, isolation and separation from the world and society. In extreme cases, the patient feels completely adrift, as if they are not really there, and they could simply dissipate.

A constrained po leads to depression with a sense of constant sadness and a tendency to weeping.

YÌ 意

The yi is the mental aspect of the Spleen and is responsible for application of mental activity to specific tasks, and for the ability to concentrate and keep the awareness (shen) focused. The yi is called into action when studying, reading, learning and meditating. Yi is also brought to bear when thinking through a problem.

A yi that is constrained by brooding or worry, leads to depression and melancholic brooding, with obsessive thinking and an inability to concentrate constructively. Patients are unable to let go of thoughts and turn the same ones over and over. When the yi is destabilized by weak Spleen qi, patients cannot concentrate, quickly lose interest and are unable to stay focused on simple tasks. There is a tendency to overeat or comfort eat, and patients may obsess about food.

ZHÌ 志

The zhi is the mental aspect of the Kidneys and is associated with memory, motivation, ambition, the willpower and determination to act, stability in the face of adversity and change, and an orienting sense of family connection and history.

Pathology of the zhi is always associated with deficiency of yin and/or yang. Deficiency of yin leads to a lack of grounding and a destabilized zhi; weak yang causes the zhi to 'freeze' in place. Instability or freezing of the zhi results in depression with despair and despondency, fearfulness, lack of drive and will to change, sexual withdrawal and loss of libido.

PATHOLOGY

Depression can be divided into two types, excess and deficient. The excess types are due to the effects of qi constraint, or stagnation of a pathogen such as phlegm damp or blood, on the anima. The deficient types are due to a lack of qi, blood, yin or yang, and the destabilizing effects of deficiency. The effects of constraint and deficiency produce different types of mental symptom. Constraint in general produces a gloomy despondency, as the free expression and movement of the animus in question is restricted. The effects of deficiency produce a depression that is an amalgamation of gloominess and anxiety, as the unanchored anima are easily scattered and thrown off balance.

Constraint of qi is more common in younger people and in those with depression of relatively recent onset. The more chronic the depression, the more likelihood of significant deficiency, with elements of constraint or stasis secondary. Acute onset of depression can occasionally be of a deficient type. This is seen in women following childbirth where blood loss has led to blood deficiency. Deficiency will gradually complicate chronic qi constraint, as the Spleen and Kidneys become progressively weaker, constrained heat damages yin, and lack of interest in food and reduced appetite leads to an inadequate diet and relative malnutrition.

The excess and deficient types of depression can appear superficially similar, but there are differences in the tone of the depression as noted above, and physical signs which can distinguish them. In general, depression due to constraint of qi, phlegm accumulation and blood stasis, reflects the pent up state of qi. The patient may appear quiet and withdrawn, but there is muscle tension and spasm, elevated shoulders, aches and pains and tension headaches. The deficiency patterns on the other hand, are due to a lack of vital energy, so the patient feels flat, exhausted and washed out. The muscles are flaccid, weak and toneless, and the posture slumped. In practice, patients who present to the Chinese medicine clinic often have multiple patterns. Combined patterns are usually linked by predictable

Figure 3.1 Pathological relationships of Liver qi constraint

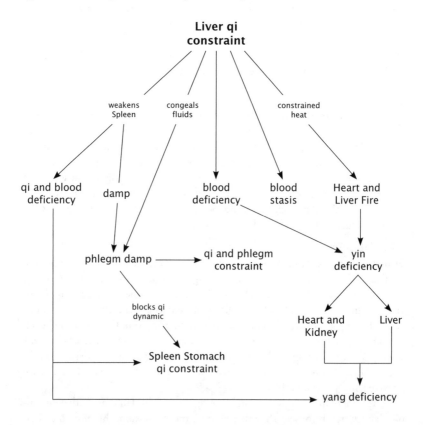

pathological relationships (Fig. 3.1).

ETIOLOGY

Emotional factors

Emotional turmoil of some type is assumed to be at least partly responsible for all depression (with the exception of depression following hemorrhage). Some patients will report a specific history that has led them to the state they are in. The traumatic events may be severe or ongoing, or their coping and recovery mechanisms may be compromised by a constitutional or acquired tendency. Others deny trauma or stress, and appear to be in supportive family and work situations. In such patients an emotional or physical trauma is assumed, but may have occurred decades before, become lost in the general run of life or was seemingly trivial and brushed off at the time. At some point, the combination of constitutional predisposition, and other non emotional contributing factors, merge and tip the patient over into depression.

Specific emotions can influence certain organ systems preferentially. Anger, rage

BOX 3.4 CONDITIONS ASSOCIATED WITH DEPRESSION

Endocrine disorders
- hypothyroidism (common)
- Cushing's disease
- reduced estrogen

Central nervous system
- stroke
- Parkinson's disease
- epilepsy
- head injury
- diabetes

Infectious diseases
- glandular fever
- hepatitis

Cancer
- both as a consequence of the tumour and/or the treatment

Cardiovascular
- recent heart attack
- anemia

Hormones and drugs
- antihypertensives
- benzodiazepines
- oral contraceptive pill
- steroids
- chemotherapy, cytotoxic agents
- substance abuse

and related emotions like resentment, frustration and bitterness cause Liver qi to become constrained when they are repressed, extreme, prolonged or unprocessed. Repression of these emotions is perhaps the most common cause of constrained qi, and some of the commonest presentations of depression can be seen as rage turned inwards.

Grief and sadness are the normal and appropriate response to bereavement and loss, but when extreme, protracted or ultimately unresolved, they can both constrain and deplete Heart and Lung qi.

Excessive or irrational worry can contribute to both constraint and deficiency. Worry can cause Spleen qi to knot, leading to obstruction of the qi dynamic and depletion of Spleen qi. This in turn gives rise to damp and phlegm, which further congest qi movement.

The Kidneys can be depleted by a severe or sudden shock or fright, and by prolonged fearfulness. The Kidney Heart axis can also be disrupted by sudden physical or emotional shock, leading to a loss of communication between the Heart and Kidneys, and disruption to the relationship between the shen and zhi (see p.781). This most commonly gives rise to depression accompanied by anxiety and insomnia, and is a factor in the depression that accompanies post traumatic stress disorder.

Constitution

Many patients with depression have a family history. A predisposition to depression may pass through the Heart and Kidneys (shaoyin), the Liver, Spleen, and Lungs, or as a tendency to phlegm accumulation. When the Heart and Kidneys are weak, depression occurs early in life, usually during late childhood or adolescence. A congenital weakness of Heart qi can lead to an anxious disposition, whereas weakness of the Kidneys leads to fearfulness, timidity and phobia which may present as withdrawal. Weakness of the Lungs contributes to a tendency to be disengaged from the world and to feelings of isolation and separation. Congenital weakness of the Spleen can lead to a tendency to excessive worry and a tendency to suppress this by overeating, compounding phlegm damp accumulation. A phlegm constitution is usually apparent from a relatively early age, with a tendency to weight problems, concentration difficulties and lack of energy. Conversely, an inherited Spleen deficiency can lead to anorexia and a persistent refusal to eat, or an obsessive or rigid attitude to food, resulting in depletion of qi and blood and a thin body.

Sleep cycle

Insufficient sleep, or a sleep cycle that is out of synchrony with the internal rhythms of the individual, is a contributing factor to the development of both qi stagnation and deficiency of yin and blood. This is seen in people who do shift work, air crew who frequently cross time zones and those who habitually stay up late into the night and sleep well into the day.

Activity levels

The increasingly sedentary work practices and leisure activities of the industrial world are a significant contributor to the rising levels of qi and blood stagnation. Regular physical activity and exercise have been shown to have a major positive impact on depression.

Depletion, overwork, exhaustion

Working excessively long hours, or laboring to the point of exhaustion, can deplete Spleen and Kidney yang qi. Any activity that excessively taxes the Spleen will lead to qi and blood deficiency, and the creation of phlegm damp.

A sudden blood loss, or increase in the demands placed upon the blood, can contribute to depression. This is seen in some cases of post–natal depression, where hemorrhage, breast feeding, inadequate rest and poor replacement of blood converge.

Diet

The diet plays a minor role in most cases of depression, but there are some cases in which diet is influential. Diets that are inadequate in some way, especially those that are too cold or raw or lacking in protein can lead to yang qi and blood deficiency. A diet rich in phlegm generating foods, sugar, fizzy drinks, carbohydrates, fats and dairy can aggravate a tendency to phlegm accumulation.

The diet becomes more influential once depression has occurred, as inattention to the diet and poor nutrition from lack of interest in food can lead to qi and blood deficiency, dampness and phlegm, which complicate the initial pathology.

TREATMENT

Successful treatment of depression requires a multifactorial approach. A regular regime of herbs and acupuncture is only one part of a comprehensive treatment plan. A combination of Chinese medical intervention, some form of psychotherapy, appropriate exercise and changes in routine lead to a better outcome than any single intervention. Acupuncture is most effective when the primary pathology is constraint of qi. With deficiency, herbs are usually required to supplement it.

There are two potential stumbling blocks which must be overcome if treatment is to succeed. The first is the nature of the illness itself, characterized as it is by a sense of hopelessness and despair. Depressed patients, as part of their pathology, can easily become disenchanted and give up treatment before it has had a chance to start working. The second problem is that real results take time to become firmly established. The challenge for the practitioner is to keep the momentum of treatment going long enough for the patient to see the benefits accruing. An ideal treatment plan involves a combination of acupuncture, herbal medicine, dietary adjustment and ongoing reinforcement, support and education, given in treatment blocks of 10–15 sessions, at twice weekly or weekly intervals. The repeated contact is an essential part of the strategy, and provides an opportunity to manage and reinforce positive habits, exercise levels and dietary changes.

Exercise

Regular exercise, especially aerobic exercise, is an important part of treatment. From a Chinese medicine point of view, exercise mobilizes qi and blood and disperses constrained qi, and is beneficial for those whose pattern includes stagnation as a significant component. A daily brisk walk of the type outlined below is an ideal way to get the qi moving and maintain its flow, but every other day will accrue significant benefit. The results of regular aerobic activity are cumulative and when a certain level of cardiovascular fitness is attained, the qi tends to be less prone to constraint, and situations that may have precipitated an episode of qi constraint and depression are tolerated better.

The most beneficial form of exercise to move qi and blood is moderate in intensity, but sustained and aerobic. The aim of the exercise is to get the heart rate up to about 50% above the resting heart rate and keep it at that level for 30–60 minutes. For example if the resting heart rate is 80 beats per minute (BPM), the target rate during exercise is 120 BPM. The person should be breathing deeply but not gasping for breath.

Yoga, taijiquan, qigong

Many patients find some form of exercise that involves mental concentration helps their mood. Yoga, taijiquan and qigong are forms of physical and mental training, involving exercises aimed at improving qi flow and the ability of the mind to maintain a point of concentration. They require a reasonable degree of effort to initiate and maintain, and may not always be the best solution for patients in the early stages of treatment, but for long term mental and emotional stability they are excellent skills to cultivate, with definite benefits on mood and other physiological parameters. A teacher is vital, and doing these sort of exercises in a group is a crucial factor in enhancing their mood elevating effects, and the encouragement to keep going. These forms of activity are more appropriate than aerobic exercise for frail or debilitated people.

Cognitive behavioral therapy (CBT)

Many people benefit from exploring and expressing their feelings in an appropriate setting. As one of the main etiological features of depression is the repression

BOX 3.5 MAIN EAR POINTS FOR DEPRESSION

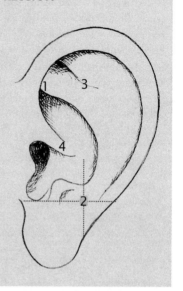

1 Sympathetic
- at the medial end of the of the inferior crus of the antihelix, where the crus of the helix and antihelix intersect (also known as Autonomic point)

2 Anti–depression
- on the ear lobe, at the intersection of a line running from the lower edge of the intertragic notch and the postantitragal fossa (AKA cheerfulness point)

3 Shenmen
- slightly above the angle formed by the superior and inferior antihelical crura

4 Zero point
- on the ascending crus of the helix as it starts to rise from the superior concha, in a small yet distinct fossa

or internalization of emotion, its expression and resolution in a safe environment can hasten recovery. Many studies have shown that therapies such as cognitive behavior therapy are effective for depression. Clinical experience suggests that the combination of acupuncture and Chinese medicine in conjunction with CBT to be even more effective.

Hot spot therapy

Hot spot therapy can be helpful for some types of depression, see Appendix 2, p.923.

Getting out of bed earlier

Many depressed patients sleep too much and at inappropriate times. Getting into bed early and rising with the sun has a beneficial effect on some depressed patients.

Ear acupuncture

Ear acupuncture is a useful addition to any treatment regime. Ear points can be left in situ for several days and provide additional support between acupuncture treatment sessions. In addition to the points selected on the basis of the organs involved, there are specific points that are especially useful for depression (Box 3.5). The best points to use are those that test positive with a point locating device.

Antidepressant medications

Many patients presenting with depression will be, or will have been, medicated with antidepressant medication. Patients present to the Chinese medicine clinic because they feel the medications are becoming less effective, they are experiencing side effects, are concerned about the long term effects, or are not happy with the sedation or flattening of the emotions that antidepressants sometimes cause.

The action of pharmaceutical antidepressants is similar to the pungent warm qi moving herbs that are used to alleviate qi constraint and phlegm damp patterns. Their pungent warmth disperses not only constrained qi and phlegm damp but also the patient's normal qi, and introduces heat into the body. When used for long periods or in high doses, qi and yin may be damaged, accounting for the common side effects of dryness and thirst. The same applies to pungent warm dispersing herbs, and similar cautions should be exercised.

The fact that pharmaceutical antidepressants mimic the action of pungent warm dispersing herbs also accounts for their relatively modest effectiveness. Various studies suggest that 35–50% of depressed patients achieve satisfactory relief with antidepressant medication. Those who fail to respond or react badly to antidepressant medications would likely be diagnosed by Chinese medicine with deficiency or mixed deficiency and excess patterns of depression for which pungent warm dispersal is contraindicated.

Managing patients taking antidepressants

The aim of Chinese medicine treatment is to relieve depression by gradually improving physiological function and the movement of qi and blood. As function improves the need for antidepressant medications should decrease, and they can be carefully withdrawn. When antidepressant medications are reduced, it should be done gradually so as to reduce the likelihood of reflex depression. When herbs are prescribed for patients already taking some form of antidepressant medication, their initial response should be carefully monitored, as qi mobilizing formulae combined with antidepressant medications can have an additive effect and increase, at least in the short term, the chance of adverse effects, such as increased heat and dryness. There are a few herbs that can help alleviate these unwanted effects to an extent, while at the same time relieving constraint and lifting the mood (Table 3.1, p.106). In patients on multiple medications, rather than prescribing more medicine, it may better to start with acupuncture, administered as frequently as possible.

Table 3.1 Herbs with an effect on the mood

Yu Jin Curcumae Radix 郁金	Turmeric root; pungent, bitter, cold; Heart, Lung, Liver, Gallbladder. Cools the Heart, moves qi and blood and relieves qi constraint. An important herb for depression and manic states from Liver qi constraint, phlegm, heat and Heart and Kidney yin deficiency. Good when there is heat, hypochondriac pain or abdominal pain.
Dan Shen Salviae miltior- rhizae Radix 丹参	Salvia root; bitter, cool; Heart, Liver. Activates qi and blood and calms the shen and hun. For depression and shen disturbances from blood stasis and heat affecting the Heart and Liver. Good when there is insomnia, agitation, irritability, hypochondriac and chest pain.
He Huan Pi Albizziae Cortex 合欢皮	Albizzia bark; sweet, neutral; Liver, Heart, Spleen. Activates qi and blood, relieves qi constraint and calms the shen and hun. For depression and mood disorders from qi and blood constraint, and Heart and Spleen deficiency. Good when there is insomnia, irritability and memory problems. Frequently combined with **ye jiao teng**.
He Huan Hua Albizziae Flos 合欢花	Albizzia flower; sweet, neutral; Liver, Stomach. Moves qi, relieves qi constraint and harmonizes the Stomach. Similar to **he huan pi**, but has a settling effect on the Stomach, and so is better when nausea or indigestion are part of the picture.
Ye Jiao Teng Polygoni multi- flori Caulis 夜交藤	Polygonum vine; sweet, neutral; Heart, Liver. Nourishes Heart blood and calms the shen and hun. A gentle herb suitable for long term use. Treats depression with anxiety and insomnia from deficiency. Frequently combined with **he huan pi**.
Mei Gui Hua Rosae rugosae Flos 玫瑰花	Chinese rose flower; sweet, slightly bitter, warm. Liver, Spleen. Activates qi and blood. A mild herb suitable for long term use in mild to moderate depression from Liver qi constraint. Can gently move qi without damaging yin.
Shi Chang Pu Acori tatarinowii Rhizoma 石菖蒲	Acorus root; bitter, pungent, warm; Heart, Spleen, Stomach. Opens the orifices and eliminates phlegm	These two are used together for mood disorders, and form a synergistic pair that resolves phlegm misting the Heart and settling over the senses. Specifically for confusion, foggy head, cloudy thinking, inability to concentrate and disordered thinking. Can be used for any pattern with phlegm. Quite dispersing, so not suitable for long term use in deficiency patterns. Often combined with **yu jin** when there is phlegm heat.
Yuan Zhi Polygalae Radix 远志	Polygala root; bitter, pungent, warm; Heart, Kidney, Lung. Calms the shen and transforms phlegm	
Bai He Lilii Bulbus 百合	Lily bulb; sweet, cool; Heart, Lung. Cools the Heart and calms the shen and po. For depression, restlessness, insomnia and irritability from Heart and Lung yin deficiency, and when yin has been damaged by long term antidepressant use or by febrile illness.

Table 3.1 Herbs with an effect on the mood (cont.)

Xiao Mai Tritici Fructus 小麦	Wheat; sweet, cool; Heart, Liver. Nourishes the Heart and calms the shen. For depression and emotional lability associated with Heart deficiency. Usually combined with **da zao** and **gan cao**.
Qing Pi Citri reticulatae viride Pericarpium 青皮	Green tangerine peel; pungent, bitter, warm; Liver, Gallbladder, Stomach. Dredges the Liver and breaks up qi constraint. A strong herb to break up and disperse constrained qi, it can provide a strong initial push to get a treatment going, but should not be overused as it can disperse qi too much.
Ba Yue Zha Akebia Fructus 八月扎	Akebia fruit; bitter, cold; Liver. Gallbladder, Stomach, Urinary Bladder. Dredges the Liver and strengthens the Kidneys. For depression from Liver qi constraint. Especially good for depression associated with menstruation.
Fo Shou Citri sarcodacylis Fructus 佛手	Finger citron; pungent, bitter, sour, warm; Liver, Spleen, Stomach, Lung. Moves qi and harmonizes the Liver and Spleen. For depression from Liver qi constraint, particularly when there are digestive symptoms such as abdominal pain, indigestion, nausea and loss of appetite. This herb is less dispersing to yin and qi than other qi moving herbs. Often used together with **xiang yuan pi**.
Xiang Yuan Pi Pericarpium Citri Medica 香橼皮	Citron; pungent, slightly bitter, sour, warm; Liver, Spleen, Lung. Moves qi and transforms phlegm. For mood disorders from qi and phlegm stagnation and Liver and Spleen disharmony. Used when there are upper digestive symptoms, nausea, indigestion, plum pit qi and chest oppression. Often used together with **fo shou**.
Xiang Fu Cyperi Rhizoma 香附	Cyperus root; pungent, slightly bitter and sweet; Liver, Triple Burner. Moves qi and alleviates constraint. Not traditionally considered a mood enhancing herb, but its qi moving effect is so reliable and well tolerated it can be added to all prescriptions, whether for stagnation or deficiency to provide mild impetus to qi movement.
Tan Xiang Santali albi Lignum 檀香	Sandalwood; pungent, warm; Spleen, Stomach, Lung. Moves qi. Not traditionally considered a mood enhancing herb, but it is effective in alleviating Heart and Lung qi constraint, and is good when there is chest oppression or pain.
Bai Shao Paeoniae Radix alba 白芍	Peony root; bitter, sour, cool; Liver, Spleen. Softens the Liver and nourishes blood. Not traditionally considered a mood enhancing herb, but an essential component of all formulas for Liver qi constraint depression. It has the unique action of softening and easing a rigid Liver and protecting it from the pungency and dispersing qualities of the qi moving herbs.

Table 3.2 Acupuncture points with a specific effect on the mood

Lu.3 tianfu	For Lung qi constraint and deficiency depression. Can be a good alternative to Lu.7 lieque when the potential for overwhelming emotional release is suspected (see below). Indicated for feeling sad all the time, weeping, confusion, speaking to oneself or not at all.
Lu.7 lieque	A major point for mood disorders from Lung and Heart qi constraint and deficiency. Diffuses the Lungs and assists descent of Lung qi to activate the po. Caution is advised in the use of this point in fragile patients since its effect can be quite powerful and it can suddenly release deeply held emotions.
Lu.9 taiyuan	Stabilizes the po. Used for Lung deficiency patterns, where the patient appears overwhelmed by sadness and grief and doesn't have enough qi to cope. The patients shoulders may be hunched, their body slumped forward and breathing shallow. Preferred to Lu.7 lieque for frail patients.
LI.4 hegu	Calms the shen and alleviates agitation, especially when combined with Liv.3 taichong and Du.20 baihui. A particularly good combination when depression is accompanied by muscle tension and stiffness, and extreme irritability or barely repressed anger.
St.36 zusanli	Calms the shen and supports the yi. Used for all mood disorders from deficiency, damp or Spleen dysfunction.
St.40 fenglong	An important point for depression from phlegm. Especially good when combined with Sp.3 taibai and PC.6 neiguan for heaviness of mind and body, clouded thinking, lack of clarity and somnolence characteristic of phlegm conditions.
St.41 jiexi	Indicated for depression, groaning, sadness and weeping, fearfulness and agitation from phlegm damp.
Sp.5 shangqiu	Indicated for depression with disturbing nightmares and somnolence, especially when damp is a factor.
Ht.3 shaohai	For depression from Heart heat or yin deficiency with a tendency to manic episodes, anxiety and restlessness.
Ht.5 tongli	For Heart and Kidney deficiency type depression, anxiety, inability to articulate or disinterest in talking and fear of people. Often combined with Kid.4 dazhong for this.
Ht.7 shenmen	Calms the shen. An important point for all shen disturbances and mood disorders. Especially good when depression is accompanied by anxiety, and for depression from Heart deficiency.

Table 3.2 Acupuncture points with a specific effect on the mood (cont.)

SI.3 houxi	Traditionally indicated for more manic types of mood disorder and seizures, but it has the ability to clear the mind and improve insight, to break through the self absorption and inward focus that characterizes some depression. Acts upon the zhi and shen via the dumai. Usually combined with Bl.62 shenmai and Du.20 baihui.
The inner Urinary Bladder channel	From Bl.13 feishu to Bl.23 shenshu, these points are used to correct the underlying pathology and should always be included in a comprehensive treatment. Select on the basis of pathology and palpation.
The outer Urinary Bladder channel	From Bl.42 pohu to Bl.52 zhishi, these points reflect the anima of their respective organ systems. Select on the basis of palpation.
Bl.62 shenmai	Clears the mind and improves insight, with SI.3 houxi.
Kid.4 dazhong	Stabilizes the zhi. Used for depression with fearfulness, anxiety, agoraphobia, disinterest in talking, somnolence and withdrawal. Often combined with Ht.5 tongli.
Kid.9 zhubin	For depression with anxiety, palpitations and a sense of too much energy in the head from Heart and Kidney deficiency. Usually combined with PC.6 neiguan for this.
Kid.25 shenzang	Indicated for 'not wishing to live'.
Kid.27 shufu	Used for sadness and unresolved grief from Lung deficiency or stagnation.
PC.4 ximen	For depression, especially when relatively acute or associated with a fresh trauma. Can be helpful for depression and flashbacks from post traumatic stress.
PC.6 neiguan	An important point for depressed mood from qi constraint with shen and hun disturbance, usually combined with Liv.3 taichong. For Heart and Kidney deficiency depression, with depression and anxiety, combined with Kid.9 zhubin. Indications for this point include frequent sighing, chest oppression, insomnia, anxiety, sadness, reflux and melancholy.
PC.7 daling	Used for conditions similar to PC.6 neiguan, but with more heat and agitation.
GB.8 shuaigu	Indicated for depression with headaches.
GB.21 jianjing	Not specifically indicated for depression, but very useful to remove some of the innate tension that accompanies qi constraint. Has a calming effect as a result, and usually combined with GB.34 yanglingquan for this.
GB.39 xuanzhong	This point has an good effect on calming the shen and hun, alleviating qi constraint and elevating the mood, especially when combined with SJ.5 waiguan. Used for depression with insomnia, anxiety and irritability. As the 'sea of Marrow' it can help in clarifying thinking.
Liv.1 dadun	Used for depression from qi constraint, and blood deficiency, treated with rice grain moxa.

Table 3.2 Acupuncture points with a specific effect on the mood (cont.)

Liv.3 taichong	Mobilizes, settles and supports the hun. A major point for depressed mood derived from qi constraint and/or yin and blood deficiency. Used in all cases with a qi constraint component. Frequently combined with LI.4 hegu and Du.20 baihui to enhance its calming effect.
Liv.5 ligou	For depression from qi constraint, especially when loss of libido and plum pit qi are features.
Ren.6 qihai	Stabilizes the zhi. Used for deficiency patterns of depression, particularly when the Kidneys are weak or cold. Usually treated with moxa.
Ren.14 juque	For depression with a tendency to manic episodes, palpitations and anxiety, from qi constraint, Heart heat or deficiency.
Ren.17 shanzhong	Not specifically indicated for depression, but one that is useful in Lung patterns to assist proper movement and descent of Lung qi. Select on the basis of tenderness.
Du.4 mingmen	For depression and exhaustion from Kidney yang deficiency. Treat with plenty of moxa.
Du.8 jinsuo	For depression with muscle tension, spasms and irritability, and when rage and frustration lurk just beneath the surface.
Du.12 shenzhu	Indicated for suppressed rage and a 'desire to kill people'.
Du.14 dazhui	For Lung weakness patterns with profound sadness and grief.
Du.20 baihui	For all patterns of depression regardless of whether from stagnation or deficiency. Elevates mood and has a strong calming effect. Specifically indicated for sadness, weeping and a lack of will to live, inability to choose words, poor memory and inability to concentrate, lack of clarity and insight.
Du.24 shenting	For depression with anxiety and insomnia.
yintang (M-HN-3)	Good as a general calming point for depression with anxiety and agitation.

肝
气
郁
结

3.1 LIVER QI CONSTRAINT

Liver qi constraint underlies many cases of recent onset depression, and will frequently complicate more chronic cases where other pathogens or deficiency states predominate. The pathology of Liver qi constraint leads to a predictable cascade (Fig. 3.1, p.100), so that qi constraint patterns are usually complicated by blood deficiency, heat, phlegm damp, food stagnation, blood stasis or a mixture thereof. Constrained Liver qi is the product of emotional repression, in particular those of the anger group. Qi can also be constrained when the internal rhythms of the body are disrupted. This is seen in shift workers, air crew and those whose routine is out of balance with their internal clock.

The depression and gloominess of Liver qi constraint is due primarily to its restrictive effects on the expression of the hun (p.98).

Clinical features
• Depression and gloominess, mood swings, feeling wound up and tense. The depression is worse in the morning and with prolonged inactivity.
• Chest, hypochondriac, epigastric and/or abdominal discomfort, aching, tightness, distension, fullness or pain. Aches and pains tend to be vague, intermittent and poorly localized.
• waking in the early hours of the morning, unable to go back to sleep
• intermittent fatigue that is worse when depressed and better for activity
• heartburn, nausea, belching, indigestion, loss of appetite, frequent sighing
• tendency to constipation, or alternating bowel habits
• neck and shoulder tightness and pain, elevated shoulders and tight trapezius; tension headaches
• premenstrual syndrome, depression is worse premenstrually
• loss of libido; impotence (but erections may be achieved during sleep)
T in early stages unremarkable, or dark or slightly mauve, with a thin coat
P wiry

Treatment Principle
Dredge the Liver and relieve qi constraint
Regulate qi and harmonize the middle burner

Prescription

CHAI HU SHU GAN SAN 柴胡疏肝散
Bupleurum Powder to Dredge the Liver, modified

chai hu (Bupleuri Radix) 柴胡 9–12g
bai shao (Paeoniae Radix alba) 白芍 12–18g
zhi shi (Fructus Immaturus Citri Aurantii) 枳实 9–12g
xiang fu (Cyperi Rhizoma) 香附 9–12g
chuan xiong (Chuanxiong Rhizoma) 川芎 6–9g
chen pi (Citri reticulatae Pericarpium) 陈皮 6–9g
zhi gan cao (Glycyrrhizae Radix preparata) 炙甘草 3–6g
he huan pi (Albizziae Cortex) 合欢皮 12–15g

mei gui hua (Rosae rugosae Flos) 玫瑰花 6–9g
Method: Decoction. **Chai hu** dredges the Liver and regulates qi, **bai shao** softens the Liver, nour-ishes yin and blood and assists **chai hu** in regulating qi; **zhi shi**, **chen pi** and **xiang fu** regulate qi; **chuan xiong** moves qi and activates blood; **zhi gan cao** strengthens the Spleen and, with **bai shao**, alleviates any cramping and spasmodic pain; **he huan pi** and **mei hui hua** activate qi and blood and relieve depression. (Source: *Shi Yong Zhong Yi Nei Ke Xue* [*Zheng Zhi Zhun Sheng*])

Modifications

- With hypochondriac aching, fullness or pain, add **qing pi** (Citri reticulatae viride Pericarpium) 青皮 9–12g and **fo shou** (Citri sarcodacylis Fructus) 佛手 9–12g.
- When depression is worse premenstrually, add **ba yue zha** (Akebiae Fructus) 八月扎 9–12g.
- With insomnia, add **dan shen** (Salviae miltiorrhizae Radix) 丹参 9–12g and **ye jiao teng** (Polygoni multiflori Caulis) 夜胶藤 15–30g.
- With belching, nausea and epigastric distension, add **xuan fu hua** (Inulae Flos) 旋复花 9–12g, **dai zhe shi** (Haematitum) 代赭石 9–12g and **zi su geng** (Perillae Caulis) 紫苏梗 6–9g.
- With abdominal distension, pain and diarrhea, add **cang zhu** (Atractylodis Rhizoma) 苍术 9–12g, **fu ling** (Poria) 茯苓 12–15g and **yi ren** (Coicis Semen) 苡仁 15–30g.
- With constipation, add **wu yao** (Linderae Radix) 乌药 6–9g and **bing lang** (Arecae Semen) 槟榔 6–9g.
- With tightness in the chest and difficulty getting a full breath, add **quan gua lou** (Trichosanthis Fructus) 全栝楼 18–24g and **qian hu** (Peucedani Radix) 前胡 6–9g.
- With food stagnation, add **shen qu** (Massa medicata fermentata) 神曲 12–15g and **shan zha** (Crataegi Fructus) 山楂 12–15g.
- With blood stasis, add **tao ren** (Persicae Semen) 桃仁 9–12g and **hong hua** (Carthami Flos) 红花 6–9g.

Variations and additional prescriptions
Postnatal depression from qi constraint with blood deficiency
The extra demands on the mother's blood during gestation and breast feeding can lead to blood deficiency. Due to the dynamics of qi and blood, Liver blood defi-ciency can allow qi to more easily become constrained. Qi constraint and blood deficiency are common in postpartum women and are significant contributors to postnatal depression. The patient is depressed, with postural dizziness, poor milk supply and low energy, pale edges on the tongue and fine and wiry pulse. In addition to ensuring adequate nutrition and rest for the patient, regulating qi, strengthening the Spleen and supplementing blood can assist. A formula such as **Xiao Yao San** (Rambling Powder 逍遥散 p.284) is ideal.

Liver qi constraint with the 'six stagnations'
Due to the pivotal nature of the Liver in the maintenance of qi and blood flow and healthy Spleen function, qi constraint is frequently complicated by one or more of the pathogens that can arise as a result of the cascade of physiological

disruption (Fig. 3.1, p.100). An effective way to address this is with Yᴜᴇ Jᴜ Wᴀɴ (Escape Restraint Pill 越鞠丸 p.126). This formula is an excellent choice for mild to moderate depression from qi constraint, especially when there are accompanying upper digestive tract symptoms such as heartburn, indigestion, belching, epigastric pain or nausea.

Prepared medicines
Concentrated powder
Chai Hu Shu Gan San (Bupleurum & Cyperus Combination)
Xiao Yao San (Bupleurum & Tangkuei Formula)
Yue Ju Tang (Cyperus & Atractylodes Combination)
Pills
Chai Hu Shu Gan Wan (Bupleurum Soothe Liver Teapills)
Shu Gan Wan (Soothe Liver Teapills, Shu Kan Wan)
  – better when there is hypochondriac or abdominal pain
Mu Xiang Shun Qi Wan (Aplotaxis Carminative Pills, Shun Qi Wan)
  – with constipation
Xiao Yao Wan (Free and Easy Wanderer Teapills, Hsiao Yao Wan)

Acupuncture (select from)
Du.20 (baihui).................these points calm the shen and lift the mood
yintang (M–HN–3)
Liv.3 (taichong –)..............the 'four gates', together these points have a strong
LI.4 (hegu –)   sedative and calming effect, mobilize qi and blood,
                                 settle the hun and shen, relieve mental cloudiness
                                 and ease muscle spasm
PC.6 (neiguan)..................regulates the Liver and alleviates constrained qi,
                                 calms the Heart and shen and settles the hun
GB.34 (yanglingquan –)......sea point of the Gallbladder, regulates qi and eases
                                 muscle tension
Bl.18 (ganshu –)................transport point of the Liver, alleviates qi constraint
• with insomnia and early waking, use GB.39 (xuanzhong) and SJ.5 (waiguan) instead of Liv.3 and LI.4.
• Ear points: shenmen, liver, anti–depression, zero point, sympathetic

Clinical notes
• Exercise is an essential component of short and long term management; see p.103 for specifics.
• A regular daily meal time, exercise and sleep routine is essential, as is avoidance of alcohol and non prescription drugs.
• A Liver qi mobilizing diet may assist. See Clinical Handbook, Vol.2, p.878.
• Hot spot therapy is helpful, see p.923.
• Getting up earlier and sleeping less is recommended.

气
郁
化
火

3.2 LIVER QI CONSTRAINT WITH HEAT

Heat is a common complication of chronic Liver qi constraint, and leads to a more volatile symptom picture, with depressed moods alternating with anger outbursts, more dryness and upper body symptoms. Antidepressant medications (which are warm and dispersing), a rich or spicy diet, alcohol and illicit drugs also contribute to heat development. Liver qi constraint with heat is more common in people in their thirties and forties, when life, family and job pressures often escalate, and may be combined with alcohol or drugs. Qi constraint also tends to transform into heat more readily in older patients, assisted by the gradual depletion of yin that is a natural consequence of ageing.

Mild degrees of heat are referred to as constrained heat, while more intense heat is described as fire. The basic pattern is often complicated by Spleen deficiency, heat in the Heart and Stomach or damp heat. Chronic heat will eventually damage yin.

Clinical features
- Depression, with marked irritability, irascibility, anger or violent outbursts.
- chest, hypochondriac, epigastric and/or abdominal oppression, tightness, distension, discomfort, fullness or pain; may be a sense of blockage in the throat
- waking in the early hours of the morning; restless sleep, excessive dreaming
- fatigue with restlessness; fatigue better after activity
- red complexion, red sore irritated eyes
- bitter taste in the mouth, dry mouth and thirst
- acid reflux, heartburn, nausea, belching, indigestion, loss of appetite
- constipation with dry stools
- tension or migraine headaches; neck and shoulder tightness and pain, elevated shoulders and tight trapezius
- premenstrual syndrome with increasing depression and irritability
- loss of libido

T red or with red edges and a thin yellow coat
P wiry and rapid

Treatment Principle
Dredge the Liver, regulate qi and relieve qi constraint
Cool the Liver and clear heat

Prescription

JIA WEI XIAO YAO SAN 加味逍遥散
Augmented Rambling Powder, modified

chai hu (Bupleuri Radix) 柴胡 9–12g
bai shao (Paeoniae Radix alba) 白芍 12–18g
dang gui (Angelicae sinensis Radix) 当归 9–12g
fu ling (Poria) 茯苓 12–15g
bai zhu (Atractylodis macrocephalae Rhizoma) 白术 9–12g
shan zhi zi (Gardeniae Fructus) 山栀子 9–12g

mu dan pi (Moutan Cortex) 牡丹皮 9–12g
zhi gan cao (Glycyrrhizae Radix preparata) 炙甘草 3–6g
yu jin (Curcumae Radix) 郁金 9–12g
he huan pi (Albizziae Cortex) 合欢皮 12–15g
Method: Decoction. **Chai hu** dredges the Liver, regulates qi and clears heat; **bai shao** softens the Liver and, with **dang gui**, nourishes Liver blood; **fu ling**, **bai zhu** and **zhi gan cao** strengthen the Spleen; **fu ling** promotes urination and drains damp; **bai zhu** dries damp; **shan zhi zi** and **mu dan pi** cool the Liver and clear heat; **yu jin** clears heat, alleviates qi constraint and lifts the mood; **he huan pi** activates qi and blood and alleviates depression. (Source: *Zhong Yi Nei Ke Xue / Nei Ke Zhai Yao*)

Modifications
• With Stomach heat, reflux and heartburn, add **huang lian** (Coptidis Rhizoma) 黄连 6–9g and **wu zhu yu** (Evodiae Fructus) 吴茱萸 2–3g.
• With insomnia, add **dan shen** (Salviae miltiorrhizae Radix) 丹参 9–12g.
• With anger outbursts, irritability, headaches and red sore eyes, add **ju hua** (Chrysanthemi Flos) 菊花 9–12g, **bai ji li** (Tribuli Fructus) 白蒺藜 9–12g and **gou teng** (Uncariae Ramulus cum Uncis) 钩藤 9–12g.
• When depression is worse premenstrually, add **ba yue zha** (Akebiae Fructus) 八月扎 9–12g and **xiang fu** (Cyperi Rhizoma) 香附 9–12g.
• With heat in the blood, acne and rashes, use **chi shao** (Paeoniae Radix rubra) 赤芍 9–12g instead of **bai shao**.
• With tightness in the chest and difficulty getting a full breath, add **quan gua lou** (Trichosanthis Fructus) 全栝楼 18–24g and **qian hu** (Peucedani Radix) 前胡 6–9g.
• With constipation, add **bing lang** (Arecae Semen) 槟榔 6–9g and **zhi shi** (Fructus Immaturus Citri Aurantii) 柴胡 9–12g.
• With food stagnation, add **shen qu** (Massa medicata fermentata) 神曲 12–15g and **lian qiao** (Forsythiae Fructus) 连翘 9–12g, or combine with the prepared medicine BAO HE WAN (Preserve Harmony Pill).
• With mild damage to Liver yin, peeled edges on the tongue, fine pulse and dry eyes, delete **bai zhu** and **sheng jiang**, and add **sheng di** (Rehmanniae Radix) 生地 12–18g, **mai dong** (Ophiopogonis Radix) 麦冬 9–12g and **shan yao** (Dioscoreae Rhizoma) 山药 9–12g. See also 3.11, p.143.

Variations and additional prescriptions
With Spleen deficiency, the primary pathological triad
When Spleen qi deficiency complicates Liver qi constraint with heat, the primary pathological triad is formed. Qi constraint, Spleen deficiency and heat commonly occur simultaneously, are tightly interlinked and mutually engendering. There are numerous solutions depending on the balance of pathology found in any individual, but a good place to start when there is a relatively equal mix of all three is XIAO CHAI HU TANG (Minor Bupleurum Decoction 小柴胡汤, p.90). See p.780 for more detail on the primary pathological triad.

Prepared medicines
Concentrated powders
Jia Wei Xiao Yao San (Bupleurum & Peony Formula)

Yue Ju Tang (Cyperus & Atractylodes Combination)
Yi Guan Jian (Linking Combination)
   – combine with one of the above when there is yin deficiency
Xiao Chai Hu Tang (Minor Bupleurum Combination)

Pills
Jia Wei Xiao Yao Wan (Free and Easy Wanderer Plus Teapills, Dan Zhi Xiao Yao Wan)
Xiao Chai Hu Wan (Minor Bupleurum Teapills)

Acupuncture (select from)
Du.20 (baihui) ....these points calm the shen and lift the mood
yintang (M–HN–3)
GB.8 (shuaigu)
Liv.3 (taichong –) ....these are the 'four gates', and together have a strong
LI.4 (hegu –)   sedative and calming effect, mobilize qi and blood,
                                     settle the hun and shen, relieve mental cloudiness
                                     and ease muscle spasm
PC.6 (neiguan)...................regulates the Liver and alleviates constrained qi,
                                     calms the Heart and shen and settles the hun
PC.7 (daling –) ....clears heat and calms the shen
Liv.2 (xingjian –).................cools the Liver and alleviates constrained qi
GB.34 (yanglingquan –).....regulates qi and clears heat
Bl.18 (ganshu –).................transport points of the Liver and Heart, regulate qi,
Bl.15 (xinshu)   clear heat and calm the shen and hun
Bl.44 (shentang).................these points calm the shen and hun
Bl.47 (hunmen)
- with insomnia and early waking, use GB.39 (xuanzhong) and SJ.5 (waiguan) instead of Liv.3 and LI.4
- With impotence and loss of libido, add Liv.5 (ligou –)
- Ear points: shenmen, liver, anti–depression, zero point, sympathetic

Clinical notes
- Liver qi constraint with heat may be diagnosed as premenstrual syndrome, reactive depression, menopausal depression or possibly attention deficit hyperactivity disorder (ADHD).
- Exercise is an essential component of short and long term management. See p.103 for specifics. A combination of physical and mental training, such as occurs in yoga, qigong or taijiquan can also assist in controlling anger outbursts.
- A regular daily meal time, exercise and sleep routine is essential, as is avoidance of alcohol and non prescription drugs.
- Hot spot therapy is helpful, see p.923.
- Getting up earlier and sleeping less is recommended..
- A Liver qi mobilizing diet may assist. See Clinical Handbook, Vol.2, p.878.

心
肝
火
盛

3.3 HEART AND LIVER FIRE

Heart and Liver fire is usually an exacerbation of Liver qi constraint with heat, and represents an acute manic episode. When heat is already present, it does not take too much extra pressure to intensify it. A sudden increase in stress, frustration, alcohol consumption or drug use can be enough to push constrained heat into fire. If this situation is allowed to persist, yin will be significantly damaged.

Clinical features

- Depression with intermittent episodes of violent outbursts, restless agitation, aggressive or manic behavior; compulsive or reckless behavior; in severe cases suicidal ideation or suicide attempts.
- red, flushed complexion and eyes; may be scleral hemorrhage
- dizziness, vertigo
- insomnia or restless sleep with violent or disturbing dreams
- palpitations, tachycardia
- tinnitus
- constipation
- mouth and tongue ulcers
- red, swollen, painful or suppurative skin lesions
- dark concentrated urine
- may be a scorched smell about the patient, like an iron left on clothes too long

T red with a thick, yellow, dry or greasy coat
P slippery, rapid, strong, surging

Treatment principle

Cool the Heart and Liver
Drain fire and sedate the hun and shen

Prescription

DANG GUI LONG HUI WAN 当归龙会丸
Tangkuei, Gentian and Aloe Pill

This prescription is selected when the heat is severe and complicated by constipation. It can quickly open the bowels and provide an outlet for the heat.

jiu dang gui (wine fried Angelicae sinensis Radix) 酒当归 30g
jiu long dan cao (wine fried Gentianae Radix) 酒龙胆草 30g
shan zhi zi (Gardeniae Fructus) 山栀子 30g
huang qin (Scutellariae Radix) 黄芩 30g
huang lian (Coptidis Rhizoma) 黄连 30g
huang bai (Phellodendri Cortex) 黄柏 30g
da huang (Rhei Radix et Rhizoma) 大黄 15g
lu hui (Aloe) 芦荟 15g
qing dai (Indigo Naturalis) 青黛 15g
mu xiang (Aucklandiae Radix) 木香 6g

Method: Pills or powder. **Huang lian**, **huang qin**, **huang bai** and **shan zhi zi** purge from all three burners; **long dan cao**, **qing dai** and **lu hui** purge fire from the Liver and Gallbladder; **huang qin** purges fire from the Lungs, **huang lian** purges fire from the Heart, **huang bai** purges fire from the

Kidneys and **jiu da huang** purges fire through the Intestines; **mu xiang** and **jiu dang gui** regulate qi and blood; **jiu da huang** and **jiu dang gui** also activate blood. The original prescription included musk [**she xiang** (Moschus) 麝香], a glandular secretion from the musk deer. This is no longer used due to the endangered status of the animal, and in modern preparations it is usually substituted with **synthetic muscone** (ren gong she xiang 人工麝香). (Source: *Xuan Ming Fang Lun*)

CHAI HU JIA LONG GU MU LI TANG 柴胡加龙骨牡蛎汤
Bupleurum plus Dragon Bone and Oyster Shell Decoction

This prescription is selected for depression with restlessness, aggression, and delusional thinking. It is commonly applied to the depression and agitation which patients can exhibit when withdrawing from narcotics or other drugs. The heat and intensity here is less than that requiring the use of the primary prescription.

chai hu (Bupleuri Radix) 柴胡 9–12g
zhi ban xia (Pinelliae Rhizoma preparatum) 制半夏 9–12g
fu ling (Poria) 茯苓 9–12g
gui zhi (Cinnamomi Ramulus) 桂枝 6–9g
sheng jiang (Zingiberis Rhizoma recens) 生姜 6–9g
huang qin (Scutellariae Radix) 黄芩 6–9g
jiu da huang (wine fried Rhei Radix et Rhizoma) 酒大黄 6–9g
ren shen (Ginseng Radix) 人参 6–9g
long gu (Fossilia Ossis Mastodi) 龙骨 15–30g
mu li (Ostreae Concha) 牡蛎 15–30g
sheng tie luo (Ferri Frusta) 生铁落 30–60g
da zao (Jujubae Fructus) 大枣 .... 4 fruit

Method: Powder is the most reliable way to deliver this formula and ensures a good quantity of the shen and hun calming minerals are ingested. In concentrated powders **sheng tie luo** is omitted. **Chai hu** dredges the Liver, regulates qi and with **huang qin**, clears heat and dispels pathogens from the shao yang; **huang qin** is especially good at clearing heat from the upper burner; **ren shen** supplements qi and moistens dryness; **zhi ban xia** transforms phlegm; **sheng tie luo**, **long gu** and **mu li** subdue and anchor yang and calm the shen; **fu ling** strengthens the Spleen and calms the shen; **gui zhi** frees up circulation of yang qi in the chest; **da huang** clears heat and open the bowels; **sheng jiang** and **da zao** harmonize the Stomach and protect it from the harsh effects of the minerals and bitter herbs. (Source: *Shang Han Lun*)

Variations and additional prescriptions
Lingering heat in the chest following an unresolved external invasion
A type of heat can persist in the chest, affecting the Heart and disturbing the shen, in the aftermath of an external invasion that has been trapped or otherwise unresolved. This may be the result of wrong treatment (over sweating, purgation or emesis) when a pathogen is on the surface. The features are relatively acute onset of depression following a cold or flu, with insomnia, agitation, restlessness and a sense of heat in the chest. The treatment is to clear lingering heat from the chest with ZHI ZI CHI TANG (Gardenia and Prepared Soybean Decoction 栀子豉汤, p.82).

Prepared medicines
Concentrated powders
Dang Gui Long Hui Wan (Tangkuei, Gentiana & Aloe Formula)

Chai Hu Jia Long Gu Mu Li Tang (Bupleurum & Dragon Bone Combination)

Pills

Chai Hu Long Gu Mu Li Tang (Bupleurum, Dragon Bone and Oyster Shell Teapills)

Long Dan Xie Gan Wan (Snake and Dragon Teapills)

Acupuncture (select from)

Du.20 (baihui) ....calms the mind

Ht.8 (shaofu –) ....fire point of the Heart, drains fire and calms the shen

Ht.9 (shaochong ↓)...........wood point of the Heart, drains Heart fire and calms the shen

SI.3 (houxi –).....................master point of the dumai, an important point for shen disturbances from heat; stabilizes the shen and zhi

LI.11 (quchi –)...................together these points clear heat systemically

LI.4 (hegu –)

GB.34 (yanglingquan –)......sea point of the Gallbladder, regulates qi, clears heat and calms ascendant Liver yang

St.40 (fenglong –) ....connecting point of the Stomach, clears heat and transforms phlegm

Liv.2 (xingjian –) ....fire point of the Liver, drains Liver fire and regulates qi

• Ear points: shenmen, heart, liver, anti–depression, zero point, sympathetic

Clinical notes

• This is usually an acute exacerbation of an existing condition, and as such is hopefully treated for a short time only. The obvious difficulties involved in treating someone who is aggressive or suicidal are obvious and such patients will usually require specialized management in a dedicated facility. Chinese medicine can be reasonably effective however, if herbs are taken correctly, acupuncture frequent and the patient closely monitored. When successful, fire can be cleared quite quickly, no more than a few weeks.

• Heart and Liver fire is often associated with an element of phlegm heat, and so overlaps with the Chinese medicine category of Mania Depression (*diān kuáng* 癫狂) and bipolar mood disorder.

• Hot spot therapy can be helpful, see p.923.

• A heat clearing diet is recommended. See Clinical Handbook, Vol.2, p.882. Alcohol and non prescription drugs should be strictly avoided.

气 3.4 QI AND PHLEGM CONSTRAINT
滞
痰
Qi and phlegm constraint is a result of constraint of Lung qi, dysfunction of the Liver and Spleen, or a combination of both. Sadness and grief may obstruct the descent and diffusion of Lung qi and fluids, which accumulate and collect in the throat. Constrained Liver qi invades and weakens the Spleen, retards fluid movement, and creates the conditions for congealing damp into phlegm. The phlegm is carried aloft along the Liver channel, to catch in the throat.

郁

The result is a sense of blockage or constriction in the throat, described as 'plum pit qi'. The throat is an energetically important area in Chinese medicine terms, a region where a number of channels converge in close proximity, and where qi and other pathogens can easily get stuck. The emotional pattern contributing to the development of plum pit qi is, like all patterns of constraint, the inability to express ones feelings in a constructive fashion. Similarly, difficulty in adapting to and accepting change can contribute to stagnation of qi and phlegm in the throat. Patients may verbalise their frustration saying –'I can't swallow any more!'

Qi and phlegm constraint may be complicated by heat, fluid damage and yin deficiency, or in long term patterns, blood stasis.

Clinical features
• Depression, nervousness, sadness, obsessive thinking and rumination; the depressed mood and anxiety are accompanied by a subjective sense of something lodged in the throat or difficulty swallowing. The sense of constriction in the throat appears and disappears according to the mood of the patient. They may have had fruitless investigations for suspected malignancy.
• frequent attempts to clear the throat
• hoarse voice or loss of voice
• heavy sleep with waking in the early hours of the morning feeling depressed and unable to sleep again
• lethargy, sluggishness, heaviness in the body and limbs; sleepiness during the day; feels worse after sleep
• chest oppression, tightness in the chest, difficulty getting a deep breath
• frequent sighing
• dizziness or vertigo
• productive cough or excessive mucus production in the sinuses, post nasal drip
• nausea or vomiting
• women may experience premenstrual breast tenderness or breast lumps
T may be swollen with a greasy, white coat
P wiry or slippery

Treatment principle
Regulate and mobilize qi and transform phlegm
Harmonize the Liver and Spleen and relieve qi constraint
Direct Lung qi downwards to activate the po

Prescription

BAN XIA HOU PO TANG 半夏厚朴汤
Pinellia and Magnolia Bark Decoction, modified

zhi ban xia (Pinelliae Rhizoma preparatum) 制半夏 9–12g
fu ling (Poria) 茯苓 9–12g
hou po (Magnoliae officinalis Cortex) 厚朴 6–9g
zi su ye (Perillae Folium) 紫苏叶 3–6g
sheng jiang (Zingiberis Rhizoma recens) 生姜 9–15g
he huan hua (Albizziae Flos) 合欢花 9–12g
yu jin (Curcumae Radix) 郁金 9–12g

Method: Decoction. **Zhi ban xia** transforms phlegm, promotes the flow of qi through areas of phlegm accumulation and downbears counterflow Stomach qi to stop nausea and vomiting; **hou po** assists **zhi ban xia** in moving qi and phlegm from the throat; **sheng jiang** disperses accumulation of phlegm and reinforces the phlegm transforming action of **zhi ban xia**; **fu ling** strengthens the Spleen and leaches damp; **zi su ye** opens up qi flow and alleviates constraint, and harmonizes the middle burner; **he huan hua** activates qi and blood and harmonizes the Stomach; **yu jin** transforms phlegm and alleviates qi constraint. (Source: *Zhong Yi Nei Ke Xue* [*Jin Gui Yao Lue*])

Modifications

- With Liver qi constraint, add **xiang fu** (Cyperi Rhizoma) 香附 9–12g and **fo shou** (Citri sarcodactylis Fructus) 佛手 9–12g or combine with **XIAO YAO SAN** (Rambling Powder 逍遥散, p.284).
- With a foggy head or clouded consciousness and somnolence, add **shi chang pu** (Acori tatarinowii Rhizoma) 石菖蒲 6–9g and **yuan zhi** (Polygalae Radix) 远志 6–9g.
- With early waking or sleep disturbance, add **mu li** (Ostreae Concha) 牡蛎 15–30g [cooked first] and **mei gui hua** (Rosae rugosae Flos) 玫瑰花 6–9g.
- With vocal cord polyps and breast lumps, add **zhe bei mu** (Fritillariae thunbergii Bulbus) 浙贝母 9–12g, **xuan shen** (Scrophulariae Radix) 玄参 12–15g and **mu li** (Ostreae Concha) 牡蛎 15–30g [cooked first].
- With yin deficiency, add **xuan shen** (Scrophulariae Radix) 玄参 12–15g and **mai dong** (Ophiopogonis Radix) 麦冬 9–12g.
- With hoarse voice or loss of voice, add **pang da hai** (Sterculiae lychnophorae Semen) 胖大海 2–3 pieces, and **mu hu die** (Oroxyli Semen) 木蝴蝶 1.5–3g.
- With heat, bitter taste, nausea and a yellow tongue coat, add **zhu ru** (Bambusae Caulis in taeniam) 竹茹 6–9g, **huang qin** (Scutellariae Radix) 黄芩 3–6g and **zhi shi** (Aurantii Fructus immaturus) 枳实 6–9g, or combine with **WEN DAN TANG** (Warm Gallbladder Decoction 温胆汤 p.87).
- With productive cough, add **pi pa ye** (Eriobotryae Folium) 枇杷叶 9–12g, **chao xing ren** (stir fried Armeniacae Semen) 炒杏仁 9–12g and **gua lou pi** (Trichosanthis Pericarpium) 栝楼皮 9–12g.
- With blood stasis, add **dan shen** (Salviae miltiorrhizae Radix) 丹参 9–12g, **jiang xiang** (Dalbergiae odoriferae Lignum) 降香 3–6g and **jiang huang** (Curcumae longae Rhizoma) 姜黄 6–9g.

Prepared medicines
Concentrated powder
Ban Xia Hou Po Tang (Pinellia & Magnolia Combination)
Si Ni San (Bupleurum & Aurantium Immaturus Formula)
 – add with marked Liver qi constraint
Pills
Ban Xia Hou Po Wan (Pinellia and Magnolia Teapills)
Si Ni San Wan (Four Pillars Teapills)
 – add with Liver qi constraint

Acupuncture (select from)
Du.20 (baihui) ....these points lift the mood
yintang (M–HN–3)
GB.8 (shuaigu)
Ren.17 (shanzhong) ....upper 'sea of qi', diffuses the Lungs and assists
                                          descent of Lung qi, use when tender
Kid.27 (shufu) ....these points help to open the chest, aid the descent
Kid.25 (shenzang)   of Lung qi and help connect the po and zhi
PC.6 (neiguan –)...............downbears counterflow Stomach qi and assists Lung
                                          qi descent, calms and shen and regulates qi
PC.5 (jianshi)....................river point of the Pericardium, transforms phlegm
Lu.7 (lieque).....................connecting point of the Lungs and master point of
                                          renmai, diffuses the Lungs, aids descent of Lung qi
                                          to activate the po; appropriate caution should be
                                          observed (see p.108)
St.40 (fenglong –) ....connecting points of the Stomach and Heart, these
Ht.5 (tongli)   points transform phlegm, calm the shen and remove
                                          stagnation from the throat
Bl.13 (feishu –) ....transport points of the Lungs and Liver respectively,
Bl.18 (ganshu –)   regulate Lung and Liver qi
• Ear points: shenmen, lungs, liver, zero point, anti–depression, sympathetic

Clinical notes
• Qi and phlegm stagnation may be diagnosed as depression, anxiety or globus hystericus.
• The phlegm in this pattern is insubstantial and thus without physical form. In prolonged cases or those complicated by heat (that congeals phlegm into substantial form) or blood stasis, the sense of obstruction may evolve into an actual blockage.
• Exercise is an essential component of treatment, see p.103.
• A phlegm transforming diet is recommended. See Clinical Handbook, Vol.2, p.880.
• Hot spot therapy can be helpful, see p.923.
• Cognitive behavioral therapy or counselling are strongly indicated to assist in verbalizing repressed emotion.

心
肺
气
郁

3.5 HEART AND LUNG QI CONSTRAINT

The Simple Questions (*Huang Di Nei Jing Su Wen*), chapter 39, tells us that 'grief and sadness cause the Lungs to overexpand and press upwards; this causes stagnation in the upper burner' (Maoshing Ni 1995). Depression associated with Heart and Lung qi constraint is due to persistent and unresolved sadness, loss or grief. A significant event, such as the loss of a loved one may trigger the depression and in the circumstances, Heart and Lung qi constraint is a perfectly normal response. In many cases, intervention at this stage is unnecessary and inappropriate, and passing time will enable the individual to gradually resolve their grief. In some individuals however, such as those with a constitutional or acquired weakness of the Lungs or Heart, the stagnation may not resolve and pathology develops. Such patients are unable to 'let go and move on', and the state of stagnation persists. These patients can benefit significantly from intervention.

Clinical features

- Persistent sadness, frequent crying, melancholia, prolonged or excessive grieving that disrupts normal life function. These patients may be hypersensitive to otherwise trivial events and feel like they are always on the verge of tears.
- sleep disturbance and early waking between 3–5am feeling sad and depressed, and unable to return to sleep
- shortness of breath, shallow breathing, sense of difficulty getting a deep breath, may be dyspnea and wheezing
- chest tightness and constriction; may feel like a weight on the chest
- the shoulders are hunched, the chest collapsed and the head falling forward
- pale, wan complexion
- cold hands and feet; pins and needles in the fingers at night (see clinical notes)
- constipation or sluggish bowels, however the stools are not dry or hard
- sensation of constriction or tightness in the throat, difficulty vocalizing

T pale and swollen on the anterior portion, or with a dip behind the tip
P weak, especially in the distal position

Treatment Principle

Regulate and mobilize Heart and Lung qi
Diffuse the Lungs, direct Lung qi downwards, calm the shen and activate the po

Prescription

SI MO TANG 四磨汤
Four Milled Herb Decoction, modified

ren shen (Ginseng Radix) 人参	3–6g
chen xiang (Aquilariae Lignum resinatum) 沉香	6–9g
bing lang (Arecae Semen) 槟榔	6–9g
wu yao (Linderae Radix) 乌药	6–9g
zi su geng (Perillae Caulis) 紫苏梗	6–9g
tan xiang (Santali albi Lignum) 檀香	3–6g
quan gua lou (Trichosanthis Fructus) 全栝楼	9–12g

Method: Decoction. **Ren shen** strengthens the Lungs, supplements qi and calms the shen; **chen xiang**, **wu yao**, **bing lang** and **zhi shi** regulate and direct qi downwards; **zi su geng**, **tan xiang** and **quan gua lou** open up qi flow through the chest, direct Lung qi downwards and diffuse the Lungs to activate the po. (Source: *Ji Sheng Fang*)

Modifications
- With sleep disturbances, add **he huan hua** (Albizziae Flos) 合欢花 6–9g and **ye jiao teng** (Polygoni multiflori Caulis) 夜胶藤 9–12g.

Prepared medicines
Concentrated powders
Ban Xia Hou Po Tang (Pinellia & Magnolia Combination)
Su Zi Jiang Qi Tang (Perilla Seed Combination)

Pills
Mu Xiang Shun Qi Wan (Aplotaxis Carminative Pills, Shun Qi Wan)
Su Zi Jiang Qi Wan (Perilla Seed Pill to Direct Qi Downward)

Acupuncture (select from)
Du.20 (baihui) .... these points lift the mood
yintang (M–HN–3)
GB.8 (shuaigu)
Lu.7 (lieque) .... connecting point of the Lungs and master point of renmai, diffuses the Lungs, aids descent of Lung qi to activate the po; appropriate caution should be observed (see below)
Lu.3 (tianfu) .... treats depression from Lung constraint, and alleviates sadness
Ht.3 (shaohai +) .... sea point of the Heart, regulates Heart qi and calms the shen
PC.6 (neiguan) .... opens up qi flow through the chest, calms the Heart and shen
Ren.17 (shanzhong) .... upper 'sea of qi', diffuses the Lungs and assists descent of Lung qi
St.36 (zusanli +) .... strengthens the Spleen and supplements qi to support the Lungs and Heart
- Caution with the use of Lu.7 (lieque) in these patients as it can sometimes lead to a sudden and uncontrolled release of the pent up grief and unprocessed emotion. Overall this is a good thing, but can be very intense and overwhelming for some people. May be best to avoid use of this point for the first few treatments until the patient is stronger and made aware of the possible effects.
- Ear points: shenmen, lungs, heart, anti–depression, sympathetic, zero point

Clinical notes
- This type of depression may be a normal response to loss and as such is not regarded as pathology, unless it is prolonged or out of proportion.
- This pattern is similar in some respects to the qi and phlegm constraint pattern. The main differences are that the etiology here is purely one of grief and

bereavement and there is more underlying Lung weakness and qi deficiency. The qi and phlegm constraint pattern may be due to factors that affect the Liver, with phlegm complicating the picture.

- A light touch is recommended here to avoid moving qi too strongly, especially in the early stages of treatment. In weaker patients or those unprepared to deal with their grief, too much qi mobilizing can cause the sudden release of pent up emotion which may be overwhelming and depleting. Note the small doses of herbs in the primary prescription.
- Pins and needles in the fingers (usually the lateral three) at night are quite common in this pattern and are due to tightness or shortening of the scalene or pectoralis minor muscles of the anterior neck and shoulder. The shortening of the muscles is due to the posture adopted by those with Lung and Heart deficiency and constraint patterns; collapsed chest, slumped and head forward. The neurovascular bundle feeding the upper limb can be constricted as it passes through or behind these muscles.
- Mild aerobic and breathing exercises are helpful. Swimming, taijiquan and singing are ideal.
- Hot spot therapy can be helpful p.923, but should be used carefully at first.
- Cognitive behavioral therapy or counselling are strongly indicated to assist in verbalizing repressed emotion.

脾
胃
气
郁

3.6 SPLEEN AND STOMACH QI CONSTRAINT

Spleen and Stomach qi constraint is due to worry, over thinking and brooding, usually in combination with a sedentary lifestyle. The yi (p.98) is inhibited, and instead of maintaining a clear outward mental focus and being able to move lightly from one topic to the next, becomes inwardly and repetitively focused. This pattern can be acquired by life circumstance and habits, or be constitutional. When acquired it may be seen in those who are involved in mentally challenging but sedentary occupations. When constitutional, there may be a lifetime tendency to worry excessively about everything.

The main pathology is disruption to the qi dynamic, the ascent of Spleen qi and descent of Stomach qi. The nature of disruption to the qi dynamic is such that it is usually complicated by other excess pathology, in particular food stagnation and phlegm damp. In prolonged cases, heat, blood stasis and deficiency may intervene.

Clinical features

- Depression, rumination, constant worry, irrational worry over trivia, obsessive thoughts; inability to let go of a thought; incessant analysis of relationships and events.
- early waking; lies awake worrying and turning the same thoughts over repeatedly
- loss of appetite and weight loss (or increased appetite and weight gain with heat)
- nausea, often in the morning
- **with food stagnation**: abdominal bloating, indigestion, acid reflux, bad breath, thick tongue coat
- **with phlegm**: daytime sleepiness, foggy head, confusion, disorientation, thick tongue coat
- **with heat**: irritability, easily distracted; over eating or comfort eating, acid reflux, red tongue with a dry yellow coat
- **with blood stasis**: black depression, focal pain

T unremarkable, or as noted above
P wiry, slippery, soggy, slightly rapid

Treatment Principle

Regulate the Spleen, Stomach and qi dynamic, relieve qi constraint
Clear heat, activate blood, transform phlegm and alleviate food stagnation

Prescription

YUE JU WAN 越鞠丸
Escape Restraint Pill

xiang fu (Cyperi Rhizoma) 香附	9–12g
cang zhu (Atractylodis Rhizoma) 苍术	9–12g
chuan xiong (Chuanxiong Rhizoma) 川芎	9–12g
shan zhi zi (Gardeniae Fructus) 山栀子	9–12g

shen qu (Massa medicata fermentata) 神曲 9–12g

Method: Grind the herbs to powder and form into 6 gram pills with water. The dose is one pill 2–3 times daily. May also be decocted with the doses as shown. **Xiang fu** dredges the Liver and alleviates constrained qi; **cang zhu** dries damp, transforms phlegm and works with **xiang fu** to improve Spleen and Stomach function and free up the qi dynamic; **chuan xiong** moves qi, activates blood and reinforces the qi regulating function of **xiang fu**; **shan zhi zi** calms the shen by clearing heat from the Liver and Heart; **shen qu** disperses stagnant food, aids digestion and harmonizes the Stomach. (Source: *Zhong Yi Nei Ke Xue [Dan Xi Xin Fa]*)

Modifications

- With marked food stagnation, halitosis and belching, add **sha ren** (Amomi Fructus) 砂仁 3–6g, **fo shou** (Citri sarcodacylis Fructus) 佛手 9–12g and **jiao shan zha** (charred Crataegi Fructus) 焦山楂 12–15g.
- With phlegm damp, somnolence and foggy head, add **shi chang pu** (Acori tatarinowii Rhizoma) 石菖蒲 6–9g and **yuan zhi** (Polygalae Radix) 远志 6–9g.
- With heat and irritability, add **yu jin** (Curcumae Radix) 郁金 9–12g.
- With blood stasis, add **he huan pi** (Albizziae Cortex) 合欢皮 9–12g and **dan shen** (Salviae miltiorrhizae Radix) 丹参 9–12g.
- With marked reflux and heartburn, add **huang lian** (Coptidis Rhizoma) 黄连 6–9g and **wu zhu yu** (Evodiae Fructus) 黄连 2–3g.
- With palpitations, add **long gu** (Fossilia Ossis Mastodi) 龙骨 15–30g, **mu li** (Ostreae Concha) 牡蛎 15–30g [both cooked first] and **ye jiao teng** (Polygoni multiflori Caulis) 夜胶藤 15–30g.
- With frontal headaches, increase the dose of **chuan xiong** (Chuanxiong Rhizoma) 川芎 by 30%, and add **bai zhi** (Angelicae dahuricae Radix) 白芷 6–9g.
- With temporal headaches and red, sore eyes, add **ju hua** (Chrysanthemi Flos) 菊花 9–12g, **bai ji li** (Tribuli Fructus) 白蒺藜 9–12g and **gou teng** (Uncariae Ramulus cum Uncis) 钩藤 9–12g.

Prepared medicines

Concentrated powders

Yue Ju Tang (Cyperus & Atractylodes Combination)

Acupuncture (select from)

Du.20 (baihui) ....these points calm the shen and lift the mood
yintang (M–HN-3)
GB.8 (shuaigu)
Ren.12 (zhongwan –) ....alarm point of the Stomach, strengthens the Stomach and activates the qi dynamic
Sp.4 (gongsun) ....master and couple points of chongmai, frees
PC.6 (neiguan)   and activates the qi dynamic to liberate the yi, calms the shen, improves digestion and lifts the mood
St.36 (zusanli) ....sea point of the Stomach, strengthens the Spleen and Stomach, supplements qi and activates the qi dynamic to liberate the yi
- With heat, add Liv.2 (xingjian –) and LI.3 (sanjian –)
- With phlegm, add St.40 (fenglong –)

- With food stagnation, add St.40 (fenglong –) and St.44 (neiting –)
- With blood stasis, add Sp.6 (sanyinjiao –) and Sp.8 (diji –)
- With Liver qi constraint, add Liv.3 (taichong –) and LI.4 (hegu –)
- With headaches, add GB.34 (yanglingquan –) and GB.20 (fengchi)
- Ear points: shenmen, spleen, stomach, zero point, anti–depression

Clinical notes

- Removing constraint from the qi dynamic and allowing middle burner qi to flow has the effect of freeing up qi flow in the rest of the body, and liberates the yi.
- This is a common pattern of mild to moderate depression, and usually responds well if the contributing lifestyle components are given attention.
- Regular daily meal times, small digestible meals, and avoidance of alcohol and non prescription drugs are helpful.
- Exercise is essential; see p.103 for specifics.
- A qi mobilizing diet is recommended. See Clinical Handbook, Vol.2, p.878.
- Hot spot therapy can be helpful p.923.

血
瘀
气
滞

3.7 BLOOD (AND QI) STASIS

The depression caused by blood stasis is severe and patients may have been de-pressed and medicated for years. The nature of the stasis profoundly restricts ex-pression of the hun (p.98), disturbs the shen and can block the movement of the po. These patients seek Chinese medical treatment because of dissatisfaction with pharmaceutical medications or concerns about side effects. Although most com-monly a chronic condition, this pattern of depression can occasionally be more acute if it follows childbirth, a severe or sudden emotional or physical trauma, or a period of high stress and anxiety. The latter is like the depression that may be associated with Post Traumatic Stress Disorder (but see also 3.12, p.147).

Blood stasis readily generates heat, which can manifest as mood swings between deep depression and sudden outbursts of anger. When heat complicates blood stasis, yin may be damaged.

Clinical features
- Chronic, recalcitrant, black depression to the point of suicidal thoughts or attempts. The patient may experience severe mood swings and loss of insight, may weep for no apparent reason, or suddenly fly off the handle with rage.
- dull, flat affect, dull eyes with no sparkle; dark complexion, dark circles around the eyes
- purplish lips, sclera, conjunctivae and nails
- persistent insomnia or early waking feeling worse
- loss of appetite, weight loss
- localized, focal pain, stabbing or boring headache, chest and hypochondriac pain; left iliac fossa pressure pain (p.925–926)
- dry mouth and throat with little desire to drink
- dry, scaly skin that may be itchy and irritated, especially in the lower limbs; patchy, brown or purple skin discolouration
- broken vessels or spider naevi on the face, trunk, inner knee and ankle; varicose veins
- loss of libido, with no nocturnal erections

T dark or purple, or with brown or purple stasis spots; sublingual veins distend-ed and dark

P deep, choppy, wiry, fine

Treatment Principle
Move qi and activate blood, transform blood stasis and relieve constraint
Alleviate depression, activate the hun and lighten the mood

Prescription

XUE FU ZHU YU TANG 血府逐瘀汤
Drive Out Stasis in the Mansion of Blood Decoction, modified

dang gui (Angelicae sinensis Radix) 当归	9–12g
sheng di (Rehmanniae Radix) 生地	9–12g
chi shao (Paeoniae Radix rubra) 赤芍	6–9g

chuan xiong (Chuanxiong Rhizoma) 川芎 6–9g
tao ren (Persicae Semen) 桃仁 9–12g
hong hua (Carthami Flos) 红花 6–9g
chai hu (Radix Bupleuri) 柴胡 6–9g
zhi ke (Aurantii Fructus) 枳壳 6–9g
gan cao (Glycyrrhizae Radix) 甘草 3–6g
chuan niu xi (Cyathulae Radix) 川牛膝 9–12g
jie geng (Platycodi Radix) 桔梗 3–6g
he huan pi (Albizziae Cortex) 合欢皮 12–15g
yu jin (Curcumae Radix) 郁金 6–9g
Method: Decoction. **Dang gui**, **sheng di**, **chuan xiong**, **chi shao**, **tao ren** and **hong hua** nourish and activate blood; **chai hu**, **zhi ke**, **gan cao** and **chi shao** dredge the Liver and regulate qi; **jie geng** frees qi in the chest and diaphragm, and raises qi; **chuan niu xi** leads blood downwards–together, **jie geng** and **chuan niu xi** seek to re–establish the qi dynamic; **he huan pi** and **yu jin** activate qi and blood and alleviate depression. (Source: *Zhong Yi Nei Ke Xue* [*Yi Lin Gai Cuo*])

Modifications

- For poor concentration and foggy head use **shi chang pu** (Acori tatarinowii Rhizoma) 石菖蒲 3–6g and **yuan zhi** (Polygalae Radix) 远志 3–6g.
- With early waking, add **dan shen** (Salviae miltiorrhizae Radix) 丹参 9–12g.
- With severe headaches, increase the dose of **chuan xiong** to as much as to 30g (see also p.421).
- With chest pain or a heavy sensation in the chest, add **quan gua lou** (Trichosanthis Fructus) 全栝楼 12–18g.
- In severe or resistent cases, a week or two of strong blood breaking herbs may assist in forcefully activating recalcitrant qi and blood. Add **e zhu** (Curcumae Rhizoma) 莪术 9–12g, **san leng** (Sparganii Rhizoma) 三棱 9–12g, or **shui zhi** (Hirudo) 水蛭 3–6g, or **di bie chong** (Eupolyphaga/Steleophaga) 地鳖虫 3–6g [the last two powdered and added to the strained decoction].
- With concerns about blood deficiency, use **shu di** (Rehmanniae Radix preparata) 熟地 instead of **sheng di**, and **bai shao** (Paeoniae Radix alba) 白芍 instead of **chi shao**, and add **ji xue teng** (Spatholobi Caulis) 鸡血藤 15–30g or **ye jiao teng** (Polygoni multiflori Caulis) 夜胶藤 15–30g.
- With heat, add **mu dan pi** (Moutan Cortex) 牡丹皮 9–12g, and increase the dose of **chi shao** to 12g.

Variations and additional prescriptions

Postnatal depression

Postnatal depression has numerous causes and is most commonly associated with blood deficiency, but in some women blood stasis occurs as a result of hemorrhage or retained birth products. Postnatal depression of a blood stasis type occurs soon after birth, and is characterized by depression, persistent crying, withdrawal, irritability, exhaustion, persistent abdominal pain and clotted discharge. The treatment is to clear the stagnation without further depleting qi and blood with a formula such as SHENG HUA TANG (Generation and Transformation Decoction 生化汤, p.919), or in severe cases with heat and a degree of mania, TAO HE CHENG QI TANG (Peach Pit Decoction to Order the Qi 桃核承气汤, p.920).

Post traumatic stress disorder

Depending on the duration of the condition, post traumatic stress disorder of a blood stasis type may lack many of the gross physical characteristics of blood stasis. A subtle approach to treatment is required as the trauma may be relatively fresh and too strong a formula can provoke overwhelming reactions. A gentle nudge to the qi and blood with a formula like TAO HONG SI WU TANG (Four Substance Decoction with Safflower and Peach Pit 桃红四物汤, p.921) is often the best place to start.

With masses

In very chronic blood stasis patterns masses are often found, in particular in the upper abdomen and Liver, or lower burner. Blood stasis formulas specific to these complications can be used as guides, instead of the primary prescription above. These include GE XIA ZHU YU TANG (Drive Out Blood Stasis Below the Diaphragm Decoction, 膈下逐瘀汤, p.13) and SHAO FU ZHU YU TANG (Drive Out Blood Stasis in the Lower Abdomen Decoction 少腹逐瘀汤, p.24).

Prepared medicines
Concentrated powder
Xue Fu Zhu Yu Tang (Persica & Carthamus Combination)
Shao Fu Zhu Yu Tang (Fennel Seed & Corydalis Combination)
   – blood stasis with cold
Ge Xia Zhu Yu Tang (Tangkuei & Corydalis Combination)
   – Liver blood stasis with masses
Tao Hong Si Wu Tang (Tangkuei Four, Persica & Carthamus Combination)
Sheng Hua Tang (Tangkuei & Ginger Combination)

Pills
Xue Fu Zhu Yu Wan (Stasis in the Mansion of Blood Teapills)
Shen Tong Zhu Yu Wan (Great Invigorator Teapills)
Shao Fu Zhu Yu Wan (Stasis in the Lower Palace Teapills)
Tao Hong Si Wu Wan (Tao Hong Si Wu Tang Teapills)

Acupuncture (select from)

Du.20 (baihui)	these points calm the mind and lift the mood
GB.8 (shuaigu)	
Sp.8 (diji –)	these points transform static blood, move qi and
Sp.10 (xuehai –)	blood and remove obstruction from the channels
Sp.6 (sanyinjiao)	and network vessels
LI.4 (hegu –)	
Liv.1 (dadun ▲)	treatment with rice grain moxa is helpful for patients with blood stasis depression
PC.6 (neiguan)	mobilizes qi and opens up qi flow through the chest, activates the hun and calms the shen
Liv.3 (taichong –)	source point of the Liver, moves Liver qi, activates blood and settles the hun
Bl.17 (geshu –)	transport point for the diaphragm, meeting point for

blood, dispels static blood

Bl.18 (ganshu –).................transport point of the Liver, dredges the Liver, activates qi and blood

Liv.14 (qimen –) ....alarm point of the Liver, dredges the Liver, activates qi and blood

- Bleeding the congested vessels that are often found around the knee and ankle can be helpful. The veins are pierced with a surgical lancet and a few drops of blood extracted. Ideally the blood should run black at first, then fresh red. This technique can be performed weekly for a few sessions, then intermittently. See Appendix 4, p.929.
- Ear points: shenmen, liver, heart, zero point, anti–depression

Clinical notes

- Blood stasis type depression is quite common in patients with concurrent chronic hepatic disease, such as the various forms of hepatitis or slow progressive cancers.
- Even though this is usually a very chronic and recalcitrant pattern, many patients nevertheless respond well, especially in the early stages of treatment. Progress may sometimes plateau or go backwards after an initial improvement, but staying the course with persistence and encouragement will generally lead to gradual and sustained benefits.
- One of the potential problems with using strong blood activating formulas is dispersal of zheng qi and blood along with the pathological blood stasis. This is seen after a few months of treatment and manifests with increasing signs of blood deficiency–postural dizziness, sleep disturbance, pallor and a fine weak pulse. Change to a milder formula or one that supplements qi and blood for a few weeks.
- Exercise is essential for the chronic pattern, but not directly after childbirth or blood loss. See p.103 for specifics.
- Hot spot therapy can be helpful p.923.
- Dietary modification, especially the avoidance of items that can aggravate constraint or irritate the Liver, such as alcohol, is helpful. See Clinical Handbook, Vol.2, pp.878 and 886.

痰
湿
郁
证

3.8 PHLEGM DAMP

Phlegm damp impedes the Spleen, weighs down the yi and hun and clouds the shen. The phlegm of this pattern is of the insubstantial type, and forms a kind of mist or veil around the consciousness. The phlegm damp may be constitutional or acquired. When constitutional, patients will usually have a long history of depression, and a family history. If the phlegm damp is acquired, diet and lifestyle factors play a significant part. In addition, the Liver may play a role, and a variation of the primary pathological triad may be seen. See p.780 and 782.

Phlegm has the tendency to coalesce and disperse periodically. It can congeal in response to increasing stress and qi constraint or changes in diet, and disperse when the patient is active and eating better.

Treatment strategy depends on the severity of the depression and the degree of Spleen deficiency. In the early stages of treatment, a relatively strong phlegm eliminating approach will be adopted, in addition to the necessary changes in dietary habits and activity levels. As the treatment progresses, a more supplementing approach is phased in to support the Spleen and prevent continual production of damp and phlegm. Due to the stagnating qualities of phlegm damp, heat may periodically be generated with an increase in symptoms of agitation and sleep disturbances.

Clinical features

- Depression, characterized by a feeling of being 'weighed down' with a passive gloominess, lack of interest or motivation, profound apathy, inertia and lethargy. During depressive episodes, inability to think clearly or concentrate, confusion, lethargy and somnolence increase. Patients are prone to obsessive thinking and irrational worry and exhibit a dull or flat affect.
- fatigue and sluggishness, heaviness in the body and limbs
- daytime desire to sleep after which the patient feels worse; may be waking early in the morning unable to return to sleep
- dizziness or vertigo which can be initiated or exacerbated by strong volatile substances such as perfume or gasoline
- morning nausea
- heartburn, reflux, abdominal bloating
- appetite may be poor, or the patient may eat for comfort
- chest oppression
- tend to be overweight; may be sinus congestion, productive cough, throat clearing or benign rubbery masses such as subcutaneous lipomas, thyroid nodules, breast cysts or ganglia

T swollen or flabby body, may or may not have a thick coat; the tongue coat thickens and becomes more greasy during depressive episodes

P slippery or wiry

Treatment Principle

Transform phlegm and regulate qi
Strengthen the Spleen, activate and free the yi

Prescription

DI TAN TANG 涤痰汤
Scour Phlegm Decoction, modified

This prescription can be used for a few months, until the phlegm has resolved. Once clear improvement is observed, a more Spleen strengthening strategy can be adopted for long term constitutional treatment.

zhi ban xia (Pinelliae Rhizoma preparatum) 制半夏 9–12g
zhu ru (Bambusae Caulis in taeniam) 竹茹 9–12g
fu ling (Poria) 茯苓 9–12g
dan nan xing (Arisaema cum Bile) 胆南星 6–9g
chen pi (Citri reticulatae Pericarpium) 陈皮 6–9g
zhi shi (Aurantii Fructus immaturus) 枳实 6–9g
shi chang pu (Acori tatarinowii Rhizoma) 石菖蒲 6–9g
ren shen (Ginseng Radix) 人参 3–6g
gan cao (Glycyrrhizae Radix) 甘草 3–6g
sheng jiang (Zingiberis Rhizoma recens) 生姜 .... 3 slices
da zao (Jujubae Fructus) 大枣 .... 4 fruit
yu jin (Curcumae Radix) 郁金 9–12g
yuan zhi (Polygalae Radix) 远志 6–9g

Method: Decoction. **Zhi ban xia** dries damp, transforms phlegm and downbears counterflow Stomach qi; **zhu ru** clears phlegm heat from the Stomach and Gallbladder, alleviates irritability and downbears counterflow Stomach qi; **fu ling** strengthens the Spleen and leaches out damp; **dan nan xing** scours phlegm and clears heat; **chen pi** dries damp, transforms phlegm and rectifies the qi dynamic; **zhi shi** breaks up stagnation in the abdomen and leads qi and phlegm downwards; **shi chang pu** and **yuan zhi** vaporize phlegm and clear the mind and senses; **ren shen** and **gan cao** strengthen the Spleen and supplement qi; **sheng jiang** and **da zao** harmonize and protect the Stomach; **yu jin** transforms phlegm and alleviates constrained qi. (Source: *Zhong Yi Nei Ke Xue [Ji Sheng Fang]*)

Modifications

• With Liver qi constraint, add **xiang fu** (Cyperi Rhizoma) 香附 9–12g and **mu xiang** (Aucklandiae Radix) 木香 9–12g.
• With Spleen deficiency, add **bai zhu** (Atractylodis macrocephalae Rhizoma) 白术 9–12g.

Variations and additional prescriptions

Phlegm heat

Obstruction caused by phlegm damp often results in the generation of heat. Such an effect is exacerbated by rich foods or alcohol, and also by stress and qi constraint. The features are increasing agitation, anxiety, irrational anger and odd or manic behavior. In addition, sleep disturbances, early waking, violent dreams, palpitations and restlessness occur. The tongue may be red, the coat becomes greasy and yellow and the pulse slippery and rapid. In its severe, but less common form, this may be akin to the manic phase of a bipolar disorder (a type of Mania Depression *diān kuáng* 癫狂). The treatment is to clear heat, transform phlegm and calm the shen with a prescription like **HUANG LIAN WEN DAN TANG** (Warm Gallbladder Decoction with Coptis 黄连温胆汤 p.915), or in severe cases with manic episodes, SHENG TIE LUO YIN (Iron Filings Decoction 生铁落饮 p.919).

Once phlegm is resolving
Strong prescriptions like the primary formula above can be used for a few months but may disperse zheng qi and damage yin. As the phlegm resolves a more supplementing approach can be phased in. The aim of treatment is to strengthen the Spleen, improve fluid metabolism and prevent phlegm formation with a formula such as XIANG SHA LIU JUN ZI TANG (Six Gentlemen Decoction with Aucklandia and Amomum 香砂六君子汤 p.618).

Prepared medicines
Concentrated powders
Ding Xian Wan (Gastrodia and Amber Combination)
– with phlegm heat, phlegm predominant
Zhu Ru Wen Dan Tang (Bamboo & Ginseng Combination)
– with phlegm heat
Chai Hu Jia Long Gu Mu Li Tang (Bupleurum & Dragon Bone Combination)
– with more severe phlegm heat, heat predominant

Pills
Hu Po Bao Long Wan (Po Lung Yuen Medical Pills)
Ban Xia Hou Po Wan (Pinellia and Magnolia Teapills)
Wen Dan Wan (Rising Courage Teapills)
Chai Hu Long Gu Mu Li Tang (Bupleurum, Dragon Bone and Oyster Shell Teapills)
Bu Nao Wan (Cerebral Tonic Pills)
Ping Wei San (Calm Stomach Teapills, Tabellae Pingwei)

Acupuncture (select from)
Du.20 (baihui) ....lift the mood and clear fogginess from the head
St.8 (touwei)
PC.4 (ximen –) ....cleft point of the Pericardium, good when there is a sense of a weight on the chest
PC.5 (jianshi –).................river point of the Pericardium, transforms phlegm and lifts the mood
PC.6 (neiguan)..................connecting point of the Pericardium, mobilizes qi and opens up qi flow through the chest, lifts the mood, activates the hun and calms the shen
St.40 (fenglong –) ....connecting and source points of the Stomach
Sp.3 (taibai +)   and Spleen, together these points resolve phlegm, activate the yi and strengthen the Spleen
St.41 (jiexi –).....................river point of the Stomach channel, resolves phlegm, activates the yi and alleviates depression
Liv.3 (taichong –)..............regulates the Liver and resolves qi constraint, activates the hun
Ren.12 (zhongwan) ....alarm point of the Stomach, strengthens the Stomach and Spleen to transform phlegm

Bl.20 (pishu) ....transport point of the Spleen, strengthens the Spleen and supplements qi to promote transformation of phlegm

• with Spleen deficiency add St.36 (zusanli +)
• with heat, add St.44 (neiting –) and PC.7 (daling –)
• with marked Liver qi constraint, add GB.34 (yanglingquan –)
• with foggy head or somnolence, add Bl.62 (shenmai)
• with cold, apply moxa to Bl.20 (pishu ▲) and Bl.21 (weishu ▲)
• with muscle aches and heaviness, add Sp.21 (dabao)
• with edema, add Sp.9 (yinlingquan –) and Sp.6 (sanyinjiao)
• with abdominal distension, add St.25 (tianshu –) and Sp.15 (daheng –)
• Ear points: shenmen, spleen, liver, zero point, anti–depression, sympathetic

Clinical notes

• The prognosis of phlegm damp depression is variable, and resolution can be difficult when there is a constitutional component. Some patients however, respond surprisingly well. In general some months of consistent work will be required to make a long lasting impact.
• The heaviness and lethargy typical of phlegm damp can be impediments to exercise, but graded exercise in groups can achieve good results.
• Hot spot therapy can be helpful, p.923.
• Diet is a crucial component of treatment. Avoidance of phlegm producing foods is important and a bland drying diet is recommended. See Clinical Handbook, Vol.2, p.880.

心
脾
两
虚

3.9 HEART AND SPLEEN DEFICIENCY

Heart blood and Spleen qi deficiency is a common cause of depression, and most commonly gives rise to depression with anxiety, irrational worry and obsessive thinking. The mechanism is associated with a failure of qi and blood to anchor and stabilize the shen, hun and yi, so they are easily agitated and thrown off balance by otherwise trivial events. This is in contrast to those patterns where the shen and other anima are weighed down by the leaden embrace of a heavy pathogen like phlegm damp, which produces a more passive gloominess.

Clinical features
- Depression with anxiety. Some patients exhibit a tendency to obsessive compulsion, obsessive thoughts, phobias or paranoia. These patients are emotionally labile, apt to dissolve into tears or be suddenly overwhelmed with unpleasant emotions and memories in response to seemingly trivial sights, sounds or smells. They may be forgetful, unable to concentrate or confused.
- lack of vitality with a feeling of perpetual exhaustion, being easily overwhelmed and unable to cope
- insomnia, with difficulty falling asleep; early waking feeling depressed and anxious; dream disturbed sleep
- palpitations, tachycardia
- postural dizziness, light–headedness
- blurred vision, spots in the visual field
- loss of appetite, weight loss
- abdominal distension after eating
- tendency to loose stools
- dry hair, eyes and skin (except the palms which may be clammy)
- pale, sallow complexion
- easy bruising, or heavy or prolonged menstrual periods
- symptoms worse with exertion or when overtired

T pale with a thin, white coat
P fine and weak

Treatment Principle
Strengthen and nourish the Heart and Spleen
Supplement qi and blood, calm and anchor the shen, yi and hun

Prescription

GUI PI TANG 归脾汤
Restore the Spleen Decoction, modified

zhi huang qi (honey fried Astragali Radix) 炙黄芪 9–12g
fu shen (Poria Sclerotium pararadicis) 茯神 9–12g
chao bai zhu (stir fried Atractylodes macrocephalae Rhizoma) 炒白术 ... 9–12g
long yan rou (Longan Arillus) 龙眼肉 3–12g
suan zao ren (Zizyphi spinosae Semen) 酸枣仁 9–12g
ren shen (Ginseng Radix) 人参 6–9g

dang gui (Angelicae sinensis Radix) 当归 3–9g
yuan zhi (Polygalae Radix) 远志 3–6g
mu xiang (Aucklandiae Radix) 木香 3–6g
zhi gan cao (Glycyrrhizae Radix preparata) 炙甘草 3–6g
ye jiao teng (Polygoni multiflori Caulis) 夜交藤 15–30g
he huan pi (Albizziae Cortex) 合欢皮 12–15g

Method: Decoction. **Zhi huang qi**, **ren shen**, **chao bai zhu** and **zhi gan cao** strengthen the Spleen and supplement qi; **dang gui** and **zhi huang qi** together have a special effect on building blood; **suan zao ren**, **long yan rou** and **yuan zhi** nourish the Heart and calm the shen and hun; **fu shen** strengthens the Spleen and calms the shen and yi; **mu xiang** regulates qi and aids the Spleen in digesting the blood supplementing herbs; **zhi gan cao** supplements qi and harmonizes the Stomach; **ye jiao teng** nourishes blood and calms the shen; **he huan pi** activates qi and blood and calms the shen. (Source: *Shi Yong Zhong Yi Nei Ke Xue* [*Ji Sheng Fang*])

Modifications

- With marked insomnia, add **wu wei zi** (Schizandrae Fructus) 五味子 6–9g and **bai zi ren** (Platycladi Semen) 柏子仁 9–12g.
- For recalcitrant insomnia, add **long chi** (Fossilia Dentis Mastodi) 龙齿 15–30g [cooked first]and **mu li** (Ostreae Concha) 牡蛎 15–30g [cooked first]. **Mai ya** (Hordei Fructus germinantus) 麦芽 9–15g can be included to protect the Stomach.
- With palpitations or tachycardia, add **long chi** (Fossilia Dentis Mastodi) 龙齿 15–30g [cooked first].
- With Liver qi constraint, add **yu jin** (Curcumae Radix) 郁金 9–12g and **fo shou** (Citri sarcodacylis Fructus) 佛手 9–12g.
- With marked Heart blood deficiency, postural dizziness and insomnia, add **shu di** (Rehmanniae Radix preparata) 熟地 6–12g, **bai shao** (Paeoniae Radix alba) 白芍 9–12g and **e jiao** (Asini Corii Colla) 阿胶 3–9g [dissolved in the strained decoction]. When the Spleen is very weak, small doses of the richer blood supplements noted above (and **long yan rou** and **dang gui**) may be better tolerated until the Spleen is strong enough to digest them properly. Combining the primary prescription with a prepared medicine such as **Bao He Wan** (Preserve Harmony Pill) or **Jian Pi Wan** (Ginseng Stomachic Pills, Spleen Digest Aid Pill) can help offset their richness and improve digestion.
- With heat, add **shan zhi zi** (Gardeniae Fructus) 山栀子 9–12g and **chai hu** (Bupleuri Radix) 柴胡 6–9g.
- With dampness and a greasy tongue coat, add **zhi ban xia** (Pinelliae Rhizoma preparata) 制半夏 6–9g and **chen pi** (Citri reticulatae Pericarpium) 陈皮 6–9g.

Variations and additional prescriptions

Postpartum blood deficiency

Postnatal depression can be due to the demands placed on blood during gestation and the blood loss experienced during delivery. When Liver blood is not quickly replenished, the hun and shen are destabilized and easily upset. The characteristic feature of this type of postnatal depression is depression with exhaustion, pallor and dizziness. The treatment is to quickly replenish blood with **Dang Gui Bu Xue Tang** (Tangkuei Decoction to Supplement the Blood 当归补血汤).

zhi huang qi (honey fried Astragali Radix) 炙黄芪 30g
dang gui (Angelicae sinensis Radix) 当归 6g
Method: Decoction. The large dose of **zhi huang qi** relative to **dang gui** is important and strengthens the Spleen to produce blood. If modifications are added the proportions of **zhi huang qi** to
dang gui should be maintained. (Source: *Nei Wai Shang Bian Huo Lun*)

Rarefied Heart and Spleen deficiency manifesting as 'Dry Organs'

This is the ancient *zàng zào* disorder 脏躁, described in some texts as 'melancholy
injuring the shen' (*yōu yù shāng shén* 忧郁伤神). It is considered to be a relatively
rarefied species of deficiency, affecting the shen and hun rather than the physical body, so mild herbs with a light touch, rather than stronger and potentially
cloying supplements are used. Zang zao is predominantly seen in women, but
occasionally also in men, and is characterized by emotional lability, hypersensitivity, weeping for no apparent reason, frequent yawning or sighing, melancholy,
absent mindedness and nervous excitability. In some cases, sudden loss of speech,
hearing or vision may occur, but otherwise physical symptoms are few. In between episodes the patient may appear normal. This is a form of Heart and Spleen
deficiency brought about by obsessive worry or prolonged anxiety, or as result of
damage from a prior illness or chronic blood loss. The recommended prescription
is **GAN MAI DA ZAO TANG** (Licorice, Wheat and Jujube Decoction 甘麦大枣汤).
gan cao (Glycyrrhizae Radix) 甘草 9–12g
xiao mai (Tritici Fructus) 小麦 30g
da zao (Jujubae Fructus) 大枣 .... 6 fruit
Method: Decoction. **Xiao mai** nourishes the Heart and calms the shen; **gan cao** strengthens the
Heart and Spleen and supplements qi; **da zao** supplements qi and moistens dryness. (Source: *Zhong
Yi Nei Ke Xue* [*Jin Gui Yao Lüe*])

Systemic qi and blood deficiency

If qi and blood deficiency is systemic, a more general supplementing prescription may be useful. Consider **REN SHEN YANG YING TANG** (Ginseng Decoction
to Nourish the Nutritive Qi 人参养营汤, p.384) or **SHI QUAN DA BU TANG** (All
Inclusive Great Supplementing Decoction 十全大补汤, p.758).

Prepared medicines
Concentrated powders
Gui Pi Tang (Ginseng & Longan Combination)
Gan Mai Da Zao Tang (Licorice & Jujube Combination)
Shi Quan Da Bu Tang (Ginseng & Dang Gui Ten Combination)
Ren Shen Yang Ying Tang (Ginseng & Rehmannia Combination)

Pills
Gui Pi Wan (Kwei Be Wan, Gui Pi Teapills)
Bai Zi Yang Xin Wan (Pai Tzu Yang Hsin Wan)
Shi Quan Da Bu Wan (Ten Flavour Teapills)
Dang Gui Ji Jing (Tang Kuei Essence of Chicken)
    – especially good for postpartum blood deficiency
Yang Xin Ning Shen Wan (Ning San Yuen Medical Pills)

Acupuncture (select from)

yintang (M–HN–3) ....these points calm the shen and alleviate anxiety and
Du.19 (houding)   depression
Du. 24 (shenting)
Ht.3 (shaohai).....................sea point of the Heart, calms the shen and lifts the
                              mood
Ht.7 (shenmen +)...............source point of the Heart, supplements and regulates
                              Heart qi and blood and calms the shen
Ren.14 (juque) ....alarm point of the Heart, calms the shen
Ren.12 (zhongwan +▲) ....alarm point of the Stomach, strengthens the Spleen
                              and Stomach and supplements qi
St.36 (zusanli +▲)...............sea point of the Stomach, strengthens the Spleen and
                              Stomach, supplements qi and blood, and stabilizes
                              the yi
Sp.6 (sanyinjiao +▲)..........strengthens the Spleen and Kidneys, regulates qi and
                              supplements qi and blood
Bl.15 (xinshu +) ....transport point of the Heart, supplements Heart qi,
                              calms the Heart and shen
Bl.20 (pishu +▲) ....transport point of the Spleen, strengthens the Spleen
                              and stabilizes the yi
Bl.25 (shenshu +▲) ....transport point of the Kidney, strengthens the
                              Kidneys to support the Spleen and fortifies the zhi

- with forgetfulness, add Bl.52 (zhishi)
- with much dreaming, add Bl.42 (pohu)
- with bruising or heavy periods, add Sp.10 (xuehai) and Sp.1 (yinbai ▲)
- with palpitations, add Ht.5 (tongli)
- with dizziness, add Du.20 (baihui ▲)
- Ear points: shenmen, heart, spleen, zero point, anti–depression, sympathetic

Clinical notes

- Heart blood and Spleen qi deficiency type depression may be diagnosed as endogenous depression, postnatal depression, obsessive compulsive disorder, thrombocytopenia or anemia.
- In general, mood disorders and anxiety states of a Heart and Spleen deficiency type respond well to treatment. When there is a constitutional component response can be slow, but a good base of qi and blood can be rebuilt over time.
- Diet is an important part of treatment; especially ensuring sufficient protein is eaten to build qi and blood. See Clinical Handbook, Vol.2, pp.870–874.
- Gentle exercises such as yoga and taijiquan are beneficial in both promoting qi flow and calming the mind.

肺
脾
气
虚

3.10. LUNG AND SPLEEN QI DEFICIENCY

Lung and Spleen qi can be dispersed by a significant bereavement, and this pattern may be found to have a constitutional component. The emotional trauma that initiated the weakness can sometimes traced to childhood, and a history of asthma or allergies may be noted.

Clinical features

- Depression with fatigue and a sense of disconnection from the world. The characteristic feature of this type of depression is the feeling of isolation and inability to interact in a meaningful and fulfilling way. Patients are withdrawn, avoid engaging, and speaking appears to exhaust them. They have an air of constant sadness. Mental processes and speaking may be slow, and they appear scattered and vulnerable.
- low weak voice, reluctance to speak
- pale translucent complexion, thin, gangly body; slumped shoulders, may appear to have difficulty holding their head up; poor muscle tone
- fatigue, weakness, breathlessness with exertion; shallow breathing
- loss of appetite, weight loss; abdominal distension with eating
- spontaneous sweating, clamminess
- increased desire to sleep during the daytime
- loose stools, diarrhea

T pale and scalloped; maybe a dip or hollow in the anterior third of the tongue
P fine and weak, or floating, big and weak, especially in the distal position

Treatment Principle

Strengthen and supplement the Lung and Spleen
Anchor and secure the po and the yi

Prescription

BU ZHONG YI QI TANG 补中益气汤
Supplement the Middle to Augment the Qi Decoction, modified

zhi huang qi (honey fried Astragali Radix) 炙黄芪	15–30g
ren shen (Ginseng Radix) 人参	9–12g
chao bai zhu (stir fried Atractylodes macrocephalae Rhizoma) 炒白术	9–12g
dang gui (Angelicae sinensis Radix) 当归	6–9g
chen pi (Citri reticulatae Pericarpium) 陈皮	6–9g
zhi gan cao (Glycyrrhizae Radix preparata) 炙甘草	3–6g
sheng ma (Cimicifugae Rhizoma) 升麻	3–6g
chai hu (Bupleuri Radix) 柴胡	3–6g
yuan zhi (Polygalae Radix) 远志	2–3g
shi chang pu (Acori tatarinowii Rhizoma) 石菖蒲	2–3g

Method: Decoction or powder. **Zhi huang qi**, **ren shen** and **chao bai zhu** strengthen the Spleen and supplement qi; **zhi huang qi** fortifies wei qi, secures the po and raises yang qi; **chai hu** and **sheng ma** raise yang qi; **dang gui** supplements blood; **chen pi** and **zhi gan cao** regulate qi and harmonize the middle burner; **yuan zhi** and **shi chang pu** clear the mind and calm the shen and clear the po without dispersing the already weak qi. (Source: *Pi Wei Lun*)

Modifications

- Some mild astringent herbs can be helpful in 'gathering together' the po and yi, preventing further scattering and dispersal. Consider **shan zhu yu** (Corni Fructus) 山茱萸 9–12g, **wu wei zi** (Schizandrae Fructus) 五味子 6–9g or **bai shao** (Paeoniae Radix alba) 白芍 6–9g.
- With yang deficiency, add **gan jiang** (Zingiberis Rhizoma) 干姜 6–9g and **zhi fu zi** (Aconiti Radix lateralis preparata) 制附子 6–9g.
- With breathlessness and spontaneous sweating, add **wu wei zi** (Schizandrae Fructus) 五味子 6–9g.
- With dryness, yin damage and chronic dry cough, add **mai dong** (Ophiopogonis Radix) 麦冬 6–9g and **wu wei zi** (Schizandrae Fructus) 五味子 6–9g.
- With loose stools, add **shan yao** (Dioscoreae Rhizoma) 山药 12–15g.

Prepared medicines
Concentrated powders
Bu Zhong Yi Qi Tang (Ginseng & Astragalus Combination)
Pills
Bu Zhong Yi Qi Wan (Central Chi Teapills)

Acupuncture (select from)
yintang (M–HN–3) ....these points calm the mind and lift the mood
Du.20 (baihui)
Lu.1 (zhongfu +) ....alarm point of the Lungs, strengthens Lung qi and stabilizes the po
Lu.9 (taiyuan +) ....source point of the Lung channel, strengthens the Lungs and supplements deficiency
Ren.17 (shanzhong –) ....mobilizes qi movement in the chest and assists in diffusing the Lungs and directing qi downwards
Bl.13 (feishu +▲)...............transport point of the Lungs, strengthens the Lungs, supplements qi and stabilizes the po
Bl.42 (pohu +▲)................strengthens the Lungs and stabilizes the po
Bl.20 (pishu +▲) ....transport point of the Spleen, strengthens the Spleen, supplements qi and stabilizes the yi
Ren.4 (guanyuan +▲)........strengthens yuan qi and supports qi systemically
St.36 (zusanli +) ....sea point of the Stomach, warms and strengthens the Spleen and Stomach and supplements qi
Sp.6 (sanyinjiao +▲)..........strengthens the Spleen and supplements qi
- Ear points: shenmen, lung, spleen, zero point, anti–depression, sympathetic

Clinical notes
- Diet is an essential component of treatment and should be appropriate for building qi and repairing the Spleen. See Clinical Handbook, Vol.2, p.870.
- Graded exercise, built up over a period of time, is an essential component to the rebuilding of Lung and Spleen qi. Breathing exercises and swimming are helpful. Some people find singing in a structured fashion, such as joining a choir to be beneficial.

肝
阴
亏
虚

3.11 LIVER YIN DEFICIENCY

Chronic Liver qi constraint with heat or fire will eventually damage Liver yin. Excessive use of bitter and pungent dispersing herbs used to alleviate constraint can have a similar effect. In practice, this pattern is usually a mixture of yin deficiency, qi constraint and sporadic ascendant yang. Patients find they swing unpredictably between apathy and withdrawal (the deficiency side) to sudden anger and temper outbursts as their yang is suddenly unleashed. The other characteristic is the counterflow of Stomach qi that often accompany episodes of depression. This is related to the chronic Liver and Stomach disharmony which typically precedes the yin damage.

Clinical features
- Depression characterized by depressed moods alternating with irritability, irascibility and restlessness; the mood swings can be unpredictable–suddenly swinging from withdrawal and apathy to flying off the handle. Patients describe themselves as aimless and lacking a sense of direction and purpose.
- insomnia or early waking with restlessness and agitation
- dull hypochondriac and epigastric pain or aching, aggravated or provoked by stress and relieved by, or made no worse by, pressing on the area
- acid reflux, heartburn, chronic indigestion
- dry, red, sore eyes; blurring or weakening vision; night blindness; dizziness
- dry mouth and throat, thirst
- headaches, distended sensation in the head
- sensation of heat in the palms and soles
- ridged or brittle nails
- muscle spasms and cramps, tics or tremors

T red with little or no coat
P fine, wiry and rapid

Treatment Principle
Nourish and enrich Liver yin and blood
Calm and stabilize the hun and shen
Soften the Liver and regulate qi

Prescription
YI GUAN JIAN 一贯煎
Linking Decoction, modified

sheng di (Rehmanniae Radix) 生地	24–30g
gou qi zi (Lycii Fructus) 枸杞子	9–15g
sha shen (Glehniae/Adenophorae Radix) 沙参	9–12g
mai dong (Ophiopogonis Radix) 麦冬	9–12g
dang gui (Angelicae sinensis Radix) 当归	9–12g
chuan lian zi (Toosendan Fructus) 川楝子	3–6g
he huan hua (Albizziae Flos) 合欢花	6–9g
mei gui hua (Rosae rugosae Flos) 玫瑰花	6–9g

Method: Decoction. **Sheng di** and **gou qi zi** enrich and nourish Liver yin and blood; **sha shen** and **mai dong** nourish yin and clear heat, moisten dryness and engender fluids; **dang gui** nourishes and moves blood; **chuan lian zi** regulates Liver qi and assists the Liver in mobilizing qi and blood; **he huan hua** and **mei gui hua** regulate qi, calm the hun and lift the mood without damaging yin. (Source: *Zhong Yi Nei Ke Xue* [*Xu Ming Yi Lei An*])

Modifications

- With ascendant Liver yang, sudden anger, headaches, muscle spasms, tics or cramps, add **gou teng** (Uncariae Ramulus cum Uncis) 钩藤 9–12g, **jue ming zi** (Cassiae Semen) 决明子 9–12g and **tian ma** (Gastrodiae Rhizoma) 天麻 6–9g.
- With insomnia or early waking, add **wu wei zi** (Schizandrae Fructus) 五味子 6–9g and **suan zao ren** (Zizyphi spinosae Semen) 酸枣仁 12–15g.
- With Stomach heat and a bitter taste in the mouth, add **jiu huang lian** (wine fried Coptidis Rhizoma) 酒黄连 1–1.5g.
- With acid reflux, add **hai piao xiao** (Sepiae Endoconcha) 海螵蛸 9–12g [as powder to the strained decoction].
- With constipation, add **huo ma ren** (Cannabis Semen) 火麻仁 9–12g or **gua lou ren** (Trichosanthis Semen) 栝楼仁 9–12g.
- With abdominal pain, add **bai shao** (Paeoniae Radix alba) 白芍 9–12g and **gan cao** (Glycyrrhizae Radix) 甘草 3–6g.
- With food stagnation and epigastric distension, add **chao mai ya** (stir fried Hordei Fructus germinantus) 炒麦芽 15–30g.
- With Stomach yin deficiency and a peeled or mirror tongue, add **yu zhu** (Polygonati odorati Rhizoma) 玉竹 12–15g.
- With night sweats or flushing, add **mu dan pi** (Moutan Cortex) 牡丹皮 9–12g and **di gu pi** (Lycii Cortex) 地骨皮 12–15g.
- With lower back and leg aching and weakness, add **he shou wu** (Polygoni multiflori Radix) 何首乌 9–12g and **shan zhu yu** (Corni Fructus) 山茱萸 9–12g, or combine with the prepared medicine **Liu Wei Di Huang Wan** (Six Flavor Teapills).

Variations and additional prescriptions
Liver and Kidney yin deficiency with more heat
With a greater degree of deficiency and more deficient heat (depression with pronounced irritability, anger outbursts, night sweats, flushed face, bitter taste, dry mouth and lower back and leg ache and weakness) a more Liver and Kidney yin enriching strategy can be adopted in the form of **Zi Shen Qing Gan Yin** (Enrich the Kidneys and Cool the Liver Decoction 滋肾清肝饮).

shu di (Rehmanniae Radix preparata) 熟地 24–30g
shan yao (Dioscoreae Rhizoma) 山药 12–15g
shan zhu yu (Corni Fructus) 山茱萸 12–15g
mu dan pi (Moutan Cortex) 牡丹皮 9–12g
fu ling (Poria) 茯苓 9–12g
ze xie (Alismatis Rhizoma) 泽泻 9–12g
chai hu (Bupleuri Radix) 柴胡 6–9g
bai shao (Paeoniae Radix alba) 白芍 9–12g
dang gui (Angelicae sinensis Radix) 当归 6–9g

suan zao ren (Ziziphi spinosae Semen) 酸枣仁 12–15g

Method. Decoction. The first six herbs constitute **Liu Wei Di Huang Wan**, the basic prescription to supplement Kidney and Liver yin; **chai hu** and **bai shao** regulate Liver qi and soften the Liver; **dang gui** and **bai shao** nourish Liver blood; **dang gui** activates Liver blood; **suan zao ren** nourishes yin and blood and calms the hun and shen. (Source: *Zhong Yi Nei Ke Xue* [*Yi Zong Ji Ren Pian*])

Prepared medicines

Concentrated powder

Yi Guan Jian (Linking Combination)

Qi Ju Di Huang Wan (Lycium, Chrysanthemum & Rehmannia Formula)

Pills

Yi Guan Jian Wan (Linking Decoction Teapills)

Qi Ju Di Huang Wan (Lycium–Rehmannia Pills)

Ming Mu Di Huang Wan (Ming Mu Di Huang Teapills)

Er Long Zuo Ci Wan (Er Ming Zuo Ci Wan, Tso–Tzu Otic Pills)

Acupuncture (select from)

yintang (M–HN–3) ....these points calm the shen and alleviate anxiety

Du.19 (houding)

Du. 24 (shenting)

Liv.14 (qimen) ....alarm point of the Liver, soothes the Liver and regulates qi

Bl.18 (ganshu +).................transport points of the Liver and Kidney,

Bl.23 (shenshu +)   supplement and nourish yin to calm the hun

PC.6 (neiguan)...................mobilizes Liver qi and opens up qi flow through the chest, lifts the mood and calms the hun and shen

Sp.6 (sanyinjiao +)..............strengthens the Spleen and Kidneys, nourishes yin and regulates qi

Kid.3 (taixi +).....................source point of the Kidneys, supplements the yin of the whole body

Liv.3 (taichong +)...............source point of the Liver, nourishes Liver yin and blood, restrains ascendant Liver yang, regulates qi and calms the hun

Liv.8 (ququan –).................sea point of the Liver, supplements Liver yin, clears heat and calms the hun

- Ear points: shenmen, liver, kidney, zero point, anti–depression, sympathetic

Clinical notes

- Depression of a Liver yin deficiency type may be diagnosed as endogenous depression, or depression subsequent to chronic hepatitis, cirrhosis or alcoholic liver disease, peptic ulcer disease, gastroesophageal reflux or bipolar mood disorder.
- Treatment usually needs to be quite prolonged, but patients can respond reasonably well.
- Care must be taken in this pattern to avoid the use of strong qi moving herbs as they can easily disperse qi and yin and aggravate the problem.
- Diet is important, in particular ensuring adequate protein and avoidance of

stimulants and items that heat and irritate the Liver, such as coffee, alcohol, chillies, unnecessary pharmaceuticals and food additives. Ensure sufficient fluids are taken to avoid dehydration. A yin nourishing diet is recommended. See Clinical Handbook, Vol.2, p.876.

- A strict regular bedtime routine can be helpful, even in patients with relatively severe sleep disturbance.
- Active pursuit of relaxation should be encouraged. This means that a gentle and positive relaxation routine should be built into the day, rather than the 'just doing nothing' type of relaxation. Activities such as taijiquan, yoga, walking and swimming are a good way to calm the hun and shen, mobilize qi and gradually build qi and yin.

心
肾
阴
虚

3.12 HEART AND KIDNEY YIN DEFICIENCY

This is a common pattern of depression and anxiety. Most patients are women over 40, and the pattern often coincides with the onset of menopause. Although more common in women, both sexes can be affected. The pattern can oscillate between dominance of the deficiency, or the heat that is created by the deficiency. The more deficiency, the more depression; the more heat, the greater the anxiety and agitation.

Heart and Kidney yin deficiency is a type of disruption to the Heart Kidney axis (see p.781). The stability of both the shen and zhi is affected. The pattern can be constitutional, with anxiety and depression reported in blood relatives. It can be of gradual onset caused by ageing, overwork, long term drug use (prescription and illicit), prolonged emotional stress and worry, or more abrupt, following a sudden severe shock or a severe febrile illness.

Clinical features

- Depression with anxiety and a sense of restlessness, unease and agitation. The depression is worse at night and is associated with fatigue or exhaustion. Patients often describe themselves as being on edge or feeling burned out, and the more tired they get the more depressed and anxious.
- insomnia, restless and fitful sleep; waking feeling more anxious and depressed
- anxiety, panic attacks, easily startled
- dryness of the skin, hair, eyes, vagina, mouth and throat
- heat in the hands and feet; warm dry palms
- facial flushing, night sweats, low grade fever in the evening
- palpitations and tachycardia with activity
- dry stools or constipation
- poor memory and inability to concentrate
- recurrent mouth and tongue ulcers
- lower back ache, aching legs
- dizziness, tinnitus, hearing loss

T red and dry with little or no coat, often redder at the tip; or with multiple surface cracks

P fine and rapid

Treatment Principle

Nourish and supplement Heart and Kidney yin and blood
Clear heat and calm the shen

Prescription

TIAN WANG BU XIN DAN 天王补心丹
Emperor of Heaven's Special Pill to Supplement the Heart

sheng di (Rehmanniae Radix) 生地	120 (24)g
tian dong (Asparagi Radix) 天冬	30 (12)g
mai dong (Ophiopogonis Radix) 麦冬	30 (12)g
chao suan zao ren (stir fried Zizyphi spinosae Semen) 炒酸枣仁	30 (12)g

dang gui (Angelicae sinensis Radix) 当归 .... 30 (9)g
wu wei zi (Schizandrae Fructus) 五味子 .... 30 (9)g
bai zi ren (Platycladi Semen) 柏子仁 .... 30 (9)g
xuan shen (Scrophulariae Radix) 玄参 .... 15 (12)g
dan shen (Salviae miltiorrhizae Radix) 丹参 .... 15 (12)g
fu ling (Poria) 茯苓 .... 15 (12)g
ren shen (Ginseng Radix) 人参 .... 15 (9)g
jie geng (Platycodi Radix) 桔梗 .... 15 (9)g
yuan zhi (Polygalae Radix) 远志 .... 15 (6)g

Method: Pills or powder. Grind herbs to a fine powder and form into 9 gram pills with honey. The dose is one pill 2–3 times daily. Can also be decocted with the doses shown in brackets. **Sheng di** and **xuan shen** supplement Kidney yin, cool the blood and stabilize the zhi; **tian dong** and **mai dong** clear heat and nourish yin; **dan shen** and **dang gui** nourish and regulate blood and prevent the supplementing herbs from contributing to blood stasis; **dan shen** also clears heat; **chao suan zao ren**, **bai zi ren** and **yuan zhi** calm the shen; **ren shen** and **fu ling** strengthen the Spleen, supplement qi and calm the shen; **wu wei zi** secures Heart qi and yin and calms the shen; **jie geng** diffuses the Lungs and directs the action of the other herbs to the upper body; **xuan shen**, **yuan zhi** and **jie geng** transform phlegm. (Source: *She Sheng Mi Pou*)

Variations and additional prescriptions

Heart yin and qi deficiency

Heart qi and yin deficiency often occur together, resulting in both instability of the shen, and a functional weakness of cardiac rhythm. In addition to the features of Heart yin deficiency, the patient has arrhythmia, which exacerbates the anxiety and depression. The treatment is to boost Heart qi and yin, unblock yang qi and restore the pulse with ZHI GAN CAO TANG (Prepared Licorice Decoction 炙甘草汤, p.811).

After a major shock or trauma

Depression and anxiety can sometimes follow weeks or months after a major shock or trauma. The patient experiences insomnia and dream or nightmare disturbed sleep, night sweats, palpitations and dizziness. This is typical of disrupted communication between the Heart and Kidneys due to shock, a form of post traumatic stress disorder. The treatment is to restore communication between the Heart and Kidneys, calm the shen and stabilize the zhi with GUI ZHI JIA LONG GU MU LI TANG (Cinnamon Twig Decoction plus Dragon Bone and Oyster Shell 桂枝加龙骨牡蛎汤, p.711).

With more Kidney yin deficiency

If the Kidney yin deficiency signs are significant (lower back ache, tinnitus, thinning or falling hair, lack of motivation), combine with LIU WEI DI HUANG WAN (Six Ingredient Pill with Rehmannia 六味地黄丸, p.192).

Prepared medicines

Concentrated powder

Tian Wang Bu Xin Dan (Ginseng & Zizyphus Formula)
Zhi Gan Cao Tang (Licorice Combination)
Gui Zhi Jia Long Gu Mu Li Tang (Cinnamon & Dragon Bone Combination)

Pills

Tian Wang Bu Xin Dan (Emperor's Teapills, Tian Wang Pu Hsin Tan)
Zhi Gan Cao Wan (Zhi Gan Cao Teapills)

Acupuncture (select from)

yintang (M–HN–3) ....these points calm the shen, lift the mood and
Du.19 (houding)   alleviate depression and anxiety
Du. 24 (shenting)
Bl.15 (xinshu +) ....transport point of the Heart, supplements Heart yin,
                              calms the Heart and shen, clears heat
Bl.23 (shenshu +) ....transport point of the Kidneys, supplements Kidney
                              yin to support systemic yin, and stabilizes the zhi
Ren.14 (juque)...................alarm point of the Heart, calms the Heart and shen
Ht.6 (yinxi).......................cleft point of the Heart, clears heat, supplements
                              Heart yin
Ht.7 (shenmen).................source point of the Heart, nourishes Heart qi and
                              yin and calms the shen
Sp.6 (sanyinjiao +).............supplements Heart and Kidney yin and with Ht.7
                              (shenmen) has a special effect on sleeplessness
Kid.3 (taixi +)....................source point of the Kidney, supplements Kidney yin,
                              clears deficiency heat and stabilizes the zhi
Kid.4 (dazhong) ....connecting point of the Kidney, stabilizes the zhi
                              and alleviates depression and anxiety
• Ear points: shenmen, heart, kidney, zero point, anti–depression, sympathetic

Clinical notes

• Heart and Kidney yin deficiency type depression and anxiety may be diagnosed
  as endogenous depression, menopausal syndrome, post traumatic stress disorder, anxiety neurosis, panic attacks or hyperthyroidism.
• Heart and Kidney yin deficiency depression usually responds quite well to treatment. For a long lasting result the yin must be replenished as far as possible and
  this takes time. Treatment with Chinese medicine will be necessary for at least
  several months and probably longer, although some signs of improvement can
  usually be expected within a few weeks.
• Diet is important, in particular ensuring adequate protein and avoidance of
  stimulants and heating or drying items like coffee and chillies. Ensure sufficient
  fluids to avoid dehydration. A yin nourishing diet is recommended. See Clinical
  Handbook Vol.2, p.876.
• Sufficient sleep is important and a strict and regular bedtime routine should be
  adhered to, even in patients with severe sleep disturbance.
• Active pursuit of relaxation should be encouraged. Pursuits such as taijiquan,
  yoga, walking and swimming are a good way to calm the mind, mobilize qi and
  gradually build qi and yin.

脾
肾
阳
虚

3.13 SPLEEN AND KIDNEY YANG DEFICIENCY

Spleen and Kidney yang deficiency depression is more common in middle aged and older patients. It represents a severe form of depression, and one in which the patient is likely to be heavily medicated, but with poor response. The depression is due to instability and weakness of the zhi (p.99).

Clinical features

- Deep depression characterized by a sense of hopelessness and exhaustion. These patients tend to be apathetic and lack the motivation and initiative to try to change as any activity is simply too much effort. They become reclusive and withdrawn.
- disabling mental and physical exhaustion, little energy reserve, any activity has to be followed by a period of recuperation
- increased desire to sleep, inability or unwillingness to get out of bed
- cold intolerance, cold extremities, feels cold to the touch
- lower back and knees sore, cold and weak
- pale puffy face with dark circles under the eyes and a flat affect
- frequent urination and nocturia, or oliguria and edema
- early morning diarrhea
- impotence, infertility, no libido

T pale, wet, swollen and scalloped

P deep and slow, especially in the proximal positions

Treatment Principle

Warm Spleen and Kidney yang

Prescription

YOU GUI WAN 右归丸
Restore the Right [Kidney] Pill

shu di (Rehmanniae Radix preparata) 熟地	24g
shan yao (Dioscoreae Rhizoma) 山药	12g
gou qi zi (Lycii Fructus) 枸杞子	12g
tu si zi (Cuscutae Semen) 菟丝子	12g
du zhong (Eucommiae Cortex) 杜仲	12g
lu jiao jiao (Cervi Cornus Colla) 鹿角胶	12g
shan zhu yu (Corni Fructus) 山茱萸	9g
dang gui (Angelicae sinensis Radix) 当归	9g
zhi fu zi (Aconiti Radix lateralis preparata) 制附子	6–12g
rou gui (Cinnamomi Cortex) 肉桂	6–12g

Method: Pills or powder. The herbs are ground to a fine powder and formed into 9 gram pills with honey. The dose is one pill twice daily. Can also be decocted, in which case **zhi fu zi** is cooked for 30 minutes before the other herbs and **lu jiao jiao** is melted into the strained decoction. **Shu di**, **gou qi zi** and **dang gui** nourish Kidney yin and blood; **shan zhu yu** supplements the Liver; **shan yao** strengthens the Spleen and Kidneys; **tu si zi** and **du zhong** supplement Kidney yang; **zhi fu zi** and **rou gui** warm yang; **lu jiao jiao** benefits yang and jing. (Source: *Zhong Yi Nei Ke Xue* ([*Jing Yue Quan Shu*])

Modifications

- With frequent urination or nocturia, add **sang piao xiao** (Mantidis Ootheca) 桑螵蛸 6–9g, **qian shi** (Euryales Semen) 芡实 9–12g and **jin ying zi** (Rosae laevigatae Fructus) 金樱子 9–12g and **yi zhi ren** (Alpiniae oxyphyllae Fructus) 益智仁 6–9g.
- With watery diarrhea, delete **shu di** and **dang gui** and add **huang qi** (Astragali Radix) 黄芪 12–15g, **chao bai zhu** (stir fried Atractylodes macrocephalae Rhizoma) 炒白术 9–12g and **yi ren** (Coicis Semen) 苡仁 15–30g.
- With urgent early morning diarrhea, add **rou dou kou** (Myristicae Semen) 肉豆蔻 3–6g and **bu gu zhi** (Psoraleae Fructus) 补骨脂 9–12g.
- With wheezing and breathing difficulty, add **bu gu zhi** (Psoraleae Fructus) 补骨脂 9–12g and **wu wei zi** (Schizandrae Fructus) 五味子 6–9g.

Variations and additional prescriptions

With marked digestive weakness

Kidney yang supports the digestive fire of Spleen yang. When Spleen yang is especially weak, the digestive symptoms are prominent and the primary prescription above may cause digestive upset, nausea and diarrhea. This can usually be addressed with a mixture of LI ZHONG WAN (Regulate the Middle Pill 理中丸, p.732) and JIN GUI SHEN QI WAN (Kidney Qi Pill from the Golden Cabinet 金匮肾气丸, p.826).

Prepared medicines

Concentrated powder

You Gui Wan (Eucommia & Rehmannia Formula)
Ba Wei Di Huang Wan (Rehmannia Eight Formula)
Jin Suo Gu Jing Wan (Lotus Stamen Formula)
– add for frequent urination and nocturia

Pills

You Gui Wan (Right Side Replenishing Teapills)
Jin Kui Shen Qi Wan (Fu Gui Ba Wei Wan, Golden Book Tea)

Acupuncture (select from)

Du.20 (baihui +▲) ....moxa can help lift yang qi and elevate the mood

Bl.23 (shenshu +▲) ....transport point of the Kidneys, warms and supports Kidney and Spleen yang, strengthens and stabilizes the zhi

Bl.20 (pishu +▲) ....transport point of the Spleen, warms Spleen yang and stabilizes the yi

Bl.52 (zhishi +▲)...............strengthens the zhi to fortify willpower and determination; strong moxa can assist in stimulating the desire to change

Ren.4 (guanyuan +▲)........supplements yuan qi, warms yang, regulates qi and stabilizes the zhi

Ren.8 (shenque ▲) ....warms yang and stabilizes the zhi; treated with moxa on salt–place a piece of thin cloth over the navel and fill it with salt, burn large cones of moxa on the salt; the cloth enables quick removal of the salt and prevents burning

Kid.7 (fuliu +) ....warms Kidney yang, an important point for exhaustion and lack of motivation

Kid.3 (taixi +).....................source point of the Kidneys, supplements and supports Kidney yang

St.36 (zusanli +▲) ....sea point of the Stomach, warms and strengthens the Spleen and Stomach and supplements yang qi

Sp.6 (sanyinjiao +▲).........strengthens the Spleen and Kidneys; warms Kidney and Spleen yang and stabilizes the yi and zhi

Du.4 (mingmen +▲).........warms and supports Kidney yang

• with edema, add Ren.9 (shuifen ▲) and Sp.9 (yinlingquan –)

• Ear points: kidney, zero point, shenmen, adrenal, anti–depression

Clinical notes

• Depression of a Spleen and Kidney yang deficiency type can be quite debilitating and difficult due to the characteristic lack of physical energy and the overwhelming feeling that everything, including treatment, is pointless. Patients simply do not seek treatment but instead tend to stay inside feeling hopeless. If a patient does seek and persist with treatment, however, they often respond reasonably well. For lasting results treatment usually needs to continue for at least a few months. Depending on the duration and severity of the initial condition, 6–12 months of treatment may be required to rebuild and sustain Spleen and Kidney yang.

• A yang warming diet is recommended. See Clinical Handbook, Vol.2, p.873.

• Movement, although difficult to initiate, is helpful; Group classes will be important to maintain motivation.

Table 3.3 Summary of depression patterns

Pattern	Depression characteristics	Other Features	Prescription
Liver qi constraint	Depression, mood swings, irritability, feeling of frustration; early waking around 1–3am. The more blood deficiency the more the fatigue and apathy aspects of the depression become apparent.	Chest, hypochondriac, abdominal discomfort or pain, sighing, heartburn, nausea, belching, loss of appetite, constipation or alternating bowel habits, neck and shoulder tight, tension headaches, irregular menses, premenstrual syndrome, mauve tongue with a thin coat and a wiry pulse	Chai Hu Shu Gan San
Liver qi constraint with blood deficiency		A common pattern of postpartum depression. In addition to the main features of Liver qi constraint there is postural dizziness, pallor, lack of milk supply, menstrual irregularity, pale edges on the tongue and a wiry, fine pulse	Xiao Yao San
Liver qi constraint with heat	The more heat there is the more irritability and anger outbursts.	In addition to the basic qi constraint symptoms, the degree of irritability and reactivity, as well as sleeplessness are greater, flushing, premenstrual acne, red edges on the tongue and a wiry, rapid pulse	Jia Wei Xiao Yao San
Heart and Liver fire	Violent anger outbursts, aggressive, manic, compulsive or reckless behavior; in severe cases suicidal ideation or suicide attempts.	Red complexion and eyes; scleral hemorrhage, dizziness, insomnia or nightmares, palpitations, tinnitus, constipation, mouth ulcers, red skin lesions, concentrated urine, scorched smell, red tongue with a thick, yellow, dry or greasy coat and a slippery, rapid, strong, surging pulse.	Dang Gui Long Hui Wan Chai Hu Jia Long Gu Mu Li Tang
Qi and phlegm constraint	Depression, anxiety, obsessive thinking; sense of blockage in the throat or difficulty swallowing.	Chest oppression, fatigue, heaviness in the limbs, somnolence, vertigo, mucus congestion, hoarse voice, nausea, a swollen tongue with a greasy, white coat and a wiry or slippery pulse	Ban Xia Hou Po Tang
Heart and Lung qi constraint	Sadness, crying, melancholia, excessive grieving, hypersensitivity to trivial events, always on the verge of tears.	Shortness of breath, wheezing, chest tightness, shoulders are hunched forward with collapse of the chest, pallor, constipation, congestion in the throat or dysphagia, pale or slightly red tongue and a weak pulse	Si Mo Tang

Table 3.3 Summary of depression patterns (cont.)

Pattern	Depression characteristics	Other Features	Prescription
Spleen and Stomach qi constraint	Depression, excessive worry over trivia, brooding and rumination.	Indigestion, heartburn, abdominal distension, loss of appetite, bad breath, chest oppression, red tongue with a thick, white or yellow coat and a wiry, slippery pulse	Yue Ju Wan
Blood and qi stasis	Black depression and despair to the point of suicidal thoughts or attempts.	Insomnia, dark complexion, purplish lips, sclera, conjunctivae and nails, localized headaches, chronic pain; dry, scaly skin; skin discolouration, vascular congestion, dark or purple tongue with stasis spots and distended sublingual veins; choppy, wiry, fine pulse	Xue Fu Zhu Yu Tang
Phlegm damp	Depression, apathy and lethargy, heaviness of spirit and body, foggy head, obsessive thinking and irrational worry.	Fatigue, somnolence, mucus congestion, masses (lipomas, thyroid nodules, breast cysts or ganglia), vertigo, nausea, heartburn, chest oppression, overweight, swollen or flabby tongue with a thick coat and a slippery or wiry pulse	Di Tan Tang
Heart blood and Spleen qi deficiency	Depression with anxiety, overwhelmed and unable to cope. Obsessive compulsion and thoughts, phobias, paranoia or suspiciousness.	Poor concentration, insomnia, palpitations, dizziness, blurred vision, loss of appetite, loose stools, dry hair, eyes and skin, clammy palms, pallor, easy bruising, heavy menstrual periods, pale tongue with a thin, white coat and a fine, weak pulse	Gui Pi Tang
Lung and Spleen qi deficiency	Depression sadness and isolation; inability to interact with others. Avoidance of engaging and speaking. Obsessive thinking or irrational worry.	Sweating, fatigue, breathlessness, weak voice, pale complexion, poor appetite, loose stools, abdominal distension, slumped shoulders, pale, scalloped tongue and a fine, weak or floating, big, weak pulse	Bu Zhong Yi Qi Tang
Liver yin deficiency (with qi constraint)	Depression with irritability; severe mood swings; aimlessness and lacking a sense of direction and purpose.	Dull hypochondriac ache, dry eyes and weak vision, night blindness, headaches, dizziness, insomnia, acid reflux, brittle nails, muscle spasms, cramps or tics, red tongue with little or no coat and a fine, wiry and rapid pulse	Yi Guan Jian

Table 3.3 Summary of depression patterns (cont.)

Pattern	Depression characteristics	Other Features	Prescription
Heart and Kidney yin deficiency	Depression with anxiety, unease and agitation, worse at night. The more tired they are the more depressed and anxious.	Insomnia, anxiety, panic attacks, general dryness; warm dry palms, flushing, night sweats, low grade fever, palpitations, constipation, poor memory, mouth ulcers, back ache, dizziness, tinnitus, hearing loss, red, dry tongue with little or no coat and a fine, rapid pulse	Tian Wang Bu Xin Dan Zhi Gan Cao Tang Gui Zhi Jia Long Gu Mu Li Tang
Spleen and Kidney yang deficiency	Profound depression characterized by a sense of hopelessness and exhaustion. Patients become reclusive and withdrawn.	Disabling mental and physical exhaustion, somnolence, lower back and knees sore, cold intolerance, frequent urination, nocturia, or oliguria and edema, early morning diarrhea, impotence, pale, wet, swollen, scalloped tongue and a deep, slow pulse	You Gui Wan

DIABETES MELLITUS

Diabetes mellitus (*táng niào bìng* 糖尿病, literally 'sweet urine disease') is an increasingly common disorder in both affluent and developing societies. Diabetes mellitus (DM) is a syndrome of impaired insulin secretion and/or resistance of cells and tissues to the influence of insulin. The end result is abnormally high blood sugar levels – hyperglycemia. Chronic diabetes is almost always complicated by other phenomena attributed to persistent hyperglycemia. It is these complications that account for the majority of the mortality and morbidity seen in chronic diabetics. The main causes of death related to diabetes are cardiovascular disease, stroke and kidney failure. Contributing to morbidity are blindness, gangrene, sensory deficit, peripheral neuropathy and chronic skin infections.

> **BOX 4.1 PATTERNS OF DIABETES MELLITUS**
>
> Lung and Stomach heat
> Spleen qi deficiency
> Phlegm damp
> Damp heat
> Liver qi constraint with heat
> Qi and yin deficiency
> Liver and Kidney yin deficiency
> Kidney yin and yang deficiency
> Blood stasis

There are two main types, type 1 (previously known as juvenile onset or insulin dependent DM) and type 2 (previously known as mature onset or non–insulin dependent DM). The old descriptions are redundant because of overlap in age group and treatment between the types. Children are increasingly being diagnosed with type 2 DM, type 2 diabetics often end up needing insulin, and type 1 DM is occasionally seen in adults.

Type 1

Type 1 DM usually occurs during adolescence and is associated with autoimmune or infectious destruction of the insulin producing ß–cells of the pancreas. A genetic susceptibility, in combination with viral or environmental exposure to triggers, starts a cascade of events resulting in destruction of ß–cells. Destruction progresses subclinically over time until few ß–cells remain, and insulin levels are too low to

Table 4.1 Comparison of type 1 and 2 diabetes

	Type 1	Type 2
Incidence	~10%	~90%
Age of onset	under 20	over 40
Onset	rapid	insidious
Weight at onset	thin	obese
Familial component	weak link	strong link
Insulin status	lacking	resistance to
Likely to develop complications	yes	yes

Table 4.2 Blood glucose level ranges and features

Blood glucose	Range	
	fasting[1]	GTT[2]
Normal	< 100 (5.6)[3]	< 140 (7.7)
Prediabetes (impaired glucose regulation)	100-125 (5.6-6.9)	140-199 (7.7 -11)
Diabetes	> 126 (7.0)	> 200 (11.1)

1 Fasting defined as no caloric intake for 8 hours
2 Glucose tolerance testing: plasma glucose concentration measured 2 hours after carbohydrate load
3 units in milligrams per decaliter-mg/dl (millimoles per liter-mmol/l)

maintain blood glucose control. Since the pancreas no longer produces insulin, the insulin must be replaced and patients are medicated with insulin injections.

Type 2

Type 2 DM is characterized by resistance of target cells to the influence of insulin. Insulin levels in the blood are high, especially in the early stages, but insulin cell receptors are insensitive and glucose is not transported into cells. The glucose remains in the blood stream, resulting in hyperglycemia. Type 2 DM usually appears in middle age, develops gradually and may take years before diagnosis, at which time around 35% of patients have developed complications. There is a strong link to obesity (see Chapter 14), however patients can be obese without developing diabetes, and not all type 2 diabetics are obese. Some people have a genetic predisposition to insulin resistance, while others develop the condition because of an unhealthy diet, lifestyle and high stress. A diet high in carbohydrate and sugar causes the pancreas to overproduce insulin. The cells of the body are overwhelmed by this excess insulin and protect themselves by reducing the number of insulin receptor sites on their surface. Consequently there are too few sites for insulin to carry out its normal function of allowing glucose to pass through the cell wall to be converted into energy.

Signs and symptoms

The classic symptoms of DM are:

- **Polydipsia**: increased thirst due to decrease in fluid volume and dehydration from excessive urination, and increased osmolarity of blood and extracellular fluids. Chinese medicine considers excessive thirst due to dryness from heat or yin deficiency, failure of Spleen qi and fluids to ascend to the mouth, blockage of the qi dynamic by damp heat or failure of Kidney yang qi to process fluids.
- **Polyphagia**: increased hunger as glucose lost in the urine is unavailable for essential metabolic activity. In Chinese medical terms this can be due to heat affecting the Stomach, or a failure of qi transformation with relative lack of qi reaching the tissues.
- **Polyuria**: increased urinary frequency and volume caused by osmotic diuresis from high levels of glucose in the urine; fluid loss leads to low blood pressure and dehydration. In Chinese medical terms this is due to failure of Kidney regulation over the lower yin (here the urethra), weakness of yang and poor

fluid metabolism, or the bodies attempt to expel accumulating dampness.

- Hyperglycemia can also cause weight loss, nausea and vomiting, blurred vision, and predisposition to bacterial or fungal infections.
- Dehydration and inability of glucose to enter cells causes weakness and fatigue, and, when severe, cognitive disturbances. Symptoms come and go as plasma glucose levels fluctuate.

Patients with type 1 DM typically present with symptoms of hyperglycemia. Patients with type 2 DM may present with symptomatic hyperglycemia, but are often asymptomatic or have atypical symptoms, or present with diabetic complications such as tiredness, blurred vision, numbness and tingling in the hands and feet, thrush or chronic infections and wounds that are slow to heal. Diagnosis is based on clinical features, if present, and measurement of blood glucose levels, tested when fasting and two hours after a 75 gram oral load of glucose, the glucose tolerance test. The diabetic and prediabetic status of many patients is detected with routine blood screening.

In practice, many patients presenting to the Chinese medicine clinic are already diagnosed, medicated and at least partly managed. They present because the side effects of the medications are troublesome, they are not achieving good blood glucose control, or are experiencing complications. The symptoms of diabetes they experienced initially will generally be controlled, but may appear sporadically during periods of stress or dietary indiscretion, when tight glucose control is lost. Even in patients with good glucose control and few symptoms, the disease process continues, albeit at a slower pace, hence the gradual onset of complications and increasing medication requirements. About 30% of patients medicated with hypoglycemic agents end up needing insulin.

Classical Chinese medicine and diabetes mellitus

The first mention of a disease resembling diabetes in China comes from the Simple Questions (*Huang Di Nei Jing Su Wen*; early Han dynasty, 1st century BCE) where the condition known as xiāo kě [1] 消渴 was described. Xiao ke is a disease state characterized by persistent thirst and hunger, copious urination and weight loss. The Simple Questions (Chapters 40 and 47) makes the observation that xiao ke is due to consuming too much fatty, sweet or rich food, usually occurs amongst the wealthy, and that such patients are reluctant to change their habits, a situation similar to that seen in type 2 DM. The disease was differentiated into three subtypes, involving the upper, middle and lower burners. The upper burner type is attributed to heat scorching the Lungs, and is characterized by thirst; the middle burner type is due to heat in the Spleen and Stomach and is characterized by hunger; the lower burner type is due to failure of the Kidneys to control the lower orifices, and is characterized by profuse urination. Contemporary Chinese internal medicine texts place diabetes within the disease diagnosis of xiao ke.

In clinic, however, we observe that many patients diagnosed with diabetes mellitus or pre–diabetic conditions are overweight and do not display the charac-

---

1 Wasting and Thirsting [Bensky] or Dispersion Thirst [Wiseman]

teristic symptoms of xiao ke. In addition, the complications of diabetes are not necessarily present in xiao ke, and diseases other than diabetes mellitus can lead to the symptoms of xiao ke, such as diabetes insipidus, hyperaldosteronism and hyperparathyroidism.

PATHOLOGY

The pathology of DM can be seen in terms of the six divisions. The majority of diabetic pathology occurs within the taiyin and shaoyin divisions. The taiyin pertains to the Spleen and Lungs, while the shaoyin pertains to the Kidneys and Heart. Hyperglycemia is common to both type 1 and 2 diabetes, and is

yang levels	taiyang shaoyang yangming	
yin levels	**taiyin shaoyin** jueyin	diabetic pathology

due to failure of Spleen transformation. In type 1 DM, failure of Spleen transformation is due to the Spleen not being supported by the Kidney; in type 2 DM it is due to direct damage to the Spleen by diet or emotional factors.

Type 2 DM starts with taiyin dysfunction, which over time, starts to involve the shaoyin. In type 1 DM, the main pathology starts in the shaoyin, which fails to support taiyin. In practice, the majority of patients have impairment of both the taiyin and shaoyin divisions to one degree or another. The more chronic and severe the disease, the more shaoyin pathology, and the more the Heart and vessels are damaged. When uncontrolled, shaoyin pathology can lapse into the final and severe jueyin division, leading to coma and death (Fig.4.2, p.162).

Taiyin (Spleen and Lungs)

The Spleen is at the centre[2] of qi production and the stability of energy supply. The main function of the Spleen is transformation of the raw materials of food into a form of qi the body can use, and distribution of the results of transformation to the rest of the body. The Spleen extracts the pure essence of food (the 'sweetness' of earth) and sends it to the Lungs for final processing

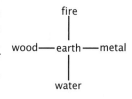

into usable forms of qi, which are then distributed to their target tissues and organs. When transformation and distribution are disrupted, the conversion of food into qi is incomplete, and the sweet precursor to qi builds up in the blood. This can happen for two reasons:

• The Spleen can be overwhelmed, and its transforming and distribution function damaged, by excessive demands placed upon it. The Spleen can be taxed by overeating, or drained by overwork and qi expenditure that exceeds the Spleens

---

2 Positioned in the middle, and as the stabilizing earth element, the Spleen is our centre of gravity, and keeps us grounded in the face of change. The Spleen is very conservative and dislikes change. When internal transformation is excessive and potentially destabilizing (as can occur when more food is consumed than can be efficiently processed), the Spleens response is to increase resistance to that change by reducing the number of insulin receptors on cell walls, thus producing insulin resistance.

ability to replace it.
- The Spleen can be critically compromised by Kidney deficiency, which fails to provide the necessary support to the Spleens demanding transformation and distribution function.

Once there is an excess of sweet in the blood several things happen. Excessive sweetness generates damp, which can condense into phlegm. Damp is sticky and obstructing, and can create heat and damp heat, which deplete yin. Damp obstructs the circulation of qi and blood leading to qi and blood stasis. The degree of blood stasis can be profound due to the combined effects of qi deficiency, yin deficiency, phlegm and damp. Qi deficiency also contributes to yin deficiency, as yin can only be acquired by efficient digestion of yin nourishing foods. As qi and yin are progressively depleted, the Kidney (shaoyin) is called upon to prop up Spleen function and a mixed taiyin shaoyin pathology emerges.

The progression from a taiyin condition seen in the early stages of type 2 DM, towards a mixture of taiyin and shaoyin pathology is consistent with what we observe in practice. Early type 2 DM and pre–diabetes is associated with Spleen qi deficiency, qi constraint, damp heat or phlegm patterns. The pathology is primarily in the middle burner. The longer the condition continues, the more the Kidney is weakened and yin depleted, until the most common chronic pattern, qi and yin deficiency, evolves. At this time, the cardiovascular complications become more significant, signalling greater shaoyin involvement. The increasing shaoyin weakness accounts for the observation that a significant proportion of type 2 diabetics end up eventually requiring insulin.

Shaoyin (Kidney and Heart)
The Kidneys are the ultimate support for all organ systems. Kidney yin supports the structural integrity of the body[3], while Kidney yang is the basis of functional activity. In the case of diabetes, a pre–existing or acquired weakness of the Kidneys leaves the Spleen vulnerable to failure when stressed by diet, Liver qi constraint or pathogenic invasion. The Kidneys can also be progressively drained in an attempt to prop up Spleen function leading to shaoyin complications.

Type 1 DM is due to pre–existing shaoyin weakness that renders the patient vulnerable to external pathogenic invasion directly into the shaoyin, or to severing of the Kidney Heart connection by a severe shock or trauma. In adolescents the shaoyin weakness is inherited; in adults it is acquired by overwork, deleterious habits, age, and temporarily, during pregnancy. The fundamental weakness is of jing. When the shaoyin is disrupted by pathogenic invasion or trauma, the already fragile yin is further depleted, and the disrupted Kidneys are unable to support the Spleens transforming function. Jing deficiency is seen in the observation that the peak onset of type 1 DM occurs around puberty, between 11–14 years of age, just at the time when jing is drawn upon to transform the child into the adult. Onset of type 1 DM is also more common in winter, the cold of which stresses the Kidney further. The shaoyin deficiency, and consequent damage that ensues from the

---

3 In the context of type 1 DM, the lack of yin substrate is reflected in the absence of insulin producing ß–cells in the pancreas.

Figure 4.1 Relative severity of DM patterns. Orderly progression through the patterns is not implied.

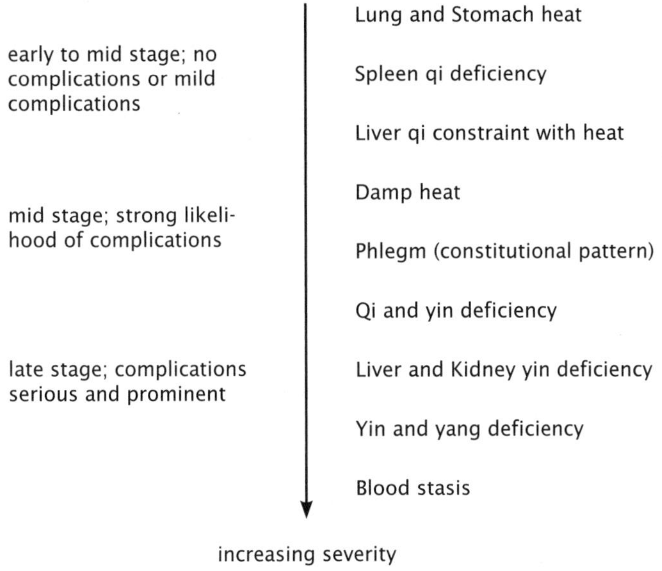

	Lung and Stomach heat
early to mid stage; no complications or mild complications	Spleen qi deficiency
	Liver qi constraint with heat
mid stage; strong likelihood of complications	Damp heat
	Phlegm (constitutional pattern)
	Qi and yin deficiency
late stage; complications serious and prominent	Liver and Kidney yin deficiency
	Yin and yang deficiency
	Blood stasis

increasing severity

trigger event in type 1 DM is profound, and before insulin replacement therapy was available, type 1 diabetics died young. Uncontrolled shaoyin pathology leads to jueyin pathology, characterized by wind, collapse, coma and death. The shaoyin (Heart and Kidney) relationship also accounts for the incidence of cardiovascular and microvascular complications observed.

Complications
Blood stasis and phlegm
Blood stasis and phlegm are almost universal complicating pathologies of chronic DM, and account for most of the morbidity and mortality – increased risk of cardiovascular disease and stroke, peripheral vascular disease and gangrene, peripheral neuropathy, diabetic retinopathy, blindness and dementia.

The blood stasis is due to the convergence of several pathologies, which accounts for its eventual severity. Spleen qi deficiency fails to lead the blood; dampness and phlegm accumulation block qi and blood flow; depletion of yin fluids causes a thickening of blood; finally yang deficiency freezes the already sluggish blood in place. Blood stasis is the most serious and frequent complication.

Phlegm accumulates when damp from qi deficiency congeals into phlegm, and because heat and dryness cooks normal fluids and damp into phlegm. The phlegm ends up clogging the large vessels of the Heart, accumulating in the tissues of the extremities causing numbness, or being deposited in the eye causing visual disturbances. Blood stasis and phlegm occur independently or together.

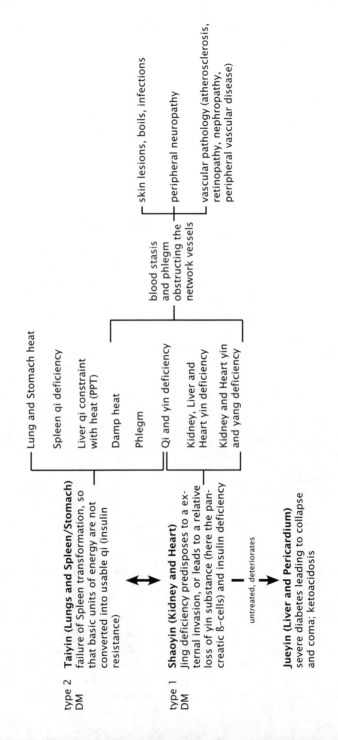

Figure 4.2 Patterns and pathology of diabetes

Figure 4.3 Etiology of type 1 DM

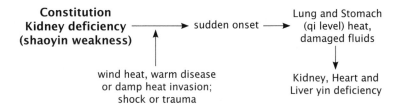

ETIOLOGY

Diet and medications

The influence of diet varies between type 1 and type 2 DM. In type 1, the diet is considered of secondary importance to the combination of the predisposing jing weakness and the trigger. The trigger is usually considered to be an external pathogenic invasion or emotional trauma, but may involve components of the diet that further weaken the already depleted jing and zheng qi. Type 1 DM is mostly seen in adolescents and children, who, by definition, have immature Spleen function, up to about the age of seven. A child's undeveloped Spleen is easily damaged by poor diet and feeding habits. Cold, raw, hard to digest or damp producing foods compromise Spleen function and may exacerbate any pre–existing deficiency. Excessive fruit and fruit juices, soft drinks, dairy products, ice cream and antibiotics can weaken the Spleen and create damp. Early exposure to cows milk and gluten during infancy has been linked to increased incidence of type 1 diabetes. Similarly, overeating and too much sugary or greasy junk food contributes to damp heat, food stagnation, accumulation disorder[4] and Spleen qi disruption. If the Kidneys are already weak, it does not take too much acquired deficiency to push the system into pathology.

In type 2 DM, an excess of food, or an overly rich, sweet, calorie dense and high carbohydrate diet, in conjunction with a decrease in physical activity, damages Spleen and Stomach qi, clogs the qi dynamic, and generates damp heat. Heat and damp heat in the middle burner gradually deplete yin and drain the Kidneys. This process is facilitated if there is an inherited Kidney deficiency. A raw, cold diet, or repeated dieting and the use of slimming agents, weakens the Spleen and leads to poor transformation and regulation of qi.

Some drugs and medications are known to contribute to diabetes. Excessive or inappropriate use of heating drugs, yang supplements or warming and drying herbs can damage Kidney yin. This includes medications that are pungent and dispersing, or heating, such as steroids, therapeutic doses of niacin, and stimulants like amphetamines. Some cooling drugs that weaken Spleen qi are implicated, including beta–blockers and protease inhibitors.

---

4 *gān jī* 疳积

Figure 4.4 Dietary factors in the development of type 2 diabetes

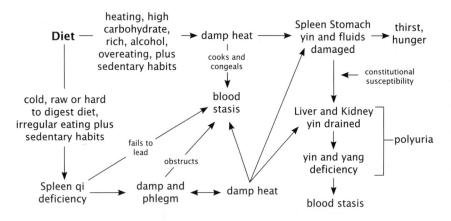

Figure 4.5 Emotional factors in the development of type 2 diabetes

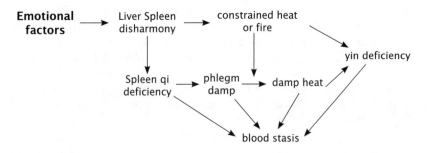

Constitutional factors

Diabetes tends to run in families. The inherited constitution can be one of Kidney weakness, Spleen deficiency, phlegm or Liver qi constraint. An inherited Kidney weakness leaves people vulnerable to invasion by external pathogens or rapid depletion of yin in response to a shock or trauma (type 1 DM, Fig. 4.3, p.163). In patients who develop type 2 DM, the Kidney deficiency is gradually exacerbated by ageing and excessive work, or the heat and Spleen deficiency created by an unhealthy diet. A phlegm type constitution can contribute to patients being overweight from an early age, while a Spleen deficient constitution is seen in thin, pale, tired children with little vim and indifference to food.

Emotional factors

Diabetes can develop subsequent to a physical or emotional trauma or shock. Severe or sudden shock disrupts the Heart and Kidney (shaoyin) which creates a weakness that can be exploited by an invading pathogen, or leads to yin or yang deficiency (see p.781). Sustained emotional conflict leads to Liver qi constraint, constrained heat and damage to qi and yin. Qi constraint weakens the Spleen, which in turn leads to the generation of damp, damp heat and phlegm (Fig. 4.5).

Exhaustion, overwork, pregnancy

Overworking, working excessively long hours, or using more energy in activity than is gained through eating (often seen in athletes) weakens the Kidneys and Spleen, and depletes yin and yang. This process is exacerbated if sleep is insufficient or disrupted by shift work, for example. When associated with physical toil, the Kidneys tend to be weakened; when associated with mental work but a sedentary occupation, the Spleen is drained.

During pregnancy, jing resources are diverted away from the mother and towards the developing fetus. Any pre–existing weakness of shaoyin can be exacerbated during this time, leading to a failure to support taiyin and Spleen transformation, with transitory gestational diabetes the result.

TREATMENT

The main aim of treatment in diabetes is to regulate blood glucose levels while correcting the imbalances that enabled it to occur. Exercise, management of the diet, and weight loss are the first line of therapy for all type 2 DM patients, and in many cases these alone are sufficient to enable the patient to manage their condition. When intervention is required, acupuncture and herbal treatment can help keep their blood sugar under control, while gradually improving their constitutional health and general well being. If treatment and management of life factors is started at an early stage of the disease, the pancreas has functional insulin producing tissue, and complications are not advanced, cure is possible.

For patients dependent on insulin, cure is not possible, but diet and exercise are important, and the addition of Chinese medicine can assist in maintaining tight blood glucose control, and sometimes in reducing insulin requirements. Tight management of blood glucose and improvement of underlying pathology helps alleviate or prevent complications.

Dietary advice

Standard diets for diabetic patients are widely available and specialist dieticians are a valuable resource for patients. Intake of carbohydrate is limited to a certain number of measured portions per day and calories from fat are restricted. Other than these basic modifications, the diet that is suitable for the pattern of the individual concerned, is recommended. For example, the diet to strengthen the Spleen and supplement qi recommends 40–60% carbohydrate, but for patients with Spleen qi deficient type diabetes, this proportion should be decreased to around 20–30%, with only complex, unprocessed carbohydrates allowed. Ideally, little or no processed or refined carbohydrate (white rice and white flour products, sugar and corn syrup, soft drinks, etc.) should be consumed.

Management of medicated patients

Treatment with oral hypoglycemic agents and insulin help maintain blood glucose levels and reduce the symptoms of diabetes. Patients may present with few clear features of diabetes, and little in the way of a clear symptom picture or pattern, although we find the tongue to be an accurate reflection of the true state of the body. Clinical experience reveals that most patients with chronic diabetes end up in between the taiyin and shaoyin ends of the spectrum, with qi and yin deficiency as their baseline pattern.

Even when patients are medicated and feel generally well, ongoing lifestyle management and Chinese medical treatment is recommended, as we know that even in patients with good blood glucose control complications can still arise.

Insulin dependent

Type 1 diabetics must inject insulin on a regular basis. Once a patient with type 2 diabetes has progressed to needing insulin, it is likely they will be dependent on it for life. After a few months any remaining functional pancreatic tissue atrophies. However, some type 2 diabetics require insulin just once in a while (for example when fighting an infection) to maintain adequate control of the blood sugar. These patients have functional pancreatic tissue that can be stimulated to perform more efficiently, and they can stop the insulin when blood sugar has stabilized. Some patients requiring regular insulin may find their requirements decreasing over time. Experienced diabetics monitoring their blood sugar levels can make the necessary adjustments to their dosage without problem.

Insulin dependent diabetics can still benefit significantly from treatment with Chinese medicine in terms of management and prevention of the common macro and microvascular complications, and general measures of increased well being and quality of life. Most benefit, however, will be gained from treatment with Chinese medicine before insulin dependence occurs.

Oral hypoglycemic agents

Patients using oral hypoglycemic agents may find their dosage requirements decreasing as their underlying condition improves with treatment and lifestyle change. The dosage can be reduced slowly in conjunction with regular blood sugar monitoring and some patients will be able to completely stop. Patients who have

BOX 4.2 ORAL MEDICATIONS FOR TYPE 2 DIABETES

The most common first line medication is Metformin, which may be augmented by a Sulphonurea if it fails to produce a satisfactory result.

Hypoglycemic agents
Metformin (Glucophage, Diabex, Diaformin)
- Metformin suppresses hepatic gluconeogenesis, increases insulin sensitivity, enhances peripheral glucose uptake, increases fatty acid oxidation and decreases absorption of glucose from the gastrointestinal tract.
- The most common adverse effect is gastrointestinal upset with symptoms that include diarrhea, cramps, nausea, vomiting and increased flatulence.
- Metformin is bitter and cooling. The bitterness dries damp and phlegm in the short term, but prolonged use damages the Spleen and depletes yin. This accounts for the observation that they are more reliably effective for the excess heat patterns, damp heat and qi constraint with heat, and that their effectiveness wanes over time.

Sulphonureas (Orinase, Diamicron, Glucotrol)
- These drugs trigger release of insulin by stimulating pancreatic beta cells.
- The most common side effect is hypoglycemia.

Alpha–glucosidase inhibitors (Glucobay, Precose)
- These drugs inhibit the enzymes needed to metabolize carbohydrate so less glucose is absorbed into the blood.
- The main side effects are due to bacterial action on the unmetabolized carbohydrates that remain in the intestines, and include flatulence, abdominal bloating and diarrhea.

made significant lifestyle changes or who have started acupuncture or herbal treatment, might experience hypoglycemia if they are taking more medication than required. Hypoglycemia is characterized by hunger, tiredness, light–headedness, tunnel vision or fainting.

Table 4.3 Herbs and combinations with a known action on blood glucose levels[1, 2]. Most are traditionally used for *xiāo kě*.

Herb	Action	
Ren Shen Ginseng Radix 人参	Ginseng root; sweet, slightly bitter, warm; Spleen, Lung. Strengthens the Lungs and Spleen, supplements qi, generates fluids and stops thirst. For all patterns with qi deficiency and fluid damage. Has a well described two dimensional blood glucose regulating effect, i.e. lowers it when too high and elevates it when too low. Extracts of ginseng enhance insulin sensitivity, promote insulin secretion, and regulate the activity of enzymes related to glucose metabolism.	
Di Huang Rehmanniae Radix 地黄	Rehmannia root; sweet, bitter, cold (raw) or sweet, slightly warm (processed). Heart, Liver, Kidney. One of the most important herbs for diabetes. The raw version clears heat and cools the blood, while the processed variety nourishes yin and blood. Often used together for yin deficiency with heat. One of the most widely used and effective herbs to lower blood glucose. Can stimulate insulin secretion when islet cells remain.	
Huang Qi Astragali Radix 黄芪	Astragalus root; sweet, warm; Spleen, Lung. Strengthens the Spleen and Lungs, supplements qi. Two dimensional regulation of blood glucose. Essential for vascular complications.	This pair is noted in many contemporary texts, and are cited as having a particular effect on lowering blood glucose in the context of Spleen deficiency. They appear together in many ancient and contemporary formulae.
Shan Yao Dioscoreae Rhizoma 山药	Dioscorea yam root; sweet, neutral; Spleen, Lung, Kidney. Strengthens the Spleen, supplements qi and yin and generates fluids. Lowers blood glucose.	
Cang Zhu Atractylodes Rhizoma 苍术	Atractylodes root; pungent, bitter, warm; Spleen, Stomach. Strengthens the Spleen and dries damp. Slow sustained hypoglycemic effect.	This pair dries damp and clears heat while nourishing and protecting yin. Their potential negative effects, excessive drying, or aggravation of damp, are balanced when combined. Considered to have a particular effect on lowering blood glucose and cholesterol, and a protective effect against accumulation of atherosclerotic plaque (phlegm).
Xuan Shen Scrophularia Radix 玄参	Scrophularia root; bitter, salty, cool; Lung, Liver. Nourishes yin, moistens dryness and clears heat.	
Huang Jing Polygonati Rhizoma 黄精	Polygonum root; sweet, neutral; Spleen, Lung, Kidney. Supplements qi and yin. Strengthens the Lungs, Kidney and Spleen. Used for chronic qi and yin deficiency patterns. Lowers blood glucose.	

Table 4.3 Herbs with a known action on blood glucose (cont.)

Herb	Action
Tian Hua Fen Trichosanthes Radix 天花粉	Trichosanthes root; sweet, slightly bitter, sour, cool; Lung, Stomach. Clears heat and generates fluids. Lowers blood glucose.
Yu Zhu Polygonati odorati Rhizoma 玉竹	Polygonum odoratum root; sweet, cool; Lung, Stomach. Nourishes Lung and Stomach yin, moistens dryness. Lowers blood glucose and may resist oxidative tissue damage.
Gui Zhi[3] Cinnamoni Ramulus 桂枝	Cinnamon twig; sweet, pungent, warm; Lung, Spleen, Heart, Urinary Bladder. Warms yang and supports Spleen qi transformation; promotes qi and blood flow through the channels and network vessels. Can lower blood glucose, triglycerides and cholesterol. For qi and yang deficiency patterns, and those with blood stasis.
Ge Gen Puerariae Radix 葛根	Kudzu root; sweet, pungent, cool; Spleen, Stomach. Generates fluids and alleviates thirst. Hypoglycemic, hypolipidemic and antioxidant effect. For hyperlipidemia and complications like retinopathy and neuropathy.
Zhi Mu Anemarrhenae Rhizoma 知母	Anemarrhena root; bitter, cold; Lung, Stomach, Kidney. Clears heat, nourishes yin, generates fluids and alleviates thirst. Lowers blood glucose and increases insulin sensitivity.
Yi Ren Coicis Semen 苡仁	Job's tears; sweet, bland, cool; Spleen. Lung, Kidney. Strengthens the Spleen and clears damp heat. Hypoglycemic and insulin stimulating effect.
Mai Dong Ophiopogonis Radix 麦冬	Ophiopogon root; sweet, slightly bitter, cool; Lung, Heart, Stomach. Nourishes Lung and Stomach yin, moistens dryness and clears heat. Lowers blood glucose. For all patterns with dryness, heat and deficiency.
Di Gu Pi Lycii Cortex 地骨皮	Lycium bark; sweet, cold, Lung, Liver, Kidney. Clears heat from the Lungs, clears deficiency heat, and cools the blood. Slow and long lasting hypoglycemic effect. For early stage patterns with dryness and heat in the Lung and Spleen/Stomach.

1. Li WL et al. (2004) Natural medicines used in the traditional Chinese medical system for therapy of diabetes mellitus. Journal of Ethnopharmacology 92:1–21
2. Jia W et al. (2003) Antidiabetic herbal drugs officially approved in China. Phytotherapy Research 17:1127–1134
3. Khan MS et al. (2003) Cinnamon Improves Glucose and Lipids of People With Type 2 Diabetes. Diabetes Care 12:3215–3218

肺
胃
燥
热

4.1 LUNG AND STOMACH HEAT WITH QI AND FLUID DAMAGE

Lung and Stomach heat is characterized by the classical features of polydipsia, polyphagia and polyuria, with the thirst and hunger predominant. This corresponds to the upper and middle burner patterns of xiao ke (p.158) and is a type of qi level heat pattern (p.516). The primary site of the pathology is the Stomach and Spleen. The heat affecting the Stomach has a secondary drying effect on the Lungs and mucous membranes as it rises. The proportion of heat and fluid damage varies, but in general the more damaged the fluids become, the more the bodies true yin is depleted. The heat originates from the diet, Liver qi constraint invading the Stomach and Spleen, or is the result of an external invasion of heat into the qi level (seen in type 1 DM).

Clinical features

- intense thirst, drinking large volumes of fluid; dryness of mucous membranes; constipation
- ravenous hunger
- frequent, copious urine, may be yellow or cloudy; glucosuria
- spontaneous sweating
- irritability, restlessness
- weakness, fatigue and weight loss
- mouth ulcers
- elevated blood glucose

T slightly pale to red body with a dry, patchy or peeled coat
P large, forceless and rapid, or fine and rapid

Treatment principle

Clear heat from the Lungs and Stomach
Generate and replenish fluids and moisten dryness

Prescription

BAI HU JIA REN SHEN TANG 白虎加人参汤
White Tiger plus Ginseng Decoction

This prescription is selected when strong thirst is a predominant feature. The heat is more pronounced, the patient is heat intolerant, sweats easily, the tongue red and pulse large and rapid. As the heat clears, a more qi and yin replenishing strategy (such as Yu Quan Wan in Variations), can be phased in.

shi gao (Gypsum fibrosum) 石膏 15–30g
zhi mu (Anemarrhenae Rhizoma) 知母 9–15g
gan cao (Glycyrrhizae Radix) 甘草 3–6g
ren shen (Ginseng Radix) 人参 6–9g
jing mi (rice) 粳米 15–30g

Method: Decoction. **Shi gao** is cooked for 30 minutes prior to the other herbs. **Shi gao** clears heat from the Lungs and Stomach and generates fluids to alleviate thirst; **zhi mu** clears heat and protects and nourishes yin; **ren shen** generates and protects fluids, and, with **gan cao**, replenishes qi; **jing**

mi and **gan cao** protect the Stomach and Spleen from damage by the coldness of the main herbs. (Source: *Zhong Yi Nei Ke Xue* [*Shang Han Lun*])

Modifications

- With dry cough, add **di gu pi** (Lycii Cortex) 地骨皮 12–15g and **sang bai pi** (Mori Cortex) 桑白皮 9–12g.
- With marked heat, a red tongue and irritability, increase the dose of **shi gao** to 60g, and add **huang lian** (Coptidis Rhizoma) 黄连 2–3g and **jiu da huang** (wine fried Rhei Radix et Rhizoma) 酒大黄 3–6g.
- With severe dryness and thirst, add **tian hua fen** (Trichosanthes Radix) 天花粉 18–30g, **lu gen** (Phragmitis Rhizoma) 芦根 30–60g, **mai dong** (Ophiopogonis Radix) 麦冬 9–12g and **sheng di** (Rehmanniae Radix) 生地 9–15g.
- With mouth ulcers add **huang lian** (Coptidis Rhizoma) 黄连 2–3g and **pu gong ying** (Taraxaci Herba) 蒲公英 18–30g.
- With low grade fever, lymphadenopathy or other hints of a lingering pathogen, a more venting strategy such as ZHU YE SHI GAO TANG (Lophatherus and Gypsum Decoction 竹叶石膏汤, p.370), may be used as guiding formula.
- With retinopathy and retinal micro hemorrhage, add **san qi fen** (powdered Notoginseng Radix) 三七粉 3–6g [taken separately], **xiao ji** (Cirsii Herba) 小蓟 12–15g and **bai mao gen** (Imperatae Rhizoma) 白茅根 15–30g.

Variations and additional prescriptions

With blazing Stomach fire draining Kidney yin

A strong heat pathogen can quickly deplete fluids and start to damage the deeper yin of the Kidneys. This is also known as concurrent heat in the qi and ying levels. The main pathology is located in the Stomach, Spleen and Kidneys, and in addition to the dryness, thirst and sweating, there is ravenous hunger, bad breath, mouth ulcers, toothache and bleeding gums, and frontal headache. The treatment is to clear fire from the Stomach and nourish Kidney yin with YU NÜ JIAN (Jade Women Decoction 玉女煎).

shi gao (Gypsum fibrosum) 石膏 15–30g
sheng di (Rehmanniae Radix) 生地 15–24g
mai dong (Ophiopogonis Radix) 麦冬 9–12g
zhi mu (Anemarrhenae Rhizoma) 知母 6–9g
xuan shen (Scrophulariae Radix) 玄参 12–18g

Method: Decoction. **Shi gao** is cooked for 30 minutes prior to the other herbs. **Shi gao** clears heat from the Lungs and Stomach and generates fluids to alleviate thirst; **zhi mu** clears heat and protects and nourishes yin; **sheng di** and **xuan shen** cool the blood, nourish and protect yin; **mai dong** clears heat and moistens dryness. (Source: *Wen Bing Tiao Bian*)

With heat in the Intestines and severe constipation

If the heat dries out the Intestines as it moves further down into the body, dry stools and constipation can become a major problem. It is essential to keep the bowels open and moving to keep the qi dynamic operational, and to ensure the heat has an exit. The treatment should focus on moistening and opening the bowels with a prescription such as ZENG YE CHENG QI TANG (Increase the Fluids and Order the Qi Decoction 增液承气汤, below). Once the bowels are moving, delete **da huang** and **mang xiao**. As the formula is bitter and cold, take care not to overuse it, and damage Spleen yang.

xuan shen (Scrophulariae Radix) 玄参 24–30g
sheng di (Rehmanniae Radix) 生地 15–24g
mai dong (Ophiopogonis Radix) 麦冬 15–24g
da huang (Rhei Radix et Rhizoma) 大黄 6–9g
mang xiao (Natrii Sulfas) 芒硝 6–9g

Method: Decoction. **Mang xiao** is dissolved in the strained decoction, **da huang** added towards the end of cooking. **Xuan shen**, **sheng di** and **mai dong** generate fluids, soften hardness and moisten the Intestines; they also reduce elevated blood sugar levels; **da huang** and **mang xiao** soften hardness, clear heat and open the bowels. (Source: *Zhong Yi Nei Ke Xue* [*Wen Bing Tiao Bian*])

With less heat and more qi and yin deficiency

Blazing heat in the Lungs and Stomach can quickly damage qi and yin. The features are similar, with dryness and thirst, urinary frequency and increased appetite but with increasing signs of deficiency such as a pale tongue, increasing fatigue and weakness and a weak pulse. The treatment is to supplement qi and yin, generate fluids and clear residual heat with YU QUAN WAN (Jade Spring Pill 玉泉丸).

tian hua fen (Trichosanthes Radix) 天花粉 45g
ge gen (Puerariae Radix) 葛根 45g
huang qi (Astragali Radix) 黄芪 30g
ren shen (Ginseng Radix) 人参 30g
fu ling (Poria) 茯苓 30g
sheng di (Rehmanniae Radix) 生地 30g
mai dong (Ophiopogonis Radix) 麦冬 30g
wu mei (Mume Fructus) 乌梅 30g
gan cao (Glycyrrhizae Radix) 甘草 30g

Method: Pills or powder. Grind the herbs into a fine powder and form into 9 gram pills with vinegar. The dose is one pill 2–3 time daily. **Tian hua fen** clears heat from the Lungs and Stomach, and generates yin fluids; **ge gen** encourages middle burner qi to ascend to the Lungs and generates fluids to alleviate thirst; **huang qi**, **ren shen** and **fu ling** supplement qi, generate fluids and regulate the water passages; **mai dong** nourishes Lung and Stomach yin and moistens dryness; the sourness of **wu mei** combines with the sweetness of **gan cao** to generate yin. (Source: *Shi Yong Zhong Yi Nei Ke Xue* [*Ren Zhai Zhi Zhi*])

Prepared medicines
Concentrated powder
Bai Hu Jia Ren Shen Tang (Ginseng & Gypsum Combination)
Yu Nü Jian (Rehmannia & Gypsum Combination)
  – note the prepared powder version has a slightly different composition to the synonymous formula above
Yu Quan Wan (Jade Source Combination)
Sha Shen Mai Men Dong Tang (Glehnia & Ophiopogon Combination)
  – less heat and more dryness

Pills
Yu Quan Wan (Jade Spring Teapills)

Acupuncture (select from)

Ren.12 (zhongwan –) ....alarm point of the Stomach, clears heat from the middle burner

yishu (M–BW–12) ....the pancreas transport point, improves pancreatic function; 1.5 cun lateral to spinous process of T8

Bl.13 (feishu –) ....transport points of the Lungs, Spleen and Stomach,
Bl.20 (pishu –)   these points clear heat, moisten dryness and
Bl.21 (weishu –)   nourish yin

LI.11 (quchi –)..................these points clear heat from yangming
St.43 (xianggu –)

St.36 (zusanli –) ....sea point of the Stomach, regulates Stomach and Intestine function, clears heat, strengthens the Spleen and Stomach and supplements qi

Sp.6 (sanyinjiao –).............clears heat, regulates the Spleen, Liver and Kidneys

• Ear points: spleen, lung, zero point, pancreas, endocrine

Clinical notes

• For type 2 DM, appropriate treatment can alleviate the symptoms, and reduce blood glucose levels and glucosuria. Type 1 diabetics with this pattern will require insulin.

• Lung and Stomach heat appears in the early stages of diabetes and is seen in type 1 DM and occasionally type 2 DM. This pattern may also sporadically appear in medicated patients with poorly regulated blood glucose. In type 1 DM, the underlying shaoyin deficiency enables this relatively superficial heat to penetrate deeper into the body and damage the deep yin of the Kidneys, so the pattern quickly evolves into a more severe deficiency pattern, and if untreated with insulin replacement, to death. In type 2 DM, it represents a stage of diabetes before irreparable damage has been done, and as such has a good probability of cure with appropriate treatment.

• Exercise is an essential component of treatment.

• In addition to the standard diet advice for diabetics, food to moisten dryness and clear heat can be helpful. See Clinical Handbook, Vol. 2, pp.882 and 887.

脾
胃
气
虚

4.2 SPLEEN AND STOMACH QI DEFICIENCY

Spleen and Stomach qi deficiency is at the root of type 2 diabetes. The Spleen deficiency is the result of poor diet and sedentary habits, prolonged damp heat, chronic Liver and Spleen disharmony, or treatment with hypoglycemic drugs for an excess pattern of diabetes.

Many people with Spleen qi deficiency present in the pre–diabetic stage, when their main complaints are general and non–specific – tiredness, digestive upsets, weight problems etc. Abnormal blood glucose levels or glucosuria are discovered during routine examination. Spleen qi deficiency type diabetes is often complicated by Kidney qi deficiency, damp, damp heat, phlegm or yin deficiency.

Clinical features
- fatigue, tiredness and weakness which tend to be worse mid afternoon and after eating
- muscle weakness and easy fatigue; poor muscle tone
- variable appetite that swings between indifference and cravings, especially for sweet foods and carbohydrates
- abdominal distension and early satiety
- dry mouth; may be thirst in some cases
- urination may be copious and frequent; urine may be turbid or frothy; maybe glucosuria
- pale complexion, pale lips
- loose stools or diarrhea; the bowels may move soon after eating
- spontaneous sweating, clamminess
- poor regulation of blood glucose levels; can fluctuate between low and high
- patients may be underweight or overweight

T pale, swollen and scalloped, with a thin or thick, possibly greasy, white coat
P weak, fine

Treatment principle
Strengthen the Spleen and Stomach
Supplement and regulate qi

Prescription

SHEN LING BAI ZHU SAN 参苓白术散
Ginseng, Poria and White Atractylodes Powder, modified

ren shen (Ginseng Radix) 人参 6–9g
bai zhu (Atractylodes macrocephalae Rhizoma) 白术 9–12g
fu ling (Poria) 茯苓 9–12g
shan yao (Dioscoreae Rhizoma) 山药 15–30g
zhi gan cao (Glycyrrhizae Radix preparata) 炙甘草 3–6g
bai bian dou (Dolichos Semen) 白扁豆 12–15g
yi ren (Coicis Semen) 苡仁 15–30g
lian zi (Nelumbinis Semen) 莲子 9–12g
jie geng (Platycodi Radix) 桔梗 6–9g

sha ren (Amomi Fructus) 砂仁.. 3–6g
huang qi (Astragali Radix) 黄芪 15–30g
Method: Decoction. **Ren shen, bai zhu, fu ling, shan yao, huang qi** and **zhi gan cao** strengthen the Spleen and supplement qi; **bai zhu** and **sha ren** dry damp; **shan yao** and **huang qi** regulate blood glucose; **fu ling** and **yi ren** leach out damp; **lian zi** stops leakage of fluids; **jie geng** assist Spleen qi to rise. (Source: *Zhong Yi Nei Ke Xue* [*Xiao Er Yao Zheng Zhi Jue*])

Modifications

- With Kidney qi deficiency and copious urination, add **shan zhu yu** (Corni Fructus) 山茱萸 12–18g and **tu si zi** (Cuscutae Semen) 菟丝子 9–12g.
- With edema, increase the dose of **fu ling** (Poria) 茯苓 to 18g, and add **ze xie** (Alismatis Rhizoma) 泽泻 9–12g and **che qian zi** (Plantaginis Semen) 车前子 9–12g [decocted in a cloth bag].
- With damp heat, a pale tongue with greasy yellow coat, taut abdominal bloating, nausea, mild sweats, and loose or bad smelling stools, add **xing ren** (Pruni Semen) 杏仁 12–15g, **yi ren** (Coicis Semen) 苡仁 18–30g, **hou po** (Magnoliae officinalis Cortex) 厚朴 6–9g and **bai dou kou** (Amomi Fructus rotundus) 白豆蔻 6–9g [added at the end of cooking].
- With damp heat pouring downwards, vaginitis, itching and skin sores, add **tu fu ling** (Smilacis glabrae Rhizoma) 土茯苓 12–15g, **cang zhu** (Atractylodis Rhizoma) 苍术 9–12g and **huang bai** (Phellodendri Cortex) 黄柏 3–6g.
- With phlegm, combine with **PING WEI SAN** (Calm the Stomach Powder, 平胃散, p.845)
- With yin deficiency, a centrally peeled tongue, and gnawing hunger, add **mai dong** (Ophiopogonis Radix) 麦冬 9–12g, **tian hua fen** (Trichosanthes Radix) 天花粉 12–15g and **huang jing** (Polygonati Rhizoma) 黄精 9–12g.
- With retinopathy, blurring vision and macular edema, increase the dose of **fu ling** (Poria) 茯苓 to 18g and add **cang zhu** (Atractylodis Rhizoma) 苍术 9–12g, **yi mu cao** (Leonurus Herba) 益母草 12–15g and **dan shen** (Salviae miltiorrhizae Radix) 丹参 9–12g.
- With numbness of the extremities, add **ji xue teng** (Spatholobi Caulis) 鸡血藤 15–30g, **qing feng teng** (Sinomenium Caulis) 清风藤 9–15g and **shen jin cao** (Lycopodii Herba) 伸筋草 9–15g.
- With cold and yang deficiency, add **gan jiang** (Zingiberis Rhizoma) 干姜 6–9g and **rou gui** (Cinnamomi Cortex) 肉桂 3–6g, or use **LI ZHONG WAN** (Regulate the Middle Pill 里中丸, p.732) as guiding prescription.
- With nighttime or intractable diarrhea, use **LI ZHONG WAN** (Regulate the Middle Pill 里中丸, p.732) and **SI SHEN WAN** (Four Miracle Pill 四神丸, p.920) as guiding prescription.
- With blood stasis, add **dan shen** (Salviae miltiorrhizae Radix) 丹参 9–12g and **ji xue teng** (Spatholobi Caulis) 鸡血藤 15–30g.
- With Liver qi constraint, add **chai hu** (Bupleuri Radix) 柴胡 6–9g and **bai shao** (Paeoniae Radix alba) 白芍 9–12g.
- With foggy head and muscle aches, add **shi chang pu** (Acori tatarinowii Rhizoma) 石菖蒲 6–9g and **yuan zhi** (Polygalae Radix) 远志 6–9g.
- With food stagnation, add **shan zha** (Crataegi Fructus) 山楂 12–15g, **chao**

mai ya (stir fried Hordei Fructus germinantus) 炒麦芽 15–30g and **chao shen qu** (stir fried Massa medicata fermentata) 炒神曲 12–15g.

Prepared medicines
Concentrated powders
Shen Ling Bai Zhu San (Ginseng & Atractylodes Formula)
Li Zhong Tang (Ginseng & Ginger Combination)
– Spleen yang deficiency
Xiang Sha Liu Jun Zi Tang (Vladmiria & Amomum Combination)
– with phlegm damp
Sheng Mai San (Ginseng & Ophiopogon Formula)
– combine with one of the above when there is yin deficiency
Yu Quan Wan (Jade Source Combination)
– Spleen qi and yin deficiency

Pills
Shen Ling Bai Zhu Wan (Absorption and Digestion Pill, Shen Ling Bai Zhu Pian)
Sheng Mai Wan (Great Pulse Teapills)
Yu Quan Wan (Jade Spring Teapills)

Acupuncture (select from)
Ren.12 (zhongwan +▲).......alarm point of the Stomach, strengthens the Spleen and Stomach, supplements qi and stimulates the qi dynamic

St.36 (zusanli +▲) ....sea point of the Stomach, strengthens the Spleen and Stomach, supplements qi and transforms damp

Sp.6 (sanyinjiao +)..............strengthens the Spleen and Kidney and supplements qi and yin

Sp.3 (taibai).......................source and connecting points of the Spleen and
St.40 (fenglong)   Stomach; these points strengthen the Spleen and have a special effect on damp and the qi dynamic

Bl.20 (pishu +▲) ....transport points of the Spleen and Stomach, warm
Bl.21 (weishu +▲)   and strengthen middle burner qi

yishu (M–BW–12) ....the pancreas transport point, improves pancreatic function; 1.5 cun lateral to spinous process of T8

- with Liver qi constraint, add Liv.3 (taichong) and PC.6 (neiguan)
- with damp heat, add St.44 (neiting –) and LI.11 (quchi –)
- with yin deficiency, add Kid.6 (zhaohai)
- with edema, add Sp.9 (yinlingquan –) and St.28 (shuidao –)
- with foggy head, add Bl.62 (shenmai)
- with diarrhea, add St.25 (tianshu) and St.37 (shangjuxu)
- with abdominal distension, add St.25 (tianshu) and Sp.15 (daheng)
- Ear points: spleen, stomach, pancreas, zero point, endocrine

Clinical notes
- This is a common pattern of pre–diabetes, poor regulation of blood sugar with episodes of high and low blood sugar, and early type 2 DM. In patients not

medicated with insulin, improvement in Spleen function and blood sugar regulation can be expected quite quickly. Sustained results may be expected within a few months, and as long as the diet and activity levels are maintained, the prognosis for full recovery is good.

- Patients are likely to be medicated with oral hypoglycemic agents, and the Spleen deficiency may be due to their side effects. Metformin (Box 4.2, p.167) in particular can aggravate weakness of the Spleen. Because of its iatrogenic effect, patients often find that Metformin becomes less effective quite quickly in this pattern.

- Treatment to strengthen the Spleen will lower blood glucose which, in combination with conventional hypoglycemic drugs, can lead to episodes of hypoglycemia. Patients should be alerted to the possibility of hypoglycemia and be educated as to the signs and symptoms to watch for. If hypoglycemia occurs the dose of conventional hypoglycemic agents should be reviewed. The ultimate aim of treatment should be to reduce the dose and need for conventional hypoglycemic agents as Spleen function and blood sugar regulation improves.

- Take care when using hot or pungent warm herbs if there are signs of cold or yang deficiency, as excessive application can promote the development of dryness, heat and yin damage.

- When thirst is a feature, it is important to clearly differentiate it from the thirst of an internal heat pattern, because use of bitter or sweet and cold heat clearing herbs will aggravate the deficiency. The mechanism of the thirst is failure of the qi dynamic, and the ascent of fluids to the upper burner, so it is an apparent thirst rather a true thirst. The more yin deficiency that complicates the qi deficiency, however, the more true dryness will be seen. The degree of yin deficiency can usually be quickly assessed by looking at the tongue, which will be thin or peeled in the centre.

- Diet and exercise are essential components of treatment. In addition to the standard diet advice suitable for diabetics, a low carbohydrate version of the diet aimed at strengthening the Spleen is recommended. See Clinical Handbook, Vol. 2, p.870.

痰
湿
阻
滞

4.3 PHLEGM DAMP

Phlegm damp diabetes is always type 2, and can be acquired by overeating and a phlegm inducing diet, or it can be constitutional. Patients with a constitutional tendency to phlegm damp will note they were overweight from an early age, and that other family members suffer diabetes or weight related problems. Occasionally, however, the patient is not overweight, and signs of phlegm are not particularly obvious, but the patient gets worse with yin, qi and blood supplementing treatments, so the diagnosis is made by default. Phlegm damp is usually complicated by Spleen qi deficiency and constrained Liver qi.

Patients with phlegm type diabetes are especially prone to the phlegm type complications of diabetes, such as cardiovascular and atherosclerotic disease. Phlegm, however, need not be a primary pattern to cause complications. It can be secondary to other pathologies, and frequently appears as a complicating factor of common deficiency patterns like qi and yin deficiency.

Clinical features

- dry mouth and thirst; sticky sensation in the mouth; thick saliva
- vertigo and dizziness; foggy head
- puffy face; thick fingers; muscles feel firm
- often overweight
- tiredness, heaviness, lassitude
- heaviness, oppression and aching in the chest
- abdominal bloating, acid reflux, belching, sweet cravings
- alternating loose and sluggish stools; or constipation (but stools not dry)
- elevated blood glucose
- may be phlegm type masses, such as polycystic ovaries, fibrocystic breast disease, lipomata or thyroid nodules
- numbness, heaviness and tingling in the feet and legs; may be edema with or without venous congestion

T normal to pale, swollen and fat, with a thin or thick greasy, white coat
P deep, wiry, slippery

Treatment Principle

Transform phlegm damp and assist the qi dynamic
Strengthen the Spleen and Stomach and supplement qi

Prescription

CANG FU DAO TAN WAN 苍附导痰丸
Guide Out Phlegm Pill with Atractylodes and Cyperus, modified

cang zhu (Atractylodis Rhizoma) 苍术	9–15g
xiang fu (Cyperi Rhizoma) 香附	6–9g
zhi ban xia (Pinelliae Rhizoma preparatum) 制半夏	9–12g
fu ling (Poria) 茯苓	9–15g
chen pi (Citri reticulatae Pericarpium) 陈皮	6–9g
gan cao (Glycyrrhizae Radix) 甘草	3–6g

dan nan xing (Arisaema cum Bile) 胆南星 6–9g

zhi ke (Aurantii Fructus) 枳壳 6–9g

sheng jiang (Zingiberis Rhizoma recens) 生姜 6–9g

shan zha (Crataegi Fructus) 山楂 9–12g

huang qi (Astragali Radix) 黄芪 12–15g

Method: Pills or powder. Grind the herbs to a fine powder and form into 6 gram pills with water. The dose is one pill 2–3 times daily. Can also be decocted with the doses as shown. **Zhi ban xia, cang zhu, fu ling, chen pi** and **gan cao** strengthen the Spleen, dry damp and transform phlegm; **xiang fu** and **zhi ke** regulate qi and alleviate qi constraint; **dan nan xing** transforms phlegm and clears heat; **sheng jiang** harmonizes the Stomach; **shan zha** improves digestion and activates blood; **huang qi** supplements qi. (Source: *Zhong Yi Fu Chan Ke Xue* [*Ye Tian Shi Nu Ke Zhi Liao Mi Fang*])

Modifications

- With chest pain, or chest oppression and breathlessness, add **quan gua lou** (Trichosanthis Fructus) 全栝楼 18–30g and **dan shen** (Salviae miltiorrhizae Radix) 丹参 9–12g.

- With phlegm masses (includes hard exudates in the retina), add **xuan shen** (Scrophulariae Radix) 玄参 9–12g, **mu li** (Ostreae Concha) 牡蛎 15–30g and **zhe bei mu** (Fritillariae thunbergii Bulbus) 浙贝母 9–12g.

- With retinopathy and macular edema, add **yi mu cao** (Leonurus Herba) 益母草 12–15g and **ze lan** (Lycopi Herba) 泽兰 9–12g.

- With numbness of the extremities, add **wei ling xian** (Clematidis Radix) 威灵仙 9–12g and **jiang huang** (Curcumae longae Rhizoma) 姜黄 9–12g.

- With amenorrhea, add **dang gui** (Angelicae sinensis Radix) 当归 6–9g, **chuan xiong** (Chuanxiong Rhizoma) 川芎 6–9g and **ji xue teng** (Spatholobi Caulis) 鸡血藤 12–15g.

- With a very dry mouth and tongue, decrease the dose of **zhi ban xia** and **dan nan xing** by 50%, and add **tian hua fen** (Trichosanthes Radix) 天花粉 12–15g and **mai dong** (Ophiopogonis Radix) 麦冬 6–9g.

- With turbid urine, add **bi xie** (Dioscoreae hypoglaucae Rhizoma) 萆薢 9–12g.

- With heat, a yellow tongue coat and flushing, add **zhi mu** (Anemarrhenae Rhizoma) 知母 6–9g and **huang lian** (Coptidis Rhizoma) 黄连 3–6g.

- With edema, increase the dose of **fu ling** to 15g and add **bi xie** (Dioscoreae hypoglaucae Rhizoma) 萆薢 9–12g.

- With blood stasis, add **dan shen** (Salviae miltiorrhizae Radix) 丹参 9–12g, **hu zhang** (Polygoni cuspidati Rhizoma) 虎杖 9–12g and **san qi fen** (powdered Notoginseng Radix) 三七粉 3–6g.

Prepared medicines

Concentrated powders

Ping Wei San (Magnolia & Ginger Formula) and Er Chen Tang (Citrus & Pinellia Combination) plus Qing Qi Hua Tang Wan (Pinellia & Scute Formula)

Wen Dan Tang (Poria & Bamboo Combination)

Xiang Sha Liu Jun Zi Tang (Vladmiria & Amomum Combination)
    – with qi deficiency

Xiao Luo Wan (Scrophularia & Fritillaria Combination)
    – add with phlegm masses

Xiang Sha Ping Wei San (Cyperus, Amomum & Atractylodes Formula)
 – with food stagnation, sluggish stools and disruption to the qi dynamic
Pills
Ping Wei San (Calm Stomach Teapills, Tabellae Pingwei)
Mu Xiang Shun Qi Wan (Aplotaxis Carminative Pills, Shun Qi Wan)
 – with Liver qi constraint
Xiang Sha Yang Wei Wan (Appetite and Digestion Pill, Hsiang Sha Yang Wei Pien)
 – with heartburn

Acupuncture (select from)

Ren.12 (zhongwan –) ....alarm point of the Stomach, strengthens the Spleen
and supplements qi to transform phlegm damp

Sp.3 (taibai).......................source and connecting points of the Spleen and
St.40 (fenglong –)   Stomach, these points transform phlegm damp,
strengthen the Spleen and correct the qi dynamic

St.36 (zusanli +▲) ....sea point of the Stomach, strengthens the Spleen and
Stomach and corrects the qi dynamic

PC.5 (jianshi)....................river point of the Pericardium, transforms phlegm

Bl.15 (xinshu) ....transport point of the Heart, activates qi and blood

Bl.18 (ganshu –).................transport point of the Liver, activates qi and blood

yishu (M–BW–12) ....the pancreas transport point, improves pancreatic
function; 1.5 cun lateral to spinous process of T8

Bl.20 (pishu) ....transport point of the Spleen, strengthens the Spleen
to transform phlegm

• with foggy head, add GB.20 (fengchi)
• with polycystic ovaries, add St.29 (guilai –)
• with sluggish stools or constipation, add SJ.6 (zhigou –) and St.37 (shangjuxu –)
• with heat, add St.41 (jiexi –) and PC.7 (daling –)
• with cold, use moxa
• Ear points: spleen, stomach, zero point, pancreas, endocrine

Clinical notes

• Resolution of phlegm, especially when there is a constitutional component, is slow. When diet is the cause, resolution can be quicker if the diet is modified. Regardless of the etiology, as the phlegm clears, a Spleen strengthening strategy should be phased in.
• These patients will usually be taking Metformin, which can weaken the Spleen and aggravate the underlying qi deficiency.
• Patients with phlegm damp and diabetes often find weight loss difficult, even when dietary moderation and increased exercise levels are maintained. Blood sugar levels, however, can be managed reasonably well with regular treatment.
• The heaviness and lethargy typical of phlegm damp can be impediments to exercise, but graded exercise in groups can achieve good results.
• In addition to the standard diet advice for diabetics, a phlegm damp resolving diet should be adopted. See Clinical Handbook, Vol. 2, p.880.

湿
热
中
阻

4.4 DAMP HEAT BLOCKING THE MIDDLE BURNER

Damp heat develops as a result of overeating and excess alcohol consumption, particularly if the diet is a rich one. It may also be caused or exacerbated by Spleen qi deficiency which allows the formation of damp and damp heat. Occasionally, this pattern of diabetes may follow an external invasion of damp or damp heat, and may be described as damp heat in the qi level (see p.516–517).

By the time a patient is diagnosed with diabetes, or found to be hyperglyce-mic, the damp heat is complicated by varying degrees of qi and yin deficiency, as heat gradually damages yin and dampness weakens Spleen qi. Treatment therefore should transform damp without excessively drying and damaging yin, and clear heat without excessive use of bitter coldness that can damage yang qi. The thirst of this pattern is usually associated with blockage of the qi dynamic and failure of fluids to ascend to the mouth, rather than as a direct effect of heat, and so tends to be moderate. As the damp heat clears, patients are left with Spleen qi and/or yin deficiency, and treatment to strengthen the Spleen and replenish yin should be gradually phased in.

Prolonged damp heat will gradually thicken further into phlegm, which lodges in the blood vessels and channels blocking qi and blood, and contributing to the common complications of chronic diabetes, in particular neuropathy, chronic in-fections and poor wound healing.

Clinical features
- moderate thirst or dryness without a great desire to drink
- sense of hunger without much desire to eat; bitter taste, bad breath
- ruddy, plethoric complexion
- epigastric and abdominal fullness and distension
- muscle aches and heaviness
- sluggish bad smelling stools, or constipation
- patients often overweight or obese, especially around the abdomen
- glucosuria, frothy, turbid or concentrated urine
- elevated blood glucose
- may be pruritus, recurrent boils, superficial infections or thrush; numbness or a burning sensation in the feet

T thick, dry or greasy, white or yellow coat
P soggy, slippery, maybe rapid

Treatment principle
Clear damp heat from the middle burner
Supplement qi and yin as necessary

Prescription
GAN LU YIN 甘露饮
Sweet Dew Drink

This prescription is selected when damp heat is moderate and complicated by a degree of qi and yin deficiency. This is a common presentation of recently diagnosed type 2 diabetes. Depending on the balance of yin deficiency and damp heat, this prescription may upset the digestion. If so, the next prescription may be better tolerated.

sheng di (Rehmanniae Radix) 生地 9–15g
shu di (Rehmanniae Radix preparata) 熟地 9–15g
tian dong (Asparagi Radix) 天冬 9–12g
mai dong (Ophiopogonis Radix) 麦冬 9–12g
pi pa ye (Eriobotryae Folium) 枇杷叶 6–12g
huang qin (Scutellariae Radix) 黄芩 9–12g
yin chen (Artemisiae scopariae Herba) 茵陈 9–12g
yu zhu (Polygonati odorati Rhizoma) 玉竹 12–15g
zhi ke (Aurantii Fructus) 枳壳 6–9g
gan cao (Glycyrrhizae Radix) 甘草 3–6g

Method: Decoction. **Huang qin** and **yin chen** clear and drain damp heat; **pi pa ye** diffuses the Lungs and assists the Lungs control of the water passages; **zhi ke** regulates middle burner qi and directs qi downwards so it can be cleared through the 'big exit'; **sheng di**, **shu di**, **tian dong**, **mai dong** and **yu zhu** nourish yin and fluids; **gan cao** clears heat and harmonizes the formula. **Sheng di**, **shu di** and **mai dong** reduce blood glucose. (Source: *Zui Xin Fang Ji Shou Ce* [*He Ji Ju Fang*])

Modifications

- With numbness, tingling or aching in the legs and feet, add **lao guan cao** (Erodii/Geranii Herba) 老鹳草 15–30g, **ren dong teng** (Lonicerae Caulis) 忍冬藤 15–30g, **xi xian cao** (Siegesbeckia Herba) 豨莶草 9–15g and **dan shen** (Salviae miltiorrhizae Radix) 丹参 9–12g, or combine with Sɪ Mɪᴀᴏ Sᴀɴ (Four Marvel Powder 四妙散 p.595).

- With suppurative lesions or recurrent infections, add **tu fu ling** (Smilacis glabrae Rhizoma) 土茯苓 12–15g, **tian hua fen** (Trichosanthes Radix) 天花粉 12–15g, **jin yin hua** (Lonicerae Flos) 金银花 15–30g and **lian qiao** (Forsythiae Fructus) 连翘 9–12g.

- With vaginitis and yellow leukorrhea, add **tu fu ling** (Smilacis glabrae Rhizoma) 土茯苓 12–15g and **bai zhi** (Angelicae dahuricae Radix) 白芷 6–9g.

- With cloudy urine, add **bi xie** (Dioscoreae hypoglaucae Rhizoma) 萆薢 9–12g.

- With marked damp, severe abdominal distension and a thick tongue coat, add **huo xiang** (Pogostemonis/Agastaches Herba) 藿香 12–15g, **sha ren** (Amomi Fructus) 砂仁 6–9g [these two added at the end of cooking] and **mu xiang** (Aucklandiae Radix) 木香 6–9g.

- With marked dryness, add **shi gao** (Gypsum fibrosum) 石膏 15–30g [cooked first] and **zhi mu** (Anemarrhenae Rhizoma) 知母 9–12g.

- With digestive upset, delete **shu di**, and add **cang zhu** (Atractylodis Rhizoma) 苍术 9–12g and **xuan shen** (Scrophulariae Radix) 玄参 9–12g.

- With sluggish bowels or constipation, add **zhi da huang** (processed Rhei Radix et Rhizoma) 制大黄 6–9g and **bing lang** (Arecae Semen) 槟榔 6–9g.

- With edema, add **han fang ji** (Stephaniae tetrandrae Radix) 汉防己 9–12g, **chi fu ling** (Poria Rubra) 赤茯苓 12–15g and **bi xie** (Dioscoreae hypoglaucae Rhizoma) 萆薢 9–12g.

HUANG QIN HUA SHI TANG 黄芩滑石汤
Scutellaria and Talcum Decoction, modified

This prescription is selected when the damp heat is more pronounced and the patient displays few signs of deficiency. These patients may appear robust, and the hyperglycemia may have been detected with a routine screen. The modifications to the previous prescription also apply.

huang qin (Scutellariae Radix) 黄芩 9–12g
hua shi (Talcum) 滑石 12–15g
fu ling pi (Poriae Cutis) 茯苓皮 9–12g
zhu ling (Polyporus) 猪苓 9–12g
tong cao (Tetrapanacis Medulla) 通草 6–9g
da fu pi (Arecae Pericarpium) 大腹皮 9–12g
bai dou kou (Amomi Fructus rotundus) 白豆蔻 6–9g
cang zhu (Atractylodis Rhizoma) 苍术 9–12g
xuan shen (Scrophulariae Radix) 玄参 9–12g

Method: Decoction. **Hua shi** is decocted in a cloth bag. **Huang qin** clears damp heat; **hua shi** drains damp heat via the urine; **fu ling pi**, **zhu ling** and **tong cao** promote urination to drain damp heat; **da fu pi** and **bai dou kou** move qi, free up the qi dynamic, transform damp and promote urination; **cang zhu** and **xuan shen** clear heat, dry damp, protect yin and reduce high blood glucose levels. (Source: *Zhong Yi Nei Ke Xue* [*Wen Bing Tiao Bian*])

Prepared medicines
Concentrated powder
Gan Lu Yin (Sweet Combination)
Gan Lu Xiao Du Dan (Forsythia & Acorus Formula)
 – with pronounced damp heat
Fang Feng Tong Sheng San (Siler & Platycodon Formula)
 – with constipation

Pills
Fang Feng Tong Sheng Wan (Ledebouriella Sagely Unblocks Teapills)

Acupuncture (select from)
yishu (M–BW–12) ....the pancreas transport point, improves pancreatic function; 1.5 cun lateral to spinous process of T8
Bl.20 (pishu –) ....transport points of the Spleen and Stomach, clear
Bl.21 (weishu –)   damp heat from the middle burner
Bl.39 (weiyang –) ....lower sea point of the triple burner, promotes urination to clear damp heat
Ren.12 (zhongwan –) ....these points clear damp heat from the middle
Sp.15 (daheng –)   burner, regulate Intestinal function and promote
St.25 (tianshu)   bowel movement to clear heat
Sp.9 (yinlingquan –)...........sea point of the Spleen, clears damp heat
Sp.6 (sanyinjiao).................clears damp heat, regulates Spleen, Liver, Kidneys
St.36 (zusanli –) ....sea point of the Stomach, regulates Stomach and Intestine function, strengthens the Spleen and Stomach and supplements qi

- with heat greater than damp, add St.45 (lidui ↓) and St.40 (fenglong −)
- with nausea, add PC.6 (neiguan −)
- with abdominal pain, add Sp.8 (diji −) and Sp.4 (gongsun −)
- Ear points: spleen, liver, zero point, pancreas, endocrine

Clinical notes

- Damp heat is a common clinical presentation of type 2 diabetes. It is usually complicated by Spleen qi and yin deficiency, but when the damp heat is predominant it must be addressed before supplementation can commence.
- An important point to remember is the use of gentle damp heat clearing herbs in this case so as to avoid exacerbating any underlying qi and yin deficiency.
- Damp heat can be cleared, or at least significantly reduced, relatively quickly, as long as the patient attends to their diet and exercises sufficiently. As the pattern changes, regular revision of the treatment strategy is necessary. Monitoring bowel habits will give some indication of the state of the Spleen qi. Some looseness is expected and desirable in the early stages of treatment as the damp heat is clearing, but persistent loose bowels suggest that the Spleen is being weakened.
- Regular aerobic exercise, and weight loss if warranted, are essential components of treatment and are a particularly effective management tool in this pattern. Weight loss alone will significantly improve blood glucose regulation.
- In addition to the standard dietary advice for diabetics, a damp heat clearing diet is recommended. See Clinical Handbook, Vol. 2, p.884.
- Hot spot therapy is helpful. See p.923.
- Patients with damp heat diabetes generally do well with the oral hypoglycemic agents, at least in the early stages of treatment. Their bitter coldness clears damp heat but gradually damages Spleen qi, and their effectiveness wanes over time.

肝
脾
郁
热

4.5 LIVER AND SPLEEN DISHARMONY WITH CONSTRAINED HEAT

This pattern describes a clinical picture which occurs when constrained Liver qi invades and weakens the Spleen and creates heat. The constrained heat and qi deficiency gradually deplete yin. This pattern is seen when glucose regulation is impaired, or in the early stage of type 2 DM. The development of diabetes or poor blood glucose regulation follows a period of high or prolonged stress. The mix of Liver qi constraint, Spleen qi deficiency and heat is known as the primary pathological triad, and the balance of pathology, and therefore the solution, can vary (see Variations).

Clinical features
- thirst, dry mouth and throat
- bitter taste in the mouth
- variable appetite, sometimes ravenous, sometimes poor
- irritability, anger
- dry, red, or sore irritated eyes
- stiff and sore neck and shoulders; tension or migraine headaches
- colicky abdominal pain and distension; sluggish bowels or constipation; maybe alternating with loose bowels; flatulence, belching, heartburn
- irregular menstruation, premenstrual symptoms
- elevated blood glucose; may be mild glucosuria
- symptoms are worse with stress
- usually normal body weight or thin; rarely overweight

T red edges, or swollen and slightly scalloped with redder edges and a thin, yellow coat

P wiry, fine, maybe rapid

Treatment principle
Harmonize the Liver and Spleen
Clear heat and cool the Liver and Stomach

Prescription

JIA WEI XIAO YAO SAN 加味逍遥散
Augmented Rambling Powder, modified

chai hu (Bupleuri Radix) 柴胡 6–9g
dang gui (Angelicae sinensis Radix) 当归 6–9g
bai shao (Paeoniae Radix alba) 白芍 9–12g
bai zhu (Atractylodis macrocephalae Rhizoma) 白术 9–12g
fu ling (Poria) 茯苓 9–12g
zhi gan cao (Glycyrrhizae Radix preparata) 炙甘草 3–6g
shan zhi zi (Gardeniae Fructus) 山栀子 6–9g
mu dan pi (Moutan Cortex) 牡丹皮 6–9g
sheng jiang (Zingiberis Rhizoma recens) 生姜 6–9g
bo he (Mentha haplocalycis Herba) 薄荷 2–3g

huang jing (Polygonati Rhizoma) 黄精 9–15g
ge gen (Puerariae Radix) 葛根 9–15g

Method: Decoction. **Chai hu** dredges the Liver and alleviates constrained qi; **dang gui** and **bai shao** nourish Liver blood and soften the Liver; **bai zhu** and **fu ling** strengthen the Spleen and dry and leach out damp through the urine; **zhi gan cao** supplements qi and, with **bai shao**, eases muscle spasms; **sheng jiang** warms and harmonizes the Stomach; **bo he** assists **chai hu** in moving Liver qi; **mu dan pi** activates and cools the blood; **shan zhi zi** clears heat from all three burners and promotes urination, to provide an exit for the heat; **huang jing** supplements qi and yin and reduces blood glucose; **ge gen** generates fluids and reduces blood glucose. (Source: *Zhong Yi Nei Ke Xue* [*Nei Ke Zhai Yao*])

Modifications

- With damp heat, add **cang zhu** (Atractylodis Rhizoma) 苍术 9–12g and **xuan shen** (Scrophulariae Radix) 玄参 9–12g.
- With dryness and yin deficiency, add **xuan shen** (Scrophulariae Radix) 玄参 12–15g, **sheng di** (Rehmanniae Radix) 生地 9–12g and **mai dong** (Ophiopogonis Radix) 麦冬 9–12g.
- With marked Spleen qi deficiency, delete **shan zhi zi** and **mu dan pi**, and add **shan yao** (Dioscoreae Rhizoma) 山药 15–30g and **huang qi** (Astragali Radix) 黄芪 15–30g.
- With blood stasis, add **dan shen** (Salviae miltiorrhizae Radix) 丹参 9–12g.
- With depression, add **he huan pi** (Albizziae Cortex) 合欢皮 12–15g and **ye jiao teng** (Polygoni multiflori Caulis) 夜胶藤 15–30g.

Variations and additional prescriptions
The primary pathological triad

Liver qi constraint with Spleen qi deficiency and heat or damp heat constitutes the primary pathological triad. These three pathologies frequently occur together, and are tightly interlinked and self perpetuating. Depending on the precise balance of the three components, the treatment strategy and prescription will change (see Figure 10.2, p.477). In practice, the balance of pathology often iterates into a more or less equal mixture of all three, in which case an equally well balanced prescription can be used to address it. This is **XIAO CHAI HU TANG** (Minor Bupleurum Decoction 小柴胡汤, p.90), which can be suitably modified with herbs drawn from Table 4.3, p.168–169. Variant formulae with slightly different therapeutic action are noted below.

Prepared medicines
Concentrated powder

Jia Wei Xiao Yao San (Bupleurum & Peony Formula) plus Yu Quan Wan (Jade Source Combination)
  – can be added proportionately, depending on damage to Stomach yin
Xiao Chai Hu Tang (Minor Bupleurum Combination)
Chai Xian Tang (Bupleurum & Scute Combination)
  – primary pathological triad with more thirst
Chai Ling Tang (Bupleurum & Poria Combination)
  – primary pathological triad with diarrhea and vomiting

Da Chai Hu Tang (Major Bupleurum Combination)
 – primary pathological triad with dryness and constipation

Pills

Jia Wei Xiao Yao Wan (Free and Easy Wanderer Plus Teapills, Dan Zhi Xiao Yao Wan)
 plus Yu Quan Wan (Jade Spring Teapills)

Xiao Chai Hu Wan (Minor Bupleurum Teapills)

Acupuncture (select from)

yishu (M–BW–12) ....the pancreas transport point, improves pancreatic function; 1.5 cun lateral to spinous process of T8

Bl.18 (ganshu –) ....transport point of the Liver, dredges the Liver and regulates qi

Bl.20 (pishu +) ....transport point of the Spleen, strengthens the Spleen and supplements qi

Liv.3 (taichong) ....source point of the Liver, dredges the Liver and regulates qi

PC.6 (neiguan) ....regulates Liver qi and the middle burner, stimulates the qi dynamic (with St.36), and calms the shen

St.36 (zusanli +) ....sea point of the Stomach, strengthens the Spleen, supplements qi and stimulates the qi dynamic

Sp.6 (sanyinjiao)................regulates the Liver, strengthens the Spleen and Kidneys, supplements qi, blood and yin, and activates qi and blood

- with marked heat, add Liv.2 (xingjian –) and St.44 (neiting –)
- with headaches, add GB.34 (yanglingquan –) and GB.21 (jianjing)
- with abdominal pain, add Ren.12 (zhongwan –) and St.34 (liangqiu –)
- Ear points: spleen, liver, zero point, pancreas, endocrine, sympathetic

Clinical notes

- Stress is the main contributor to this pattern, so the influence of the diet may not be as significant as it is in the other patterns. However, patients should be educated as to the standard diabetic approach to the diet, and an appropriate diet for maintaining qi flow. See Clinical Handbook, Vol. 2, p.876 and 878.
- Exercise is an essential component of treatment, with aerobic exercise the most beneficial. The aim should be to do at least an 1–2 hours per day of sustained activity. For those with significant deficiency, working up to this level slowly as their qi improves, over a period of weeks to months, is recommended. Walking and weight training are ideal. Patients exhibiting this pattern will find that when undertaken regularly, this level of exercise alone will maintain their blood glucose levels, and keep the qi and blood moving. See p.103 for specifics.
- Hot spot therapy is helpful. See p.923.

气
阴
两
虚

4.6 QI AND YIN DEFICIENCY

This is the most common pattern of chronic diabetes, and may be seen in both type 1 and type 2 diabetes. It reflects the progressive relationship between the two main centres of pathology, the middle burner (taiyin) and the lower burner (shaoyin). The qi deficiency reflects the fundamental weakness of the Spleen, while the yin deficiency is of the Kidneys. The symptoms of diabetes can be muted or absent, as qi deficiency and yin deficiency can moderate each other's effects, and patients are usually medicated with either insulin, hypoglycemic agents or both. Patients who are medicated and reasonably well managed with hypoglycemic agents or insulin will have few of the typical symptoms noted below, but the disease process is still present and progressive. Qi and yin deficiency is usually the default pattern of patients who present, exhibiting few symptoms, with chronic managed diabetes. Patients with qi and yin deficiency almost always have complications of varying degrees, either phlegm or blood stasis, or both.

Clinical features
- dry mouth, throat, skin, hair and mucous membranes
- increased urinary frequency; nocturia
- fatigue and weakness
- pale complexion with red cheeks
- breathlessness and palpitations
- lower back and legs weak and aching
- spontaneous sweating; mild night sweats
- sense of heat in the hands and feet
- digestive weakness, easy abdominal distension, nausea, constipation
- may be numbness and tingling in the extremities; visual weakness or blurring, mild facial and peripheral edema
- may be elevated blood glucose and glucosuria

T slightly red, swollen, scalloped tongue, with a thin white, dry or patchy coat; or dry and swollen with multiple surface cracks

P deep, weak, fine

Treatment principle
Strengthen the Spleen and Kidney
Supplement qi and yin

Prescription

SHENG MAI SAN 生脉散
Generate the Pulse Powder, plus
ZENG YE TANG 增液汤
Increase the Fluids Decoction, modified

---

ren shen (Ginseng Radix) 人参 6–9g
mai dong (Ophiopogonis Radix) 麦冬 9–15g
wu wei zi (Schizandrae Fructus) 五味子 6–9g
xuan shen (Scrophulariae Radix) 玄参 15–24g

sheng di (Rehmanniae Radix) 生地 18–30g
shan yao (Dioscoreae Rhizoma) 山药 18–30g
huang qi (Astragali Radix) 黄芪 15–30g
cang zhu (Atractylodis Rhizoma) 苍术 9–12g
dan shen (Salviae miltiorrhizae Radix) 丹参 9–12g

Method: Pills or powder. Grind the herbs to a fine powder and take 6–9 grams as a draft with water twice daily. **Ren shen, shan yao** and **huang qi** strengthen the Spleen, supplement qi and regulate blood glucose; **mai dong, xuan shen** and **sheng di** nourish Spleen and Kidney yin and regulate blood glucose; **cang zhu** balances the cloying nature of the rich yin supplements and assists Spleen transformation; **dan shen** activates blood. (Source: *Shi Yong Zhong Yi Nei Ke Xue* [*Nei Wai Shang Bian Huo Lun / Wen Bing Tiao Bian*])

Modifications

- With blood stasis and peripheral vascular disease, add **dang gui** (Angelicae sinensis Radix) 当归 6–9g, **chi shao** (Paeoniae Radix rubra) 赤芍 9–12g and **di long** (Pheretima) 地龙 6–9g, or combine with Bᴜ Yᴀɴɢ Hᴜᴀɴ Wᴜ Tᴀɴɢ (Supplement Yang to Restore Five Tenths Decoction 补阳还五汤, p.600).
- With numbness and neuropathy, add **qin jiao** (Gentianae macrophyllae Radix) 秦艽 9–12g and **qiang huo** (Notopterygii Rhizoma seu Radix) 羌活 9–12g.
- With retinal microaneurysm and macular edema, add **yi mu cao** (Leonurus Herba) 益母草 15–20g, **fu ling** (Poria) 茯苓 12–15g and **che qian zi** (Plantaginis Semen) 车前子 9–12g [cooked in a cloth bag], or combine with Gᴜɪ Zʜɪ Fᴜ Lɪɴɢ Wᴀɴ (Cinnamon Twig and Poria Pill 桂枝茯苓丸, p.27).
- With retinal hemorrhage, add **san qi fen** (powdered Notoginseng Radix) 三七粉 3–6g [taken separately], **ce bai ye** (Platycladi Cacumen) 侧柏叶 9–12g and **han lian cao** (Ecliptae Herba) 旱莲草 9–12g.
- With blurring vision and hard retinal exudates from phlegm accumulation, combine with Wᴇɴ Dᴀɴ Tᴀɴɢ (Warm Gallbladder Decoction 温旦汤, p.87).
- With visual weakness or blurring vision from Liver yin deficiency, combine with Qɪ Jᴜ Dɪ Hᴜᴀɴɢ Wᴀɴ (Lycium Fruit, Chrysanthemum and Rehmannia Pill 杞菊地黄丸, p.467).
- With angina, add **dan shen** (Salviae miltiorrhizae Radix) 丹参 9–12g, **quan gua lou** (Trichosanthis Fructus) 全栝楼 18–30g and **jiang xiang** (Dalbergiae odoriferae Lignum) 降香 9–12g.
- With high cholesterol and triglycerides, add **shan zha** (Crataegi Fructus) 山楂 12–15g, **he shou wu** (Polygoni multiflori Radix) 何首乌 9–12g, **hu zhang** (Polygoni cuspidati Rhizoma) 虎杖 9–12g and **san qi fen** (powdered Notoginseng Radix) 三七粉 3–6g [taken separately].
- With high blood pressure, add **gou teng** (Uncariae Ramulus cum Uncis) 钩藤 9–12g, **chuan niu xi** (Cyathulae Radix) 川牛膝 12–15g and **dan shen** (Salviae miltiorrhizae Radix) 丹参 9–12g.
- With impaired renal function, nephropathy, proteinuria and edema, add **yi mu cao** (Leonurus Herba) 益母草 15–20g, **hu zhang** (Polygoni cuspidati Rhizoma) 虎杖 9–12g, **dan shen** (Salviae miltiorrhizae Radix) 丹参 9–12g and **xian ling pi** (Epimedii Herba) 仙灵脾 12–15g.

- With recurrent boils and skin infections, combine with WEN QING YIN (Warming and Clearing Drink 温请饮, p.400).
- If glucosuria does not decrease, add **tian hua fen** (Trichosanthes Radix) 天花粉 30g and **wu mei** (Mume Fructus) 乌梅 15–24g.
- With ketonuria, add **huang lian** (Coptidis Rhizoma) 黄连 3–6 and **huang qin** (Scutellariae Radix) 黄芩 3–6g.
- With mild edema, combine with WU LING SAN (Five Ingredient Powder with Poria 五苓散, p.219–220); with significant edema, combine with JI SHENG SHEN QI WAN (Kidney Qi Pill from Formulas to Aid the Living 济生肾气丸, p.248).
- With diarrhea, add **xian ling pi** (Epimedii Herba) 仙灵脾 12–15g and **bu gu zhi** (Psoraleae Fructus) 补骨脂 9–12g.
- For constipation with dry stools, add **tao ren** (Persicae Semen) 桃仁 9–12g, and take a decoction of **da huang** (Rhei Radix et Rhizoma) 大黄 6–12g [cooked for a few minutes] and **mang xiao** (Natrii Sulfas) 芒硝 3–6g [dissolved in the strained decoction] until the bowels move regularly.
- For constipation and sluggish stools from lack of peristalsis, add **zhi shi** (Aurantii Fructus immaturus) 枳实 9–12g and **mu xiang** (Aucklandiae Radix) 木香 9–12g.

Variations and additional prescriptions
Heart and Kidney qi and yin deficiency
When the shen disturbance aspects of a qi and yin deficiency pattern are prominent, with sleep disturbances, palpitations and anxiety, a more shen calming strategy should be adopted. An excellent choice is TIAN WANG BU XIN DAN (Emperor of Heaven's Special Pill to Supplement the Heart 天王补心丹, p.147) with a double dose of **xuan shen** (Scrophulariae Radix) 玄参, and the addition of **huang qi** (Astragali Radix) 黄芪.

Prepared medicines
Concentrated powder
Liu Wei Di Huang Wan (Rehmannia Six Formula) plus Sheng Mai San (Ginseng & Ophiopogon Formula)
Tian Wang Bu Xin Dan (Ginseng & Zizyphus Formula)

Pills
Liu Wei Di Huang Wan (Six Flavor Teapills) plus Sheng Mai Wan (Great Pulse Teapills)
Tian Wang Bu Xin Dan (Emperor's Teapills, Tian Wang Pu Hsin Tan)

Acupuncture (select from)
yishu (M–BW–12) ....the pancreas transport point, improves pancreatic function; 1.5 cun lateral to spinous process of T8
Bl.20 (pishu +) ....transport point of the Spleen, strengthens the Spleen and supplements qi
Bl.23 (shenshu +) ....transport point of the Kidney, strengthens the Kidney and nourishes yin

Liv.3 (taichong)..................source point of the Liver, dredges the Liver and regulates qi

PC.6 (neiguan)..................regulates Liver qi, stimulates the qi dynamic (with St.36), and calms the shen

St.36 (zusanli +) ....sea point of the Stomach, strengthens the Spleen, supplements qi and stimulates the qi dynamic

Sp.6 (sanyinjiao)..................regulates the Liver, Spleen and Kidneys, supplements qi and activates qi and blood

- with marked heat, add Liv.2 (xingjian –) and St.44 (neiting –)
- with edema, add Kid.7 (fuliu –)
- with night sweats, add Ht.6 (yinxi –)
- with constipation, add St.25 (tianshu –) and St.37 (shangjuxu –)
- with palpitations and shen disturbance, add Ht.7 (shenmen)
- with visual disturbance, add GB.20 (fengchi) and qiuhou (M–HN–8)
- with numbness in the extremities, add LI.11 (quchi) and St.40 (fenglong)
- with chest pain, add PC.5 (jianshi –), Bl.15 (xinshu –) and Ren.17 (shanzhong)
- Ear points: spleen, kidney, zero point, pancreas, endocrine, adrenal, shenmen

Clinical notes

- Qi and yin deficiency is the most common pattern of chronic diabetes. Most patients will be medicated with oral hypoglycemic agents, and some with occasional insulin. Patients will often note their medication requirements are increasing.
- Exercise is an essential feature of management, but in this case should initially be graded and built up over time. The ultimate aim is to work up to at least an hour per day of sustained aerobic activity. Walking and weight training are ideal. When the deficiency is significant, it is best to start with some mild form of activity such as taijichuan or yoga, and increase it as the patients energy allows.
- Diet is an essential component of treatment. In addition to the standard diet advice for diabetics, a low carbohydrate version of the diet aimed at supplementing qi and yin is recommended. See Clinical Handbook, Vol. 2, p.870 and 876.

肾心肝阴虚 4.7 KIDNEY, HEART AND LIVER YIN DEFICIENCY

This pattern represents a predominance of shaoyin pathology. It usually occurs late in the course of type 2 diabetes as the disease process shifts from taiyin into shaoyin. It may also be seen in recent onset diabetes occurring in older patients with pre–existing Kidney deficiency, and in adolescents with type 1 diabetes.

The yin deficiency is now the primary pathology. Heat from the yin deficiency becomes more prominent, the yin may fail to restrain yang leading to ascendant yang and an increased risk of wind stroke. Other shaoyin complications (microvascular, cardiovascular, nephropathy) are more advanced by the time this pattern has evolved. Patients with type 2 DM will be medicated with hypoglycemic agents and sporadic or regular insulin, so the classic DM symptoms may be muted.

Clinical features
- Frequent, copious urination; nocturia. The urine may be cloudy and turbid or leave a sediment; glucosuria and albuminuria.
- thirst, dry mouth and tongue; dry skin, hair and mucous membranes
- facial flushing; heat in the hands and feet; night sweats
- lower back pain and weakness; weak, sore knees
- dry eyes, visual weakness or blurring vision
- dizziness and tinnitus
- generalized pruritus
- impotence; scanty menses or amenorrhea
- frequent or persistent skin infections; slow healing; chronic thrush
- weight loss, emaciation

T red and dry, with little or no coat
P fine and rapid

Treatment principle
Nourish and supplement Liver and Kidney yin

Prescription

LIU WEI DI HUANG WAN 六味地黄丸
Six Ingredient Pill with Rehmannia, modified

This is an important and effective prescription for chronic diabetes, and serves to gradually strengthen the Kidneys and regulate blood sugar.

shu di (Rehmanniae Radix preparata) 熟地 15–30g
shan yao (Dioscoreae Rhizoma) 山药 24–30g
shan zhu yu (Corni Fructus) 山茱萸 12–15g
mu dan pi (Moutan Cortex) 牡丹皮 9–12g
fu ling (Poria) 茯苓 9–12g
ze xie (Alismatis Rhizoma) 泽泻 9–12g
dan shen (Salviae miltiorrhizae Radix) 丹参 9–15g

Method: Decoction or pills. Decoction is recommended in the early stages of treatment until the condition stabilizes, then pills may be used. **Shu di** supplements Kidney yin and blood and augments the jing; **shan zhu yu** warms and supplements the Liver and Kidneys and restrains leakage of fluids; **shan yao** strengthens the Spleen and, with **shan zhu yu**, restrains excessive urination; **ze**

xie clears heat; **mu dan pi** cools and activates the blood; **fu ling** strengthens the Spleen and leaches damp; **dan shen** activates the blood. (Source: *Zhong Yi Nei Ke Xue* [*Xiao Er Yao Zheng Zhi Jue*])

Modifications

- With marked thirst, add **xuan shen** (Scrophulariae Radix) 玄参 15–24g, **tian hua fen** (Trichosanthes Radix) 天花粉 15–30g, **sheng di** (Rehmanniae Radix) 生地 9–12g and **bai shao** (Paeoniae Radix alba) 白芍 9–12g.
- With visible blood stasis, add **san qi fen** (powdered Notoginseng Radix) 三七粉 3–6g [taken separately].
- With retinopathy and pin point hemorrhage, add **bai mao gen** (Imperatae Rhizoma) 白茅根 15–30g and **huai hua** (Sophora Flos immaturus) 槐花 12–15g.
- With blurring vision and red irritated eyes, add **gou qi zi** (Lycii Fructus) 枸杞子 12–15g and **ju hua** (Chrysanthemi Flos) 菊花 9–12g.
- With cataracts, add **dang gui** (Angelicae sinensis Radix) 当归 6–9g, **bai shao** (Paeoniae Radix alba) 白芍 9–12g, **bai ji li** (Tribuli Fructus) 白蒺藜 6–9g and **shi jue ming** (Haliotidis Concha) 石决明 9–12g [cooked first].
- With numbness and neuropathy, add **qin jiao** (Gentianae macrophyllae Radix) 秦艽 9–12g and **ji xue teng** (Spatholobi Caulis) 鸡血藤 15–30g.
- With high blood pressure, add **gou teng** (Uncariae Ramulus cum Uncis) 钩藤 9–12g and **chuan niu xi** (Cyathulae Radix) 川牛膝 12–15g.
- With albuminuria, increase **shan zhu yu** to 30g, and add **huang qi** (Astragali Radix) 黄芪 15–30g and **chuan xiong** (Chuanxiong Rhizoma) 川芎 6–9g.
- With nocturia, add **duan long gu** (calcined Fossilia Ossis Mastodi) 煅龙骨 15–30g, **duan mu li** (calcined Ostreae Concha) 煅牡蛎 15–30g [both cooked first] and **tu si zi** (Cuscutae Semen) 菟丝子 9–12g.
- With night sweats, flushing and heat intolerance, add **zhi mu** (Anemarrhenae Rhizoma) 知母 9–12g and **huang bai** (Phellodendri Cortex) 黄柏 9–12g.
- With bone steaming fever or low grade fever, add **di gu pi** (Lycii Cortex) 地骨皮 12–15g, **yin chai hu** (Stellariae Radix) 银柴胡 9–12g, **bie jia** (Trionycis Carapax) 鳖甲 12–15g and **gui ban** (Testudinis Plastrum) 龟板 12–15g.
- With ascendant Liver yang, headaches, dizziness, visual disturbances, pressure in the eyes and hypertension, add **shi jue ming** (Haliotidis Concha) 石决明 15–30g, **zhen zhu mu** (Margaritiferae Concha usta) 珍珠母 15–30g and **huai niu xi** (Achyranthis bidentatae Radix) 怀牛膝 12–15g.
- With Lung and Spleen qi and yin deficiency, add **ren shen** (Ginseng Radix) 人参 6–12g and **huang qi** (Astragali Radix) 黄芪 15–30g or combine with SHENG MAI SAN (Generate the Pulse Powder 生脉散, p.278).
- With insomnia, add **long gu** (Fossilia Ossis Mastodi) 龙骨 15–30g and **mu li** (Ostreae Concha) 牡蛎 15–30g [both cooked first].
- With high cholesterol and triglycerides, add **shan zha** (Crataegi Fructus) 山楂 12–15g and **he shou wu** (Polygoni multiflori Radix) 何首乌 9–12g.

Prepared medicines
Concentrated powder
Liu Wei Di Huang Wan (Rehmannia Six Formula)
Zhi Bai Di Huang Wan (Anemarrhena, Phellodendron & Rehmannia Formula)

– with a lot of heat, sweats and flushing

Sheng Mai San (Ginseng & Ophiopogon Formula)

    – add to the primary formula when there is qi and yin deficiency

Yu Nu Jian (Rehmannia & Gypsum Combination)

    – add to the primary formula when there is Stomach yin deficiency

Pills

Liu Wei Di Huang Wan (Six Flavor Teapills)

Sheng Mai Wan (Great Pulse Teapills)

Yu Quan Wan (Jade Spring Teapills)

Ming Mu Di Huang Wan (Ming Mu Di Huang Teapills)

    – with visual disturbances and ascendant yang

Acupuncture (select from)

yishu (M–BW–12) ....the pancreas transport point, improves pancreatic function; 1.5 cun lateral to spinous process of T8

Bl.18 (ganshu +).................transport point of the Liver, regulates the Liver and supplements Liver yin and blood

Bl.20 (pishu +) ....transport point of the Spleen, strengthens the Spleen and supplements qi

Bl.23 (shenshu +) ....transport point of the Kidneys, strengthens the Kidneys and nourishes Liver and Kidney yin

Ren.4 (guanyuan +)............strengthens the Kidneys, yuan qi and yin

Sp.6 (sanyinjiao)................regulates the Spleen, Liver and Kidneys, supplements qi and yin

Kid.2 (rangu –) ....spring and fire point of the Kidneys, clears deficient heat

Kid.3 (taixi +)....................source and stream point of the Kidneys, supplements yin, clears deficient heat

Kid.6 (zhaohai +) ....master point of yinqiaomai, clears heat, nourishes yin and moistens dryness

• Ear points: spleen, kidney, zero point, pancreas, endocrine, adrenal

Clinical notes

• Liver and Kidney yin deficiency is a common pattern of mid to late stage diabetes. It can respond well to treatment, with better regulation and stabilization of blood sugar levels, and alleviation of complications.

• Diet and appropriate exercise are essential components of treatment. In addition to the standard diet advice for diabetics, food to nourish yin can be helpful. See Clinical Handbook, Vol. 2, p.876. As these patients are quite deficient and easily fatigued, exercise should be modest initially and interspersed with appropriate yin replenishing rest periods.

阴阳两亏 4.8 KIDNEY AND HEART YANG AND YIN DEFICIENCY

Kidney and Heart yang and yin deficiency is a late stage of chronic diabetes, with the primary location of the disorder in the Kidneys. The signs and symptoms reflect weakness of both yin and yang, often with the yang deficiency apparent in the lower body and the yin deficiency in the upper body. The usual shaoyin diabetic complications, in particular nephropathy and microvascular pathology, are advanced.

Clinical features
- frequent, copious urination; nocturia; ingested fluids pass straight through and are immediately urinated; incontinence; glucosuria and albuminuria
- pale and puffy, or flushed complexion
- dry mouth and tongue; may be thirst
- lower back and legs cold, aching and weak; cold pale or purple feet
- hearing loss, tinnitus; dry withered ears
- may be signs of heat in the upper body – hot flushes, sweating and insomnia
- cold intolerance, cold in the lower body (although the hands and face may be warm)
- diarrhea with undigested food, often soon after eating; in severe cases may be fecal incontinence
- impotence, infertility

T pale, swollen and dry, with a white coat; dark distended sublingual veins
P deep, fine, weak

Treatment principle
Warm and supplement Kidney yang
Support Kidney yin and fluids

Prescription

JIN GUI SHEN QI WAN 金匮肾气丸
Kidney Qi Pill from The Golden Cabinet, modified

shu di (Rehmanniae Radix preparata) 熟地	15–30g
shan yao (Dioscoreae Rhizoma) 山药	24–30g
shan zhu yu (Corni Fructus) 山茱萸	12–15g
fu ling (Poria) 茯苓	12–15g
mu dan pi (Moutan Cortex) 牡丹皮	9–12g
ze xie (Alismatis Rhizoma) 泽泻	9–12g
zhi fu zi (Aconiti Radix lateralis preparata) 制附子	3–6g
gui zhi (Cinnamomi Ramulus) 桂枝	3–6g
huai niu xi (Achyranthis bidentatae Radix) 怀牛膝	9–12g

Method: Pills or powder. Grind the herbs to a fine powder and form into 9 gram pills with vinegar. The dose is one pill twice daily. **Shu di**, nourishes yin and Blood, supplements the Kidneys and regulates blood glucose; **shan zhu yu** supplements the Liver and Kidneys and restrains urination; **shan yao** strengthens the Spleen and Kidneys, supplements qi and reduces high blood glucose; **zhi fu zi** and **gui zhi** support and warm Kidney yang, dispel cold and promote qi transformation; **ze xie** promotes urination and drains damp; **fu ling** strengthens the Spleen and leaches damp; **mu dan pi** and **huai niu xi** activate blood. (Source: *Zhong Yi Nei Ke Xue* [*Jin Gui Yao Lue*])

Modifications

- Depending on the mixture of yin and yang deficiency, it is wise in the initial stages to use small doses of the pungent hot herbs (**zhi fu zi** and **gui zhi**), and monitor the patient for any signs of increasing thirst, sleep disturbance or restlessness. Yin deficiency can be masked by yang deficiency, and pungent warm herbs can aggravate it. The dose can be gradually increased if all is well.
- With marked blood stasis, add **ji xue teng** (Spatholobi Caulis) 鸡血藤 12–15g and **dan shen** (Salviae miltiorrhizae Radix) 丹参 9–15g.
- With retinopathy and macular edema, add **che qian zi** (Plantaginis Semen) 车前子 9–12g [cooked in a cloth bag], **tu si zi** (Cuscutae Semen) 菟丝子 9–12g and **gou qi zi** (Lycii Fructus) 枸杞子 9–12g.
- With retinal bleeding and loss of vision, add **san qi fen** (powdered Notoginseng Radix) 三七粉 3–6g [taken separately].
- With aching and weakness of the lower back, legs and knees, add **du zhong** (Eucommiae Cortex) 杜仲 12–15g and **xu duan** (Dipsaci Radix) 续断 12–15g.
- With cold, numb extremities, add **lu jiao jiao** (Cervi Cornus Colla) 鹿角胶 9–12g and **hu lu ba** (Trigonellae Semen) 胡芦巴 6–9g.
- With diarrhea, add **bu gu zhi** (Psoraleae Fructus) 补骨脂 9–12g and **yi zhi ren** (Alpiniae oxyphyllae Fructus) 益知仁 9–12g, or combine with Sɪ Sʜᴇɴ Wᴀɴ (Four Miracle Pill 四神丸, p.920).
- With urinary and fecal incontinence, increase the dose of **shan zhu yu** to 30g, add **bu gu zhi** (Psoraleae Fructus) 补骨脂 9–12g and **wu wei zi** (Schizandrae Fructus) 五味子 6–9g.
- With albuminuria, increase **shan zhu yu** to 30g, and add **huang qi** (Astragali Radix) 黄芪 15–30g and **chuan xiong** (Chuanxiong Rhizoma) 川芎 6–9g.
- With marked edema, increase the dose of **fu ling** to 30 grams, and add **yi mu cao** (Leonurus Herba) 益母草 12–15g, **ze lan** (Lycopi Herba) 泽兰 12–15g and **huang qi** (Astragali Radix) 黄芪 15–30g.
- With blood deficiency, add **he shou wu** (Polygoni multiflori Radix) 何首乌 9–12g and **gou qi zi** (Lycii Fructus) 枸杞子 9–12g.

Prepared medicines
Concentrated powder
Ba Wei Di Huang Wan (Rehmannia Eight Formula) plus Fu Tu Dan (Poria & Cuscuta Formula)
You Gui Wan (Eucommia & Rehmannia Formula)
Jin Suo Gu Jing Wan (Lotus Stamen Formula)
 – add with frequent urination and nocturia
Ji Sheng Shen Qi Wan (Cyathula & Plantago Formula)
 – with edema

Pills
Jin Kui Shen Qi Wan (Fu Gui Ba Wei Wan, Golden Book Teapills)
You Gui Wan (Right Side Replenishing Teapills)

Acupuncture (select from)

yishu (M–BW–12) ....the pancreas transport point, improves pancreatic function; 1.5 cun lateral to spinous process of T8

Bl.23 (shenshu +▲) ....transport point of the Kidneys, warms and supports yang

Du.4 (mingmen +▲) ....warms and supports Kidney yang

Ren.6 (qihai +▲) ....regulates qi and supports Kidney yang

Ren.4 (guanyuan +▲)........alarm point of the Small Intestine, supplements source qi, warms yang and regulates qi

Ren.8 (shenque ▲) ....warms yang; treated with moxa on salt; place a piece of thin cloth over the navel and fill it with salt; burn cones of moxa on the salt. The cloth enables quick removal of the salt and prevents excessive burning.

Kid.3 (taixi +)....................source point of the Kidneys, supplements and supports Kidney yang

St.36 (zusanli +▲) ....sea point of the Stomach, strengthens the Spleen and supplements yang qi

Sp.6 (sanyinjiao +▲).........strengthens the Spleen and Kidneys

• a moxa box over the abdomen is useful
• with edema, add Kid.7 (fuliu –), Ren.9 (shuifen ▲) and Sp.9 (yinlingquan –)
• Ear points: spleen, kidney, zero point, pancreas, endocrine, adrenal

Clinical notes

• Diabetes of a yin and yang deficiency type is debilitating, but patients can respond symptomatically to prolonged treatment. The main aim of treatment at this stage is to support and restore Kidney function as much as possible and prevent or arrest complications.

• Diet and appropriate exercise are an essential component of treatment. In addition to the standard diet advice for diabetics, a yang warming, low carbohydrate diet, is recommended. See Clinical Handbook, Vol. 2, p.873. As these patients are quite deficient and easily fatigued, exercise should be modest initially and balanced by appropriate yin replenishing rest periods.

• Some caution should be exercised initially with the doses of **zhi fu zi** and **gui zhi**. In some patients, the yin deficiency can be quite masked by the yang weakness, but still be aggravated by pungent hot herbs. Signs to watch for are increasing thirst, agitation and insomnia. A small dose at the low end of the range to start with is recommended. When using concentrated powders, to decrease the proportion of the pungent hot herbs, Ba Wei Di Huang Wan can be combined 50:50 with Liu Wei Di Huang Wan.

血
瘀
阻
络

4.9 BLOOD STASIS

Blood stasis is the main complications of long term diabetes, even when blood glucose is well managed. The majority of diabetic patients end up with some degree of blood stasis, and many will experience significant cardiovascular disease, atherosclerosis, peripheral vascular disease and diabetic retinopathy. The prescriptions for the patterns most likely to result in blood stasis already have some element of blood activation built in to them. The preferred approach to dealing with mild to moderate blood stasis is to augment the primary constitutional prescription as necessary. In some cases, however, when the blood stasis is severe, it becomes necessary to address it as the main pathology, while attending to the underlying pathology secondarily.

Treatment should proceed cautiously at first, because the underlying deficiency can be aggravated with too much blood activation. Keep a close eye on blood glucose levels and for signs of increasing deficiency (increasing fatigue, dizziness, thirst, insomnia etc.).

Clinical features
- numbness and tingling of the extremities, with dark, purple or brown discoloration; may be mild edema
- chronic non healing ulcers with dark margins, slow healing cuts and abrasions
- vascular congestion, spider veins and nevi
- chest pain, angina
- visual weakness, partial loss of vision or blindness

T purple or mauve, or with purple patches or stasis spots; dark congested sublingual veins

P choppy or irregular and intermittent

Treatment principle
Activate blood and qi, free the channels and network vessels
Support qi, blood, yin and yang as necessary

Prescription

JIANG TANG HUO XUE FANG 降糖活血方
Sugar Reducing Blood Activating Decoction

This is a good starting point for activating blood. It is well tolerated and unlikely to cause aggravation of underlying deficiency.

dan shen (Salviae miltiorrhizae Radix) 丹参 9–12g
chi shao (Paeoniae Radix rubra) 赤芍 9–12g
dang gui (Angelicae sinensis Radix) 当归 9–12g
chuan xiong (Chuanxiong Rhizoma) 川芎 9–12g
yi mu cao (Leonurus Herba) 益母草 12–15g
mu xiang (Aucklandiae Radix) 木香 6–9g
ge gen (Puerariae Radix) 葛根 12–15g
Method: Decoction. **Dan shen**, **chuan xiong** and **yi mu cao** activate blood and disperse static blood; **dang gui** and **chi shao** nourish and activate blood; **mu xiang** moves qi and enhances the

stasis transforming effect of the primary herbs; **ge gen** reduces blood sugar, generates fluids and alleviates dryness and thirst. (Source: *Shi Yong Zhong Yi Nei Ke Xue*)

Modifications

- With numbness and tingling in the upper limbs, add **gui zhi** (Cinnamomi Ramulus) 桂枝 9–12g, **sang zhi** (Mori Ramulus) 桑枝 15–30g and **ji xue teng** (Spatholobi Caulis) 鸡血藤 15–30g.
- With numbness and tingling in the lower limbs, add **chuan niu xi** (Cyathulae Radix) 川牛膝 9–12g, **du zhong** (Eucommiae Cortex) 杜仲 9–12g and **ji xue teng** (Spatholobi Caulis) 鸡血藤 15–30g.
- With chest oppression or angina, add **quan gua lou** (Trichosanthis Fructus) 全栝楼 18–30g and **jiang xiang** (Dalbergiae odoriferae Lignum) 降香 9–12g.
- With retinopathy, visual weakness or loss of vision, add **san qi fen** (powdered Notoginseng Radix) 三七粉 3–6g, **gou qi zi** (Lycii Fructus) 枸杞子 9–12g and **bai ji li** (Tribuli Fructus) 白蒺藜 9–12g.
- With cataracts, add **gou qi zi** (Lycii Fructus) 枸杞子 9–12g and **bai ji li** (Tribuli Fructus) 白蒺藜 9–12g.
- With chronic ulceration of the lower legs that exudes a thin inoffensive fluid, add **huang qi** (Astragali Radix) 黄芪 30–45g.
- With chronic purple ulceration of the lower legs that exudes a thick turbid fluid, add **san qi fen** (powdered Notoginseng Radix) 三七粉 3–6g, **xuan shen** (Scrophulariae Radix) 玄参 15–24g, **jin yin hua** (Lonicerae Flos) 金银花 15–30g and **gan cao** (Glycyrrhizae Radix) 甘草 9–12g.
- With phlegm, add **cang zhu** (Atractylodis Rhizoma) 苍术 9–12g and **xuan shen** (Scrophulariae Radix) 玄参 9–12g.
- With qi and yin deficiency, combine with Sᴴᴇɴɢ Mᴀɪ Sᴀɴ (Generate the Pulse Powder 生脉散, p.278).
- With yin deficiency, flushing and night fever, add **nu zhen zi** (Ligustri Fructus) 女贞子 9–12g and **han lian cao** (Ecliptae Herba) 旱莲草 9–12g.
- With yin deficiency and ascendant yang, add **mu li** (Ostreae Concha) 牡蛎 15–30g, **shi jue ming** (Haliotidis Concha) 石决明 15–30g [both cooked first], **tian dong** (Asparagi Radix) 天冬 9–12g and **mai dong** (Ophiopogonis Radix) 麦冬 9–12g.
- With Spleen qi deficiency and marked fatigue, add **shan yao** (Dioscoreae Rhizoma) 山药 15–30g, **huang qi** (Astragali Radix) 黄芪 15–30g and **ren shen** (Ginseng Radix) 人参 6–9g.
- With marked dryness, add **xuan shen** (Scrophulariae Radix) 玄参 12–15g, **sheng di** (Rehmanniae Radix) 生地 9–12g and **mai dong** (Ophiopogonis Radix) 麦冬 9–12g.
- With blood deficiency and dry, itchy or scaly skin, add **gou qi zi** (Lycii Fructus) 枸杞子 9–12g and **bai shao** (Paeoniae Radix alba) 白芍 9–12g and **he shou wu** (Polygoni multiflori Radix) 何首乌 9–12g.
- With edema, add **yi mu cao** (Leonurus Herba) 益母草 12–15g and **ze lan** (Lycopi Herba) 泽兰 12–15g.

Variations and additional prescriptions

The guiding prescription can be varied depending on the location of the blood stasis and the major underlying pathology. The modifications above apply.

Blood stasis with qi deficiency

For blood stasis with qi deficiency use **Bu Yang Huan Wu Tang** (Supplement Yang to Restore Five Tenths Decoction 补阳还五汤, p.600) as guiding prescription. Mostly used for peripheral neuropathy and retinopathy.

Blood stasis with cold

For blood stasis with cold, **Gui Zhi Fu Ling Wan** (Cinnamon Twig and Poria Pill 桂枝茯苓丸, p.27) is helpful. This prescription is especially useful as it is gentle enough for prolonged use, and effectively lowers blood glucose. Used for blood stasis retinopathy.

Blood and qi stasis

For relatively robust patients with qi and blood stasis, use **Xue Fu Zhu Yu Tang** (Drive Out Stasis in the Mansion of Blood Decoction 血府逐瘀汤, p.303). This prescription is quite strong and should be used with care in those with any deficiency. It is best used in short bursts of 2–3 weeks interspersed with the appropriate constitutional treatment.

Severe blood stasis with constipation

Chronic qi and yin deficiency is often complicated by relatively severely blood stasis and recalcitrant constipation. The constipation is compounded by weak peristalsis (qi deficiency) and dryness (yin deficiency), and the poor elimination aggravates the blood stasis further. The solution is to use a prescription that activates blood and keeps the Intestines free. This can be achieved with **Tao He Cheng Qi Tang** (Peach Pit Decoction to Order the Qi 桃核承气汤, p.920). This prescription is strong and can aggravate Spleen deficiency, so just enough should be used, in combination with appropriate qi and yin supplements, to enable a smooth bowel movement. It should be given separately to the supplementing herbs so the dose can be easily adjusted.

Prepared medicines

Concentrated powders

Bu Yang Huan Wu Tang (Astragalus & Peony Combination)
Gui Zhi Fu Ling Wan (Cinnamon & Poria Formula)
Dang Gui Si Ni Tang (Tangkiei & Jujube Combination)
Xue Fu Zhu Yu Tang (Persica & Carthamus Combination)
Tao He Cheng Qi Tang (Persica & Rhubarb Combination)
Tao Hong Si Wu Tang (Tangkuei Four, Persica & Carthamus Combination)
    – with blood deficiency

Pills

Bu Yang Huan Wu Wan (Great Yang Restoration Teapills)
Gui Zhi Fu Ling Wan (Cinnamon and Poria Teapills)

Xue Fu Zhu Yu Wan (Stasis in the Mansion of Blood Teapills)
Tao Hong Si Wu Wan (Tao Hong Si Wu Tang Teapills)
San Shen Jian Kang Wan (Sunho Multi Ginseng Tablets)

Acupuncture (select from)

Acupuncture should be performed with extra care on the limbs, as the combination of blood stasis and higher than normal blood glucose makes patients susceptible to infection. Areas of gross stasis (cool, dark and discolored) should be avoided. Acupuncture can be helpful, but in general herbs are required to make the most significant inroads into advanced blood stasis.

General treatment

Bl.15 (xinshu −) ....transport point of the Heart, strengthens the Heart
and activates blood

Bl.17 (geshu −)..................meeting point for blood, dispels stagnant blood

yishu (M−BW−12) ....the pancreas transport point, improves pancreatic
function; 1.5 cun lateral to spinous process of T8

Bl.18 (ganshu)...................transport point of the Liver, dredges the Liver and
rectifies qi, activates blood

Bl.20 (pishu +) ....transport point of the Spleen, strengthens the Spleen
and supplements qi

Bl.23 (shenshu +) ....transport point of the Kidneys, warms and strengthen the Kidneys to support the Spleen

Ren.4 (guanyuan +)...........strengthens yuan qi and supports qi systemically

Sp.10 (xuehai −) ....this point activates blood and dispels static blood

Sp.6 (sanyinjiao)................strengthens the Spleen and Kidneys, regulates the
liver and activates qi and blood

Liv.3 (taichong)................source point of the Liver, nourishes and activates
Liver blood

• moxa or warm needle should be used when there is cold or qi deficiency
• Ear points: liver, kidney, pancreas, zero point, sympathetic, endocrine

Peripheral neuropathy and peripheral vascular disease

The main points are selected from the yangming channels along the affected limbs. Points proximal to the discolored or numb area are selected.

LI.15 (jianyu) .... these points access the yangming channels, the

LI.11 (quchi)   repository of qi and blood

LI.10 (shousanli)

LI.4 (hegu)

St.36 (zusanli)

St.40 (fenglong)

• Congested veins may be cautiously bled (see p.929)
• Additional ear points: points related to the affected area

Retinopathy, visual disturbance

qiuhou (M−HN−8)...........local points for the eyes

Bl.1 (jingming)
GB.20 (fengchi) ....main point for eye disease
GB.37 (guanming) ....connecting point of the Gallbladder, treats all eye
                                disease
• Additional ear points: eye

Cardiovascular
PC.4 (ximen –) ....these points alleviate chest oppression
PC.6 (neiguan –)
Ren.17 (shanzhong) ....upper 'sea of qi', opens up qi flow through the chest
St.40 (fenglong –) ....transforms phlegm
• Additional ear points: heart

Nephropathy
Bl.52 (zhishi +)..................strengthens the Kidneys
Kid.3 (taixi +)...................source point of the Kidneys, supplements Kidney
                                yin and yang
Kid.7 (fuliu –)...................with edema
St.28 (shuidao –)
• Additional ear points: adrenal

Clinical notes
• Blood stasis can respond reasonably well to treatment if caught early enough,
  and if qi and yin are effectively maintained.
• Exercise is important, and should be tailored to the capacity of the patient. Any
  activity is better than none.
• Massage and hot and cold foot baths can be helpful in stimulating blood flow.

4.10 MANAGEMENT OF COMMON COMPLICATIONS

In both insulin dependent and non–insulin dependent diabetics, the complications of high or unregulated blood sugar levels are common. The complications are due to blood stasis and phlegm which block the channels and network vessels in the chest, extremities, skin and eyes. In most cases, blood stasis is the principal component in the development of complications, and even when phlegm is seemingly the most obvious pathogen, there will always be some blood stasis requiring attention. In rare cases, a deficiency state may be the primary pathology behind a complication. These are noted under the headings below.

The primary strategy to alleviate and prevent the complications of diabetes is to maintain tight control of blood sugar levels. Complications generally develop gradually, and when mild to moderate, management can be achieved by treatment of the constitutional pathology, with the integration of additional herbs or acupuncture points to activate blood or transform phlegm damp.

In some patients, the complications become the major component of the pathology, and the risk of permanent damage or serious consequences escalates. In patients in imminent danger of blindness, gangrene or renal failure, the complication must be addressed as the priority. In such cases, the prescriptions noted in the blood stasis section above can be used on their own, with modification as necessary from Tables 4.4, p.205 and 4.5, p.206. The blood stasis prescriptions can also be used in conjunction with other suitable constitutional treatment, with the blood stasis treatment the main proportion, for example in a 3:1 or 2:1 ratio.

4.10.1 RETINOPATHY

Diabetic retinopathy develops gradually and may progress without the patient being aware of visual loss until the pathology is quite advanced. Retinal damage is characterized by aneurysms in the capillary network, spot hemorrhages and infarction, exudates and edema. Blurred vision, black spots or flashing lights in the field of vision, and partial or total loss of vision may be the first symptoms.

In Chinese medicine, this type of visual loss is due to blockage of the network vessels of the eye by blood stasis and phlegm damp. The physical presence of these pathogens can be observed by examination of the retina by ophthalmoscope. The more aneurysms and spot hemorrhages, the greater the degree of blood stasis; the more edema and exudate, the more phlegm damp. Blood stasis and phlegm damp usually occur together, and patients will exhibit varying degrees of qi and yin deficiency.

Occasionally retinopathy and retinal bleeding may be associated with qi and blood deficiency without blood stasis, in which case a formula such as GUI PI TANG (Restore the Spleen Decoction 归脾汤, p.387) is selected as the guiding prescription.

4.10.2 VASCULAR DISEASE

This includes cardiac and peripheral vascular disease. The main manifestations are angina, myocardial infraction and stroke, claudication, nocturnal leg pain and vascular ulcers. In most cases, adequate management can be achieved with herbs to activate blood and transform phlegm added to the primary constitutional prescription.

With non healing vascular ulcers and ischaemia, to the point of necrosis or gangrene, a vigorous strategy of blood stasis activation and toxic heat clearing is necessary. This can be achieved with the prescription below. Progress should be closely monitored to determine whether the blood circulation improves within a few weeks. If deterioration of circulation or necrosis occurs, surgery is required. For patients taking Warfarin, **dan shen**, which specifically interferes with INR[5] determination, should be deleted and replaced with **san qi fen** (powdered Notoginseng Radix) 三七粉.

Prescription

SI MIAO YONG AN TANG 四妙勇安汤
Four Valiant Decoction for Well Being, modified

jin yin hua (Lonicerae Flos) 金银花..60–90g
xuan shen (Scrophulariae Radix) 玄参 60–90g
dang gui (Angelicae sinensis Radix) 当归..30–60g
gan cao (Glycyrrhizae Radix) 甘草...15–30g
dan shen (Salviae miltiorrhizae Radix) 丹参..9–15g
hu zhang (Polygoni cuspidati Rhizoma) 虎杖..9–15g
Method: Decoction. **Jin yin hua** resolves toxic heat, reduces swelling and inflammation; salty and cold **xuan shen** resolves toxic heat, cools the blood and nourishes yin; **dang gui** nourishes and activates the blood, gently disperses blood stasis and reduces swelling; **gan cao** enhances the ability of **jin yin hua** to resolve toxic heat, while protecting the Spleen and Stomach and boosting anti–pathogenic qi; **dan shen** and **hu zhang** activate blood and clear heat. (Source: *Yan Fang Xin Bian*)

4.10.3 PERIPHERAL NEUROPATHY

Peripheral neuropathy is due to nerve ischemia from microvascular disease, increased viscosity of blood, and the effect of elevated blood glucose on neurons. Peripheral neuropathy is characterized by numbness, tingling and burning in the hands and feet, or loss of sensitivity to temperature and touch. There may also be muscle weakness and atrophy. Standard management is applied, with constitutional treatment and maintenance of blood glucose the primary goal. Additional herbs from Table 4.4 and 4.5 are added as necessary. When severe, a strategy directed toward blood activation (p.198) is recommended.

Occasionally, the neuropathy can be associated with qi and blood deficiency, with little blood stasis, in which case a prescription such as SHI QUAN DA BU TANG (All Inclusive Great Supplementing Decoction 十全大补汤, p.758) can be used as the guide.

4.10.4 NEPHROPATHY

Diabetic nephropathy is a serious late stage complication characterized by thick-

---

5 International Normalization Ratio, a measure of the clotting tendency of blood used to titrate the correct dose of warfarin.

Table 4.4 Herbs with a specific effect on blood stasis[1, 2] complications

Dan Shen Salviae miltiorrhizae Radix 丹参	Salvia root; bitter, cool; Heart, Lung. Activates blood and dispels blood stasis. For all microvascular and macrovascular complications. Lowers blood glucose, reduces blood viscosity, increases levels of antioxidants (superoxide dismutase), resists vascular injury by lipid peroxidation and stimulates growth of microcirculation.
San Qi Notoginseng Radix 三七	Tianqi ginseng root; sweet, slightly bitter, warm; Liver, Stomach. Disperses static blood and stops bleeding. For cardiovascular, retinal, renal and peripheral vascular complications of chronic diabetes. Regulatory effect on blood glucose, reduces blood viscosity and improves microcirculation.
Hu Zhang Polygoni cuspidati Rhizoma 虎杖	Polygonum cuspidatum root; Slightly bitter, sour, neutral; Liver, Kidney. Clears heat and activates blood. Improves microcirculation. For peripheral neuropathy and blood stasis complications.
Shui Zhi Hirudo 水蛭	Leech; salty, bitter; Liver. Breaks up blood stasis, reduces blood viscosity, blood cholesterol and triglycerides. For relatively advanced microangiopathy, peripheral vascular disease, nephropathy and retinopathy.
Yi Mu Cao Leonuri Herba 益母草	Motherwort; pungent, slightly bitter, cool; Liver, Heart, Kidney. Activates blood, reduces blood viscosity and reduces edema. For nephropathy and retinopathy from blood stasis with edema.
Da Huang Rhei Radix et Rhizoma 大黄	Rhubarb root; bitter, cold; Heart, Liver, Stomach, Large Intestine. Activates blood when well cooked, reduces blood lipids and blood glucose. For nephropathy in patients with constipation. The dose can be adjusted until the bowels move smoothly.
Shan Zha Crategi Fructus 山楂	Hawthorn fruit; sweet, sour, warm; Spleen, Stomach, Liver. Improves digestion, activates blood and lowers cholesterol. For cardiovascular complications from blood and phlegm stasis.
Bai Ji Li Tribuli Fructus 白蒺藜	Tribulus fruit; pungent, bitter, slightly warm; Liver, Lung. Dispels wind, dredges the Liver and activates qi and blood. Lowers blood glucose and increases insulin secretion. For retinopathy from blood stasis.

1. Li WL et al. (2004) Natural medicines used in the traditional Chinese medical system for therapy of diabetes mellitus. Journal of Ethnopharmacology 92:1–21
2. Jia W et al. (2003) Antidiabetic herbal drugs officially approved in China. Phytotherapy Research 17:1127–1134

ening and sclerosis of the glomerular network, with decline in renal capacity, eventual renal failure and dialysis. This complication is asymptomatic until significant damage has occurred. Albuminuria suggests renal damage.

Treatment with Chinese medicine is aimed at slowing the progress of the nephropathy. In advanced cases, a mixture of Western medicine (usually ACE inhibitors) and Chinese medicine can produce a better outcome, in terms of quality of life and retarded deterioration, than either used alone. There are two broad

Table 4.5 Herbs for phlegm complications

Wei Ling Xian Clematidis Radix 威灵仙	Chinese clematis root; pungent, salty, warm; enters all organs and channels. Dispels wind damp, dissipates phlegm and blood stasis, and opens up qi flow through the channels. For numbness and peripheral neuropathy, limb pain. Only used for short periods of time, as it can disperse qi and yin.
Zao Jiao Gleditsiae Fructus 皂角	Chinese honeylocust fruit; pungent, salty, warm, slightly toxic; Lung, Large Intestine. Transforms phlegm and breaks through obstruction. For numbness and peripheral neuropathy.
Mu Li Ostreae Concha 牡蛎	Oyster shell; salty, astringent, cool; Liver, Kidney. Softens hardness and disperses phlegm. For phlegm accumulation in the channels causing numbness (with zhe bei mu and xuan shen), and excessive urination.
Zhe Bei Mu Fritillaria thunbergii Bulbus 浙贝母	Zhejiang fritillaria tuber; bitter, cold; Heart, Lung. Transforms phlegm. For phlegm accumulation anywhere in the body, usually in combination with **mu li** and **xuan shen** (Xɪᴀᴏ Lᴜᴏ Wᴀɴ 消瘰丸 Reduce Scrophula Pill, p.921).

patterns observed when nephropathy becomes an issue, qi and yin deficiency, and yang deficiency, both with marked blood stasis. Treatment proceeds in the conventional way, with suitable blood activating herbs (in particular **da huang**, or a small proportion of a blood activating prescription such as Tᴀᴏ Hᴇ Cʜᴇɴɢ Qɪ Tᴀɴɢ [Peach Pit Decoction to Order the Qi 桃核承气汤, p.920]) added to the appropriate constitutional prescription. The dose of **da huang** or the **da huang** containing prescription can be adjusted until a smooth bowel movement occurs.

4.10.5 SKIN INFECTIONS, BOILS AND SORES

Diabetics are especially prone to recurrent suppurative sores. In general these are associated with damp heat or toxic heat lingering in the skin as a result of the educed ability of anti–pathogenic to expel pathogens. When persistent or recurrent, but relatively low grade, prescription No.1 can be incorporated into the primary constitutional formula. When lesions are widespread or when associated with systemic signs of toxic heat (malaise, fever, etc.), a more focused toxic heat clearing, blood sugar reducing and blood activating strategy is called for. Prescription No.2 can be used for a week or two to quickly resolve the lesions before resuming constitutional treatment.

Prescription 1

WU WEI XIAO DU YIN 五味消毒饮

Five Ingredient Decoction to Eliminate Toxin

jin yin hua (Lonicerae Flos) 金银花 15–30g
pu gong ying (Taraxaci Herba) 蒲公英 15–30g
zi hua di ding (Violae Herba) 紫花地丁 15–30g
ye ju hua (Chrysanthemi indici Flos) 野菊花 9–12g
zi bei tian kui (Begonia fimbristipulata Herba) 紫背天葵 9–12g

Method: Decoction. **Jin yin hua**, the main herb, clears toxic heat from the qi and blood levels to treat suppurative sores; **pu gong ying, zi hua di ding, ye ju hua** and **zi bei tian kui** resolve toxic heat, cool the blood and disperse local accumulations. (Source: *Shi Yong Zhong Yi Nei Ke Xue* [*Yi Zong Jin Jian*]).

Prescription 2

XIAN FANG HUO MING YIN 仙方活命饮
Sublime Formula for Sustaining Life

jin yin hua (Lonicerae Flos) 金银花.. 15–30g
tian hua fen (Trichosanthes Radix) 天花粉 12g
dang gui wei (rootlets of Angelicae sinensis Radix) 当归尾 9g
chi shao (Paeoniae Radix rubra) 赤芍.. 9g
zhe bei mu (Fritillariae thunbergii Bulbus) 浙贝母 9g
bai zhi (Angelicae dahuricae Radix) 白芷 9g
zao jiao ci (Gleditsiae Spina) 皂角刺 9g
zhi ru xiang (Olibanum preparata) 制乳香 6g
zhi mo yao (Myrrha preparata) 制没药 6g
wang bu liu xing (Vaccariae Semen) 王不留行...................................... 12g
fang feng (Saposhnikovae Radix) 防风 6g
chen pi (Citri reticulatae Pericarpium) 陈皮 6g
gan cao (Glycyrrhizae Radix) 甘草.. 6g

Method: Decoction. **Jin yin hua** clears heat and resolves toxin; **bai zhi** dispels wind, dries damp and aids in the discharge of pus; **dang gui, chi shao, ru xiang** and **mo yao** activate blood, dispel blood stasis and stop pain; **zhe bei mu** and **tian hua fen** clear heat, transform phlegm and dissipate nodules and swellings; **chen pi** regulates qi and harmonizes the Stomach; **wang bu liu xing** and **zao jiao ci**, along with the blood activating herbs, assist in penetrating the lesion, enabling the other herbs to gain access. **Wang bu liu xing** is used instead of the endangered **chuan shan jia** (Squama Manitis 穿山甲) that appears in the original prescription. (Source: *Jiao Zhu Fu Ren Liang Fang*)

Table 4.6 Summary of diabetes mellitus patterns

Pattern	Features	Prescription
Lung and Stomach heat	Strong thirst and hunger, copious urination, weight loss, glucosuria, dry yellow tongue coat, surging rapid pulse	Bai Hu Jia Ren Shen Tang
Spleen qi deficiency	Fatigue, muscle weakness, dry mouth, variable appetite, frequent urination, glucosuria, diarrhea, sweating, pale swollen tongue, weak fine pulse	Shen Ling Bai Zhu San
Phlegm	Dry mouth and thirst, vertigo, foggy head, lassitude, glucosuria, phlegm masses, numbness of the extremities, abdominal bloating, fat tongue, slippery pulse	Cang Fu Dao Tan Wan
Damp heat	Moderate thirst or dryness, hunger, bitter taste, abdominal distension, muscle aches, sluggish bowels, overweight, itchy skin, boils and sores, glucosuria, red tongue with a greasy yellow coat, slippery rapid pulse	Gan Lu Yin Huang Qin Hua Shi Tang
Liver and Spleen disharmony with heat	Thirst, dry mouth and throat, variable appetite, dry sore eyes, stiff neck and shoulders, alternating bowel habits, menstrual irregularity, glucosuria, symptoms worse with emotional upset, red edges on the tongue, wiry pulse	Jia Wei Xiao Yao San Xiao Chai Hu Tang
Qi and yin deficiency	Thirst and dryness, frequent urination, fatigue, breathlessness, sweating, heat in the hands and feet, glucosuria, red or pink swollen tongue with surface cracks, weak pulse	Sheng Mai San plus Zeng Ye Tang
Kidney, Heart and Liver yin deficiency	Frequent copious urination, nocturia, glucosuria, thirst, lower back and legs aching, visual weakness, flushed face, dry itchy skin, red dry tongue with little or no coat, fine rapid pulse	Liu Wei Di Huang Wan
Kidney and Heart yin and yang deficiency	Frequent copious urination, nocturia, glucosuria, thirst, sallow or dark complexion, cold intolerance and cold extremities, lower back ache, diarrhea, facial flushing, visual weakness and hearing loss, impotence, pale swollen tongue, deep, weak pulse.	Jin Gui Shen Qi Wan
Blood stasis	Vascular congestion, dark discolored skin peripheral neuropathy and vascular disease, retinopathy, chest pain, purple tongue and choppy pulse	Jiang Tang Huo Xue Fang

EDEMA

Edema, (*shuǐ zhŏng*[1] 水肿) is the abnormal accumulation of fluid in the extracellular spaces and interstitial tissues of the body. Extracellular fluid is a normal component of the matrix in which cells bathe. It serves to transport nutrients into, and waste products away from, cells. Normally, the balance of extracellular fluid volume is maintained by capillary permeability, the relationship between arterial and venous pressures, the osmotic pressure exerted by the fluids themselves and the volume of water in the body. When extracellular fluid volume is increased, edema becomes apparent. In biomedical terms, edema may be caused by one or more of the following (see also Box 5.3, p213):

(see also Box 5.3, p213)

BOX 5.1 PATTERNS OF EDEMA

External wind
 – wind cold
 – wind heat
Toxic heat in the skin
Damp heat
Spleen damp
Liver qi constraint
Blood stasis
Qi deficiency
Spleen and Kidney yang
 deficiency
Kidney and Heart yang
 deficiency
Qi and yin deficiency

1. Increased capillary permeability
Capillaries can become more permeable to fluid, allowing plasma to leak into the extracellular space, as a result of inflammation or allergy.

2. Increased sodium concentration in extracellular fluid
High levels of sodium increases the osmotic pressure of the extracellular fluids, drawing more fluid into the extracellular spaces. The sodium may come from the diet, or be the result of kidney disorders where the retention and excretion of sodium and potassium are abnormal.

3. Increased fluid volume
Increased fluid volume may result from high sodium levels that increase the osmotic pressure of the extracellular fluids, or poor excretion from kidney pathology such as renal failure and nephrotic syndrome, or endocrine disease.

4. Decreased osmotic pressure due to hypoproteinemia
Decreased osmotic pressure within the vessels from low serum protein can cause fluids to escape into the extracellular space. Protein levels in the blood can be low due to malnutrition, decreased manufacture of proteins due to liver disease or loss in the urine in some renal diseases.

5. Reduction of venous and lymphatic drainage
Reduced venous or lymphatic drainage of a limb by scarring, tumor, parasites or loss of lymph nodes following surgery, can lead to increased pressure in the venous and lymphatic systems of the affected area. Edema of this type tends to be unilateral.

---

1 Practical Dictionary of Chinese Medicine (1998) – 'water swelling'

BOX 5.2 KEY DIAGNOSTIC POINTS

Location
- face and mucous membranes of the respiratory passages – Lungs
- eyelids, fingers, abdomen, lower body – Spleen
- below the waist, especially knees and ankles – Kidneys
- unilateral or localized – toxic heat, blood stasis

Aggravation, onset
- premenstrual – qi constraint
- exertion – yang qi deficiency
- menopause – yin deficiency, yang deficiency

Pitting
- yes – deficiency, the more deficient the longer lasting the indentation
- no – excess

Yang edema
- may be acute, rapid onset (not always), starts in the upper body, non (or minimal) pitting, excess pathology primarily
- wind, damp, toxic heat, damp heat, qi constraint, blood stasis (most common are mixtures of yin and yang edema)

Yin edema
- chronic, gradual onset, starts in the lower body, pitting, deficient pathology
- Spleen and Kidney yang qi deficiency; qi and yin deficiency

Models for the analysis of edema appear as early as the Han dynasty (206BC–220AD), and descriptions can be found in the Simple Questions (*Huang Di Nei Jing Su Wen*). The ancient writers referred to a variety of 'water' diseases, including wind water, stone water, skin water, Heart water, Liver water, Lung water, Spleen water and so on. Zhu Dan Xi[2] classified edema into yin edema and yang edema, and this analysis was adopted by later authors. Yang edema is acute, rapid in onset and usually affects the upper body first. Yin edema is chronic, of gradual onset, pitting, and associated with deficiency of one or more internal organ systems. Today we differentiate a variety of distinct patterns within the categories of yin and yang edema (Box 5.2).

In Chinese medicine, edema is caused by pathogenic obstruction to the movement of fluids, blockage to and disruption of the organs of fluid metabolism, or to functional weakness of the organs of fluid metabolism (Figure 5.2, p.212).

FLUID PHYSIOLOGY IN CHINESE MEDICINE

Successful treatment of edema is based on a sound understanding of fluid physiology. The organ systems fundamental to the metabolism of fluids are the Lungs, Spleen and Kidneys.

The Spleen is central to fluid metabolism, and the driving force, with the Stomach, of the qi dynamic. The qi dynamic is the pivotal dynamo behind the movement of qi and fluids through the triple burner, and is essential for the normal transformation and distribution of fluids. The Spleen extracts usable qi from the

---

2 Essential Teachings of Dan Xi (*Dan Xi Xin Fa* 丹溪心法 1481)

Figure 5.1 Diagnostic flowchart for edema. No pitting here indicates that deep and persistent pitting is not observed, but negligible and short lasting indents (along sock lines for example) may be seen.

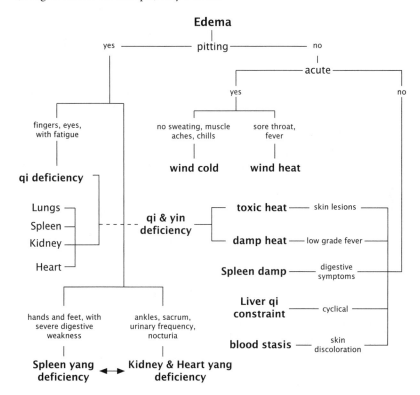

raw materials of food and drink, then sends these extracts up to the Lungs for final processing into the various types of physiological qi. The residual wastes left from this initial extraction are discharged downwards to be excreted. Failure to efficiently extract and distribute the usable ('pure') part of the food and fluids can allow the unprocessed portions to accumulate in the flesh and surface tissues. Once the pathological fluids and damp have accumulated, they further hamper the Spleen, creating a vicious cycle of Spleen weakness, accumulation of damp and edema.

The Lungs govern the 'water passages', and are the 'upper source of water'. This means that the Lungs process the fluids they receive from the Spleen and diffuse them outwards to the skin, and downwards to the Kidneys and Urinary Bladder for refining and reprocessing. The descent of Lung qi provides the motive force for the downward movement of waste fluids through the triple burner. The Lungs are also contiguous with the skin, so a pathogen lodged in either the skin or Lungs can interfere with the descent and diffusion of Lung qi and the normal excretion of fluids as sweat.

Figure 5.2 Pathology of edema

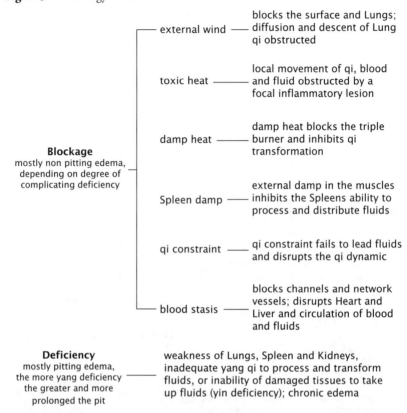

blocks the surface and Lungs;
external wind —— diffusion and descent of Lung
qi obstructed

local movement of qi, blood
toxic heat —————— and fluid obstructed by a
focal inflammatory lesion

damp heat blocks the triple
damp heat —————— burner and inhibits qi
transformation

Blockage
mostly non pitting edema,
depending on degree of
complicating deficiency

external damp in the muscles
Spleen damp —— inhibits the Spleens ability to
process and distribute fluids

qi constraint —— qi constraint fails to lead fluids
and disrupts the qi dynamic

blocks channels and network
vessels; disrupts Heart and
blood stasis —————— Liver and circulation of blood
and fluids

Deficiency
mostly pitting edema,
the more yang deficiency
the greater and more
prolonged the pit

weakness of Lungs, Spleen and Kidneys,
inadequate yang qi to process and transform
fluids, or inability of damaged tissues to take
up fluids (yin deficiency); chronic edema

The Kidney, in particular Kidney yang, is the foundation of qi transformation and all fluid metabolism. Kidney yang underpins the yang functions of the Lungs and Spleen, and their ability to transform and distribute fluids efficiently. Kidney yang provides the metabolic heat required to transform fluids into 'steam', the first step in refining and separating the pure usable fluids from impure wastes. Yang qi also underpins the function of the qi dynamic to ensure continuous and free movement of fluids through the triple burner.

The triple burner is the pathway for the distribution of yuan qi and fluids from the Kidneys to the Spleen and Lungs. The triple burner links the Lungs, Spleen, Stomach, Intestines and Kidneys into a functional unit of qi and fluid movement, and drains into the Urinary Bladder. The triple burner assists the Urinary Bladder's role of excreting waste fluids. This is achieved by draining all waste fluids from qi transformation processes elsewhere in the body, and by carrying the recovered pure fluids back up through the body once qi transformation is complete. For an excellent and thorough discussion of fluid metabolism, see Clavey (2003).

ETIOLOGY

External pathogens

Pathogens invading the body can disrupt fluid metabolism and generate edema in several ways. When a pathogen invades the Lungs, it disrupts the Lungs diffusion and descent of qi and fluids. When descent of Lung qi and fluid are obstructed, the occluded fluids accumulate in the face and upper burner first, then, if the condition persists, throughout the superficial tissues of the limbs and trunk. The presence of a pathogen on the surface, blocks the pores and the taiyang level, hindering the normal elimination of sweat from the skin and urine from the Urinary Bladder.

Prolonged exposure to damp conditions, such as living in a damp house, humid climate or working in contact with water, can result in damp seeping into the body and permeating the muscles and flesh. Because the muscles and skin are associated with taiyin (Spleen and Lungs), the saturating damp reduces the Spleen and Lungs ability to transform and distribute fluids properly; more damp is generated and a vicious cycle ensues. The edema is gradual and usually begins in the limbs. Prolonged or unresolved Spleen damp will invariably lead to Spleen qi and/or yang deficiency.

Trauma, boils and toxic lesions

Trauma, surgery and scarring can obstruct the channels and network vessels and lead to poor circulation or stasis of qi, blood and fluids. The resulting edema is usually unilateral and seen distal to the site of the trauma.

Toxic heat and damp heat can accumulate focally in the skin and muscles as boils and other skin infection. Once a lesion has formed, it blocks the local movement of qi, blood and fluids, leading to localized edema. Depending on the extent of the toxic heat the edema can be mild and confined to the region around the lesion and the affected limb, or extensive and systemic. Chronic superficial sores and boils can gradually affect the Lungs and Spleen through their influence on the skin and muscles.

BOX 5.3 BIOMEDICAL CAUSES OF EDEMA

Bilateral

Cardiac
- right ventricular failure
- biventricular failure
- pericardial effusion

Hypoalbuminemic states
- nephrotic syndrome
- malnutrition
- malabsorption
- chronic liver disease

Renal
- acute and chronic renal failure
- acute and chronic glomerulonephritis
- nephrotic syndrome

Endocrine
- hypothyroidism
- Cushing's syndrome

Drug induced
- calcium antagonists
- non steroidal anti-inflammatories (NSAIDs)
- corticosteroids
- estrogens

Unilateral
- postoperative (following bypass surgery or saphenous vein harvesting)
- venous or lymphatic obstruction from scarring, parasites, lymphadenectomy, or tumors
- thrombophlebitis
- deep venous thrombosis
- allergic reaction
- local inflammation, cellulitis

Figure 5.3 Etiology of edema

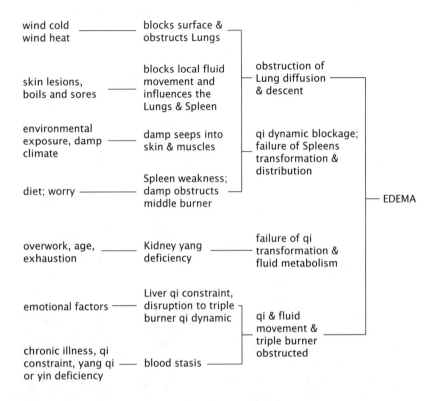

Diet and medications

The dietary factors that are most likely to contribute to edema are those that weaken the Spleen and Kidneys and deplete yang qi. Commonly seen are restrictive or fad diets that rely on single food items, raw or uncooked foods, or very low caloric intake. Missing meals, inappropriate fasting, or irregular meal times weakens the Spleen and depletes qi. The use of appetite suppressants and slimming aids weaken the Spleen and damage qi, including over the counter medicines that contain bitter cold purgative herbs such as rhubarb root and senna.

Some commonly used herbs and medications can damage the Spleen, deplete qi and contribute to edema. These include purgative laxatives, antibiotics, antihypertensive drugs and heat clearing herbs.

Excessive amounts of salt in the diet can damage the Kidneys and impair fluid metabolism. The habit of drinking large quantities of water every day in an attempt to 'flush the kidneys' can cause problems. If the volume ingested is more than Kidney yang can process, yang is overwhelmed and weakened and the unprocessed fluids ends up in the tissues as edema.

Emotional factors

The emotions that constrain the Liver, and weaken the Spleen and Kidneys, are those most likely to lead to edema. Emotional repression and chronic stress are important causes of disruption to the Liver, Spleen and qi dynamic. Any emotional factor, if prolonged or extreme, may disrupt the function of the Liver and Spleen, or provoke the Liver to invade the Spleen. Dysfunction of either organ system can influence the qi dynamic, impairment of which affects the movement and distribution of fluids, initially through the triple burner, then later through the limbs. Chronic Liver qi constraint can generate heat, which may combine with damp from the weakened Spleen to create damp heat.

Worry, obsessive thinking and prolonged concentration weaken the Spleen, especially when combined with a sedentary lifestyle and poor diet. Chronic fear or a sudden severe fright or shock can weaken the Kidneys, and deplete yang qi.

Overwork, exhaustion

Factors that deplete Spleen and Kidney yang qi are those likely to contribute to edema. Working excessively long hours or laboring to the point of exhaustion can deplete Spleen and Kidney yang qi. Using more qi in activity than is harvested by eating is commonly seen, and a problem that often affects professional athletes. In athletes the high expenditure of energy is often compounded by restrictive diets aimed at maintaining competition weight. Academics and those involved in highly concentrated mental pursuits are prone to Spleen weakness, especially when combined with too much sitting.

Constitution

Some people inherit a tendency to edema. This is mediated through a constitutional weakness of the organs of fluid metabolism, usually the Kidneys and Spleen. Patients with such a weakness will report a history of fluid problems and intermittent edema from an early age.

PITTING AND NON–PITTING EDEMA

One of the key features in differentiating edema is whether or not it is pitting. When finger pressure leaves a persistent indentation in the edematous area this is pitting. The ability of tissues to fill out following focal pressure depends on the flow of yang qi in the flesh and skin. In excess patterns, the still intact yang qi in the tissues will 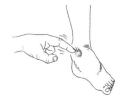 move fluids back into the indentation made by the pressing finger. When yang qi is deficient, it is unable to mobilize qi and fluids, so the pit fills slowly and the indent remains. The rate of filling of the indent reflects the degree of deficiency; the slower to rebound the greater the deficiency.

TREATMENT

There are two components to the treatment of edema, eliminating the fluids and correcting the underlying pathology, but the principle of treatment can change depending on the severity and duration of the edema. When edema is severe or dangerous, the focus of treatment is to vigorously alleviate the edema, regardless of the deficient state of the patient. In most chronic cases, the primary aim of treatment is to improve the strength and function of the affected organs. In this way, the edema resolves more slowly, but the prospects for long term recovery are significantly better. In addition to herbal and acupuncture treatment, evaluation and correction of the diet, assessment of salt intake and other herbs, medications, slimming aids, and exercise levels are important in long term management.

Treatment of the edema involves active elimination of the pathological fluids through one or more of the pathways of elimination, while promoting normal function of the Lungs, Spleen and Kidneys and maintaining the free flow of qi.

Eliminating edema

There are three techniques utilized to eliminate the edema, depending on the location and pathology.

1. Promote Lung function

This method is used for edema in the upper burner and face, and when the edema is concentrated close to the surface (as in the toxic heat pattern, p.224). The aim is to stimulate the diffusion (*xuān* 宣) of Lung qi and fluids to the surface, so the edema can be dissipated as sweat, and to promote normal descent of Lung qi and maintenance of the 'water passages', which assists in maintaining normal urinary output. Diaphoretic herbs are combined with those that strengthen the Lungs and direct Lung qi downwards (Table 5.1, p.217).

2. Strengthen the Spleen and rectify the qi dynamic

This method is aimed at removing impediments to the normal ascent of Spleen qi and descent of Stomach qi (the qi dynamic), and promoting Spleen function to improve the processing and distribution of fluids. This technique is useful when edema affects the upper extremities, fingers and abdomen. Pungent and bitter herbs are combined to free the qi dynamic. Pungency disperses and lifts damp off the Spleen and allows Spleen qi to rise, while bitterness dries damp and assists the descent of Stomach qi. The combined effect of pungent and bitter herbs is to free the qi dynamic so it can operate properly, which in turn improves the transformation and distribution of fluids. Freeing the qi dynamic, the pivot for triple burner qi movement, has ramifications beyond the middle burner. By encouraging normal qi movement it assists organ function in all three burners.

3. Promote urination

Promoting urination (diuresis) is the mainstay of alleviating edema, especially when the edema is concentrated below the waist. There are two methods of promoting diuresis. The first is to ensure the water passages of the lower burner remain open and clear, and gently assist Kidney and Urinary Bladder function to promote urination. Diuretic acupuncture techniques and bland natured, damp draining herbs are used. This method is well tolerated, but when used inappropriately or to excess can damage qi and yin. The second method is to vigorously warm and stimulate yang qi, and the transformation and mobilization of physiological and pathological fluids.

Caution when using diuretic substances

The temptation to use diuresis alone should be avoided. Herbs and pharmaceutical drugs that force expulsion of fluids may temporarily relieve edema, but clinical experience shows that the edema recurs and tends to be worse than before. Prolonged use of diuretics can weaken or further aggravate Spleen and Kidney yang.

Diuretic medications

Conventional diuretics, such as frusemide (Lasix), are the standard medical treatment for edema. They work by inhibiting the resorption of sodium chloride and water in the kidneys. Increased renal excretion of salt and water causes a reduction in plasma volume and thus a relative increase in plasma protein concentration. Increased plasma protein concentrations exert an osmotic force on the extracellular fluids, drawing them back into the capillaries and general circulation.

In Chinese medicine terms, the common diuretics tend to be cool or cold and bland. Prolonged use can deplete yin, weaken the Spleen and damage Kidney yang qi. Many patients presenting to the Chinese medicine clinic for treatment of an edema problem are already taking a diuretic medication of some type. In most cases these medicines are similar in fluid leaching action to the bland herbal diuretics. When prescribing herbs for a patient taking a pharmaceutical diuretic, the dose of the bland herbs can be adjusted to compensate, while the herbs to correct the underlying condition are emphasized. The aim is to gradually reduce the dose of the diuretic medicine as the condition improves.

Table 5.1 Methods of eliminating edema

	Method	Herb examples	Acupoints
Lungs	Diffuse the Lungs with pungency	ma huang	Lu.7 lieque LI.4 hegu
	promote descent of Lung qi with bitter herbs	jie geng xing ren	LI.6 pianli Lu.6 kongzui BI.13 feishu
Spleen	dry damp and rectify the qi dynamic with pungent and bitter herbs	cang zhu hou po	Ren.12 zhongwan Sp.6 sanyinjiao Sp.9 yinlingquan St.36 zusanli BI.20 pishu
	Strengthen Spleen function to promote fluid movement and transformation	huang qi bai zhu	
Kidneys	gentle diuresis with bland herbs	fu ling zhu ling che qian zi	Ren.9 shuifen (moxa) St.28 shuidao BI.23 shenshu BI.28 pangguangshu BI.39 weiyang Sp.6 sanyinjiao Sp.9 yinlingquan Kid.7 fuliu
	vigorous stimulation of qi transformation with pungency and heat	zhi fu zi gui zhi	

风
水
泛
滥

5.1 WIND EDEMA

1. Wind cold
2. Wind heat

Edema due to invasion of wind is an acute pattern, in which the wind, plus cold or heat, disrupts the normal diffusion and descent of Lung qi and fluids. The fluids that should be directed to the skin and the Kidneys though the water passages of the triple burner, back up and accumulate in the face and upper burner.

These patterns may follow an upper respiratory tract infection or other superficial infection such as suppurative skin lesions, or a procedure such as tooth extraction. Wind edema predominantly affects younger people. This is a yang type of edema.

风
寒
遏
肺

5.1.1 WIND COLD

Wind cold obstructs the diffusion and descent of Lung qi and fluids. Edema of a wind cold type is less common than edema from wind heat, but the edema itself is more pronounced as the pores are shut tight and the fluids more constrained.

Clinical features

- Sudden onset of orbital and facial edema. In the early stages edema is seen around the eyes and then the face. The edema develops quickly, and over the course of days, may become generalized.
- muscle and joint aches
- cold intolerance
- aversion to wind
- no sweating
- chills, mild fever
- scanty urination
- dyspnea or wheezing
- cough

T thin, white coat
P floating, slippery or tight (when edema is severe the pulse may appear deep)

Treatment Principle

Dispel wind cold
Diffuse the Lungs and direct Lung qi downwards
Promote sweating and urination to drain damp and relieve edema

Prescription

MA HUANG JIA ZHU TANG 麻黄加术汤
Ephedra Decoction plus Atractylodes

ma huang (Ephedra Herba) 麻黄 3–9g
gui zhi (Cinnamomi Ramulus) 桂枝 3–9g
xing ren (Armeniacae Semen) 杏仁 6–12g
bai zhu (Atractylodes macrocephalae Rhizoma) 白术 9–15g

zhi gan cao (Glycyrrhizae Radix preparata) 炙甘草................................. 3–6g
Method: Decoction. **Ma huang** and **gui zhi** dispel wind cold from the surface and promote sweating; **ma huang** dispels wind cold and promotes sweating, diffuses the Lungs and directs Lung qi downwards to promote the Lungs' regulation of the water passages. **Xing ren** directs Lung qi downwards and stops cough. **Bai zhu** strengthens the Spleen and metabolism of fluids, and dries damp; **zhi gan cao** supports the Spleen and prevents the pungent herbs from excessive dispersal of qi. (Source: Fluid Physiology and Pathology in Traditional Chinese Medicine [*Shang Han Lun*])

Modifications

* The diuretic action of the prescription can be enhanced with bland damp leaching herbs such as **fu ling pi** (Poriae Cutis) 茯苓皮 12–15g, **zhu ling** (Polyporus) 猪苓 9–12g, **ze xie** (Alismatis Rhizoma) 泽泻 9–12g and **che qian zi** (Plantaginis Semen) 车前子 9–12g.
* With wheezing or productive cough and watery or clear sputum, add **chen pi** (Citri reticulatae Pericarpium) 陈皮 9–12g, **su zi** (Perillae Fructus) 苏子 6–9, and **ting li zi** (Lepidii/Descurainiae Semen) 葶苈子 6–9g.
* With severe chills and muscle aches, add **qiang huo** (Notopterygii Rhizoma seu Radix) 羌活 9–12g, **fang feng** (Saposhnikovae Radix) 防风 9–12g and **zi su ye** (Perillae Fructus) 紫苏叶 9–12g.

Variations and additional prescriptions

Wind invasion with exterior deficiency

If the above treatment fails to increase urinary output and decrease the edema within a few days, or if the patient is increasingly lethargic, feels heavy and starts sweating freely without decrease in edema, the indications are that qi is too weak to move fluids adequately. The treatment is to fortify wei qi, strengthen the Spleen and relieve edema with FANG JI HUANG QI TANG (Stephania and Astragalus Decoction 防己黄芪汤).

han fang ji (Stephaniae tetrandrae Radix) 汉防己 9–12g
huang qi (Astragali Radix) 黄芪 15–30g
bai zhu (Atractylodes macrocephalae Rhizoma) 白术 9–12g
zhi gan cao (Glycyrrhizae Radix preparata) 炙甘草............................... 3–6g
sheng jiang (Zingiberis Rhizoma) 生姜... 9–12
da zao (Jujubae Fructus) 大枣 3pce
Method: Decoction. **Han fang ji** dispels wind and promotes urination to relieve edema; **huang qi** boosts qi and secures the exterior and promotes urination; **bai zhu** supplements qi, strengthens the Spleen, dried damp and secures wei qi; **zhi gan cao** supplements qi and harmonizes the middle burner; **sheng jiang** and **da zao** harmonize ying and wei and support the Spleen. (Source: *Zhong Yi Nei Ke Xue* [*Shang Han Lun*])

Blockage of taiyang and the Urinary Bladder organ by wind cold

A wind cold pathogen may influence the taiyang organ as well as the taiyang channel, especially when there is a pre–existing Kidney deficiency. The Urinary Bladder organ is obstructed leading to a backing up of fluids through the triple burner. The symptoms are acute edema of the lower body with oliguria or anuria, nausea or vomiting. There may also be fever, headache and a floating pulse. The treatment is to promote urination and leach out damp with WU LING SAN (Five Ingredient Powder with Poria 五苓散).

ze xie (Alismatis Rhizoma) 泽泻 12–15g
fu ling (Poria) 茯苓 9–12g
zhu ling (Polyporus) 猪苓 9–12g
bai zhu (Atractylodes macrocephalae Rhizoma) 白术 9–12g
gui zhi (Cinnamomi Ramulus) 桂枝 6–9g
Method: Decoction. **Ze xie** promotes urination to drain damp; **fu ling** leaches damp and strengthens the Spleen; **zhu ling** leaches damp; **bai zhu** strengthens the Spleen, supplements qi and dries damp; **gui zhi** assists Urinary Bladder qi transformation and the metabolism of fluids, while clearing wind cold from the exterior. (Source: *Shang Han Lun*)

Prepared medicines
Concentrated powders
Ma Huang Tang (Ephedra Combination)
Fang Ji Huang Qi Tang (Stephania & Astragalus Combination)
Xiao Qing Long Tang (Minor Blue Dragon Combination)
 – acute edema in the limbs with watery cough
Wu Ling San (Poria Five Herb Formula)

Pills
Ma Huang Tang Wan (Ma Huang Tang Teapills)
Fang Ji Huang Qi Wan (Stephania and Astragalus Teapills)
Xiao Qing Long Wan (Minor Blue Dragon Teapills)
Wu Ling San Wan (Wu Ling San Teapills)

Acupuncture (select from)
Lu.7 (lieque) .... connecting point of the Lungs; dispels wind cold, diffuses the Lungs and directs Lung qi downwards to free the water passages and promote urination

LI.4 (hegu –) .... source point of the Large Intestine, diffuses the Lungs and dispels wind

LI.6 (pianli –) .... connecting point of the Large Intestine, diffuses the Lungs, frees and regulates the water passages

Sp.9 (yinlingquan –) .... sea point of the Spleen, promotes urination to relieve edema

Bl.13 (feishu –Ω) .... transport point of the Lungs, diffuses the Lungs and directs Lung qi downward, dispels wind

Bl.22 (sanjiaoshu –) .... transport point of the triple burner, regulates the water passages of the triple burner, promotes urination and assists in qi transformation and fluid metabolism

Bl.39 (weiyang –) .... lower sea point of the triple burner, regulates the water passages and promotes urination to relieve edema

Ren.9 (shuifen ▲) .... promotes urination and qi transformation, metabolism and elimination of fluids

Ren.3 (zhongji) .... alarm point of the Urinary Bladder, promotes urination to relieve edema

Du.26 (renzhong) ....for facial edema
- with cough, add Lu.9 (taiyuan −)
- with significant wheezing, use dingchuan (M−BW−1)
- with copious sputum, add St.40 (fenglong −)
- Ear points: lungs, kidney, subcortex, endocrine, adrenal

Clinical notes
- Edema of a wind cold type may be diagnosed as post−streptococcal glomeru-lonephritis, Bright's disease, acute nephritis, allergic edema or angioneurotic edema.

风
热
遏
肺

5.1.2 WIND HEAT
The pathology of wind heat edema is similar to that of wind cold, but the wind heat variety is more commonly seen. Both wind heat and wind cold disrupt the normal diffusion and descent of Lung qi.

Clinical features
- Sudden onset of orbital and facial edema. In the early stages edema is seen around the eyes and then the face. The edema develops quickly, and over the course of days, may become generalized.
- mild fever, or fever and chills
- red, sore, swollen throat
- mild sweating, spontaneous sweating
- aversion to wind
- cough
- scanty concentrated urine

T red tip and edges, with a thin, yellow coat
P floating, slippery, rapid, when edema is severe the pulse may appear deep

Treatment Principle
Dispel wind and clear heat
Diffuse the Lungs and direct Lung qi downwards
Promote urination and sweat to relieve edema

Prescription

YUE BI JIA ZHU TANG 越婢加术汤
Maidservant from Yue Decoction plus Atractylodes

ma huang (Ephedrae Herba) 麻黄	6–12g
bai zhu (Atractylodes macrocephalae Rhizoma) 白术	9–12g
shi gao (Gypsum fibrosum) 石膏	15–30g
gan cao (Glycyrrhizae Radix) 甘草	3–6g
sheng jiang (Zingiberis Rhizoma) 生姜	9–12g
da zao (Jujubae Fructus) 大枣	4 fruit

Method: Decoction. **Shi gao** is decocted for 30 minutes prior to the other herbs. **Ma huang** diffuses the Lungs, promotes sweating, directs Lung qi downward and promotes the Lungs' regulation of the water passages to promote urination; **bai zhu** strengthens the Spleen and dries damp; **shi gao** clears heat; **gan cao** supports the Spleen and prevents the pungent herbs from causing excessive dispersal of qi; **sheng jiang** promotes sweating and clears the exterior; **da zao** prevents excessive sweating and, with **sheng jiang**, supports and protects the middle burner. (Source: *Zhong Yi Nei Ke Xue* [*Shang Han Lun*])

Modifications

- With marked edema, add **che qian zi** (Plantaginis Semen) 车前子 12–15g and **bai mao gen** (Imperatae Rhizoma) 白茅根 15–30g.
- With sore, swollen throat, delete **sheng jiang**, and add **ban lan gen** (Isatidis/Baphicacanthis Radix) 板蓝根 12–18g, **she gan** (Belamacandae Rhizoma) 射干 12–15g, **huang qin** (Scutellariae Radix) 黄芩 9–12g and **niu bang zi** (Arctii Fructus) 牛蒡子 9–12g.
- With wheezing or coughing, add **xing ren** (Armeniacae Semen) 杏仁 9–12g, **chen pi** (Citri reticulatae Pericarpium) 陈皮 9–12g, **su zi** (Perillae Fructus) 苏子 6–9g and **ting li zi** (Lepidii/Descurainiae Semen) 葶苈子 6–9g.
- With pruritus, add **bai xian pi** (Dictamni Cortex) 白藓皮 9–12g, **di fu zi** (Kochiae Fructus) 地肤子 9–12g and **ku shen** (Sophorae flavescentis Radix) 苦参 9–12g.
- With hematuria, add **xiao ji** (Cirsii Herba) 小蓟 12–15g and **bai mao gen** (Imperatae Rhizoma) 白茅根 15–30g.
- With boils, abscesses or superficial sores, add **jin yin hua** (Lonicerae Flos) 金银花 15–30g, **pu gong ying** (Taraxici Herba) 蒲公英 15–30g and **zi hua di ding** (Violae Herba) 紫花地丁 15–30g. See also 5.2 Toxic Heat, p.224.
- With damage to yin, dry mouth, red, dry tongue and thirst, add **sheng di** (Rehmanniae Radix) 生地 15–18g and **xuan shen** (Scrophulariae Radix) 玄参 12–18g.

Variations and additional prescriptions

Wind invasion with exterior deficiency

If the above treatment fails to increase urinary output and decrease the edema within a few days, or if the patient is lethargic, feels heavy and starts sweating freely without decrease in edema, the indication is that qi is too weak to move fluids adequately. The treatment is to fortify wei qi, strengthen the Spleen and promote urination to relieve edema with FANG JI HUANG QI TANG (Stephania and Astragalus Decoction 防己黄芪汤, p.219).

Prepared medicines

Concentrated powders

Yue Bi Jia Zhu Tang (Atractylodes Combination)

Pills

Yin Qiao Jie Du Pian (Yin Chiao Chieh Tu Pien) plus Wu Ling San Wan (Wu Ling San Teapills)

Acupuncture (select from)

LI.4 (hegu –).....................source point of the Large Intestine, diffuses the Lungs, dispels wind heat

LI.6 (pianli –)....................connecting point of the Large Intestine, clears heat and diffuses the Lungs, regulates the water passages

SJ.5 (waiguan –) ....connecting point of the triple burner, dispels wind heat and promotes triple burner qi transformation

Du.14 (dazhui – Ω) ....meeting point of the yang channels, an important point for clearing heat from the exterior

Sp.9 (yinlingquan –)...........sea point of the Spleen, promotes urination to relieve edema

Bl.13 (feishu – Ω) ....transport point of the Lungs, diffuses the Lungs, directs Lung qi downwards and dispels wind

Bl.22 (sanjiaoshu –)............transport point of the triple burner, regulates the water passages of the triple burner, promotes urination and stimulates qi transformation and fluid metabolism

Bl.39 (weiyang –) ....lower sea point of the triple burner, regulates the water passages and promotes urination

Ren.9 (shuifen ▲)..............promotes urination and the transformation, metabolism and elimination of fluids

Ren.3 (zhongji) ....alarm point of the Urinary Bladder, clears damp heat and promotes urination

Du.26 (renzhong) ....for facial edema

- with cough, add Lu.5 (chize –)
- with wheezing, use dingchuan (M–BW–1)
- with sore throat, add Lu.11 (shaoshang ↓) and SI.17 (tianrong –)
- Ear points: lungs, kidney, tonsils, subcortex, endocrine, adrenal

Clinical notes

- Edema of a wind heat type may be diagnosed as post–streptococcal glomerulonephritis, Bright's disease, acute nephritis, allergic edema or angioneurotic edema.

热
毒
侵
淫

5.2 TOXIC HEAT IN THE SKIN

Toxic heat is highly concentrated damp heat which disrupts the circulation of qi, blood and fluids at some locus, causing destruction of local tissues, suppuration and localized edema. This is a yang type of edema.

Clinical features
- Edema associated with suppurative and inflammatory sores and ulcerations. The edema may be localized to the area around the lesion, or may be more systemic and extensive. When the edema is systemic, it is also seen in parts of the body at a distance from the lesion, typically beginning in the face and upper body.
- scanty, concentrated urination
- fever, or fever and chills

T red, with a thin, yellow coat
P floating and rapid or slippery and rapid

Treatment Principle
Clear and resolve toxic heat
Promote urination to relieve edema

Prescription

MA HUANG LIAN QIAO CHI XIAO DOU TANG 麻黄连翘赤小豆汤
Ephedra, Forsythia and Phaseolus Calcaratus Decoction, plus
WU WEI XIAO DU YIN 五味消毒饮
Five Ingredient Decoction to Eliminate Toxin

chi xiao dou (Phaseoli Semen) 赤小豆	15–30g
lian qiao (Forsythiae Fructus) 连翘	9–12g
ma huang (Ephedra Herba) 麻黄	6–9g
xing ren (Armeniacae Semen) 杏仁	9–12g
sang bai pi (Mori Cortex) 桑白皮	12–15g
zhi gan cao (Glycyrrhizae Radix preparata) 炙甘草	3–6g
jin yin hua (Lonicerae Flos) 金银花	15–30g
pu gong ying (Taraxici Herba) 蒲公英	15–30g
zi hua di ding (Violae Herba) 紫花地丁	15–30g
ye ju hua (Chrysanthemi indici Flos) 野菊花	9–12g
zi bei tian kui (Begoniae fimbristipulatae Herba) 紫背天葵	9–12g

Method: Decoction. **Chi xiao dou** promotes urination and relieves edema; **lian qiao** clears heat and dissipates focal accumulation and hot masses; **ma huang**, **xing ren** and **sang bai pi** diffuse the Lungs and move fluids; **zhi gan cao** supports and protects the middle burner; **jin yin hua**, **pu gong ying**, **ye ju hua**, **zi hua di ding** and **zi bei tian kui** clear toxic heat. (Source: *Zhong Yi Nei Ke Xue* [*Shang Han Lun*/*Yi Zong Jin Jian*])

Modifications
- With copious pus, double the dose of **pu gong ying** and **zi hua di ding**.
- With weeping ulcerations, add **ku shen** (Sophorae flavescentis Radix) 苦参 9–12g and **tu fu ling** (Smilacis glabrae Rhizoma) 土茯苓 18–30g.

- With severe pruritus, add **bai xian pi** (Dictamni Cortex) 白蘚皮 9–12g and **chi shao** (Paeoniae Radix rubra) 赤芍 9–12g.
- With constipation, add **da huang** (Rhei Radix et Rhizoma) 大黄 3–9g and **mang xiao** (Natrii Sulfas) 芒硝 3–9g.

Prepared medicines
Concentrated powders
Wu Wei Xiao Du Yin (Dandelion & Wild Chrysanthemum Combination) plus Wu Ling San (Poria Five Herb Formula)

Pills
Wu Wei Xiao Du Wan (Five Flavor Teapills) plus Wu Ling San Wan (Wu Ling San Teapills)

Acupuncture (select from)
ahshi points........................above and below the lesion and edematous region
LI.4 (hegu –).....................source point of the Large Intestine, diffuses the Lungs, dispels wind heat, clears heat and activates qi and blood
LI.11 (quchi –)...................sea point of the Large Intestine, clears heat
Du.10 (lingtai –)................these points clear heat and treat skin lesions
Du.12 (shenzhu –)
Sp.9 (yinlingquan –)...........sea point of the Spleen, promotes urination and relieves edema
Bl.22 (sanjiaoshu –)............transport point of the triple burner, regulates the water passages of the triple burner, promotes urination and assists in qi transformation and fluid metabolism
Bl.40 (weizhong – ↓).........lower sea and earth point of the Urinary Bladder, clears heat and cools the blood, treats toxic skin lesions
Ren.3 (zhongji –) ....alarm point of the Urinary Bladder, clears heat and promotes urination to relieve edema
- Ear points: lungs, large intestine, zero point, subcortex, sympathetic

Clinical notes
- Edema of a toxic heat type may be diagnosed as abscesses and carbuncles, cellulitis, erysipelas, diabetic ulcers and tropical ulcers, post–streptococcal glomerulonephritis or Bright's disease.

湿
热
壅
盛

5.3 DAMP HEAT

There are several presentations of damp heat edema, ranging from mild to severe. The damp heat can be concentrated in the legs and feet, in the lower burner or throughout the triple burner. In all cases the damp heat can be introduced with the diet (including alcohol), or be the result of external invasion that affects the Liver and Spleen, qi level, or Urinary Bladder.

When concentrated in the feet, the damp heat sinks down from the triple burner and there are generally only mild systemic signs of damp heat. When concentrated in the lower burner and Urinary Bladder, qi transformation and the passage of urine are blocked and urinary symptoms accompany the edema. In the severe form, damp heat is lodged throughout the triple burner, blocking the qi dynamic and the distribution of qi and fluids, and the edema is more generalized, affecting the limbs and abdomen. All variants are types of yang type edema.

Clinical features

- Non pitting edema that is worse below the waist, and may be most apparent in the lower legs and feet, but in severe cases may be seen in the abdomen and upper body. The edematous areas feel warm and taut.
- the skin over the edematous area appears tight, shiny or greasy; may be suppurative or ulcerated sores
- may be numbness or burning in the feet
- drum like abdominal distension and chest oppression
- low grade afternoon fever, or contained fever (p.367); night sweats
- thirst and dry mouth, but with little desire to drink
- scanty, concentrated urine, dysuria, or cloudy urine
- constipation or difficult, sluggish stools

T red with a thick, yellow coat
P deep, slippery and rapid, or soggy and rapid

Treatment Principle

Separate damp and heat, and clear both
Promote expulsion of edema through Urinary Bladder and Large Intestine

Prescription

SI MIAO SAN 四妙散
Four Marvel Powder, modified

This prescription is selected for edema and numbness in the feet with mild systemic symptoms of damp heat.

cang zhu (Atractylodis Rhizoma) 苍术 15–30g
huang bai (Phellodendri Cortex) 黄柏 9–12g
yi ren (Coicis Semen) 苡仁.. 30–60g
huai niu xi (AchyranthisRadix) 怀牛膝.. 12–15g
han fang ji (Stephaniae tetrandrae Radix) 汉防己 9–12g
chi fu ling (Poria Rubra) 赤茯苓 12–15g
bi xie (Dioscoreae hypoglaucae Rhizoma) 萆薢 9–12g

lu lu tong (Liquidambaris Fructus) 路路通 6–12g
Method: Decoction. **Huang bai** clears damp heat, **cang zhu** and **yi ren** dry and leach out dampness and strengthen the Spleen and thus support **huang bai** in clearing damp heat; **huai niu xi** activates the flow of qi and blood through the legs; **han fang ji** and **bi xie** promote urination to drain damp; **chi fu ling** clears damp heat; **lu lu tong** activates blood and promotes urination. (Source: *Cheng Fang Bian Du*)

Modifications (to San Miao San)
- With redness and heat in the feet, add **shan zhi zi** (Gardeniae Fructus) 山栀子 9–12g and **shi gao** (Gypsum fibrosum) 石膏 15–30g [cooked first].
- With a degree of yin damage, burning in the soles of the feet and peeled tongue coat on the root of the tongue, add **sheng di** (Rehmanniae Radix) 生地 12–15g and **mai dong** (Ophiopogonis Radix) 麦冬 9–12g.

TONG LING SAN 通苓散
Akebia and Poria Powder

This formula is selected when damp heat congests the lower burner and blocks the Urinary Bladders' qi transformation function. Edema is seen in the legs and feet, and urinary symptoms are prominent, with cloudiness, burning or sediment.

mu tong (Akebiae Caulis) 木通 6–9g
zhu ling (Polyporus) 猪苓 12–15g
fu ling (Poria) 茯苓 9–12g
ze xie (Alismatis Rhizoma) 泽泻 9–12g
che qian zi (Plantaginis Semen) 车前子 9–12g
qu mai (Dianthi Herba) 瞿麦 9–12g
yin chen (Artemisiae scopariae Herba) 茵陈 9–15g
bai zhu (Atractylodes macrocephalae Rhizoma) 白术 12–15g
Method: Decoction. **Mu tong** and **qu mai** clear heat, promote urination and ease painful urination; **fu ling**, **zhu ling**, **ze xie** and **che qian zi** promote urination and relieve edema; **yin chen** promotes urination and clears damp heat; **bai zhu** strengthens the Spleen and dries damp. (Source: *Shi Yong Zhong Yi Nei Ke Xue* [*Shi Yi De Xiao Fang*])

Modifications (to Tong Ling San)
- With lower back ache, cloudy urine, or urine that leaves a sediment, delete **bai zhu** and add **huang bai** (Phellodendri Cortex) 黄柏 9–12g, **cang zhu** (Atractylodis Rhizoma) 苍术 9–12g, **bi xie** (Dioscoreae hypoglaucae Rhizoma) 萆薢 9–12g and **tu fu ling** (Smilacis glabrae Rhizoma) 土茯苓 18–30g.
- With hematuria, add **bai mao gen** (Imperatae Rhizoma) 白茅根 15–30g and **sheng di** (Rehmanniae Radix) 生地 9–15g.
- With dizziness, insomnia, lower back ache and other signs of yin damage with ascendant yang, add **ju hua** (Chrysanthemi Flos) 菊花 12–15g and **shi jue ming** (Haliotidis Concha) 石决明 15–30g. See also qi and yin deficiency, p.253.

SHU ZAO YIN ZI 疏凿饮子
Dispersing Chisel Decoction

This is a purging prescription and is selected for relatively severe cases with damp heat blocking the triple burner. The edema affects the limbs and abdomen, and systemic signs of damp heat are marked.

shang lu (Phytolaccae Radix) 商陆 3–6g
 – Substitute: **ting li zi** (Lepidii/Descurainiae Semen) 葶苈子 9–12g
bing lang (Arecae Semen) 槟榔 9–12g
chi xiao dou (Phaseoli Semen) 赤小豆 15–30g
chuan jiao mu (Zanthoxyli Fructus) 川椒目 3–9g
mu tong (Akebiae Caulis) 木通 6–12g
fu ling pi (Poriae Cutis) 茯苓皮 12–30g
da fu pi (Arecae Pericarpium) 大复皮 6–15g
ze xie (Alismatis Rhizoma) 泽泻 6–12g
qiang huo (Notopterygii Rhizoma seu Radix) 羌活 6–12g
qin jiao (Gentiana macrophylla Radix) 秦艽 6–12g
sheng jiang pi (Zingiberis Rhizomatis Cortex) 生姜皮 6–12g

Method: Decoction. **Shang lu** purges damp through the urine and bowels; **chi xiao dou**, **chuan jiao mu** and **mu tong** clear heat, promote urination and reduce edema; **fu ling pi**, **da fu pi** and **ze xie** leach out damp; **bing lang** and **da fu pi** move qi and drain damp; **qiang huo** and **sheng jiang pi** promote sweating to provide another outlet for the edema; **qin jiao** clears damp heat.

*NB. **Shang lu** is toxic and must only be used in robust patients for short periods of time until fluids are moving. In practice, it is usually better to err on the side of caution and select a less potentially harmful purging agent, such as **ting li zi** (Lepidii/Descurainiae Semen) 葶苈子 9–12g. (Source: *Zhong Yi Nei Ke Xue* [*Ji Sheng Fang*])

Modifications (to Shu Zao Yin Zi)

• An alternative to using one of the strong cathartic substances, **shang lu** or **ting li zi**, is to use a large dose of **ze xie** (Alismatis Rhizoma) 泽泻, up to 30 grams.
• With constipation, add **da huang** (Rhei Radix et Rhizoma) 大黄 3–9g.
• With painful urination or blood in the urine, add **xiao ji** (Cirsii Herba) 小蓟 12–15g and **bai mao gen** (Imperatae Rhizoma) 白茅根 15–30g.
• With suppurative sores, add **jin yin hua** (Lonicerae Flos) 金银花 15–30g, **lian qiao** (Forsythiae Fructus) 连翘 9–12g, **pu gong ying** (Taraxici Herba) 蒲公英 15–30g and **ye ju hua** (Chrysanthemi indici Flos) 野菊花 9–12g.
• With weeping ulcerations, add **ku shen** (Sophorae flavescentis Radix) 苦参 9–12g and **tu fu ling** (Smilacis glabrae Rhizoma) 土茯苓 18–30g.

Prepared medicines
Concentrated powders
Dang Gui Nian Tong San (Tangkuei & Anemarrhena Combination)
 – damp heat with edema and numbness in the feet
Yin Chen Wu Ling San (Capillaris & Poria Five Formula) plus Ba Zheng San (Dianthus Formula)
 – damp heat concentrated in the lower burner
Mu Xiang Bing Lang Wan (Vladmiria & Areca Seed Formula)
 – severe systemic damp heat with strong heat and blood stasis
Fen Xiao Tang (Poria & Alisma Combination) plus San Miao San (Atractylodes & Phellodendron Formula)
 – severe systemic damp heat with abdominal distension

Pills

Bi Xie Sheng Shi Wan (Subdue the Dampness Teapills)
 – suitable for mild types

Long Dan Xie Gan Wan (Snake and Dragon Teapills) plus Wu Ling San Wan
(Wu Ling San Teapills)
 – damp heat affecting the Liver and Spleen

Acupuncture (select from)

LI.11 (quchi –)..................clears damp heat from the qi level

SJ.6 (zhigou –) ....river point of the triple burner, promotes movement
through the triple burner to dispel damp heat

Bl.22 (sanjiaoshu –)............transport point of the triple burner, frees the water
passages of the triple burner and promotes urina-
tion, and stimulates qi transformation and fluid
movement

Bl.28 (pangguangshu –) .....transport point of the Urinary Bladder, clears damp
heat from the Urinary Bladder

Ren.3 (zhongji –) ....alarm point of the Urinary Bladder, promotes urination and clears damp heat

Ren.4 (guanyuan –)............alarm point of the Small Intestine, clears damp heat

Ren.5 (shimen –)...............alarm point of the triple burner, clears damp heat

Sp.9 (yinlingquan –)...........sea point of the Spleen, promotes urination and
clears damp heat from the lower burner

Kid.7 (fuliu –) ....river point of the Kidney, clears damp heat and
relieves edema

• with hypochondriac pain, add Liv.14 (qimen –)
• with nausea add PC.6 (neiguan)
• Ear points: liver, spleen, kidney, zero point, lower extremities, subcortex,
endocrine, adrenal

Clinical notes

• Edema of a damp heat type may be diagnosed as chronic urinary tract infection, cystitis, pyelonephritis, hepatic cirrhosis or post–streptococcal glomerulonephritis.
• For dietary recommendations, see Clinical Handbook, Vol.2, p.884.

脾
湿
侵
渍

5.4 SPLEEN DAMP

Prolonged exposure to a humid or wet environment, or prolonged immersion in water enables dampness to permeate the body and seep into the muscles. As the muscles are part of the Spleen organ system, saturation with damp disrupts Spleen function and overwhelms its ability to process food and fluids. Failure to transform and distribute food and fluids results in a vicious cycle of more damp, increased Spleen dysfunction and depletion of qi. Unprocessed fluids are shunted from the Spleen back to the muscles and skin resulting in edema. This is a yang type of edema, but the longer it persists, the more Spleen deficiency starts to intervene, and the more yin type the edema becomes.

Clinical features
- Gradual onset of edema, usually starting in the extremities and over time involving the trunk. The edema may be severe enough to hide a pressing finger, but is generally non pitting or moderately pitting (depending on the degree of complicating deficiency).
- heavy sensation in the head and body
- lethargy, lassitude, fatigue
- fullness and distension in the epigastrium and abdomen
- loss of appetite, yet weight gain is noted
- nausea, reflux, heartburn
- chest oppression
- scanty, clear urine
T thick, white coat
P soggy and moderate

Treatment Principle
Promote urination to relieve edema
Dry damp and activate the qi dynamic to support the Spleen

Prescription

WU PI SAN 五皮散
Five Peel Powder, plus
WEI LING TANG 胃苓汤
Calm the Stomach and Poria Decoction

fu ling pi (Poriae Cutis) 茯苓皮 12–15g
sang bai pi (Mori Cortex) 桑白皮 12–15g
sheng jiang pi (Zingiberis Rhizomatis Cortex) 生姜皮 6–9g
chen pi (Citri reticulatae Pericarpium) 陈皮 9–12g
da fu pi (Arecae Pericarpium) 大复皮 12–15g
ze xie (Alismatis Rhizoma) 泽泻 9–12g
gui zhi (Cinnamomi Ramulus) 桂枝 6–9g
cang zhu (Atractylodis Rhizoma) 苍术 12–15g
hou po (Magnoliae officinalis Cortex) 厚朴 6–9g
bai zhu (Atractylodes macrocephalae Rhizoma) 白术 12–15g

zhu ling (Polyporus) 猪苓 12–15g
sheng jiang (Zingiberis Rhizoma) 生姜 9–12g
da zao (Jujubae Fructus) 大枣 .... 4 fruit
Method: Decoction. **Fu ling pi, sang bai pi, sheng jiang pi, ze xie** and **zhu ling** promote urination to reduce edema; **gui zhi** promotes Urinary Bladder qi transformation and frees the flow of yang qi; **cang zhu** and **bai zhu** strengthen the Spleen and dry damp; **hou po** directs qi downward and transforms damp; **chen pi** and **da fu pi** regulate the qi dynamic, move qi and promote urination; **sheng jiang** and **da zao** supplement and support the Spleen and Stomach. (Source: *Zhong Yi Nei Ke Xue* [*Zhong Zang Jing* / *Dan Xi Xin Fa*])

Modifications

- With wheezing or productive cough, add **xing ren** (Armeniacae Semen) 杏仁 9–12g, **ma huang** (Ephedra Herba) 麻黄 6–9g, **su zi** (Perillae Fructus) 苏子 6–9g and **ting li zi** (Lepidii/Descurainiae Semen) 葶苈子 6–9g.
- With cold, add **gan jiang** (Zingiberis Rhizoma) 干姜 6–9g and **chuan jiao** (Zanthoxyli Pericarpium) 川椒 6–9g.
- With spontaneous sweating and aversion to wind, add **huang qi** (Astragali Radix) 黄芪 15–30g.

Prepared medicines

Concentrated powders
Wei Ling Tang (Magnolia & Poria Combination) plus Wu Pi Yin (Poria & Areca Combination)
Fen Xiao Tang (Poria & Alisma Combination)

Pills
Wu Pi Yin (Five Peel Teapills)
Ping Wei San (Calm Stomach Teapills, Tabellae Pingwei)
Wu Ling San Wan (Wu Ling San Teapills)

Acupuncture (select from)

Bl.22 (sanjiaoshu –) .... transport point of the triple burner, regulates the water passages of the triple burner, promotes urination and stimulates qi transformation and fluid metabolism

Ren.6 (qihai +▲) .... supplements qi and activates lower burner qi transformation

Ren.9 (shuifen ▲) .... frees the water passages, promotes urination, qi transformation and the metabolism and elimination of fluids

Ren.12 (zhongwan +) .... alarm point of the Stomach, strengthens the Spleen to dry damp

Sp.6 (sanyinjiao) .... strengthens the Spleen and Kidneys to transforms damp and promote urination

Sp.9 (yinlingquan –) .... sea point of the Spleen, promotes urination to relieve edema

St.36 (zusanli +) .... sea point of the Stomach, strengthens the Spleen and Stomach, supplements qi and corrects the qi dynamic

Bl.20 (pishu +▲) ....transport point of the Spleen, strengthens the Spleen
to promote fluid metabolism

• with severe edema, add Sp.8 (diji –)
• Ear points: spleen, kidney, lungs, zero point, subcortex, endocrine, adrenal

Clinical notes

• Spleen damp type edema may be diagnosed as idiopathic edema, protein deficiency edema or chronic nephritis.
• When persistent, Spleen damp is usually complicated by Spleen qi or yang deficiency. The clinical features are similar and the first indication of increasing deficiency is seen in the edema as it becomes more and more pitting.
• A diet that strengthens the Spleen and Kidneys and assists fluid metabolism is recommended. See, Clinical Handbook, Vol.2, pp.870– 873.

气
郁
水
停

5.5 LIVER QI CONSTRAINT

The Liver ensures smooth and regular distribution of qi, blood and fluids, and regulates the qi dynamic. When the harmonious function of the Liver is impaired, the free movement of qi and fluids through the triple burner is obstructed and pathological fluid accumulates as edema. The pattern often occurs with, or is complicated by, Spleen qi deficiency, blood deficiency, heat or blood stasis.

Clinical features
- Cyclical edema that comes and goes with the patients emotional state, and is worse before the menstrual cycle. The edema primarily affects the lower abdomen, breasts and lower limbs.
- moodiness, depression, easily angered, irritability
- hypochondriac aching, distension or pain
- abdominal and epigastric distension and fullness
- poor appetite, belching, heartburn
- sallow or darkish complexion
- scanty, clear urine
- premenstrual syndrome, breast tenderness

T normal or pale, or pale edges, with a thin, white coat
P wiry

Treatment Principle
Dredge the Liver and regulate Liver qi
Promote urination to relieve edema
Support the Spleen and correct the qi dynamic

Prescription
CHAI HU SHU GAN SAN 柴胡疏肝散
Bupleurum Powder to Dredge the Liver, plus
WEI LING TANG 胃苓汤
Calm the Stomach and Poria Decoction

chai hu (Radix Bupleuri) 柴胡 9–12g
bai shao (Paeoniae Radix alba) 白芍 12–15g
zhi ke (Aurantii Fructus) 枳壳 9–12g
chen pi (Citri reticulatae Pericarpium) 陈皮 6–9g
xiang fu (Cyperi Rhizoma) 香附 9–12g
chuan xiong (Chuanxiong Rhizoma) 川芎 6–9g
zhi gan cao (Glycyrrhizae Radix preparata) 炙甘草 3–6g
fu ling (Poria) 茯苓 9–15g
zhu ling (Polyporus) 猪苓 9–12g
ze xie (Alismatis Rhizoma) 泽泻 9–15g
bai zhu (Atractylodes macrocephalae Rhizoma) 白术 9–12g
cang zhu (Atractylodis Rhizoma) 苍术 9–12g
gui zhi (Cinnamomi Ramulus) 桂枝 6–9g
hou po (Magnoliae officinalis Cortex) 厚朴 6–9g

Method: Decoction. **Chai hu** dredges the Liver and relieves qi constraint; **xiang fu** regulates Liver qi; **bai shao** softens the Liver and nourishes blood; **zhi ke** and **chen pi** regulate qi; **chuan xiong** activates the blood and stops pain; **zhi gan cao** harmonizes the other herbs in the prescription; **fu ling, zhu ling** and **ze xie** leach out damp and relieve edema; **cang zhu** dries damp; **bai zhu** strengthens the Spleen and dries damp; **gui zhi** assists in the transformation of qi to promote urination; **hou po** directs qi downward and alleviates distension. (Source: *Zhong Yi Nei Ke Xue* [*Jing Yue Quan Shu* / *Dan Xi Xin Fa*])

Modifications

- With qi deficiency, add **dang shen** (Codonopsis Radix) 党参 12–15g and **huang qi** (Astragali Radix) 黄芪 15–30g.
- With blood deficiency, use **XIAO YAO SAN** (Rambling Powder 逍遥散, p.284) as guiding prescription, instead of **CHAI HU SHU GAN SAN**.
- With heat, add **yin chen** (Artemisiae scopariae Herba) 茵陈 9–15g, **hu zhang** (Polygoni cuspidati Rhizoma) 虎杖 9–12g and **huang lian** (Coptidis Rhizoma) 黄连 3–6g, or select **JIA WEI XIAO YAO SAN** (Augmented Rambling Powder 加味逍遥散, p.713) as guiding prescription.
- With blood stasis, add **yi mu cao** (Leonurus Herba) 益母草 12–15g, **tao ren** (Persicae Semen) 桃仁 9–12g, and **hong hua** (Carthami Flos) 红花 6–9g.
- With abdominal distension, add **mu xiang** (Aucklandiae Radix) 木香 9–12g, **qing pi** (Citri reticulatae Viride Pericarpium) 青皮 6–9g and **mai ya** (Hordei Fructus germinantus) 麦芽 9–15g.
- With cold, add **gan jiang** (Zingiberis Rhizoma) 干姜 6–9g and **bu gu zhi** (Psoraleae Fructus) 补骨脂 9–12g.

Variations and additional prescriptions

Premenstrual edema from Liver and Spleen disharmony

A common type of edema is seen in women with Liver and Spleen disharmony with qi and blood deficiency and damp. They suffer from premenstrual edema, abdominal bloating, dysmenorrhea and back ache. The treatment is to harmonize the Liver and Spleen, supplement qi and blood, promote urination and relieve edema with **DANG GUI SHAO YAO SAN** (Tangkuei and Peony Powder 当归芍药散). This is a useful prescription for all fluid metabolism disorders associated with menstruation. It can also be used for abdominal pain, scanty urination and mild edema during pregnancy.

dang gui (Angelicae sinensis Radix) 当归 9–12g
bai shao (Paeoniae Radix alba) 白芍 9–15g
chuan xiong (Chuanxiong Rhizoma) 川芎 6–9g
bai zhu (Atractylodes macrocephalae Rhizoma) 白术 9–12g
ze xie (Alismatis Rhizoma) 泽泻 9–15g
fu ling (Poria) 茯苓 12–15g

Method: Grind the herbs to a powder and take 6 grams three times daily with yellow wine or water. May also be decocted with the doses as shown. **Dang gui, bai shao** and **chuan xiong** nourish and activate blood and soften the Liver; **bai zhu** strengthens the Spleen, supplements qi and dries damp; **ze xie** and **fu ling** promote urination to relieve edema. In cases with severe edema, combine with **Wu Ling San** (Five Ingredient Powder with Poria 五苓散, p.219–220). (Source: *Zhong Yi Nei Ke Xue* [*Jin Gui Yao Lüe*])

Prepared medicines
Concentrated powders
Chai Hu Shu Gan San (Bupleurum & Cyperus Combination) plus Wu Ling San (Poria Five Herb Formula)

Xiao Yao San (Bupleurum & Tangkuei Formula) plus Wu Ling San (Poria Five Herb Formula)

Jia Wei Xiao Yao San (Bupleurum & Peony Formula) plus Wu Ling San (Poria Five Herb Formula)

Dang Gui Shao Yao San (Tangkuei & Peony Formula)

Pills
Chai Hu Shu Gan Wan (Bupleurum Soothe Liver Teapills) or Xiao Yao Wan (Free and Easy Wanderer Teapills, Hsiao Yao Wan) plus Wu Ling San Wan (Wu Ling San Teapills) or Wu Pi Yin (Five Peel Teapills)

Acupuncture (select from)
Sp.9 (yinlingquan –)..........these points strengthen the Spleen and promote

Sp.6 (sanyinjiao) ....urination to relieve edema

Liv.3 (taichong –)...............source, stream and earth point of the Liver, dredges the Liver and regulates qi

GB.34 (yanglingquan –).....sea point of the Gallbladder, dredges the Liver and regulates qi

St.28 (shuidao –)................promotes urination and frees the water passages

Bl.18 (ganshu –)................transport point of the Liver, soothes the Liver and regulates qi

Bl.22 (sanjiaoshu –)...........transport point of the triple burner, frees and regulates the triple burner, promotes urination and assists in qi transformation and fluid movement

- with premenstrual edema, use Sp.4 (gongsun) and PC.6 (neiguan) to harmonize the Liver and Spleen
- with heat, add Liv.2 (xingjian –)
- with qi deficiency, add St.36 (zusanli +)
- with blood deficiency, add Bl.20 (pishu +) and Sp.10 (xuehai)
- with blood stasis and dysmenorrhea, add Sp.8 (diji –) and St.29 (guilai –)
- Ear points: liver, kidney, zero point, sympathetic, subcortex, shenmen

Clinical notes
- Edema of a qi stagnation type may be diagnosed as idiopathic edema, hormonal edema or premenstrual syndrome.
- Exercise is an essential component of treatment, p.103.
- Hot spot therapy is helpful, p.923.
- A qi mobilizing diet is recommended. See Clinical Handbook, Vol.2, p.878. Salt intake should be minimized.

瘀
血
阻
络

5.6 BLOOD STASIS

Edema associated with blood stasis can be caused by systemic pathology or localized trauma. When part of a systemic pattern, it is the result of other long term pathologies that have weakened or obstructed the circulation of qi and blood. This is a chronic and serious disorder, where static blood has permeated the network vessels impairing the free passage of qi, blood and fluids, which accumulate and spill out into the tissues. The organ systems most commonly involved are the Heart and Liver, with qi constraint or yang qi deficiency the most likely underlying pathology, although heat is sometimes seen. This type of edema may be bilateral or unilateral, and most often a mixed pattern of yin and yang edema with aspects of both excess and deficiency.

When localized, the edema follows disruption to the local channels and network vessels by trauma, surgery or scarring. The edema is likely to be unilateral, affecting one limb.

Clinical features
- Chronic non pitting or mildly pitting bilateral or unilateral edema, usually of the lower limbs. The skin over and around the edematous area is firm and may be thickened, dry, scaly or dark and discolored. There may be chronic ulcerations. When post traumatic or post surgical only one limb is affected, and the systemic signs of blood stasis may be minimal or absent.
- hypochondria fullness and pain; may be palpable masses under the ribs
- dark or purplish spider naevi or broken vessels over the abdomen (caput medusae), ribs and on the face
- abdominal distension, chest oppression, chest pain
- left iliac fossae pressure pain (p.925–926)
- dull, sallow or darkish complexion; dark rings around the eyes; dark or purplish lips and conjunctiva and nail beds
- dark clotted menses, amenorrhea, dysmenorrhea

T purplish or with purple or brown stasis spots; little or no coat; sublingual vessels are congested and dark

P deep, wiry, choppy, or irregular or intermittent

Treatment Principle
Activate qi and blood and free the network vessels and mobilize fluids
Promote urination to relieve edema

Prescription

XUE FU ZHU YU TANG 血府逐瘀汤
Drive Out Stasis in the Mansion of Blood Decoction, modified

tao ren (Persicae Semen) 桃仁	9–12g
hong hua (Carthami Flos) 红花	6–9g
dang gui (Angelicae sinensis Radix) 当归	9–12g
chuan xiong (Chuanxiong Rhizoma) 川芎	6–9g
chi shao (Paeoniae Radix rubrae) 赤芍	9–12g

chuan niu xi (Cyathulae Radix) 川牛膝 9–12g
chai hu (Radix Bupleuri) 柴胡 6–9g
zhi ke (Aurantii Fructus) 枳壳.. 6–9g
gan cao (Glycyrrhizae Radix) 甘草 3–6g
chi xiao dou (Phaseoli Semen) 赤小豆.. 15–30g
huang qi (Astragali Radix) 黄芪 15–30g
yi mu cao (Leonuri Herba) 益母草 9–15g
ze lan (Lycopi Herba) 泽兰.. 9–15g
ma bian cao (Verbenae Herba) 马鞭草 9–12g

Method: Decoction. **Tao ren** and **hong hua** activate blood, dispel blood stasis and free the network vessels; **chuan xiong**, **dang gui** and **chi shao** nourish and activate blood and free the network vessels; **chuan niu xi** supplements the Liver and Kidneys, activates blood and directs it downward; **chai hu** and **zhi ke** regulate qi; **gan cao** supplements qi, eliminates toxin and protects the Stomach; **chi xiao dou** clears heat, promotes urination and reduces swelling; **huang qi** promotes movement of fluids, strengthens the Spleen, and promotes qi flow through the network vessels; **yi mu cao**, **ze lan** and **ma bian cao** activate blood, dispel stasis, promote urination and free the network vessels. (Source: *Zhong Yi Nei Ke Xue* [*Yi Lin Gai Cuo*])

Modifications

- With severe or unresponsive edema, add **lu lu tong** (Liquidambaris Fructus) 路路通 9–12g and **che qian zi** (Plantaginis Semen) 车前子 12–15g [cooked in a cloth bag].
- With severe blood stasis, add one or two of the following substances: **san qi fen** (powdered Notoginseng Radix) 三七粉 3–6g, **di bie chong** (Eupolyphaga/Steleophaga) 地鳖虫 3–6g, **wu gong** (Scolopendra) 蜈蚣 1–2g, **quan xie** (Scorpio) 全蝎 1–2g, [all powdered and added to the strained decoction] or **di long** (Pheretima) 地龙 6–9g.
- With heat, add **sheng di** (Rehmanniae Radix) 生地 9–12g, **mu dan pi** (Moutan Cortex) 牡丹皮 9–12g and **xuan shen** (Scrophulariae Radix) 玄参 12–15g.
- With ulceration, increase the dose of **dang gui** to 15g, **gan cao** to 12g, and add **jin yin hua** (Lonicerae Flos) 金银花 15–30g and **xuan shen** (Scrophulariae Radix) 玄参 15–30g.
- With qi deficiency, add **dang shen** (Codonopsis Radix) 党参 15–24g.
- With yang deficiency, add **xian ling pi** (Epimedii Herba) 仙灵脾 12–15g, **zi he che** (Hominis Placenta) 紫河车 6g [powdered and taken separately] and **chao bai zhu** (stir fried Atractylodes macrocephalae Rhizoma) 炒白术 9–15g.
- With Heart yang deficiency and an imperceptible pulse, add **zhi fu zi** (Aconiti Radix lateralis preparata) 制附子 6–12g [cooked first] and **gui zhi** (Cinnamomi Ramulus) 桂枝 6–12g.
- With yin deficiency, add **mai dong** (Ophiopogonis Radix) 麦冬 9–12g.
- With pain in the legs, add **zhi mo yao** (Myrrha preparata) 炙没药 6–9g and **zhi ru xiang** (Olibanum preparata) 炙乳香 6–9g.
- With hypochondric or abdominal pain, add **yan hu suo** (Corydalis Rhizoma) 延胡索 9–12g and **yu jin** (Curcumae Radix) 郁金 9–12g.
- With Liver cirrhosis, add **dan shen** (Salviae miltiorrhizae Radix) 丹参 9–12g [contraindicated for patients using warfarin or heparin].

Variations and additional prescriptions

Edema following trauma or surgery

Edema that occurs after a trauma or surgical procedure is usually unilateral, affecting the limb or region below the site of the trauma or scarring. A common example is edema of the arm after axillary lymphadenectomy. In the absence of pre–existing blood stasis, there may be few of the systemic signs of blood stasis. The treatment is to gently activate blood and relieve edema with a formula such as GUI ZHI FU LING WAN (Cinnamon Twig and Poria Pill 桂枝茯苓丸) modified.

gui zhi (Cinnamomi Ramulus) 桂枝 9–12g
fu ling (Poria) 茯苓 12–15g
mu dan pi (Moutan Cortex) 牡丹皮 9–12g
chi shao (Paeoniae Radix rubra) 赤芍 9–12g
tao ren (Semen Persicae) 桃仁 6–9g
yi mu cao (Leonuri Herba) 益母草 9–12g
ze lan (Lycopi Herba) 泽兰 9–12g
lu lu tong (Liquidambaris Fructus) 路路通 9–12g
ji xue teng (Spatholobi Caulis) 鸡血藤 18–30g

Method: Decoction is preferred in this case. **Gui zhi** warms yang, promotes movement of yang qi and stimulates qi transformation; **fu ling** strengthens the Spleen and leaches out dampness; **tao ren**, **mu dan pi** and **chi shao** activate blood and transform blood stasis; **yi mu cao**, **ze lan** and **lu lu tong** activate blood, dispel stasis, promote urination and free the network vessels; **ji xue teng** nourishes blood and activates blood circulation through the network vessels. (Source: *Shang Han Lun*)

Prepared medicines

Concentrated powder

Xue Fu Zhu Yu Tang (Persica & Carthamus Combination)
Gui Zhi Fu Ling Wan (Cinnamon & Poria Formula)
Bu Yang Huan Wu Tang (Astragalus & Peony Combination) plus Wu Pi Yin
   (Poria & Areca Combination)
   – edema from blood stasis and qi deficiency

Pills

Xue Fu Zhu Yu Wan (Stasis in the Mansion of Blood Teapills)
Gui Zhi Fu Ling Wan (Cinnamon and Poria Teapills)
Sheng Tian Qi Pian 生田七片 (Raw Tian Qi Ginseng Tablets)

Acupuncture (select from)

Liv.14 (qimen –) ....alarm point of the Liver, dredges the Liver and
                                regulates qi, dispels stagnant blood
Liv.13 (zhangmen –) ....alarm point of the Spleen and meeting point of the
                                internal organs, strengthens the Spleen to assist fluid
                                metabolism and promotes Liver function
Bl.17 (geshu –) ....meeting point for blood, dispels stagnant blood
Bl.18 (ganshu –) ....transport point of the Liver, regulates Liver qi and
                                activates blood
Sp.10 (xuehai –) ....activates and cools blood
Sp.9 (yinlingquan –) ....together these points strengthen the Spleen and

Sp.6 (sanyinjiao)   promote urination to relieve edema, and activate qi
                           and blood flow through the legs
Ren.9 (shuifen ▲)..............promotes urination and transformation of fluids
St.28 (shuidao –)..............promotes urination and frees the water passages
Liv.3 (taichong –)..............source, stream and earth point, activates qi and
                           blood

- for scarring, insert needles on both sides of the scar obliquely towards the scar at 1–2 cm intervals
- with pain, add LI.4 (hegu –) and Liv.6 (zhongdu –)
- with qi deficiency, add Ren.12 (zhongwan), St.36 (zusanli)
- with heat, add Liv.2 (xingjian –)
- with spasms or cramping pain, add Du.8 (jinsuo –)
- Ear points: liver, spleen, kidney, zero point, lower extremities or affected region, adrenal, subcortex, endocrine

Clinical notes

- Edema of a blood stasis type may be diagnosed as thrombophlebitis, deep venous thrombosis, post surgical edema, lymph edema following lymphadenectomy, hepatic cirrhosis or cancer, chronic nephritis, chronic hepatitis, congestive cardiac failure or coronary heart disease.
- The edema of a blood stasis type can respond relatively well depending on the primary location of the pathogen. Blood stasis in the Liver can respond reasonably well to prolonged treatment. Heart blood stasis and blood stasis associated with masses or tumors can be more difficult to treat and often require a combined Western and Chinese medical approach. Blood stasis in the limbs will often respond well, with edema clearing as the circulation is gradually restored. As a general rule, however, the underlying blood stasis requires lengthy treatment for a lasting result.
- Pay close attention to the clotting status of the patient, as some patients will often be medicated with pharmaceuticals such as warfarin or heparin. While Chinese herbs and blood activating formulae can be used in conjunction with blood thinning medications, herbs such as **dan shen** (Salviae miltiorrhizae Radix) 丹参 should be avoided.
- A qi and blood mobilizing diet is recommended. See Clinical Handbook, Vol.2, 886. Salt intake should be minimized.

气
虚
水
溢

5.7 QI DEFICIENCY

Qi deficiency impairs the ability of the Lungs, Spleen and Kidneys to process fluids. Depending on the organ systems affected, the clinical features and treatments vary. When Lung qi deficiency is predominant, the edema is concentrated in the upper body and face. When Spleen function is impaired, the edema affects the eyes, fingers and abdomen. When the Kidneys are involved, the edema is seen below the waist. This type of edema is chronic and mild to moderate. The location of the edema gives clues as to the organ system most affected. The Heart can also be affected, and although it is not specifically involved in fluid metabolism, weak Heart qi can be a factor in dependent edema.

Clinical features
- Persistent or intermittent mild edema. The edema is moderately pitting.
- tiredness, fatigue, weakness
- waxy, pale complexion
- **Lung qi deficiency**: edema more prominent in the face, breathlessness with exertion, weak voice, spontaneous sweating, scanty urine
- **Spleen qi deficiency**: edema prominent in the eyelids and orbits, fingers and hands in the morning. Edema in the ankles increases in the afternoon; loss of appetite, poor muscle tone, abdominal distension, loose stools, scanty, frequent, occasionally profuse urination
- **Kidney qi deficiency**: edema in the ankles when standing, and over the sacrum when lying down, lower back aching and weakness, aching legs, scanty, profuse or frequent urine, nocturia
- **Heart qi deficiency**: edema of the ankles, palpitations, arrhythmia, chest oppression, intermittent or irregular pulse

T pale and scalloped and a thin, white coat
P fine and weak

Treatment Principle
Supplement qi, drain damp and strengthen fluid metabolism to transform damp
Promote urination to relieve edema

Prescription

FANG JI HUANG QI TANG 防己黄芪汤
Stephania and Astragalus Decoction, plus
SHEN LING BAI ZHU SAN 参苓白术散
Ginseng, Poria and White Atractylodes Powder, modified

This prescription is suitable for patients with Lung and Spleen qi deficiency and scanty urination.

huang qi (Astragali Radix) 黄芪 15–60g
han fang ji (Stephaniae tetrandrae Radix) 汉防己 9–12g
ren shen (Ginseng Radix) 人参 6–9g
chao bai zhu (stir fried Atractylodes macrocephalae Rhizoma) 炒白术 ... 9–15g
fu ling pi (Poriae Cutis) 茯苓皮 12–15g

yi ren (Coicis Semen) 苡仁.. 15–30g
shan yao (Dioscoreae Rhizoma) 山药................................. 12–15g
che qian zi (Plantaginis Semen) 车前子.............................. 9–12g
du zhong (Eucommiae Cortex) 杜仲 12–15g
zhi gan cao (Glycyrrhizae Radix preparata) 炙甘草.............................. 3–6g
Method: Decoction. **Che qian zi** is cooked in a cloth bag. **Huang qi** and **ren shen** strengthen the Spleen, supplement qi and stimulate qi transformation to move fluids and relieve edema; **han fang ji** drains damp and promotes urination; **shan yao** and **chao bai zhu** strengthen the Spleen and dry damp; **fu ling pi**, **yi ren** and **che qian zi** promote urination and reduce edema; **du zhong** supplements Kidney yang qi; **zhi gan cao** supplements qi and harmonizes the other herbs. (Source: *Zhong Yi Nei Ke Xue* [*Shang Han Lun* / *He Ji Ju Fang*])

Modifications
- With copious urination, delete **han fang ji** and **che qian zi**, and add **gui zhi** (Cinnamomi Ramulus) 桂枝 3–9g to promote qi transformation.
- With fluid in the abdominal cavity, add **da fu pi** (Arecae Pericarpium) 大复皮 9–12g, **sheng jiang pi** (Zingiberis Rhizomatis Cortex) 生姜皮 6–9g, **chen pi** (Citri reticulatae Pericarpium) 陈皮 6–9g and **ji nei jin** (Gigeriae galli Endothelium corneum) 鸡内金 5g [as powder added to the strained decoction].
- With qi stagnation, disruption to the qi dynamic and abdominal bloating, add **mu xiang** (Aucklandiae Radix) 木香 9–12g, **xiang yuan pi** (Citri Pericarpium) 香橼皮 9–12g, **fo shou** (Citri sarcodactylis Fructus) 佛手 9–12g and **da fu pi** (Arecae Pericarpium) 大复皮 9–12g.

Variations and additional prescriptions
Kidney qi deficiency
With prominent Kidney qi deficiency the edema is predominant in the ankles and urinary symptoms such as frequency and nocturia feature. The aim of treatment is to warm and supplement Kidney qi and promote urination to relieve edema. When urination is scanty and edema pronounced **JI SHENG SHEN QI WAN** (Kidney Qi Pill from Formulas to Aid the Living 济生肾气丸, p.248) is selected to focus on relieving the edema. When edema is mild and urination frequent or copious, warming the Kidneys is the priority, and the formula to do so is **JIN GUI SHEN QI WAN** (Kidney Qi Pill from the Golden Cabinet 金匮肾气丸, p.826).

Heart qi deficiency
The Heart can be affected by systemic qi deficiency, and the circulation of qi, blood and fluids is further compromised. There are two variants. Heart, Lung and Spleen qi deficiency gives rise to edema in the face, hands and feet, sleep disturbance, palpitations and anxiety. The treatment is to supplement qi and blood, calm the shen and promote urination with **GUI PI TANG** (Restore the Spleen Decoction 归脾汤, p.387) as guiding prescription.

With Heart and Kidney qi deficiency, ankle edema is accompanied by arrhythmias, chest oppression and an irregular or intermittent pulse. The treatment is to supplement qi and blood, restore the pulse and promote urination with **ZHI GAN CAO TANG** (Prepared Licorice Decoction 炙甘草汤, p.811) as guiding prescription. Both prescriptions can be augmented with bland, diuretic herbs such as **chi xiao dou** (Phaseoli Semen) 赤小豆, **yi mu cao** (Leonurus Herba) 益母草, **ze xie** (Alismatis Rhizoma) 泽泻 and **che qian zi** (Plantaginis Semen) 车前子, or combined with **Wu Ling San** (Five Ingredient Powder with Poria 五苓散, p.219–220).

Premenstrual edema

Premenstrual edema can be caused by Spleen and Kidney qi deficiency. The main symptoms are edema that is worse between ovulation and menstruation, with progressive abdominal bloating, diarrhea, scanty urination, lower back ache, a pale, swollen tongue with a thick coat and a moderate, deep and wiry pulse. The basal body temperature chart may reveal a low or short luteal (yang) phase. The treatment is to warm the Kidneys, strengthen the Spleen and reduce edema with **Xiao Zhong Tang** (Disperse Swelling Decoction 消肿汤).

xian ling pi (Epimedii Herba) 仙灵脾 12–15g
ba ji tian (Morindae Radix) 巴戟天 12–15g
zhu ling (Polyporus) 猪苓 9–12g
ze xie (Alismatis Rhizoma) 泽泻 9–12g
hou po (Magnoliae officinalis Cortex) 厚朴 9–12g
cang zhu (Atractylodis Rhizoma) 苍术 9–12g
bai dou kou (Amomi Fructus rotundus) 白豆蔻 3–6g
chao zhi shi (stir fried Aurantii Fructus immaturus) 炒枳实 6–9g
chuan xiong (Chuanxiong Rhizoma) 川芎 6–9g
hong hua (Carthami Flos) 红花 6–9g
yu jin (Curcumae Radix) 郁金 6–9g

Method: Decoction. **Bai dou kou** is added towards the end of cooking. **Xian ling pi** and **ba ji tian** warm and supplement Kidney qi to stimulate fluid metabolism; **zhu ling** and **ze xie** promote urination and reduce edema; **hou po** and **chao zhi shi** move qi and alleviate distension; **cang zhu**, **hou po** and **bai dou kou** dry damp and rectify the qi dynamic; **chuan xiong**, **hong hua** and **yu jin** activate qi and blood. (Source: *Zhong Yi Zhi Liao Yi Nan Za Bing Mi Yao*)

With blood stasis in the network vessels

Occasionally patients do not respond to qi supplementation as expected, even when clearly qi deficient. If the prescription selected does not reduce the edema significantly within a week or two, it may be that the disease has entered the blood level. Blood stasis is not always obvious symptomatically, and may only be surmised from the lack of effect of the initial treatment strategy. Try addressing the blood level by combining the primary prescription above (p.240) with a blood activating, network vessel freeing prescription such as **Tao Hong Si Wu Tang** (Four Substance Decoction with Safflower and Peach Pit 桃红四物汤, p.921).

During pregnancy

Edema during pregnancy is often caused by Spleen and Kidney qi deficiency. The symptoms are edema of the ankles, face and hands, loss of appetite and nausea, lower back ache, a pale swollen tongue and a moderate, slippery or weak pulse. The treatment is to strengthen the Spleen and Kidney, while gently promoting urination with **Bai Zhu San** (White Atractylodes Powder 白术散). Caution with excessive diuresis during pregnancy as this can reduce amniotic fluid.

bai zhu (Atractylodes macrocephalae Rhizoma) 白术 9–12g
fu ling pi (Poriae Cutis) 茯苓皮 15–30g
da fu pi (Arecae Pericarpium) 大复皮 9–12g
sheng jiang pi (Zingiberis Rhizomatis Cortex) 生姜皮 9–12g
chen pi (Citri reticulatae Pericarpium) 陈皮 6–9g

Method: Decoction. **Bai zhu**, **fu ling pi** and **sheng jiang pi** strengthen the Spleen, dry damp and promote urination; **da fu pi** directs qi and damp downward; **chen pi** regulates qi and harmonizes the middle burner. With severe edema, add **che qian zi** (Plantaginis Semen) 车前子 6–9g, **sang bai pi** (Mori Cortex) 桑白皮 9–12g and **chi xiao dou** (Phaseoli Semen) 赤小豆 15–30g; with hypertension, add **gou teng** (Uncariae Ramulus cum Uncis) 钩藤 12–15g and **ju hua** (Chrysanthemi Flos) 菊花 9–12g. (Source: *Shi Yong Zhong Yi Fu Ke Xue*)

To strengthen the Spleen and Lungs following resolution

Following resolution of the edema, a supplementing strategy should be adopted to consolidate and rebuild qi. A variety of suitable prescriptions are available, in convenient prepared pill and powder form for long term use. For example, Yu Ping Feng Wan (Jade Screen Teapills) or Bu Zhong Yi Qi Wan (Central Chi Teapills) can be used when the Lungs and wei qi are weak; Shen Ling Bai Zhu Wan (Absorption and Digestion Pill, Shen Ling Bai Zhu Pian) or Si Jun Zi Wan (Four Gentlemen Teapills) are used for Spleen qi deficiency; Jin Kui Shen Qi Wan (Fu Gui Ba Wei Wan, Golden Book Teapills) or Ba Ji Yin Yang Wan (Ba Ji Yin Yang Teapills) are suitable for Kidney qi deficiency; Sheng Mai Wan (Great Pulse Teapills) is used for qi and yin deficiency.

Prepared medicines
Concentrated powders
Shen Ling Bai Zhu San (Ginseng & Atractylodes Formula) plus Fang Ji Huang
  Qi Tang (Stephania & Astragalus Combination)

Pills
Shen Ling Bai Zhu Wan (Absorbtion and Digestion Pill, Shen Ling Bai Zhu Pian)
  plus Fang Ji Huang Qi Wan (Stephania and Astragalus Teapills)

Acupuncture (select from)

Sp.9 (yinlingquan –)	together these points strengthen the Spleen and
Sp.6 (sanyinjiao +)	promote urination to relieve edema, and activate qi and blood flow through the legs
Lu.7 (lieque)	diffuses the Lungs and directs Lung qi downward to free the water passages and promote urination
Kid.7 (fuliu –)	metal point of the Kidneys, strengthens Kidney qi and stimulates fluid metabolism to relieve edema
Ren.9 (shuifen ▲)	frees and regulates the water passages, promotes urination, qi transformation and elimination of fluids
Ren.12 (zhongwan +)	alarm point of the Stomach, strengthens the Spleen and supplements qi
St.36 (zusanli +)	sea point of the Stomach, strengthens the Spleen and Stomach, supplements qi and corrects the qi dynamic

Bl.22 (sanjiaoshu)...............transport point of the triple burner, frees and regulates the water passages of the triple burner, promotes urination and stimulates qi transformation and fluid metabolism

- Ear points: spleen, lungs, kidney, heart, zero point, subcortex, endocrine, adrenal

Clinical notes

- Edema of a qi deficiency type may be diagnosed as nephrotic syndrome, idiopathic edema, hormonal edema, preeclampsia, premenstrual syndrome, ovarian hyper stimulation syndrome, allergy or chronic nephritis.
- Edema from qi deficiency is common, especially amongst women of reproductive years. In general it responds well to treatment.
- A qi supplementing diet is recommended. See Clinical Handbook, Vol.2, p.870. In addition to a warming and Spleen strengthening diet, certain foods can assist in managing edema from qi deficiency. For example, a rice porridge or congee (*zhōu* 粥) cooked with **huang qi** (Astragali Radix) 黄芪 30–60g, **yi ren** (Coicis Semen) 苡仁 30g and **chi xiao dou** (Phaseoli Semen) 赤小豆 15g makes a relatively tasty diuretic breakfast, which also strengthens the Spleen. Salt intake should be minimized.
- Take careful note of how much fluid the patient is drinking. Many people drink too much fluid in an attempt to 'flush their kidneys' or because they have been led to believe they must drink several liters of water per day. If fluid metabolism is already weak, this practice will overload the Kidneys and Spleen. It is sufficient to drink enough water for the urine to run clear (although some substances such as the B group of vitamins, will color of urine no matter how much you drink).

脾
阳
虚
衰

5.8 SPLEEN YANG DEFICIENCY

Edema from Spleen yang deficiency is common, and usually the result of dietary factors. Spleen yang is easily damaged by inappropriate weight loss programs, fasting and excessive use of slimming aids. It can also be weakened by bitter cold herbs and medications used in the treatment of damp heat conditions. Weak yang is unable to process and distribute fluids, which accumulate in the tissues and sink into the abdomen and lower body. This failure of processing is compounded by the cold which restricts the vessels and further slows qi, blood and fluid movement. This is a yin type of edema. Spleen yang deficiency edema is usually complicated by varying degrees of Kidney yang deficiency.

Clinical features
- Chronic pitting edema that begins gradually, starting on the limbs and around the eyes, eventually affecting the whole body. Orbital and upper limb edema are worse in the morning, with increasing ankle edema as the day progresses.
- Urine may be scanty or copious. When the edema is severe the urine will be scanty. Occasionally, however, the weakened Spleen is unable to maintain muscle tone, the urethral sphincter becomes lax or the bladder prolapses, and the patient experiences frequency or incontinence or urine.
- loss of appetite, anorexia; patients may report they eat little and still gain weight
- loose stools or watery diarrhea with undigested food; occasionally constipation with dry stools (if fluids are drawn away from the Intestines into the tissues)
- marked abdominal distension; abdominal pain better for warmth
- upper abdomen feels toneless and cool to the touch; poor muscle tone, tissues feel soggy and waterlogged
- pale, waxy or sallow complexion
- cold intolerance, cold abdomen, cold extremities
- fatigue and weakness

T pale and swollen with teeth marks and a thin, white or greasy coat
P deep and moderate or deep and weak

Treatment Principle
Warm and strengthen Spleen yang and stimulate fluid metabolism
Promote urination to relieve edema

Prescription

SHI PI YIN 实脾饮
Bolster the Spleen Drink

zhi fu zi (Aconiti Radix lateralis preparata) 制附子 6–9g
gan jiang (Zingiberis Rhizoma) 干姜 6–9g
fu ling (Poria) 茯苓 9–12g
chao bai zhu (stir fried Atractylodes macrocephalae Rhizoma) 炒白术 ... 9–12g
mu gua (Chaenomelis Fructus) 木瓜 9–12g
hou po (Magnoliae officinalis Cortex) 厚朴 6–9g

mu xiang (Aucklandiae Radix) 木香..6–9g
da fu pi (Arecae Pericarpium) 大复皮 6–9g
cao guo (Tsaoko Fructus) 草果..6–9g
zhi gan cao (Glycyrrhizae Radix preparata) 炙甘草............................3–6g
sheng jiang (Zingiberis Rhizoma) 生姜...6–9g
da zao (Jujubae Fructus) 大枣 ....3 fruit

Method: Decoction. **Zhi fu zi** is cooked for 30 minutes prior to the other herbs. **Zhi fu zi** and **gan jiang** warm Spleen yang and stimulate fluid metabolism; **fu ling** and **chao bai zhu** strengthen the Spleen and dry damp; **mu gua**, **hou po**, **mu xiang**, **da fu pi** and **cao guo** direct qi downwards, transform damp and promote urination; the combination of the ascending pungent heat of **zhi fu zi** and **gan jiang** with the bitter descent of **hou po** and **da fu pi** rectifies the qi dynamic; **sheng jiang**, **zhi gan cao** and **da zao** strengthen and protect the Stomach. (Source: *Zhong Yi Nei Ke Xue* [*Shi Yi De Xiao Fang*])

Modifications

- With severe abdominal distension and scanty urination, delete **da zao** and **zhi gan cao**, and add **ze xie** (Alismatis Rhizoma) 泽泻 9–12g, **gui zhi** (Cinnamomi Ramulus) 桂枝 9–12g and **zhu ling** (Polyporus) 猪苓 9–12g.
- With watery diarrhea, add **bu gu zhi** (Psoraleae Fructus) 补骨脂 6–9g and **shan yao** (Dioscoreae Rhizoma) 山药 9–12g.
- With constipation, add **suo yang** (Cynomorii Herba) 锁阳 12–15g.
- With damp and a thick white tongue coat, add **cang zhu** (Atractylodis Rhizoma) 苍术 9–12g.
- With organ prolapse and incontinence of urine, add **huang qi** (Astragali Radix) 黄芪 15–30g and **ren shen** (Ginseng Radix) 人参 6–9g.
- With wheezing or productive cough, delete **da zao** and **zhi gan cao**, and add **sha ren** (Amomi Fructus) 砂仁 3–6g, **chen pi** (Citri reticulatae Pericarpium) 陈皮 6–9g and **zi su ye** (Perillae Fructus) 紫苏叶 9–12g.

Prepared medicines
Concentrated powders
Fu Zi Li Zhong Tang (Aconite, Ginseng and Ginger Combination) plus Hou Po Wen Zhong Tang (Magnolia & Vladmiria Combination)

Pills
Fu Zi Li Zhong Wan (Fu Tzu Li Chung Wan, Li Chung Yuen Medical Pills) or Li Zhong Wan (Li Chung Wan) plus Wu Ling San Wan (Wu Ling San Teapills)

Acupuncture (select from)
Ren.9 (shuifen ▲)..............promote urination and transformation of fluids
St.28 (shuidao ▲)
Ren.4 (guanyuan +▲) ....these points warm Kidney yang to promote
Ren.6 (qihai +▲)   transformation and metabolism of fluids
Sp.9 (yinlingquan –)...........together these points strengthen the Spleen and
Sp.6 (sanyinjiao +)   promote urination to relieve edema
Kid.7 (fuliu –) ....river and metal point of the Kidneys, strengthens
                                Kidney qi to stimulate fluid metabolism and relieve
                                edema

St.36 (zusanli +▲) ....sea point of the Stomach, strengthens the Spleen and Stomach, supplements qi and corrects the qi dynamic

Bl.20 (pishu +▲) ....transport points of the Spleen, triple burner, Kidney
Bl.22 (sanjiaoshu +▲)   and Urinary Bladder respectively, together these
Bl.23 (shenshu +▲)   points warm Spleen and Kidney yang, free and
Bl.28 (pangguangshu +▲) regulate the water passages of the triple burner and promote urination, assist in qi transformation and promote fluid metabolism

• with organ prolapse, add Du.20 (baihui ▲)
• with marked abdominal bloating or pain, add St.25 (tianshu ▲)
• Ear points: spleen, kidney, zero point, adrenal, subcortex, endocrine

Clinical notes

• Spleen yang deficiency edema may be diagnosed as idiopathic edema, nephrotic syndrome, chronic nephritis, chronic hepatitis, early stage of hepatic cirrhosis or cardiac edema.
• This is a common pattern of recurrent and chronic edema, with a lengthy course that fluctuates depending on diet, work and the energy levels of the patient, and in some cases the weather. The edema often responds quite quickly to correct treatment, however long term success varies depending on the length and severity of the condition. Some months of dedicated treatment and dietary modification may be necessary to rebuild Spleen yang.
• A yang warming diet is recommended. See Clinical Handbook, Vol.2, p.873. Salt intake should be minimized.
• Take careful note of how much fluid the patient is drinking. Many people drink too much fluid because they have been led to believe they must drink several liters of water per day. If fluid metabolism is weak, this practice will overload the Kidneys and Spleen. It is sufficient to drink enough water for the urine to run clear (although some substances such as the B group of vitamins, will color of urine no matter how much you drink).
• Harsh fluid purging cathartic herbs must be avoided in deficiency patterns unless absolutely necessary. They effectively eliminate fluids in the short term, but may aggravate yang deficiency with repeated or prolonged use.

肾
阳
衰
微

5.9 KIDNEY YANG DEFICIENCY

• Kidney and Heart yang deficiency

Kidney yang deficiency is common cause of chronic edema. Kidney yang is the foundation of fluid metabolism, and it is Kidney yang that supplies yang to and supports the function of, the Spleen, Lungs and Heart. Any chronic edema pattern will eventually involve the Kidneys to some degree. This is a yin type of edema.

Clinical features
• Chronic pitting edema that is worse below the waist. Edema is most obvious in the ankles and knees while ambulant, and may accumulate in the scrotum and sacrum when recumbent. In severe cases the whole body is affected.
• When the edema is severe the urine will be scanty. When Kidney yang is unable to process fluids at all, or loses control of the 'lower yin', the urethral sphincter, and the patient can experience frequent nocturia or incontinence. The urine may be frothy or cloudy.
• weak, cold, aching lower back and knees; the abdomen is flaccid and cold below the umbilicus
• cold intolerance, cold extremities
• pale sallow complexion, dark circles under the eyes
• weakness, lethargy, exhaustion
• loss of libido, impotence
• **Heart yang deficiency**: severe edema, pulmonary edema, palpitations, arrhythmia, breathlessness, icy cold extremities, irregular or imperceptible pulse
T swollen, pale and scalloped and a thin, white coat
P deep, fine, weak; or irregular and intermittent

Treatment Principle
Warm and supplement Kidney yang and stimulate fluid metabolism
Promote urination to relieve edema

Prescription

JI SHENG SHEN QI WAN 济生肾气丸
Kidney Qi Pill from Formulas to Aid the Living

ze xie (Alismatis Rhizoma) 泽泻	30g
fu ling (Poria) 茯苓	30g
che qian zi (Plantaginis Semen) 车前子	30g
shan zhu yu (Corni Fructus) 山茱萸	30g
shan yao (Dioscoreae Rhizoma) 山药	30g
mu dan pi (Moutan Cortex) 牡丹皮	30g
zhi fu zi (Aconiti Radix lateralis preparata) 制附子	15g
gui zhi (Cinnamomi Ramulus) 桂枝	15g
shu di (Rehmanniae Radix preparata) 熟地	15g
chuan niu xi (Cyathulae Radix) 川牛膝	15g

Method: Grind herbs to a fine powder and form into 9 gram pills with honey. The dose is one pill 2–3 times daily. May also be decocted with a 50% reduction in dosage. When decocted **zhi fu zi** is cooked for 30 minutes before the other herbs, **rou gui** is added towards the end of cooking and **che qian zi** is decocted in a cloth bag. **Ze xie**, **fu ling** and **che qian zi** promote urination and relieve edema; **zhi fu zi** and **gui zhi** warm Kidney yang, dispel cold, promote the transformation of qi and improve fluid metabolism; **shu di** and **shan zhu yu** nourish and protect Liver and Kidney yin and improve Kidney function; **shan yao** strengthens the Spleen and Kidneys and supplements qi; **mu dan pi** activates the blood; **chuan niu xi** supplements the Kidneys and directs the action of the formula to the lower burner. (Source: *Shi Yong Zhong Yi Nei Ke Xue* [*Ji Sheng Fang*])

Modifications (to Ji Sheng Shen Qi Wan)

- With profuse urination or nocturia, delete **ze xie** and **che qian zi**, and add **tu si zi** (Cuscutae Semen) 菟丝子 30g and **bu gu zhi** (Psoraleae Fructus) 补骨脂 30g.
- With cloudy or frothy urine, add **tu si zi** (Cuscutae Semen) 菟丝子 30g and **bi xie** (Dioscoreae hypoglaucae Rhizoma) 萆薢 15g.
- With low back and leg ache, add **du zhong** (Eucommiae Cortex) 杜仲 30g and **xu duan** (Dipsaci Radix) 续断 30g.
- With icy cold limbs and severe yang deficiency, delete **mu dan pi** and add **hu lu ba** (Trigonellae Semen) 胡芦巴 15g and **ba ji tian** (Morindae officinalis Radix) 巴戟天 15g.
- With ascites and severe abdominal distension, add **da fu pi** (Arecae Pericarpium) 大腹皮 30g and **hou po** (Magnoliae officinalis Cortex) 厚朴 15g.
- With Spleen deficiency, add **chao bai zhu** (stir fried Atractylodes macrocephalae Rhizoma) 炒白术 30g.
- With blood stasis, add **pu huang** (Typhae Pollen) 蒲黄 15g and **dan shen** (Salviae miltiorrhizae Radix) 丹参 15g.
- With wheezing, shortness of breath or orthopnea, add **ren shen** (Ginseng Radix) 人参 15g and **wu wei zi** (Schizandrae Fructus) 五味子 10g.
- With frequent nocturia, add **wu wei zi** (Schizandrae Fructus) 五味子 15g.
- With impotence, add **ba ji tian** (Morindae Radix) 巴戟天 30g, **rou cong rong** (Cistanches Herba) 肉苁蓉 30g and **gou qi zi** (Lycii Fructus) 枸杞子 30g.

ZHEN WU TANG 真武汤
True Warrior Decoction

This prescription is selected when Heart and Kidney yang are deficient. The weak Heart is unable to move the unprocessed fluids and severe edema results. The treatment is to vigorously transform and drain the edema, while warming Heart yang. This prescription can be used until fluids are moving, urinary output increases and the patient is more stable (a few weeks), after which time a supplementing strategy (see Variations) can be adopted.

zhi fu zi (Aconiti Radix lateralis preparata) 制附子 9–15g
bai zhu (Atractylodis macrocephalae Rhizoma) 白术 9–12g
fu ling (Poria) 茯苓 12–30g
sheng jiang (Zingiberis Rhizoma Recens) 生姜 9–15g
bai shao (Paeoniae Radix alba) 白芍 12–18g
Method: Decoction. **Zhi fu zi** is cooked for 30 minutes prior to the other herbs. **Zhi fu zi** strength-

ens the Heart, warms yang, scatters cold and vigorously stimulates fluid metabolism; **bai zhu** and **fu ling** strengthen the Spleen, dry damp and promote urination; **sheng jiang** warms and scatters cold; **bai shao** protects yin and prevents excessive dispersal of the weak yang qi. (Source: *Shi Yong Zhong Yi Nei Ke Xue* [*Shang Han Lun*])

Modifications (to Zhen Wu Tang)

- With pulmonary edema, add **ting li zi** (Lepidii/Descurainiae Semen) 葶苈子 6–9g, **ze xie** (Alismatis Rhizoma) 泽泻 9–12g and **zhu ling** (Polyporus) 猪苓 9–12g.
- With blood stasis, add **gui zhi** (Cinnamomi Ramulus) 桂枝 9–12g, **zhi gan cao** (Glycyrrhizae Radix preparata) 炙甘草 9–12g, **dan shen** (Salviae miltiorrhizae Radix) 丹参 9–15g and **hong hua** (Carthami Flos) 红花 6–9g.
- In severe Heart yang deficiency, the yang may be on the point of collapse. The patient is cold and clammy, cyanotic, pale white and has icy extremities and a fibrillating pulse. The dose of **zhi fu zi** can be increased to as much as 30 grams (see Clinical notes), **gan jiang** (Zingiberis Rhizoma) 干姜 6–9g substituted for **sheng jiang**, and **gui zhi** (Cinnamomi Ramulus) 桂枝 9–12g and **zhi gan cao** (Glycyrrhizae Radix preparata) 炙甘草 9–12g added.

Variations and additional prescriptions

Collapsing Heart yang

- If Heart yang collapses and the patient loses consciousness, the treatment is to administer an emergency medicine such as GUAN XIN SU HE XIANG WAN (Liquid Styrax Pills for Coronary Heart Disease 冠心苏合香丸), and institute emergency acupuncture techniques (next page) until paramedic assistance arrives. An alternative approach used in hospitals in China is SHEN FU TANG (Ginseng and Prepared Aconite Decoction 参附汤, p.919 and 263) administered intravenously.

After the edema has subsided

- Once the edema has subsided, a more general Kidney yang warming and supplementing prescription, such as YOU GUI WAN (Restore the Right [Kidney] Pill 右归丸, p.394) or JIN GUI SHEN QI WAN (Kidney Qi Pill from the Golden Cabinet 金匮肾气丸, p.826) may be phased in for long term rebuilding of yang.

Prepared medicines

Concentrated powder

Ji Sheng Shen Qi Wan (Cyathula & Plantago Formula)
Zhen Wu Tang (Ginger, Aconite, Poria & Peony Combination)
Ba Wei Di Huang Wan (Rehmannia Eight Formula)

Pills

Jin Gui Shen Qi Wan (Fu Gui Ba Wei Wan, Golden Book Teapills)
Zhen Wu Tang Wan (True Warrior Teapills)

Acupuncture (select from)

Ren.9 (shuifen ▲)..............these points free the water passages, promote

St.28 (shuidao ▲)   urination and transformation of fluids

Ren.4 (guanyuan +▲)........these points warm Kidney yang

Ren.6 (qihai +▲)

Sp.9 (yinlingquan –)...........sea point of the Spleen, promotes urination and
relieves

Sp.6 (sanyinjiao ▲)...........warms and strengthens the Spleen and Kidney

Kid.7 (fuliu –) ....river and metal point of the Kidneys, strengthens
Kidney qi and stimulates fluid metabolism to relieve
edema

St.36 (zusanli +▲) ....sea point of the Stomach, strengthens the Spleen and
supplements qi

Bl.15 (xinshu +▲) ....transport points of the Heart, triple burner, Kidney

Bl.22 (sanjiaoshu +▲)   and Urinary Bladder respectively, together these

Bl.23 (shenshu +▲)   points warm Heart and Kidney yang, free the

Bl.28 (pangguangshu ▲)   water passages of the triple burner to promote urination and fluid metabolism

- Ear points: kidney, heart, triple burner, zero point, adrenal, subcortex,
endocrine

Emergency management of Heart yang collapse

During an acute episode of collapsing Heart yang, emergency management may
be necessary until paramedic assistance is available. If a pulse cannot be detected
Cardio–Pulmonary Resuscitation (CPR) should be started immediately.

Main points

- PC.6 (neiguan –), PC.4 (ximen –), Bl.15 (xinshu –)
- Huatuo Jiaji points around T4–T5, Ren.17 (shanzhong –)
- All points are treated with strong reducing stimulation, with the needle sensation radiating up the arm or to the chest. The points can be needled or pressed
with strong finger pressure or other appropriate instrument.

Secondary points

- Ht.5 (tongli –) – arrhythmia
- PC.5 (jianshi –) – chest oppression
- St.36 (zusanli –) – severe sweating, collapse

Clinical notes

- Edema of a Kidney and Heart yang deficiency type may be diagnosed as nephrotic syndrome, congestive cardiac failure, left ventricular failure, chronic
nephritis, hypothyroidism, prostatic hypertrophy or hepatic cirrhosis.
- Take careful note of how much fluid the patient is drinking. Many people drink
too much fluid because they have been led to believe they must drink several
liters of water per day. If fluid metabolism is weak, this practice will overload
the Kidneys and Heart and aggravate the edema. It is sufficient to drink enough
water for the urine to run clear (although some substances such as the B group
of vitamins, will color of urine no matter how much you drink).

- When yin edema is extreme, causing breathing difficulties and imminent collapse, quickly mobilizing and eliminating fluids is imperative. In such cases, up to 30 grams of **zhi fu zi** (Aconiti Radix lateralis preparata) 制附子, boiled for at least an hour, can be used to promote diuresis for a few days. This may seem like an excessively high dose, but is safe when used properly and can be life saving in the correct circumstance. Once urinary output increases, the dose of **zhi fu zi** is reduced until the patient is stable and a maintenance dose reached.
- A yang warming diet is recommended. See Clinical Handbook, Vol.2, p.873. Salt intake should be minimized.
- Harsh fluid purging cathartic herbs must be avoided in deficiency patterns unless absolutely necessary. They effectively eliminate fluids in the short term, but seriously aggravate yang deficiency with repeated or prolonged use.
- This is a relatively serious pattern, especially when Heart yang is weak, and may require months of persistent treatment for stabilization and sustained results.

气阴两虚 | 5.10 QI AND YIN DEFICIENCY

气
阴
两
虚

Qi and yin deficiency edema often starts as a qi or yang deficiency pattern that is poorly treated or untreated. Excessive or inappropriate diuresis in the treatment of a pre–existing pattern of edema can damage yin. Excessive or improper use of pungent warm or hot dispersing herbs and pharmaceuticals (**zhi fu zi**, steroids) may also be implicated. Qi and yin deficiency type edema can also follow pregnancy, or be the result of chronic heat pathogen in the lower burner.

The mechanism of the edema is based on the fact that yin deficiency reflects a failure of cells and tissues to absorb and hold onto physiological fluids. The tissues become desiccated, normal physiological fluids are not incorporated into cells and remain in the interstitial space. The process can be likened to the effects of rain on ground long parched by drought–instead of soaking into the ground it skates off the surface and accumulates in stagnant pockets.

Clinical features
• Mild to moderate edema in a patient with general dryness. The edema is mostly lower body, but may be seen in the face and eyes in the morning.
• dryness of the mouth, throat, skin and hair
• dry stools or constipation
• scanty, concentrated urine; uncomfortable urination
• sensation of heat in the palms and soles
• insomnia or restless dream disturbed sleep; wakes feeling hot
• spontaneous sweating or night sweats
• shortness of breath with exertion
• dizziness, light–headedness
• irritability and restlessness; anxiety
• weakness, fatigue with difficulty settling to rest
• lower back ache
T red with little or no coat, or pink, swollen and scalloped with multiple surface cracks and little coat
P fine and rapid or fine and weak

Treatment Principle
Supplement qi and nourish Kidney yin
Support fluid metabolism and the absorption of fluids to relieve edema

Prescription
FANG JI HUANG QI TANG 防己黄芪汤
Stephania and Astragalus Decoction, plus
LIU WEI DI HUANG WAN 六味地黄丸
Six Ingredient Pill with Rehmannia, modified

huang qi (Astragali Radix) 黄芪	15–60g
han fang ji (Stephaniae tetrandrae Radix) 汉防己	9–12g
shu di (Rehmanniae Radix preparata) 熟地	9–12g
sheng di (Rehmanniae Radix) 生地	9–12g

shan yao (Dioscoreae Rhizoma) 山药 12–15g
shan zhu yu (Corni Fructus) 山茱萸 9–12g
fu ling pi (Poriae Cutis) 茯苓皮 12–15g
gou qi zi (Lycii Fructus) 枸杞子 12–15g
han lian cao (Ecliptae Herba) 旱莲草 12–15g
nu zhen zi (Ligustri Fructus) 女贞子 12–15g
tai zi shen (Pseudostellariae Radix) 太子参 12–15g
yi ren (Coicis Semen) 苡仁 15–30g
xu duan (Dipsaci Radix) 续断 9–12g
che qian zi (Plantaginis Semen) 车前子 12–15g
lu gen (Phragmitis Rhizoma) 芦根 15–30g
bai mao gen (Imperatae Rhizoma) 白茅根 12–18g

Method: Decoction. **Che qian zi** is decocted in a cloth bag. **Huang qi** supplements Lung qi to free and regulate the water passages; **han fang ji** promotes urination and drains damp; **sheng di** and **shu di** supplement Kidney yin; **tai zi shen** assists **huang qi** in strengthening the Spleen; **shan yao**, **gou qi zi**, **shan zhu yu**, **han lian cao** and **nu zhen zi** supplement Kidney yin; **fu ling pi**, **yi ren** and **che qian zi** promote urination and reduce edema; **bai mao gen** and **lu gen** clear heat and generate fluids to moisten dryness; **xu duan** supports Kidney yang to promote yin. (Source: *Zhong Yi Nei Ke Xue* [*Shang Han Lun* / *Xiao Er Yao Zheng Zhi Jue*])

Modifications

- The doses of the main herbs can be adjusted to allow for the balance of qi and yin deficiency. For example, if qi deficiency is relatively severe, with pale tongue, fatigue, spontaneous sweating and shortness of breath, use a large dose of **huang qi** and **tai zi shen** and decrease the dose of the yin supplements. With relatively severe yin deficiency, the opposite applies, but pay attention to Spleen function as the yin supplements can overload the Spleen and aggravate damp.
- With severe dryness and thirst, add **sha shen** (Glehniae/Adenophorae Radix) 沙参 12–18g and **mai dong** (Ophiopogonis Radix) 麦冬 9–12g.
- With copious sweating or night sweats, add **duan long gu** (calcined Fossilia Ossis Mastodi) 煅龙骨 15–30g, **duan mu li** (calcined Ostreae Concha) 煅牡蛎 15–30g and **fu xiao mai** (Tritici Fructus levis) 浮小麦 12–18g.

Variations and additional prescriptions

Kidney yin deficiency with edema and urinary discomfort

Chronic heat or damp heat in the lower burner and Urinary Bladder can damage Kidney yin. The symptoms are mild yet persistent edema of the feet and ankles, with urinary discomfort, inhibited urination, thirst, a red dry tongue with little or no coat and a fine pulse. The treatment is to gently promote urination and nourish yin with Zhu Ling Tang (Polyporus Decoction 猪苓汤), modified.

zhu ling (Polyporus) 猪苓 15g
fu ling (Poria) 茯苓 15g
ze xie (Alismatis Rhizoma) 泽泻 15g
hua shi (Talcum) 滑石 24g
e jiao (Asini Corii Colla) 阿胶 9g
che qian zi (Plantaginis Semen) 车前子 15g
sheng di (Rehmanniae Radix) 生地 30g

Method: Decoction. **E jiao** is melted before being added to the strained decoction, **che qian zi** is decocted in a cloth bag. **Zhu ling, fu ling, ze xie** and **che qian zi** promote urination and relieve edema; **hua shi** clears heat from the Urinary Bladder; **e jiao** nourishes and protects yin and moistens dryness; **sheng di** cools the blood and nourishes yin. (Source: *Nei Ke Chang Jian Bing Zheng Zhen Zhi Zhi Nan* [*Shang Han Lun*])

Spleen and Stomach yin deficiency

Spleen and Stomach yin deficiency causes edema in the extremities and face, along with a thirst, a robust appetite, or gnawing hunger and red dry tongue. The mechanism is peculiar to the Spleen Stomach complex, with qi deficiency causing poor metabolism and distribution of fluids, and yin deficiency poor absorption of fluids. The treatment is to nourish Spleen and Stomach yin, and supplement qi to promote fluid metabolism and relieve edema. SHEN LING BAI ZHU SAN (Ginseng, Poria and White Atractylodes Powder 参苓白术散), modified, is effective.

bai ren shen (Ginseng Radix) 白人参 9–12g
bai zhu (Atractylodis macrocephalae Rhizoma) 白术 6–9g
fu ling (Poria) 茯苓 9–12g
shan yao (Dioscoreae Rhizoma) 山药 15–18g
bai bian dou (Dolichos Semen) 白扁豆 12–15g
yi ren (Coicis Semen) 苡仁 15–30g
lian zi (Nelumbinis Semen) 莲子 12–15g
zhi gan cao (Glycyrrhizae Radix preparata) 炙甘草 3–6g
yu zhu (Polygonati odorati Rhizoma) 玉竹 12–15g
tian hua fen (Trichosanthes Radix) 天花粉 12–15g

Method: Grind the herbs to a powder and take 9 grams, 2–3 times daily with warm water. May be decocted with quantities as shown. **Bai ren shen, bai zhu, yi ren, fu ling, bai bian dou, shan yao, qian shi** and **zhi gan cao** strengthen the Spleen and Stomach and nourish and supplement yin and qi; **yi ren, fu ling** and **bai bian dou** promote urination to resolve edema; **bai zhu** strengthens the Spleen and dries damp; **lian zi** astringes the Intestines and stops diarrhea; **yu zhu, shan yao** and **tian hua fen** nourish Spleen and Stomach yin and improve the ability of those organs to absorb and hold fluids. (Source: *He Ji Ju Fang*)

Prepared medicines

Concentrated powder
Liu Wei Di Huang Wan (Rehmannia Six Formula) plus Fang Ji Huang Qi Tang
    (Stephania & Astragalus Combination)
Shen Ling Bai Zhu San (Ginseng & Atractylodes Formula)

Pills
Liu Wei Di Huang Wan (Six Flavor Teapills) plus Fang Ji Huang Qi Wan
    (Stephania and Astragalus Teapills)
Zhi Bai Ba Wei Wan (Eight Flavor Rehmannia Teapills)
    – with heat
Sheng Mai Wan (Great Pulse Teapills)
Shen Ling Bai Zhu Wan (Absorbtion and Digestion Pill, Shen Ling Bai Zhu Pian)

Acupuncture (select from)
Ren.12 (zhongwan +) ....alarm point of the Stomach, strengthens the Spleen
                    and supplements qi

Ren.4 (guanyuan +)............these points supplement Kidney yin and qi to
Ren.6 (qihai +)   promote fluid metabolism
Sp.9 (yinlingquan –)...........sea point of the Spleen, promotes urination to
                                relieve edema
Sp.6 (sanyinjiao)................strengthens the Spleen and Kidney and supplements
                                qi and yin
Ren.9 (shuifen ▲)..............frees the water passages, promotes urination qi
                                transformation and elimination of fluids
Kid.7 (fuliu –) ....river and metal point of the Kidneys, strengthens
                                Kidney qi and yin and stimulates fluid metabolism
                                to relieve edema
St.36 (zusanli +) ....sea point of the Stomach, strengthens the Spleen and
                                Stomach and supplements qi
Bl.20 (pishu +) ....transport points of the Spleen, triple burner, Kidney
Bl.22 (sanjiaoshu)   and Urinary Bladder, these points strengthen Spleen
Bl.23 (shenshu +)   and Kidney qi, nourish yin, free the water passages
Bl.28 (pangguangshu)   of the triple burner and promote urination

- Ear points: spleen, kidney, triple burner, zero point, adrenal, subcortex, endocrine

Clinical notes

- Edema of a qi and yin deficiency type may be diagnosed as menopausal or postpartum edema, interstitial cystitis, chronic urinary tract infection, chronic nephritis or nephrotic syndrome.
- This can be a stubborn type of edema, but will generally respond to prolonged and persistent treatment.
- Keep a careful eye on the signs and symptoms of yin deficiency when using diuretic substances, as excessive application to alleviate symptoms quickly can further deplete yin.
- A qi and yin supplementing diet is recommended., see Clinical Handbook, Vol.2, p.870 and 876. Salt intake should be minimized.

Table 5.1 Summary of edema patterns

Pattern		Features	Prescription
External wind	wind cold	Acute facial edema, with fever & chills (chills predominant), scanty urine, no sweating, muscle aches, floating tight pulse	Ma Huang Jia Zhu Tang
	wind heat	Acute facial edema, with red, sore throat, fever & chills (fever predominant), floating rapid pulse	Yue Bi Jia Zhu Tang
Toxic heat		Edema associated with sores & ulcerations. May be localized around the lesion or systemic. A red tongue with a thin yellow coat and floating & rapid or slippery & rapid pulse	Ma Huang Lian Qiao Chi Xiao Dou Tang plus Wu Wei Xiao Du Yin
Spleen damp		Gradual onset of non pitting edema with scanty urine, heaviness, lethargy, loss of appetite, nausea, a thick, white tongue coat and a soggy, moderate pulse	Wu Pi San plus Wei Ling Tang
Damp heat		Non pitting edema of the legs and feet. The skin appears shiny and taut; night sweats, afternoon fever, scanty, concentrated or cloudy urine, lethargy, a thick, yellow tongue coat and deep & rapid, or soggy & rapid pulse	Shu Zao Yin Zi
Qi constraint		Cyclical edema worse before a period with change in the emotional state, wiry pulse	Chai Hu Shu Gan San plus Wei Ling Tang
Blood stasis		Chronic bilateral or unilateral edema, dark skin discoloration, chronic pain, clotted menses, vascular congestion, palpable liver, purple tongue or dark sublingual veins, deep, wiry, choppy, irregular or intermittent pulse	Xue Fu Zhu Yu Tang
Qi deficiency		Mild pitting edema of the face, orbits, fingers, lower limbs & abdomen. Fatigue, weakness, pale complexion, digestive & immune weakness, pale, scalloped tongue with a thin white coat and a fine weak pulse	Shen Ling Bai Zhu San plus Fang Ji Huang Qi Tang
Spleen yang deficiency		Chronic pitting edema with severe digestive weakness, prolapse, anorexia, diarrhea or constipation, cold intolerance, fatigue, pale, swollen & scalloped tongue with a white coat and a deep weak pulse	Shi Pi Yin

Table 5.1 Summary of edema patterns (cont.)

Pattern	Features	Prescription
Kidney yang deficiency	Chronic pitting edema below the waist, scanty or frequent urine, nocturia or incontinence of urine; cold aching lower back & knees, cold intolerance, pale complexion, pale, swollen & scalloped tongue with a white coat and a deep, weak, imperceptible, irregular or intermittent pulse	Ji Sheng Shen Qi Wan (mild) Zhen Wu Tang (severe)
Qi and yin deficiency	Mild edema, with signs of heat & dryness. Spontaneous sweating or night sweats, fatigue, insomnia, irritability, heat in the palms and soles, constipation, red tongue with no coat, or pink, swollen & scalloped with multiple surface cracks, fine, rapid pulse or fine & weak pulse	Fang Ji Huang Qi Tang plus Liu Wei Di Huang Wan

FAINTING AND FUNNY TURNS

Fainting is a sudden, brief loss of consciousness. The episode may be preceded by a variety of symptoms such as dizziness, hyperventilation, the feeling that one is sinking, or that everything is getting louder. Fainting may also occur without warning, in which case it is known as a drop attack. A 'funny turn' or 'turn' is a colloquial term used by patients to describe an event involving a sudden change of consciousness, without loss of consciousness. A funny turn can refer to a wide variety of subjective experiences, including sudden giddiness and loss of balance, disturbed proprioception and spatial disorientation, feeling on the edge of losing consciousness or of suddenly sinking, dimming or tunnel vision, a sense of waves of energy rushing up from the abdomen, sudden transitory weakness of the muscles and limbs or transient amnesia.

> **BOX 6.1 PATTERNS OF FAINTING AND FUNNY TURNS**
>
> Instability of the anima
> Spleen qi deficiency with damp
> Sinking da qi
> Qi and yin deficiency
> Qi and blood deficiency
> Heart yang deficiency
> Liver qi constraint with blood deficiency
> Ascendant Liver yang, Liver fire
> Liver and Kidney yin deficiency with
>   ascendant yang
> Phlegm blocking the head and muscles
> Wind phlegm
> Food stagnation, Stomach heat
> Blood stasis

Fainting (also known as syncope) in Chinese medicine is known as *jué zhèng*[1] 厥证, and was first mentioned in the Simple Questions (*Huang Di Nei Jing Su Wen*), Chapter 45, where two types, hot and cold, are described. The analysis and management described in the Su Wen focused on acute care and restoration of consciousness. In modern practice, unconscious patients are managed with appropriate first aid, and our treatment is aimed at correction of the underlying pathology.

Fainting can be distinguished from other conditions that may be associated with sudden loss of consciousness such as wind stroke, by the absence of sequelae. Epilepsy (*diān xián* 癫痫, Clinical Handbook, Vol.1) can cause disturbances of consciousness, and in the absence of the typical tonic clonic seizure, can look like a faint or funny turn. Atypical or partial seizures are often associated with phlegm and can be analyzed according to the patterns described in this chapter.

PATHOLOGY

The pathology of fainting and turns can be divided into excess and deficient types. Both the excess and deficient patterns are chronic, with the exception of those due to trauma or hemorrhage. In general, the deficient patterns are more likely to cause fainting and loss of consciousness, while the excess patterns are more likely to produce the various altered states of consciousness described as funny turns. This distinction should be applied flexibly, however, because there are often exceptions, and

---

1 Practical Dictionary of Chinese Medicine (1998) – 'reversal pattern'

mixed patterns of excess and deficiency are common. The mechanism of fainting and turns is due to one or more of the following factors:

1. The head and brain are suddenly starved of qi and blood

Qi and blood can fail to reach the head and brain because:

- their volume is insufficient to meet the demands of positional change and increasing exertion
- qi and blood are adequate, but their distribution is obstructed, or the Heart is too weak to propel them
- qi sinks into the lower body away from the chest and head

2. There is too much yang qi in the upper body and head

- too much yang qi in the upper body is an imbalance in yang qi distribution caused by sudden release and upward counterflow of pent up qi
- yin deficiency is unable to counterbalance and anchor yang

3. The shen or other anima (p.97) are suddenly scattered or constrained

- an unstable shen (or hun, zhi, or po) is easily unbalanced by external events
- there is insufficient blood or yin to anchor the anima
- sudden constraint of qi can impede the expression of the shen and hun
- the anima can be scattered by shock or trauma

4. The head, senses or Heart are blocked by a pathogen

- phlegm, blood stasis and qi constraint block the distribution of qi and blood to the head or Heart
- phlegm clogs the head and senses (Heart orifices)
- blood stasis blocks local circulation of qi and blood in the head or Heart
- heat or stagnant food disrupt the qi dynamic and disturb the shen

---

BOX 6.2 KEY DIAGNOSTIC POINTS

Initiating factors
- emotion, anger – qi constraint, ascendant yang
- fright, panic – Heart and Gallbladder qi deficiency
- upon standing – qi and blood deficiency
- after eating – food stagnation, Stomach heat
- with exertion – qi and blood deficiency, yin and yang deficiency
- strong smells, perfume, gasoline – phlegm

Accompanying symptoms
- excessive sleepiness – phlegm
- foggy head, confusion – phlegm
- sweating, hunger – Spleen deficiency
- palpitations – qi, blood and yin deficiency
- visual disturbances – ascendant Liver yang, yin and blood deficiency
- speech problems – Heart and Gallbladder qi deficiency, ascendant yang
- throat clearing, sinus congestion – phlegm
- tinnitus and nausea – wind phlegm, ascendant yang
- pounding headache – qi constraint, fire, ascendant yang, phlegm
- dull headache – deficiency

BOX 6.3 BIOMEDICAL CAUSES OF FAINTING AND FUNNY TURNS

Syncope
• vasovagal syncope
• anxiety, hysteria, hyperventilation

Seizures
• epilepsy, complex partial seizure
(temporal lobe epilepsy) and atonic
or absence seizures

Cardio and cerebrovascular
• arrhythmias
– Stokes–Adams attacks
– sick sinus syndrome
– ventricular tachycardia
• postural hypotension
• aortic stenosis
• vertebrobasilar insufficiency
• transient ischemic attack (TIA)
• anemia
• carotid sinus sensitivity

Labyrinthine
• vertigo
• Meniere's disease

Other
• hypoglycemia
• narcolepsy, catalepsy
• atypical migraine
• drug or alcohol effects/intoxication
– narcotics, anti–depressants,
anti–hypertensives, peripheral
vasodilators, anticonvulsants, ACE
inhibitors
– sudden cessation of medications
• electrolyte disturbance
• cervical spondylosis
• space occupying lesion
• atypical infection, endocarditis
• choking
• pregnancy

ETIOLOGY

Emotional factors

Emotional factors that can result in fainting or funny turns are those that impact on the shen and other anima (p.97), and influence the functions of the internal organ systems, especially the Liver, Spleen and Heart. The anima can be congenitally unstable due to parental jing deficiency, maternal illness or trauma during gestation or delivery. The anima can also be destabilized by acquired deficiency of blood and yin.

Repression of emotion and excessive worry constrain Liver and Spleen qi and disrupt the qi dynamic. This in turn leads to pent up qi, Spleen deficiency, weakness of qi and blood, the creation of damp and phlegm, or the generation of heat. Persistent heat will damage yin and contribute to ascendant yang.

Diet and medications

An inadequate diet, especially one lacking in protein can lead to blood deficiency, a common cause of fainting and turns. An erratic diet, or one biased towards raw or sweet foods, will weaken the Spleen and create damp and phlegm, as will repeated courses of antibiotics and other cold natured or Spleen weakening medications, such as Metformin (Box 4.2, p.167). An overly rich, sweet or fatty diet can lead to phlegm, while a heating diet and alcohol promote ascendant yang and fire.

Exhaustion

Chronic illness, extended periods of overwork, lack of sleep and any excessive demand on qi and blood, or yin and yang, can lead to deficiency. Any factors that

BOX 6.4 MANAGEMENT OF ACUTE FAINTING OR LOSS OF CONSCIOUSNESS

In most cases of fainting discussed in this section, consciousness is quickly restored and there are no lasting after effects from the episode. The basic principles of first aid are the most appropriate until the patient is ambulant and cognizant, or until paramedic assistance is available. In situations where paramedic help is unavailable and the patient remains unconscious, basic first aid is primary, but certain acupuncture points can sometimes assist in restoration of consciousness or prevention of circulatory collapse and death.

Acupuncture
Distinguishing between yang and yin types of collapse is the most important aspect of acute management. Yang collapse is characterized by heat, redness, muscle spasm, and no incontinence of urine or feces. Yin collapse is characterized by flaccidity, incontinence, cold extremities and pallor.

Yang collapse, main points
• Du.26 (renzhong) or Du.25 (suliao), PC.6 (neiguan −)
• With heat or fever, bleed the points on the finger tips, shixuan (M–UE–11), or the jing well points
• All points are treated with strong stimulation. The points can be needled or pressed with strong finger pressure or other appropriate instrument.

Yin collapse, main points
• Du.20 (baihui), treated with finger pressure or a heat source of some type
• Ren.8 (shenque), Ren.4 (guanyuan) with a strong heat source
• St.36 (zusanli), LI.4 (hegu)

Additional points
• Tremor or convulsions – LI.11 (quchi), LI.4 (hegu), GB.34 (yanglingquan)
• Confusion, clouded consciousness – Kid.1 (yongquan)

Other
In China, a number of herbal preparations are available for intravenous infusion or intramuscular injection, see Box 6.5. These preparations are generally administered in hospital.

deplete the Kidneys, Heart or Spleen can predispose to fainting or turns. Working excessively long hours or laboring to the point of exhaustion can deplete Spleen and Kidney yang qi. Any activity that excessively taxes the Spleen will lead to qi and blood deficiency, and may lead to the generation of phlegm damp. The Spleen is weakened by excessive, concentrated mental activity and sedentary habits. Lack of sleep depletes yin. Heart qi and yin are depleted by profuse sweating or other fluid loss, as well as an excessively busy and hectic life with insufficient rest.

Trauma and hemorrhage
A traumatic injury to the head can cause disturbances of consciousness and fainting. In acute cases, it is an alarming sign suggesting bleeding in the brain, a medical emergency. In less dramatic cases, the fainting or turns occur sporadically for some time following the initial injury. The trauma can cause blood stasis which

> ## BOX 6.5 INJECTABLE PREPARATIONS
>
> **Qing Kai Ling Zhu She Ye** 清开灵注射液
> Cooling & Opening [Orifices] Injection
> The main components are:
> **niu huang** (Bovis Calculus) 牛黄
> **shui niu jiao** (Bubali Cornu) 水牛角
> **huang qin** (Scutellariae Radix) 黄芩
> **jin yin hua** (Lonicerae Flos) 金银花
> **shan zhi zi** (Gardeniae Fructus) 山栀子
> Clears toxic heat, transforms phlegm and restores consciousness. For high fever
> with delirium, consciousness disturbance and loss of consciousness from warm
> disease, wind stroke and other heat and yang patterns.
>
> **Shen Fu Zhu She Ye** 参附注射液
> Aconite and Ginseng Injection
> **hong shen** (Ginseng Radix) 红参
> **zhi fu zi** (Aconiti Radix lateralis preparata) 制附子
> Warms and supports collapsing yang and restores consciousness and is used for
> collapse from yang deficiency. Yang collapse is similar to biomedical conditions
> such as hypovolemic shock, cardiogenic shock and collapse following blood loss
> and certain infections.
>
> **Sheng Mai Zhu She Ye** 生脉注射液
> Restore the Pulse Injection
> **hong shen** (Ginseng Radix) 红参
> **mai dong** (Ophiopogonis Radix) 麦冬
> **wu wei zi** (Schizandrae Fructus) 五味子
> Supplements qi and yin, supports the pulse and restores consciousness. Used for
> the treatment of cardiogenic shock, hypovolemic shock, myocardial infarction
> and post infectious shock.

disrupts the local circulation of qi and blood in the head, or may disrupt the Heart
Kidney axis (p.781) and destabilize the anima. Physical trauma to the body resulting in severe pain can lead to loss of consciousness and shock. A sudden blood loss
can lead to fainting.

External pathogens

Acute invasion of summerheat can cause sudden fainting or collapse. This is a seasonal pathology, and occurs as a one off event, not requiring any specific treatment
other than standard first aid and rehydration.

DIAGNOSIS

A detailed history and thorough physical examination is essential. All current and
previous medications, drugs and alcohol intake should be noted. The questioning
around the actual episode or episodes should focus on three phases:
1. Events and sensations occurring immediately preceding the episode
2. An account of the episode (usually from a witness)
3. The events thereafter, as the patient regains senses

In addition to the standard Chinese medical diagnostic routine, the physical examination should include assessment of the neck, with particular attention paid to the sternocleidomastoid muscles, and cervical spine. A careful cardiovascular and cerebrovascular assessment should be made, with particular attention paid to the carotid arteries. A standing and seated blood pressure measurement should be performed.

TREATMENT

If a person collapses or has a blackout, the treatment during the unconscious state is standard first aid; maintenance of the airway, breathing and circulation. Paramedic assistance should be sought. There are some acupuncture and acupressure techniques that can be of assistance (Box 6.4, p.262).

Patients present to Chinese medicine practitioners in between episodes. Our role is to deal with the constitutional pathology underlying the episodes, thereby preventing them, or at least making them less frequent and more manageable.

265

Figure 6.1 Mechanism and possible triggers of fainting and funny turns

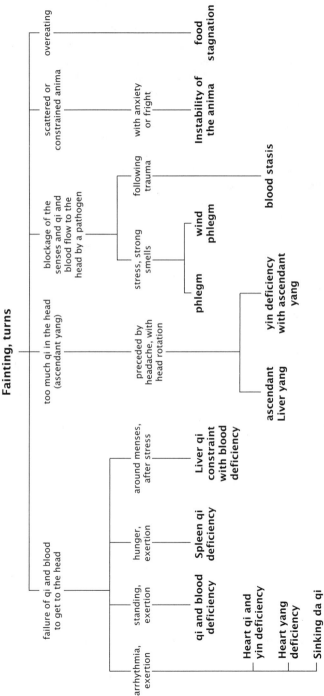

五
神
不
稳
定
的

6.1 INSTABILITY OF THE ANIMA

The anima (p.97) referred to here are the shen, hun, po, yi and zhi. The pathology derives from their lack of grounding, without which they are easily destabilized and scattered by external events. The traditional description of this disorder is Heart and Gallbladder qi deficiency (*xīn dǎn qì xū* 心胆气虚). The Heart and Gallbladder (and by convention the shen and hun) are designated as the primary site of the pathology, and it describes a patient with a constitutional or acquired tendency to nervousness and anxiety. The Gallbladder qi deficiency is a reference to the timidity and 'lack of gall' (that is, fearfulness) which characterizes people with this pattern. In the Chinese language (as in English) there is an implicit understanding of the relationship between the Gallbladder and courage, indeed to be bold and courageous is to have a 'big Gallbladder' (*dà dǎn* 大胆). In practice, any or all the anima may be affected, and the manifestations vary accordingly.

Instability of the anima is a state in which the patient is hypersensitive to external influences, perceived threats and sudden change, and have insufficient protection or boundary. Their response to an anticipated or current event is out of proportion, and because the anima are already tenuously grounded, trivial events are enough to unhinge them sufficiently to disturb consciousness, resulting in sudden fainting.

Clinical features
- Sudden fainting in response to social or psychological stress of some type, preceded by flushing, hyperventilation, palpitations and sweating. There may be tunnel vision, loss of bladder control, sleep disturbances and disturbing nightmares or agoraphobia.
- Long term tendency to nervousness and timidity, fearfulness and anxiety, poor self image and emotional instability

T unremarkable or variable depending on complicating pathology
P generally fine, but may be variable, depending on complicating pathology

Treatment principle
Stabilize the shen and anima
Strengthen the Heart and Kidney (as foundation of the other anima)

Prescription

DING ZHI WAN 定志丸
Settle the Emotions Pill, plus
GAN MAI DA ZAO TANG 甘麦大枣汤
Licorice, Wheat and Jujube Decoction

This prescription is used for fainting episodes and congenital instability of the anima in a timid anxious individual. It is suitable for long term use.

ren shen (Ginseng Radix) 人参 90g
fu ling (Poria) 茯苓 90g
shi chang pu (Acori tatarinowii Rhizoma) 石菖蒲 60g
yuan zhi (Polygalae Radix) 远志 60g

gan cao (Glycyrrhizae Radix) 甘草 60g
xiao mai (Tritici Fructus) 小麦 60g
da zao (Jujubae Fructus) 大枣 60g
Method: Pills or powder. Grind herbs to a powder and form into 9 gram pills with honey. The dose is 1 pill twice daily. May also be decocted with a 90% reduction in dosage. **Ren shen** and **fu ling** supplement Heart qi and calm the shen; **shi chang pu** and **yuan zhi** calm the shen, and clear the mind; **gan cao**, **xiao mai** and **da zao** nourish qi and blood and calm the shen and hun. (Source: *Qian Jin Yao Fang / Jin Gui Yao Lüe*)

Modifications

- With fearfulness and loss of bladder control, add **shan zhu yu** (Corni Fructus) 山茱萸 90g, **tu si zi** (Cuscutae Semen) 菟丝子 90g, **he shou wu** (Polygoni multiflori Radix) 何首乌 60g and **gou qi zi** (Lycii Fructus) 枸杞子 60g to anchor the zhi.
- With anxiety about social situations, isolation and aversion to interact with others, add **huang qi** (Astragali Radix) 黄芪 90, **mai dong** (Ophiopogonis Radix) 麦冬 60g and **wu wei zi** (Schizandrae Fructus) 五味子 30g to stabilize the po.
- With sleep disturbance and disturbing dreams or even waking dreams, add **bai shao** (Paeoniae Radix alba) 白芍 90g, **suan zao ren** (Ziziphi spinosae Semen) 酸枣仁 90g and **bai zi ren** (Platycladi Semen) 柏子仁 90g to stabilize the hun.
- In very agitated patients, add **long gu** (Fossilia Ossis Mastodi) 龙骨 60g and **hu po** (Succinum) 琥珀 30g.
- With marked qi deficiency, add **zhi huang qi** (honey fried Astragali Radix) 炙黄芪 120g and **huang jing** (Polygonati Rhizoma) 黄精 90g.
- With blood deficiency, add **dang gui** (Angelicae sinensis Radix) 当归 60g and **bai shao** (Paeoniae Radix alba) 白芍 60g.
- With phlegm, add **zhi ban xia** (Pinelliae Rhizoma preparatum) 制半夏 60g and **zhu li** (Bambusae Succus) 竹沥 60g.

GUI ZHI JIA LONG GU MU LI TANG 桂枝加龙骨牡蛎汤
Cinnamon Twig Decoction plus Dragon Bone and Oyster Shell

This formula is selected when fainting episodes or turns follow a major shock or trauma without head injury or concussion (see blood stasis for post concussion fainting). Episodic fainting may be triggered by a sight, smell or sound associated with the initial event. These symptoms are typical of severed communication between the Heart and Kidneys due to shock.

gui zhi (Cinnamomi Ramulus) 桂枝 9–12g
bai shao (Paeoniae Radix alba) 白芍 9–15g
long gu (Fossilia Ossis Mastodi) 龙骨 15–30g
mu li (Ostreae Concha) 牡蛎 15–30g
gan cao (Glycyrrhizae Radix) 甘草 3–6g
sheng jiang (Zingiberis Rhizoma) 生姜 6–9g
da zao (Jujubae Fructus) 大枣 .... 4 fruit
Method: Decoction. **Long gu** and **mu li** are decocted for 30 minutes prior to the other herbs. **Gui zhi** warms and mobilizes yang and supports fire, while **bai shao** preserves yin, nourishes blood and maintains water. Together they balance each other in such a way as to harmonize and regulate yin

and yang, both in the narrow context of ying wei imbalance on the surface, and in the deeper context of a Heart Kidney imbalance (a disconnection between water and fire, the zhi and shen). The heaviness of **long gu** and **mu li** draws the action of the principal herbs away from the surface and into the body, and at the same time anchors yang, stop sweating and calms the shen. **Sheng jiang**, **da zao** and **gan cao** support the Spleen and qi production. (Source: *Shang Han Lun*)

Variations and additional prescriptions

With a sensation of energy rushing up to the head

Fainting may be preceded by a sensation of energy rushing upwards from the epigastrium or abdomen. This sensation is described as 'running piglet qi' (*bèn tūn qì* 奔豚气), and is precipitated by instability of the Heart and Kidneys. A sudden fright or shock, or even a sudden loud noise, can be sufficient to disrupt Heart Kidney communication, leading to acute qi counterflow. The treatment is to reconnect the Heart and Kidneys, lead the ascendant qi down and support qi and blood with a prescription such as **BEN TUN TANG** (Running Piglet Decoction 奔豚汤).

bai shao (Paeoniae Radix alba) 白芍 15–24g
dang gui (Angelicae sinensis Radix) 当归 12–15g
chuan xiong (Chuanxiong Rhizoma) 川芎 9–12g
zhi ban xia (Pinelliae Rhizoma preparatum) 制半夏 9–12g
chen pi (Citri reticulatae Pericarpium) 陈皮 9–12g
dang shen (Codonopsis Radix) 党参 9–12g
yu jin (Curcumae Radix) 郁金 9–12g
sang bai pi (Mori Cortex) 桑白皮 9–12g
fu ling (Poria) 茯苓 9–12g
shi chang pu (Acori tatarinowii Rhizoma) 石菖蒲 6–9g
yuan zhi (Polygalae Radix) 远志 6–9g
chai hu (Bupleuri Radix) 柴胡 6–9g

Method: Decoction. **Dang gui**, **bai shao** and **chuan xiong** nourish and activate blood; **zhi ban xia** and **chen pi** transform phlegm; **dang shen** and **fu ling** supplement qi; **shi chang pu** and **yuan zhi** transform phlegm and calm the shen; **yu jin** alleviates constraint; **sang bai pi** cools the Lungs and directs Lung qi downwards; **chai hu** regulates the Liver and moves Liver qi. (Source: *Zhong Yi Nei Ke Shou Ce* / *Jin Gui Yao Lüe*)

Prepared medicines

Concentrated powders

Gan Mai Da Zao Tang (Licorice & Jujube Combination)
Gui Zhi Jia Long Gu Mu Li Tang (Cinnamon & Dragon Bone Combination)

Pills

Bu Nao Wan (Cerebral Tonic Pills)
An Shen Bu Xin Wan (Calm the Shen and Supplement the Heart Pill)
Ding Xin Wan (Calm the Heart Pill)
Yang Xin Ning Shen Wan (Ning San Yuen Medical Pills)

Acupuncture (select from)

Du.19 (houding)................these points calm the shen
Du.20 (baihui)
Du.24 (shenting)
yintang (M–HN–3)
Ren.14 (juque)...................alarm point of the Heart, calms the Heart and shen
Bl.15 (xinshu +) ....transport point of the Heart, supplements Heart qi,
                               calms the Heart and shen
Ht.7 (shenmen +)...............source point of the Heart, calms the shen, regulates
                               and supplements Heart qi
Bl.23 (shenshu +) ....these points supplement the Kidneys and stabilize
Bl.52 (zhishi +)   the zhi

- with anxiety and aversion to social interaction, add Lu.3 (tianfu), Bl.13 (feishu ▲) and B.42 (pohu)
- with fearfulness and loss of bladder control, add Kid.4 (dazhong) and Ren.4 (guanyuan ▲)
- with disturbing dreams, add Bl.47 (hunmen), Bl.18 (ganshu) and Liv.8 (ququan)
- with tightness in the chest and palpations, add PC.6 (neiguan)
- Ear points: heart, shenmen, sympathetic

Clinical notes

- Fainting of this type may be associated with personality type, autonomic nervous system dysfunction, hyperventilation, conversion reactions, hysteria or vasovagal syncope.
- The prognosis for fainting from an unstable animus is variable. When constitutional, the prognosis is poorer than from when the condition is acquired later in life. However, some patients do surprisingly well, and become much more confident and self assured. Regardless of the etiology, treatment needs to be consistent and prolonged. Regular, long term acupuncture seems to be the most effective intervention.
- For dietary recommendations, see Clinical Handbook, Vol. 2, p.870.

脾
气
虚
弱

6.2 SPLEEN QI DEFICIENCY

The Spleen is responsible for the harvesting and maintenance of adequate levels of qi and blood. When the Spleen is weak and qi levels low, even a slight increase in usage of qi can lead to a failure of Spleen qi's ascent and inadequate qi getting to the head.

Clinical features
- Sudden light–headedness, tunnel vision, feeling of not being present or fainting, usually in response to hunger or following a period of increased activity. Episodes are more likely to occur in the afternoon, and are accompanied by pallor, sweating, palpitations and hunger. Recovery may be gradual with the patient quite groggy for a while.

In between episodes–
- fatigue and tiredness that are better for rest and worse at the end of the day
- appetite that varies between indifference to food and gnawing hunger; sweet cravings
- abdominal distension, early satiety
- loose stools
- muscles easily fatigued and tired; muscle weakness, poor muscle tone
- spontaneous sweating

T pale, swollen and scalloped and a thin white coat
P weak, fine

Treatment principle
Strengthen the Spleen and supplement qi

Prescription

SHEN LING BAI ZHU SAN 参苓白术散
Ginseng, Poria and White Atractylodes Powder

ren shen (Ginseng Radix) 人参	100g
bai zhu (Atractylodes macrocephalae Rhizoma) 白术	100g
fu ling (Poria) 茯苓	100g
shan yao (Dioscoreae Rhizoma) 山药	100g
zhi gan cao (Glycyrrhizae Radix preparata) 炙甘草	100g
bai bian dou (Dolichos Semen) 白扁豆	75g
yi ren (Coicis Semen) 苡仁	50g
lian zi (Nelumbinis Semen) 莲子	50g
jie geng (Platycodi Radix) 桔梗	50g
sha ren (Amomi Fructus) 砂仁	50g

Method: Grind the herbs to a fine powder and take in doses of 9 grams, two or three times daily. May also be decocted with an 85–90% reduction in dosage, in which case **sha ren** is added towards the end of cooking. **Ren shen, bai zhu, yi ren, fu ling, bai bian dou, shan yao** and **zhi gan cao** strengthen the Spleen and supplement qi; **bai zhu** dries damp; **yi ren, fu ling** and **bian dou** leach out damp and promote urination; **lian zi** astringes the Intestines and stops diarrhea; **jie geng** assists the ascent of Spleen qi; **sha ren** transforms damp and regulates qi. (Source: *He Ji Ju Fang*)

Modifications

- With foggy head and inability to concentrate, add **shi chang pu** (Acori tatarinowii Rhizoma) 石菖蒲 60g and **yuan zhi** (Polygalae Radix) 远志 60g.
- With Liver qi constraint, add **chai hu** (Bupleuri Radix) 柴胡 60g and **bai shao** (Paeoniae Radix alba) 白芍 60g.
- To assist ascent of Spleen qi, add **chai hu** (Bupleuri Radix) 柴胡 30g, **sheng ma** (Cimicifugae Rhizoma) 升麻 30g and **zhi huang qi** (honey fried Astragali Radix) 炙黄芪 100g.
- With Stomach yin deficiency, dry mouth, centrally peeled tongue and gnawing hunger, add **mai dong** (Ophiopogonis Radix) 麦冬 75g, **tian hua fen** (Trichosanthes Radix) 天花粉 75g and **huang jing** (Polygonati Rhizoma) 黄精 60g.
- With edema, use 150g of **fu ling** (Poria) 茯苓, and add **ze xie** (Alismatis Rhizoma) 泽泻 60g and **che qian zi** (Plantaginis Semen) 车前子 60g [cooked in a cloth bag when decocted].
- With persistent diarrhea, **bai zhu**, **yi ren**, **bian dou** and **shan yao** can be stir fried (*chao* 炒) to enhance their warmth and anti–diarrheal effect.
- With yang deficiency, add **gan jiang** (Zingiberis Rhizoma) 干姜 60g and **rou gui** (Cinnamomi Cortex) 肉桂 15g.
- With wei qi deficiency, add **zhi huang qi** (honey fried Astragali Radix) 炙黄芪 100g and **wu wei zi** (Schizandrae Fructus) 五味子 30g.

Variations and additional prescriptions
Spleen qi deficiency with damp

Spleen qi deficiency is often complicated by damp. The damp settles like a mist over the mind, so foggy head and difficulty in concentration are more pronounced, sometimes to the point of disorientation, or a momentary lapse of consciousness ('spacing out') in the middle of a conversation. The lack of energy resulting from qi deficiency is compounded by a sense of heaviness. The patient will want to lie down and sleep, especially after eating and more so in the mid afternoon, but will wake feeling worse. The tongue is pale and swollen with a thick, greasy, white coat. The treatment is to strengthen the Lungs and Spleen, supplement qi and transform damp with a prescription such as Xiang Sha Liu Jun Zi Tang (Six Gentlemen Decoction with Aucklandia and Amomum 香砂六君子汤) modified.

ren shen (Ginseng Radix) 人参 6–9g
bai zhu (Atractylodis macrocephalae Rhizoma) 白术 9–12g
fu ling (Poria) 茯苓 12–15g
zhi ban xia (Pinelliae Rhizoma preparata) 制半夏 9–12g
chen pi (Citri reticulatae Pericarpium) 陈皮 9–12g
mu xiang (Aucklandiae Radix) 木香 6–9g
sha ren (Amomi Fructus) 砂仁 6–9g
zhi gan cao (Glycyrrhizae Radix preparata) 炙甘草 3–6g
cang zhu (Atractylodis Rhizoma) 苍术 9–12g
shi chang pu (Acori tatarinowii Rhizoma) 石菖蒲 6–9g
yuan zhi (Polygalae Radix) 远志 6–9g

Method: Decoction. **Sha ren** is added towards the end of cooking. **Ren shen** and **zhi gan cao** supplement qi and strengthen the Spleen; **bai zhu** strengthens the Spleen and dries damp; **fu ling** strengthens the Spleen and leaches damp out through the urine; **zhi ban xia** transforms phlegm and damp, downbears counterflow Stomach qi and corrects the qi dynamic; **chen pi** dries damp and corrects the qi dynamic; **sha ren** and **mu xiang** rectify and mobilize qi in the middle burner, alleviate distension and stimulate the appetite; **cang zhu**, **shi chang pu** and **yuan zhi** dry damp, and clear the mind. (Source: *Yi Fang Ji Jie*)

Prepared medicines
Concentrated powders
Shen Ling Bai Zhu San (Ginseng & Atractylodes Formula)
Xiang Sha Liu Jun Zi Tang (Vladmiria & Amomum Combination)
Sheng Mai San (Ginseng & Ophiopogon Formula)
 – combine with one of the above when there is yin deficiency

Pills
Shen Ling Bai Zhu Wan (Absorption and Digestion Pill, Shen Ling Bai Zhu Pian)
Xiang Sha Liu Jun Zi Wan (Aplotaxis–Ammomum Pills, Six Gentlemen Tea Pills)
Sheng Mai Wan (Great Pulse Teapills)

Acupuncture (select from)
Ren.12 (zhongwan +▲).......alarm point of the Stomach, strengthens the Spleen and Stomach and supplements qi
St.36 (zusanli +▲) ....sea point of the Stomach, strengthens the Spleen and Stomach and supplements qi
Sp.3 (taibai)......................these points strengthen the Spleen and transform
St.40 (fenglong)   damp and phlegm
Du.20 (baihui ▲) ....clears the head and elevates qi
Bl.20 (pishu +▲) ....transport points of the Spleen and Stomach, warm
Bl.21 (weishu +▲)   and strengthen middle burner qi
• with foggy head, add Bl.62 (shenmai)
• with edema, add Sp.9 (yinlingquan –) and Sp.6 (sanyinjiao)
• with abdominal pain, add Sp.4 (gongsun)
• with diarrhea, add St.25 (tianshu)
• with abdominal distension, add St.25 (tianshu) and Sp.15 (daheng)
• Ear points: spleen, stomach, pancreas, zero point, endocrine, sympathetic

Clinical notes
• Fainting and funny turns from Spleen qi deficiency are common, and may be diagnosed as hypoglycemia or poor blood sugar regulation. Spleen qi deficiency, with or without damp is a common starting point for the development of type 2 diabetes mellitus.
• Spleen qi deficiency responds reliably to treatment. In most cases, the patient should expect some improvement within a few weeks, then restoration of digestive function and regulation of blood sugar levels over several months. Regulation of the diet is a crucial factor in long term maintenance.
• For dietary recommendations, see Clinical Handbook, Vol. 2, p.870.
• Moderate aerobic exercise, in particular walking, swimming, yoga, taijiquan and qi gong are beneficial in strengthening the Spleen and Lungs.

6.3 SINKING DA QI (Collapse of Heart and Lung qi)

大
气
下
陷

Sinking da qi is the result of failure of the Spleen, Heart and Lungs to maintain the integrity of qi against the pull of gravity. The da qi (which is synonymous with zong qi, the qi of the Heart and Lungs) is unable to maintain its position in the upper burner and slumps into the lower body, which impairs the function of the Heart and Lungs, and leads to compromised circulation of qi and blood. Qi and blood fail to reach the head and sudden fainting or scattered consciousness occur. Sinking da qi usually begins with transitory turns characterized by sweating, palpitations and light–headedness. As the qi becomes weaker and sinks for longer periods, fainting and drop attacks start to occur.

Da qi is weakened by factors that influence the Heart and Lungs. These include acute and chronic emotional stress (intense grief and sadness or loss, periods of extreme excitement or over–stimulation), physical exhaustion, excessive sweating, chronic diarrhea and excessive use of substances that disperse or direct qi downwards, such as medications for asthma.

Clinical features
- Sudden, transitory disturbance of consciousness, fainting or drop attacks. Episodes may be initiated by periods of increased or unaccustomed activity. Pallor, hyperventilation, sweating, confusion, disorientation or 'feeling distant' may precede an episode. There may be incontinence of urine or feces. Recovery is gradual, with lingering fatigue and grogginess.
- breathlessness, rapid or laboured breathing, dyspnea, panting
- pale or ashen complexion
- copious spontaneous sweating
- empty feeling in the chest; chest pain
- lower abdominal fullness, distension and discomfort
- palpitations, bradycardia

T pale

P weak, fine, or imperceptible, especially in the distal (cun) position and clearly stronger in the proximal (chi) position; or irregular and intermittent

Treatment principle
Supplement and raise sinking yang qi

Prescription
SHENG XIAN TANG 升陷汤
Raise the Sunken Decoction

huang qi (Astragali Radix) 黄芪 18–24g
zhi mu (Anemarrhenae Rhizoma) 知母 9–12g
jie geng (Platycodi Radix) 桔梗 3–6g
chai hu (Bupleuri Radix) 柴胡 3–6g
sheng ma (Cimicifugae Rhizoma) 升麻 3–6g

Method: Decoction. **Huang qi** supplements and raises yang qi; **jie geng, chai hu** and **sheng ma** support the lifting action of **huang qi**; **zhi mu** cools and moistens any heat and dryness that may be present. (Source: *Yi Xue Zhong Zhong Can Xi Lu*)

Modifications

- With severe qi deficiency, add **ren shen** (Ginseng Radix) 人参 9–12g.
- With profuse sweating, add **shan zhu yu** (Corni Fructus) 山茱萸 9–12g.
- With fullness in the lower abdomen, double the dose of **sheng ma**.
- With yang deficiency, cold extremities, ashen complexion and blue lips, delete **zhi mu** and add **gan jiang** (Zingiberis Rhizoma) 干姜 6–9g and **gui zhi** (Cinnamomi Ramulus) 桂枝 6–9g.
- With chest pain, add **quan gua lou** (Trichosanthis Fructus) 全栝楼 18–24g.
- With blood stasis, add **hong hua** (Carthami Flos) 红花 6–9g, **ji xue teng** (Spatholobi Caulis) 鸡血藤 12–15g and **dan shen** (Salviae miltiorrhizae Radix) 丹参 9–12g.

Prepared medicines

Concentrated powders
Bu Zhong Yi Qi Tang (Ginseng & Astragalus Combination)

Pills
Bu Zhong Yi Qi Wan (Central Chi Teapills)

Acupuncture (select from)

Du.20 (baihui +▲) ....lifts yang qi to the upper body
Bl.13 (feishu +▲)...............transport points of the Lungs and Heart, these
Bl.15 (xinshu +▲)   points supplement zong qi
Du.14 (dazhui +▲)............meeting point of the yang channels, an important
                       point elevating yang qi to the upper body
Ren.17 (shanzhong +) ....these points promote correct movement of qi in the
Ren.12 (zhongwan +)   triple burner and supplement qi
Ren.4 (guanyuan +▲)
Lu.9 (taiyuan +) ....source point of the Lungs, meeting point for the
                       vessels, strengthens Lung qi and yin
St.36 (zusanli +▲) ....sea point of the Stomach, strengthens the Spleen and
                       Stomach and supplements qi
Sp.6 (sanyinjiao +)..............strengthens the Spleen and supplements qi
Bl.62 (shenmai)..................master and couple points of yangqiaomai, can
SI.3 (houxi)   assist in elevating qi to the upper body
- with spontaneous sweating, add LI.4 (hegu) and Kid.7 (fuliu)
- with thin, watery sputum, add St.40 (fenglong –) and Sp.3 (taibai +)
- with palpitations or bradycardia, add Ht.5 (tongli +)
- Ear points: lung, heart, spleen, zero point, shenmen, sympathetic

Clinical notes

- Fainting and blackouts associated with collapsing da qi may be a serious condition associated with cardiac weakness or failure, cardiopulmonary disease, cor pulmonale, emphysema, atrial fibrillation, ventricular tachycardia or sick sinus syndrome.
- Light exercise, especially swimming and easy walking, are recommended.
- For dietary recommendations, see Clinical Handbook, Vol. 2, p.870.

气
血
虚
弱

6.4 QI AND BLOOD DEFICIENCY

Fainting and turns associated with qi and blood deficiency are common. Fainting and turns may occur because there is not enough qi and blood to maintain adequate pressure in the head when changing position. Fainting may also occur because the supply of qi and blood to the Heart is insufficient, and any extra load on the Heart causes arrhythmia and a sudden drop in circulation.

Clinical features

- Sudden fainting or transitory disturbance of consciousness, usually upon rising from a recumbent position. Episodes are associated with palpitations, spots or blurring in the visual field, weakness or loss of vision. The patient usually recovers quickly.
- dry skin and hair
- pale complexion, nails and conjunctivae
- palpitations, arrhythmia, tachycardia brought on by exertion
- insomnia, dream disturbed sleep
- forgetfulness, poor memory, poor concentration
- spontaneous sweating and/or night sweats
- fatigue and weakness
- breathlessness
- dry stools or constipation

T pale and maybe swollen with a thin coat
P fine and weak, or irregular

Treatment principle

Strengthen the Spleen and supplement qi and blood

Prescription

BA ZHEN TANG 八珍汤
Eight Treasure Decoction

---

shu di (Rehmanniae Radix preparata) 熟地 12–18g
dang gui (Angelicae sinensis Radix) 当归 9–12g
bai shao (Paeoniae Radix alba) 白芍 6–9g
chuan xiong (Chuanxiong Rhizoma) 川芎 3–6g
bai zhu (Atractylodes macrocephalae Rhizoma) 白术 9–12g
ren shen (Ginseng Radix) 人参 3–6g
fu ling (Poria) 茯苓 6–9g
zhi gan cao (Glycyrrhizae Radix preparata) 炙甘草 3–6g

Method: Decoction or powdered extracts. **Shu di** nourishes yin and blood and supplements the Kidneys; **dang gui** and **bai shao** supplement blood and soften the Liver; **dang gui** and **chuan xiong** activate blood and move qi; **ren shen** supplements yuan qi and strengthens the Spleen; **bai zhu** strengthens the Spleen, dries damp, and alleviates the cloying nature of the blood supplements; **fu ling** strengthens the Spleen and leaches out damp; **zhi gan cao** supplements qi, harmonizes the action of the other herbs, and with **bai shao,** alleviates spasmodic pain. (Source: *Zhong Yi Zhi Liao Yi Nan Za Bing Mi Yao* [*Zheng Ti Lei Yao*])

Modifications

- With loose stools, abdominal bloating and loss of appetite, use **chao dang gui** (stir fried Angelicae sinensis Radix) 炒当归, and add **shan yao** (Dioscoreae Radix) 山药 12–15g and **shen qu** (Massa medicata fermentata) 神曲 9–12g.
- With marked blood deficiency, add **e jiao** (Asini Corii Colla) 阿胶 9–12g [dissolved in the hot strained decoction].
- With low grade fever, add **yin chai hu** (Stellariae Radix) 银柴胡 9–12g and **bai wei** (Cynanchi atrati Radix) 白薇 9–12g.
- With night sweats, add **wu wei zi** (Schizandrae Fructus) 五味子 3–6g and **fu xiao mai** (Semen Tritici Aestivi Levis) 浮小麦 12–15g.
- With cold, add **zhi huang qi** (honey fried Astragali Radix) 炙黄芪 15–24g and **rou gui** (Cinnamomi Cortex) 肉桂 3–6g.
- With blurring vision or spots before the eyes, add **jue ming zi** (Cassiae Semen) 决明子 9–15g and **chu shi zi** (Broussonetiae Fructus) 楮实子 6–9g.
- With anxiety, fearfulness and palpitations, add **long chi** (Fossilia Dentis Mastodi) 龙齿 15–30g and **yuan zhi** (Polygalae Radix) 远志 6–9g.
- With dream disturbed sleep or nightmares, add **he huan pi** (Albizziae Cortex) 合欢皮 12–15g, **ye jiao teng** (Polygoni multiflori Caulis) 夜交藤 15–30g and **long chi** (Fossilia Dentis Mastodi) 龙齿 15–30g.
- With Liver qi constraint, add **xiang fu** (Cyperi Rhizoma) 香附 9–12g.
- With muscle spasm, fasiculation, tremors or numbness, add **mu gua** (Chaenomelis Fructus) 木瓜 6–9g and **tian ma** (Gastrodiae Rhizoma) 天麻 6–9g.
- With blood stasis, add **tao ren** (Persicae Semen) 桃仁 9–12g and **hong hua** (Carthami Flos) 红花 6–9g.
- With bleeding, heavy periods or tarry stools, add **ce bai ye** (Platycladi Cacumen) 侧柏叶 9–12g, **ou jie** (Nelumbinis Nodus rhizomatis) 藕节 9–12g and **xian he cao** (Agrimoniae Herba) 仙鹤草 12–15g.

Variations and additional prescriptions
Heart qi deficiency with arrhythmia
Heart qi deficiency causes fainting associated with sudden arrhythmia or ventricular tachycardia. Depending on the degree of deficiency, arrhythmias of a qi deficiency type can be sporadic and difficult to detect, occurring only when the patient is tired or suffering periods of stress. In such cases the arrhythmia may only be evident prior to fainting. When fainting is frequent however, the degree of deficiency is usually more profound, and irregularities will be noted on the pulse. The more irregular the heartbeat the greater the deficiency. The treatment is to supplement qi and blood, unblock yang qi and restore the pulse with ZHI GAN CAO TANG (Prepared Licorice Decoction 炙甘草汤, p.811).

With chronic bleeding
Chronic bleeding can lead to significant qi and blood deficiency. It may go undetected, especially when occurring in the upper digestive tract. The bleeding may only be detected by a stool test. Bleeding of a qi deficient type may also be seen in easy bruising or heavy periods. The treatment is to supplement Heart blood and

Spleen qi, and stop bleeding with **GUI PI TANG** (Restore the Spleen Decoction 归脾汤, p.387).

Prepared medicines
Concentrated powders
Ba Zhen Tang (Tangkuei & Ginseng Eight Combination)
Shi Quan Da Bu Tang (Ginseng & Dang Gui Ten Combination)
  – with cold
Ren Shen Yang Ying Tang (Ginseng & Rehmannia Combination)
Gui Pi Tang (Ginseng & Longan Combination)
  – with bleeding
Zhi Gan Cao Tang (Licorice Combination)
  – with arrhythmia

Pills
Ba Zhen Wan (Women's Precious Pills, Nu Ke Ba Zhen Wan)
Shi Quan Da Bu Wan (Ten Flavour Teapills)
Gui Pi Wan (Kwei Be Wan, Gui Pi Teapills)
Dang Gui Ji Jing (Tang Kuei Essence of Chicken)
  – a liquid extract especially good for postpartum qi and blood deficiency

Acupuncture (select from)
Du.20 (baihui +▲) ....elevates yang qi and blood to the head
Ren.12 (zhongwan +▲) ......alarm point of the Stomach, strengthens the Spleen and Stomach and supplements qi and blood
St.36 (zusanli +▲) ....sea point of the Stomach, strengthens the Spleen and Stomach and supplements qi and blood
Sp.6 (sanyinjiao +▲).........strengthens the Spleen and Kidneys, and supplements qi and blood
Bl.20 (pishu +▲) ....transport point of the Spleen, strengthens the Spleen and supplements qi and blood
Ren.4 (guanyuan +▲)........supplements yuan qi
Ren.6 (qihai +▲) ....boosts the Kidneys and regulates qi
• with bruising, heavy periods or occult bleeding, add Sp.1 (yinbai ▲)
• with sweating, add Ht.6 (yinxi +)
• with arrhythmia, add Ht.5 (tongli) and Bl.15 (xinshu +)
• with insomnia, add Ht.7 (shenmen +) and anmian (N–HN–54)
• Ear points: heart, spleen, shenmen, sympathetic, adrenal

Clinical notes
• Fainting and funny turns of a qi and blood deficiency type may be diagnosed as anemia, pregnancy, postural hypotension, hypoglycemia, cardiac arrhythmias, Stokes–Adams attacks or mitral valve prolapse.
• Qi and blood deficiency generally responds well to treatment, in combination with an appropriate supplementing diet. See Clinical Handbook, Vol 2, p.870–874. Treatment should be sustained for several months for a satisfactory result.

心
气
阴
两
虚

6.5 HEART QI AND YIN DEFICIENCY

Fainting from Heart qi and yin deficiency can be caused by damage to fluids and qi by a prolonged or serious febrile illness, or dehydration caused by vomiting, diarrhea or inadequate fluid intake. Heart qi and yin can also be depleted by chronic use of heating, dispersing or stimulant drugs such as amphetamines, cocaine, antihypertensives and steroids. The weakened circulation of qi and blood that is characteristic of Heart qi deficiency is compounded by lack of yin fluids and increased viscosity of blood. This pattern is often complicated by blood stasis.

Clinical features
- Fainting, drop attacks or transitory disturbances of consciousness preceded by dizziness, light–headedness, flushing and hyperventilation.
- palpitations, tachycardia, bradycardia
- breathlessness
- spontaneous sweating and/or night sweats
- dry mouth and throat
- fatigue, lethargy and weakness
- anxiety
- insomnia
- dry stools or constipation

T reddish, swollen and dry with little or no coat, or with multiple surface cracks
P fine, weak, or intermittent or irregular

Treatment principle
Supplement Heart qi and yin
Strengthen the Heart and restore the pulse

Prescription

SHENG MAI SAN 生脉散
Generate the Pulse Powder

---

ren shen (Ginseng Radix) 人参 9–15g
mai dong (Ophiopogonis Radix) 麦冬 15–24g
wu wei zi (Schizandrae Fructus) 五味子 6–9g
Method: Decoction. **Ren shen** supplements Heart qi; **mai dong** nourishes yin and clears heat; **wu wei zi** secures the exterior, stops sweating and preserves yin. (Source: *Nei Wai Shang Biao Huo Lun*)

Modifications
- With marked qi deficiency, add **huang jing** (Polygonati Rhizoma) 黄精 12–15g and **huang qi** (Astragali Radix) 黄芪 15–24g.
- With marked yin deficiency, add **yu zhu** (Polygonati odorati Rhizoma) 玉竹 12–15g.
- With tachycardia, add **zhi gan cao** (Glycyrrhizae Radix preparata) 炙甘草 12–15g and **dan shen** (Salviae miltiorrhizae Radix) 丹参 9–12g.
- With anxiety, add **bai he** (Lilii Bulbus) 百合 12–15g.
- With blood stasis, add **dan shen** (Salviae miltiorrhizae Radix) 丹参 9–12g and **hong hua** (Carthami Flos) 红花 6–9g.

- With profuse sweating, add **mu li** (Ostreae Concha) 牡蛎 18–30g, **ma huang gen** (Ephedrae Radix) 麻黄根 9–12g, **xiao mai** (Tritici Fructus) 小麦 12–15g.
- With insomnia, add **ye jiao teng** (Polygoni multiflori Caulis) 夜胶藤 18–30g and **long chi** (Fossilia Dentis Mastodi) 龙齿 15–30g.

Variations and additional prescriptions
With marked arrhythmia
When irregularity of the pulse is marked, ZHI GAN CAO TANG (Prepared Licorice Decoction 炙甘草汤, p.811) can be used to supplement Heart qi and yin, unblock yang qi and regulate the pulse.

With shen disturbance, sleep disorder and anxiety
When shen disturbances are marked, with anxiety, panic attacks and hyperventilation preceding episodes, TIAN WANG BU XIN DAN (Emperor of Heaven's Special Pill to Supplement the Heart 天王补心丹, p.147) can be used to nourish qi and yin and calm the shen.

Prepared medicines
Concentrated powders
Sheng Mai San (Ginseng & Ophiopogon Formula)
Zhi Gan Cao Tang (Licorice Combination)
Tian Wang Bu Xin Dan (Ginseng & Zizyphus Formula)
Pills
Sheng Mai Wan (Great Pulse Teapills)
Zhi Gan Cao Wan (Zhi Gan Cao Teapills)
Tian Wang Bu Xin Dan (Emperor's Teapills, Tian Wang Pu Hsin Tan)

Acupuncture (select from)
Ht.7 (shenmen +)...............source point of the Heart, calms the shen, regulates and supplements Heart qi

Ren.4 (guanyuan +)............supplements yuan qi

St.36 (zusanli +) ....sea point of the Stomach, strengthens the Spleen and Stomach and supplements qi

Sp.6 (sanyinjiao +)..............strengthens the Spleen and Kidneys, nourishes qi and yin

Ren.17 (shanzhong) ....regulates qi in the chest

Bl.15 (xinshu +) ....transport point of the Heart, supplements Heart qi and yin, calms the Heart and shen

Bl.23 (shenshu +) ....transport point of the Kidney, supplements source qi and yin and supports the qi and yin of the whole body

yintang (M–HN–3) ....calms the shen

- with arrythmia, add Ht.5 (tongli +)
- with spontaneous sweating, add Bl.43 (gaohuangshu) and Du.14 (dazhui ▲)
- with night sweats, add Ht.6 (yinxi) and Kid.7 (fuliu)
- with chest oppression, add PC.6 (neiguan –)

- Ear points: heart, shenmen, spleen, stomach, sympathetic

Clinical notes

- Fainting and turns of a Heart qi and yin deficiency type may be associated with hypotension, atrial fibrillation, arrhythmias and sick sinus syndrome.
- For dietary recommendations, see Clinical Handbook, Vol. 2, p.870 and 876.
- Mild aerobic exercise is important to help rebuild qi and yin. Especially good are taijiquan, qigong and yoga.
- A review of the patients medications may be warranted. Illicit stimulant drugs should be strictly prohibited.

心
阳
虚
弱

6.6 HEART YANG DEFICIENCY

Heart yang deficiency causes fainting and turns because Heart function is seriously compromised. The Heart is too weak to adequately propel blood to the head, and the Heart is liable to sudden arrhythmia, further weakening the already poor circulation. Heart yang deficiency is frequently complicated by Kidney yang deficiency, blood stasis and/or phlegm.

Clinical features
- Frequent fainting or drop attacks
- pale or ashen complexion; purple lips
- chest oppression, chest pain
- bradycardia, arrythmia, palpitations
- breathlessness; in severe cases dyspnea or orthopnea
- spontaneous sweating
- fatigue, weakness, exhaustion
- icy cold extremities, blue or purple discolouration of the extremities
- edema of the lower limbs
- all symptoms aggravated by exertion
- **with blood stasis**: stabbing chest pain, angina, purple or mauve tongue with dark distended sublingual veins
- **with phlegm**: marked chest oppression, thick tongue coat

T pale, swollen and scalloped
P deep, weak or imperceptible, or slow and irregular or irregularly irregular

Treatment principle
Warm and supplement Heart yang

Prescription

REN SHEN SI NI TANG 人参四逆汤
Frigid Extremities Decoction with Ginseng

This prescription is selected when episodes are frequent and Heart yang markedly weak. It is not suitable for prolonged use. As Heart yang is restored and cardiac function improves, a more yang supplementing approach can be adopted for long term treatment (see Variations, below).

hong ren shen (red Ginseng Radix) 红人参 9–15g
zhi fu zi (Aconiti Radix lateralis preparata) 制附子 12–15g
gan jiang (Zingiberis Rhizoma) 干姜 6–9g
zhi gan cao (Glycyrrhizae Radix preparata) 炙甘草 6–12g
gui zhi (Cinnamomi Ramulus) 桂枝 9–12g
chao bai zhu (stir fried Atractylodes macrocephalae Rhizoma) 炒白术 ... 9–12g
fu ling (Poria) 茯苓 9–12g

Method: Decoction. **Hong ren shen** supplements yuan qi and strengthens the Heart; **zhi fu zi** warms Heart yang and mobilizes fluids; **gan jiang** warms the Spleen and dispels cold; **fu ling** and **chao bai zhu** strengthen the Spleen and dry damp; **gui zhi** unblocks Heart yang; **zhi gan cao** alleviates arrhythmia and protects against excessive dispersal of qi by the pungent warmth of **zhi fu zi** and **gan jiang**. (Source: *Zhong Yi Zhi Liao Yi Nan Za Bing Mi Yao* [*Shang Han Lun*])

Modifications

- With chest oppression or pain and a thick or greasy tongue coat from phlegm obstruction, add **quan gua lou** (Trichosanthis Fructus) 全栝楼 15–24g, **zhi ban xia** (Pinelliae Rhizoma preparatum) 制半夏 9–12g and **xie bai** (Allii macrostemi Bulbus) 薤白 6–9g.
- With blood stasis, add **chuan xiong** (Chuanxiong Rhizoma) 川芎 6–9g, **san qi fen** (powdered Notoginseng Radix) 三七粉 3–6g and **hong hua** (Carthami Flos) 红花 6–9g.
- With marked yang deficiency and an imperceptible pulse, up to 30 grams of **zhi fu zi** (Aconiti Radix lateralis preparata) 制附子 may be used (see clinical notes, p.251–252).
- In very severe cases the patient is cold and clammy, cyanotic, pale white and has icy extremities and a fibrillating pulse, indicating imminent collapse of Heart yang. The treatment strategy is to administer an emergency medicine such as GUAN XIN SU HE XIANG WAN (Liquid Styrax Pills for Coronary Heart Disease 冠心苏合香丸), and institute emergency acupuncture techniques (Box 6.4, p.262) until paramedic assistance arrives.

Variations and additional prescriptions

Kidney yang deficiency

Once Heart yang is responding to treatment and getting stronger, a more supplementing approach can be phased in. The aim is to strengthen the source of yang qi, the Kidneys and thereby support the Heart. The treatment is to warm and supplement Kidney and Heart yang with a prescription such as JIN GUI SHEN QI WAN (Kidney Qi Pill from the Golden Cabinet 金匮肾气丸, p.826). This prescription is suitable for long term, systemic yang supplementation.

Prepared medicines

Concentrated powder

Si Ni Tang (Aconite, Ginger and Licorice Combination)
Zhen Wu Tang (Ginger, Aconite, Poria & Peony Combination)
 – Heart yang deficiency with edema and orthopnea
Ba Wei Di Huang Wan (Rehmannia Eight Formula)
 – for long term yang supplementation

Pills

Zhen Wu Tang Wan (True Warrior Teapills)
Jin Kui Shen Qi Wan (Fu Gui Ba Wei Wan, Golden Book Teapills)
 – for long term yang supplementation

Acupuncture (select from)

Bl.15 (xinshu +▲) ....transport point of the Heart, warms and activates
                               circulation of Heart yang
Bl.23 (shenshu +▲) ....transport point of the Kidneys, warms Kidney yang
                               to support Heart yang
Du.4 (mingmen +▲) ....warms and supplements Kidney yang to support
                               yang systemically

Ren.17 (shanzhong) ....improves circulation of yang qi through the chest

PC.6 (neiguan –)................connecting point of the Pericardium, opens up the
flow of yang qi through the chest

Ren.4 (guanyuan +▲)........warms Kidney yang to support Heart yang

St.36 (zusanli +▲) ....sea point of the Stomach, strengthens the Spleen and
Stomach and supplements yang qi

• with arrhythmia, add Ht.7 (shenmen +) and Ht.5 (tongli)
• with chest pain, add PC.4 (ximen –)
• with blood stasis, add Bl.17 (geshu) and Bl.18 (ganshu)
• with sweating, add Du.14 (dazhui ▲)
• with edema or watery cough, add Ren.9 (shuifen ▲) and St.28 (shuidao ▲)
• for emergency management of collapsing Heart yang, see Box 6.4, p.262.
• Ear points: heart, kidneys, shenmen, adrenal, sympathetic

Clinical notes

• Fainting of a Heart yang deficiency type may be associated with cardiac arrhythmia, atherosclerosis, arteriosclerosis, cardiomyopathy, congestive cardiac failure, sick sinus syndrome, mitral valve prolapse or Stokes–Adams attacks.
• For dietary recommendations, see Clinical Handbook, Vol. 2, p.873.
• Exercise is difficult for patients with yang deficiency, but can be helpful when undertaken in a controlled fashion. Gentle physiotherapy in a warm pool is a good way to begin.

肝郁血虚 6.7 LIVER QI CONSTRAINT WITH BLOOD DEFICIENCY

Liver qi constraint with blood deficiency is more likely to cause funny turns than fainting. There are two mechanisms at play. The pent up qi can suddenly be released and counterflow to the head. The blood deficiency compounds the likelihood of developing qi constraint, can fail to rise to the head and not anchor the hun (p.98). The more blood deficiency, the more the likelihood of fainting. There is a clear stress component to this pattern but, paradoxically, turns or fainting of this type often occur some time (weeks to a couple of months) after the stress has subsided. Patients are often able to 'soldier on' through a difficult time, but as soon as they relax, the effects of the qi constraint on the body become apparent and turns occur.

Qi constraint is a precursor to other pathology implicated in fainting and funny turns. Prolonged qi constraint can slow and congeal fluids into phlegm, slow and stagnate blood, and generate heat and fire which damage yin and lead to ascendant yang or wind.

Clinical features
- Turns with sudden loss of balance, giddiness, blurring vision, disturbed proprioception and spatial disorientation, or rarely fainting. Restoration of normal consciousness is usually quick. Turns can be preceded by sudden rotation of the head, stress or emotional upset, or occur around the menstrual period.
- postural dizziness, light–headedness
- fatigue, lethargy, worse in the morning and with inactivity
- irritability, depression
- muscular stiffness and tightness in the upper back and neck
- tension headaches; occipital and temporal headaches
- shallow breathing; tightness in the chest; frequent sighing
- sleep disturbance; typically waking between 1–3am
- constipation and sluggish stools, or alternating constipation and diarrhea
- heartburn, reflux, belching, abdominal bloating, loss of appetite

T normal color or mauve, or with pale or orangey edges and a thin coat
P wiry and fine

Treatment Principle
Dredge the Liver and relieve qi constraint
Strengthen the Spleen and supplement qi and blood

Prescription

XIAO YAO SAN 逍遥散
Rambling Powder

chai hu (Bupleuri Radix) 柴胡	9–12g
dang gui (Angelicae sinensis Radix) 当归	9–12g
bai shao (Paeoniae Radix alba) 白芍	12–18g
bai zhu (Atractylodis macrocephalae Rhizoma) 白术	9–12g

fu ling (Poria) 茯苓 12–15g
zhi gan cao (Glycyrrhizae Radix preparata) 炙甘草 3–6g
wei jiang (Zingiberis Rhizoma preparata) 煨姜 3–6g
bo he (Mentha haplocalycis Herba) 薄荷 3–6g
Method: Decoction. **Bo he** is added a few minutes before the end of cooking. **Chai hu** dredges the
Liver and regulates Liver qi; **dang gui** and **bai shao** soften the Liver and nourish Liver blood; **bai
zhu** and **fu ling** strengthen the Spleen and dry damp; **zhi gan cao** supplements qi and, with **bai
shao**, eases muscle spasm; **wei jiang** warms and harmonizes the Stomach; **bo he** assists **chai hu** in
moving Liver qi. (Source: *He Ji Ju Fang*)

Modifications

- With heat, add **shan zhi zi** (Gardeniae Fructus) 山栀子 6–9g and **mu dan pi** (Moutan Cortex) 牡丹皮 6–9g.
- With marked blood deficiency, add **shu di** (Rehmanniae Radix preparata) 熟地 9–15g.
- With depression, add **he huan pi** (Albizziae Cortex) 合欢皮 12–15g, **yu jin** (Curcumae Radix) 郁金 9–12g and **ye jiao teng** (Polygoni multiflori Caulis) 夜交藤 18–30g.
- With tightness in the chest, add **gua lou** (Trichosanthis Fructus) 栝楼 15–24g.
- With muscle spasm and pain, increase the dose of **bai shao** to 30g and the dose of **zhi gan cao** to 12g
- With abdominal or hypochondriac pain, add two or three of the following herbs: **chuan lian zi** (Toosendan Fructus) 川楝子 9–12g, **yu jin** (Curcumae Radix) 郁金 9–12g, **mu xiang** (Aucklandiae Radix) 木香 6–9g and **yan hu suo** (Corydalis Rhizoma) 延胡索 9–12g or **fo shou** (Citri sarcodactylis Fructus) 佛手 9–12g.
- With constipation, add **hou po** (Magnoliae officinalis Cortex) 厚朴 9–12g, **bing lang** (Arecae Semen) 槟榔 6–9g and **zhi shi** (Aurantii Fructus immaturus) 枳实 6–9g.
- With alternating bowel habits and colicky abdominal pain, increase the dose of **bai shao** to 30g and add **chen pi** (Citri reticulatae Pericarpium) 陈皮 6–9g and **fang feng** (Saposhnikovae Radix) 防风 9–12g.
- With belching, add **zhu ru** (Bambusae Caulis in taeniam) 竹茹 6–9g and **zhi ban xia** (Pinelliae Rhizoma preparatum) 制半夏 6–9g.
- With heartburn and acid reflux, add **huang lian** (Coptidis Rhizoma) 黄连 3–6g and **wu zhu yu** (Evodiae Fructus) 吴茱萸 2–3g.
- With abdominal bloating, add **hou po** (Magnoliae officinalis Cortex) 厚朴 9–12g.
- With flatulence, add **hou po** (Magnoliae officinalis Cortex) 厚朴 9–12g and **sha ren** (Amomi Fructus) 砂仁 3–6g.
- With constriction or tightness in the throat, or difficulty swallowing, combine with **BAN XIA HOU PO TANG** (Pinellia and Magnolia Bark Decoction 半夏厚朴汤, p.858).

Prepared medicines
Concentrated powder
Xiao Yao San (Bupleurum & Tangkuei Formula)
Pills
Xiao Yao Wan (Free and Easy Wanderer Teapills, Hsiao Yao Wan)

Acupuncture (select from)
Du.20 (baihui) .... these points regulate qi, subdue ascendant yang qi
GB.20 (fengchi –)   and clear the mind
Ren.12 (zhongwan –) .... alarm point of the Stomach, strengthens the Spleen and supplements qi
PC.6 (neiguan –) .... regulates Liver qi and downbears counterflow qi
GB.34 (yanglingquan –) ..... regulates the Liver and subdues ascendant yang qi
Sp.6 (sanyinjiao +) .... strengthens the Spleen and supplements blood, dredges the Liver
Liv.3 (taichong –) .... source point of the Liver, regulates Liver qi and blood, and nourishes Liver blood
Bl.18 (ganshu –) .... transport point of the Liver, mobilizes Liver qi and activates blood
Bl.20 (pishu +) .... transport point of the Spleen, supplements qi and blood
ahshi points .... tender points on the upper back and neck (sternocleidomastoid, trapezius)
• with Spleen deficiency, add St.36 (zusanli +)
• with tight neck and shoulders, add GB.21 (jianjing –)
• with blurring vision, add GB.37 (guanming)
• with marked dizziness, add GB.43 (xiaxi –)
• with insomnia, add SJ.5 (waiguan) and GB.39 (xuanzhong)
• Ear points: shenmen, liver, zero point, sympathetic

Clinical notes
• Fainting of a Liver qi constraint type may be diagnosed as autonomic nervous system imbalance, vasovagal syncope, anemia or transient ischemic attack.
• Trigger points in the sternocleidomastoid muscle are a common contributor to dizziness and turns, and are commonly found in patients with Liver pathology. The posterior neck muscles and trapezius should also be assessed for tightness and trigger point activity, and treated if necessary.
• Exercise is an important component of treatment, p.103.
• Hot spot therapy is helpful, p.923.
• Dietary modification is important when there is blood deficiency. See Clinical Handbook, Vol. 2, p.874.

6.8 ASCENDANT LIVER YANG, LIVER FIRE

肝
阳
上
亢

Ascendant Liver yang is a severe form of counterflow Liver qi. Ascendant Liver yang or Liver fire are seen in younger patients without significant deficiency. As the patient ages or the condition persists, yin deficiency usually starts to intervene and the ascendant yang becomes more severe. In patients over 40, it is unusual to see ascendant yang without some underlying deficiency. In practice, the distinction between pent up Liver qi, ascendant Liver yang or fire and Liver yin deficiency with ascendant yang is rarely clear cut. Many patients will have elements of all patterns.

In this pattern, Liver yang ascends rapidly when severely constrained qi is suddenly released. Fire rises because it is its nature to do so. Fire is hotter and drier and may cause hemorrhages. Liver fire is more likely to develop if there is pre–existing internal heat or a heating diet.

Clinical features
• Fainting, disturbances of proprioception and spatial orientation, vertigo, sense of heat rushing to the head, visual disturbances or loss of balance initiated or aggravated by stress, anger or emotional upset, alcohol consumption, or sudden rotation of the head. The episode may be preceded or followed by migraine, fullness and distension in the head and eyes and nausea and vomiting.
• tension or migraine headaches; distending sensation in the head
• blurring vision, red, sore, gritty eyes
• irritability, short temper, anger outbursts, easily 'flies off the handle'
• red complexion or facial flushing
• sensation of heat rushing to the head; sensation of heat in the chest
• right sided hypochondriac pain
• insomnia, dream disturbed sleep; waking between 1–3am
• muscle spasms and tics
• **Liver fire**: scleral hemorrhage, epistaxis, bitter taste in the mouth, dry mouth and thirst, red sore eyes, pain in the ears
T red, or with red edges and a yellow coat
P wiry, strong and rapid

Treatment principle
Calm the Liver and subdue ascendant yang
Clear heat and fire

Prescription
TIAN MA GOU TENG YIN 天麻钩藤饮
Gastrodia and Uncaria Drink

This prescription is selected when there is too much yang in the head, and the patient is not especially hot.
tian ma (Gastrodiae Rhizoma) 天麻 6–9g
gou teng (Uncariae Ramulus cum Uncis) 钩藤 9–12g
shi jue ming (Haliotidis Concha) 石决明 15–30g

shan zhi zi (Gardeniae Fructus) 山栀子 6–9g
huang qin (Scutellariae Radix) 黄芩... 6–9g
du zhong (Eucommiae Cortex) 杜仲 9–12g
chuan niu xi (Cyathulae Radix) 川牛膝...................................... 9–15g
sang ji sheng (Taxilli Herba) 桑寄生... 9–12g
fu shen (Poriae Sclerotium pararadicis) 茯神 9–12g
ye jiao teng (Polygoni multiflori Caulis) 夜交藤 15–30g
yi mu cao (Leonuri Herba) 益母草 9–12g

Method: Decoction. **Shi jue ming** is cooked for 30 minutes before the other herbs are added, **gou teng** is added near the end of cooking. **Tian ma**, **gou teng** and **shi jue ming** calm the Liver and subdue yang; **shan zhi zi** and **huang qin** clear heat; **yi mu cao** activates blood and promotes urination to provide an outlet for the heat; **sang ji sheng**, **du zhong** and **chuan niu xi** supplement the Liver and Kidneys, and assist in leading qi and blood downwards; **ye jiao teng** and **fu shen** calm the Heart and shen. (Source: *Za Bing Zheng Zhi Xin Yi*)

LONG DAN XIE GAN TANG 龙胆泻肝汤
Gentian Decoction to Purge the Liver, modified

This prescription is selected for Liver fire.

long dan cao (Gentianae Radix) 龙胆草 6–9g
huang qin (Scutellariae Radix) 黄芩... 6–12g
shan zhi zi (Gardeniae Fructus) 山栀子 6–12g
ze xie (Alismatis Rhizoma) 泽泻 6–12g
mu tong (Akebiae Caulis) 木通 3–6g
che qian zi (Plantaginis Semen) 车前子 9–15g
sheng di (Rehmanniae Radix) 生地 9–15g
dang gui (Angelicae sinensis Radix) 当归 6–12g
chai hu (Bupleuri Radix) 柴胡 3–9g
gan cao (Glycyrrhizae Radix) 甘草 3–6g
shi jue ming (Haliotidis Concha) 石决明...................................... 15–30g
gou teng (Uncariae Ramulus cum Uncis) 钩藤 9–12g

Method: Decoction. **Che qian zi** is decocted in a cloth bag, **shi jue ming** cooked for 30 minutes prior to the other herbs. **Long dan cao** clears Liver fire; **shan zhi zi** and **huang qin** clear heat from the Heart, Stomach and Liver; **chai hu** dredges the Live and clears heat; **ze xie**, **che qian zi** and **mu tong** promote urination and provide an escape route for the heat; **sheng di** cools the blood; **dang gui** nourishes and protects blood; **gan cao** protects the Stomach; **gou teng** calms the Liver and subdues yang; **shi jue ming** calms the Liver and subdues ascendant Liver yang. (Source: *Yi Fang Ji Jie*)

Modifications (apply to both prescriptions)
- With visual disturbances and loss of balance, add **xia ku cao** (Prunellae Spica) 夏枯草 15–18g and **ju hua** (Chrysanthemi Flos) 菊花 9–12g.
- With constipation, add **da huang** (Rhei Radix et Rhizoma) 大黄 6–9g and **mang xiao** (Natrii Sulfas) 芒硝 6–9g, or use **DANG GUI LONG HUI WAN** (Dang Gui, Gentian and Aloe Pill 当归龙荟丸 p.117) to clear Liver heat through the bowels.

Prepared medicines
Concentrated powders
Tian Ma Gou Teng Yin (Gastodia & Gambir Combination)

Long Dan Xie Gan Tang (Gentiana Combination)
Dang Gui Long Hui Wan (Tangkuei, Gentiana & Aloe Formula)
Pills
Tian Ma Gou Teng Wan (Tian Ma Gou Teng Teapills)
Long Dan Xie Gan Wan (Snake and Dragon Teapills)
Yang Yin Jiang Ya Wan (Nourish Yin and Reduce [Blood] Pressure Pill)
 – for ascendant yang and hypertension

Acupuncture (select from)
Du.20 (baihui –)................these points subdue ascendant Liver yang
St.8 (touwei)
GB.20 (fengchi –) ....calms the Liver and subdues ascendant yang
Liv.3 (taichong –)..............source point of the Liver, activates Liver qi, subdues
                              Liver yang, extinguishes wind and alleviates spasms
GB.34 (yanglingquan –).....soothes the Liver and subdues yang
GB.43 (xiaxi –) ....clears heat and subdues yang
Bl.18 (ganshu)...................transport point of the Liver, moves Liver qi
Bl.23 (shenshu +) ....transport point of the Kidney, nourishes Kidney yin
                              to restrain and anchor yang
ahshi points ....tender points on the upper back and neck (sterno-
                              cleidomastoid, trapezius)
* with Liver fire, add Liv.2 (xingjian –)
* with muscle spasm in the neck, add GB.21 (jianjing –) and Du.9 (zhiyang –)
* with blurring vision, add GB.37 (guanming)
* with anxiety or headache, add yintang (M–HN–3)
* with insomnia and headache, add SJ.5 (waiguan –) and GB.39 (xuanzhong –)
* with nausea, add PC.6 (neiguan –)
* Ear points: liver, kidney, ear apex ↓, lowering blood pressure groove ↓

Clinical notes
* The fainting and turns associated with ascendant Liver yang or fire may be diagnosed as transitory ischemic attacks, migraine or cluster headaches, an impending stroke, hypertension, eclampsia, puerperal fever or Meniere's disease.
* Fainting or turns of an ascendant yang or fire type may represent a potentially dangerous condition or an impending catastrophe.
* Trigger points in the sternocleidomastoid muscle are a common contributor to dizziness and problems with proprioception, and are commonly found in patients with Liver pathology. The posterior neck muscles and trapezius should also be assessed for tightness and trigger point activity, and treated if necessary.
* Hot spot therapy in the region of T7–T10 can be helpful, p.923.
* A cooling diet can be helpful. For dietary recommendations, see Clinical Handbook, Vol. 2, p.882.
* Regular exercise (p.103) and stress management are essential components of successful long term treatment.

6.9 LIVER AND KIDNEY YIN DEFICIENCY WITH ASCENDANT YANG OR WIND

肝
肾
阴
虚，
风
阳
上
扰

Liver and Kidney yin deficiency with ascendant yang is a mixture of deficiency and excess, and depending on their balance, the nature and intensity of symptoms varies. The pattern can oscillate between the background yin deficiency and the sudden manifestation of the ascendant yang. Patients have periods when the yang is more unanchored, fainting and turns are frequent, and active steps to subdue it are required. When the yang is more stable, the focus of treatment shifts to rebuilding the yin.

Liver yang rises because the yin is unable to anchor it, and provide a counter-weight to its active and rising nature. The yang loses its mooring and becomes excessively mobile, rising suddenly to the head. When ascendant yang reaches a certain level of intensity, it may be redefined as wind. The instability of the un-anchored yang here is such that minor triggers are sufficient to cause it to ascend. Liver and Kidney yin deficiency with ascendant yang is often complicated by phlegm, phlegm heat or blood stasis.

Clinical features
- Fainting or drop attacks, or frequent disturbances of proprioception and spatial orientation, dizziness and vertigo, sense of heat rushing to the head, visual disturbances or loss of balance. Symptoms can be initiated or aggravated by stress, or emotional upset, sexual activity or sudden rotation of the head. The episode may be preceded or followed by migraine, distension in the head and eyes, and nausea and vomiting.
- tics, tremors, muscle spasms and fasciculation; numbness in the extremities
- blurred vision or visual disturbances, pressure behind the eyes
- temporal or vertex headaches; distending sensation in the head
- insomnia or restless sleep with much dreaming
- palpitations, anxiety, irritability and restlessness
- red complexion, facial flushing or malar flushing
- sensation of heat in the chest, palms and soles; night sweats
- weakness, fatigue, exhaustion
- lower back ache and weakness; tinnitus

T red and dry with little or no coat
P wiry, fine and rapid

Treatment principle
Subdue and anchor Liver yang and extinguish wind
Nourish and supplement Liver and Kidney yin to anchor yang

Prescription

ZHEN GAN XI FENG TANG 镇肝熄风汤
Sedate the Liver and Extinguish Wind Decoction

This prescription is used when yang is unstable and rising frequently. It can be used until the yang is pacified (no more than 6–8 weeks), and should be gradually replaced with a more yin supplementing prescription as the condition improves.

huai niu xi (Achyranthis bidentatae Radix) 怀牛膝...............................15–30g
dai zhe shi (Haematitum) 代赭石..15–30g
long gu (Fossilia Ossis Mastodi) 龙骨 9–15g
mu li (Ostreae Concha) 牡蛎 9–15g
gui ban (Testudinis Plastrum) 龟板..9–15g
bai shao (Paeoniae Radix alba) 白芍...9–15g
xuan shen (Scrophulariae Radix) 玄参 9–15g
tian dong (Asparagi Radix) 天冬...9–15g
chuan lian zi (Toosendan Fructus) 川楝子 6–9g
mai ya (Hordei Fructus germinantus) 麦芽...6–9g
yin chen (Artemisiae scopariae Herba) 茵陈..6–9g
gan cao (Glycyrrhizae Radix) 甘草...3–6g

Method: Decoction. The mineral and shell ingredients are decocted for 30 minutes prior to the other herbs. The large dose of **huai niu xi** leads qi and blood away from the head, while supplementing the Liver and Kidneys to anchor yang; **dai zhe shi** pacifies the Liver, subdues yang and extinguishes wind; **long gu**, **mu li** and **gui ban** subdue and anchor yang and calm the Liver; **xuan shen**, **tian dong** and **bai shao** enrich the yin, nourish blood and soften the Liver; **yin chen**, **chuan lian zi** and **mai ya** cool the Liver and rectify Liver qi; **mai ya** and **gan cao** assist in protecting and harmonizing the Stomach. (Source: *Yi Xue Zhong Zhong Can Xi Lu*)

Modifications

- With heat in the chest, add **shi gao** (Gypsum fibrosum) 石膏 15–30g and **shan zhi zi** (Gardeniae Fructus) 山栀子 9–12g.
- With blood stasis, add **dan shen** (Salviae miltiorrhizae Radix) 丹参 9–12g and **yu jin** (Curcumae Radix) 郁金 9–12g.
- With phlegm or phlegm heat, add **dan nan xing** (Arisaemae cum Bile) 胆南星 6–9g and **tian zhu huang** (Bambusae Concretio silicea) 天竺黄 6–9g.
- For focal headache, add **dan shen** (Salviae miltiorrhizae Radix) 丹参 12–15g and **chuan xiong** (Chuanxiong Rhizoma) 川芎 9–12g.
- With hypertension, add **xia ku cao** (Prunellae Spica) 夏枯草 15–18g, **gou teng** (Uncariae Ramulus cum Uncis) 钩藤 9–12g, **ju hua** (Chrysanthemi Flos) 菊花 9–12g and **di long** (Pheretima) 地龙 6–9g.
- With loose stools, use **chi shi zhi** (Halloysitum rubrum) 赤石脂 15–24g instead of **dai zhe shi**.

Variations and additional prescriptions

With gradual improvement

As the ascendant yang is subdued and the symptoms improve, the heaviness of the mineral sedatives in the primary prescription can weigh the yang down too much and weaken the Spleen. The strategy should be gradually shifted to a more balanced approach that addresses the yin deficiency directly while still attending to subduing and anchoring the yang. This can be achieved with a prescription such as **DA DING FENG ZHU** (Major Arrest Wind Pearl 大定风珠).

sheng di (Rehmanniae Radix) 生地...9–15g
bai shao (Paeoniae Radix alba) 白芍..12–18g
mai dong (Ophiopogonis Radix) 麦冬..12–18g

mu li (Ostreae Concha) 牡蛎 15–30g
bie jia (Trionycis Carapax) 鳖甲 9–15g
gui ban (Testudinis Plastrum) 龟板 9–15g
zhi gan cao (Glycyrrhizae Radix preparata) 炙甘草 6–9g
e jiao (Asini Corii Colla) 阿胶 6–9g
huo ma ren (Cannabis Semen) 火麻仁 6–9g
wu wei zi (Schizandrae Fructus) 五味子 3–6g
ji zi huang (egg yolk) 鸡子黄 2

Method: Decoction. The shells are decocted for 30 minutes prior to the other herbs, **e jiao** is pulverized to a powder, and, with the eggs, added to the strained decoction. **E jiao** and the **egg yolks** nourish yin and blood; **bai shao**, **sheng di** and **mai dong** nourish yin and blood, soften the Liver and 'generate fluids to water wood'; **gui ban** and **bie jia** nourish yin and subdue and anchor the yang; **huo ma ren** moistens dryness and lubricates the Intestines to keep the bowels open and encourages the downwards movement of qi; **mu li** calms the Liver and subdues yang; **wu wei zi** preserves yin, and, with **zhi gan cao**, combines sweet and sour flavors to create yin; **zhi gan cao** also protects the Stomach and balances the other herbs in the formula. (Source: *Wen Bing Tiao Bian*)

Follow up treatment

When the symptoms are under control, a yin nourishing prepared medicine such as QI JU DI HUANG WAN (Lycium Fruit, Chrysanthemum and Rehmannia Pill 杞菊地黄丸, p.467) or ZHI BAI DI HUANG WAN (Anemarrhena, Phellodendron and Rehmannia Pill 知柏地黄丸, p.922) may be used to nourish Liver and Kidney yin and anchor yang over a prolonged period.

Prepared medicines

Concentrated powders

Zhen Gan Xi Feng Tang (Hematite & Scrophularia Combination)
Qi Ju Di Huang Wan (Lycium, Chrysanthemum & Rehmannia Formula)
Zhi Bai Di Huang Wan (Anemarrhena, Phellodendron & Rehmannia Formula)

Pills

Zhen Gan Xi Feng Wan (Zhen Gan Xi Feng Teapills)
Yang Yin Jiang Ya Wan (Nourish Yin and Reduce [Blood] Pressure Pill)
Er Long Zuo Ci Wan (Er Ming Zuo Ci Wan, Tso–Tzu Otic Pills)

Acupuncture (select from)

Du.20 (baihui –) ....these points subdue ascendant Liver yang
St.8 (touwei)
GB.20 (fengchi –) ....calms the Liver and subdues ascendant yang
Bl.18 (ganshu +).................transport points of the Liver and Kidney, nourish
Bl.23 (shenshu +)   Liver and Kidney yin to secure and anchor yang
Ren.4 (guanyuan +)............supplements Kidney yin to anchor yang
Kid.3 (taixi +)....................source point of the Kidneys, supplements Kidney
                                        yin and clears heat from deficiency
Kid.6 (zhaohai +) ....supplements Kidney yin and clears heat from
                                        deficiency
GB.34 (yanglingquan –).....dredges the Liver and subdues yang
Liv.3 (taichong –)...............source point of the Liver, subdues ascendant yang,

extinguishes wind and alleviates spasms

ahshi points ....tender points on the upper back and neck (sterno-cleidomastoid, trapezius)

- with muscle spasm in the neck, add GB.21 (jianjing –) and Du.9 (zhiyang –)
- with blurring vision, add GB.37 (guanming)
- with anxiety or headache, add yintang (M–HN–3)
- with insomnia and headache, add SJ.5 (waiguan –) and GB.39 (xuanzhong –)
- with nausea, add PC.6 (neiguan –)
- Ear points: liver, kidney, ear apex ↓, lowering blood pressure groove ↓

Clinical notes

- The fainting and turns associated with yin deficiency and ascendant yang may be associated with transitory ischemic attacks, vertebrobasilar insufficiency, atherosclerosis, arteriosclerosis, hypertension, post concussion syndrome or disorders of the cerebellum.
- This pattern can respond well to treatment, however persistent fainting or disturbances of consciousness requires thorough investigation. This can be a potentially dangerous situation indicating an impending stroke in some patients, so frequent monitoring of subjective and objective signs, including blood pressure, is necessary.
- In many cases, patients will be taking some form of antihypertensive medication. Interactions between antihypertensives and the prescriptions recommended above are uncommon. However, the additive effect on blood pressure can be significant and low blood pressure may result. Patients should be alerted to the signs of low blood pressure–postural dizziness being the main one–and referred to their physician for a review of medication.
- Trigger points in the sternocleidomastoid muscle are a common contributor to dizziness and problems with proprioception, and are commonly found in patients with Liver pathology. The posterior neck muscles and trapezius should also be assessed for tightness and trigger point activity, and treated if necessary.
- Hot spot therapy in the region of T7–L2 can be helpful, p.923.
- Regular exercise (p.103) and stress management are essential components of successful long term treatment.
- A yin nourishing diet is recommended. See Clinical Handbook, Vol. 2, p.876.

痰
湿
阻
头

6.10 PHLEGM DAMP BLOCKING THE CHANNELS OF THE HEAD AND MUSCLES

Phlegm damp causes disturbances of consciousness and turns in two ways. It clogs up the channels and impedes the normal circulation of yang qi to the head and muscles, and it sits like a veil over the senses. Without adequate yang qi getting to the head and muscles, and with the senses clouded, the patient experiences mental dullness, somnolence or sudden loss of muscle function.

Turns and disturbances of consciousness of a phlegm damp type can be intermittent, appearing in clusters for a period of time, after which the patient is comparatively normal until the episodes begin again. This sporadic course is due to the alternate congealing and dispersal of phlegm, which occurs in response to changes in diet or increases in emotional tension.

Clinical features

- Sudden loss of muscle function causing collapse without loss of consciousness. In mild cases there may only be limpness of the neck or knees, sagging facial muscles or inability to speak clearly. The collapse may be triggered by emotion. Episodes last from seconds to minutes, after which normal function is restored.
- Irresistible sleepiness during the day, often worse in the afternoon and after eating. The patient may fall asleep without warning. After restoration of consciousness the patient may be quite groggy for a period of time.
- foggy head, difficulty concentrating; dizziness and vertigo
- heaviness and lethargy
- headaches, dull distension in the head
- fullness in the abdomen, chest oppression
- mucus congestion, throat clearing
- loss of appetite, loss of sense of taste
- nausea, vomiting, belching, acid reflux
- loose stools, or occasionally constipation (but stools are not dry)
- even though the condition is chronic, the patient appears robust and may be overweight

T thick, greasy, white coat, possible swollen or flabby tongue body
P slippery or wiry or moderate

Treatment principle

Dry damp and transform phlegm
Strengthen the Spleen and correct the qi dynamic

Prescription

DAO TAN TANG 导痰汤
Guide Out Phlegm Decoction

zhi ban xia (Pinelliae Rhizoma preparatum) 制半夏 12–15g
ju hong (Citri reticulatae Exocarpium rubrum) 橘红 3–6g
fu ling (Poria) 茯苓 3–6g
zhi shi (Aurantii Fructus immaturus) 枳实.. 3–6g

dan nan xing (Arisaema cum Bile) 胆南星.. 3–6g
sheng jiang (Zingiberis Rhizoma recens) 生姜 3–6g
zhi gan cao (Glycyrrhizae Radix preparata) 炙甘草............................... 3–6g
Method: Decoction. **zhi ban xia** and **ju hong** transform phlegm and rectify the qi dynamic; **ju hong** and **zhi shi** regulate qi and direct qi downward; **fu ling** strengthens the Spleen and improves fluid metabolism to drain damp; **dan nan xing** scours out phlegm; **sheng jiang** transforms phlegm, moderates the toxicity of **zhi ban xia** and **dan nan xing** and alleviates nausea; **zhi gan cao** moderates the harsh drying nature of the principal herbs, and protects the Stomach. (Source: *Zhong Yi Nei Ke Xue* [*He Ji Ju Fang*])

Modifications
- With foggy head and mental dullness, add **shi chang pu** (Acori tatarinowii Rhizoma) 石菖蒲 6–9g, **yuan zhi** (Radix Polygalae Tenuifoliae) 远志 6–9g and **yu jin** (Curcumae Radix) 郁金 6–9g to vaporize phlegm.
- With headache and dizziness, add **bai zhu** (Atractylodes macrocephalae Rhizoma) 白术 6–9g and **tian ma** (Gastrodiae Rhizoma) 天麻 6–9g.
- With hypersalivation or drooling, add **bai jie zi** (Sinapsis Semen) 白芥子 3–6g and **su zi** (Perillae Fructus) 苏子 3–6g.
- With cold, add **rou gui** (Cinnamomi Cortex) 肉桂 3–6g and **gan jiang** (Zingiberis Rhizoma) 干姜 6–9g.
- With heat, add **yu jin** (Curcumae Radix) 郁金 9–12g, **huang qin** (Scutellariae Radix) 黄芩 3–6g and **huang lian** (Coptidis Rhizoma) 黄连 2–3g.
- With constipation, add **lai fu zi** (Raphani Semen) 莱菔子 6–9g and **da fu pi** (Arecae Pericarpium) 大腹皮 6–9g.
- With Spleen deficiency, add **bai zhu** (Rhizoma Atractylodis Macrocephalae) 白术 9–12g.
- If abdominal discomfort or distension increases with ingestion of the prescription, delete **zhi gan cao**, and add **shen qu** (Massa medicata fermentata) 神曲 9–12g and **lai fu zi** (Raphani Semen) 莱菔子 6–9g.

Prepared medicines
Concentrated powders
Er Chen Tang (Citrus & Pinellia Combination)
Ding Xian Wan (Gastrodia and Amber Combination)
Ping Wei San (Magnolia & Ginger Formula)

Pills
Er Chen Wan (Pinellia Pachyma Pills, Erh Chen Wan)
Ping Wei San (Calm Stomach Teapills, Tabellae Pingwei)
Xiang Sha Liu Jun Zi Wan (Aplotaxis–Ammomum Pills, Six Gentlemen Tea Pills) – with qi deficiency

Acupuncture (select from)
Du.20 (baihui –) ....clears phlegm from the head
GB.20 (fengchi –) ....calms the Liver, clears the head and subdues yang
PC.5 (jianshi –)..................river point of the Pericardium, transforms phlegm
Sp.3 (taibai)........................source and connecting point of the Spleen and
St.40 (fenglong –)   Stomach to strengthen and transform phlegm damp

Bl.62 (shenmai) ....master points of dumai and yinqiaomai, used
Kid.6 (zhaohai)   on alternate sides for inability to keep the eyes open
St.41 (jiexi –).....................river and fire point of the Stomach, strengthens the
                                Spleen and Stomach to transform phlegm damp
St.36 (zusanli +▲) ....sea point of the Stomach, warms and strengthens the
                                Spleen and Stomach, supplements yang qi
Bl.20 (pishu) ....transport point of the Spleen, strengthens and
                                supplements Spleen qi and yang to promote trans-
                                formation of damp and phlegm
• with Liver qi constraint, add GB.34 (yanglingquan –) and Liv.3 (taichong –)
• with cold, apply moxa cones to Bl.20 (pishu ▲) and Bl.21 (weishu ▲)
• with muscle aches, add Sp.21 (dabao)
• with abdominal distension, add St.25 (tianshu –) and Sp.15 (daheng –)
• Ear points: spleen, zero point, liver, subcortex, sympathetic, shenmen, lowering blood pressure groove ↓

Clinical notes

• Turns and disturbances of consciousness associated with phlegm damp may
  be diagnosed as narcolepsy, catalepsy, food allergies, hypoglycemia or chronic
  fatigue syndrome.
• This pattern can respond to treatment, but depending on the duration of the
  condition and the age of the patient can take a long time to achieve a satisfactory result.
• The heaviness and lethargy typical of phlegm damp can be impediments to
  exercise, but graded exercise in groups can achieve good results.
• Hot spot therapy can be helpful, p.923.
• Diet is an important part of phlegm damp treatment. Avoidance of certain
  foods is important if there is intolerance or allergy. For dietary recommendations, see Clinical Handbook, Vol. 2, p.880.

风
痰
上
扰

6.11 WIND PHLEGM

Wind phlegm is a pattern that combines the sudden onset and involuntary move-ment of wind with the consciousness clouding of phlegm. There are two types of consciousness disturbance associated with wind phlegm, depending on the bal-ance of wind and phlegm. The first is associated with severe vertigo and spatial disorientation to the point of falling but without loss of consciousness, and occurs when the phlegm component is greater than the wind. The second is associated with fainting, involuntary movement, spasms or convulsions, and is due to the dominance of the wind over the phlegm.

Phlegm causes consciousness disturbances by clogging the senses, like a 'mist'. When fainting occurs, the phlegm is carried swiftly to the head by wind. This pat-tern is often complicated by Spleen qi deficiency and ascendant Liver yang.

Clinical features
- **Phlegm dominant**: Confusion, befuddlement, vertigo, disordered proprioception and spatial disorientation, or sudden collapse, usually preceded by vertigo and headaches. Episodes may be triggered by movement of the head, exposure to strong smells like perfume and gasoline or emotional upheaval. After the episode the patient is groggy, sick and disoriented.
- **Wind dominant**: abrupt impairment of consciousness and muscle twitching without collapse ('absence' seizure), loss of voluntary control over a limb or collapse and convulsions.
- dull headaches and head distension
- tinnitus
- heaviness in the body, lethargy, fatigue
- nausea or vomiting; nausea may precede episodes
- abdominal distension, chest oppression

T swollen, with a thick, greasy, white coat
P slippery and wiry or soft and soggy

Treatment principle
Transform and disperse phlegm and extinguish wind
Strengthen the Spleen and Stomach and regulate qi

Prescription
BAN XIA BAI ZHU TIAN MA TANG 半夏白术天麻汤
Pinellia, Atractylodes Macrocephala, and Gastrodia Decoction, modified

This formula is selected when phlegm is dominant.
zhi ban xia (Pinelliae Rhizoma preparatum) 制半夏 9–12g
bai zhu (Atractylodes macrocephalae Rhizoma) 白术 12–15g
tian ma (Gastrodiae Rhizoma) 天麻 9–12g
chen pi (Citri reticulatae Pericarpium) 陈皮 6–9g
fu ling (Poria) 茯苓 9–15g
gan cao (Glycyrrhizae Radix) 甘草 3–6g
sheng jiang (Zingiberis Rhizoma recens) 生姜 9–12g

da zao (Jujubae Fructus) 大枣 .... 3 fruit
cang zhu (Atractylodis Rhizoma) 苍术 9–12g
shi chang pu (Acori tatarinowii Rhizoma) 石菖蒲 6–9g
yuan zhi (Polygalae Radix) 远志 6–9g
Method: Decoction. **Zhi ban xia** transforms phlegm, dries damp, downbears counterflow Stomach qi and stops nausea and vomiting; **tian ma** calms the Liver and extinguishes wind; **bai zhu** and **fu ling** strengthen the Spleen and transform phlegm; **chen pi** transforms phlegm and corrects the qi dynamic; **sheng jiang** transforms phlegm and assists the other herbs in stopping nausea and vomiting; **da zao** and **gan cao** strengthen the Spleen and harmonize the Stomach; **cang zhu** dries damp and transforms phlegm; **shi chang pu** and **yuan zhi** vaporize phlegm and clear the senses. (Source: *Yi Xue Xin Wu*)

Modifications

- With marked Spleen qi deficiency, add **dang shen** (Codonopsis Radix) 党参 12–15g and **huang qi** (Astragali Radix) 黄芪 12–15g.
- With Liver qi constraint, add **zi su ye** (Perillae Folium) 紫苏叶 9–12g, **zhi shi** (Aurantii Fructus immaturus) 枳实 6–9g and **hou po** (Magnoliae officinalis Cortex) 厚朴 9–12g.
- With ascendant Liver yang, add **gou teng** (Uncariae Ramulus cum Uncis) 钩藤 12–15g and **shi jue ming** (Haliotidis Concha) 石决明 15–30g [cooked first].
- With heat, add **huang qin** (Scutellariae Radix) 黄芩 6–9g, **huang lian** (Coptidis Rhizoma) 黄连 3–6g and **shan zhi zi** (Gardeniae Fructus) 山栀子 6–9g.
- With severe vertigo and nausea, increase the dose of **tian ma**, and add one or two of the following herbs: **dai zhe shi** (Haematitum) 代赭石 12–18g, **xuan fu hua** (Inulae Flos) 旋覆花 9–15g, **bai jiang can** (Bombyx Batryticatus) 白僵蚕 9–12g or **dan nan xing** (Arisaemae cum Bile) 胆南星 6–9g.
- With edema, combine with **WU LING SAN** (Five Ingredient Powder with Poria 五苓散, p.219).
- With frontal headache, add **bai zhi** (Angelicae dahuricae Radix) 白芷 9–12g.
- With epigastric fullness and loss of appetite, add **bai dou kou** (Amomi Fructus rotundus) 白豆蔻 6–9g and **sha ren** (Amomi Fructus) 砂仁 6–9g.

Variations and additional prescriptions

Wind phlegm, with wind dominant

Wind phlegm, with wind dominant, can cause seizures. When seizures or loss of consciousness are frequent, it is important to concentrate on reducing the seizures as quickly as possible. The manifestation of the seizures can vary from sudden loss of conscious awareness (an 'absence'), loss of voluntary control of one limb, to collapse and convulsions. The treatment is to eliminate phlegm and extinguish wind with **DING XIAN WAN** (Arrest Seizures Pill 定痫丸). Once the seizures have been alleviated somewhat a more constitutional approach (Spleen and Kidney strengthening, as appropriate) should be phased in. This prescription is not suitable for prolonged use, and may damage yin and fluids if used excessively.

tian ma (Gastrodiae Rhizoma) 天麻 30g
chuan bei mu (Fritillariae cirrhosae Bulbus) 川贝母 30g
zhi ban xia (Pinelliae Rhizoma preparatum) 制半夏 30g
fu ling (Poria) 茯苓 30g

fu shen (Poria Sclerotium pararadicis) 茯神 30g
dan nan xing (Arisaemae cum Bile) 胆南星 15g
shi chang pu (Acori tatarinowii Rhizoma) 石菖蒲 15g
quan xie (Scorpio) 全蝎 15g
bai jiang can (Bombyx Batryticatus) 白僵蚕 15g
hu po (Succinum) 琥珀 15g
deng xin cao (Junci Medulla) 灯心草 15g
chen pi (Citri reticulatae Pericarpium) 陈皮 21g
yuan zhi (Polygalae Radix) 远志 21g
dan shen (Salviae miltiorrhizae Radix) 丹参 60g
mai dong (Ophiopogonis Radix) 麦冬 60g

Method: Grind the herbs into a fine powder and form into 6 gram pills by decocting the powder with 120g of **gan cao** (Glycyrrhizae Radix) 甘草, 100mls of **zhu li** (Bambusae Succus) 竹沥, 50 mls of ginger juice and sufficient water to form a thick paste. The dose is one pill 2–3 times daily. The original prescription used the toxic and now obsolete **zhu sha** (Cinnabaris) 朱砂 to coat the pills. **Tian ma** extinguishes wind; **chuan bei mu, zhi ban xia, dan nan xing** and **chen pi** transform and eliminate phlegm; **shi chang pu** and **yuan zhi** transform phlegm and open the orifices; **fu shen** and **fu ling** calm the shen and promote urination; **quan xie** and **bai jiang** can extinguish wind; **hu po** and **deng xin cao** clear heat and calm the shen; **dan shen** activates blood; **mai dong** protects yin against the drying effects of the principle herbs. (Source: *Yi Xue Xin Wu*)

Prepared medicines
Concentrated powders
Ban Xia Bai Zhu Tian Ma Tang (Pinellia & Gastrodia Combination)
Ding Xian Wan (Gastrodia & Amber Combination)

Pills
Ban Xia Bai Zhu Tian Ma Wan (Head Clear Pill)
Wen Dan Wan (Rising Courage Teapills)
  – phlegm heat
Xiang Sha Liu Jun Zi Wan (Aplotaxis–Ammomum Pills, Six Gentlemen Tea Pills)
  – with Spleen qi deficiency

Acupuncture (select from)
Du.20 (baihui –) ....these points clear phlegm from the head
St.8 (touwei)
GB.20 (fengchi –) ....clears the head, regulates qi and subdues yang
Ren.12 (zhongwan) ....alarm point of the Stomach, strengthens Stomach
                              and Spleen function to transform phlegm
Liv.13 (zhangmen –) ....alarm point of the Spleen and meeting point of the
                              internal organs, strengthens the Spleen and improves
                              digestion, promotes Liver function
PC.5 (jianshi –) ....river point of the Pericardium, transforms phlegm
GB.34 (yanglingquan –).....subdues yang and wind
Sp.3 (taibai +)....................source and connecting points of the Spleen and
St.40 (fenglong –)   Stomach, transform phlegm
Sp.5 (shangqiu –) ....metal point of the Spleen, transforms damp,
                              strengthens the Spleen

St.41 (jiexi –).....................fire point of the Stomach, strengthens the Spleen
and Stomach to transform phlegm

Bl.20 (pishu +) ....transport point of the Spleen, strengthens the Spleen
to promote transformation of phlegm

- with Spleen deficiency add St.36 (zusanli +)
- with Liver qi constraint, add GB.34 (yanglingquan –) and Liv.3 (taichong –)
- with foggy head, add Bl.62 (shenmai)
- with cold, apply moxa cones to Bl.20 (pishu ▲) and Bl.21 (weishu ▲)
- with muscle aches, add Sp.21 (dabao)
- with edema, add Sp.9 (yinlingquan –) and Sp.6 (sanyinjiao)
- with somnolence, add Kid.6 (zhaohai) and Bl.62 (shenmai)
- Ear points: stomach, spleen, zero point, subcortex, sympathetic, shenmen

Clinical notes

- Fainting or turns of this type are likely to be diagnosed as Meniere's disease, labyrinthine disorders or epilepsy.
- Wind phlegm can respond reasonably well to persistent treatment and provide some symptom control.
- Diet is an important part of phlegm treatments. For dietary recommendations, see Clinical Handbook, Vol. 2, p.880.

食滞胃热 6.12 FOOD STAGNATION, STOMACH HEAT

Fainting from food stagnation is associated with overeating or ingestion of specific foods. As a result of overeating, qi is drawn away from the periphery and head, the qi dynamic and qi distribution are disrupted. Certain foods can trigger episodic fainting or turns in susceptible patients, in particular items such as aged cheese, fermented foods, chocolate, red wine and sulfites used as preservatives.

The main treatment is to avoid overeating and the known food triggers, but in some chronic cases even small amounts of food can initiate an episode.

Clinical features
• Fainting after eating a large meal or specific foods. Episodes may be preceded by visual disturbances, facial flushing, breathing difficulty or food cravings. Recovery can be gradual and accompanied by pallor, nausea, vomiting and throbbing headache.
• abdominal and epigastric distension or pain, relieved by belching or flatulence
• constipation, difficult or irregular stools, or occasional diarrhea
• halitosis
• acid reflux, heartburn
• nausea or vomiting
• copious foul flatulence

T thick, white or yellow, greasy coat
P wiry and slippery or slippery and rapid

Treatment principle
Disperse accumulated food, resolve stagnation and clear heat

Prescription

ZHI SHI DAO ZHI WAN 枳实导滞丸
Unripe Bitter Orange Pill to Guide Out Stagnation

da huang (Rhei Radix et Rhizoma) 大黄	30g
zhi shi (Aurantii Fructus immaturus) 枳实	15g
shen qu (Massa medicata fermentata) 神曲	15g
huang qin (Scutellariae Radix) 黄芩	9g
huang lian (Coptidis Rhizoma) 黄连	9g
fu ling (Poria) 茯苓	9g
bai zhu (Atractylodis macrocephalae Rhizoma) 白术	9g
ze xie (Alismatis Rhizoma) 泽泻	6g

Method: Grind the herbs to powder and form into 9 gram pills with water. The dose is one pill 2–3 times daily. May also be decocted, with the **da huang** reduced to 6–9 grams and added towards the end of cooking. Use this prescription for a few days or weeks only, then, when the heat is clearing, switch to something less bitter and cold (such as the prepared medicine **BAO HE WAN**). **Da huang** purges accumulations and heat from the Stomach and Intestines; it is assisted in this by **zhi shi** which also rectifies qi and alleviates epigastric distension; **shen qu** alleviates food stagnation; **huang qin** and **huang lian** clear damp heat; **fu ling** and **ze xie** promote urination to clear damp heat; **bai zhu** and **fu ling** strengthen the Spleen and dry damp. (Source: *Nei Wai Shang Bian Huo Lun*)

Modifications
• With severe distension and discomfort, add **hou po** (Magnoliae officinalis Cortex) 厚朴 9–12g.

Prepared medicines
Concentrated powders
Mu Xiang Bing Lang Wan (Vladmiria & Areca Seed Formula)
Bao He Wan (Red Tangerine Peel & Crategus Formula)

Pills
Bao He Wan (Preserve Harmony Pill)
Mu Xiang Shun Qi Wan (Aplotaxis Carminative Pills, Shun Qi Wan)
Zi Sheng Wan (Zi Sheng Stomachic Pills)
Xiang Sha Yang Wei Wan (Appetite and Digestion Pill, Hsiang Sha Yang Wei Pien)
Jian Pi Wan (Ginseng Stomachic Pills, Spleen Digest Aid Pill)
   – with Spleen deficiency

Acupuncture (select from)
Ren.12 (zhongwan –) ....alarm point of the Stomach, clears heat and disperses food stagnation
St.25 (tianshu –).................alarm point of the Large Intestine, regulates Intestinal function
Ren.6 (qihai –) ....regulates qi and alleviates distension
St.36 (zusanli –) ....sea point of the Stomach, regulates and strengthens the Stomach and Intestines
LI.10 (shousanli –) ....benefits digestion and regulates gastrointestinal function
St.44 (neiting –) ....water point of the Stomach, clears heat from the Stomach and Intestines and disperses stagnant food
• with constipation, add St.37 (shangjuxu –) and SJ.6 (zhigou –)
• with abdominal pain, add St.34 (liangqiu –) and Sp.4 (gongsun –)
• with nausea, add PC.6 (neiguan –)
• with Spleen deficiency, add Sp.6 (sanyinjiao)
• with borborygmus, add Sp.5 (shangqiu –)
• Ear points: zero point, spleen, stomach, liver, abdomen

Clinical notes
• Fainting associated with food stagnation may be diagnosed as allergy, gastro-esophageal reflux or migrainous syncope.
• The main treatment is regulation of the diet and avoidance of known triggers. Even though the etiology is overeating or food allergy, it is the heat that has been generated that must be cleared, and this can take a while. Treatment should persist for at least two to three weeks, in conjunction with appropriate dietary modification.

瘀
血
阻
络

6.13. BLOOD STASIS

Fainting and funny turns due to blood stasis may be acute or chronic. When acute, there will usually be a history of head trauma; when chronic, there is often a long history of constrained Liver and Heart qi. The presence of static blood obstructs the free movement of qi and blood in the network vessels, and obstructs the distribution of yin and yang in the head and sensory orifices.

Clinical features
- Loss of balance, dizziness, disturbed proprioception and spatial disorientation, blurring vision, amnesia, or fainting
- purplish complexion, lips, sclera, conjunctiva and nail beds
- dark rings around the eyes
- palpitations, chest pain and/or persistent localized headaches
- insomnia, fitful sleep disturbed by low grade or hectic fever
- depression, mood swings
- dry, scaly skin
- broken vessels or spider naevi on the face, trunk, inner knee and ankle
- pressure pain in the left iliac fossa

T in acute cases following head trauma the tongue body may be unremarkable; in chronic cases it will be mauve or purple, or with brown or purple stasis spots and a thin, white coat; sublingual veins are congested and dark

P deep, fine, choppy, wiry or intermittent

Treatment principle
Activate qi and blood and dispel blood stasis

Prescription

XUE FU ZHU YU TANG 血府逐瘀汤
Drive Out Stasis in the Mansion of Blood Decoction

dang gui (Angelicae sinensis Radix) 当归	9–12g
sheng di (Rehmanniae Radix) 生地	9–12g
chi shao (Paeoniae Radix rubrae) 赤芍	9–12g
chuan xiong (Chuanxiong Rhizoma) 川芎	6–9g
tao ren (Persicae Semen) 桃仁	9–12g
hong hua (Carthami Flos) 红花	6–9g
chai hu (Bupleuri Radix) 柴胡	6–9g
zhi ke (Aurantii Fructus) 枳壳	6–9g
gan cao (Glycyrrhizae Radix) 甘草	3–6g
chuan niu xi (Cyathulae Radix) 川牛膝	9–15g
jie geng (Platycodi Radix) 桔梗	3–6g

Method: Decoction. **Dang gui, sheng di, chuan xiong, chi shao, tao ren** and **hong hua** nourish, and activate blood; **chai hu, zhi ke, gan cao** and **chi shao** regulate the Liver and mobilize qi; **jie geng** frees the movement of qi through the chest and diaphragm, and elevates qi to the upper body; the large dose of **chuan niu xi** leads blood downwards–together they re–establish the correct ascent and descent of qi and blood. (Source: *Yi Lin Gai Cuo*)

Modifications

- With severe headache, increase the dose of **chuan xiong** to up to 30g.
- With qi deficiency, add **huang qi** (Astragali Radix) 黄芪 30–60g.
- With cold, add **zhi fu zi** (Aconiti Radix latealis preparata) 制附子 6–9g cooked for 30 minutes prior to the other herbs and **gui zhi** (Cinnamomi Ramulus) 桂枝 9–12g.
- With low grade fever, delete **jie geng** and **zhi ke**, increase the dose of **sheng di** to 18g, and add **mu dan pi** (Moutan Cortex) 牡丹皮 9–12g, **zhi mu** (Anemarrhenae Rhizoma) 知母 9–12g and **huang bai** (Phellodendri Cortex) 黄柏 9–12g.
- If the blood stasis follows a head trauma, add **zi ran tong** (Pyritum) 自然铜 6–9g, **su mu** (Sappan Lignum) 苏木 6–9g and **xue jie** (Daemonoropis Resina) 血竭 1–1.5g.

Variations and additional prescriptions

With severe headache or migraine

Sudden disturbance or loss of consciousness of a blood stasis type can accompany severe migraine or post traumatic headache. Although the principal prescription is effective, a more vigorous and focused approach may be considered. This is appropriate when there are recurrent fainting episodes with severe pain, and the patient is familiar enough with the warning signs to take the following prescription before fainting occurs. The treatment is to activate blood circulation in the head, local channels and network vessels, with XIONG LONG TANG (Ligusticum and Earthworm Decoction 芎龙汤). The large doses are aimed at producing a swift and decisive result, and are not suitable for more than a week at a time.

chuan xiong (Chuanxiong Rhizoma) 川芎 30g
ge gen (Puerariae Radix) 葛根 30g
yan hu suo (Corydalis Rhizoma) 延胡索 30g
huai niu xi (Achyranthis bidentatae Radix) 怀牛膝 30g
di long (Pheretima) 地龙 15g
bai zhi (Angelicae dahuricae Radix) 白芷 9g
xi xin (Asari Herba) 细辛 3g

Method: Decoction. **Chuan xiong** moves qi and blood and alleviates headache in general and blood stasis headache in particular; **ge gen** alleviates occipital headaches; **yan hu suo** stops pain; **huai niu xi** activates blood and directs blood away from the head; **di long** burrows through stagnation and opens up circulation in the network vessels; the pungent warmth of **bai zhi** and **xi xin** alleviate frontal and temporal headaches. (Source: *Zhong Yi Zhi Liao Yi Nan Za Bing Mi Yao*)

Prepared medicines

Concentrated powders

Xue Fu Zhu Yu Tang (Persica & Carthamus Combination)
Tong Qiao Huo Xue Tang (Persica & Ligusticum Combination)

Pills

Xue Fu Zhu Yu Wan (Stasis in the Mansion of Blood Teapills)
Tong Qiao Huo Xue Tang (Tong Qiao Huo Xue Teapills)
Sheng Tian Qi Pian (Raw Tian Qi Ginseng Tablets)

Acupuncture (select from)

Du.20 (baihui –) ....clears the head

GB.20 (fengchi –) ....dispels and extinguishes wind, calms the Liver and subdues Liver yang, clears the mind

ahshi points ....tender points on the head, upper back and neck

SI.3 (houxi –).....................the master and couple points of dumai, these

Bl.62 (shenmai)   points open up the circulation of dumai qi to assist in moving blood through the head

Bl.17 (geshu –)..................meeting point for blood, transforms and dispels stagnant blood

Sp.6 (sanyinjiao –)..............these points activate blood and dispel static blood

Sp.10 (xuehai –)

LI.4 (hegu –)

Liv.3 (taichong –) ....source point of the Liver, dredges the Liver and activates qi and blood

- with trauma, add points of pain on the head (ahshi)
- with depression, add LI.4 (hegu) and Liv.3 (taichong)
- Ear points: head, brain, liver, heart, sympathetic, shenmen

Clinical notes

- Fainting and turns of a blood stasis type may be diagnosed as the sequelae of concussion, tumors in the head, cerebellar lesions, cardiac arrhythmias, sick sinus syndrome, Stokes–Adams attacks, vertebrobasilar insufficiency, congestive cardiac failure or angina.
- A qi and blood mobilizing diet is appropriate. See Clinical Handbook, Vol. 2, pp.878.

6.14 MISCELLANEOUS

There are a variety of fainting and syncope patterns described in the literature. Most of these are isolated episodes for which the cause is obvious, such as fainting as a result of sunstroke, excessive alcohol intake, intense pain or food poisoning. There are also some that are unusual and rarely seen, such as fainting associated with sexual activity or increased respiratory pressure. When fainting is recurrent, management involves addressing the underlying cause.

6.14.1 ORGASM SYNCOPE (*sè jué* 色厥)

This involves a sudden alteration of consciousness or mild tonic seizures with orgasm. While relatively rare, it tends to be more common in young women. It may be accompanied by sweating, shortness of breath or epistaxis. It is thought to be due to weakness of yang qi and blood and failure of blood to anchor the shen, which is easily scattered during climax. The treatment is based on the constitutional findings, but aims to supplement qi and blood, secure jing and stabilize the shen. Recommended prescriptions include GUI PI TANG (Restore the Spleen Decoction 归脾汤, p.387) for Heart blood and Spleen qi deficiency; GUI ZHI JIA LONG GU MU LI TANG (Cinnamon Twig Decoction plus Dragon Bone and Oyster Shell 桂枝加龙骨牡蛎汤, p.267) for loss of connection between the Heart and Kidneys, ZUO GUI WAN (Restore the Left [Kidney] Pill 左归丸, p.900) for Kidney yin deficiency, YOU GUI WAN (Restore the Right [Kidney] Pill 右归丸, p.394) with yang deficiency.

6.14.2 ALCOHOL SYNCOPE (*jiǔ jué* 酒厥)

Fainting and disturbances of consciousness can occur with binge drinking or serious alcohol abuse. Treatment requires a multifactorial approach, but Chinese medicine can offer some assistance for those determined to beat the bottle, both in reducing desire and in correcting the various pathologies (damp heat, Spleen deficiency etc.), that may result from heavy drinking. A representative prescription that has been recommended for excessive alcohol intake for over 700 years is CHAI GE JIE CHENG SAN (Pueraria Flower Decoction to Resolve Hangover 柴葛解酲散). It is used in the early stages of alcohol withdrawal, the first 4–6 weeks or so, or 15–20 packets of herbs. Following this period, treatment, if required, is applied according to the constitutional findings.

ge hua (Puerariae Flos) 葛花.. 15g
bai dou kou (Amomi Fructus rotundus) 白豆蔻.................................... 15g
sha ren (Amomi Fructus) 砂仁... 15g
qing pi (Citri reticulatae viride Pericarpium) 青皮 6g
chen pi (Citri reticulatae Pericarpium) 陈皮....................................... 4.5g
ren shen (Ginseng Radix) 人参 4.5g
bai zhu (Atractylodis macrocephalae Rhizoma) 白术........................... 6g
fu ling (Poria) 茯苓.. 4.5g
shen qu (Massa medicata fementata) 神曲 6g
gan jiang (Zingiberis Rhizoma) 干姜 6g

zhu ling (Polyporus) 猪苓 4.5g
ze xie (Alismatis Rhizoma) 泽泻 6g
mu xiang (Aucklandiae Radix) 木香 4.5g

Method: Decoction. **Ge hua** has a unique effect on alleviating the after effects of excessive alcohol consumption; **sha ren, bai dou kou, qing pi, chen pi** and **mu xiang** regulate qi, dry damp, harmonize the middle burner and stimulate the qi dynamic; **ren shen** and **bai zhu** strengthen the Spleen and supplement qi; **zhu ling, fu ling** and **ze xie** promote urination and drain damp; **gan jiang** warms the Spleen and supports yang; **shen qu** alleviates food stagnation. With significant damp heat, add **huang bai** (Phellodendri Cortex) 黄柏 9g and **huang qin** (Scutellariae Radix) 黄芩 9g. (Source: *Zhong Yi Nei Ke Xue / Lan Shi Mi Cang*)

6.14.3 URINATION SYNCOPE (*niào jué* 尿厥)

Urination Syncope occurs in older men who feel faint or collapse while urinating. It happens at night after leaving a warm bed to urinate. The treatment is to warm and supplement Kidney yang with a prescription such as JIN GUI SHEN QI WAN (Kidney Qi Pill from the Golden Cabinet 金匮肾气丸, p.826).

6.14.4 RESPIRATORY SYNCOPE

Fainting can be associated with increased respiratory pressure during a severe episode of coughing, weight lifting or playing a wind instrument. The mechanism involves an acute disruption of Lung diffusion and descent, leading to stagnation of Lung and Heart qi and blockage to the ascent of yang qi to the head. Treatment requires alleviation of the cough, or learning more efficient breathing techniques.

6.14.5 FOOD POISONING (*huì jué* 秽厥)

Fainting or collapse from food poisoning is an isolated event. The condition is self limiting and treatment is palliative, aimed at dispelling residual turbid damp with a formula such as HUO XIANG ZHENG QI SAN (Agastache Powder to Rectify the Qi 藿香正气散 p.916).

6.14.6 PAIN (*tòng jué* 痛厥)

Fainting or collapse from pain can be a complicated issue, and can be associated with any event that causes sufficiently severe pain or the perception of severe pain. When pain is a trigger for an episode of fainting the treatment is to identify the cause of the pain and alleviate it.

6.14.7 SUMMERHEAT (*shǔ jué* 暑厥)

This is collapse associated with heatstroke, is an isolated event, and best managed by appropriate first aid, cooling and rehydration.

Table 6.1 Summary of fainting and funny turn patterns

Pattern	Features	Prescription
Instability of the anima (p.97)	Sudden fainting in response to social or psychological stress, preceded by flushing, hyperventilation, palpitations and sweating. Patients tend to be constitutionally nervous and anxious	Ding Zhi Wan + Gan Mai Da Zao Tang Gui Zhi Jia Long Gu Mu Li Tang
Spleen qi deficiency	Sudden light-headedness, tunnel vision in response to hunger or following a period of increased activity. Episodes occur in the afternoon, with pallor, palpitations and hunger. Fatigue, sweet cravings, abdominal distension, loose stools, muscle weakness, pale scalloped tongue with a thin or thick white coat, weak fine pulse	Shen Ling Bai Zhu San
Sinking da qi	Sudden, transitory disturbance of consciousness, fainting or drop attacks preceded by hyperventilation, sweating, or 'feeling distant'. May be incontinence of urine or feces. Empty feeling in the chest or chest pain, breathlessness, lower abdominal discomfort, pale tongue, weak fine intermittent or imperceptible pulse	Sheng Xian Tang
Qi and blood deficiency	Sudden fainting or transitory disturbance of consciousness with rising from a recumbent position. Episodes associated with palpitations, spots or blurring in the visual field and weakness. Postural dizziness, insomnia, poor memory, and concentration, fatigue, pale tongue with a thin coat, fine weak or intermittent pulse	Ba Zhen Tang
Qi and yin deficiency	Fainting, drop attacks or transitory disturbances of consciousness preceded by dizziness, light-headedness, flushing and hyperventilation. Arrhythmia, sweating or night sweats, dryness, fatigue, anxiety, insomnia, constipation, reddish swollen dry or cracked tongue with no coat, fine weak or intermittent pulse	Sheng Mai San
Heart yang deficiency	Frequent fainting or drop attacks, pale or ashen complexion; blue lips, chest pain, bradycardia or arrythmia, breathlessness, cold extremities, purple discolouration of the extremities, edema, pale or blue scalloped tongue, deep weak irregular or imperceptible pulse	Ren Shen Si Ni Tang
Liver qi constraint with blood deficiency	Sudden loss of balance, giddiness, blurring vision, or rarely, fainting. Fatigue, depression, muscle tension and headaches, tightness in the chest, heartburn, normal or mauve tongue, or with pale or orangey edges and a thin coat, wiry fine pulse	Xiao Yao San

Table 6.1 Summary of fainting and funny turn patterns (cont.)

Pattern	Features	Prescription
Ascendant Liver yang, Liver fire	Fainting, vertigo, sense of heat rushing to the head, visual disturbances or loss of balance. Migraines, eye distension, nausea and vomiting, blurring vision, short temper, red complexion, muscle spasms and tics, red tongue or with red edges and a yellow coat, wiry rapid pulse	Tian Ma Gou Teng Yin Long Dan Xie Gan Tang
Liver and Kidney yin deficiency with ascendant yang and wind	Fainting or drop attacks, dizziness and vertigo, sense of heat rushing to the head, blurring vision, eye distension, irritability, headache, tinnitus, heat in the palms and soles, night sweats, lower backache, muscle spasms and tics; numbness, red dry tongue with little or no coat, wiry fine rapid pulse	Zhen Gan Xi Feng Tang
Phlegm damp	Sudden loss of muscle function causing collapse without loss of consciousness, irresistible sleepiness during the day, foggy head, dizziness, heaviness, nausea, acid reflux, thick greasy white tongue coat, slippery wiry pulse	Dao Tan Tang
Wind phlegm	Confusion, befuddlement, vertigo, sudden collapse, or abrupt impairment of consciousness and muscle twitching. Dull headaches, tinnitus, poor concentration, foggy head, heaviness, lethargy, nausea or vomiting, swollen tongue with a thick greasy white coat, slippery wiry or soft and soggy pulse	Ban Xia Bai Zhu Tian Ma Tang Ding Xian Wan
Food stagnation	Fainting after eating a large meal or specific foods	Zhi Shi Dao Zhi Wan
Blood stasis	Loss of balance, blurring vision, amnesia, or fainting; purple complexion, focal headaches, broken vessels and spider nevi; pressure pain in left iliac fossa, mauve or purple with brown or purple stasis spots and a thin white coat; fine choppy or intermittent pulse	Xue Fu Zhu Yu Tang Xiong Long Tang

ACUTE FEVER

Acute fevers are most commonly caused by invasion of an external pathogen. Traditionally, such fevers are analyzed according to the guidelines laid out in the classic texts that deal with the consequences of external pathogenic invasion, the Shang Han Lun and Wen Re Lun. While there are many causes of acute fever, there are certain patterns that are more frequently encountered in the Chinese medicine clinic and these are the patterns discussed in this chapter. The nature, frequency and specific features of acute fever vary depending on the pathogen involved, the season and the geographical location. Fever patterns due to pathogens associated with particular geographical regions are tabulated in the appendix, p.355.

The fevers described in this chapter are usually of no more than 7–10 days duration. Fever that persists beyond 14 days is considered chronic. The manifestation of acute fever can vary considerably, from the continuous high fever of a qi level pathogen, to the afternoon and evening fevers or alternating fever and chills patterns of damp heat and shaoyang pathogens. The traditional designation of fever of this type is 'external damage' (wài shāng fā rè [1] 外伤发热).

> **BOX 7.1 ACUTE FEVER PATTERNS**
>
> Wei level
> – wind heat
> Qi level
> – Lung heat
> – yangming channel syndrome
> – yangming organ syndrome
> – damp heat
> Shaoyang
> Toxic heat
> Epidemic toxic wind damp heat
> Liver Gallbladder damp heat
> Spleen Stomach damp heat
> Large Intestine damp heat
> Urinary Bladder damp heat
> Damp heat or toxic heat in the Uterus
> Heat in the ying level
> Heat in the blood level

The biomedical view

Normal body temperature, measured orally around mid morning is 36–37.2⁰C (96.8–99⁰F), with an average of 36.8⁰C (98.2⁰F). There is a normal diurnal variation in body temperature of 0.5–1⁰C, with basal body temperature lowest in the morning and highest in the late afternoon. In infectious processes fever plays an important physiological and defensive role. Elevated body temperature makes the environment hostile to the pathogen, inhibits viral replication, speeds metabolic processes and enhances T–cell production.

Not all fevers need to be treated, and the fever of many common and benign illnesses is beneficial for the reasons noted above. Many acute fevers will run a predictable self limiting course without undue interference. Treatment of mild acute fever is discouraged. Unnecessary suppression of a fever with antipyretics or antibiotics can lead to a lingering pathogen. Treatment is mandatory when the fever is high and damage to yin and fluids likely, when the patient appears to deteriorate

---

1 Practical Dictionary of Chinese Medicine (1998) – 'external damage heat effusion'

and when there are complicating factors that are likely to lead to a worsening of the condition (see Box 7.3, p.312).

Childhood fevers are always of concern to parents and anything over 38.5⁰C requires close attention. Fever is not considered dangerous until it reaches 40⁰C. Complications include dehydration and convulsions which are alarming, but are generally not harmful.

ETIOLOGY

External pathogens

Acute fevers are usually due to invasion by one or more of the external pathogens–wind, cold, heat, dampness, damp heat, dryness or summerheat. Regardless of the initial pathogen, however, once it is in the body and struggling with the anti–pathogenic qi, it is transformed into heat or damp heat by the intensity of the battle, and relatively high fever is the result. This only occurs when the patients anti–pathogenic qi is robust. In patients with feeble defenses such as the elderly, debilitated or very young, an invading pathogen may meet little resistance, so a fever, the most obvious feature of the battle, is not seen.

> **BOX 7.2 BIOMEDICAL CAUSES OF ACUTE FEVER (TO 14 DAYS DURATION)**
>
> - influenza
> - viral infections, usually upper respiratory tract or urinary tract
> - sinusitis
> - Glandular fever
> - Cytomegalovirus infection
> - Lyme disease
> - dental infection/abscess
> - hepato–biliary infections
>   – hepatitis, cholecystitis, empyema of the gall bladder
> - pelvic inflammatory disease
> - tropical or travel acquired
>   – malaria, dengue fever, hepatitis, dysentery, typhoid
> - drug reaction
> - rare–psittacosis, brucellosis, leptospirosis

The type of pathogen an individual ends up with is partly geographically determined and partly determined by the constitution and initial condition of the patient. In warm or cool dry climates, wind heat and qi level heat pathogens prevail. In hot humid climates, damp heat and summerheat pathogens are more frequently encountered. Patients with a damp constitution or pre–existing damp heat from the diet are more likely to develop damp heat fevers in response to pathogenic invasion, regardless of the initial pathogen. Patients with a yang constitution or pre–existing yin deficiency are more likely to develop heat or fire. These are only general trends, as the interaction of the initial pathogen, the constitution, diet, air conditioning and climate control all have a bearing on how a pathogen presents.

Internal causes

Acute fever can occasionally be due to internal causes. In most cases there will be a history of a pre–existing condition that has been suddenly exacerbated by diet, stress or an external invasion. Factors that lead to persistent internal heat, dampness or damp heat can predispose someone to development of an acute fever. Prolonged qi constraint with constrained heat due to chronic stress, heat, dampness or damp heat introduced in the diet, and a yang constitution, are most common. When a patient is so primed, a sudden escalation of stress levels, or increase in alcohol consumption and heating foods can be sufficient to amplify the heat suf-

BOX 7.3 RED FLAGS

All practitioners need to be aware of their limitations, especially when serious and rapidly progressive disease is a possibility. The following may suggest potentially severe illness requiring special attention or appropriate referral. In most patients the existence of a life threatening illness is obvious. In others the diagnosis is not clear cut and there are warning signs to be aware of.

Very high fever
- Fever of 40°C (104°F) and above may indicate severe disease. The patient's resistance is strong and the struggle fierce, but yin and fluids may be damaged to the point of collapse.

Moderate fever
- Fever of 37.2–39°C (99–100°F) may indicate a mild or early stage of an infectious process, or may be the muted response of weak anti–pathogenic qi in a compromised, very young or elderly individual.

Accompanying symptoms
- Incessant vomiting, diarrhea and sweating can lead to swift dehydration and rapid deterioration, especially in young children and the elderly. Skin rashes, drenching night sweats, severe pain anywhere, marked pallor, respiratory distress and disturbances of consciousness are major red flags.

Location of the pathogen
- The deeper the pathogen, the more serious the condition. Heat in the blood is the most dangerous, even though the fever may not be extreme. The fever of a qi level pathogen can be very high but generally responds quickly to treatment.

Progression
- A pathogen heading deeper is potentially dangerous.

ficiently to cause fever.

DIFFERENTIATING FEVER TYPES

Types of fever

A variety of distinct fever types are recognized in Chinese medicine. Acute fevers of short duration as discussed in this chapter tend to be relatively high and objective (a thermometer will register an elevated body temperature). Chronic fevers tend to be low grade, may be subjective (body temperature only mildly elevated, normal or even low), and are analyzed in the chapter on chronic fever, p.364).

Simultaneous fever and chills

This is an objective fever, as measured by an independent hand or thermometer, while the patient feels cold, has goose bumps or shivers. It is caused by an external wei or tai yang pathogen. This type of fever pattern is caused by the struggle between a pathogen, usually wind cold or wind heat, and a robust wei qi. The cold on the surface causes the chills, while the heat of battle between the pathogen and the wei qi generates the fever. This type of fever is differentiated in Acute exterior disorders (Clinical Handbook Vol.1).

Fever without chills

Fever without chills is a continuous fever with no chill or aversion to cold. It is experienced when a pathogen has broached the surface defenses of the body and entered the interior – the qi level, yangming, ying or blood. The battle at this point is usually fierce and this is reflected in the vigorous nature of the fever. These are the fevers differentiated in this chapter.

Alternating fever and chills

Distinct episodes of fever followed by chills or shivering in a sequential pattern. Depending on the actual pathology and duration of the illness, this fever pattern can be quite dramatic or rather subtle. In acute cases, and in those with strong pathogens and robust anti–pathogenic qi, patients may flush, sweat and remove layers of clothing, then a few minutes later replace them as they start to shiver. When chronic, and in those with a degree of underlying deficiency, the fever and chill episodes can be somewhat muted, appearing sporadically when the patient is run down. Regardless of the intensity of the manifestation, the location of the pathogen is in the shaoyang level, in–between the surface and the deeper yin levels of the body. The alternating nature of the fever pattern reflects the changing fortunes of the pathogen and the anti–pathogenic qi. As the pathogen moves further into the interior of the body, the yangming or qi level, the fever builds. As the anti–pathogenic qi responds and pushes the pathogen back out towards the surface, wei qi is recruited and diverted away from warming the surface, and chills ensue.

Low grade fever

Low grade fever is seen predominantly in cases that continue for more than two weeks, and is the characteristic chronic fever pattern. Low grade fevers are described on p.367.

TREATMENT

The Chinese medical treatment of acute fevers can be effective, but intervention needs to be frequent and vigorous. The main aim of treatment, other than clearing heat, is prevention of possible complications, such as damage to yin and fluids, and the creation of a lingering pathogen.

Acupuncture is valuable and effective for acute fever, but usually needs to be applied frequently. Ideally, one or two treatments are given daily. If this is possible, the effect is likely to be quick, and the condition resolved in a few days.

With herbs, a dose taken every couple of hours or so is best. Decoctions are generally recommended for their swift action and flexibility. Concentrated powders are effective, but the recommended daily dose should be increased by 30–50%. It is essential to keep a careful eye on the progress of patients with acute fever because the situation can change quickly, and treatment must be adapted. Patients should be counselled to take sufficient fluids to maintain hydration. A good rule of thumb to determine adequate hydration is the clarity of the urine.

Medications

Antibiotics

Antibiotics kill bacteria or inhibit their replication. They are cold in nature, and

Figure 7.1 Common patterns of acute fever

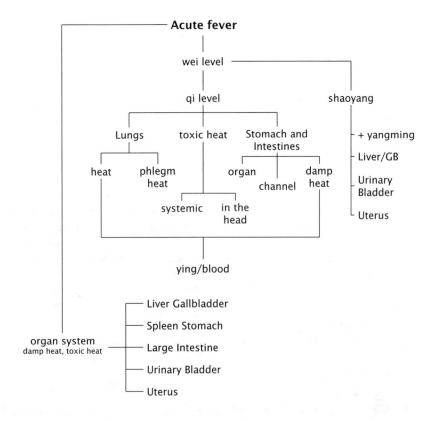

can in some circumstances damage Spleen yang, leading to damp accumulation. When used appropriately, they are well tolerated and a valuable tool, quickly reducing heat and preventing damage to yin. They have no ability to disperse and clear away any residue remaining after the heat has abated, and in certain circumstances this can cause problems. Practitioners will be familiar with patients who are prescribed course after course of antibiotics, only to have the initial problem recur once a course is completed. Repeated use of antibiotics, especially when inappropriate, weakens the Spleen and digestive function, alters gut flora and impacts on the immune response.

Antipyretics

Aspirin, paracetamol, ibuprofen, acetaminophen (Panadol, Tylenol) and other non steroidal anti–inflammatory (NSAID) drugs are commonly used to allay a fever. This can be helpful when the fever is very high and the patient in pain or distress. In mild fevers the use of these drugs is not recommended as they can inhibit the body's attempts to throw off the pathogen.

7.1 WEI LEVEL

7.1.1 WIND HEAT

风
热
袭
表

Wind heat is a common presentation of acute fever, sore throat and cough, and tends to occur in clusters during the warmer months, although it may appear at any time of the year.

Wind heat enters the body through the nose and mouth. Wind and heat are both yang pathogens, so symptoms are concentrated in the upper body. The heat aspect rises upwards affecting the head, throat and chest, and dries fluids and yin, leading to thickened, colored secretions. A severe wind heat invasion may interact with pre–existing damp or damp heat and intensify into toxic heat (7.4, p.332) or toxic wind damp heat (7.5, p.335).

Clinical features

- Acute fever of 1–4 days duration which may be mild or moderate; may be mild chills (in practice often absent), aversion to wind and changes of temperature.
- sore, dry or scratchy throat, often the first symptom noted by the patient
- headache, usually frontal
- dry mouth and throat, mild thirst
- sweating
- cough with hard to expectorate, thick or sticky, yellow sputum
- nasal obstruction, or a nasal discharge which is thick and yellow or green
- mild cervical lymphadenopathy

T normal or red tipped with a thin, yellow coat
P floating and slightly rapid

Treatment principle

Dispel and vent wind heat from the surface

Prescription

YIN QIAO SAN 银翘散
Honeysuckle and Forsythia Powder

jin yin hua (Lonicerae Flos) 金银花	12–18g
lian qiao (Forsythia Fructus) 连翘	9–12g
lu gen (Phragmitis Rhizoma) 芦根	15–30g
dan zhu ye (Lophateri Herba) 淡竹叶	9–12g
niu bang zi (Arctii Fructus) 牛蒡子	9–12g
jing jie (Schizonepetae Herba) 荆芥	9–12g
jie geng (Platycodi Radix) 桔梗	6–9g
dan dou chi (Sojae Semen preparatum) 淡豆豉	6–9g
bo he (Menthae haplocalycis Herba) 薄荷	3–6g
gan cao (Glycyrrhizae Radix) 甘草	3–6g

Method: Decoction, powder or pills. When decocted, the herbs should be simmered for no longer than 20 minutes and **bo he** is added at the end of cooking. Take cool or at room temperature. **Jin yin hua** and **lian qiao** vent wind heat from the exterior and resolve toxic heat; **niu bang zi** dispels wind heat and with **gan cao**, cools and eases the sore throat; **bo he** and **dan dou chi** dispel wind heat; **jing jie** disperses wind without drying; **jie geng** transforms phlegm, stops cough and eases the throat; **dan zhu ye** and **lu gen** clear heat, and, with **gan cao**, generate fluids and stop thirst. (Source: *Shi Yong Zhong Yao Xue [Wen Bing Tiao Bian]*)

Modifications

- With a red, sore, swollen throat, add **shan dou gen** (Sophorae tonkinensis Radix) 山豆根 18g and **da qing ye** (Isatidis Folium) 大青叶 30g.
- With a ticklish, itchy or scratchy throat, add **chan tui** (Cicadae Periostracum) 蝉蜕 9–12g.
- With stiff neck and occipital headache, add **ge gen** (Puerariae Radix) 葛根 9–12g.
- With nasal congestion, add **cang er zi** (Xanthii Fructus) 苍耳子 6–9g.
- With headache, add **sang ye** (Mori Folium) 桑叶 9–12g, **ju hua** (Chrysanthemi Flos) 菊花 12–15g and **man jing zi** (Viticis Fructus) 蔓荆子 9–12g.
- With cough, add **qian hu** (Peucedani Radix) 前胡 9–12g, **chuan bei mu** (Fritillariae cirrhosae Bulbus) 川贝母 9–12g and **quan gua lou** (Trichosanthis Fructus) 栝楼仁 12–18g.
- With thick, sticky, yellow sputum, add **yu xing cao** (Houttuyniae Herba) 鱼腥草 18–24g, **zhe bei mu** (Fritillariae thunbergii Bulbus) 浙贝母 9–12g and **gua lou ren** (Trichosanthis Semen) 栝楼仁 9–12g.
- With epistaxis, add **bai mao gen** (Imperatae Rhizoma) 白茅根 30g and **ou jie** (Nelumbinis Nodus rhizomatis) 藕节 9–12g.

Prepared medicines

Concentrated powder

Yin Qiao San (Lonicera & Forsythia Formula)

Pills

Yin Qiao Jie Du Pian (Yin Chiao Chieh Tu Pien)
Gan Mao Ling (Miraculous Common Cold Pills)
Ban Lan Gen Chong Ji (Isatidis Granules)

Acupuncture (select from)

Du.14 (dazhui – Ω) ....meeting point of the yang channels, clears wind and heat from the exterior
LI.11 (quchi –)...................sea point of the Large Intestine, dispels wind heat
Bl.12 (fengmen – Ω) ....dispels wind heat from the exterior
GB.20 (fengchi –) ....dispels wind heat from the exterior, clears the nose and alleviates headache
Bl.13 (feishu – Ω) ....transport point of the Lungs, diffuses the Lungs and directs Lung qi downward
LI.4 (hegu –) ....dispels wind heat (with SJ.5 [waiguan]), diffuses the Lungs and stops pain
SJ.5 (waiguan –) ....connecting point of the triple burner, dispels wind heat
Lu.10 (yuji).......................fire point of the Lungs, clears heat from the Lungs and eases the throat

- with sore throat, add Lu.11 (shaoshang ↓) and SI.17 (tianrong –)
- with cough add Lu.5 (chize –)
- Ear points: lung, large intestine, tonsils, ear apex ↓, zero point
- Light guasha (p.426) along the Urinary Bladder channel until the area becomes red is helpful, especially in children.

Clinical notes

- Wind heat in the wei level is a common pattern of acute fever that responds well to timely treatment. It may be diagnosed as the common cold, tonsillitis, viral infection, upper respiratory tract infection, acute bronchitis, and the early stage of measles, encephalitis or meningitis. While usually self limiting, treatment is recommended for vulnerable individuals and those prone to Lung heat, so as to prevent the deeper penetration of the pathogen.
- Acupuncture can be applied twice daily in severe cases. When treated early enough (within a day or two of onset) results should be swift.
- The patient should be advised to stay warm and well covered, especially the neck, even though there is fever.

7.2 QI LEVEL HEAT

1. Lung heat
2. Yangming syndrome
3. Yangming organ syndrome
4. Damp heat
5. Summerheat

The qi level lies between the surface and the deep internal organs. It is in the qi level that the body mounts its most robust defense against invading pathogens. The fever of acute qi level pathogenic invasion is intense, reflecting to heat of battle. In terms of depth, the qi level corresponds primarily to the more superficial and exposed organ systems, the Lungs, Spleen, Stomach and Intestines. Qi level pathology reflects the presence of a heat pathogen in these organs systems and related tissues, so in addition to the fever, respiratory, gastrointestinal, skin and muscle symptoms are seen.

肺
热
发
热

7.2.1 LUNG HEAT

Lung heat is a common type of fever that follows some days after an unresolved or improperly treated wei level wind heat pattern. It can also follow a wind cold pathogen that turns hot once in the Lungs.

Clinical features
- continuous fever that may be quite high, with or without sweating
- loud dry, unproductive cough; if there is a small amount of sputum, it is sticky and hard to expectorate and may be blood streaked
- dyspnea and wheezing
- maybe night sweats
- chest oppression and pain
- sensation of heat in the chest
- dry mouth and thirst
- swollen tender lymph nodes

T red or with a red tip and a dry, yellow coat
P surging and rapid, or wiry and rapid

Treatment principle
Clear heat from the Lungs
Diffuse the Lungs and direct Lung qi downwards
Stop cough and wheezing

Prescription

MA XING SHI GAN TANG 麻杏石甘汤
Ephedra, Apricot Kernel, Gypsum and Licorice Decoction

zhi ma huang (honey fried Ephedra Herba) 炙麻黄 6–9g
xing ren (Armeniacae Semen) 杏仁 9–12g
shi gao (Gypsum fibrosum) 石膏 15–30g

zhi gan cao (Glycyrrhizae Radix preparata) 炙甘草 3–6g

Method: Decoction. **Shi gao** is decocted for 30–60 minutes prior to the other herbs. **Zhi ma huang** directs Lung qi downwards, stops cough and alleviates wheezing–its pungent warmth is balanced by the pungent cold **shi gao**; **xing ren** directs Lung qi downwards and stops cough; **shi gao** vents and clears heat from the Lungs; **zhi gan cao** protects the Stomach and prolongs the action of the other herbs. (Source: *Zhong Yi Nei Ke Xue [Shang Han Lun]*)

Modifications

- Keeping the bowels moving is an essential component of treatment. Free moving Large Intestine qi enables the Lung qi to descend, and an open bowel is an important escape route for heat. With constipation or sluggish bowels, add **da huang** (Rhei Radix et Rhizoma) 大黄 3–9g. See also Variations.

- When severe, the basic prescription can be augmented with additional Lung cooling herbs, such as **yu xing cao** (Houttuyniae Herba) 鱼腥草 18–24g, **huang qin** (Scutellariae Radix) 黄芩 9–12g, **jin yin hua** (Lonicera Flos) 金银花 12–18g, **zhi sang bai pi** (honey fried Mori Cortex) 炙桑白皮 9–12g and **zhi mu** (Anemarrhenae Rhizoma) 知母 9–12g.

- With residual surface pathogen and no sweating, use unprocessed **ma huang** (Ephedra Herba) 麻黄, and add **jing jie** (Schizonepetae Herba) 荆芥 9–12g, **bo he** (Menthae haplocalycis Herba) 薄荷 3–6g, **dan dou chi** (Sojae Semen preparatum) 淡豆豉 6–9g and **niu bang zi** (Arctii Fructus) 牛蒡子 6–9g.

- With copious sweating and thirst, use **shi gao** (Gypsum fibrosum) 石膏 at the upper end of the dosage range and add **tian hua fen** (Trichosanthis Radix) 天花粉 9–12g.

- With severe cough, add **zhi pi pa ye** (honey fried Eriobotryae Folium) 炙枇杷叶 9–12g.

- With hemoptysis or blood streaked sputum, add **qian cao tan** (charred Rubiae Radix) 茜草炭 9–12g, **bai mao gen** (Imperatae Rhizoma) 白茅根 9–15g and **ce bai ye tan** (charred Platycladi Cacumen) 侧柏叶炭 12–15g.

- With sore throat, add **she gan** (Belamcandae Rhizoma) 射干 9–12g and **xuan shen** (Scrophulariae Radix) 玄参 15–18g.

Variations and additional prescriptions

Lung heat with constipation

Constipation is a common complication of Lung heat due to the Lung / Large Intestine connection. The blockage of Lung qi by a pathogen impedes the downwards movement of Large Intestine qi, and the heat dries the surface tissues of the Large Intestine. When constipation occurs, it further blocks descent of Lung qi, aggravates the heat and increases the fever. The treatment is to clear heat from the Lungs and open the bowel with XUAN BAI CHENG QI TANG (Diffuse the White [Lungs] and Order the Qi Decoction 宣白承气汤).

shi gao (Gypsum fibrosum) 石膏 30–60g

quan gua lou (Trichosanthis Fructus) 全栝楼 18–30g

da huang (Rhei Radix et Rhizoma) 大黄 6–9g

xing ren (Armeniacae Semen) 杏仁 9–12g

Method: Decoction. **Shi gao** is decocted for 30–60 minutes prior to the other herbs; **da huang** is added towards the end of cooking. **Shi gao** vents and clears heat from the Lungs; **quan gua lou** cools the Lungs and clears Phlegm heat, and with **xing ren**, diffuses the Lungs, directs Lung qi downward and moistens the Intestines; **da huang** purges heat and stimulates peristalsis to open the bowels. (Source: *Zhong Yi Nei Ke Xue* [*Wen Bing Tiao Bian*])

Phlegm heat

Phlegm heat can develop when a patient with pre–existing phlegm is invaded by a heat pathogen. It can also develop when there is a blockage of the Lungs diffusion and the descent of fluids by the pathogen. In both cases, a dry hacking cough becomes more productive over the course of a few days as the phlegm accumulates. Initially the phlegm tends to be thick, sticky and hard to expectorate, gradually loosening as the heat subsides. When phlegm heat is significant, the treatment focuses on clearing phlegm heat with QING QI HUA TAN TANG (Clear the Qi and Transform Phlegm Decoction 清气化痰汤).

gua lou (Trichosanthis Fructus) 栝楼 30–45g
huang qin (Scutellariae Radix) 黄芩 9–12g
chen pi (Citri reticulatae Pericarpium) 陈皮 6–9g
zhi shi (Aurantii Fructus immaturus) 枳实 9–12g
xing ren (Armeniacae Semen) 杏仁 9–12g
fu ling (Poria) 茯苓 9–12g
dan nan xing (Arisaema cum Bile) 胆南星 6–9g
zhi ban xia (Pinelliae Rhizoma preparatum) 制半夏 6–9g

Method: Concentrated powder is the best format as **dan nan xing** is particularly unpleasant when decocted. **Dan nan xing** clears heat, transforms phlegm heat and unbinds the chest; **gua luo** transforms phlegm heat and unbinds the chest; **huang qin** clears heat from the Lungs; **chen pi** and **zhi shi** regulate qi and assist in mobilizing sticky phlegm; **xing ren** diffuses the Lungs and directs Lung qi downward; **zhi ban xia** transforms phlegm; **fu ling** strengthens the Spleen, leaches out damp and assists **xing ren** in maintaining free flow in the water passages, to facilitate dispersal of the phlegm. (Source: *Yi Fang Kao*)

Prepared medicines

Concentrated powder

Ma Xing Shi Gan Tang (Ephedra & Apricot Seed Combination)
Qing Qi Hua Tang Wan (Pinellia & Scute Formula)
  – with copious sputum
Chai Xian Tang (Bupleurum & Scute Combination)
  – with alternating fever and chills

Pills

Qing Fei Yi Huo Pian (Ching Fei Yi Huo Pien)
Chuan Xin Lian Kang Yan Pian (Chuan Xin Lian Antiphlogistic Tablets)
Niu Huang Qing Huo Wan (Cattle Gallstone Pills to Clear Fire)
  – Lung fire
Qing Qi Hua Tan Wan (Clean Air Teapills, Pinellia Expectorant Pills)

Acupuncture (select from)

Lu.5 (chize) ....sea point of the Lungs, clears Lung heat and directs Lung qi down to stop cough and bleeding
Lu.6 (kongzui) ....cleft point of the Lungs, clears Lung heat, directs Lung qi down, stops pain and bleeding

Lu.10 (yuji).......................brook and fire point of the Lungs, clears heat from the Lungs and benefits the throat

Bl.13 (feishu –Ω) ....transport point of the Lungs, diffuses the Lungs and directs Lung qi downwards, clears heat

Lu.1 (zhongfu)..................alarm point of the Lungs, clears heat from the Lungs

Ren.17 (shanzhong –) ....opens and promotes correct movement of qi in the chest, directs Lung qi downwards to stop cough

LI.4 (hegu –).....................source point of the Large Intestine, clears heat, stops pain and diffuses the Lungs

Du.14 (dazhui –Ω) ....clears heat

- with marked heat, add Du.12 (shenzhu –) and Du.10 (lingtai –)
- Ear points: ear apex ↓, lung, large intestine, tonsils, zero point

Clinical notes
- Lung heat type fever may be diagnosed as upper respiratory tract infection, pneumonia, bronchitis or tracheitis.
- This pattern responds reliably to correct treatment, and patients should be feeling significantly better within a few days. Make sure the patient is adequately hydrated, see clinical notes, p.328.

阳
明
经
证

7.2.2 YANGMING CHANNEL SYNDROME (without constipation)

This pattern is classically attributed to the progress of a cold pathogen through the superficial layers into the interior of the body, where, confronted by strong resistance from anti–pathogenic qi, it transforms from cold to heat. Yangming channel syndrome is so called because at this stage of the invasion, the heat is 'formless', and the yangming organs, the Stomach and Large Intestine, are not yet obstructed by constipation. The main features of yangming channel syndrome reflect the intensity of the struggle between a strong pathogen and the anti–pathogenic qi of a robust patient. These are the 'four bigs' (*sì dà* 四大) – high fever, great thirst, copious sweating and a surging, rapid pulse.

Even though the four 'bigs' are considered a prerequisite for the use of the following prescription, they may not all be present in every patient. For example, in some cases fluids may be damaged by the heat, so there is no sweating. As long as there is severe heat in yangming without constipation, the prescription is applicable.

Clinical features
- acute high fever
- profuse sweating, or no sweating and hot dry skin
- great thirst for cold fluids
- irritability
- red complexion
- frontal headache
- toothache, bleeding gums, oral ulceration
- swollen tender lymph nodes

T dry, yellow tongue coat
P surging and rapid

Treatment principle
Clear and vent heat from yangming
Generate fluids and protect the Stomach

Prescription

BAI HU TANG 白虎汤
White Tiger Decoction

---

shi gao (Gypsum fibrosum) 石膏 30–90g
zhi mu (Anemarrhenae Rhizoma) 知母 9–15g
jing mi (Oryzae Semen) 粳米... 15–30g
gan cao (Glycyrrhizae Radix) 甘草 3–6g
Method: Decoction. **Shi gao** is broken into small pieces and cooked for 30 minutes in 300–400ml of water. Add the other herbs, including the rice, and boil until the rice is cooked. Strain off the dregs and divide the remaining liquid into two doses (around 150ml each dose). Take one dose twice daily. In severe cases, two packets of herbs can be used per day, in four doses. When used correctly only a few doses should be necessary. If the condition is unchanged after 2–3 days, stop treatment and reassess the diagnosis. **Shi gao**, clears heat from the Lungs, Stomach and Intestines, generates fluids and alleviates thirst; **zhi mu** clears heat and protects yin; **gan cao** and **jing mi** protect the Stomach. (Source: *Zhong Yi Nei Ke Xue* [*Shang Han Lun*])

Modifications
- With severe heat or toxic heat, add **jin yin hua** (Lonicera Flos) 金银花 15–30g, **lian qiao** (Forsythia Fructus) 连翘 9–12g, **ban lan gen** (Isatidis/Baphicacanthis Radix) 板蓝根 15–30g, and **da qing ye** (Isatidis Folium) 大青叶 15–30g.
- With marked fluid damage, add **yu zhu** (Polygonati odorati Rhizoma) 玉竹 12–15g, **tian hua fen** (Trichosanthes Radix) 天花粉 9–12g and **lu gen** (Phragmitis Rhizoma) 芦根 30–60g.
- With disorientation, irritability and restlessness, add **huang lian** (Coptidis Rhizoma) 黄连 3–6g, **huang qin** (Scutellariae Radix) 黄芩 9–12g, **huang bai** (Phellodendri Cortex) 黄柏 9–12g and **shan zhi zi** (Gardeniae Fructus) 山栀子 9–12g.
- With red eyes and headache, add **huang lian** (Coptidis Rhizoma) 黄连 3–6g and **huang qin** (Scutellariae Radix) 黄芩 9–12g.

Prepared medicines
Concentrated powder
Bai Hu Tang (Gypsum Combination)
Bai Hu Jia Ren Shen Tang (Ginseng & Gypsum Combination)
    – with fluid damage

Pills
Bai Hu Tang Wan (White Tiger Teapills)

Acupuncture (select from)
Du.14 (dazhui –)................meeting point of the yang channels, clears heat and
                    drains fire

LI.11 (quchi –)....................these points clear heat from yangming
St.44 (neiting –)
LI.4 (hegu –)
- with severe heat, bleed the finger tips
- Ear points: ear apex ↓, lungs, stomach, large intestine, zero point

Clinical notes
- Yangming channel syndrome may be diagnosed as the apogee of an acute infection such as influenza, encephalitis, meningitis, measles or lobar pneumonia.
- Fluids can be significantly damaged in this pattern, so make sure the patient is adequately hydrated. See clinical notes, p.328.

7.2.3 YANGMING ORGAN SYNDROME (with constipation)

阳
明
腑
证

Yangming organ syndrome is a complication of yangming channel syndrome. The two patterns appear similar but should be carefully differentiated, as the treatment strategy is quite different. In the organ syndrome, heat has dried out the Intestines and the stools, leading to constipation. On rare occasions, patients may have watery diarrhea (spurious diarrhea), where Intestinal fluids are forced around an impacted stool. The obstructed stool increases the heat, and is an impediment to clearing the heat, so the priority of treatment is to clear the constipated stool, and with it, the heat.

Clinical features
- fever which may be tidal or high and continuous
- constipation with abdominal pain, fullness and distension that is worse for pressure; a hard mass will be palpable in the left iliac fossa; occasionally watery diarrhea may occur, but a fecal mass will still be palpable
- dry mouth, thirst
- restlessness, irritability
- sweating, either whole body or hands and feet
- concentrated urine
- swollen tender lymph nodes

T red or with red spots and a greasy or dry, brown or yellow coat
P strong, surging, rapid, slippery, or deep and strong

Treatment principle
Open the bowel to purge and clear heat

Prescription

DA CHENG QI TANG 大承气汤
Major Order the Qi Decoction

da huang (Rhei Radix et Rhizoma) 大黄..9–12g
mang xiao (Natrii Sulphas) 芒硝..6–9g
zhi shi (Aurantii Fructus immaturus) 枳实...9–12g
hou po (Magnoliae officinalis Cortex) 厚朴 12–15g
Method: Decoction. **Da huang** is added a few minutes before the end of cooking, and **mang xiao**

is dissolved in the strained decoction. **Da huang** purges accumulation and heat from the Intestines; **mang xiao** softens hard dry stools, easing their passage; **zhi shi** and **hou po** regulate qi and direct it downwards, and alleviate the cramps that **da huang** can sometimes cause. (Source: *Shang Han Lun*)

Modifications
- With marked dryness and fluid damage, add **sheng di** (Rehmanniae Radix) 生地 12–15g, **xuan shen** (Scrophulariae Radix) 玄参 12–15g and **mai dong** (Ophiopogonis Radix) 麦冬 9–12g.
- With high fever, a burning sensation in the chest and mouth ulcers, add **shan zhi zi** (Gardeniae Fructus) 山栀子 9–12g, **lian qiao** (Forsythiae Fructus) 连翘 9–12g, **dan zhu ye** (Lophatheri Herba) 淡竹叶 6–9g and **huang bai** (Phellodendri Cortex) 黄柏 9–12g.

Prepared medicines
Concentrated powder
Da Cheng Qi Tang (Major Rhubarb Combination)
Pills
Liang Ge Wan (Cool Valley Teapills)
Qing Fei Yi Huo Pian (Ching Fei Yi Huo Pien)
Niu Huang Qing Huo Wan (Cattle Gallstone Pills to Clear Fire)

Acupuncture (select from)
LI.11 (quchi –)...................these points clear heat from yangming
LI.4 (hegu –)
St.44 (neiting –)
SJ.6 (zhigou –) ....fire point of the Triple Burner, opens the Intestines and disperses obstruction
St.25 (tianshu –).................alarm point of the Large Intestine, regulates Intestinal function and clears heat
St.37 (shangjuxu –) ....lower sea point of the Large Intestine, clears heat and stagnation from yangming
St.39 (xiajuxu –).................lower sea point of the Small Intestine, clears heat and stagnation from yangming
Bl.25 (dachangshu –) ....transport point of the Large Intestine, opens the bowels and clears heat
- with abdominal pain, add St.34 (liangqiu –)
- Ear points: ear apex ↓, lungs, large intestine, zero point, shenmen

Clinical notes
- Yangming organ syndrome may be diagnosed as influenza, encephalitis, meningitis, bacterial dysentery, acute hepatitis, cholecystitis, pancreatitis or lobar pneumonia.
- Fluids can be significantly damaged in this pattern, so make sure the patient is adequately hydrated. See clinical notes, p.328.
- Once the bowels are moving, the heat will usually subside. If the bowels are moving but the heat persists, this is usually due to fluid and yin damage. A prescription that vents heat and supplements qi and fluids, such as ZHU YE SHI

GAO TANG (Lophatherus and Gypsum Decoction 竹叶石膏汤 p.370), can be used to clear the remnant heat.

湿
热
在
气
分

7.2.4 DAMP HEAT

Damp heat invades the qi level most commonly during hot humid weather and is a common pattern in hot humid tropical and subtropical climates. Damp heat, with the yin heaviness of damp, sinks deep into the qi level and primarily influences the Spleen and its associated tissues, especially the muscles.

Clinical features
- acute fever, persistent during the day but worse in the afternoon and early evening
- no sweating, or a sticky oozing sweat that fails to break the fever
- muscle aches, usually the large proximal muscles of the limbs
- heaviness and lethargy; headache or heavy head, like 'being wrapped in a damp towel'
- abdominal distension
- foul diarrhea, or sluggish stools
- nausea and vomiting; loss of appetite
- chest oppression
- scanty, concentrated or cloudy urine
- sore, swollen throat; dry mouth and throat
- swollen tender lymph nodes

T thick, dry or greasy, yellow tongue coat
P slippery, rapid pulse

Treatment principle
Clear damp heat from the qi level
Promote urination to provide an outlet for the damp heat

Prescription

GAN LU XIAO DU DAN 甘露消毒丹
Sweet Dew Special Pill to Eliminate Toxin

hua shi (Talcum) 滑石 18–21g
yin chen (Artemisiae scopariae Herba) 茵陈 24–30g
lian qiao (Forsythiae Fructus) 连翘 12–15g
huang qin (Scutellariae Radix) 黄芩 12–15g
mu tong (Akebiae Caulis) 木通 9–12g
huo xiang (Pogostemonis/Agastaches Herba) 藿香 9–12g
she gan (Belamcandae Rhizoma) 射干 9–12g
shi chang pu (Acori tatarinowii Rhizoma) 石菖蒲 6–9g
chuan bei mu (Fritillariae cirrhosae Bulbus) 川贝母 6–9g
bo he (Mentha haplocalycis Herba) 薄荷 6–9g
bai dou kou (Amomi Fructus rotundus) 白豆蔻 6–9g

Method: Decoction. The herbs should be simmered for no longer than 20 minutes. **Bo he** and **bai dou kou** are added at the end of cooking. Take cool or at room temperature. **Yin chen, mu tong** and **hua shi** clear damp heat by promoting urination; **huang qin**, **lian qiao** and **bo he** clear heat from the upper body; **she gan** and **chuan bei mu** clear heat from the Lungs; **bai dou kou**, **shi chang pu** and **huo xiang** fragrantly transform damp. (Source: *Shi Yong Zhong Yi Nei Ke Xue* [*Wen Re Jing Wei*])

Modifications

- With high fever, jaundice, and constipation, delete **bai dou kou** and add **shi gao** (Gypsum fibrosum) 石膏 15–30g, **da huang** (Rhei Radix et Rhizoma) 大黄 6–9g, **shan zhi zi** (Gardeniae Fructus) 山栀子 9–12g and **bai mao gen** (Imperatae Rhizoma) 白茅根 15–30g.
- With severe nausea and vomiting, add **chen pi** (Citri reticulatae Pericarpium) 陈皮 6–9g, **zhi ban xia** (Pinelliae Rhizoma preparatum) 制半夏 9–12g and **zhu ru** (Bambusae Caulis in taeniam) 竹茹 9–12g.

Prepared medicines

Concentrated powder
Gan Lu Xiao Du Dan (Forsythia & Acorus Formula)

Acupuncture (select from)

Du.14 (dazhui –)................meeting point of the yang channels, clears heat
LI.11 (quchi –)...................clears damp heat and alleviates fever
Lu.6 (kongzui) ....cleft point of the Lungs, diffuses the Lungs and directs Lung qi downwards to regulate the water passages, promote urination and clear damp heat
Sp.9 (yinlingquan –)...........water and metal points of the Spleen, these points
Sp.5 (shangqiu –)   promote urination and clear damp heat
SJ.6 (zhigou –) ....fire point of the Triple Burner, promotes elimination of damp and heat through the bowel
SI.4 (wangu –) ....source point of the Small Intestine, clears damp heat
Ren.5 (shimen –)................alarm point of the triple burner, clears damp heat
Ren.12 (zhongwan –).........alarm point of the Stomach, activates the qi dynamic
- with nausea add PC.6 (neiguan)
- with diarrhea add zhixie (N–CA–3) and Bl.25 (tianshu)
- with myalgia add Sp.21 (dabao)
- Ear points: ear apex ↓, spleen, stomach, zero point, shenmen

Clinical notes

- Damp heat in the qi level acute fever may be diagnosed as acute gastroenteritis, summer flu, early stage of chicken pox, typhoid fever, acute icteric hepatitis, cholecystitis and cholangitis or leptospirosis.
- This pattern generally responds well to early treatment, but has a tendency to drag on or become recurrent if neglected. Continuing treatment for a week or so after the symptoms have cleared is recommended to ensure all damp is eliminated.

暑热 7.2.5 SUMMERHEAT

Summerheat is an acute disorder that occurs during hot weather. There are two main variations. The first is associated with prolonged exposure to direct sun or a very hot environment, and is a type of heatstroke. The body is unable to cool itself sufficiently and overheats, producing an elevated body temperature and dehydration. The second type is due to an invasion of a summerheat pathogen. This is similar to a damp heat invasion, with the heat component considerably stronger, but still with an element of dampness that blocks the qi dynamic and urinary flow. The pattern described here is the second type.

Clinical features
- acute, high, unrelenting fever
- pounding frontal headache
- red complexion
- profuse sweating initially, then less as the patient becomes dehydrated
- hot, dry, flushed skin
- thirst and dry throat
- scanty clear urine, or concentrated urine
- may be vomiting and explosive, foul, burning diarrhoea
- irritability
- vesicular, itchy skin lesions
- swollen tender lymph nodes

T dry, yellow or patchy tongue coat
P rapid and strong, or rapid and fine

Treatment principle
Expel summerheat, clear heat and damp

Prescription

GUI LING GAN LU YIN 桂苓甘露饮
Cinnamon and Poria Sweet Dew Decoction

hua shi (Talcum) 滑石	15–30g
han shui shi (Glauberitum) 寒水石	15–30g
shi gao (Gypsum fibrosum) 石膏	15–30g
fu ling (Poria) 茯苓	6–15g
ze xie (Alismatis Rhizoma) 泽泻	6–15g
zhu ling (Polyporus) 猪苓	6–15g
bai zhu (Atractylodes macrocephalae Rhizoma) 白术	6–12g
gan cao (Glycyrrhizae Radix) 甘草	3–9g
rou gui (Cinnamomi Cortex) 肉桂	2–3g

Method: Decoction. **Shi gao** and **han shui shi** are decocted for 30 minutes prior to the other herbs. **Hua shi** leads heat out through the urine; **shi gao** and **han shui shi** are sweet and cold, and the large doses clear heat from the qi level while preserving fluids; **fu ling**, **ze xie**, **zhu ling**, **bai zhu** and **rou gui** encourage transformation of qi and fluids and keep the urinary passages open to facilitate elimination of the pathogen; the warmth of **rou gui** moderates the coldness of the mineral substances; **bai zhu**, **fu ling** and **gan cao** strengthen the Spleen; **gan cao** clears heat and protects the Stomach, and with **hua shi** clears damp heat and summerheat. (Source: *Xuan Ming Lun Fang*)

Modifications

- With marked dryness and dark urine, reduce the dose of **ze xie** and **zhu ling** to 3 grams, and use **fu ling** and **bai zhu** at the low end of the dosage range.
- With vesicular skin lesions, add **tu fu ling** (Smilacis glabrae Rhizoma) 土茯苓 12–15g.

Prepared medicines

Concentrated powder

Bai Hu Jia Ren Shen Tang (Ginseng & Gypsum Combination)

Qing Shu Yi Qi Tang (Astragalus & Atractylodes Combination)
  – this formula is recommended in the latter stages of a summerheat invasion when the qi and fluids have been damaged

Acupuncture (select from)

Du.14 (dazhui –)................these points clear heat and dispel external pathogens
LI.11 (quchi –)   from the surface and yangming
LI.4 (hegu –)
SJ.5 (waiguan –).................connecting point of the triple burner, clears heat and facilitates qi flow through the triple burner
PC.3 (quze ↓).....................sea point of the Pericardium and Urinary Bladder
Bl.40 (weizhong ↓)   respectively, these points cool the blood and clear heat; useful for heatstroke as well
Kid.6 (zhaohai +) ....to replenish fluids
- Ear points: ear apex ↓, lungs, large intestine, zero point

Clinical notes

- Summerheat fever may be diagnosed as acute gastroenteritis, food poisoning, gastric flu, influenza, acute colitis or heatstroke.
- When heat exposure is the cause of the fever, ice packs at critical points such as the axillae, neck and groin can help cool the patient quickly.
- Acute summerheat patterns respond well to early treatment, but have a tendency to drag on or become recurrent if neglected.
- Fluid and electrolyte replacement is important, as dehydration is likely to occur. This is especially so in infants and young children, who can become dangerously dehydrated quite quickly. Oral isotonic fluid replacement solution should be administered in small amounts frequently. Isotonic solution can be made by adding 3.5 grams of household salt (NaCl), 2.5 grams of sodium bicarbonate, 1.5 grams of potassium chloride (KCl) and 20 grams of sugar to one liter of water. Isotonic drinks are commercially available. Alternatively use lemonade with a teaspoon of salt.

少
阳
证

7.3 SHAOYANG SYNDROME

Pathogenic invasion into the shaoyang level can lead to both acute fever and a more lingering pattern. When acute, it follows an external wei level surface disorder. Penetration into the shaoyang level can happen quite quickly, a day or so, if the pathogen is strong or the patient is weak or postpartum. It may develop over the course of a week or so if the external pathogen is unresolved, ignored and poorly treated or if the patient soldiers on through the illness or attempts to 'sweat or purge it out'.

Shaoyang type fever patterns can also appear when heat or damp heat affects specific organ systems, especially the Liver, Gallbladder and Urinary Bladder. These are dealt with under those headings. The presentation here is not organ specific, but may appear in the early stage of infections such as acute mastitis, acute otitis and acute atypical upper respiratory tract infections.

Clinical features
• Acute alternating fever and chills; with the fever and chill episodes quite distinct. In illness of relatively short duration, the fever pattern may be so prominent that the patient flushes, sweats and removes clothing, then begins to shiver and replace it in quick succession.
• reduced appetite or anorexia
• bitter taste in the mouth; food tastes bad
• nausea, vomiting; heartburn
• hypochondriac pain, distension or tenderness
• chest oppression; difficulty getting a deep breath
• dizziness
• irritability
• swollen lymph nodes
T normal or slightly red and coated on the left side, or red on the edges
P wiry

Treatment principle
Harmonize shaoyang

Prescription
XIAO CHAI HU TANG 小柴胡汤
Minor Bupleurum Decoction

chai hu (Bupleuri Radix) 柴胡 9–15g
huang qin (Scutellariae Radix) 黄芩 9–12g
zhi ban xia (Pinelliae Rhizoma preparatum) 制半夏 6–9g
ren shen (Ginseng Radix) 人参 6–9g
zhi gan cao (Glycyrrhizae Radix preparata) 炙甘草 3–6g
sheng jiang (Zingiberis Rhizoma recens) 生姜 6–9g
da zao (Jujubae Fructus) 大枣 .... 4 fruit

Method: Decoction. **Chai hu** vents heat from the shaoyang, and with **huang qin** clears heat from the Liver and Gallbladder. **Zhi ban xia** and **sheng jiang** harmonize the Stomach, downbear counterflow Stomach qi and stop nausea; **ren shen** and **zhi gan cao** strengthen and support zheng qi; **sheng jiang** and **da zao** support **zhi ban xia** in harmonizing the Stomach and stopping nausea and vomiting. (Source: *Shang Han Lun*)

Modifications

- For acute mastitis with shaoyang symptoms, add **xiang fu** (Cyperi Rhizoma) 香附 9–12g, **pu gong ying** (Taraxaci Herba) 蒲公英 30g and **jin yin hua** (Lonicerae Flos) 金银花 15–30g. The herb dregs left over after cooking can be applied topically to the affected breast as a poultice.
- For acute cystitis or pyelonephritis with shaoyang symptoms, combine with **Ba Zheng San** (Eight Herb Powder for Rectification 八正散 p.345).
- For acute upper respiratory tract infection with cough and shaoyang symptoms, add **yu xing cao** (Herba Houttuyniae) 鱼腥草 18–30g **quan gua lou** (Trichosanthis Fructus) 全栝楼 18–24g, **jie geng** (Platycodi Radix) 荆芥 6–9g and **qian hu** (Peucedani Radix) 前胡 9–12g.
- For acute otitis, add **zao jiao ci** (Gleditsiae Spina) 皂角刺 6–9g, **jin yin hua** (Lonicerae Flos) 金银花 15–30g and **lian qiao** (Forsythiae Fructus) 连翘 9–12g.

Variations and additional prescriptions

Shaoyang / yangming syndrome

A strong pathogen can quickly drive deeper, causing pathogenic influence in both the shaoyang and yangming levels. This is usually a more intense pattern than the simple shaoyang pattern, characterized by strong alternating fever and chills with high fever, nausea and vomiting, abdominal and epigastric pain and constipation or urgent diarrhea. There may be jaundice. Penetration of a pathogen into yangming may be facilitated by improper treatment, usually purgation during the initial illness when the pathogen is on the surface. The treatment is to harmonize shaoyang and purge heat from yangming with **Da Chai Hu Tang** (Major Bupleurum Decoction 大柴胡汤).

chai hu (Bupleuri Radix) 柴胡 9–15g
huang qin (Scutellariae Radix) 黄芩 9–12g
bai shao (Paeoniae Radix alba) 白芍 6–9g
zhi ban xia (Pinelliae Rhizoma preparatum) 制半夏 6–9g
zhi shi (Aurantii Fructus immaturus) 枳实 6–9g
da huang (Rhei Radix et Rhizoma) 大黄 6–9g
sheng jiang (Zingiberis Rhizoma recens) 生姜 6–9g
da zao (Jujubae Fructus) 大枣 .... 4 fruit

Method: Decoction. **Chai hu** vents heat from the shaoyang, and with **huang qin** clears heat from the Liver and Gallbladder; **da huang** and **zhi shi** purge heat and constipation from yangming, and open the 'big exit' to provide another escape route out of the body; **bai shao** cools and softens the Liver, assisting **chai hu** and **huang qin** in clearing Liver and Gallbladder heat, and alleviating spasmodic pain; **zhi ban xia**, **sheng jiang** and **da zao** downbear counterflow Stomach qi and stop vomiting. (Source: *Shang Han Lun*)

Prepared medicines

Concentrated powders

Xiao Chai Hu Tang (Minor Bupleurum Combination)

Da Chai Hu Tang (Major Bupleurum Combination)

Pills

Xiao Chai Hu Wan (Minor Bupleurum Teapills)

Da Chai Hu Wan (Major Bupleurum Teapills)

Acupuncture (select from)

SJ.5 (waiguan –)................these points vent pathogens from shaoyang, dredge
GB.41 (zulinqi –)   the Liver and Gallbladder and regulate qi
GB.39 (xuanzhong –)
GB.34 (yanglingquan –)

- with mastitis, add SI.1 (shaoze ↓), Liv.3 (taichong –) and St.39 (xiajuxu –)
- with otitis, add GB.2 (tinghui –) and LI.4 (hegu –)
- with cough, add Lu.5 (chize –)
- with constipation, add SJ.6 (zhigou –), St.37 (shangjuxu –) and St.25 (tianshu –)
- Ear points: ear apex ↓, liver, gall bladder, spleen, zero point, shenmen

Clinical notes

- Shaoyang syndrome may be diagnosed as influenza, mastitis, hepatitis, otitis medic and ear infections, bronchitis, pneumonia, malaria, postpartum fever or cholecystitis.
- Shaoyang syndrome is a common cause of acute fever. Typically patients will have had an acute exterior wind cold or wind heat pattern, that was for some reason unresolved. The initial symptoms of the acute exterior disorder quickly give way to feelings of heat and cold, fatigue, and loss of appetite. If the shaoyang pathogen is unresolved, it may linger in the shaoyang for weeks, months or even years.
- When correctly identified, acute shaoyang patterns generally respond quickly (within hours to a few days) to treatment.

热
毒

7.4 TOXIC HEAT

Toxic heat refers to two types of disorder, both of which are characterized by severe heat. In the first, a severe localized accumulation of heat or damp heat reaches a degree of focal intensity sufficient to destroy tissue and create pus, at which point it is defined as toxic heat. Lesions of this type are often recurrent and due to the persistent presence of a damp heat pathogen in the qi level. The qi level involves the Lungs and skin, Spleen, Stomach and muscles. The low grade damp heat can be suddenly exacerbated and brought out by changes of diet, increasing humidity, or stress.

The second type of toxic heat is associated with external invasion of a strong, and usually epidemic, heat pathogen that overwhelms the bodies defenses and quickly overruns the qi and blood levels.

Clinical features
- high fever
- thirst, dry mouth
- suppurative skin lesions; red lines running along a limb (lymphangitis)
- restlessness, irritability and insomnia
- nausea and vomiting; malaise
- red complexion
- concentrated, smelly urine; painful urination
- swollen tender lymph nodes
- may be constipation or explosive diarrhea
- may be jaundice

P rapid, slippery, strong pulse
T red tongue with a thick, yellow coat

Treatment principle
Clear toxic heat and fire

Prescription

HUANG LIAN JIE DU TANG 黄连解毒汤
Coptis Decoction to Resolve Toxicity

huang qin (Scutellariae Radix) 黄芩	6–12g
huang lian (Coptidis Rhizoma) 黄连	3–9g
huang bai (Phellodendri Cortex) 黄柏	6–12g
shan zhi zi (Gardeniae Fructus) 山栀子	6–12g

Method: Decoction. **Huang qin, huang lian, huang bai** and **shan zhi zi** clear toxic heat and damp heat from the Triple Burner. **Huang qin** clears heat from the upper burner; **huang lian** clears heat from the Heart and Stomach, **huang bai** clears heat from the lower burner; **shan zhi zi** clears heat from all, and promotes urination to provide an escape route for the heat. (Source: *Wai Tai Yi Bao*)

Modifications
- For boils, carbuncles and abscesses, add **pu gong ying** (Taraxaci Herba) 蒲公英 15–30g, **lian qiao** (Forsythiae Fructus) 连翘 9–12g and **zi hua di ding** (Violae Herba) 紫花地丁 12–15g.

- With painful urination, add **ze xie** (Alismatis Rhizoma) 泽泻 9–12g, **che qian zi** (Plantaginis Semen) 车前子 9–12g [cooked in a cloth bag] and **mu tong** (Akebiae Caulis) 木通 6–9g.
- With constipation, add **da huang** (Rhei Radix et Rhizoma) 大黄 6–9g.
- For diarrhea with pus and blood, add **bai tou weng** (Pulsatillae Radix) 白头翁 12–18g, **mu xiang** (Aucklandiae Radix) 木香 6–9g and **bing lang** (Arecae Semen) 槟榔 6–9g.
- With jaundice, add **yin chen** (Artemisiae scopariae Herba) 茵陈 15–30g and **da huang** (Rhei Radix et Rhizoma) 大黄 6–9g [added at the end].

Variations and additional prescriptions
Epidemic toxic heat in the qi and blood levels
A toxic heat pathogen can inhabit multiple levels simultaneously. This occurs when an virulent epidemic pathogen clashes with robust anti–pathogenic qi. The fierce battle produces great heat and a raging fever. The heat quickly moves deeper into the body. The heat is still in the qi level, seen in the continuous high fever and intense thirst, while pushing deeper into the blood, seen in maculopapular rash, petechial hemorrhage and bleeding, delirium and disturbances of consciousness. In addition there are general signs of systemic toxicity–generalized malaise, nausea, vomiting and severe headache. The tongue is dark red or scarlet and the pulse surging and rapid. The treatment is to clear heat from the qi level and cool the blood, resolve toxic heat and nourish yin with QING WEN BAI DU YIN (Clear Epidemics and Overcome Toxin Decoction 清瘟败毒饮).

shi gao (Gypsum fibrosum) 石膏 30–60g
shui niu jiao (Cornu Bubali) 水牛角 30–60g
sheng di (Rehmanniae Radix) 生地 18–30g
huang qin (Scutellariae Radix) 黄芩 3–9g
huang lian (Coptidis Rhizoma) 黄连 3–9g
shan zhi zi (Gardeniae Fructus) 山栀子 6–12g
zhi mu (Anemarrhenae Rhizoma) 知母 6–12g
chi shao (Paeoniae Radix rubra) 赤芍 6–12g
xuan shen (Scrophulariae Radix) 玄参 6–12g
lian qiao (Forsythiae Fructus) 连翘 6–12g
mu dan pi (Moutan Cortex) 牡丹皮 6–12g
jie geng (Platycodi Radix) 桔梗 3–6g
dan zhu ye (Lophatheri Herba) 淡竹叶 3–6g
gan cao (Glycyrrhizae Radix) 甘草 3–6g

Method: Decoction. **Shi gao** and **shui niu jiao** are broken up or shaved and cooked for 30 minutes prior to the other herbs. **Shi gao**, **zhi mu** and **dan zhu ye** vent and clear heat from the qi level; **sheng di**, **shui niu jiao**, **xuan shen**, **chi shao** and **mu dan pi** cool the blood; **chi shao** and **mu dan pi** activate the blood and prevent the blood stasis that can result from intense heat congealing blood, and the coldness of the principle herbs; **huang qin**, **huang lian** and **shan zhi zi** clear toxic heat and damp heat. **Huang qin** clears heat from the upper burner; **huang lian** clears heat from the Heart and Stomach; **shan zhi zi** clears heat from all three burners and promotes urination to provide an escape route for the heat; **lian qiao** clears toxic heat; the ascending action of **jie geng** balances the descending nature of the bitter cold herbs and provides a counterbalance to power the qi dynamic; **gan cao** clears toxicity and harmonizes the prescription. (Source: *Yi Zhen Yi De*)

Prepared medicines

Concentrated powders

Huang Lian Jie Du Tang (Coptis & Scute Combination)
Pu Ji Xiao Du Yin (Scute & Cimicifuga Combination)

Pills

Huang Lian Jie Du Wan (Huang Lian Jie Du Teapills)
Pu Ji Xiao Du Wan (Universal Benefit Teapills)
Niu Huang Jie Du Pain (Peking Niu Huang Jie Du Pian)
Da Bai Du Jiao Nang (DBD Capsule)

Acupuncture (select from)

PC.3 (quze ↓)....................sea points of the Pericardium and Urinary Bladder,
Bl.40 (weizhong ↓)   these points cool the blood, clear toxic heat and
                             reduce fever
Du.14 (dazhui –)...............meeting point of the yang channels, clears heat and
                             drains fire
shixuan ↓ (M–UE–1).........clears heat when bled; used when there is severe heat
                             and disturbance of consciousness
LI.11 (quchi –)..................these points clear heat from yangming
St.44 (neiting –)
LI.4 (hegu –)

- Ear points: ear apex ↓, zero point, lung
- treatment can be given every 6–8 hours
- with confusion or delirium add Du.26 (renzhong)

Clinical notes

- Toxic heat fever is a serious condition that may be diagnosed as abscesses and carbuncles, lymphangitis, lymphadenitis, bacteremia, septicemia, blood poisoning, acute appendicitis, diverticulitis, dysentery, encephalitis or meningococcal meningitis. In its severe form, it should be managed in hospital.
- In severe cases, and in elderly, frail or debilitated patients, concurrent use of antibiotics may be necessary to quickly cool the heat. Herbs and acupuncture support the swift action of the antibiotics, and finish the job by expelling the pathogen, clearing residual heat, strengthening resistance and replenishing damaged qi and yin.

7.5 EPIDEMIC TOXIC WIND DAMP HEAT

大头瘟

Epidemic toxic wind damp heat is a seasonal pathogen that primarily affects children and young adults during winter and spring. It is characterized by abrupt onset of high fever and pronounced heat symptoms in the head and throat. The pathogen is described as toxic because of its severity. This is a type of warm disease (*wēn bìng* 温病), and corresponds to the presentation of a variety of childhood febrile illnesses. The Chinese characters to the left are *dà tóu wēn*, the original description of the illness, literally meaning massive febrile disease of the head.

Clinical features
- acute high fever, chills and rigors
- redness, swelling and burning pain in the face, head, throat and upper body
- sore, red, swollen throat, with or without suppuration; with suppuration the tonsils may be dotted with white spots of pus
- splitting headache
- cough with sticky, yellow sputum and chest pain
- thirst, dryness; maybe constipation
- swollen tender cervical lymph nodes

T red with a dry, yellow coat
P floating, rapid, surging

Treatment principle
Clear and resolve wind damp heat toxin

Prescription

PU JI XIAO DU YIN 普济消毒饮
Universal Benefit Drink to Eliminate Toxin

jiu huang qin (wine fried Scutellariae Radix) 酒黄芩 6–12g
jiu huang lian (wine fried Coptidis Rhizoma) 酒黄连 3–9g
ban lan gen (Isatidis/Baphicacanthis Radix) 板蓝根 9–15g
lian qiao (Forsythia Fructus) 连翘 6–12g
xuan shen (Scrophulariae Radix) 玄参 6–12g
chao jiang can (stir fried Bombyx Batryticatus) 炒僵蚕 3–9g
ma bo (Lasiosphaera/Calvatia) 马勃 2–3g
niu bang zi (Arctii Fructus) 牛蒡子 9–15g
chen pi (Citri reticulatae Pericarpium) 陈皮 3–6g
jie geng (Platycodi Radix) 桔梗 3–6g
sheng ma (Rhizoma Cimicifugae) 升麻 3–6g
chai hu (Bupleuri Radix) 柴胡 3–9g
bo he (Menthae haplocalycis Herba) 薄荷 3–6g
gan cao (Glycyrrhizae Radix) 甘草 3–6g

Method: Decoction. **Bo he** is added at the end of cooking, **ma bo** is cooked in a cloth bag. **Jiu huang lian** and **jiu huang qin** clear heat from the upper body; **ban lan gen**, **lian qiao** and **ma bo** clear toxic heat; **chao jiang can**, **niu bang zi**, **sheng ma**, **bo he** and **chai hu** dispel wind heat; **sheng ma** and **chai hu** conduct the action of the herbs to the head; **xuan shen** cools the blood; **xuan shen**, **gan cao**, **jie geng**, **niu bang zi** and **ma bo** clear heat from the throat and stop pain; **chen pi** rectifies qi. (Source: *Wei Sheng Bao Jian*)

Modifications
- With constipation, add **da huang** (Rhei Radix et Rhizoma) 大黄 3–6g.
- With less obvious internal heat and more external symptoms, reduce the dose of **huang qin** and **huang lian**, and add **jing jie** (Schizonepetae Herba) 荆芥 9–12g, **fang feng** (Saposhnikovae Radix) 防风 9–12g and **chan tui** (Cicadae Periostracum) 蝉蜕 9–12g.
- With less obvious external symptoms and more internal heat, delete **chai hu** and **bo he**, and add **jin yin hua** (Lonicerae Flos) 金银花 12–18g.

Prepared medicines
Concentrated powder
Pu Ji Xiao Du Yin (Scute & Cimicifuga Combination)

Pills
Pu Ji Xiao Du Wan (Universal Benefit Teapills)
Huang Lian Shang Qing Pian (Huang Lien Shang Ching Pien)
Niu Huang Jie Du Pian (Peking Niu Huang Jie Du Pian)
Shuang Liao Hou Feng San (Superior Sore Throat Powder)
  – for topical use in the throat

Acupuncture (select from)
Du.14 (dazhui –)................clears heat and drains fire
LI.11 (quchi –)...................these points clear heat from yangming and have a
LI.4 (hegu –)   special effect on heat lesions of the face
St.44 (neiting –)
Lu.10 (yuji).......................fire point of the Lungs, clears heat from the Lungs
                                  and eases the throat
Lu.11 (shaoshang ↓)...........wood point of the Lungs, clears heat from the
                                  Lungs, dispels wind heat and eases the throat
Du.10 (lingtai –).................these points have a special effect on pyogenic lesions
Du.12 (shenzhu –)
- with severe heat, bleed the jing points of the finger tips
- Ear points: ear apex ↓, lungs, throat, tonsils ↓

Clinical notes
- Epidemic toxic wind damp heat may be diagnosed as epidemic parotitis, acute bacterial tonsillitis, streptococcal infection, cellulitis of the head and face, erysipelas, measles, scarlet fever, lymphadenitis or suppurative otitis media.
- An eyedropper can be used to deliver small amounts of the prescription. A dose should be taken cold, as often as the patient will allow it.
- This pattern is potentially dangerous, and should only be managed by experienced practitioners. In severe cases, concurrent use of antibiotics may be necessary to quickly cool the heat. Herbs and acupuncture support the swift action of the antibiotics, and finish the job by expelling the pathogen, clearing residual damp, fortifying resistance and nourishing damaged yin.

肝 | 7.6 LIVER AND GALLBLADDER DAMP HEAT
胆
湿
热

Damp heat in the Liver and Gallbladder causing fever can be due to external invasion of a damp heat pathogen (most common), or internally generated damp heat. External invasion of damp heat is more common in hot and humid climates, although it may occur in temperate zones via transmission of damp heat through contaminated food and water, sexual intercourse, blood transfusion, and intravenous drug use. In biomedical terms, it frequently corresponds to viral hepatitis.

Damp heat generated internally through physiological dysfunction may be an acute episode. However, there will usually be a chronic history of gastrointestinal dysfunction, alcohol consumption, a diet of rich heating foods and high stress.

Fever of a damp heat type is the product of two opposing pathogens, yin damp and yang heat. This produces a variable fever pattern depending on the mix of damp and heat. In general, the presence of the damp obscures or 'wraps' the heat, preventing its full expression. When damp is ascendant, the fever tends to be low grade or tidal, rising in the afternoon. When heat is dominant, the fever will be higher and more continuous.

Clinical features
- Acute fever, or alternating fever and chills. The fever tends to be moderate, but may be high, and is apparent all day, but rises in the afternoon; night sweats.
- hypochondriac distension, heat and pain, right sided and worse for pressure
- irritability, restlessness, easily angered
- insomnia and fitful sleep
- loss of appetite, nausea and vomiting; aversion to fats and oils
- bitter or bad taste in the mouth
- abdominal distension and chest oppression
- maybe jaundice
- dark, concentrated or painful urination
- constipation or loose and sluggish stools; stools may be pasty or clay like
- swollen lymph nodes

T red with a thick, greasy, yellow coat
P floating and rapid, or wiry and rapid

Treatment principle
Clear damp heat from the Liver and Gallbladder

Prescription

LONG DAN XIE GAN TANG 龙胆泻肝汤
Gentian Decoction to Purge the Liver

jiu long dan cao (wine fried Gentianae Radix) 酒龙胆草	3–9g
huang qin (Scutellariae Radix) 黄芩	6–12g
shan zhi zi (Gardeniae Fructus) 山栀子	6–12g
ze xie (Alismatis Rhizoma) 泽泻	6–12g
mu tong (Akebiae Caulis) 木通	3–6g
che qian zi (Plantaginis Semen) 车前子	9–15g

sheng di (Rehmanniae Radix) 生地 9–15g
dang gui (Angelicae sinensis Radix) 当归 6–12g
chai hu (Bupleuri Radix) 柴胡 3–9g
gan cao (Glycyrrhizae Radix) 甘草 3–6g

Method: Decoction. **Che qian zi** is cooked in a cloth bag. **Jiu long dan cao** cools the Liver and clears damp heat; **shan zhi zi** and **huang qin** clear heat from all three burners; **chai hu** clears heat, dredges the Liver and alleviates qi constraint; **ze xie, che qian zi** and **mu tong** promote urination to provide an escape route for the heat; **sheng di** cools the blood; **dang gui** nourishes and protects blood; **gan cao** protects the Stomach. (Source: *Zhong Yi Nei Ke Xue* [*Yi Fang Ji Jie*])

Modifications

- The balance of heat and damp can vary. When the heat is mild and the damp pronounced, the dose of **long dan cao**, **huang qin** and **shan zhi zi** should be at the low end of the range, and damp drying herbs, such as **bai zhu** (Atractylodes macrocephalae Rhizoma) 白术 9–12g and **fu ling** (Poria) 茯苓 12–15g, added.
- With jaundice, add **yin chen** (Artemisiae scopariae Herba) 茵陈 18–30g and **huang bai** (Phellodendri Cortex) 黄柏 9–12g or combine with YIN CHEN HAO TANG (Virgate Wormwood Decoction 茵陈蒿汤 p.922).
- With constipation, add **da huang** (Rhei Radix et Rhizoma) 大黄 6–9g and **mang xiao** (Natrii Sulfas) 芒硝 6–9g.
- With difficult or sluggish stools, add **zhi ke** (Aurantii Fructus) 枳壳 9–12g and **bai zhu** (Atractylodes macrocephalae Rhizoma) 白术 30g.
- With abdominal distension, add **zhi shi** (Aurantii Fructus immaturus) 枳实 9–12g, **hou po** (Magnoliae officinalis Cortex) 厚朴 9–12g and **da fu pi** (Arecae Pericarpium) 大复皮 9–12g.
- With concentrated or painful urination, add **bai mao gen** (Imperatae Rhizoma) 白茅根 12–18g and **hua shi** (Talcum) 滑石 9–12g.
- With hypochondriac pain, add **chuan lian zi** (Toosendan Fructus) 川楝子 9–12g and **yan hu suo** (Corydalis Rhizoma) 延胡索 9–12g.
- With viral hepatitis, add **ji gu cao** (Abri Herba) 鸡骨草 15–30g.

Variations and additional prescriptions

Damp heat in the Gallbladder with pain and jaundice

Sudden onset of fever, hypochondriac and abdominal pain, pain radiating to the tip and back of the right shoulder, jaundice, dark urine, nausea and vomiting and pale clay like stools suggest a damp heat pathogen in the Gallbladder. This may complicate chronic Liver and Gallbladder pathology, or occur suddenly as the result of dietary indiscretion, excessive alcohol intake, gallstones or an unresolved low grade infection or parasite infestation. The treatment is to clear damp heat from the Gallbladder, and promote elimination to drain damp heat with a mixture of DA CHAI HU TANG (Major Bupleurum Decoction 大柴胡汤, p.330) and YIN CHEN HAO TANG (Virgate Wormwood Decoction 茵陈蒿汤, p.921–922).

Toxic heat

Toxic heat can accumulate in the Liver or Gallbladder, and form a focal lesion. This relatively uncommon situation can be a complication and intensification of damp heat, or follow a few weeks after an episode of dysentery or an Intestinal abscess. The fever is high, with rigors and profuse sweating, and an exquisitely tender mass is palpable in the right hypochondrium. See Abdominal masses, p.40.

Prepared medicines
Concentrated powders
Long Dan Xie Gan Tang (Gentiana Combination)
Da Chai Hu Tang (Major Bupleurum Combination)

Pills
Long Dan Xie Gan Wan (Snake and Dragon Teapills)
Li Dan Pian 利胆片 (Lidan Tablets)

Acupuncture (select from)
Liv.14 (qimen –) ....alarm point of the Liver, dredges the Liver and clears damp heat

SJ.6 (zhigou –) ....these points clear damp heat and promote qi move–
GB.34 (yanglingquan)   ment through the lateral aspect of the body

GB.24 (riyue –)..................alarm point of the Gallbladder, clears damp heat

Liv.3 (taichong –) ....source point of the Liver, dredges the Liver and clears damp heat

GB.41 (zulinqi –) ....clears damp heat from the Gallbladder

Bl.18 (ganshu)....................transport point of the Liver, dredges the Liver and clears damp heat

Bl.19 (danshu –) ....transport point of the Gallbladder, clears damp heat

- with high fever add Du.14 (dazhui –) and LI.11 (quchi –)
- with alternating fever and chills, add SJ.5 (waiguan –) and GB.39 (xuanzhong –)
- with abdominal distension, add Ren.12 (zhongwan –) and St.25 (tianshu –)
- with constipation, add St.25 (tianshu –) and St.37 (shangjuxu –)
- with nausea add PC.6 (neiguan –)
- with jaundice add Du.9 (zhiyang –)
- with gallstones, add dannangxue (M–LE–23)
- Ear points: ear apex ↓, liver, gallbladder, spleen, shenmen

Clinical notes
- Acute fever of a Liver Gallbladder damp heat type may be diagnosed as acute viral hepatitis, alcoholic hepatitis, acute cholecystitis, pancreatitis, gallstones, shingles and round worms in the bile duct.
- An important principle to observe in the treatment of Liver Gallbladder damp heat is to keep the bowels moving and urination flowing to provide an escape route. An increase in both should be observed following ingestion of medicine or acupuncture. When **da huang** is used, it should be reduced in dosage or deleted once the bowels are moving satisfactorily to avoid iatrogenic damage to Spleen yang.
- Acute external damp heat in the Liver and Gallbladder is relatively easy to treat. Acute exacerbations of chronic conditions also tend to respond quite well. Chronic damp heat is more difficult to resolve, and usually involves significant modifications to diet and lifestyle, in addition to herbs, for adequate results.

脾
胃
湿
热

7.7 SPLEEN AND STOMACH DAMP HEAT

Spleen and Stomach damp heat often follows ingestion of spoiled food. The main pathology is blockage of the qi dynamic by damp heat. Damp heat in the Spleen and Stomach is similar to, but can be can be distinguished from, damp heat in the qi level (p.325), by the absence of muscle aches, sore throat and other qi level symptoms. In contrast to damp heat in the Large Intestine, where the focus of pathology is the lower digestive tract, in this pattern the upper digestive tract is the focus.

Clinical features

- abrupt onset of afternoon fever that is unrelieved by sweating, with vomiting, nausea and diarrhea
- chest oppression
- fullness, distension and pain in the epigastrium and abdomen
- irritability and restlessness
- concentrated, dark or cloudy urine
- swollen lymph nodes

T greasy, yellow tongue coat
P slippery, rapid pulse

Treatment principle

Clear damp heat from the Spleen and Stomach

Prescription

LIAN PO YIN 连朴饮
Coptis and Magnolia Bark Drink

huang lian (Coptidis Rhizoma) 黄连 3–6g
hou po (Magnoliae officinalis Cortex) 厚朴 6–9g
shan zhi zi (Gardeniae Fructus) 山栀子 9–12g
dan dou chi (Sojae Semen preparatum) 淡豆豉 9–12g
shi chang pu (Acori tatarinowii Rhizoma) 石菖蒲 6–9g
zhi ban xia (Pinelliae Rhizoma preparatum) 制半夏 6–9g
lu gen (Phragmitis Rhizoma) 芦根 30–60g

Method: Decoction. **Huang lian** and **shan zhi zi** clear damp heat. Being bitter and descending, they combine well with the pungent warmth of **zhi ban xia** and the downbearing nature of **hou po**, to correct the qi dynamic; **zhi ban xia** transforms damp, downbears counterflow and stops vomiting; **dan dou chi** and **shan zhi zi** clear heat from the qi level and alleviate irritability; **shi chang pu** rouses the Spleen and transforms damp; **lu gen** clears heat from the Stomach and stops vomiting. (Source: *Shi Yong Fang Ji Xue [Huo Luan Lun]*)

Modifications

- With high fever, add **huang bai** (Phellodendri Cortex) 黄柏 9–12g and **huang qin** (Scutellariae Radix) 黄芩 9–12g.
- With severe nausea and vomiting, add **huo xiang** (Pogostemonis/Agastaches Herba) 藿香 12–15g and **pei lan** (Eupatorii Herba) 佩兰 9–12g.
- With frequent diarrhea, add **yi ren** (Coicis Semen) 苡仁 15–30g and **che**

qian zi (Plantaginis Semen) 车前子 9–12g [cooked in a cloth bag].

Prepared medicines
Concentrated powders
Gan Lu Xiao Du Dan (Forsythia & Acorus Formula)
Pills
Bi Xie Sheng Shi Wan (Subdue the Dampness Teapills)

Acupuncture (select from)
Du.14 (dazhui –)................meeting point of the yang channels, clears heat and alleviates fever
LI.11 (quchi –)...................sea point of the Large Intestine, clears heat from yangming
PC.6 (neiguan –)................activates the qi dynamic and alleviates nausea and vomiting
Ren.12 (zhongwan –).........alarm point of the Stomach, clears heat and damp
St.25 (tianshu –).................alarm point of the Large Intestine, activates the qi dynamic and clears damp heat
St.36 (zusanli –) ....sea point of the Stomach, activates and rectifies the qi dynamic to clear damp heat
Sp.9 (yinlingquan –)...........water and metal points of the Spleen, these points
Sp.5 (shangqiu –)   promote urination and clear damp heat
- with diarrhea, add zhixie (N–CA–3)
- with severe fever, vomiting and diarrhea, bleed PC.3 (quze ↓) and Bl.40 (weizhong ↓) with a lancet and extract a few drops of blood; may also be needled with a reducing method
- Ear points: ear apex ↓, spleen, stomach, lung, zero point, shenmen

Clinical notes
- Damp heat in the Spleen and Stomach may be diagnosed as acute gastroenteritis, food poisoning, 'Bali belly', summer flu, cholera or typhoid fever.
- This pattern shares characteristics with damp heat in the qi level, damp heat in the Liver and damp heat in the Large Intestine. The main difference is simply the location of the pathogen. The prescriptions for qi level damp heat and Spleen and Stomach damp heat are interchangeable.
- This pattern can respond well to treatment. Diseases like typhoid and cholera should be managed in hospital. Treatment should continue for a few days to a week or so after cessation of symptoms to ensure that damp heat is completely eliminated.

大肠湿热 7.8 DAMP HEAT IN THE LARGE INTESTINE

Damp heat in the Large Intestine pattern can be caused by external invasion of damp heat or internally generated damp heat. External damp heat is more common in hot humid weather, but can occur at any time of the year. Internally generated damp heat can be due to the diet or physiological disruptions such as the primary pathological triad (p.780). Internally generated damp heat is less likely to cause a significant fever. Occasionally, damp heat in the Large Intestine may also be the result of inappropriate purgation during an acute external wei level disorder. The purge weakens the Spleen and Stomach, facilitating invasion by the pathogen into yangming.

Clinical features
- fever or afternoon fever which is unrelieved with sweating
- acute, frequent, urgent, foul smelling, hot diarrhea, with a burning anus and tenesmus
- restlessness and irritability
- cramping abdominal pain
- concentrated, scanty urine
- thirst
- warm, tender lower abdomen
- swollen lymph nodes

T greasy yellow coat; may be red tongue body
P slippery and rapid

Treatment principle
Clear damp heat from the Intestines
Stop diarrhea

Prescription
GE GEN HUANG QIN HUANG LIAN TANG 葛根黄芩黄连汤
Kudzu, Coptis and Scutellaria Decoction

wei ge gen (roasted Puerariae Radix) 煨葛根 12–15g
huang qin (Scutellariae Radix) 黄芩 9–12g
huang lian (Coptidis Rhizoma) 黄连 6–9g
gan cao (Radix Glycyrrhizae Uralensis) 甘草 3–6g

Method: Decoction. **Wei ge gen** dispels heat and alleviates diarrhea; **huang qin** and **huang lian** clear damp heat from the Intestines, **gan cao** protects the Stomach. (Source: *Shi Yong Zhong Yi Nei Ke Xue* [*Shang Han Lun*])

Modifications
- With high fever and severe heat, add **jin yin hua** (Lonicerae Flos) 金银花 15–30g, **lian qiao** (Forsythia Fructus) 连翘 9–12g and **shan zhi zi** (Gardeniae Fructus) 山栀子 9–12g.
- With marked damp and heaviness, add **cang zhu** (Atractylodis Rhizoma) 苍术 12–15g, **fu ling** (Poria) 茯苓 12–15g and **yi ren** (Coicis Semen) 苡仁 15–30g.
- For diarrhea with pus and blood, add **ma chi xian** (Portulacae Herba) 马齿苋 15–18g.

- With cramping abdominal pain, add **mu xiang** (Aucklandiae Radix) 木香 6–9g and **bai shao** (Paeoniae Radix alba) 白芍 9–12g.
- With rectal bleeding, add **di yu** (Sanguisorbae Radix) 地榆 9–12g and **huai hua mi** (Sophora Flos immaturus) 槐花米 9–12g.
- With nausea or vomiting, add **zhi ban xia** (Pinelliae Rhizoma preparatum) 制半夏 9–12g and **zhu ru** (Bambusae Caulis in taeniam) 竹茹 12–15g.
- With abdominal distension, add **hou po** (Magnoliae officinalis Cortex) 厚朴 9–12g and **zhi ke** (Aurantii Fructus) 枳壳 9–12g.
- With difficult or scanty urination, add **hua shi** (Talcum) 滑石 12–18g.
- With residual wind heat, or damp heat in the Intestines that is stirred up by a wind heat attack, add **jin yin hua** (Lonicerae Flos) 金银花 15–30g, **lian qiao** (Forsythia Fructus) 连翘 9–12g and **bo he** (Mentha haplocalycis Herba) 薄荷 6g [added at the end of cooking].
- With evidence of infection by the parasite *Giardia lamblia* or other amoebic organisms, add **qing hao** (Artemisiae annuae Herba) 青蒿 15g and **da suan** (Allii sativi Bulbus) 大蒜 6–9g. These herbs can also be decocted separately and given as an enema.

Variations and additional prescriptions
With umbilical and right iliac fossa pain
High fever accompanied by abdominal pain that begins around the navel then concentrates in the right iliac fossa, is worse with pressure and is associated with rebound tenderness and abdominal guarding, is an Intestinal abscess. Additional symptoms include nausea, constipation or diarrhea, a greasy, yellow tongue coat and slippery, rapid pulse. The treatment is to open the bowels to clear and purge heat, move qi and disperse blood stasis with **DA HUANG MU DAN TANG** (Rhubarb and Moutan Decoction 大黄牡丹汤, p.51).

Prepared medicines
Concentrated powders
Ge Gen Huang Qin Huang Lian Tang (Pueraria, Coptis & Scute Combination)
Pills
Huang Lian Jie Du Wan (Huang Lian Jie Du Teapills)
Chuan Xin Lian Kang Yan Pian (Chuan Xin Lian Antiphlogistic Tablets)
Bao Ji Wan (Po Chai Pills)
Huang Lian Su Pian (Coptis Teapills, Tabellae Berberini)

Acupuncture (select from)
LI.11 (quchi –)...................these points clear damp heat from the Stomach and
LI.4 (hegu –)   Large Intestine
St.44 (neiting –)
zhixie (N–CA–3)...............extra point for diarrhea, located halfway between
                                 Ren.8 (shenque) and the pubic bone
St.25 (tianshu –).................alarm point of the Large Intestine, clears damp heat
                                 and stops diarrhea

Sp.9 (yinlingquan –)...........sea point of the Spleen, promotes urination and
                                drains damp heat
St.37 (shangjuxu –) ....lower sea point of the Large Intestine, clears damp
                                heat

- with high fever, add Du.14 (dazhui –)
- with nausea, add PC.6 (neiguan)
- with sudden severe diarrhea, vomiting and fever, bleed PC.3 (quze ↓) and Bl.40 (weizhong ↓) with a lancet and extract a few drops of blood; may also be needled with a reducing method
- Ear points: ear apex ↓, large intestine, spleen, zero point, sympathetic

Clinical notes

- Damp heat in the Large Intestine may be diagnosed as acute gastroenteritis, enteritis, colitis, food poisoning, giardiasis or bacillary dysentery.
- This pattern responds well to treatment. Treatment should continue for a few days to a week or so after cessation of symptoms to ensure that damp heat is completely eliminated.

膀
胱
湿
热

7.9 DAMP HEAT IN THE URINARY BLADDER

Damp heat in the Urinary Bladder is most commonly due to invasion of a pathogen directly into the Bladder organ via the local network vessels, but may be introduced through the taiyang channels. Invasion by external pathogens into the Urinary Bladder is facilitated by pre–existing Kidney deficiency.

Clinical features
- acute fever, afternoon fever, or alternating fever and chills; in severe cases the patient may experience fever and rigors
- painful, frequent and urgent urination; the urine is dark, concentrated and strong smelling and may be accompanied by a feeling of incomplete emptying or dripping
- suprapubic fullness and discomfort
- lower back and loin pain
- swollen inguinal lymph nodes

T greasy, yellow coat, especially on the root
P slippery and rapid or soft and rapid

Treatment principle
Clear heat and promote urination to clear damp heat from the Urinary Bladder

Prescription

BA ZHENG SAN 八正散
Eight Herb Powder for Rectification

hua shi (Talcum) 滑石 12–30g
che qian zi (Plantaginis Semen) 车前子 9–15g
qu mai (Dianthi Herba) 瞿麦.. 9–12g
bian xu (Polygoni avicularis Herba) 萹蓄 9–12g
shan zhi zi (Gardeniae Fructus) 山栀子 6–9g
zhi da huang (processed Rhei Radix et Rhizoma) 制大黄 6–9g
mu tong (Akebiae Caulis) 木通 3–6g
gan cao shao (tips of Glycyrrhizae Radix) 甘草稍 3–6g
deng xin cao (Junci Medulla) 灯心草 3–6g

Method: Powder or decoction. Grind equal quantities of all herbs to a fine powder, and take 9 grams as a draft. Can be decocted with the doses as shown. When decocted, **che qian zi** and **hua shi** are cooked in a cloth bag. and a dose may be taken every two hours. **Hua shi, che qian zi, bian xu, qu mai, mu tong** and **deng xin cao** clear heat and promote urination; **shan zhi zi** clears damp heat from all three burners; **zhi da huang** clears heat and drains fire, and provides an escape route for heat through the bowel; **gan cao shao** clears heat and harmonizes the other herbs in the prescription. (Source: *Zhong Yi Nei Ke Xue* [*He Ji Ju Fang*])

Modifications
- With high fever, add **pu gong ying** (Taraxaci Herba) 蒲公英 18–30g, **bai hua she she cao** (Hedyotis diffusae Herba) 白花蛇舌草 15–30g and **jin yin hua** (Lonicerae Flos) 金银花 15–30g.
- With alternating fever and chills, add **chai hu** (Bupleuri Radix) 柴胡 9–12g and **huang qin** (Scutellariae Radix) 黄芩 6–9g, or combine with **XIAO CHAI**

Hu Tang (Minor Bupleurum Decoction 小柴胡汤, p.329).
- With hematuria, add **bai mao gen** (Imperatae Rhizoma) 白茅根 15–30g, **xiao ji** (Cirsii Herba) 小蓟 12–15g and **han lian cao** (Ecliptae Herba) 旱莲草 9–12g.
- With urinary calculi, add **jin qian cao** (Lysimachiae/Desmodii Herba) 金钱草 30g and **hai jin sha** (Lygodii Spora) 海金沙 15g [cooked in a cloth bag].
- With dry stools or constipation use unprocessed **da huang**.
- With loose stools or diarrhea, delete **zhi da huang**.

Prepared medicines
Concentrated powders
Ba Zheng San (Dianthus Formula)

Pills
Ba Zheng San Wan (Eight Righteous Teapills)
Da Bai Du Jiao Nang (DBD Capsule)
Long Dan Xie Gan Wan (Snake and Dragon Teapills)
Qing Re Qu Shi Chong Ji (Qing Re Qu Shi Tea)

Acupuncture (select from)
Du.14 (dazhui –)................meeting point of the yang channels, clears heat
LI.11 (quchi –)...................sea point of the Large Intestine, clears heat
Ren.3 (zhongji –) ....alarm point of the Urinary Bladder, promotes urination, clears damp heat from the Urinary Bladder
Liv.5 (ligou –)....................connecting point of the Liver, clears heat from the lower burner
Sp.9 (yinlingquan –)...........sea point of the Spleen, promotes urination and clears damp heat from the lower burner
Bl.28 (pangguangshu –) .....transport point of the Urinary Bladder, clears damp heat from the Urinary Bladder
Bl.32 (ciliao –) ....clears heat, regulates the lower burner
Bl.40 (weizhong –) ....lower sea point of the Urinary Bladder, clears heat and cools the blood
- with alternating fever and chills, add GB.41 (zulinqi –) and SJ.5 (waiguan –)
- with Kidney deficiency, add Bl.23 (shenshu +)
- with hematuria, add Sp.10 (xuehai –)
- Ear points: ear apex ↓, kidney, urinary bladder, shenmen, subcortex, endocrine

Clinical notes
- Damp heat in the Urinary Bladder may be diagnosed as acute urinary tract infection, cystitis, pyelonephritis or urinary calculi.
- This pattern responds well to treatment, depending on complicating factors. It is recommended to continue treatment for a few days to a week after cessation of symptoms to ensure all damp heat is eliminated. When there is urinary calculi, the main symptoms can be alleviated, but long term treatment is needed to resolve the calculi and prevent recurrence.

子宮熱毒 7.10 TOXIC HEAT IN THE UTERUS

Toxic heat can enter the Uterus by direct injection, as may occur during menstruation or childbirth, a surgical procedure or with sexual contact. Less commonly, it can be the result of damp heat generated by the diet, alcohol or physiological dysfunction (see primary pathological triad, p.780) that sinks in to the lower burner, where it gradually condenses and intensifies into toxic heat.

Clinical features
- high fever with chills or rigors
- acute lower abdominal or suprapubic pain that is warm or hot to touch, and is worse for pressure; may be muscle guarding
- profuse, malodorous vaginal discharge with blood and/or pus
- dry mouth and thirst
- constipation
- concentrated urine
- swollen inguinal lymph nodes
- **T** thick, greasy, yellow tongue coat
- **P** slippery, wiry, rapid

Treatment principle
Clear toxic heat and activate blood

Prescription
YIN QIAO HONG JIANG JIE DU TANG 银翘红酱解毒汤
Lonicera, Forsythia, Sargentodoxae and Patrinia Decoction to Eliminate Toxin

jin yin hua (Lonicerae Flos) 金银花 15–30g
lian qiao (Forsythiae Fructus) 连翘 15–30g
bai jiang cao (Patriniae Herba) 败将草 15–30g
hong teng (Sargentodoxae Caulis) 红藤 15–30g
shan zhi zi (Gardeniae Fructus) 山栀子 15–30g
chi shao (Paeoniae Radix rubra) 赤芍 12–15g
yi ren (Coicis Semen) 苡仁 12–15g
mu dan pi (Moutan Cortex) 牡丹皮 9–12g
tao ren (Persicae Semen) 桃仁 9–12g
yan hu suo (Corydalis Rhizoma) 延胡索 9–12g
chuan lian zi (Toosendan Fructus) 川楝子 9–12g

Method: Decoction. **Jin yin hua**, **lian qiao**, **bai jiang cao** and **hong teng** clear toxic heat; **yi ren** aids the discharge of pus; **shan zhi zi** clears heat from the triple burner; **tao ren** activates blood and disperses stagnant blood; **chi shao**, **mu dan pi** and **hong teng** cool and activate the blood, and disperse static blood; **yan hu suo**, **chuan lian zi** move qi, activate blood and stop pain. (Source: *Zhong Yi Fu Chan Ke Xue*)

Modifications
- With severe pain, add **pu huang** (Typhae Pollen) 蒲黄 9–12g and **wu ling zhi** (Trogopterori Faeces) 五灵脂 9–12g.
- With constipation, add **da huang** (Rhei Radix et Rhizoma) 大黄 6–9g and

mang xiao (Natrii Sulfas) 芒硝 6–9g [dissolved in the strained decoction].
- With abdominal distension, add **xiang fu** (Cyperi Rhizoma) 香附 9–12g, **mu xiang** (Aucklandiae Radix) 木香 6–9g and **sha ren** (Fructus Amomi) 砂仁 3–6g.
- With palpable masses, add **san leng** (Sparganii Rhizoma) 三棱 9–12g, **e zhu** (Curcumae Rhizoma) 莪术 9–12g and **dan shen** (Salviae miltiorrhizae Radix) 丹参 15–30g.

Prepared medicines
Concentrated powders
Huang Lian Jie Du Tang (Coptis & Scute Combination) plus Wu Wei Xiao Du Yin (Dandelion & Wild Chrysanthemum Combination)
Dang Gui Long Hui Wan (Tangkuei, Gentiana & Aloe Formula)

Pills
Da Bai Du Jiao Nang (DBD Capsule)
Huang Lian Jie Du Wan (Huang Lian Jie Du Teapills) plus Wu Wei Xiao Du Wan (Five Flavor Teapills)

Acupuncture (select from)
Du.14 (dazhui –) ....these points clear heat and alleviate fever
LI.11 (quchi –)
LI.4 (hegu –)
zigong – (M–CA–18) ....extra point for the Uterus, clears heat from the Uterus
GB.26 (daimai –) ....clears damp heat from the lower burner
Sp.8 (diji –) ....cleft point of the Spleen, regulates and activates blood and clears heat
Liv.5 (ligou –).....................connecting point of the Liver, clears damp heat from the lower burner
Kid.7 (fuliu –) ....river point of the Kidneys, clears damp heat from the lower burner
ahshi points.......................between Bl.31 (shangliao) and Bl.34 (xialiao), treated with a strong reducing technique
- with alternating fever and chills, add GB.39 (xuanzhong –), SJ.5 (waiguan –) and GB.34 (yanglingquan –)
- with nausea, add PC.6 (neiguan)
- with vulval redness and swelling, add Liv.2 (xingjian –)
- Ear points: ear apex ↓, uterus, ovary, sympathetic, adrenal, shenmen

Clinical notes
- Toxic heat in the Uterus may be diagnosed as pelvic inflammatory disease, salpingitis, endometritis or adnexitis. This is a serious condition that can quickly congeal blood and cause blood stasis, scarring and infertility. In severe cases it may be best to employ antibiotics to quickly cool the heat before utilizing Chinese medicine to clear any residual pathogens, restore qi and blood flow and support the Kidneys.

热入营分 | 7.11 HEAT IN THE YING LEVEL

An acute fever associated with heat in the ying level is a serious disorder caused by a strong pathogen. In practice, there can be elements of qi, ying and blood level pathogens simultaneously, as a pathogen strong enough to penetrate the body's defenses usually moves quickly from the qi level deeper into the body. At the ying level stage, the pathogen can still be vented back to the surface with specific light natured herbs. Once heat reaches the blood, it is too deep to be vented and must be cooled in situ, but the basic picture and strategy are similar and the prescription below can be effective in both ying and blood level patterns.

In clinical practice it is unusual to see heat in the ying level when it is the result of an invasion of an external pathogen into the body – these patients are quickly hospitalized, and the Chinese medicine practitioner sees them after the acute phase, for recuperation. Heat in the ying level can, however, be a more chronic pattern of disharmony with acute flare–ups on top of a persistent background of lingering heat. This is the situation observed in some types of connective tissue disease–systemic lupus erythematosus or Behçets disease for example.

Clinical features
- acute onset of moderate to high fever which is worse at night
- irritability and restlessness
- faint erythema, purpura or maculopapular rash
- thirst or dryness without thirst
- insomnia, restlessness at night
- may be confusion or mild delirium
- joint pain and inflammation
- swollen, tender lymph nodes

T dry red or scarlet with thorns, and little or no coat
P fine and rapid

Treatment principle
Clear and vent heat from the ying level
Nourish and enrich yin

Prescription

QING YING TANG 清营汤
Clear the Nutritive Level Decoction

shui niu jiao (Cornu Bubali) 水牛角	30–60g
sheng di (Rehmanniae Radix) 生地	15–30g
xuan shen (Scrophulariae Radix) 玄参	9–18g
mai dong (Ophiopogonis Radix) 麦冬	6–12g
jin yin hua (Lonicerae Flos) 金银花	9–15g
lian qiao (Forsythiae Fructus) 连翘	6–15g
dan zhu ye (Lophatheri Herba) 淡竹叶	3–6g
huang lian (Coptidis Rhizoma) 黄连	3–6g
dan shen (Salviae miltiorrhizae Radix) 丹参	6–15g

Method: Decoction. **Shui niu jiao** is shaved into fine strips and cooked for 30 minutes prior to the other herbs. **Shui niu jiao** clears heat from the ying level and cools the blood; **xuan shen** and **sheng di** cool the blood and protect yin; **mai dong** clears heat, nourishes yin and moistens dryness; **jin yin hua**, **lian qiao**, **dan zhu ye** clear and vent heat from the qi and ying levels; **huang lian** clears heat from the Heart and Stomach; **dan shen** clears heat, activates the blood, and helps prevent the blood stasis that may complicate both heat and the use of cold herbs. **Shui niu jiao** is used instead of **xi jiao** (Rhinocerotis Cornu) 犀角, the horn of the critically endangered rhinoceros. (Source: *Wen Bing Tiao Bian*)

Modifications

- With severe heat, add **da qing ye** (Isatidis Folium) 大青叶 15–30g and **ban lan gen** (Isatidis/Baphicacanthis Radix) 板蓝根 15–30g.
- With constipation, add **zhi da huang** (processed Rhei Radix et Rhizoma) 制大黄 6–9g and **mang xiao** (Natrii Sulfas) 芒硝 6–9g [dissolved in the strained decoction].
- With spasms or convulsions, add **gou teng** (Ramulus Uncariae cum Uncis) 钩藤 9–12g and **di long** (Pheretima) 地龙 9–12g.

Prepared medicines

Concentrated powders

Wen Qing Yin (Tangkuei and Gardenia Combination) plus Wu Wei Xiao Du Yin (Dandelion & Wild Chrysanthemum Combination)

Pills

Huang Lian Jie Du Tang (Coptis & Scute Combination) plus Si Wu Wan (Four Substances for Women Teapills) and Wu Wei Xiao Du Yin (Dandelion & Wild Chrysanthemum Combination)

Acupuncture (select from)

PC.3 (quze ↓).....................sea points of the Pericardium and Urinary Bladder
Bl.40 (weizhong ↓)   channels, these points clear heat from the ying and blood levels
LI.11 (quchi –)...................sea point of the Large Intestine, clears heat
PC.1 (zhongchong ↓) ....well point of Pericardium channel, clears heat and cools the Heart and Pericardium
Ht.9 (shaochong ↓)............well point of Heart channel, clears heat, cools the Heart and calms the shen
Kid.7 (fuliu –)....................clears and vents heat from the ying and blood levels
Kid.2 (rangu –) ....clears heat from shaoyin
- Ear points: ear apex ↓, liver, heart, kidney, shenmen, sympathetic, subcortex

Clinical notes

- Heat in the ying level may be diagnosed as bacteremia, septicemia, heatstroke, meningitis, meningococcal meningitis, encephalitis, thrombocytopenic purpura, or an acute flare up of connective tissue disease.
- This is a serious illness, and when associated with a major and potentially fatal or debilitating infection should be managed in hospital.

热
盛
动
血

7.12 HEAT IN THE BLOOD

Heat in the blood is in the deepest level of the body and is potentially the most dangerous. There are two broad varieties of heat in the blood, the first being the end result of an acute pathogenic invasion, the second being heat generated internally in the Liver that is transferred to the blood. Acute fever as described here is associated with a pathogenic invasion, and therefore represents a serious and potentially dangerous infectious illness.

The frenetic movement that characterizes heat in the blood can force the blood out of the vessels as bleeding or purpura. Because the heat 'cooks and congeals' the blood, blood stasis is always a complication.

Clinical features
- acute onset of fever which is worse at night
- purpura or maculopapular rash; rashes are usually dark or purplish
- sudden, often violent bleeding–subcutaneous hemorrhage, hematemesis, epistaxis, scleral hemorrhage, abnormal uterine bleeding, rectal bleeding
- disturbances of consciousness, delirium, mania
- thirst and dryness
- swollen, tender lymph nodes

T red, scarlet or purple tongue with raised prickles
P fine, rapid pulse

Treatment principle
Clear heat from the blood

Prescription

SHUI NIU JIAO DI HUANG TANG 水牛角地黄汤
Water Buffalo Horn and Rehmannia Decoction

shui niu jiao (Cornu Bubali) 水牛角 30–120g
sheng di (Rehmanniae Radix) 生地...15–30g
chi shao (Paeoniae Radix rubra) 赤芍..9–12g
mu dan pi (Moutan Cortex) 牡丹皮 9–12g

Method: Decoction. **Shui niu jiao** should be shaved and cooked for 30 minutes prior to the other herbs. **Shui niu jiao** cools the blood and clears toxic heat; **sheng di** cools the blood, protects yin and reinforces the action of **shui niu jiao**; **chi shao** and **mu dan pi** cool the blood and Liver, activate blood and disperse blood stasis. **Shui niu jiao** is used instead of **xi jiao** (Rhinocerotis Cornu) 犀角, the horn of the critically endangered rhinoceros. (Source: *Qian Jin Yao Fang*)

Modifications
- When there is bleeding and damage to yin and blood, use **bai shao** (Paeoniae Radix alba) 白芍 9–12g instead of **chi shao**.
- With severe heat, add **da qing ye** (Isatidis Folium) 大青叶 15–30g and **ban lan gen** (Isatidis/Baphicacanthis Radix) 板蓝根 15–30g.
- With petechial hemorrhage, add **qian cao gen** (Rubiae Radix) 茜草根 9–12g, **zi cao** (Arnebiae/Lithospermi Radix) 紫草 9–12g and **xuan shen** (Scrophulariae Radix) 玄参 15–18g.

- With qi constraint and Liver fire (inflammation of the eyes, temporal head-ache, scleral hemorrhage), add **chai hu** (Bupleuri Radix) 柴胡 9–12g and **huang qin** (Scutellariae Radix) 黄芩 9–12g.
- With confusion, delirium or psychosis, add **shi chang pu** (Acori tatarinowii Rhizoma) 石菖蒲 6–9g, **dan nan xing** (Arisaema cum Bile) 胆南星 6–9g and **tian zhu huang** (Bambusae Concretio silicea) 天竺黄 6–9g.
- With epistaxis, add **bai mao gen** (Imperatae Rhizoma) 白茅根 15–30g and **huai niu xi** (Achyranthis bidentatae Radix) 怀牛膝 12–15g.
- With rectal bleeding, add **di yu** (Sanguisorbae Radix) 地榆 9–12g and **huai hua** (Sophora Flos immaturus) 槐花 12–15g.
- With hematuria, add **bai mao gen** (Imperatae Rhizoma) 白茅根 15–30g and **xiao ji** (Cirsii Herba) 小蓟 12–15g.
- With jaundice, combine with YIN CHEN HAO TANG (Virgate Wormwood De-coction 茵陈蒿汤, p.922).

Prepared medicines
See heat in the ying level p.350.

Acupuncture (select from)
PC.3 (quze ↓).....................sea points of the Pericardium and Urinary Bladder
Bl.40 (weizhong ↓)   channels respectively, these points clear heat from the blood
LI.11 (quchi –)...................sea point of the Large Intestine, clears heat
PC.1 (zhongchong ↓) ....well point of Pericardium channel, clears heat and cools the Heart and Pericardium
Ht.9 (shaochong ↓)............well point of Heart channel, clears heat, cools the Heart and calms the shen
Kid.7 (fuliu –)....................clears and vents heat from the ying and blood levels
Kid.2 (rangu –) ....clears heat from shaoyin
- with serious confusion or delirium, add Du.26 (renzhong –) and bleed the tips of all ten fingers, or the well points on each finger
- with bleeding, add Sp.10 (xuehai –)
- Ear points: ear apex ↓, shenmen, sympathetic, adrenal

Clinical notes
- Heat in the blood may be diagnosed as hemorrhagic fever, septicemia, menin-gococcal meningitis, encephalitis, thrombocytopenic purpura, acute leukemia, hepatic encephalopathy, or acute flare up of connective tissue disease such as systemic lupus erythematosus or Behçet's disease.
- This is a serious illness, and when associated with a major and potentially fatal or debilitating infection, should be managed in hospital.

Table 7.1 Summary of common acute fever patterns

Pattern		Fever and common features	Specific features	Prescription
Wei level		usually mild to moderate; rarely high	Aversion to wind, sore throat, headache, nasal congestion, cough, slight sweat, red tipped tongue, floating pulse. Classically associated with simultaneous chills, but in practice this is often absent, or so mild that it is not seen.	Yin Qiao San
Qi level	Lung heat	high continuous fever, or tidal fever	loud painful cough, dyspnea	Ma Xiang Shi Gan Tang
	yangming channel syndrome	thirst and dryness sweating	severe thirst, copious sweating, surging, rapid pulse	Bai Hu Tang
	yangming organ syndrome		constipation, abdominal pain, palpable mass in the left iliac fossa	Da Cheng Qi Tang
	damp heat	afternoon fever	lethargy, muscles aches, sore throat	Gan Lu Xiao Du Yin
Shaoyang level		distinct alternating periods of fever and chills	fatigue, dizziness, bitter or bad taste in the mouth, nausea, wiry pulse	Xiao Chai Hu Tang / Da Chai Hu Tang
Toxic heat	toxic heat, systemic	high fever or fever and rigors	general malaise, suppurative skin lesions, lymphangitis, severe restlessness	Huang Lian Jie Du Tang / Qing Wen Bai Du Yin
	toxic heat, localized in the head and throat	red tongue	severe sore throat, swelling, redness and pain in the head and face, general malaise	Pu Ji Xiao Du Yin

Table 7.1 Summary of common acute fever patterns (cont.)

	Pattern	Fever and common features	Specific features	Prescription
Internal organs	Liver Gallbladder damp heat	moderate afternoon fever; occasionally high fever or fever and rigors greasy yellow tongue coat	hypochondriac pain, bitter taste, jaundice	Long Dan Xie Gan Tang
	Spleen Stomach damp heat		nausea, vomiting	Lian Po Yin
	Large Intestine damp heat		urgent burning diarrhea	Ge Gen Huang Qin Huang Lian Tang
	Urinary Bladder damp heat		painful or burning urination, suprapubic or lower back and loin pain	Ba Zheng San
	damp heat or toxic heat in the Uterus		lower abdominal pain with muscle guarding, offensive discharge	Yin Qiao Hong Jiang Jie Du Tang
Heat in the ying level		moderate to high fever, worse at night deep red or scarlet tongue	faint rashes, mild disturbance of consciousness	Qing Ying Tang
Heat in the blood			purpura, hemorrhage, delirium	Shui Niu Jiao Di Huang Tang

APPENDIX: CLASSIFICATION OF PATHOGENS THAT CAN CAUSE FEVER

There are many illnesses that can produce acute fever. In the traditional literature a great deal of attention was paid to the analysis and treatment of fever, due to the fact that in pre–modern times, diseases with fever were the major cause of death and morbidity, both in China and the rest of the world. Numerous analytical systems were developed in different parts of China in response to local climactic and environmental conditions. These models share some overlapping characteristics, but are distinguished on the basis of the primary pathogen. These systems are still of clinical value and can be adapted to the prevailing climate in which one practices.

There are 6 models described in standard texts.
1. Wind warmth/heat (*fēng wēn* 风温)
2. Damp warmth/heat (*shī wēn* 湿温)
3. Summer warmth (*shǔ wēn* 暑温)
4. Heat stroke (*zhōng shǔ* 中暑)
5. Autumn dryness (*qiū zào* 秋燥)
6. Spring warmth (*chūn wēn* 春温)

In addition to seasonal pathogens, Chinese texts place several other major illnesses with fever in the external pathogenic invasion category. These are Dysenteric disorder (*lì jí* 痢疾, Clinical Handbook, Vol.2), Sudden Turmoil Disorder (*huò luàn* 霍乱, Clinical Handbook, Vol.2) and Acute Exterior disorders (*gǎn mào* 感冒, Clinical Handbook, Vol.1).

Table 7.2 Wind warmth [*fēng wēn* 风温 wind heat fevers]

Wind warmth is caused by invasion of a wind heat pathogen. These patterns can occur at any time of the year, and in all climates but are more common in hot, dry environments. This group may be diagnosed as illnesses as diverse as the common cold, influenza, tracheitis, acute bronchitis and pneumonia, (bacterial and viral), and infectious encephalomeningitis. (Source: *Shi Yong Zhong Yi Nei Ke Xue*)

	Pattern	Features	Prescription
Wei level		fever, mild chills, aversion to wind, sore throat, headache, nasal congestion, cough, no sweat or slight sweat, red tipped tongue, floating pulse	Yin Qiao San San Ju Yin
Qi level	Heat in the Lungs	fever, dry hacking cough with scant yellow or blood streaked sputum, dyspnea, thirst, yellow tongue coat, rapid pulse	Ma Xing Shi Gan Tang
	Phlegm heat in the Lungs with constipation	fever, productive cough with copious sticky yellow or green sputum, constipation, greasy yellow tongue coat, slippery rapid pulse	Xuan Bai Cheng Qi Tang
	Yangming heat	high fever, sweating, thirst, surging pulse	Bai Hu Tang
	Phlegm heat knotting in the chest	fever, focal chest pain, barking painful cough with sticky yellow sputum, bitter taste, yellow tongue coat	Xiao Xian Xiong Tang
	Yangming heat with constipation	fever or tidal fever, sweating, constipation or impacted stool with a hard mass palpable in the left iliac fossa, abdominal pain, tension and fullness, clammy hands and feet, delirium or confusion	Da Cheng Qi Tang Xiao Cheng Qi Tang Tiao Wei Cheng Qi Tang Zeng Ye Cheng Qi Tang
	Heat lingering in the chest and diaphragm	fever, insomnia, fitful sleep, thirst and dryness, restlessness and irritability, sense of heat in the chest, thin, yellow tongue coat	Zhi Zi Chi Tang
Ying level	Heat affecting the Pericardium	fever worse at night, dry mouth with little desire to drink, insomnia, restlessness, faint skin rash, mild delirium or confusion, scarlet tongue, fine, rapid pulse	Qing Ying Tang
	Heat blocking the Pericardium	as for heat affecting the Pericardium with more severe disturbance of consciousness	An Gong Niu Huang Wan Zhi Bao Dan

Table 7.2 Wind warmth (cont.)

	Pattern	Features	Prescription
Blood level	Heat causing blood to move recklessly	fever which may be relatively high or tidal, distinct maculopapular rash or subcutaneous hemorrhage, bleeding from various sites	Shi Niu Jiao Di Huang Wan Hua Ban Tang Qing Wen Bai Du Yin
	Heat and blood stagnation	tidal fever, lower abdominal pain, constipation or black, sticky stools (melena), disturbances of consciousness, red or purple tongue, deep strong pulse	Tao He Cheng Qi Tang
Post acute phase	Lung and Stomach yin and qi damage	low grade fever, dry unproductive cough, dry mouth and thirst, dry tongue with little or no coat	Sha Shen Mai Men Dong Tang
	Liver and Kidney yin damage	low grade fever, heat in the palms and soles, dry mouth and teeth, exhaustion, tinnitus, spasms or tremors in the extremities, scarlet red tongue with no coat, fine rapid pulse	San Jia Fu Mai Tang
	Qi collapse	copious, incessant sweating, ashen complexion, respiratory distress, restlessness, cold extremities, imperceptible or irregular pulse	Sheng Mai San

Table 7.3 Damp warmth [*shi wen* 濕溫 – damp heat fevers]
Acute febrile illness from damp or damp and heat in varying proportions. This system of analysis was devised for the febrile illness of the humid and tropical parts of China, the south and south east. Damp heat fevers may be diagnosed as a variety of tropical and subtropical infections, including gastroenteritis, summer flu, typhoid fever, infectious encephalitis, acute icteric hepatitis, cholecystitis and cholangitis or leptospirosis. (Source: *Shi Yong Zhong Yi Nei Ke Xue*)

	Pattern	Features	Prescription
Wei level		low grade fever and chills, muscle aches, no sweat, heaviness and foggy head, chest oppression, no thirst, lethargy, greasy white tongue coat, soggy pulse, greasy white tongue coat	Huo Po Xia Ling Tang
Qi level	Damp heat; damp predominant	low grade fever or contained fever that rises in the afternoon, heavy head, muscle aches, headache, chest oppression, diarrhea, abdominal distension, greasy white or yellow tongue coat	San Ren Tang
	Damp and heat more or less equal	distinct afternoon fever with a sticky sweat that does not break the fever, dry mouth without a desire to drink, irritability, chest oppression, nausea and vomiting, concentrated urine, diarrhea, vesicular skin rash, jaundice, thick, greasy, yellow coat, slippery, rapid pulse	Lian Po Yin Gan Lu Xao Du Yin Chang Pu Yu Jin Tang
	Damp heat with heat predominant	high fever, thirst, red complexion, sweating, breathlessness, greasy, yellow tongue coat	Bai Hu Jia Cang Zhu Tang
	Damp heat transforming into dryness	high fever, profuse sweating, dehydration, red complexion, intense thirst, surging pulse	Bai Hu Tang
Ying and blood levels	Damp heat in the ying/blood	fever worse at night, irritability and restlessness, confusion or delirium, muscle spasms, tics or febrile convulsions, petechial skin rash, scarlet tongue with little or no coat	Qing Ying Tang

Table 7.4 Summerheat warmth [*shǔ wēn* 暑温 – summerheat fevers]
Summerheat illnesses occur during the height of summer. Depending on the climate, summerheat illnesses can be complicated by varying degrees of damp. One of the characteristic features of summerheat disorders is their ability to damage qi and yin very quickly. (Source: *Shi Yong Zhong Yi Nei Ke Xue, Zhong Yi Nei Ke Shou Ce*)

Pattern	Features	Prescription
Summerheat in the qi level	fever, mild thirst, foggy head or light-headedness, pink tongue with a thin white coat	Qing Luo Yin
Summerheat attacking the Lungs and surface	fever with sweating, slight aversion to wind, cough, head distension, joint aches, dry mouth, chest oppression, heaviness in the body, greasy tongue coat	Huang Lian Xiang Ru Yin
Summerheat affecting the Stomach and Intestines	high fever with copious sweating, irritability, pounding headache, red complexion, thirst, constipation, dry yellow tongue coat, big surging pulse	Bai Hu Jia Ren Shen Tang
Summerheat damaging fluids and qi	high fever, breathlessness, irritability, thirst, copious sweating, lethargy, concentrated urine, red dry tongue with yellow coat, fine weak pulse	Wang Shi Qing Shu Yi Qi Tang
Summerheat in the ying and blood levels	fever, irritability, insomnia, dry mouth, delirium, rashes, bleeding, scarlet tongue with a dry brown or black coat	Qing Ying Tang Shui Niu Jiao Di Huang Tang
Summerheat generating wind	high fever, spasms or tremor in the extremities and neck, convulsions, disturbances of consciousness, scarlet tongue, fine rapid wiry pulse	Qing Ying Tang + Ling Jiao Gou Teng Tang Da Ding Feng Zhu San Jia Fu Mai Tang
Summerheat causing collapse	high fever, delirium, copious oily sweat, surging pulse – this may quickly progress into loss of consciousness, respiratory distress, icy cold extremities, imperceptible pulse	Zi Xue Dan An Gong Niu Huang Wan Shen Fu Long Mu Tang
Summerheat with damp	high fever, thirst, heaviness in the head and body, joint aches, nausea, sweating, abdominal distension, red tongue with a greasy yellow tongue coat, soggy, rapid pulse	Bai Hu Jia Cang Zhu Tang

Table 7.5 Heatstroke [*zhòng shǔ* 中暑]

Heatstroke is the response of the body to exposure to the sun. After prolonged exposure, the body is unable to shed heat and cool itself, internal body temperature rises, excessive fluid is lost in sweat and severe dehydration and hypovolemic shock can occur. (Source: *Shi Yong Zhong Yi Nei Ke Xue*)

Pattern	Features	Prescription
Heatstroke of a yang type (severe heat in the qi level)	high fever, copious sweating, great thirst, scanty concentrated urine, red dry tongue, surging pulse	Bai Hu Tang Bai Hu Jia Ren Shen Tang Zhu Ye Shi Gao Tang
	with damp: fever with aversion to cold, irritability, thirst, diarrhea, headache, concentrated urine or dysuria, nausea and vomiting, greasy yellow tongue coat, surging pulse	Huang Lian Xiang Ru Yin Gui Ling Gan Lu Yin Bai Hu Jia Cang Zhu Tang
Heatstroke of a yin type (hypovolemic shock)	This stage occurs as a result of transformation of the yang type, which having reached its maxima, suddenly switches to the yin type. Low fever, copious sweating, lassitude, cold limbs, respiratory distress, diarrhea, pallor, fading consciousness, imperceptible pulse	Sheng Mai San + Shen Fu Long Mu Tang
Summerheat harassing the Heart	high fever with mania, disturbances of consciousness and delirium	An Gong Niu Huang Wan Zhi Bao Dan Zi Xue Dan
Liver wind generated by the heat	high fever with muscle spasms, tremors and convulsions	San Jia Fu Mai Tang

Table 7.6 Autumn dryness [*qiū zào* 秋燥 – dryness with heat or cold]
This system was devised for the febrile illnesses of the north and west of China, where the prevailing climate is windy, dry and desiccating.
(Source: *Shi Yong Zhong Yi Nei Ke Xue*)

Pattern	Features	Prescription
Cool dryness	mild fever, aversion to wind and cold, headache, no sweating, nasal congestion with dry mucus membranes, dry lips and mouth, dry unproductive cough, floating pulse	Xing Su San
Warm dryness	mild fever, aversion to wind, headache, mild sweating, dry unproductive cough, dry mucus membranes, thirst, red tongue tip with thin dry white coat, floating rapid pulse	Sang Xing Tang
Dryness transforming into heat	fever, hacking unproductive cough, or cough with scant blood streaked sputum, breathlessness, chest pain, irritability, thirst, dry mucous membranes, constipation, red tongue with a thin dry white or yellow tongue coat, rapid fine pulse	Qing Zao Jiu Fei Tang
Lung and Stomach yin damage	low grade fever, dryness of mucous membranes, red tongue with a peeled centre, fine pulse	Sha Shen Mai Dong Tang

Table 7.7 Spring warmth [chūn wēn 春溫]

Spring warmth fevers start abruptly with the features of a deep level heat pattern (qi, ying or blood). The typical progression from the wei level is absent. Spring warmth is thought to be due to invasion of a cold pathogen during winter, into a compromised patient. The weakness of the hosts defenses leads to a poor response on the surface, which enables the pathogen to quickly gain access to the deeper levels of the body. Once the pathogen has gained access, the host zheng qi is unable to expel it, and the pathogen goes into hiding. In the spring, a new invasion, or the ascendancy of wood energy and arousal of Liver and Gallbladder qi, reactivates the pathogen. This is a 'lurking pathogen' that is, one that invades in one season, sits quietly, then emerges in another season fully formed, without the typical sequential invasion through the shallower levels. Even though these disorders are called spring warmth, they can occur at other times of the year. They may be diagnosed as diseases such as infectious or viral encephalitis or meningitis, bacteremia or septicemia. (Source: *Zhong Yi Nei Ke Shou Ce*)

	Pattern		Features	Prescription
Qi level	Heat in the chest and diaphragm		mild fever, or a sensation of heat in the chest, irritability and restlessness, thirst, dry red lips, flushed complexion, constipation, red tongue with a dry yellow coat, slippery rapid pulse	Liang Ge San
	Heat accumulating in the Gallbladder		fever, bitter taste, irritability, thirst, headache, nausea and vomiting, right hypochondriac pain, red tongue with a yellow coat, wiry rapid pulse	Huang Qin Tang
	Heat in the yangming channels		high fever, copious sweating, great thirst, flushed complexion, irritability, red dry tongue with a yellow coat, surging or slippery and rapid pulse	Bai Hu Tang
	Heat in the Stomach and Intestines (yangming organ syndrome)	with fluid damage	fever or tidal fever, abdominal distension and pain, constipation, dry mouth, thick dry yellow or brown tongue coat, deep fine rapid pulse	Zeng Ye Cheng Qi Tang
		with qi and yin deficiency	afternoon fever, abdominal distension and pain, constipation or foul watery diarrhea, dryness, lethargy, delirium, deep weak pulse	Huang Long Tang
		with heat in the Small Intestine	fever, abdominal distension and pain, thirst, constipation, dysuria with dark scanty burning urine, yellow tongue coat, rapid slippery pulse	Dao Chi Cheng Qi Tang

Table 7.7 Spring warmth (cont.)

Pattern		Features	Prescription
Ying level	Heat in the ying level	fever worse at night, irritability and restlessness, mild disturbances of consciousness, faint rashes, dry mouth and throat without desire to drink, deep red or scarlet tongue without coat, fine rapid pulse	Qing Ying Tang
	Heat disturbing the Pericardium	blocking the Pericardium	as for heat in the ying level with severe delirium	Qing Xin Wan
		with collapse	delirium or loss of consciousness, panting, cold extremities, copious sweat, fine rapid pulse	Sheng Mai San
Blood level	Heat in the blood	fever worse at night, irritability and restlessness, obvious febrile rashes, bleeding, purpura, deep red or scarlet tongue with little or no coat, fine rapid pulse	Shui Niu Jiao Di Huang Tang
	Heat congealing the blood	tidal fever, acute lower abdominal pain and fullness worse for pressure, constipation, delirium or manic behavior, purple red tongue with stasis spots, deep strong or rough pulse	Tao He Cheng Qi Tang
	Heat in the qi and blood levels	high fever, thirst, headache, skin rashes, bleeding, scarlet tongue with a yellow coat, rapid pulse	Yu Nu Jian
	Heat generating wind	high fever, headache and head distension, muscle spasms in the extremities, tremors or convulsions, scarlet tongue, wiry rapid pulse	Ling Yang Jiao Tang
	Heat consuming yin	yin deficiency with fire	fever, insomnia, restlessness, red tongue with dry yellow coat, fine rapid pulse	Huang Lian E Jiao Tang
		Kidney yin consumed	low grade fever, heat in the palms and soles, thirst and dryness, lower back ache, lethargy and restlessness, tinnitus, thin dry red tongue with no coat, fine or intermittent pulse	Jia Wei Fu Mai Tang

CHRONIC FEVER

Chronic fever is defined as a fever that persists or reoccurs over an extended period of time. The duration of a chronic fever may be from several weeks to years. Fever of this type is generally low grade, and the fever may be continuous or follow a cyclical pattern, occurring in a regular and predictable fashion. The cyclical pattern of the fever can gives clues as to its origin, both in Chinese medicine and biomedical terms (Figure 8.1). In Chinese medicine, fever of this type is generally considered to be caused by 'internal damage' (*nèi shāng fā rè*[1] 内伤发热). Internal damage type fevers are traditionally due to internally generated pathology such as deficiencies of qi, blood, yin or yang, or excess pathology such

as damp heat, qi and blood stasis. In clinical practice, however, chronic fevers are often the result of lingering pathogens.

Fever in Chinese medicine

In Chinese medicine, fever can be broadly classified into three groups. These are:

1. Acute fever due to pathogens on the surface, i.e. the wei or taiyang level
2. Acute fever due to pathogens in the deeper parts of the body, the qi level, shaoyang, yangming, ying and blood levels or organ systems
3. Low grade, persistent fevers associated with physiological deficiency, lingering pathogens and internal organ system dysfunction

The first type is described in the chapter on acute exterior disorders (Clinical Handbook, Vol.1), the second in acute fever (p.310), and the low grade persistent fevers described in this chapter and in lingering pathogens (p.500).

PATHOLOGY

The mechanism of chronic fever can be divided into excess and deficient types. The excess types are due to the lingering presence of a pathogen, or to internal organ dysfunction. Fever associated with a lingering pathogen occurs as a result of the body's anti–pathogenic qi continuing to exert resistance. The ongoing battle between the weakened opponents creates a low grade fever. In the case of fever from organ system dysfunction, the heat is generated by prolonged stagnation of qi, blood or damp.

The deficiency types of fever are the result of the lack of a physiological sub-

---

1 Practical Dictionary of Chinese Medicine (1998) – 'internal damage heat effusion'

strate, and the resulting pathological imbalance that ensues. Heat of a deficient type is considered to be 'false' heat, that is, the illusion of heat due to a failure of the cooling systems of the body rather than an actual surplus of heat in the system. Yin and blood deficiency can give rise to false heat, due to the relative surplus of yang that is implicit in yin deficiency. Qi and yang deficiency are uncommon causes of fever, and when seen, reflect a relatively severe illness. The appearance of heat is due to the relative inefficiency of the feeble yang qi, the power of which goes into the creation of waste heat rather than useful work, in the same way as an underpowered engine overheats when climbing a steep hill.

Heat derived from deficiency may affect the whole body, or be localized to a specific area, such as the hands and feet, or chest and head. The patient may feel relatively hot or easily overheated, but objective findings may reveal only moderately elevated temperature, normal or even low body temperature. Fever associated with deficiency can fluctuate with the patients energy levels and emotional state.

ETIOLOGY

Lingering pathogens

A persistent low grade fever is common

> **BOX 8.2 BIOMEDICAL CAUSES OF CHRONIC FEVER**
>
> **Infectious**
> * pyogenic abscess (liver, subphrenic, pelvic)
> * urinary tract infection
> * biliary infection (cholangitis)
> * chronic septicemia
> * endocarditis
> * tuberculosis
> * Lyme disease
> * brucellosis
> * osteomyelitis
> * Epstein Barr mononucleosis
> * cytomegalovirus
> * psittacosis
> * Q fever
> * HIV
> * malaria
> * toxoplasmosis
> * amoebiasis
>
> **Malignant**
> * lymphoma
> * leukemia
> * localized tumors
>
> **Other**
> * autoimmune disorders (lupus, rheumatoid arthritis, giant cell arteritis etc.)
> * hyperthyroidism
> * drugs (see Box 8.3, p.366)
> * Crohn's disease
> * familial Mediterranean fever

in the aftermath of an acute febrile illness. The fever may persist because the pathogen responsible for the initial episode has not been completely expelled, or because its presence has damaged qi and/or yin, or congealed fluids into phlegm heat or damp heat. The probability of developing a persistent problem is greater in those who were treated inappropriately or failed to rest during the acute phase. Improper use of purgation, emesis or bitter cold herbs or antibiotics when the pathogen is on the surface will encourage heat to be trapped in the qi level. Persistent fever may follow some immunizations. Immunizations introduce pathogens directly into the muscles and qi level, ying and blood levels. For a more detailed look at the pathology of lingering pathogens, see Chapter 11, p.500.

Overwork, exhaustion

Any factor that exhausts qi or depletes yin and blood can contribute to chronic fever. Working too hard or excessive hours for prolonged periods weakens the Kidneys and depletes Kidney yin and yang. Blood and yin deficiency may be associated with ageing and the onset of menopause, or occur in the aftermath of childbirth or a major blood loss. Yin deficiency is aggravated by insufficient sleep or disrupted sleep cycles. Blood deficiency also occurs in patients with insufficient protein in their diets and in women who breast feed for prolonged periods.

Diet and medications

There are several ways that the diet can contribute to chronic fever. The classic case, described by Li Dong–Yuan in his Treatise on the Spleen and Stomach (*Pí Wèi Lùn* 13th century), describes chronic fever associated with qi deficiency. The qi deficiency was the result of severe malnutrition suffered by citizens of a besieged city. This degree of malnutrition is uncommon today, although similar pathological conditions can be created by fad or starvation diets, the use of slimming aids, as well as anorexia and bulimia nervosa, all of which may seriously damage Spleen qi and yang.

An excess of heating foods such as chillies, coffee, spirits, spices, fats and meat can introduce heat and damp into the body, or damage yin. The inappropriate or profligate use of supplementing or hot herbs, such as aconite or red ginseng can contribute to internal heat and yin depletion.

A number of common pharmaceutical drugs are implicated in persistent fevers. These are noted in Box 8.3.

Emotional factors

Any emotional factor that leads to the generation of heat, damages qi, blood and yin, or reduces their production, may lead to chronic fever. Emotional stress is an important cause of disruption to the Liver, Spleen and qi dynamic. Chronic Liver qi constraint contributes to constrained heat, damp heat, blood stasis and qi, blood and yin deficiency (see Figure 9.1, p.411).

BOX 8.3 MEDICATIONS THAT CAN CAUSE CHRONIC FEVER

Antibiotics
- Carbapenems
- Cephalosporins
- Minocycline HCl
- Nitrofurantoin
- Penicillins
- Rifampin
- Sulfonamides

Anticonvulsants
- Barbiturates
- Carbamazepine
- Phenytoin

Antihistamines

Cardiovascular drugs
- Hydralazine HCl
- Procainamide HCl
- Quinidine

Histamine2 (H2) blockers
- Cimetidine
- Ranitidine HCl

Iodides

Nonsteroidal anti–inflammatory drugs
- Ibuprofen
- Sulindac

Phenothiazines

Salicylates

A consequence of these pathological interactions is the development of the primary pathological triad (PPT). The PPT is at the basis of many common conditions characterized by heat and deficiency seen in the Chinese medicine clinic, including chronic fever. See p.780, for more detail.

Blood stasis

Fever due to blood stasis may be acute or chronic. Acute fever from blood stasis may follow trauma, hemorrhage or surgery. Chronic blood stasis fever may be caused by unresolved blood stasis from an acute trauma, heat from a lingering pathogen congealing the blood or long term qi constraint failing to lead the blood. Chronic blood stasis fever is often associated with tumors or malignancy.

Menopause

Easy overheating, a sense of elevated body temperature, hot flushing and night sweats are a common feature of menopause. The pathology can be complex but often involves depletion of yin and blood (as well as qi and yang) due to the unique aspects of female physiology, the menstrual cycle, childbirth and breast feeding. This is exacerbated by the natural decline of yin that occurs due to ageing.

LOW GRADE FEVER

Chronic fevers are mostly low grade. A low grade fever is a recurrent, tidal elevation in body temperature, or a subjective feeling of heat even though the body temperature is normal or even low. A low grade fever may be obvious, or subtle and not immediately recognized as a fever. Flushing episodes, night sweats, localized heat in parts of the body or restless, fitful sleep may be signs of a low grade fever. There are several subtypes:

Afternoon fever (tidal fever)

An afternoon fever rises in the afternoon, between 3–6pm. Patients may feel relatively normal in the morning, and begin to deteriorate in the early afternoon as the fever rises. The gradual increase and predictability of the fever at this time resembles an incoming tide, and hence this fever type is also known as a tidal fever. Fever rising in the mid afternoon (around 3pm) is more likely to be due to damp heat, while fever rising in the later afternoon (after 5pm), is more likely due to yin deficiency. This is a type of quotidian fever (p.368).

Contained fever

This type of fever is characterized by a sense of heat detected during palpation. Also described as unsurfaced fever, at first touch the skin temperature feels normal or only slightly hot, but the sense of heat increases as palpation proceeds and deepens. The patient may not subjectively feel hot, but may have an objectively elevated temperature. Even when the fever is not clear, there will usually be other corroborating signs of heat, red tongue with a yellow coat, dry mouth and so on. Contained fevers are characteristic of damp heat patterns with damp predominant. The damp gets into the muscles and its sticky viscosity blocks the full expression of the heat on the surface.

Bone steaming fever

A bone steaming fever (*gǔ zhēng* 骨蒸) is a subjective sense of heat emanating from deep within the body, while the skin is not especially warm to the touch. In contrast to contained fever, the patient feels hot. Mostly experienced in the late afternoon and evening and characteristic of relatively severe yin deficiency.

Hectic fever

A hectic fever is a low grade fever that recurs each night and leads to fitful sleep. The fever pattern is of irregular spikes in body temperature, perhaps preceded by chills, but usually without sweating. Also known as tumor fever, a hectic fever is characteristic of blood stasis.

Cyclical fever

Many low grade fevers are cyclical, rising repeatedly at specific times of the day. The type of fever pattern can give clues as to the pathology.

- A quotidian fever (Figure 8.1.a) rises around same time every day. A recurrent fever that spikes in the morning may indicate qi deficiency; fever rising in the mid afternoon suggests damp heat; fever that rises in the late afternoon and evening may suggest yin deficiency; fever that occurs at night may indicate heat in the qi or ying level, or blood stasis. Biomedical diseases with a quotidian fever pattern include localized collections of pus (e.g. pelvic or subphrenic abscess, or empyema of the gall bladder), cytomegalovirus and pseudomonas infection.

- An intermittent fever (Figure 8.1.b) rises for a few hours then returns to normal, usually every few days. This is characteristic of some types of lingering pathogen, of which Malarial disorder (*nüè bìng* 疟病) is the classic example, spiking every three or four days. Biomedical diseases that display an intermittent fever pattern include malaria, Epstein Barr mononucleosis and cytomegalovirus.

- An undulant fever (Figure 8.1.c) is characterized by bouts of continuous fever for several days followed by an afebrile remission lasting a variable number of days or weeks. It is seen in some types of lingering pathogen and blood stasis patterns. Biomedical diseases that display an undulant fever pattern include lymphoma, Hodgkins lymphoma and brucellosis.

PROGNOSIS

The prognosis of chronic fever can be quite variable, and depends on the duration of the problem, the age and overall vitality of the patient, the pattern or patterns involved and the biomedical condition underlying the fever. For example, blood stasis fevers of a traumatic origin in a relatively young individual generally respond reliably and quickly to correct treatment, whereas blood stasis type fever in an older person with malignancy is more difficult and a successful outcome less likely. Similarly, simple yin deficiency fever in a middle aged patient generally responds well, but yin deficiency associated with tuberculosis or in an elderly patient is more difficult. Heat in the blood associated with chronic qi constraint is usually easy to treat, while the prognosis for heat in the blood associated with a connective tissue disease such as Systemic Lupus Erythematosus (SLE) or Beçhets' syndrome is less certain.

Figure 8.1 Chronic fever patterns

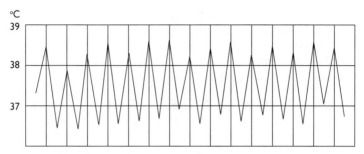

Fig. 8.1.a Quotidian fever pattern (remittent fever, tidal fever)

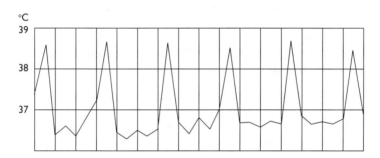

Fig. 8.1.b Intermittent fever pattern

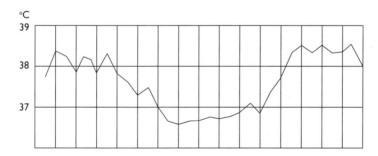

Fig. 8.1.c Undulant fever pattern

8.1 LINGERING PATHOGENS

1. Lingering heat in the qi level (Lungs and Stomach)
2. Shaoyang syndrome
3. Damp heat
4. Summerheat
5. Heat in the ying/blood

热
留
气
分

8.1.1 LINGERING HEAT IN THE QI LEVEL

This common pattern may follow an acute upper respiratory tract infection associated with a wind heat pathogen, a warm disease or Lung heat, or it can be introduced by ingestion of toxic substances or hot natured pharmaceuticals such as chemotherapeutic agents. If the heat pathogen is not cleared, it can linger in the qi level, the Lungs and/or Stomach, consuming fluids and yin and damaging qi.

Depending on whether the Lungs of Stomach are most affected, the main features (in addition to the fever) will vary. When the Lungs are affected, the cough is prominent; when the Stomach is affected, nausea, vomiting and indeterminate gnawing hunger are prominent.

Clinical features
- lingering low grade fever, of weeks to several months duration
- persistent, dry, irritating cough, worse at night
- thirst, dry mouth, lips and throat
- sweating, night sweats
- insomnia, restlessness, fitful sleep
- fatigue, tiredness
- chest oppression
- irritability
- sore throat, loss of voice
- nausea, vomiting
- swollen lymph nodes

T red and dry with little or no coat
P weak, fine, rapid

Treatment principle
Vent heat from the qi level
Supplement qi and generate and replenish fluids

Prescription

ZHU YE SHI GAO TANG 竹叶石膏汤
Lophatherus and Gypsum Decoction

dan zhu ye (Lophateri Herba) 淡竹叶	9–15g
shi gao (Gypsum fibrosum) 石膏	15–30g
zhi ban xia (Pinelliae Rhizoma preparatum) 制半夏	6–9g
mai dong (Ophiopogonis Radix) 麦冬	6–15g
ren shen (Ginseng Radix) 人参	3–9g

zhi gan cao (Glycyrrhizae Radix preparata) 炙甘草 3–9g
jing mi (Oryzae Semen) 粳米 9–15g
Method: Decoction. **Shi gao** is decocted for 30 minutes prior to the other herbs. **Dan zhu ye** and **shi gao** clear heat from the qi level; **ren shen** supplements qi and supports the Spleen, and, with **mai dong**, generates fluids and protects yin; **mai dong** assists in clearing heat; **zhi ban xia** downbears counterflow Stomach qi to stop nausea and vomiting; **zhi gan cao** and **jing mi** assist in strengthening the Spleen and protecting the Stomach. (Source: *Shang Han Lun*)

Modifications

- For Stomach qi and yin damage with nausea and vomiting following chemotherapy, add **yu zhu** (Polygonati odorati Rhizoma) 玉竹 12–15g and **xuan fu hua** (Inulae Flos) 旋复花 12–15g.

Variations and additional prescriptions

Lingering heat in the chest

A mild, yet relatively common variant of the above pattern involves the lingering heat affecting the Heart and shen with little damage to qi or yin. Again following an upper respiratory tract infection, the heat upsets the Heart causing restlessness and irritability, fitful sleep, mild but persistent fever, fatigue and a burning or stifling sensation in the chest. Occasionally the agitation can border on depression and despair. The tongue is not especially red, reflecting the mild nature of the heat, and the pulse is strong and floating in the distal position (reflecting the upper burner). The treatment is to clear and vent heat from the qi level and alleviate irritability with ZHI ZI CHI TANG (Gardenia and Prepared Soybean Decoction 栀子豉汤).

shan zhi zi (Gardeniae Fructus) 山栀子 6–9g
dan dou chi (Sojae Semen preparatum) 淡豆豉 9–12g
Method: Decoction. Boil the **dan dou chi** for 8–10 minutes than add the **shan zhi zi** and cook for a further 5 minutes. **Shan zhi zi** clears heat from all three burners and alleviates irritability; **dan dou chi** drains constrained heat from the chest. (Source: *Shang Han Lun*)

Prepared medicines

Concentrated powders

Zhu Ye Shi Gao Tang (Bamboo Leaves & Gypsum Combination)

Acupuncture (select from)

Lu.7 (lieque –) ....diffuses the Lungs and vents pathogens from the qi level
LI.11 (quchi –) ....these points clear heat from the qi level and Stomach
St.44 (neiting –)
Du.14 (dazhui –) ....meeting point of the yang channels, an important point for clearing lingering pathogens
Du.12 (shenzhu –) ....these points diffuse the Lungs, and clear residual
Du.13 (taodao –)   heat from the chest and Lungs
- with severe irritability, add PC.7 (daling –) and PC.8 (laogong –)
- with dryness and thirst, add Kid.6 (zhaohai +)
- with cough, add Lu.5 (chize –) and Ren.17 (shanzhong)
- with sore throat, add Lu.10 (yuji –)

- with nausea and vomiting, add PC.6 (neiguan –) and Ren.12 (zhongwan)
- with constipation, add Kid.6 (zhaohai +) and St.37 (shangjuxu –)
- Ear points: lung, stomach, zero point, shenmen

Clinical notes

- Lingering heat in the qi level is a common cause of persistent night time fever, cough and nausea in the aftermath of an acute upper respiratory tract infection or gastrointestinal infection. It is especially common in children, and may persist for weeks to months following the initial event.
- When correctly identified, residual pathogenic influences in the qi level can be reliably dispelled, and the qi and fluids quickly replenished. Only a few days to a week or so of treatment is usually necessary.
- Residual heat in the qi level may be diagnosed as the convalescent phase of an upper respiratory or gastrointestinal tract infection, post viral syndrome or the side effects of chemotherapy.

少
阳
证

8.1.2 SHAOYANG SYNDROME

The shaoyang level is the transitional zone between the surface and the interior of the body where pathogens can persist for long periods of time. An equilibrium state is created whereby the zheng qi is unable to eject the pathogen, and the pathogen is contained and unable to penetrate further. The containment process consumes qi and the heat damages yin. Depending on the initial pathogen the intensity of fever may vary. When heat alone is involved the fever will tend to be more prominent. When damp heat is involved the fever episodes are cyclical, low grade or contained.

Clinical features

- Alternating fever and chills; depending on the duration of the pattern, the fever and chills episodes may be quite distinct or subtle. In conditions of relatively short duration, the fever pattern may be so prominent that the patient removes and replaces clothing during the consultation. In more chronic cases, the deficiency aspects may mask the distinctive features of the fever pattern, so that it is expressed in a subtler form. Typical of this is the patient who complains of 'flu like feelings' or getting 'hot and cold' when tired or run down.
- reduced appetite or anorexia
- nausea, often worse in the morning
- fatigue
- hypochondriac pain, distension or tenderness
- fullness in the chest
- dizziness
- irritability
- bitter taste in the mouth; food tastes bad
- swollen lymph nodes

T maybe unremarkable, or coated on the left side, or slightly red on the edges
P wiry

Treatment principle

Harmonize shaoyang

Prescription

XIAO CHAI HU TANG 小柴胡汤

Minor Bupleurum Decoction

chai hu (Bupleuri Radix) 柴胡	12–24g
huang qin (Scutellariae Radix) 黄芩	6–12g
zhi ban xia (Pinelliae Rhizoma preparatum) 制半夏	6–9g
ren shen (Ginseng Radix) 人参	6–9g
zhi gan cao (Glycyrrhizae Radix preparata) 炙甘草	3–6g
sheng jiang (Zingiberis Rhizoma recens) 生姜	6–9g
da zao (Jujubae Fructus) 大枣	4 fruit

Method: Decoction. **Chai hu** vents pathogens from shaoyang and regulates qi; **huang qin** clears heat from the Liver, Gallbladder and shaoyang. Together these two herbs are the main pair for dispelling pathogens from the shaoyang level. **Zhi ban xia** and **sheng jiang** harmonize the Stomach, downbear counterflow Stomach qi and stop nausea; **ren shen** and **zhi gan cao** strengthen anti–pathogenic qi and assist in preventing the pathogen from penetrating further; **sheng jiang** and **da zao** support **zhi ban xia** in harmonizing the Stomach and stopping nausea and vomiting. (Source: *Shang Han Lun*)

Modifications

- With damp (muscle aches, alternating fever and chills, with chills greater than fever, heaviness and a thick white tongue coat) add **cang zhu** (Atractylodis Rhizoma) 苍术 12–15g, **hou po** (Magnoliae officinalis Cortex) 厚朴 9–12g and **chen pi** (Citri reticulatae Pericarpium) 陈皮 9–12g.

Variations and additional prescriptions

Damp heat lodged in the shaoyang level

Depending on locality and climate, different pathogens can lodge in the shaoyang. In tropical or warm humid climates, the prevailing pathogen is damp heat, which produces a somewhat different clinical picture than that above. In addition to the characteristic alternating fever and chill pattern with fever predominant, there is night sweats, nausea and vomiting, aching and heaviness in the muscles, heavy and foggy head, a thick, greasy, yellow tongue coat and a wiry, rapid, slippery pulse. The treatment is to clear damp heat from shaoyang and harmonize the Stomach with **HAO QIN QING DAN TANG** (Sweet Wormwood and Scutellaria Decoction to Clear the Gallbladder 蒿芩清胆汤).

qing hao (Artemisiae annuae Herba) 青蒿	12–15g
huang qin (Scutellariae Radix) 黄芩	6–9g
zhu ru (Bambusae Caulis in taeniam) 竹茹	9–12g
zhi ban xia (Pinelliae Rhizoma preparatum) 制半夏	9–12g
chi fu ling (Poria Rubra) 赤茯苓	9–12g
chen pi (Citri reticulatae Pericarpium) 陈皮	3–6g
zhi ke (Aurantii Fructus) 枳壳	6–9g
qing dai (Indigo naturalis) 青黛	1.5–3g
hua shi (Talcum) 滑石	12–18g

gan cao (Glycyrrhizae Radix) 甘草 3–6g
Method: Decoction. **Hua shi** is decocted in a cloth bag; **qing hao** is added towards the end of cooking; **qing dai** is added to the strained decoction. **Qing hao** and **huang qin** clear damp heat from shaoyang and cool the Liver and Gallbladder; **qing hao** is especially good at finding and expelling deeply rooted pathogens; **zhu ru** clears heat and stops vomiting, and with **zhi ban xia** transforms phlegm and downbears counterflow Stomach qi; **chen pi** and **zhi ke** harmonize the Stomach, transform damp and rectify the qi dynamic; **chi fu ling, qing dai** and **hua shi** promote urination to provide an outlet for damp heat; **gan cao** harmonizes the other herbs in the prescription. Source: (*Chong Ding Tong Su Shang Han Lun*)

Prepared medicines
Concentrated powders
Xiao Chai Hu Tang (Minor Bupleurum Combination)
Pills
Xiao Chai Hu Wan (Minor Bupleurum Teapills)

Acupuncture (select from)
SJ.5 (waiguan –).................these points vent pathogens from shaoyang, and
GB.39 (xuanzhong –)   regulate Liver qi
GB.41 (zulinqi –)
GB.34 (yanglingquan –)
• with marked fever, add Du.14 (dazhui –)
• with damp or damp heat, add Sp.9 (yinlingquan –) and Kid.7 (fuliu –)
• with qi deficiency, add St.36 (zusanli +) and Liv.13 (zhangmen +)
• with nausea, add PC.6 (neiguan –) and Bl.21 (weishu)
• with hypochondriac pain, add Liv.14 (qimen –) and Bl.19 (danshu –)
• with dizziness, add GB.20 (fengchi) and GB.43 (xiaxi –)
• Ear points: liver, gall bladder, stomach, zero point, shenmen, sympathetic

Clinical notes
• Shaoyang syndrome may be diagnosed as post viral or chronic fatigue syndrome, influenza, the convalescent phase of an upper respiratory tract infection, glandular fever, postpartum fever or cholecystitis.
• Shaoyang syndrome is a common cause of persistent fever. Typically patients will have had an acute exterior wind cold, wind heat or damp heat pattern that was for some reason unresolved. The initial symptoms of the acute exterior disorder give way to feelings of heat and cold, fatigue and loss of appetite. Patients may harbor pathogens in the shaoyang for weeks, months or even years.
• When correctly identified, shaoyang patterns respond well to treatment. Patterns of weeks to a few months duration can be resolved within a few days. The more deficiency there is, the slower the resolution, but even pathogens of many months duration can often be resolved in a couple of weeks. Once the pathogen is expelled, the strategy should focus on rebuilding damaged qi and yin.

湿
热

8.1.3 DAMP HEAT

Chronic fever of a damp heat type is common, especially in humid climates, and may be the result of an invasion of damp heat, summerheat or a warm disease that was never fully resolved. Damp heat fever will occasionally follow a surgical procedure that inadvertently introduces a pathogen. This is seen in post–operative abscess and wound infection.

Damp heat being sticky and viscous, can linger for long periods of time, and may appear to resolve only to reappear during periods of humid weather, over-work, poor diet or stress. The damp heat may affect the qi level or a specific organ system such as the gastrointestinal, Liver Gallbladder and Urinary Bladder sys-tems. Damp heat can also accumulate in the sinuses and inner ears (parts of the body aligned with the qi level and shaoyang respectively). The fever described here is due to damp heat in the qi level.

Clinical features

- Lingering or recurrent low grade fever which rises or reaches a peak mid afternoon. The fever may be accompanied by a sticky or oily sweat that begins as the fever reaches its peak. When damp is predominant, the fever may not be obvious at first, instead the heat is felt upon palpation. At first touch the skin temperature feels normal or slightly hot, but the sense of heat increases as palpation proceeds. This is a contained fever. See p.367.
- night sweats, warm clammy palms
- muscle aches, especially the large proximal muscles
- heaviness in the limbs, head and body; foggy head
- fatigue, lethargy
- fullness in the chest and abdomen, chest oppression
- loss of appetite, nausea
- loose stools, or sticky or difficult to pass stools
- no thirst
- swollen lymph nodes

T thick, greasy, white or yellow coat
P slippery, wiry or soft; maybe rapid

Treatment Principle

Clear damp heat from the qi level
Harmonize the middle burner and rectify the qi dynamic
Promote urination to provide an outlet for the damp heat

Prescription

SAN REN TANG 三仁汤
Three Nut Decoction, modified

xing ren (Pruni Semen) 杏仁	12–15g
yi ren (Coicis Semen) 苡仁	18–30g
bai dou kou (Amomi Fructus rotundus) 白豆蔻	6–9g
zhi ban xia (Pinelliae Rhizoma preparata) 制半夏	9–12g

hou po (Magnoliae officinalis Cortex) 厚朴 6–9g
dan zhu ye (Lophatheri Herba) 淡竹叶 6–9g
hua shi (Talcum) 滑石 18g
huang qin (Scutellariae Radix) 黄芩 6–9g
huang lian (Coptidis Rhizoma) 黄连 3–6g
gua lou (Trichosanthis Fructus) 栝楼 15–24g
ge gen (Puerariae Radix) 葛根 12–18g

Method: Decoction. **Bai dou kou** is added towards the end of cooking; **hua shi** is cooked in a cloth bag. The pungent bitterness of **xing ren** diffuses the Lungs, directs Lung qi downwards, and assists the Lungs control over the water passages to facilitate urination; **bai dou kou** fragrantly transforms damp and stimulates the qi dynamic; **yi ren** promotes urination to clear damp heat; **zhi ban xia** and **hou po** are bitter, warm, drying and descending, and assist **xing ren** and **bai dou kou** in moving qi and freeing up the qi dynamic; **dan zhu ye** and **hua shi** promote urination to clear damp heat; **huang qin** and **huang lian** clear damp heat; **gua lou** clears heat and transforms phlegm, unbinds the chest and promotes qi movement; **ge gen** promotes dispersal of pathogenic heat to the exterior and elevates yang qi to balance the descending of the bitter herbs, thus stimulating the qi dynamic. (Source: *Zhong Yi Nei Ke Xue* [*Wen Bing Tiao Bian*])

Modifications

- With less heat and a white tongue coat, delete **huang qin** and **huang lian**.
- With an alternating fever and chill pattern, indicating damp heat affecting the shaoyang level, add **qing hao** (Artemisiae annuae Herba) 青蒿 9–15g [added towards the end].
- With jaundice, add **yin chen** (Artemisiae scopariae Herba) 茵陈 12–18g and **shan zhi zi** (Gardeniae Fructus) 山栀子 9–12g.
- With nausea and vomiting, add **chen pi** (Citri reticulatae Pericarpium) 陈皮 6–9g, **sheng jiang** (Zingiberis Rhizoma recens) 生姜 6–9g and **zhu ru** (Bambusae Caulis in taeniam) 竹茹 9–12g.
- With prominent damp, muscle aches and foggy head, add **huo xiang** (Pogostemonis/Agastaches Herba) 藿香 12–15g and **shi chang pu** (Acori tatarowii Rhizoma) 石菖蒲 6–9g.
- With sluggish or difficult stools, add **chao bai zhu** (stir fried Atractylodes macrocephalae Rhizoma) 炒白术 6–9g and **zhi shi** (Aurantii Fructus immaturus) 枳实 6–9g, or **bing lang** (Arecae Semen) 槟榔 6–9g and **lai fu zi** (Raphani Semen) 莱菔子 6–9g.
- With epigastric distension, add **chao shan zha** (stir fried Crataegi Fructus) 炒山楂 12–15g and **zhi shi** (Aurantii Fructus immaturus) 枳实 6–9g.
- With headache or heaviness in the head, add **bai zhi** (Angelicae dahuricae Radix) 白芷 6–9g, **qiang huo** (Notopterygii Rhizoma seu Radix) 羌活 6–9g and **chuan xiong** (Chuanxiong Rhizoma) 川芎 6–9g.

Variations and additional prescriptions

Damp heat, with heat predominant, concentrated in the digestive system

This prescription is selected for damp heat or summerheat invasion with heat predominant. The main features are relatively high, persistent afternoon fever that is unrelieved by sweating, accompanied by nausea, vomiting and diarrhea, fullness in the chest and epigastrium, irritability and restlessness, concentrated urine, a greasy yellow tongue coat and slippery, rapid pulse. There may also be small, itchy, fluid filled vesicular eruptions on the neck and trunk (miliaria crystallina), a sign of damp heat in the muscles. The treatment is to clear damp heat, move qi and transform turbidity with LIAN PO YIN (Coptis and Magnolia Bark Drink 连朴饮).

huang lian (Coptidis Rhizoma) 黄连 3–6g
hou po (Magnoliae officinalis Cortex) 厚朴.. 6–9g
shan zhi zi (Gardeniae Fructus) 山栀子 9–12g
dan dou chi (Sojae Semen preparatum) 淡豆豉 9–12g
shi chang pu (Acori tatarinowii Rhizoma) 石菖蒲 6–9g
zhi ban xia (Pinelliae Rhizoma preparatum) 制半夏 6–9g
lu gen (Phragmitis Rhizoma) 芦根 30–60g

Method: Decoction. Lu gen is soaked for 60 minutes before cooking to rehydrate. **Huang lian** and **shan zhi zi** clear damp heat and, being bitter and descending, combine well with the ascending pungent warmth of **zhi ban xia** and **shi chang pu** to correct the qi dynamic; **zhi ban xia** transforms dampness, downbears counterflow Stomach qi and stops vomiting; **hou po** directs qi downwards and alleviates distension; **dan dou chi** and **shan zhi zi** clear heat from the qi level and alleviate irritability; **shi chang pu** rouses the Spleen and transforms dampness; **lu gen** clears heat from the Stomach and stops vomiting. (Source: *Shi Yong Fang Ji Xue* [*Huo Luan Lun*])

Other locations and presentations of damp heat

There are different approaches to the treatment of chronic damp heat fever, depending on the location of the damp heat. If the organ system or structure where the damp heat is located can be identified, prescriptions that specifically target these areas can be selected. For xample, if the damp heat is concentrated in the Liver Gallbladder system, consider LONG DAN XIE GAN TANG (Gentian Decoction to Purge the Liver 龙胆泻肝汤 p.337). If there is jaundice use YIN CHEN HAO TANG (Virgate Wormwood Decoction 茵陈蒿汤, p.922). For damp heat in the Large Intestine consider SHAO YAO TANG (Peony Decoction 芍药汤, p.918). See also the relevant section in Hypochondriac Pain (Vol. 1), Abdominal Pain (Vol. 2) or Painful Urination (Vol. 1).

Prepared medicines

Concentrated powders

San Ren Tang (Triple Nut Combination)
Gan Lu Xiao Du Dan (Forsythia & Acorus Formula)
    – with heat greater than damp

Pills

Bi Xie Sheng Shi Wan (Subdue the Dampness Teapills)
Long Dan Xie Gan Wan (Snake and Dragon Teapills)
    – damp heat affecting the Liver
Ba Zheng San Wan (Eight Righteous Teapills)
    – damp heat in the Kidney and Urinary Bladder
Huang Lian Jie Du Wan (Huang Lian Jie Du Teapills)
    – damp heat in the Intestines
Chuan Xin Lian Kang Yan Pian (Chuan Xin Lian Antiphlogistic Tablets)
Huang Lian Su Pian (Coptis Teapills, Tabellae Berberini)

Acupuncture (select from)

Lu.7 (lieque –)....................diffuses the Lungs and vents pathogens from the qi level

SJ.5 (waiguan –).................connecting point of the triple burner, clears heat and facilitates qi flow through the triple burner

SI.4 (wangu –) ....source point of the Small Intestine, clears damp heat

Sp.9 (yinlingquan –)...........water and metal points of the Spleen, these points

Sp.5 (shangqiu –)   clear heat and promote urination to drain damp heat

Ren.5 (shimen –).................alarm point of the triple burner, clears damp heat

Kid.7 (fuliu –)....................promotes urination and vents pathogens

- with high fever add Du.14 (dazhui –)
- with muscle aches, add Sp.21 (dabao –)
- with nausea add PC.6 (neiguan)
- with diarrhea add zhixie (N–CA–3) and Bl.25 (tianshu)
- Ear points: spleen, stomach, lung, zero point, shenmen

Clinical notes

- Damp heat chronic fever may be diagnosed as a chronic infection, such as cytomegalovirus, glandular fever, chronic fatigue syndrome, fibromyalgia, cholangitis, enteric fever, pyelonephritis, hepatic, pelvic or subphrenic abscess or undulant fever.
- The source of the damp heat should be investigated thoroughly to rule out pathologies better suited to surgical or biomedical intervention, such as abscesses that should be opened and drained.

暑伤津气   8.1.4 SUMMERHEAT WITH QI AND FLUID DAMAGE

In hot climates, the middle and late period of summer brings clusters of summerheat disorders, characterized by high fever, profuse sweating, restlessness and thirst. The summerheat pathogen is yang in nature, and easily damages fluids and qi. This pattern can progress quite rapidly, and if poorly treated or incompletely resolved, may lead to a lingering summerheat pathogen that can persist following the initial episode. This pattern is differentiated from the acute summerheat episode, described in Acute exterior disorders (Vol.1), by the complication of severe fluid damage and qi deficiency which compounds the body's inability to expel the pathogen and initiate recovery.

Clinical features

- persistent or recurrent low grade fever
- profuse sweating; constant clamminess
- scanty, concentrated urine
- thirst
- irritability
- fatigue, listlessness, low spirits
- shortness of breath
- weakness of the limbs
- epigastric and abdominal distension

- loss of appetite
- swollen lymph nodes

T dry, yellow or geographic, peeled coat
P weak, fine and slightly rapid

Treatment Principle

Clear and vent summerheat
Supplement qi, replenish fluids and nourish yin

Prescription

WANG SHI QING SHU YI QI TANG 王氏清暑益气汤
Master Wang's Clear Summerheat and Augment the Qi Decoction

xi gua pi (Citrulli Exocarpium) 西瓜皮 15–30g
xi yang shen (Panacis quinquefolii Radix) 西洋参 6–9g
yu zhu (Polygonati odorati Rhizoma) 玉竹 9–15g
mai dong (Ophiopogonis Radix) 麦冬 9–12g
huang lian (Coptidis Rhizoma) 黄连 3–6g
dan zhu ye (Lophateri Herba) 淡竹叶 6–9g
he geng (Nelumbinis Caulis) 荷梗 6–9g
zhi mu (Anemarrhenae Rhizoma) 知母 6–9g
gan cao (Glycyrrhizae Radix) 甘草 3–6g
jing mi (Oryzae Semen) 粳米 15–30g

Method: Decoction. **Xi gua pi** clears summerheat, generates fluids and stops thirst; it is assisted in this by **he geng**, which also opens up qi flow; **xi yang shen** supplements qi, generates fluids and clears heat; sweet cold **yu zhu** (instead of **shi hu**) and **mai dong** clear heat, nourish yin and generate fluids; the bitter coldness of **huang lian** cools the Heart and Stomach and balances the moistening herbs; **zhi mu** cools the Lungs and Stomach; **dan zhu ye** vents pathogens from the qi level and alleviates irritability; **jing mi** and **gan cao** supplement qi, harmonize and protect the Stomach. (Source: *Zhong Yi Nei Ke Xue* [*Wen Re Jing Wei*]).

Modifications

- With marked heat, add **shi gao** (Gypsum fibrosum) 石膏 15–30g.
- If the qi deficiency is relatively pronounced with fatigue and shortness of breath, reduce the dose of **huang lian** to 1–2g, and add **huang qi** (Astragali Radix) 黄芪 15–30g and **ren shen** (Ginseng Radix) 人参 6–9g.
- In children with persistent summerheat fever, substitute **huang lian** and **zhi mu** with **bai wei** (Cynanchi atrati Radix) 白薇 6–9g and **chan tui** (Cicadae Periostracum) 蝉蜕 6–9g to safeguard the Stomach.

Prepared medicines
Concentrated powders
Qing Shu Yi Qi Tang (Astragalus & Atractylodes Combination)

Acupuncture (select from)
Lu.7 (lieque –) .... diffuses the Lungs, vents pathogens from the qi level
Kid.6 (zhaohai +) .... supplements yin and moistens dryness
Bl.40 (weizhong –) .... sea point of the Urinary Bladder, clears summerheat
PC.3 (quze –) .... sea point of the Pericardium, clears summerheat

LI.11 (quchi −)..................these points clear heat from the qi level and Stomach
St.44 (neiting −)
St.36 (zusanli +) ....sea point of the Stomach, strengthens the Spleen and
                  Stomach and supplements qi
• with severe irritability, add PC.7 (daling −)
• with sweating, add Ht.6 (yinxi −)
• with nausea, add PC.6 (neiguan)
• with diarrhea add zhixie (N–CA–3) and Bl.25 (tianshu)
• Ear points: spleen, stomach, lung, zero point, sympathetic

Clinical notes
• Summerheat type chronic or recurrent fever may be diagnosed as post heat
  stroke, fever of unknown origin, or post viral syndrome.
• Ensure adequate hydration in patients with summerheat patterns.

热
灼
营
血

8.1.5 HEAT IN THE YING/BLOOD LEVEL
In the aftermath, or latter stages of, a relatively severe febrile illness or warm disease, heat can persist in the deepest levels of the body, the ying and blood levels.
In contrast to the previous patterns, the degree of fluid damage is more severe and
starts to deplete the true yin of the Kidneys. Because of the depth of the pathogen,
it is more difficult to expel.

There are two ways that heat can infiltrate the ying and blood levels. It can come
from the outside, as is the case here, or it can be created by Liver qi constraint. The
latter is discussed in 8.6, p.398. When heat is of external origin, it can be related
to a specific infectious event from which the patient never completely recovered.
The fever and symptoms of ying and blood level heat may also appear suddenly,
with no apparent cause. This is a type of lurking pathogen (fu xie 伏邪, p.501),
which is able to breach the body's superficial defenses, get deep into the body and
lie dormant for a period of time, reemerging sporadically.

Clinical features
• Recurrent low grade fever which is worse at night. The fever recedes in the
  early hours of the morning and is followed by feeling cold and an inability
  to maintain body temperature. The fever may be continuous or sporadic,
  recurring at changes of season, when the patient is run down or stressed, or in
  response to a secondary external invasion.
• fatigue and exhaustion, compounded by agitation and insomnia
• heat in the palms and soles; warm, dry palms; facial flushing
• transitory red, itchy skin rashes that flare at night; dry skin
• may or may not be sweating
• weight loss, emaciation
• restlessness and irritability; may be irrational behavior or personality change
• swollen lymph nodes
T deep or scarlet red and dry with thorns, and little or no coat
P fine and rapid

Treatment Principle
Clear and vent heat from the ying and cool the blood
Nourish and supplement yin and fluids

Prescription

QING HAO BIE JIA TANG 青蒿鳖甲汤
Sweet Wormwood and Soft–Shelled Turtle Shell Decoction, modified

qing hao (Artemisiae annuae Herba) 青蒿 6–15g
bie jia (Trionycis Carapax) 鳖甲 9–15g
sheng di (Rehmanniae Radix) 生地... 9–15g
zhi mu (Anemarrhenae Rhizoma) 知母 6–12g
mu dan pi (Moutan Cortex) 牡丹皮 6–9g
xuan shen (Scrophulariae Radix) 玄参 12–15g
dan dou chi (Sojae Semen preparatum) 淡豆豉 9–12g
Method: Decoction. **Qing hao** is added towards the end of cooking; **bie jia** is cooked first. **Qing hao** clears heat, and is especially good at uncovering and evicting to the surface deeply hidden pathogens; salty cold **bie jia** enriches yin and clears deeply rooted heat and deficiency heat; **sheng di** cools the blood and nourishes yin; **zhi mu** clears heat and nourishes yin; **mu dan pi** reaches deep into the blood to clear heat; **xuan shen** cools the blood, nourishes yin and its saltiness draws fluid back into the ying and blood; **dan dou chi** vents heat from the ying level. (Source: *Wen Bing Tiao Bian*)

Modifications
• In persistent cases, add **yin chai hu** (Stellariae Radix) 银柴胡 9–12g, **di gu pi** (Lycii Cortex) 地骨皮 12–15g and **bai wei** (Cynanchi atrati Radix) 白薇 9–12g.

Prepared medicines
Concentrated powders
Qing Hao Bie Jia Tang (Artemesia & Turtle Shell Combination)

Acupuncture (select from)
Kid.7 (fuliu –) ....vents pathogens form the ying level
PC.3 (quze) ....together these points cool and activate the blood
Bl.40 (weizhong –)
Sp.10 (xuehai –)
Kid.3 (taixi +).....................replenishes damaged yin
Bl.23 (shenshu +) ....these points clear heat and replenish damaged yin
Bl.18 (ganshu +)   and fluids
• Ear points: liver, kidney, heart, shenmen, endocrine, sympathetic

Clinical notes
• Fever of this type may be diagnosed as persistent fever following meningitis or other serious infection, fever of unknown origin or post surgical fever.
• Heat in the ying/blood can be a prolonged condition, and take some time to resolve.
• Although related to the yin deficiency pattern, it is distinguished from it by the presence of the lingering pathogen and the history.

气虚发热 8.2 QI DEFICIENCY

Qi deficiency fevers are persistent and recurrent. The fever, or subjective sense of heat, waxes and wanes with the patients energy. The degree of qi deficiency required to produce a fever is relatively severe, and the product of privation, prolonged illness, extreme overwork or qi depletion from resisting or containing an external pathogen.

The mechanism of the heat experienced in this pattern is the result of significant weakness of the Spleen and Lung. Because the qi generating organ systems are weak and working inefficiently, much of their effort is wasted and lost as heat. The situation can be likened to the struggle a small underpowered car has in climbing a steep hill. The engine labors to produce sufficient power to climb the hill, and in doing so starts to overheat. In those with significant qi deficiency any exertion can produce heat instead of useful work, and low grade fever results.

Clinical features

- Recurrent low grade fever which is aggravated or initiated with exertion, and when the patient is fatigued and overtired. The fever may be subjective (the body temperature is normal or even slightly low), or objective (body temperature measurably higher than normal). The heat may be felt primarily in the face. The fever tends to be more noticeable in the morning, rising as the patient starts the activity of the day. The fever generally follows a quotidian pattern (see p.368). On light touch the skin of the head and trunk may feel warm while the extremities feel cool; on firm pressure, however, the heat appears to decrease.
- even through there is fever, the patient may feel cold in general
- fatigue, weakness, lack of endurance and vitality
- waxy pale or sallow complexion
- spontaneous sweating
- shortness of breath, reluctance to speak or soft, weak voice
- poor appetite, early satiety, abdominal distension, loose stools, diarrhea
- poor muscle tone, muscle weakness, organ prolapses, slumped posture
- susceptibility to repeated upper respiratory tract infections
- weight loss

T pale, swollen and scalloped; thin white coat
P fine and weak

Treatment Principle

Strengthen the Lungs and Spleen and supplement qi

Prescription

BU ZHONG YI QI TANG 补中益气汤
Supplement the Middle to Augment the Qi Decoction

zhi huang qi (honey fried Astragali Radix) 炙黄芪 12–30g
ren shen (Ginseng Radix) 人参 6–9g
bai zhu (Atractylodis macrocephalae Rhizoma) 白术................................9–12g

dang gui (Angelicae sinensis Radix) 当归 6–9g
chen pi (Citri reticulatae Pericarpium) 陈皮 6–9g
sheng ma (Cimicifugae Rhizoma) 升麻 3–6g
chai hu (Bupleuri Radix) 柴胡 3–6g
zhi gan cao (Glycyrrhizae Radix preparata) 炙甘草 3–6g

Method: Decoction, or powdered and taken in doses of 9–grams as a draft. **Zhi huang qi** strengthens the Spleen, supplements and reinforces yang qi and raises Spleen qi; **ren shen, bai zhu** and **zhi gan cao** strengthen the Spleen and supplement qi; **chai hu** and **sheng ma** support these principal herbs in elevating qi and by doing so assist in correcting the qi dynamic and the distribution of yang qi; **dang gui** nourishes and activates blood; **chen pi** rectifies qi. (Source: *Zhong Yi Nei Ke Xue* [*Pi Wei Lun*])

Modifications

- If the fever persists beyond a few weeks following commencement of treatment, add **yin chai hu** (Stellariae Radix) 银柴胡 9–12g, **bai wei** (Cynanchi atrati Radix) 白薇 9–12g, **xian he cao** (Agrimoniae Herba) 仙鹤草 9–12g and **shi da gong lao ye** (Mahoniae Folium) 十大功劳叶 15–18g.
- With concurrent yin deficiency, chronic dry cough and a dry tongue, add **mai dong** (Ophiopogonis Radix) 麦冬 6–9g and **wu wei zi** (Schizandrae Fructus) 五味子 3–6g.
- With abdominal distension and a greasy tongue coat, reduce the dose of **zhi huang qi** by 50–75%, delete **dang gui**, and add **cang zhu** (Atractylodis Rhizoma) 苍术 6–9g and **hou po** (Magnoliae officinalis Cortex) 厚朴 6–9g.
- With copious spontaneous sweating, add **duan mu li** (calcined Ostreae Concha) 煅牡蛎 18–30g [cooked first], **fu xiao mai** (Tritici Fructus levis) 浮小麦 12–18g and **ma huang gen** (Ephedrae Radix) 麻黄根 9–12g.
- With diarrhea, add **chao yi ren** (stir fried Coicis Semen) 炒苡仁 15g, **chao bian dou** (stir fried Dolichos Semen) 炒扁豆 12–15g and **chao shan yao** (stir fried Dioscoreae Rhizoma) 炒山药 15–18g.
- With aversion to wind and mild sweating, add **gui zhi** (Cinnamomi Ramulus) 桂枝 6–9g and **bai shao** (Paeoniae Radix alba) 白芍 9–12g.
- With cough, add **xing ren** (Armeniacae Semen) 杏仁 6–9g and **qian hu** (Peucedani Radix) 前胡 6–9g.
- With cold extremities and diarrhea, add **gan jiang** (Zingiberis Rhizoma) 干姜 6–9g and **rou gui** (Cinnamomi Cortex) 肉桂 3g.
- With mild internal heat, bitter taste and yellow tongue coat, delete **ren shen**, decrease the dose of **huang qi**, and add **huang qin** (Scutellariae Radix) 黄芩 3–6g and **huang lian** (Coptidis Rhizoma) 黄连 1–3g.
- If the patient experiences a negative reaction to the unmodified primary prescription, such as increased fatigue or abdominal bloating, the probability is that there is a lingering pathogen or subclinical damp. Expelling the pathogen or resolving damp is required before qi supplementation can proceed with formula such as Xiao Chai Hu Tang (Minor Bupleurum Decoction 小柴胡汤, p.329) or San Ren Tang (Three Nut Decoction 三仁汤, p.375 and 84). See also Chapter 11 Lingering pathogens for more.

Variations and additional prescriptions
Qi and blood deficiency
Qi deficiency is frequently complicated by blood deficiency, as the Spleen is important in the manufacture of blood. In severe qi and blood deficiency patterns, the significant features are fever, heat sensations or easy overheating with exertion, palpitations, fatigue and exhaustion, weight loss, shortness of breath, digestive weakness, sweating, hair loss and back ache. Situations such as this may occur in the aftermath of a severe or prolonged illness or following surgery or chemotherapy. The treatment is to supplement qi and blood, nourish the Heart and calm the shen with a formula such as REN SHEN YANG YING TANG (Ginseng Decoction to Nourish the Nutritive Qi 人参养营汤).

ren shen (Ginseng Radix) 人参 3–6g
bai zhu (Atractylodis macrocephalae Rhizoma) 白术 6–9g
fu ling (Poria) 茯苓 6–9g
zhi gan cao (Glycyrrhizae Radix preparata) 炙甘草 3–6g
huang qi (Astragali Radix) 黄芪 12–15g
shu di (Rehmanniae Radix preparata) 熟地 9–12g
bai shao (Paeoniae Radix alba) 白芍 6–9g
dang gui (Angelicae sinensis Radix) 当归 6–9g
wu wei zi (Schizandrae Fructus) 五味子 3–6g
chen pi (Citri reticulatae Pericarpium) 陈皮 3–6g
yuan zhi (Polygalae Radix) 远志 3–6g
rou gui (Cinnamomi Cortex) 肉桂 2–3g
sheng jiang (Zingiberis Rhizoma recens) 生姜 3–6g
da zao (Jujubae Fructus) 大枣 .... 3 fruit

Method. Pills or Powder. Grind the herbs to a fine powder and take 6–12 grams as a draft with warm water twice daily. May also be decocted. When qi and blood are weak enough to create fever, the Spleen may be unable to process large doses of the rich herbs. Small doses are used initially until the Spleen is functioning better. **Ren shen, bai zhu, fu ling, huang qi** and **zhi gan cao** strengthen the Spleen and supplement qi; **huang qi** raises yang qi, fortifies wei qi and secures the exterior; **dang gui, bai shao** and **shu di** nourish blood and yin; **rou gui** warms the interior, supports yang qi and stimulates yang transformation and the production of blood; **yuan zhi** calms the Heart and shen; **wu wei zi** astringes the Lungs and Kidneys, stops leakage and assists **huang qi** in securing the exterior; **chen pi** regulates qi and harmonizes the middle burner; **sheng jiang** and **da zao** warm and nourish the Spleen and Stomach. (Source: *He Ji Ju Fang*)

Qi deficiency following summerheat invasion
Qi and fluids can be damaged by summerheat or summerdamp invasion, which occurs during hot humid weather towards the end of Summer. Depending on the mixture of qi deficiency and residual pathogen, the fever pattern can vary, and may not follow the typical qi deficiency morning rise. See 8.1.4, p.378.

Prepared medicines
Concentrated powders
Bu Zhong Yi Qi Tang (Ginseng & Astragalus Combination)
Ren Shen Yang Ying Tang (Ginseng & Rehmannia Combination)

Pills

Bu Zhong Yi Qi Wan (Central Chi Teapills)

Shen Ling Bai Zhu Wan (Absorption and Digestion Pill, Shen Ling Bai Zhu Pian)
 – with diarrhea

Shi Quan Da Bu Wan (Ten Flavour Teapills)
 – qi and blood deficiency

Acupuncture (select from)

Du.14 (dazhui +▲)............meeting point of the yang channels, reinforces yang qi and secures the exterior

LI.11 (quchi +)..................sea point of the Large Intestine, supplements qi and blood (with St.36) and clears heat

LI.4 (hegu +).....................source point of the Large Intestine, clears heat from yangming, fortifies wei qi and secures the exterior

Ren.12 (zhongwan +).........alarm point of the Stomach, strengthens the Spleen to supplement qi

Ren.4 (guanyuan +▲)........warms and supplements source qi

St.36 (zusanli +▲)..............sea point of the Stomach, strengthens the Spleen and Stomach and supplements qi and blood

Du.20 (baihui +)................assists in raising Spleen yang qi to correct the qi dynamic

Bl.20 (pishu +▲)...............transport point of the Spleen, warms and supplements Spleen qi and yang

Bl.21 (weishu +▲)..............transport point of the Stomach, warms and strengthens the Stomach

- with phlegm damp, add St.40 (fenglong) and Sp.3 (taibai)
- with diarrhea, add St.25 (tianshu +▲) and St.37 (shangjuxu)
- with abdominal distension, add Sp.3 (taibai –) and Sp.15 (daheng –)
- Ear points: spleen, stomach, lung, zero point, shenmen adrenal

Clinical notes

- Chronic fever of a qi deficiency type may be diagnosed as debility in the aftermath of a serious illness, convalescence from serious infection, malnutrition, malabsorption or fever of unknown origin.
- A degree of caution with herb dosage is required when Spleen function is significantly compromised. In the early stages of treatment, it is often better to use smaller doses of the Spleen supplements, so as not to overwhelm digestive function, and thus gradually restore its activity. Large doses of **huang qi** may be better tolerated after a few weeks of treatment. In addition, qi deficiency is frequently complicated by an excess pattern of some type, such as phlegm damp, or a lingering pathogen. If symptoms increase, especially heat sensation and abdominal discomfort following administration of the principal prescription, it is likely that there is an excess pattern still unresolved.
- On occasion, qi deficiency fever may appear to be relatively high and the patient may report feeling quite hot. This can occur when there is severe deficiency, or when there are other complications, such as yin deficiency or a lingering

pathogen. The temptation to use bitter cold heat clearing herbs in such situations should be resisted, as further damage to the Spleen and Stomach, and yin may result. When a lingering pathogen is suspected, it must be identified and expelled with the techniques described in Chapter 11.

• Diet and proper rest are an important part of the process of recovery. A qi supplementing diet is recommended, see Clinical Handbook, Vol. 2, p.870.

• Breathing exercises and graded exercise programs are useful to help in rebuilding Lung and Spleen qi.

血
虚
发
热
8.3 BLOOD DEFICIENCY

Blood deficiency causes fever by failing to securely anchor yang qi, which drifts to the surface and manifests as heat. The mechanism is similar to that for yin deficiency fever, and indeed the fever of blood deficiency can be just as marked. The degree of blood deficiency required to produce heat is usually quite severe. Blood deficiency fevers commonly occur in postpartum women, and may follow significant hemorrhage. It may also afflict those with relative degrees of malnourishment, a low protein or otherwise inadequate diet, or significant digestive weakness.

Clinical features
- Continuous, persistent low grade fever; the heat may be predominantly felt in the face and hands. The fever may be more prominent after menstruation.
- pale, sallow, lusterless complexion, but cheeks, forehead and lips may be blotchy red; pale conjunctiva, lips and nail beds
- blurring vision, floaters before the eyes; dry, tired eyes
- exhaustion, fatigue, weakness, lethargy; tired aching limbs
- postural dizziness, light–headedness
- depression, anxiety, feeling of inability to cope
- forgetfulness, poor concentration
- insomnia
- palpitations, tachycardia
- possibly night sweats
- tendency to constipation
- dry skin and hair
- numbness or tingling in the extremities
- scanty periods or amenorrhea

T pale, or with pale or orangey edges
P fine and weak, or choppy and weak

Treatment Principle
Supplement and nourish qi and blood
Strengthen the Spleen and calm the Heart

Prescription

GUI PI TANG 归脾汤
Restore the Spleen Decoction

zhi huang qi (honey fried Astragali Radix) 炙黄芪 9–12g
ren shen (Ginseng Radix) 人参 6–9g
fu shen (Poria Sclerotium pararadicis) 茯神 9–12g
bai zhu (Atractylodes macrocephalae Rhizoma) 白术 9–12g
dang gui (Angelicae sinensis Radix) 当归 3–6g
long yan rou (Longan Arillus) 龙眼肉 3–6g
suan zao ren (Zizyphi spinosae Semen) 酸枣仁 3–9g
yuan zhi (Polygalae Radix) 远志 3–6g

mu xiang (Aucklandiae Radix) 木香 3–6g
zhi gan cao (Glycyrrhizae Radix preparata) 炙甘草 3–6g
sheng jiang (Zingiberis Rhizoma recens) 生姜 3–6g
da zao (Jujubae Fructus) 大枣 .... 3 fruit

Method: Decoction. **Zhi huang qi**, **ren shen**, **bai zhu** and **zhi gan cao** strengthen the Spleen and supplement qi; **dang gui** and **zhi huang qi** taken together stimulate blood production; **suan zao ren**, **long yan rou** and **yuan zhi** nourish the Heart and calm the shen; **fu shen** strengthens the Spleen and calms the shen; **mu xiang** regulates qi and aids the Spleen in digesting the blood supplementing herbs; **zhi gan cao** supplements qi and harmonizes the Stomach; **sheng jiang** and **da zao** assist **mu xiang** in digestion of the cloying supplements. (Source: *Zhong Yi Nei Ke Xue* [*Ji Sheng Fang*])

Modification

- With marked blood deficiency, very pale tongue and amenorrhea, add **shu di** (Rehmanniae Radix preparata) 熟地 6–12g, **bai shao** (Paeoniae Radix alba) 白芍 6–12g, **gou qi zi** (Lycii Fructus) 枸杞子 6–12g, or **e jiao** (Asini Corii Colla) 阿胶 6–9g [dissolved in the strained decoction]. **Shu di** and **e jiao** can cause digestive upset, so **sha ren** (Amomi Fructus) 砂仁 3–6g may be added to offset their cloying effects.
- With persistent fever, add **yin chai hu** (Stellariae Radix) 银柴胡 9–12g, **di gu pi** (Lycii Cortex) 地骨皮 12–15g, **bai wei** (Cynanchi atrati Radix) 白薇 9–12g and **mu dan pi** (Moutan Cortex) 牡丹皮 9–12g.
- If the blood supplements cause symptoms of loose stools, abdominal bloating and loss of appetite, use **chao dang gui** (stir fried Angelicae sinensis Radix) 炒当归, and add **shan yao** (Dioscoreae Rhizoma) 山药 12–15g, **shen qu** (Massa medicata fermentata) 神曲 9–12g and **sha ren** (Amomi Fructus) 砂仁 3–6g [added at the end of cooking].
- With mild blood stasis (lower abdominal pain, dysmenorrhea, clotted menstrual flow, dark spots on the tongue or dark sublingual veins), add **chuan xiong** (Chuanxiong Rhizoma) 川芎 6–9g, **hong hua** (Carthami Flos) 红花 6–9g and **tao ren** (Persicae Semen) 桃仁 6–9g.

Variations and additional prescriptions

Following a hemorrhage

If the fever follows soon after a significant hemorrhage (either postpartum or post traumatic), the treatment is to quickly replenish qi and blood with **DANG GUI BU XUE TANG** (Tangkuei Decoction to Supplement the Blood 当归补血汤).

huang qi (Astragali Radix) 黄芪 30g
dang gui (Angelicae sinensis Radix) 当归 6g

Method: Decoction. **Huang qi** supplements qi; **dang gui** nourishes blood. The important feature of this prescription is the proportion of **huang qi** to **dang gui**–this ratio helps the Spleen to rapidly replenish blood loss. (Source: *Nei Wai Shang Bian Huo Lun*)

Prepared medicines

Concentrated powders

Gui Pi Tang (Ginseng & Longan Combination)

Pills

Gui Pi Wan (Kwei Be Wan, Gui Pi Teapills)

Dang Gui Ji Jing (Tang Kuei Essence of Chicken)
 – an excellent blood supplement, particularly good for postpartum and
   breast feeding women, enhanced by the richness of the medicinal black
   boned chicken
Wu Ji Bai Feng Wan (Black Chicken White Phoenix Pill)
 – A popular and common prepared medicine based on the medicinal black
   boned chicken. Comes in the form of a large black pill encased in a plastic
   and wax sealed ball. The dose is 1–2 pills daily.
Shi Quan Da Bu Wan (Ten Flavour Teapills)
 – qi and blood deficiency with cold

Acupuncture (select from)

Sp.6 (sanyinjiao +▲).........strengthens the Spleen, nourishes and regulates qi
                             and blood, calms the shen
St.36 (zusanli +▲) ....sea point of the Stomach, warms and strengthens the
                             Spleen and Stomach and supplements qi and blood
LI.11 (quchi).....................sea point of the Large Intestine, strengthens qi and
                             blood, clears heat
Ren.12 (zhongwan +▲) ....alarm point of the Stomach, warms and strengthens
                             the Spleen and Stomach
Ren.4 (guanyuan +▲)........boosts the Kidneys, supplements source qi and
                             regulates qi
Bl.17 (geshu +▲)...............meeting point of the blood, supplements and
                             replenishes blood
Bl.20 (pishu +▲) ....transport point of the Spleen, warms and strength-
                             ens the Spleen and supplements qi and blood
yintang (M–HN–3) ....calms the shen
 • with insomnia, add Ht.7 (shenmen –)
 • with night sweats, add Ht.6 (yinxi –) and Kid.7 (fuliu +)
 • with dizziness, add Du.20 (baihui ▲)
 • with forgetfulness and poor concentration, add Bl.52 (zhishi)
 • with dream disturbed sleep, add Bl.42 (pohu)
 • with anxiety, add Du.19 (houding) and Du.24 (shenting)
 • Ear points: heart, shenmen, spleen, zero point, sympathetic

Clinical notes

 • Fever of a blood deficiency type may be diagnosed as anemia, thrombocytopenia, neurasthenia, chronic fatigue syndrome, chronic leukemia, postpartum
   hemorrhage or malnutrition.
 • Blood deficiency fever is responsive to treatment, but this needs to be continued until the Spleen is strong enough to make sufficient blood. In the case of
   postpartum fever from blood deficiency, treatment should begin promptly and
   continue during breast feeding. Attention to diet and adequate protein are essential (see Clinical Handbook, Vol. 2, p.874). Iron supplements (predigested
   iron is easier on the Spleen) are also useful. A strictly regular bedtime routine
   should be adhered to.

阴虚发热 | 8.4 YIN DEFICIENCY

Chronic fever from yin deficiency is common, and may appear gradually as a consequence of ageing, life habits and menopause, or may occur suddenly in the aftermath of a major febrile illness. Yin deficiency fever can also intervene when chronic qi and blood stasis creates heat, which in turn damages yin.

The mechanism of the fever is the generation of heat from deficiency. When yin is insufficient, it is unable to moisten and cool the body and balance the heat of yang qi. Heat starts to accumulate internally, in the same way an car engine can overheat when the radiator is empty.

The presentation of the heat can vary in degree and location. In mild cases or in the early stages of yin depletion, it may simply manifest as hot feet at night. In advanced or severe cases, with marked deficiency and unrestrained yang the heat may rage into a relatively high fever with flushing and frequent night sweats.

The treatment strategy focuses on clearing the heat, as persistent heat will continue to deplete yin. As the heat signs diminishes the cooling herbs can be reduced and replaced with more supplementing herbs. More fundamental yin supplementing formulae can be phased in depending on the location and nature of the yin deficiency.

Clinical features
- Chronic low grade or 'bone steaming' fever that rises in the afternoon or evening. This is a quotidian type of fever (see p.368). The heat may be experienced all over the body or localized in the face and periphery. Body temperature may be elevated or normal.
- Sensation of heat in the palms, soles and chest. The sensation of heat in the "five hearts" can be obvious or subtle. In mild cases the patient may only be aware of kicking the bedclothes off his or her feet at night. The palms are generally warm and dry.
- Tiredness or exhaustion, compounded by a sense of jitteriness, agitation and over stimulation that makes resting difficult. The patient may complain of being without energy or completely exhausted at the end of the day, but are unable to relax or sleep at night.
- facial flushing, malar flushing; red lips and cheeks
- night sweats
- insomnia and fitful sleep
- irritability, restlessness
- thirst, dry mouth and throat
- dry stools or constipation
- scanty, concentrated urine
- scanty menses, amenorrhea
- all symptoms tend to be worse in the afternoon and evening

T red and dry with little or no coat; the tongue may appear peeled, or have multiple surface cracks

P fine and rapid

Treatment Principle

Clear deficient heat and alleviate bone steaming
Supplement and enrich yin

Prescription

QING GU SAN 清骨散
Cool the Bones Powder

---

qing hao (Artemisiae annuae Herba) 青蒿 9–12g
di gu pi (Lycii Cortex) 地骨皮 9–15g
bie jia (Trionycis Carapax) 鳖甲 9–15g
yin chai hu (Stellariae Radix) 银柴胡 6–12g
hu huang lian (Picrorhizae Rhizoma) 胡黄连 6–9g
zhi mu (Anemarrhenae Rhizoma) 知母 6–12g
qin jiao (Gentianae macrophyllae Radix) 秦艽 6–9g
gan cao (Glycyrrhizae Radix) 甘草 3–6g

Method: Decoction. **Yin chai hu, hu huang lian, zhi mu** and **di gu pi** clear heat from yin deficiency and alleviate bone steaming; **qing hao** and **qin jiao** vent deeply lying heat to the surface to
facilitate dispersal; **bie jia** clears heat, enriches yin to anchor yang, and leads the other herbs into
the deep levels of the body; **gan cao** protects the middle burner and harmonizes the other herbs in
the prescription. (Source: *Zhong Yi Nei Ke Xue* [*Zheng Zhi Zhun Sheng*])

Modifications

• With dryness and thirst, add **sheng di** (Rehmanniae Radix) 生地 12–18g,
  tian dong (Asparagi Rhizoma) 天冬 9–12g and **mai dong** (Ophiopogonis
  Radix) 麦冬 9–12g.
• With severe heat, add **huang bai** (Phellodendri Cortex) 黄柏 6–9g and **xuan
  shen** (Scrophulariae Radix) 玄参 12–15g.
• With frequent night sweats, add **duan mu li** (calcined Ostreae Concha) 煅牡
  蛎 18–30g [cooked first], **fu xiao mai** (Tritici Fructus levis) 浮小麦 12–15g
  and **ma huang gen** (Ephedrae Radix) 麻黄根 9–12g.
• With blood stasis, add **dan shen** (Salviae miltiorrhizae Radix) 丹参 12–15g.
• With insomnia, add **suan zao ren** (Ziziphi spinosae Semen) 酸枣仁 12–15g,
  bai zi ren (Platycladi Semen) 柏子仁 9–12g, **ye jiao teng** (Polygoni multiflori
  Caulis) 夜交藤 15–30g and **he huan pi** (Albizziae Cortex) 合欢皮 12–15g.
• With poor temperature regulation (often described by patients as feeling hot
  all night but cold in the early hours of the morning) from ying wei disharmo-
  ny, combine with **Gui Zhi Tang** (Cinnamon Twig Decoction 桂枝汤, p.76).
• With qi deficiency, shortness of breath and spontaneous sweating, combine
  with **Sheng Mai San** (Generate the Pulse Powder 生脉散, p.278).

Variations and additional prescriptions

Yin deficiency affecting specific organ systems

When the main feature of a yin deficiency pattern is the fever, the primary prescription above is most appropriate, and can be used until the heat has abated.
This should not take longer than a few weeks. Following reduction of the heat,
however, a more yin supplementing approach should be adopted. Rebuilding yin
can be a relatively lengthy process, and a prescription better suited to long term

supplementation of specific organ systems can be selected. The deficiency may be concentrated in the Heart, Lungs, Liver, Kidney or Stomach and Spleen. Pills or concentrated extracts are convenient and effective for long term supplementation.

- For Heart and Kidney yin deficiency (palpitations, insomnia, anxiety, raw tender tongue or mouth ulcers), select TIAN WANG BU XIN DAN (Emperor of Heaven's Special Pill to Supplement the Heart 天王补心丹, p.147).

- For Kidney yin deficiency (weak sore lower back, chronic sore throat, malar flush, heat in the palms and soles, hair loss), select either LIU WEI DI HUANG WAN (Six Ingredient Pill with Rehmannia 六味地黄丸, p.192), ZHI BAI DI HUANG WAN (Anemarrhena, Phellodendron and Rehmannia Pill 知柏地黄丸, p.922) or DA BU YIN WAN (Great Supplement the Yin Pill 大补阴丸, p.914).

- For Liver and Kidney yin deficiency (dizziness, headaches, irritability, visual weakness or dry eyes, muscle spasms or tics) select QI JU DI HUANG WAN (Lycium Fruit, Chrysanthemum and Rehmannia Pill 杞菊地黄丸, p.467), MING MU DI HUANG WAN (Improve Vision Pill with Rehmannia 明目地黄丸, p.917), YI GUAN JIAN (Linking Decoction 一贯煎, p.816) or GUI SHAO DI HUANG WAN (Tangkuei and Rehmannia Pill 归芍地黄丸, p.915).

- For Lung yin deficiency (dry cough, hoarse raspy voice), select BAI HE GU JIN TANG (Lily Bulb Decoction to Preserve the Metal 百合固金汤, p.705) or MAI WEI DI HUANG WAN (Schizandra, Ophiopogon and Rehmannia Pill 麦味地黄丸, p.917).

- For Spleen and Stomach yin deficiency (dry mouth, thirst, sore gums, no appetite, dry stools), select SHEN LING BAI ZHU SAN (Ginseng, Poria and White Atractylodes Powder 参苓白术散 p.270) or ZENG YE TANG (Increase the Fluids Decoction 增液汤, p.922).

- Occasionally, long term yin supplementation fails to substantially increase yin, and the heat recurs as soon as treatment ceases. One reason for this may be that there is insufficient yang to spark the transformation and manufacture of yin. Hence when supplementing yin, it can sometimes be helpful to include one or two yang supplementing herbs, even when there is heat. The yang supplements selected are generally those that are warming but not especially drying, such as **tu si zi** (Cuscutae Semen) 菟丝子, **rou cong rong** (Cistanches Herba) 肉苁蓉, **suo yang** (Cynomorii Herba) 锁阳, **ba ji tian** (Morindae officinalis Radix) 巴戟天 or **xian ling pi** (Epimedii Herba) 仙灵脾.

Prepared medicines
Concentrated powders
Qing Hao Bie Jia Tang (Artemisia & Turtle Shell Combination)
  – used until the heat abates

Pills
Da Bu Yin Wan (Abundant Yin Teapills)
  – Kidney yin deficiency with heat
Zhi Bai Ba Wei Wan (Eight Flavor Rehmannia Teapills)
  – Kidney yin deficiency with heat

Liu Wei Di Huang Wan (Six Flavor Teapills)
- Kidney yin deficiency
Zuo Gui Wan (Left Side Replenishing Teapills)
- Kidney yin deficiency
Tian Wang Bu Xin Dan (Emperor's Teapills, Tian Wang Pu Hsin Tan)
- Heart and Kidney yin deficiency
Mai Wei Di Huang Wan (Ba Xian Chang Shou Wan, Eight Immortals Teapills)
- Lung and Kidney yin deficiency
Qi Ju Di Huang Wan (Lycium Rehmannia Teapills)
- Liver and Kidney yin deficiency

Acupuncture (select from)

Kid.3 (taixi +)....................source point of the Kidneys, supplements Kidney yin and clears deficiency heat

Kid.7 (fuliu).....................connecting point of the Kidney, supplements Kidney yin and clears heat

Lu.7 (lieque).....................master and couple points of renmai, supplement
Kid.6 (zhaohai)   Kidney yin, moisten dryness and clear deficiency heat

Ren.4 (guanyuan +)...........these points supplement Kidney yin and yuan qi
Ren.6 (qihai +)

Sp.6 (sanyinjiao)................nourishes Kidney, Liver and Spleen yin

Bl.23 (shenshu +) ....transport point of the Kidneys, supplements Kidney yin

Bl.15 (xinshu +) ....transport point of the Heart, supplements Heart yin, calms the Heart and shen, clears heat

- with insomnia, add Ht.7 (shenmen) and PC.6 (neiguan)
- with night sweats, add Ht.6 (yinxi)
- with anxiety, add yintang (M–HN–3) and Du.20 (baihui)
- with forgetfulness, add Du.20 (baihui) and Bl.52 (zhishi)
- with palpitations or arrhythmias add Ht.5 (tongli)
- with dizziness, add Du.20 (baihui)
- Ear points: kidney, liver, lung, shenmen, adrenal, subcortex, endocrine

Clinical notes

- Persistent fever of a yin deficiency type may be diagnosed as fever of unknown origin (FUO), post–menstrual fever, tuberculosis, blood dyscrasia, leukemia, chronic infection or endocrine disorder such as hyperthyroidism and meno-pause, or old age.
- Fever and heat from yin deficiency generally responds well to persistent treat-ment. Low doses of herbs, such as in prepared pill form, over a long period of time are adequate to produce a good sustained response. Depending on the degree of deficiency, 6–12 months of treatment may be necessary. In the case of old age, ongoing treatment without a time limit, is recommended.
- For dietary recommendations see Clinical Handbook, Vol. 2, p.876.

阳虚发热 | 8.5 YANG DEFICIENCY

Yang deficiency is an uncommon cause of fever, and reflects a serious degree of deficiency. The fever, or subjective sense of heat, is due to the preponderance of internal yin cold which displaces yang qi and forces it to the surface where it is experienced as a low grade fever. In addition, the feeble yang qi is unable to performs its functional tasks efficiently, so what yang there is, is dissipated as waste heat rather than as useful work. This is similar to the mechanism of qi deficiency fever (p.382).

Clinical features

- Low grade subjective fever which is aggravated or initiated when fatigued or after exertion. The heat is experienced in the face and upper body, while the lower body (lower abdomen in particular) and extremities are cold. The patient may notice a damp pillow from sweating on the head and neck.
- fatigue, exhaustion and weakness; somnolence; low energy reserve; slow recovery after exertion
- waxy, pale, sallow complexion; rarely the face may appear flushed
- cold intolerance, cold abdomen and extremities
- lower back, legs and knees aching, weak and cold
- edema of the lower extremities, or generalized edema
- frequent, copious clear urination, nocturia (or scanty urination when there is edema)
- frequent or watery stools with undigested food; early morning ('cockcrow') diarrhea
- loss of appetite, abdominal distension

T pale, swollen, scalloped and wet, with a white coat
P deep, fine, weak, imperceptible, or floating and large without strength

Treatment Principle

Warm and supplement Kidney yang
Preserve and protect yin

Prescription

YOU GUI WAN 右归丸
Restore the Right [Kidney] Pill

shu di (Rehmanniae Radix preparata) 熟地	12–24g
shan yao (Dioscoreae Rhizoma) 山药	9–12g
gou qi zi (Lycii Fructus) 枸杞子	9–12g
tu si zi (Cuscutae Semen) 菟丝子	9–12g
du zhong (Eucommiae Cortex) 杜仲	9–12g
lu jiao jiao (Cervi Cornus Colla) 鹿角胶	9–12g
shan zhu yu (Corni Fructus) 山茱萸	6–9g
dang gui (Angelicae sinensis Radix) 当归	6–9g
zhi fu zi (Aconiti Radix lateralis preparata) 制附子	6–12g
rou gui (Cinnamomi Cortex) 肉桂	6–9g

Method: Pills or powder. The herbs are ground to a fine powder and formed into 9 gram pills with honey. The dose is one pill twice daily. When decocted, **zhi fu zi** is cooked for 30 minutes before the other herbs and **lu jiao jiao** is melted in the hot strained decoction. **Shu di, gou qi zi** and **dang gui** nourish Kidney yin and blood; **shan zhu yu** supplements the Liver; **shan yao** strengthens the Spleen and Kidneys; **tu si zi** and **du zhong** supplement Kidney yang; **zhi fu zi** and **rou gui** warm yang; **lu jiao jiao** warms yang and benefits jing. (Source: *Zhong Yi Nei Ke Xue* ([*Jing Yue Quan Shu*]))

Modification

- With Spleen yang deficiency, loose stools, loss of appetite, early satiety and abdominal distension, add **gan jiang** (Zingiberis Rhizoma) 干姜 6–9g, or combine the primary prescription with Lɪ Zʜᴏɴɢ ᴡᴀɴ (Regulate the Middle Pill 理中丸, p.732).
- With early morning diarrhea, add **rou dou kou** (Myristicae Semen) 肉豆蔻 6–9g and **bu gu zhi** (Psoraleae Fructus) 补骨脂 9–12g.
- With frequent urination or nocturia, add **qian shi** (Euryales Semen) 芡实 9–12g and **jin ying zi** (Rosae laevigatae Fructus) 金樱子 9–12g.
- With qi deficiency, add **huang qi** (Astragali Radix) 黄芪 12–15g and **dang shen** (Codonopsis Radix) 党参 9–12g.

Variations and additional prescriptions

With the appearance of significant heat

When yang qi is especially weak, the illusion of significant heat can be created, which may be mistaken for a true fever from excess. This is known as 'true cold, false heat', and indicates a relatively severe and dangerous degree of yang deficiency. The patient appears flushed and irritable, but at the same time can be lethargic and sleepy, cold in the lower body or with a lower than normal body temperature. There may be watery diarrhea or vomiting, and the pulse imperceptible. In extreme cases the yin and yang may be on the point of separation. This is a serious condition and should be managed in hospital. The treatment is to warm and restore yang with Sɪ Nɪ Tᴀɴɢ (Frigid Extremities Decoction 四逆汤). In China this formula is prepared as an intravenous infusion for emergency use.

zhi fu zi (Aconiti Radix lateralis preparata) 制附子 9–15g
gan jiang (Zingiberis Rhizoma) 干姜 9g
zhi gan cao (Glycyrrhizae Radix preparata) 炙甘草 12g
Method: Decoction. **Zhi fu zi** warms Kidney yang and mobilizes yang qi; **gan jiang** warms the Spleen and dispels cold from the middle burner. The heat and yang invigorating function of **zhi fu zi** is enhanced when combined with **gan jiang**. **Zhi gan cao** strengthens the Spleen and moderates the toxicity of **zhi fu zi** and the drying tendency of the primary herbs. (Source: *Shang Han Lun*)

With cold and deficiency of the chongmai and renmai

A low grade fever rising in the evening and accompanied by heat in the palms and soles may can be due to yang and blood deficiency affecting the lower burner. The deficiency is of the chongmai and renmai, and thus the Uterus, Kidneys and reproductive system. This is a common cause of infertility and menopausal symptoms. The heat in the upper body and palms reflects the displacement of yang qi from the lower burner by cold. There may be abdominal pain that is better for warmth, irregular or scanty menses with clotting and persistent spotting or uterine bleeding. Lower back and sacral pain are worse following menstruation or when tired, the tongue is pale and the pulse deep and slow. The treatment is to warm chongmai and renmai, dispel cold, and nourish and activate blood with **WEN JING TANG** (Flow Warming Decoction 温经汤).

wu zhu yu (Evodiae Fructus) 吴茱萸 3–6g
gui zhi (Cinnamomi Ramulus) 桂枝 6–9g
dang gui (Angelicae sinensis Radix) 当归 6–9g
bai shao (Paeoniae Radix alba) 白芍 6–9g
chuan xiong (Chuanxiong Rhizoma) 川芎 3–6g
e jiao (Asini Corii Colla) 阿胶 6–9g
mu dan pi (Moutan Cortex) 牡丹皮 6–9g
mai dong (Ophiopogonis Radix) 麦冬 6–9g
zhi ban xia (Pinelliae Rhizoma preparatum) 制半夏 6–9g
ren shen (Ginseng Radix) 人参 6–9g
gan cao (Glycyrrhizae Radix) 甘草 3–6g
sheng jiang (Zingiberis Rhizoma recens) 生姜 3–6g

Method: Decoction. **E jiao** is melted in the hot strained decoction. **Wu zhu yu** and **gui zhi** warm the Uterus, chongmai and renmai, dispel cold and invigorate the circulation of lower burner qi; **dang gui**, **bai shao** and **chuan xiong** nourish and activate blood, and regulate menstruation; **e jiao** nourishes yin and blood and stops bleeding; **zhi ban xia** and **sheng jiang** warm and harmonize the Stomach and dry dampness and phlegm; **mai dong** nourishes yin and clears deficiency heat; **mu dan pi** activates blood and disperses blood stasis; **ren shen** and **gan cao** strengthen the Spleen and supplement qi; **bai shao** and **gan cao** alleviate spasmodic pain. (Source: *Jin Gui Yao Lue*)

Prepared medicines
Concentrated powders
You Gui Wan (Eucommia & Rehmannia Formula)
Ba Wei Di Huang Wan (Rehmannia Eight Formula)
    – Kidney yang deficiency
Li Zhong Tang (Ginseng & Ginger Combination)
    – Spleen yang deficiency
Wen Jing Tang (Tangkuei & Evodia Combination)

Pills
You Gui Wan (Right Side Replenishing Teapills)
Jin Kui Shen Qi Wan (Fu Gui Ba Wei Wan, Golden Book Tea)
    – Kidney yang deficiency
Fu Zi Li Zhong Wan (Fu Tzu Li Chung Wan, Li Chung Yuen Medical Pills)
    – Spleen yang deficiency
Wen Jing Wan (Warm Cycle Teapills)

Acupuncture (select from)
Ren.8 (shenque ▲) ....moxa on salt; place a piece of thin cloth over the navel and fill it with salt; burn large cones of moxa on the salt. The cloth enables quick removal of the salt and prevents burning; this method warms yang and 'returns the dragon to the sea', i.e. guides the errant yang qi back to it source in the Kidneys.
Ren.4 (guanyuan +▲) ....warms and supplements source qi and Kidney yang

Du.4 (mingmen +▲).........warms Kidney yang
St.36 (zusanli +▲) ....sea point of the Stomach, warms and strengthens the
Spleen and Stomach to supplement yang qi
Sp.6 (sanyinjiao +▲).........strengthens the Spleen and Kidneys and supple-
ments yang qi and yin
Kid.3 (taixi +▲).................source point of the Kidneys, warms Kidney yang
Bl.23 (shenshu +▲) ....transport point of the Kidneys, warms and stimu-
lates Kidney yang
• Ear points: kidney, adrenal, shenmen, sympathetic

Clinical notes
• Yang deficiency fever is uncommon, and when it does occur reflects a severe
weakness of yang qi.
• Yang deficiency fever may be diagnosed as nephrotic syndrome, congestive cardiac failure, left ventricular failure, chronic nephritis, hypothyroidism, prostatic
hypertrophy, hepatic cirrhosis, chronic colitis, chronic dysentery, malabsorption syndrome, or post intestinal surgery.
• A degree of caution with herb dosage is required when Spleen yang is compromised. In the early stages of treatment, it is often better to use smaller doses,
say ¼ – ½ of the target dose, so as not to overwhelm the Spleen, and assist in
gradually restoring its activity and ability to assimilate the herbs.
• Treatment will need to be lengthy and regular to achieve a satisfactory and
sustained result. Although the fever may subside in a reasonable time (a few
weeks), rebuilding yang may take some months.
• Diet and proper rest are clearly an important part of the process of recovery. See
Clinical Handbook, Vol. 2, p.873 for dietary suggestions.

肝
郁
发
热

8.6 LIVER QI CONSTRAINT

Chronic fever from constrained Liver qi with heat is a common reaction to persistent or extreme emotional turmoil. The fever is initiated or aggravated when the patient is upset or angry. The constraint of qi leads to a build up of pressure, which at a certain critical intensity, transforms into heat (or fire when severe). Once heat has been generated, it can rise to the head and upper body, accumulate in the Liver, heat the blood or damage yin.

Clinical features

- Chronic low grade fever or feelings of heat that come and go according to the emotional state or stage of the menstrual cycle. When associated with menstruation, the fever occurs premenstrually and subsides after menstruation commences. The heat is often experienced as easy overheating or flushing in the upper body.
- When associated with menstruation there are symptoms such as irregular menstruation, premenstrual breast tenderness and swelling, facial acne, red skin or rashes on the neck and face and increasing irritability.
- irritability, easy anger, depression
- bitter taste in the mouth, dry mouth
- red, sore, irritated eyes
- tightness in the chest, described as difficulty in drawing a satisfying breath
- dizziness, light–headedness
- sluggishness and fatigue which is better with activity or exercise
- abdominal bloating and flatulence
- alternating constipation and diarrhea
- all symptoms aggravated by stress

T red with redder edges with a thin, yellow coat
P wiry and rapid

Treatment Principle

Dredge the Liver and relieve qi constraint
Cool the Liver and clear heat

Prescription

JIA WEI XIAO YAO SAN 加味逍遥散
Augmented Rambling Powder, modified

chai hu (Bupleuri Radix) 柴胡 9–12g
bai shao (Paeoniae Radix alba) 白芍 12–18g
dang gui (Angelicae sinensis Radix) 当归 9–12g
fu ling (Poria) 茯苓 12–15g
bai zhu (Atractylodes macrocephalae Rhizoma) 白术 9–12g
shan zhi zi (Gardeniae Fructus) 山栀子 9–12g
mu dan pi (Moutan Cortex) 牡丹皮 9–12g
gan cao (Glycyrrhizae Radix) 甘草 3–6g
bo he (Menthae haplocalycis Herba) 薄荷 3–6g

yu jin (Curcumae Radix) 郁金 9–12g
Method: Decoction. **Chai hu** and **yu jin** dredge the Liver qi, alleviate qi constraint and cool the Liver; **dang gui** and **bai shao** nourish blood and soften the Liver; **dang gui** also activates blood and moves stagnation; **shan zhi zi** and **mu dan pi** cool the Liver and clear constrained heat; **mu dan pi** cools and activates the blood and dispels blood stasis; **fu ling**, **bai zhu** and **gan cao** strengthen and protect the Spleen; **bo he** assists in relieving constraint of qi and clearing heat. (Source: *Zhong Yi Nei Ke Xue* [*Nei Ke Zhai Yao*])

Modifications

- With relatively high fever, add **huang qin** (Scutellariae Radix) 黄芩 9–12g and **long dan cao** (Gentianae Radix) 龙胆草 3–6g.
- With fever that rises at night and skin rashes (mild heat in the blood), add **qing hao** (Artemisiae annuae Herba) 青蒿 9–15g **yin chai hu** (Stellariae Radix) 银柴胡 9–12g and **di gu pi** (Lycii Cortex) 地骨皮 12–15g.
- With constipation, add **bing lang** (Arecae Semen) 槟榔 6–9g and **zhi shi** (Aurantii Fructus immaturus) 枳实 6–9g.
- With hypochondriac pain, add **chuan lian zi** (Toosendan Fructus) 川楝子 9–12g and **yan hu suo** (Corydalis Rhizoma) 延胡索 9–12g.
- With headache or fullness and distension in the head, add **sang ye** (Mori Folium) 桑叶 9–12g, **ju hua** (Chrysanthemi Flos) 菊花 12–15g and **man jing zi** (Viticis Fructus) 蔓荆子 9–12g.
- With premenstrual breast tenderness, add **he huan pi** (Albizziae Cortex) 合欢皮 12–15g, **xiang fu** (Cyperi Rhizoma) 香附 9–12g and **qing pi** (Citri reticulatae viride Pericarpium) 青皮 9–12g.
- With premenstrual edema, add **ze lan** (Lycopi Herba) 泽兰 9–15g and **yi mu cao** (Leonurus Herba) 益母草 12–15g.
- With loss of appetite or food stagnation, add **shan zha** (Crataegi Fructus) 山楂 12–15g and **mai ya** (Hordei Fructus germinantus) 麦芽 12–15g.
- With plum pit qi, add **su geng** (Perillae Caulis) 苏梗 6–9g and **jie geng** (Platycodi Radix) 桔梗 6–9g.
- With Liver and Stomach disharmony (belching, nausea, epigastric distension), add **zhu ru** (Bambusae Caulis in taeniam) 竹茹 6–9g and **zhi ban xia** (Pinelliae Rhizoma preparatum) 制半夏 6–9g.
- With abdominal distension, add **hou po** (Magnoliae officinalis Cortex) 厚朴 9–12g.
- With flatulence or belching, add **hou po** (Magnoliae officinalis Cortex) 厚朴 9–12g, **mu xiang** (Aucklandiae Radix) 木香 6–9g and **sha ren** (Amomi Fructus) 砂仁 3–6g.
- With damp, add **cang zhu** (Atractylodis Rhizoma) 苍术 9–12g and **hou po** (Magnoliae officinalis Cortex) 厚朴 9–12g.
- With yin deficiency, a peeled tongue and fine rapid pulse, add **sheng di** (Rehmanniae Radix) 生地 12–15g and **gou qi zi** (Lycii Fructus) 枸杞子 9–12g, or combine with YI GUAN JIAN (Linking Decoction 一贯煎, p.816).

Variations and additional prescriptions

Heat in the blood

The Liver stores blood, so when the Liver is hot, heat can be easily transferred to the blood. The combination of qi constraint and hot blood are behind some common types of chronic fever, abnormal bleeding and skin rash associated with menstruation. Symptoms include evening fever and flushing, menorrhagia and premenstrual nosebleed, acne and red dry itchy eczema on the upper body. The treatment is to clear heat, cool the blood, dredge the Liver and nourish blood with **WEN QING YIN** (Warming and Clearing Drink 温清饮). This treatment need only continue until the heat has abated and any bleeding ceases, then a qi regulating approach (such as the primary prescription above) can be adopted.

sheng di (Rehmanniae Radix) 生地 12–18g
chi shao (Paeoniae Radix rubra) 赤芍 9–12g
dang gui (Angelicae sinensis Radix) 当归 9–12g
chuan xiong (Chuanxiong Rhizoma) 川芎 6–9g
huang qin (Scutellariae Radix) 黄芩 6–9g
huang bai (Phellodendri Cortex) 黄柏 6–9g
huang lian (Coptidis Rhizoma) 黄连 3–9g
shan zhi zi (Gardeniae Fructus) 山栀子 6–9g

Method: Decoction. **Sheng di** and **chi shao** cool the blood; **dang gui**, **chi shao** and **chuan xiong** nourish and activate blood; **huang lian**, **huang qin**, **huang bai** and **shan zhi zi** clear heat; **huang qin** clears heat from the upper body; **huang lian** clears heat from the Heart and chest; **huang bai** clears heat from the lower burner; **shan zhi zi** clears heat from all three burners via the urine. (Source: *Wan Bing Hui Chun*)

Prepared medicines

Concentrated powders
Jia Wei Xiao Yao San (Bupleurum & Peony Formula)
Wen Qing Yin (Tangkuei & Gardenia Combination)
 – qi constraint with heat in the blood

Pills
Jia Wei Xiao Yao Wan (Dan Zhi Xiao Yao Wan, Free and Easy Wanderer Plus Teapills)
Si Wu Wan (Four Substances for Women Teapills) plus Huang Lian Jie Du Wan
 (Huang Lian Jie Du Teapills)
 – heat in the blood

Acupuncture (select from)
Liv.14 (qimen –) ....alarm point of the Liver, cools the Liver and regulates qi
GB.34 (yanglingquan –).....sea point of the Gallbladder, regulates Liver qi and clears heat
Liv.2 (xingjian –) ....brook and fire point of the Liver, cools the Liver
Liv.3 (taichong –) ....source, transport and earth point of the Liver, dredges the Liver and activates qi and blood
Sp.6 (sanyinjiao)..................strengthens the Spleen and Kidney, regulates Liver qi, supplements qi and yin
PC.6 (neiguan –) ....connecting point of the Pericardium, regulates Liver qi and corrects the qi dynamic

Bl.18 (ganshu)...................transport points of the Liver and Gallbladder,
Bl.19 (danshu)   regulates Liver and Gallbladder qi, relieves qi
                              constraint and clears heat
- with lateral headaches and neck tension, GB.41 (zulinqi −) and SJ.5 (waiguan −)
- with constipation, add Sp.15 (daheng −) and St.37 (shangjuxu −)
- with heat in the blood, add Sp.10 (xuehai −) and PC.3 (quze −)
- with phlegm or plum pit qi, add PC.5 (jianshi −) and St.40 (fenglong −)
- with Spleen deficiency, add Bl.20 (pishu +) and St.36 (zusanli +)
- with dizziness, add GB.20 (fengchi −) and GB.43 (xiaxi −)
- with yin deficiency, add Bl.23 (shenshu +) and Kid.3 (taixi +)
- In most cases, points to calm the shen can be helpful: select one or two of the following: Ht.7 (shenmen), yintang (M–HN–3), Du.19 (houding), Du. 24 (shenting)
- Ear points: liver, spleen, shenmen, subcortex, sympathetic

Clinical Notes
- Liver qi constraint fever may be diagnosed as premenstrual syndrome, menopausal syndrome, neurodermatitis and eczema and autonomic nervous system dysfunction.
- This is a common pattern of fever and flushing, and one that often requires diligence to resolve completely. Identification and, if possible, rectification of the emotional and stress triggers is essential for long term success, as are suitable strategies designed to minimize their impact. These tools include meditation, yoga, active relaxation and exercise (p.103). Treatment often needs to be prolonged (several month minimum) to effect long term change. Acupuncture, given regularly, can facilitate 'physiological retraining', modifying the way the patient responds to the stress triggers.
- For dietary recommendations, see Clinical Handbook, Vol. 2, p878.
- Hot spot therapy is helpful, p.923.

瘀
血
发
热

8.7 BLOOD STASIS

Chronic fever from blood stasis is most often a complication of some other protracted pathology, such as Liver qi constraint, yang or yin deficiency or chronic heat. This type of fever may also follow an unresolved or poorly managed physical trauma, childbirth, hemorrhage, or severe emotional trauma.

The mechanism of the fever is due to both the propensity of stasis to generate heat, and the diminished capacity of the blood to lubricate and moisten the tissues of the body.

Clinical features
- Low grade, hectic or undulant fever which rises in the afternoon and is more prominent at night. The heat may be subjective (body temperature normal or even low) or localized to one part of the body, often the chest or upper body. The fever is rarely accompanied by night sweats.
- fitful sleep with much dreaming and restlessness
- irritability, anger, depression
- focal or recurrent pain that recurs in the same location
- hard immobile masses felt on palpation (usually in the abdomen)
- left iliac fossa pressure pain (p.925–926)
- dry mouth and throat with little desire to drink
- dry, scaly, itchy skin, especially in the lower limbs
- broken vessels or spider naevi on the face, trunk, inner knee and ankle
- purplish lips, sclera, conjunctivae and nails
- dark rings around the eyes
- sallow or grey complexion

T dark or red purple, or with brown or purple stasis spots; sublingual veins are distended and dark

P deep and choppy or wiry and fine

Treatment Principle
Activate blood and qi and dispel stagnant blood
Clear heat and cool the blood
Regulate the Liver and invigorate qi

Prescription

XUE FU ZHU YU TANG 血府逐瘀汤
Drive Out Stasis in the Mansion of Blood Decoction

tao ren (Persicae Semen) 桃仁	9–12g
hong hua (Carthami Flos) 红花	6–9g
sheng di (Rehmanniae Radix) 生地	9–12g
dang gui (Angelicae sinensis Radix) 当归	9–12g
chi shao (Paeoniae Radix rubra) 赤芍	9–12g
chuan xiong (Chuanxiong Rhizoma) 川芎	6–9g
chai hu (Bupleuri Radix) 柴胡	6–9g
zhi ke (Aurantii Fructus) 枳壳	6–9g

gan cao (Glycyrrhizae Radix) 甘草 3–6g
chuan niu xi (Cyathulae Radix) 川牛膝 9–15g
jie geng (Platycodi Radix) 桔梗 6–9g

Method: Decoction. **Tao ren, hong hua, chi shao, chuan xiong** and **chuan niu xi** activate blood and disperse stagnant blood; **sheng di, dang gui, chi shao** and **chuan xiong** nourish and regulate blood; **sheng di** and **chi shao** cool the blood and clear heat from stagnation; **chai hu** and **zhi ke** dredge the Liver and regulate qi; **chai hu, chuan xiong, jie geng** and **chuan niu xi** and **zhi ke** combine ascending and descending actions to stimulate the flow of qi and blood and rectify the qi dynamic; **gan cao** protects the Stomach. (Source: *Zhong Yi Nei Ke Xue* [*Yi Lin Gai Cuo*])

Modification

- If fever is persistent, add **qin jiao** (Gentianae macrophyllae Radix) 秦艽 6–9g, **bai wei** (Cynanchi atrati Radix) 白薇 9–12g, **zhi mu** (Anemarrhenae Rhizoma) 知母 9–12g and **yin chai hu** (Stellariae Radix) 银柴胡 6–12g.
- With high fever, increase the dose of **chi shao** to 15g and add **mu dan pi** (Moutan Cortex) 牡丹皮 9–12g.
- With chest or hypochondriac pain, add two or three of the following herbs: **yu jin** (Curcumae Radix) 郁金 9–12g, **chuan lian zi** (Toosendan Fructus) 川楝子 9–12g, **mo yao** (Myrrha) 没药 6–9g, **ru xiang** (Olibanum) 乳香 9g or **xie bai** (Allii macrostemi Bulbus) 薤白 6–9g.
- With amenorrhea, add **yi mu cao** (Leonurus Herba) 益母草 12–15g and **ze lan** (Lycopi Herba) 泽兰 9–12g.
- With palpable masses beneath the ribs, or if the liver is enlarged and nodular, add **dan shen** (Salviae miltiorrhizae Radix) 丹参 12–15g, **e zhu** (Curcumae Rhizoma) 莪术 9–12g, **san leng** (Sparganii Rhizoma) 三棱 9–12g and **bie jia** (Trionycis Carapax) 鳖甲 12–15g. See also Table 1.3. p.9.
- With qi deficiency, add **huang qi** (Astragali Radix) 黄芪 15–30g, **dang shen** (Codonopsis Radix) 党参 15–30g and **bai zhu** (Atractylodis macrocephalae Rhizoma) 白术 12–15g.
- With blood deficiency, add **huang qi** (Astragali Radix) 黄芪 15–30g and **shu di** (Rehmanniae Radix preparata) 熟地 18–24g.
- With phlegm damp, add **cang zhu** (Atractylodis Rhizoma) 苍术 9–12g, **yi ren** (Coicis Semen) 苡仁 15–30g and **fu ling** (Poria) 茯苓 12–18g.
- With fluid in the peritoneal cavity (ascites) and scanty urination, add **hou po** (Magnoliae officinalis Cortex) 厚朴 12–15g, **che qian zi** (Plantaginis Semen) 车前子 12–15g and **da fu pi** (Arecae Pericarpium) 大复皮 12–15g.

Variations and additional prescriptions

Blood stasis following trauma

A persistent, low grade, hectic fever may follow a significant physical trauma. The patient may experience ongoing pain and swelling, insomnia or dream disturbed sleep. The treatment is to activate blood, disperse static blood and clear heat with FU YUAN HUO XUE TANG (Revive Health by Activating the Blood Decoction 复元活血汤), modified. The prescription is usually used only for a few weeks, depending on how severe the trauma was. The patient should experience loose stools or diarrhea initially as the blood stasis resolves.

jiu da huang (wine fried Rhei Radix et Rhizoma) 酒大黄 9–12g

dang gui (Angelicae sinensis Radix) 当归 9–12g
tian hua fen (Trichosanthes Radix) 天花粉 9–12g
tao ren (Persicae Semen) 桃仁 6–9g
hong hua (Carthami Flos) 红花 6–9g
chai hu (Bupleuri Radix) 柴胡 6–9g
gan cao (Glycyrrhizae Radix) 甘草 3–6g
wang bu liu xing (Vaccariae Semen) 王不留行 9–12g

Method: Decoction. Often taken with a little yellow wine (*shaoxing jiu* 绍兴酒) or vodka. **Jiu da huang** clears heat, breaks up and moves static blood, stimulates metabolism of old blood and provides an outlet for heat and static blood through the bile and the bowel; **dang gui**, **tao ren**, **hong hua** and **wang bu liu xing** activate blood, reduce swelling, disperse stagnant blood and stop pain; **mu dan pi** cools the blood and clears heat; **wang bu liu xing** frees the channels and network vessels; **chai hu** dredges the Liver and regulates qi to lead blood; **tian hua fen** reduces swelling and stimulates healing; **gan cao** protects the Stomach and eases spasms. **Wang bu liu xing** is substituted for **chuan shan jia** (Squama Manitis) 穿山甲, the scales of the endangered pangolin that appeared in the original prescription. (Source: *Shi Yong Fang Ji Xue [Yi Xue Fa Ming]*).

Postpartum blood stasis in the Uterus with heat

Following a difficult or traumatic labor and delivery, blood stasis can be left in the Uterus for some time. The stasis creates heat and leads to hectic nighttime fever, lower abdominal pain, dark clotted vaginal discharge or menstrual flow, amenorrhea, irritability or disturbances of consciousness, constipation and a choppy pulse. The treatment is to drain heat and break up blood stasis with Tao He Cheng Qi Tang (Peach Pit Decoction to Order the Qi 桃核承气汤, p.920). Following administration, the patient should pass large clots and have diarrhea, after which all symptoms should diminish. The formula should not be used for longer than 2–3 weeks.

Blood stasis complicated by other pathology

Blood stasis patterns can have numerous causes and may be complicated by other pathologies for which other prescriptions may be better suited. For example, when blood stasis with cold in the lower burner is a feature, Shao Fu Zhu Yu Tang (Drive Out Blood Stasis in the Lower Abdomen Decoction 少腹逐瘀汤, p.24) is preferred. With masses or nodules in the Liver, or swelling of the Liver and Spleen, Ge Xia Zhu Yu Tang (Drive Out Blood Stasis Below the Diaphragm Decoction 膈下逐瘀汤 p.13) can be used.

Prepared medicines

Concentrated powder

Xue Fu Zhu Yu Tang (Persica & Carthamus Combination)
Shao Fu Zhu Yu Tang (Fennel Seed & Corydalis Combination)
Ge Xia Zhu Yu Tang (Tangkuei & Corydalis Combination)
Tao He Cheng Qi Tang (Persica & Rhubarb Combination)
Fu Yuan Huo Xue Tang (Tangkuei & Persica Combination)

Pills

Xue Fu Zhu Yu Wan (Stasis in the Mansion of Blood Teapills)
Shao Fu Zhu Yu Wan (Stasis in the Lower Palace Teapills)

Ge Xia Zhu Yu Wan (Stasis in the Lower Chamber Teapills)

Acupuncture (select from)

LI.11 (quchi –)...................these points activate and cool the blood
LI.4 (hegu –)
Sp.10 (xuehai –)
Sp.6 (sanyinjiao)
Bl.15 (xinshu +) ....strengthens the Heart and activate blood circulation
Bl.17 (geshu –)...................meeting point for blood, dispels static blood
Bl.18 (ganshu –).................transport point of the Liver, dredges the Liver and
                                activates qi and blood
Liv.14 (qimen –) ....alarm point of the Liver, dredges the Liver and
                                activates qi and blood
Liv.2 (xingjian –)................brook and fire point of the Liver, clears heat from
                                the Liver and cools the blood
Liv.3 (taichong –)...............source, transport and earth point, activates blood,
                                regulates the channels

- Blooding letting can be helpful in activating blood and clearing heat. Congested vessels found around the knee, popliteal fossa or ankle can be pierced with a surgical lancet and a few drops of blood extracted. Ideally the blood should run black at first, then fresh red. This technique can be performed weekly for a few sessions, then intermittently thereafter. See also p.929.
- with Spleen deficiency, add Ren.12 (zhongwan +) and St.36 (zusanli +)
- with spasm or cramping pain, add Du.8 (jinsuo –)
- with depression, apply rice grain moxa to Liv.1 (dadun)
- Ear points: liver, heart, shenmen, sympathetic, subcortex

Clinical notes

- Chronic fever from blood stasis may be diagnosed as autoimmune conditions such as Systemic Lupus Erythematosus (SLE) and Behçets syndrome, or tumors, lymphoma or leukemia. When the diagnosis is cancer, a combination of Western and Chinese medicine is required.
- Treatment usually needs to be prolonged. The primary prescription can be used for some months, but blood activating treatment can also disperse healthy blood. The patient should be monitored for signs of increasing blood deficiency and a break from the main treatment every 2–3 months may be required. Mild blood activating supplements or prepared medicines to supplement blood can be used during this time. In fever patterns following trauma or childbirth, treatment should not be required for longer than 2–3 weeks.

Table 8.1 Summary of chronic fever patterns

Pattern		Features	Prescription
Lingering pathogens	heat in the qi level	Low grade fever, night sweating, insomnia, restlessness, persistent dry cough, thirst, nausea, irritability, fatigue, swollen cervical lymph nodes, red dry tongue with little or no coat, weak fine rapid pulse	Zhu Ye Shi Gao Tang
	shaoyang	Alternating episodes of fever & chills, loss of appetite, nausea, hypochondriac pain, fullness in the chest, dizziness, irritability, bitter taste in the mouth, wiry pulse	Xiao Chai Hu Tang
	damp heat	Low grade fever rising mid afternoon, night sweats, muscle aches, fatigue, abdominal distension, loss of appetite, loose stools, nausea, swollen cervical lymph nodes, thick greasy white or yellow tongue coat, slippery wiry slightly rapid pulse	San Ren Tang
	summerheat	Low grade fever, copious sweating, thirst, irritability, scanty urine, fatigue, shortness of breath, weakness, loss of appetite, swollen cervical lymph nodes, dry tongue with yellow or geographic coat, weak soggy slightly rapid pulse	Wang Shi Qing Shu Yi Qi Tang
	heat in the blood	Low grade fever at night, weight loss, fatigue, heat in the palms & soles, red itchy skin rashes, flushing, swollen lymph nodes, red dry tongue with little or no coat, fine rapid pulse	Qing Hao Bie Jia Tang
Qi deficiency		Low grade fever which is worse in the morning and when overtired. Fatigue, pale complexion, spontaneous sweating, breathlessness, poor appetite, muscle weakness, slumped posture, susceptibility to infections, pale swollen scalloped tongue with a thin white coat, fine weak pulse	Bu Zhong Yi Qi Tang
Blood deficiency		Continuous low grade fever; the heat may be felt mainly in the face & hands, postural dizziness, blurring vision, fatigue, pallor; pale conjunctiva, lips & nail beds, insomnia, palpitations, forgetfulness, night sweats, constipation, dry skin & hair, scanty periods; anxiety, pale tongue with orangey edges, fine weak pulse	Gui Pi Tang
Yin deficiency		Low grade fever, hot flushes, night sweats, heat in the palms & soles, tiredness & agitation, malar flushing, insomnia, irritability, dry mouth & throat, constipation, concentrated urine, red dry or cracked tongue with no coat, fine rapid pulse	Qing Gu San

Table 8.1 Summary of chronic fever patterns (cont.)

Pattern	Features	Prescription
Yang deficiency	Low grade fever, worse when tired and after exertion. Heat is felt in upper body, while the lower body & extremities are cold. Exhaustion, pallor, cold intolerance, lower back, legs & knees aching, edema, frequent urination, nocturia, early morning ('cockcrow') diarrhea, pale swollen scalloped tongue, deep, fine, weak, imperceptible pulse	You Gui Wan
Liver qi constraint with heat	Low grade fever related to emotional state or stage of menstrual cycle. Premenstrual syndrome, red skin or rashes on the neck & face, flushing, irritability, depression, bitter taste, dry mouth, red sore eyes, hypochondriac discomfort, abdominal bloating, flatulence, alternating constipation & diarrhea, red tongue with redder edges and a thin yellow coat, wiry rapid pulse	Jia Wei Xiao Yao San
Blood stasis	Low grade fever worse at night, fitful sleep, irritability, depression, focal pain or hard immobile lumps, dry, scaly itchy skin hair loss, broken vessels or spider naevi, purplish lips, sclera, conjunctivae & nails, sallow or dark complexion, purple tongue with brown or purple stasis spots, distended & dark sublingual veins, choppy wiry fine pulse	Xue Fu Zhu Yu Tang

HEADACHE

Headache (*tóu tòng* 头痛) is pain in the head. Almost everyone will experience a headache at one time or another. As an isolated event in response to some postural, physical or emotional state, a headache is part and parcel of life. When persistent or recurrent, or when they interfere with normal functioning, headaches suggests chronic imbalance that requires intervention.

The headaches likely to bring a patient into the Chinese medicine clinic are the chronic, recurrent types. Most chronic headaches have an internal and an external component. What this means is that the underlying internal imbalance is frequently complicated by pathological (myofascial) lesions in the soft tissues of the neck and upper back. These lesions are associated with specific changes in muscle architecture, and can be felt as tight knots or painful bands of tissue. These lesions can cause pain to be referred to various areas of the head, and are commonly known as trigger points (p.410–411). Trigger points in the muscles of the neck and upper back are a common finding in patients with chronic headaches. Trigger points can develop in response to the underlying pathology, or may develop independently due to mechanical and postural forces. In either case, successful treatment of chronic headaches usually involves both constitutional treatment and the removal of as much tension and trigger point activity as possible.

> **BOX 9.1 PATTERNS OF HEADACHE**
>
> External invasion
> – wind cold
> – wind heat
> – wind damp
> – summerheat
> Liver qi constraint
> Liver fire
> Ascendant Liver yang and wind
> Cold affecting the Liver and Stomach
> Phlegm damp
> Wind phlegm
> Blood stasis
> Stomach heat
> Stomach and Gallbladder disharmony
> Qi deficiency
> Blood deficiency
> Kidney deficiency
> – yin deficiency
> – yang deficiency

ETIOLOGY

External pathogens

Invasion by external pathogens is a common cause of acute, usually self limiting headaches. Wind, cold, damp and heat, either singly or in combination may be involved. The taiyang channels of the back of the neck are most commonly targeted as they are the most exposed to the environment and the first point of contact between the pathogen and the host. In most cases, these headaches will be accompanied by exterior signs and symptoms, but occasionally the headache may appear before the onset of other symptoms. Each pathogen produces a characteristic type of headache, and may affect different parts of the head. The headache is the result of disruption to the distribution of qi and blood through the superficial tissues of the head and neck by the pathogen.

BOX 9.2 BIOMEDICAL CAUSES OF HEADACHE

General
- tension/stress
- referred pain from trigger points in neck and upper body muscles
- infection/fever
  - sinus
  - otitis
  - dental infection, gum disease
  - meningitis/encephalitis

Cardiovascular
- subarachnoid hemorrhage
- cerebral hemorrhage
- temporal arteritis

Neurological
- migraine/cluster headaches
- trigeminal neuralgia

Drugs (use or withdrawal from)
- alcohol
- aspirin and codeine (rebound from)
- antibiotics and anti–fungal agents
- antihypertensives

- caffeine
- corticosteroids
- ergotamine (rebound from)
- MAO inhibitors
- nicotine
- oral contraceptives
- vasodilators

Other
- occupational or environmental toxins and chemicals
- post traumatic, concussion
- anemia
- hypoglycemia
- herpes zoster (pre–eruption)
- glaucoma

Caution: Sudden severe headaches or steadily increasing headaches may hint at a sinister malady such as meningitis, a subdural hematoma or a cerebral tumor.

Emotional factors

Emotions are significant contributors to both acute and chronic headaches. Liver qi constraint from unexpressed frustration, anger, worry or other internalized emotion, leads directly to the common tension headaches that afflict a large proportion of humanity. Chronic qi constraint, in turn, sets the scene for the development of more serious pathology, such as blood stasis, yin deficiency with ascendant yang and Liver wind. In addition, chronic qi constraint can weaken the Spleen and lead to qi and blood deficiency, damp and phlegm (Fig. 9.1, p.411). Prolonged qi constraint also contributes to the chronic muscle tension in the upper back and neck that leads to the development of trigger points.

Some emotional states may weaken the Spleen and Lungs and lead to qi deficiency. Qi deficiency, in turn, can be complicated by excess pathology in the form of phlegm damp or qi constraint. Worry, obsessive thinking or rumination deplete Spleen qi or cause Liver Spleen disharmony. Grief, prolonged sadness or bereavement can weaken the Lungs and deplete Lung qi. Weak Lung qi loses the ability to restrain the Liver through the controlling cycle (metal controlling wood) which encourages both qi constraint and the chaotic ascent of qi.

Diet

The diet is a common contributor to headaches. Insufficient food or lack of protein can lead to qi and blood deficiency. Foods or dietary habits that weaken the Spleen, such as raw and cold foods, and restrictive or rigid diets, can lead to qi and blood deficiency and the generation of damp and phlegm. An excess of sweet, oily, rich food and dairy products directly introduces

> **BOX 9.3 COMPREHENSIVE ASSESSMENT**
>
> - Constitutional diagnosis
> - Assessment of the neck and upper back for trigger point activity
> - Postural and ergonomic assessment, including bed and pillow, work habits, desk, keyboard and screen height
> - Miscellaneous causes – dehydration, drugs, eyestrain, exposure to the sun

phlegm damp into the body. Some medications weaken the Spleen, deplete Spleen yang qi, or create damp and phlegm when used inappropriately. These include heat clearing herbs, hypoglycemic agents, antihypertensive drugs, laxatives and antibiotics. Excessive reliance on analgesics can damage Stomach and Liver yin.

Overconsumption of heating foods, in particular red wine and spirits, chocolate, coffee, shellfish, chillies, cheese and some spices can heat the Stomach, Liver and Gallbladder, leading to heat or fire patterns.

A common and often overlooked cause of headache is dehydration. This is seen in those who do manual or outdoor work, as well as those who work in hot environments or in the desiccating environment of air conditioned buildings.

Overwork

Working excessively long hours or laboring to the point of exhaustion depletes Spleen and Kidney yang qi. Insufficient sleep depletes Heart and Kidney yin. Headaches are quite common in people who expend lots of mental energy while being largely sedentary, a frequent finding in students, academics and office workers. This is due to the combined effects of qi and blood deficiency, the creation of damp as a result of qi deficiency, and the postural stresses associated with prolonged sitting. In addition, excessive use of the eyes, in combination with working long hours or working at night, depletes Liver blood.

Constitution

Chronic headaches can be associated with constitutional or inherited imbalances. Migraine headaches often run in families, and many patients report a history of headaches that start from a young age. This may involve aspects of Kidney jing deficiency and subsequent yin deficiency causing ascendant yang, or an inherited tendency to phlegm damp, qi constraint or qi and blood deficiency.

Trauma

A fall or blow to the head is a common cause of blood stasis type headaches. The headaches may not necessarily appear immediately following the trauma, but can occur months or years later, initiated by another illness, or a decline in general health and circulation.

Trigger points and mechanical stress

Trigger points (TPs) are focal contracted and irritated areas within a muscle that produce pain signals. Pain is referred to a location some distance from the site of

Figure 9.1 Pathological relationships of Liver qi constraint relating to headache

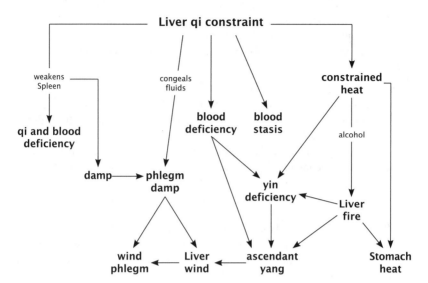

the trigger point. Muscles of the neck and upper back are especially prone to develop trigger points and frequently refer pain to specific regions of the head. TP's are characterized by an area of focal tenderness and knots within a tight band of contracted muscle and can be easily located by palpation.

Many chronic types of headache have both a constitutional and muscular component. Some conditions, notably the Liver patterns (qi constraint, ascendant yang and wind) and yin and blood deficiency patterns, predispose patients to the formation of trigger points. The resulting trigger points then become a source of pain in the head themselves, and overlapping patterns of pain may emerge. For a thorough discussion of trigger points, see Travel and Simons (1983), Legge (2010) and Baldry (1993).

Trigger points can develop because of mechanical stress, as the result of internal pathology, or a mixture of both. The pathology most likely to produce TPs is associated with the Liver, in particular Liver qi constraint and its related complications, and deficiency of Liver blood and yin which fails to nourish the muscles and sinews, leaving them prone to mechanical strain and injury.

The mechanical causes of TP formation include sudden unaccustomed overload of a muscle, traumatic injury, repetitive activity or postural stress. Mechanical stresses that specifically give rise to headaches include postural stress associated with poorly designed furniture, sitting hunched for hours in front of a computer, a cramped sleeping position, an excessively soft or high and hard pillow, or prolonged head extension while engaged in a task requiring an awkward orientation. The muscles implicated in headaches are noted in Boxes 9.5–9.8, pp.415–418.

Once trigger points have formed, they generally persist unless actively treated. Many people harbor latent TPs that can be activated by seemingly trivial events such as coughing or sneezing, overexertion, a long drive or sudden rotation of the head.

PATHOLOGY

There are two mechanisms of headache production, those associated with deficiency and those associated with excess. These two types produce quite different types of headache.

The excess types of headache are more severe, and can be debilitating. They are caused by obstruction to the circulation of qi and blood by a pathogen. The nature of the obstructing pathogen has a direct bearing on the quality of the pain. The more substantial the obstruction, the more intense the headache. Trigger point activity in associated tissues is common.

The deficient types of headache are due to insufficient qi, blood, yin or yang reaching the head. They are mild to moderate and dull, and are associated with mental and physical fatigue. Mixed deficiency and excess headaches are common, with some patients experiencing both at the same time, or sequentially. A common example is the persistent dull headache of yin and blood deficiency which occasionally yields to the intense and splitting headache of ascendant yang.

TREATMENT

Treatment of the acute headache aims at immediate relief with the use of acupuncture to disperse stagnation, deactivate trigger points, dispel wind and so forth, or with swift acting herb decoctions and prepared medicines. Between episodes the treatment focuses on the underlying condition. As a general rule, headaches due to deficiency, in particular blood and yin deficiency, respond best to herbal therapy, while the Liver patterns respond well to regular acupuncture, massage and deactivation of associated trigger points. Blood stasis patterns can do well with acupuncture, but will often need herbs to obtain a sustained result. Headaches due to external pathogens usually respond quickly to both herbs and acupuncture.

Biomechanical and ergonomic factors need to be addressed. Sleeping position, pillow height, computer keyboard and screen placement, office furniture and couch design are frequent factors in chronic headaches, regardless of the systemic pathology also present.

Selection of acupuncture points

Acupuncture points are selected on the basis of the pattern involved, the location of the headache and the presence of trigger points. During a headache, the main points will be selected from those that influence the location of the headache (Boxes 9.5–9.8, pp.415–418). In between headaches, points are selected primarily on the basis of the diagnostic pattern. Points can be selected on the basis of their specific effects on headache (Table 9.1, p.419–420). Trigger points, when present, should be treated until they resolve.

BOX 9.4 KEY DIAGNOSTIC POINTS

Nature
- throbbing, pounding, splitting – ascendant Liver yang, Liver fire, Stomach and Gallbladder disharmony, toxic heat
- distending – ascendant Liver yang, Liver fire, wind heat
- focal, stabbing, boring – blood stasis
- heavy, as if wrapped in a wet cloth – phlegm damp
- like a tight band around the head – Liver qi constraint
- dull, background, all over ache – blood deficiency, Kidney deficiency

Onset
- premenstrual – Liver qi constraint, ascendant yang, blood stasis
- after menstruation or when breast feeding – blood deficiency
- when hungry – Spleen qi deficiency
- with eating – Stomach heat, phlegm damp
- first thing in the morning, waking with – phlegm damp, qi constraint, biomechanical stress on neck with trigger point activation from poor pillow height
- soon after getting out of bed – blood deficiency, Liver qi constraint
- with activity, at end of the day – qi and blood deficiency
- evening, at night – yin and blood deficiency, blood stasis
- weekends, holidays – Liver qi constraint, ascendant yang

Aggravation
- with emotional upset, anger – Liver pathology
- with prolonged standing – blood deficiency, Kidney deficiency
- with prolonged sitting or lying – phlegm damp, qi constraint, ascendant yang
- alcohol, fatty food – Stomach and Gallbladder disharmony, Liver fire
- with changes of weather – wind damp, phlegm damp
- with massage of the neck – blood deficiency, yin deficiency
- waking with headache during the night – blood deficiency, Liver qi constraint ascendant yang (between 1–3am), Stomach and Gallbladder disharmony
- with strong smells – phlegm damp
- with use of the eyes – blood deficiency
- after sex – Kidney deficiency

Amelioration
- with exercise – Liver qi constraint, phlegm damp
- with rest – deficiency
- with eating – Spleen qi deficiency
- with a cold compress – Stomach heat, Liver fire, ascendant yang, wind heat
- after vomiting – Stomach and Gallbladder disharmony, phlegm damp, ascendant yang, Liver fire

Accompanying features
- nausea, vomiting – Stomach and Gallbladder disharmony, cold affecting the Liver and Stomach, phlegm damp, Liver fire, ascendant Liver yang
- eye distension and pain – ascendant yang, Liver fire
- dizziness, vertigo – phlegm damp, ascendant yang, Liver wind
- postural dizziness – blood deficiency, yin deficiency
- cold extremities – cold affecting the Liver and Stomach, Liver qi constraint

Manual therapy

Massage and passive mobilization of the neck and upper back are helpful for alleviating muscular tension and deactivating trigger points. Strong massage is most suitable for the excess patterns. Patients with blood or yin deficiency patterns should be treated gently, as deep massage can irritate the muscles, aggravate tension and trigger points, and worsen the headache.

Hot Spot therapy

Hot spot therapy (see Appendix 2, p.923) is a method of self treatment of trigger points done at home in between formal treatment sessions. Hot spot therapy is particularly useful for Liver qi constraint and ascendant yang patterns. The most common location to find active trigger points potentially contributing to headache, is in the paraspinal muscles between T3–T10.

Hot spot therapy is not suitable for yin and blood deficiency due to the characteristic irritability of the tissues of the neck and upper back. Headaches and muscular pain of a deficiency type can be aggravated by hot spot therapy.

Medications

The following pharmaceutical medications are commonly used for headaches. Patients with chronic headaches will often be taking multiple medications, both preventively and for acute episodes. The use of preventive medication may mask the underlying pattern and can impede diagnosis and treatment. As treatment progresses, the aim should be to reduce all medications, including Chinese herbs, but this should be done slowly, following the patients decreasing requirements as their condition improves. Withdrawal of some medications can lead to rebound headaches if done too quickly.

Analgesics and Non–Steroids Anti–inflammatory Drugs (NSAIDS)

This group includes aspirin, paracetamol, indomethacin, iboprufen, naproxen and diclofenac, the most common medications used for common headaches, and widely available over the counter. In Chinese medical terms they tend to be cooling and dispersing to qi, yin and blood. Overuse may damage Liver and Stomach yin.

Ergotamine (Cafergot, Ergodryl)

Ergotamine is used at the onset of a migraine headache. It produces vasoconstriction peripherally, and in high doses can damage peripheral epithelium and contribute to blood stasis, thrombosis and gangrene.

Pizotifen (Sandomigran)

Used to prevent migraine headaches, pizotifen is a serotonin antagonist and also has some activity as an antihistamine. Side effects include dry mouth, drowsiness, increased appetite and weight gain. Pizotifen is pungent, warm and dispersing, and may disperse and damage zheng qi and yin.

Sumatriptin (Imigran)

A strong drug used at the onset of migraine. Used frequently, it can lead to increased frequency of headache. Sumatriptin is pungent, warm and dispersing to qi and yin. Side effects include flushing, feelings of heat, weakness and fatigue.

BOX 9.5 YANGMING DISTRIBUTION (FRONTAL)

Frontal headaches may be associated with trigger point activity in the muscles noted below, and with disorders of the Stomach, Spleen, Large Intestine, Liver and Gallbladder. Common pathology includes Stomach heat, Stomach and Gallbladder disharmony, Spleen qi deficiency, phlegm damp, qi constraint, wind heat and sinus congestion (see Sinusitis and Nasal Congestion, Vol. 1).

Common points

Local
- yintang (M–HN–3)
- Du.23 (shangxing)
- GB.14 (yangbai)
- Bl.2 (zanzhu)
- GB.20 (fengchi)

Distal
- LI.4 (hegu)
- St.36 (zusanli)
- St.44 (neiting)
- St.41 (jiexi)

Herbs that target the yangming area
- bai zhi (Angelicae dahuricae Radix)
- cang er zi (Xanthii Fructus)
- man jing zi (Viticis Fructus)
- ju hua (Chrysanthemi Flos)
- sheng ma (Cimicifugae Rhizoma)
- chuan xiong (Chuanxiong Rhizoma)

Referred pain from trigger points
- sternocleidomastoid
- semispinalis capitis
- frontalis
- zygomaticus major
- masseter
- splenius cervicus

Characteristic

Dull
- phlegm damp
- wind damp
- qi deficiency

Tight, constant
- Liver qi constraint

Splitting, pounding, throbbing
- wind heat
- toxic heat
- summerheat
- Stomach heat
- GB and Stomach disharmony
- Liver fire

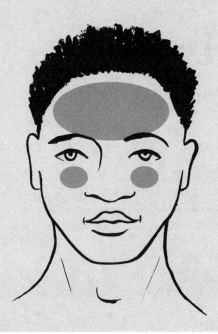

BOX 9.6 SHAOYANG DISTRIBUTION (TEMPORAL)

Temporal headaches are associated with trigger point activity in the muscles noted below (especially sternocleidomastoid), and disorder of the Liver and Gallbladder, and qi and blood stasis. Ascendant yang, Liver fire, and Gallbladder and Stomach disharmony may be unilateral or bilateral. Blood stasis is usually unilateral. Temporal headaches often concentrate behind the eyes.

Common points

Local
- GB.20 (fengchi)
- taiyang (M–HN–5)
- St.8 (touwei)
- GB.1 (tongziliao)
- GB.8 (shuaigu)

Distal
- SJ.5 (waiguan) + GB.41 (zulinqi)
- Liv.3 (taichong) + LI.4 (hegu)
- GB.34 (yanglingquan) + GB.21 (jianjing)
- Lu.7 (lieque)

Herbs that target the shaoyang area
- chuan xiong (Chuanxiong Rhizoma)
- chai hu (Bupleuri Radix)
- ju hua (Chrysanthemi Flos)
- gou teng (Uncariae Ramulus cum Uncis)
- bai ji li (Tribuli Fructus)
- shi jue ming (Haliotidis Concha)

Referred pain from trigger points
- sternocleidomastoid, [mastoid end of the sternal head, near SI.17 (tianrong)]
- trapezius [upper fibres, near GB.21 (jianjing)]
- temporalis
- semispinalis capitis [near GB.20 (fengchi)]
- suboccipital group

Characteristic

Dull, background
- blood deficiency

Tight, constant
- Liver qi constraint

Splitting, pounding, throbbing
- ascendant Liver yang
- Liver fire
- GB and Stomach disharmony

Stabbing, boring focal
- blood stasis

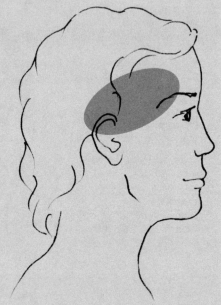

BOX 9.7 TAIYANG DISTRIBUTION (OCCIPITAL)

Occipital headaches can be caused by trigger point activity in the muscles noted below, or be associated with invasion of an external pathogen, Kidney deficiency, Liver qi constraint and pathology of the Urinary Bladder, Small Intestine and du channels.

Common points

Local
- GB.20 (fengchi)
- Du.16 (fengfu)
- Bl.10 (tianzhu)

Distal
- SI.3 (houxi) + Bl.62 (shenmai)
- Lu.7 (lieque)
- GB.41 (zulinqi)
- Bl.60 (kunlun)

Herbs that target the taiyang area
- qiang huo (Notopterygii Rhizoma seu Radix)
- gao ben (Ligustici Rhizoma)
- ge gen (Puerariae Radix)
- chuan xiong (Chuanxiong Rhizoma)

Referred pain from trigger points
- low and middle fibres of trapezius
- sternocleidomastoid
- semispinalis
- splenius
- suboccipital group
- multifidus

Characteristic

Dull, heavy
- wind damp

Dull, empty
- Kidney deficiency

Tight, constant
- wind cold
- Liver qi constraint

Splitting, pounding, throbbing
- ascendant Liver yang

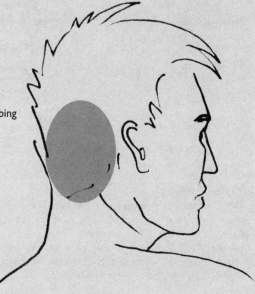

BOX 9.8 JUEYIN DISTRIBUTION (VERTEX)

Vertex headaches are associated with the pathology of the Liver (Liver qi constraint, ascendant yang, cold in the Liver and Stomach), and deficiency of qi and blood. A vertex headache is distinct and localized, and should be distinguished from a headache that involves the Urinary Bladder and du channels and which extends down to the occiput and neck.

Common points

Local
- Du.20 (baihui)
- Bl.7 (tongtian)
- GB.20 (fengchi)
- Du.23 (shangxing)

Distal
- Liv.3 (taichong)
- Bl.67 (zhiyin)
- SI.3 (houxi)
- Bl.60 (kunlun)

Herbs that target the jueyin area
- wu zhu yu (Evodiae Fructus)
- gao ben (Ligustici Rhizoma)
- gou teng (Uncariae Ramulus cum Uncis)
- tian ma (Gastrodiae Rhizoma)
- shi jue ming (Haliotidis Concha)
- chuan xiong (Chuanxiong Rhizoma)

Referred pain from trigger points
- sternocleidomastoid
- splenius capitus

Characteristic

Dull
- qi and blood deficiency
- Liver qi constraint

Tight, boring
- ascendant Liver yang
- cold in the Liver and Stomach

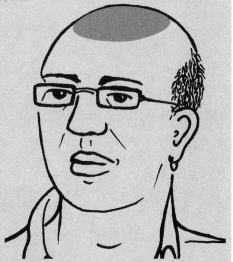

WHOLE HEAD

When a headache involves the whole head it extends down to the eyes in front and the hairline on the rest of the head. It may feel superficial, with sensitivity on the scalp, or feel deep inside the head. When acute it is usually due to an external invasion. When chronic, dull, heavy or 'empty', it may be due to prolonged Kidney deficiency or the clogging effects of phlegm damp; when splitting, ascendant Liver yang, Liver fire or toxic heat are implicated.

Table 9.1 Commonly used acupuncture points with specific effects on headaches

	Point	Attributes
L O C A L	taiyang (M-HN-9)	For excess headaches focusing in the temples, especially ascendant Liver yang or blood stasis. Be careful to avoid the temporal artery.
	yintang (M-HN-3)	For frontal headache, or any headache associated with qi constraint, stress and tension.
	yuyao (M-HN-6)	For frontal headache and orbital pain.
	St.8 (touwei)	Convergent point of the Stomach, Gallbladder and yangwei channels. For frontal and temporal headaches from ascendant yang or phlegm damp, especially when there are visual disturbances and eye pain.
	GB.1 (tongziliao)	For temporal headache from wind heat, Liver and Gallbladder pathology, with eye pain and visual disturbance.
	GB.8 (shuaigu)	For temporal and vertex headaches, and pain felt inside the head from Liver qi constraint or ascendant yang.
	GB.14 (yangbai)	A point where the Gallbladder, Stomach and Large Intestine channels converge. For frontal headaches from ascendant yang, headache with eye involvement and sinus congestion.
	GB.20 (fengchi)	An important point for all types of headache and facial pain. Dispels wind, pacifies ascendant yang and clears the head.
	BL.2 (zanzhu)	For frontal headache, pain above the orbital ridge and sinus headaches.
	Bl.7 (tongtian)	For vertex headache.
	Bl.10 (tianzhu)	For occipital headaches, pain behind the eyes and neck pain.
	SJ.23 (sizhukong)	For temporal and lateral orbital pain from wind heat, Liver and Gallbladder pathology.
	Du.16 (fengfu)	For all headaches associated with wind, both internal and external. Mostly for occipital pain, but can be used for temporal and frontal headaches as well.
	Du.20 (baihui)	An important point for all types of headache, and one that will be quite tender to palpation. In excess patterns, needling can move stagnation and pacify ascendant yang, and in deficient patterns light needling or moxa can help elevate qi and blood.
	Du.23 (shangxing)	For frontal and vertex headaches, especially when accompanied by nasal or sinus congestion.

Table 9.1 Commonly used acupuncture points (cont.)

Point		Attributes
	Liv.3 (taichong)	The main point for dredging the Liver, regulating qi and blood, and subduing ascendant yang. Combines well with PC.6 (neiguan) for headaches with nausea or vomiting, with GB.21 (jianjing) when the muscles of the neck and shoulders are tight, and GB.20 (fengchi) for all other patterns.
	PC.6 (neiguan)	For all types of Liver and Stomach related headaches. Especially good when digestive symptoms and sleep disturbances are part of the picture. Combines well with Liv.3 (taichong).
	GB.41 (zulinqi) + SJ.5 (waiguan)	For temporal headaches from qi constraint or ascendant yang. Works by rebalancing the distribution of yin and yang through opening daimai, which helps to drag yang qi downwards and out of the head. Also for premenstrual headaches.
	SJ.5 (waiguan) + GB.39 (xuanzhong)	For qi constraint, Liver heat and ascendant yang, especially when there is insomnia and a feeling as if the 'head is on fire'.
D I S T A L	Lu.7 (lieque)	For occipital headache from wind cold and temporal headache from Liver qi constraint or ascendant yang. Works to restrain ascendant yang by strengthening metal to control wood through the controlling cycle. Also used for yang qi deficiency headaches, as it can assist yang qi in getting to the head.
	LI.4 (hegu)	Important point for frontal and temporal headache, especially when associated with external pathogens, sinus congestion, Liver qi constraint [with Liv.3 (taichong)] or Stomach heat [with St.44 (neiting)].
	SI.3 (houxi) + Bl.62 (shenmai)	Major combination for occipital headache, especially good when there is stiffness and spasm of the neck with painful rotation and extension.
	SJ.10 (tianjing) + GB.38 (yangfu)	Reducing points of their respective channels, used for ascendant Liver yang headaches that concentrate behind the eye and at the lateral aspect of the eyebrow, with stiffness of the neck and shoulders.
	GB.34 (yanglingquan)	For temporal headaches from all Liver pathology, good when there is muscle spasm and tension in the neck. Combines well with GB.21 (jianjing).
	St.40 (fenglong)	For headaches from phlegm damp or ascendant yang with phlegm.
	St.41 (jiexi)	For frontal headaches from phlegm or Stomach heat.
	Bl.60 (kunlun)	For occipital or all over headaches from ascendant yang, wind heat or Kidney deficiency.
	Kid.1 (yongquan)	For vertex headaches with dizziness or fainting.

Table 9.2 Herbs with specific effects on headache

Herb	Attributes
Chuan Xiong Chuanxiong Rhizoma 川芎	Cnidium root; pungent, warm; Liver, Heart. Activates qi and blood, dispels wind. The premier herb for headaches. Can be used for all excess types of headache. For severe headaches it can be used in doses of 30–50 grams. When used at these large doses, it is only used for the duration of the headache, and should be combined with proportional doses of **bai shao** (Paeoniae Radix alba) 白芍 and **huai niu xi** (Achyranthis bidentatae Radix) 怀牛膝 to balance its rising pungent warmth and prevent excessive dispersal of qi and blood. For blood stasis headaches, up to 50 grams can be used in short bursts, always in combination with **dang gui** (Angelicae sinensis Radix) 当归 to enhance its blood activating effects while preventing excessive dispersal of yin and blood.
Bai Zhi Angelicae dahuricae Radix 白芷	Angelica dahurica root; pungent, warm; Stomach, Large Intestine. Dispels wind cold and stops pain. For frontal and temporal headaches, facial pain and toothache from wind cold, wind heat or phlegm damp. Good when there is sinus congestion.
Cang Er Zi Xanthii Fructus 苍耳子	Cocklebur fruit; pungent, bitter, warm; Lung, Spleen. Dispels wind and stops pain. For frontal headaches, especially those associated with sinus congestion.
Gao Ben Ligustici Rhizoma 藁本	Ligusticum root; pungent, warm; Urinary Bladder. Dispels wind cold damp. Used for occipital and vertical headaches, and headache from external invasion.
Qiang Huo Notopterygii Rhizoma seu Radix 羌活	Notopterygium root; pungent, bitter, warm; Urinary Bladder, Liver, Kidney. Dispels wind cold damp and stops pain. For occipital headaches from external invasion or protracted wind damp in the taiyang channels.
Ge Gen Puerariae Radix 葛根	Kudzu root; sweet, pungent, cool; Stomach, Spleen. Eases the muscles and dispels wind. For neck and occipital pain from a variety of causes, including external pathogens, ascendant yang and qi constraint.
Man Jing Zi Viticis Fructus 蔓荆子	Vitex fruit; pungent, bitter, cool; Urinary Bladder, Liver, Stomach. Dispels wind heat and damp and targets the face and eyes. For frontal and temporal headache and eye pain from wind heat and Liver heat patterns.
Ju Hua Chrysanthemi Flos 菊花	Chrysanthemum flower; sweet, slightly biter, cool; Lung, Liver. Dispels wind heat, calms the Liver. For wind heat and ascendant yang headaches. Targets the eyes, forehead and temporal area.
Chai Hu Bupleuri Radix 柴胡	Bupleurum root; pungent, bitter, cool; Liver, Gallbladder. Dispels wind heat, harmonizes shaoyang, dredges the Liver and alleviates qi constraint. For temporal and vertex headaches from qi constraint, ascendant yang, Gallbladder and Stomach disharmony and wind heat.

Table 9.2 Herbs with specific effects on headache (cont.)

Herb	Attributes
Sheng Ma Cimicifugae Rhizoma 升麻	Cimicifuga root; sweet, pungent, cool; Spleen, Stomach, Lung, Large Intestine. Clears heat. For frontal headache from Stomach heat and qi deficiency headache (in small doses with chai hu).
Tian Ma Gastrodiae Rhizoma 天麻	Gastrodia root; sweet, slightly pungent; Liver. Extinguishes wind, alleviates spasm and stops pain. An important herb for temporal, vertex and entire cranium headache from ascendant yang and phlegm damp.
Gou Teng Uncariae Ramulus cum Uncis 钩藤	Uncaria twigs; sweet, cool; Liver, Pericardium. Extinguishes wind, alleviates spasm, calms the Liver and clears heat. For temporal and vertex headaches from Liver heat and wind. Good when there is spasm and tension in the neck.
Bai Ji Li Tribuli Fructus 白蒺藜	Tribulus fruit; pungent, bitter, warm; Liver, Lung. Dispels wind, dredges the Liver, activates qi and blood. For temporal headaches from Liver qi constraint and ascendant yang, especially when there is dizziness and redness or pain in the eyes.
Ci Shi Magnetitum 磁石	Magnetite; pungent, salty, cool; Liver, Kidney. Subdues ascendant Liver yang. For headache from Liver yin deficiency with ascendant yang.
Shi Jue Ming Haliotidis Concha 石决明	Abalone shell; salty, cool; Liver, Lung. Calms the Liver and restrains yang. For temporal and vertex headache from ascendant yang. Good when there is visual disturbances and aura.
Wu Gong Scolopendra 蜈蚣 **Quan Xie** Scorpio 全蝎	Centipede and scorpion; pungent, slightly toxic; Liver. Extinguish wind, alleviate spasms and stop pain. Used together for relatively severe, stubborn or neuralgic pain. Best powdered and added to the strained decoction or in concentrated powder form.
Di Long Lumbricus 地龙	Earthworm; salty, cold; Liver, Kidney, Lung. Frees the channels and network vessels. For stubborn headache and loss of function from blood stasis.
Zhi Bai Fu Zi Typhonii Rhizoma preparatum 制白附子	Typhonium root; pungent, sweet, hot, toxic; Liver, Spleen. Dispels wind phlegm and stops pain. A strong dispersing and slightly toxic herb used for stubborn headaches and facial pain associated with phlegm or blood stasis.

423

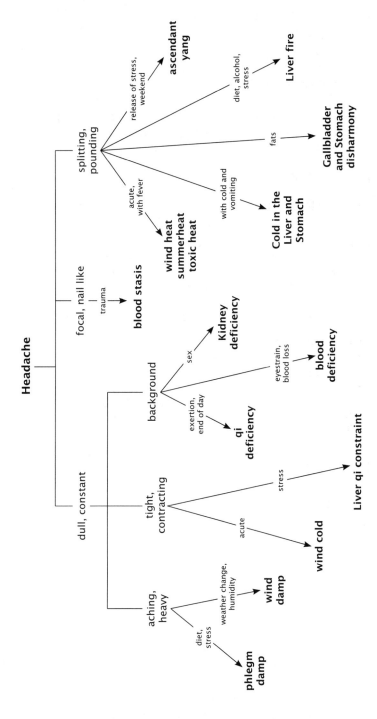

Figure 9.2 Headaches and some common triggers

9.1. HEADACHE FROM EXTERNAL INVASION
1. Wind cold
2. Wind heat
3. Wind damp
4. Summerheat

All headaches in this category are acute and associated with exposure to a sudden change of weather or an external pathogen. They are usually self limiting, but can turn into more protracted disorders if the pathogen is not dispelled. The headache may precede the onset of the classical symptoms of a wind invasion by a couple of days.

风
寒
头
痛

9.1.1 WIND COLD
Wind cold headaches are due to exposure to wind and cold, as may occur for example, from getting chilled as the weather changes, sleeping in a draught or having air conditioning blowing on the head and neck area. The wind cold penetrates into the taiyang channels, constricting and obstructing the circulation of qi and blood, resulting in pain. See Box 9.7, p.417.

Migraine type headaches and facial pain may be of a wind cold type, especially those triggered by exposure to wind or sudden changes of temperature.

Clinical features
• Acute headache, most commonly occipital, but which may involve other parts of the head and face.
• Aversion to wind and cold; exposure to wind may aggravate or initiate the headache or facial pain. Covering the head and neck in a scarf or some protective covering can provide some degree of comfort and relief.
• muscle aches and stiffness, especially neck and upper back
• simultaneous chills and fever, with chills predominant
• no sweating
• nasal obstruction or a runny nose with thin watery mucus
T thin, white coat
P floating, or floating and tight

Treatment principle
Dispel wind cold and stop pain

Prescription
CHUAN XIONG CHA TIAO SAN 川芎茶调散
Chuanxiong Powder to be Taken with Green Tea

chuan xiong (Chuanxiong Rhizoma) 川芎 120g
jing jie (Schizonepetae Herba) 荆芥 120g
bo he (Menthae haplocalycis Herba) 薄荷 240g
bai zhi (Angelicae dahuricae Radix) 白芷 60g
qiang huo (Notopterygii Rhizoma seu Radix) 羌活 60g

gan cao (Glycyrrhizae Radix) 甘草 60g
fang feng (Saposhnikovae Radix) 防风 45g
xi xin (Asari Herba) 细辛 30g
Method: Grind the herbs to a powder and take six grams with green tea or ginger tea every two hours. May also be decocted with a 90% reduction in dosage, in which case the formula is cooked for no longer than 20 minutes, and **bo he** (6g) is added at the end of cooking. **Chuan xiong** dispels wind, activates blood and stops pain; **bai zhi** alleviates frontal headache and dispels wind cold; **qiang huo**, dispels wind cold and alleviates occipital headache. **Jing jie** and **fang feng** dispel wind from the exterior; **bo he** dispels wind and regulates qi. **Xi xin** dispels wind cold and stops pain; **gan cao** harmonizes the formula and prevents the pungent dispersal of the primary herbs from damaging qi; **gan cao** protects qi and blood against excessive dispersal and drying. (Source: *Zhong Yi Nei Ke Xue* [*He Ji Ju Fang*])

Modifications

- With marked frontal headache, add **man jing zi** (Viticis Fructus) 蔓荆子 60g.
- With marked temporal headache, add **chai hu** (Bupleuri Radix) 柴胡 60g.
- With marked vertex headache, add **gao ben** (Ligustici Rhizoma) 藁本 60g.
- With damp, add **cang zhu** (Atractylodis Rhizoma) 苍术 60g, **gao ben** (Ligustici Rhizoma) 藁本 60g, **zhi ban xia** (Pinelliae Rhizoma preparatum) 制半夏 45g and **chen pi** (Citri reticulatae Pericarpium) 陈皮 45g.
- With stiff neck, add **gao ben** (Ligustici Rhizoma) 藁本 60g and **ge gen** (Puerariae Radix) 葛根 60g.
- For facial pain, including trigeminal neuralgia initiated by cold, add **quan xie** (Scorpio) 全蝎 1–3g and **wu gong** (Scolopendra) 蜈蚣 1–3g [both powdered and taken separately].
- With productive cough, add **xing ren** (Armeniacae Semen) 杏仁 60g, **su zi** (Perillae Fructus) 苏子 60g and **zhi ban xia** (Pinelliae Rhizoma preparatum) 制半夏 60g.

Variations and additional prescriptions
With yang deficiency / shaoyin syndrome

A wind cold pathogen may penetrate through the Urinary Bladder channel and affects its yin partner, the Kidney, especially when there is pre–existing Kidney qi or yang deficiency. This is mediated through the taiyang–shaoyin channel relationship. The features are acute onset of occipital or facial pain, with marked cold intolerance and possibly mild fever. In addition, pre–existing Kidney deficiency symptoms are aggravated, resulting in increasing nocturia or urinary frequency, fatigue and exhaustion, sleepiness and pallor. The tongue is pale and scalloped and the pulse deep and weak. The treatment is to support yang, dispel wind cold and stop pain with MA HUANG FU ZI XI XIN TANG (Ma Huang, Asarum and Prepared Aconite Decoction 麻黄附子细辛汤), modified.

ma huang (Ephedrae Herba) 麻黄 6g
zhi fu zi (Radix Aconiti Carmichaeli Praeparata) 制附子 9g
xi xin (Herba cum Radice Asari) 细辛 6g
bai zhi (Radix Angelicae Dahuricae) 白芷 9g
chuan xiong (Radix Ligustici Chuanxiong) 川芎 9g
Method: Decoction. **Zhi fu zi** should be cooked for 30 minutes prior to the other herbs. **Ma huang**, **xi xin** and **bai zhi** dispel wind cold; **zhi fu zi** warms yang and stops pain; **chuan xiong** stops head-

ache and supports **bai zhi** and **xi xin** alleviate facial pain. (Source: *Shi Yong Zhong Yi Nei Ke Xue* [*Shang Han Lun*])

Prepared medicines
Concentrated powders
Chuan Xiong Cha Tiao San (Ligusticum & Tea Formula)
Pills
Chuan Xiong Cha Tiao Wan (Ligusticum Teapills)

Acupuncture
GB.20 (fengchi –) ....dispels wind and alleviates neck pain and headache
LI.4 (hegu –) ....source point of the Large Intestine, clears wind cold
                                  and diffuses the Lungs (with Lu.7 [lieque])
Lu.7 (lieque –)....................connecting point of the Lungs, diffuses the Lungs
                                  and directs Lung qi downwards, dispels wind cold
Bl.12 (fengmen – Ω).........dispels wind
Bl.13 (feishu – Ω) ....transport point of the Lungs, diffuses the Lungs
Du.14 (dazhui – Ω) ....meeting point of the yang channels, clears pathogens
                                  from the exterior
- with marked stiff neck and severe occipital pain, add SI.3 (houxi) and Bl.60 (kunlun)
- with frontal headache, add yintang (M–HN–3)
- with temporal headache, add St.8 (touwei)
- with cough, add Lu.9 (taiyuan –)
- with wheezing, use dingchuan (M–BW–1)
- with copious sputum, add St.40 (fenglong –)
- with nasal congestion, add Du.23 (shangxing) and LI.20 (yingxiang)
- with a weak pulse, add St.36 (zusanli +)
- Ear points: lung, large intestine
- Treat 1–2 times daily if possible

Gua Sha
Scraping the taiyang channels of the back of the neck with a coin, or more conveniently and comfortably, a chinese soup spoon or plate, (*guā shā* 刮痧) is effective for headaches due to wind. The lubricated implement is dragged from GB.20 (fengchi) to around GB.21 (jianjing) until red blotches appear.

Clinical notes
- Wind cold type headaches are most commonly associated with the common cold, influenza or upper respiratory tract infection, but may also be diagnosed as a migraine headache or trigeminal neuralgia. Migraines or facial pain of this type are not associated with the classic wind cold signs and symptoms. Instead, the headache is triggered by exposure to wind or sudden changes of environment, such as going from a warm to cold room.
- Simple measures, like covering the neck with a scarf during changeable weather, can help to prevent wind cold headaches.

风
热
头
痛

9.1.2 WIND HEAT

Wind heat headache is caused by invasion of wind and heat. Wind heat, being a purely yang pathogen, tends to rise and expand affecting the forehead or the whole head.

Clinical features

- Acute distending headache which affects the frontal area or the whole head. The headache may be quite severe and accompanied by a feeling of heat, and is alleviated by the application of a cold compress.
- fever, with or without mild chills
- red face and eyes
- aversion to wind
- thirst with a desire for cool fluids
- maybe a dry cough or cough with sticky, yellow sputum
- sore swollen throat

T red tip with a yellow coat
P floating and rapid

Treatment principle

Dispel wind heat and stop pain

Prescription

XIONG ZHI SHI GAO TANG 芎芷石膏汤
Chuanxiong, Angelica Dahurica and Gypsum Decoction

chuan xiong (Chuanxiong Rhizoma) 川芎 9–12g
bai zhi (Angelicae dahuricae Radix) 白芷 9–12g
shi gao (Gypsum fibrosum) 石膏 15–30g
ju hua (Chrysanthemi Flos) 菊花 9–12g
gao ben (Ligustici Rhizoma) 藁本 9–12g
qiang huo (Notopterygii Rhizoma seu Radix) 羌活 6–9g

Method: Decoction. **Shi gao** is decocted for 30 minutes prior to the other herbs. **Chuan xiong** dispels wind and stops pain; **shi gao** and **ju hua** vent wind heat from the head and eyes; **bai zhi** dispels wind and stops frontal pain; **gao ben** and **qiang huo** dispel wind and stop occipital and vertex pain. (Source: *Zhong Yi Nei Ke Xue* [*Yi Zong Jin Jian*])

Modifications

- With sore throat, add **niu bang zi** (Arctii Fructus) 牛蒡子 9–12g and **huang qin** (Scutellariae Radix) 黄芩 6–9g.
- With damp, nausea, heavy head, chest oppression, afternoon fever and thick tongue coat, add **huo xiang** (Pogostemonis/Agastaches Herba) 藿香 12–15g, **pei lan** (Eupatorii Herba) 佩兰 9–12g and **huang lian** (Coptidis Rhizoma) 黄连 3–6g.
- With high fever, decrease the dose of **gao ben** and **qiang huo** and add **jin yin hua** (Lonicerae Flos) 金银花 15–30g and **shan zhi zi** (Gardeniae Fructus) 山栀子 9–12g.
- With constipation, add a small dose of **da huang** (Rhei Radix et Rhizoma) 大黄 3–6g.

- With irritability and restlessness, add **mu dan pi** (Moutan Cortex) 牡丹皮 9–12g and **shan zhi zi** (Gardeniae Fructus) 山栀子 9–12g.

Variations and additional prescriptions
Severe toxic wind heat
Severe wind heat may be concentrated enough to generate toxic heat. Acute toxic heat in the head is characterized by sudden onset of severe pounding headache, with high fever and chills or rigors, and redness, swelling and pain in the throat and/or other structures of the head (the parotid and salivary glands, subcutaneous connective tissues). The tongue is red and dry and the pulse rapid strong or rapid and floating. This is known as 'thunder head wind' (*léi tóu fēng* 雷头风) and represents diseases such as acute mumps or meningitis, and localized bacterial infections with redness and swelling, like tonsillitis, erysipelas and cellulitis. The treatment is to clear toxic wind heat and alleviate swelling and suppuration with **Pu Ji Xiao Du Yin** (Universal Benefit Drink to Eliminate Toxin 普济消毒饮)

jiu huang qin (Scutellariae Radix) 酒黄芩 6–12g
xuan shen (Scrophulariae Radix) 玄参 6–12g
niu bang zi (Arctii Fructus) 牛蒡子 9–15g
lian qiao (Forsythiae Fructus) 连翘 6–12g
ban lan gen (Isatidis/Baphicacanthis Radix) 板蓝根 9–15g
jiu huang lian (Coptidis Rhizoma) 酒黄连 3–9g
jie geng (Platycodi Radix) 桔梗 3–6g
chai hu (Bupleuri Radix) 柴胡 3–9g
gan cao (Glycyrrhizae Radix) 甘草 3–6g
chen pi (Citri reticulatae Pericarpium) 陈皮 3–6g
ma bo (Lasiosphaerae/Calvatiae) 马勃 2–3g
bai jiang can (Bombyx Batryticatus) 白僵蚕 3–9g
bo he (Mentha haplocalycis Herba) 薄荷 3–6g
sheng ma (Cimicifugae Rhizoma) 升麻 3–6g

Method: Decoction. **Jiu huang qin** and **jiu huang lian** clear heat and toxic heat from the upper burner; the wine processing focuses the action of these herbs on the upper body and head; **niu bang zi**, **lian qiao**, **bo he** and **bai jiang can** dispel wind heat from the head and upper burner; **xuan shen**, **ma bo**, **ban lan gen**, **jie geng** and **gan cao** clear toxic heat from the throat; **chen pi** regulates qi and assists in moving stagnant qi and alleviating pain; the ascending action of **sheng ma** and **chai hu** help the formula target the upper body, while clearing heat from the face and head. (Source: *Zhong Yi Nei Ke Xue* [*Dong Yuan Shi Xiao Fang*])

Prepared medicines
Concentrated powders
Yin Qiao San (Lonicera & Forsythia Formula)
Sheng Ma Ge Gen Tang (Cimicifuga & Pueraria Combination)
Pu Ji Xiao Du Yin (Scute & Cimicifuga Combination)

Pills
Yin Qiao Jie Du Pian (Yin Chiao Chieh Tu Pien)
Pu Ji Xiao Du Wan (Universal Benefit Teapills)

Acupuncture (select from)

Bl.7 (tongtian)....................dispels wind from the head

yintang (M–HN–3) ....alleviates frontal headache or sinus pain

Bl.2 (zanzhu).....................dispels wind heat; for frontal headache

GB.20 (fengchi –) ....dispels wind from the exterior, alleviates headache

LI.11 (quchi –)...................these points dispel wind heat and stop pain

LI.4 (hegu –)

SJ.5 (waiguan –)

Du.14 (dazhui – Ω) ....clears wind heat

Bl.12 (fengmen – Ω) ....dispels wind from the exterior

Bl.13 (feishu – Ω) ....transport point of the Lungs, diffuses the Lungs and directs Lung qi downwards

- with sore throat, add Lu.11 (shaoshang ↓) and SI.17 (tianrong –)
- with cough add Lu.5 (chize –)
- Ear points: lung, large intestine, tonsils
- Treat 1–2 times daily if possible

Gua Sha

See p.426.

Clinical notes

- Wind heat headaches may be associated with the common cold, influenza, tonsillitis, acute bronchitis and other upper respiratory tract infection, and the early stage of measles, mumps, encephalitis or meningitis.
- The patient should be advised to stay warm and well covered even though there is fever.

9.1.3 WIND DAMP

风湿头痛

Wind damp headaches may be acute, or chronic and recurrent. Damp can quickly gain access to the body on the back of wind via the taiyang channels when the pores are open and the patient sweating, or gradually by prolonged exposure to damp or humid conditions or contact with water. Once in the body, damp has an affinity for the Spleen and muscles, and blocks qi and blood flow through the muscles and middle burner. The blockage of qi and blood flow through the muscles, compounded by obstruction of the qi dynamic and accumulation of damp in the head lead to the heaviness and dull ache in the head and muscles.

Clinical features

- Dull occipital, frontal or generalized headache, with heavy or woolly head as if 'the head is wrapped in a damp cloth'. Stiffness, heaviness and pain of the lower or upper back, neck and occipital region. The headache is worse in the morning, in humid or rainy weather, or with exposure to moulds and mildews.
- muscle and joint aches
- sinus and nasal congestion
- fullness and discomfort in the chest and epigastrium
- loss of appetite and nausea

- loose stools
- sticky cloying sensation in the mouth
- urinary disturbance, scanty urine
- may be chills with mild fever when acute

T may be pale, with a thick, greasy, white coat
P floating, soft, soggy

Treatment principle
Dispel wind damp and stop pain

Prescription

QIANG HUO SHENG SHI TANG 羌活胜湿汤
Notopterygium Decoction to Overcome Dampness

qiang huo (Notopterygii Rhizoma seu Radix) 羌活 6–9g
du huo (Angelicae pubescentis Radix) 独活 6–9g
gao ben (Ligustici Rhizoma) 藁本 6–9g
man jing zi (Fructus Viticis) 蔓荆子 9–12g
fang feng (Saposhnikovae Radix) 防风 9–12g
chuan xiong (Chuanxiong Rhizoma) 川芎 3–6g
zhi gan cao (Glycyrrhizae Radix preparata) 炙甘草 3–6g

Method: Decoction. **Qiang huo** and **du huo** dispel wind damp from the taiyang channels and the muscles, **qiang huo** targets the upper body and **du huo** the lower body; **gao ben**, **man jing zi** and **fang feng** dispel wind from the exterior and stop pain; **chuan xiong** activates blood, dispels wind, and eases headache; **zhi gan cao** protects the Stomach and zheng qi. (Source: *Zhong Yi Nei Ke Xue* [*Nei Wai Shang Bian Huo Lun*])

Modifications

- For sinus congestion and frontal pain, add **bai zhi** (Angelicae dahuricae Radix) 白芷 6–9g and **cang er zi** (Xanthii Fructus) 苍耳子 6–9g.
- For temporal or vertex headache, add **bai ji li** (Tribuli Fructus) 白蒺藜 9–12g and **man jing zi** (Viticis Fructus) 蔓荆子 9–12g.
- With Spleen qi deficiency, add **dang shen** (Codonopsis Radix) 党参 12–15g and **huang qi** (Astragali Radix) 黄芪 12–15g.
- With marked nausea, add **cang zhu** (Atractylodis Rhizoma) 苍术 12–15g and **huo xiang** (Pogostemonis Herba) 藿香 12–15g.
- With abdominal distension, add **chen pi** (Citri reticulatae Pericarpium) 陈皮 6–9g and **hou po** (Magnoliae officinalis Cortex) 厚朴 9–12g.
- With loose stools or diarrhea, add **yi ren** (Coicis Semen) 苡仁 15–24g and **bai dou kou** (Amomi Fructus rotundus) 白豆蔻 3–6g [added at the end].
- With cough, add **xing ren** (Armeniacae Semen) 杏仁 9–12g, **jie geng** (Platycodi Radix) 桔梗 6–9g and **qian hu** (Peucedani Radix) 前胡 9–12g.

Prepared medicines
Concentrated powder
Qiang Huo Sheng Shi Tang (Notopterygium & Tuhuo Combination)
Pills
Juan Bi Wan (Clear Channel Teapills)

Acupuncture (select from)
St.8 (touwei) ....dispels wind damp from the head
GB.20 (fengchi –) ....dispels wind from the upper body, alleviates
headache and neck pain
Du.14 (dazhui – Ω) ....meeting point of the yang channels, clears pathogens
from the exterior
SI.3 (houxi).......................dispels wind damp and relaxes the muscle channels;
for occipital headache and stiff neck
Bl.60 (kunlun –) ....dispels wind damp from the upper portion of the
taiyang channel network and alleviates pain
Bl.12 (fengmen – Ω)..........dispels wind from the exterior
SJ.5 (waiguan –).................dispels wind damp from the shaoyang channels
• with foggy head, add Bl.62 (shenmai)
• with nausea, add PC.6 (neiguan –)
• with marked muscle aches and heaviness, add Sp.21 (dabao)
• with edema, add Sp.9 (yinlingquan –) and Sp.6 (sanyinjiao)
• Ear points: lung, large intestine, spleen, zero point

Gua Sha
See p.426.

Clinical notes
• Acute wind damp headaches may be diagnosed as the common cold, influenza, stomach flu, viral gastroenteritis or rheumatic fever.
• Wind damp patterns can be slower to resolve than wind cold and wind heat patterns. The stickiness of damp adheres more tightly to tissues and has a tendency to get locked in if not treated properly and fully. It is recommended to continue treatment for a week or so after the symptoms have cleared to ensure complete elimination of the damp.
• When nausea and vomiting are a feature, strong tasting decoctions can be difficult to ingest. A useful technique in such situations involves strong needling or finger pressure on PC.6 (neiguan), prior to taking the herbs. Gently patting the spine around T7–T12 or cupping of Ren.8 (shenque) may also help some patients. The herbs should be taken in tiny sips as frequently as possible. Sipping through a straw placed at the back of the tongue may help.

9.1.4 SUMMERHEAT
暑热头痛

Summerheat is an acute disorder that occurs during hot weather. There are two main variations. In the first, prolonged exposure to direct sun or a hot environment can lead to a type of heatstroke, where the body is unable to cool itself sufficiently and overheats producing an elevated body temperature and dehydration. The second type is due to an invasion of a summerheat pathogen. This is similar to a damp heat invasion, with the heat component considerably stronger than the damp in this case. The pattern discussed here is the second variation.

Clinical features
- acute, pounding, frontal headache accompanied by high unrelenting fever
- red, flushed complexion
- profuse sweating initially, then less as the patient becomes dehydrated
- hot, dry, flushed skin
- severe dryness and thirst
- scanty, concentrated urine
- may be vomiting and explosive, foul, burning diarrhoea

T dry, yellow tongue coat
P rapid and strong, or rapid and fine

Treatment principle
Expel summerheat and stop pain

Prescription

XIN JIA XIANG RU YIN 新加香薷饮
Newly Augmented Elsholtzia Decoction, modified

xiang ru (Herba Elsholtzia seu Moslae) 香薷 9–12g
jin yin hua (Lonicerae Flos) 金银花 15–24g
lian qiao (Forsythia Fructus) 连翘 9–12g
bai bian dou (Semen Dolichos Lablab) 白扁豆 12–15g
hou po (Magnoliae officinalis Cortex) 厚朴 9–12g
sang ye (Mori Folium) 桑叶 9–12g
ju hua (Chrysanthemi Flos) 菊花 9–12g
bai zhi (Angelicae dahurica Radix) 白芷 6–9g

Method: Decoction. The herbs should be simmered for no longer than 20 minutes in a pot with a tight fitting lid. This formula should be taken cool as **xiang ru** can aggravate vomiting when taken hot. **Xiang ru** clears the exterior, harmonizes the qi dynamic and dispels summerheat; **bai bian dou** and **hou po** harmonize the Stomach, downbear counterflow Stomach qi and transform damp to alleviate distension and stop vomiting; **jin yin hua** and **lian qiao** clear heat and summerheat from the exterior; **sang ye** and **ju hua** clear heat and stop headache; **bai zhi** dispels wind, dries damp and stops frontal headache. (Source: *Shi Yong Zhong Yi Nei Ke Xue* [*Wen Bing Tiao Bian*])

Modifications
- With marked nausea or vomiting, add **chen pi** (Citri reticulatae Pericarpium) 陈皮 6–9g, **zhi ban xia** (Pinelliae Rhizoma preparatum) 制半夏 9–12g and **zhu ru** (Bambusae Caulis in taeniam) 竹茹 9–12g.
- With Heart fire, irritability, concentrated urine and mouth ulcers, add **dan zhu ye** (Lophateri Herba) 淡竹叶 6–9g, **chi fu ling** (Poria Rubrae) 赤茯苓 12–15g and **hua shi** (Talcum) 滑石 9–12g.

Prepared medicines
Concentrated powder
Bai Hu Jia Ren Shen Tang (Ginseng & Gypsum Combination)
Qing Shu Yi Qi Tang (Astragalus & Atractylodes Combination)
  – this formula is recommended in the latter stages of a summerheat invasion when the qi and fluids have been damaged.

Acupuncture (select from)

St.8 (touwei) ....dispels wind and damp from the head, an important point for headache

GB.20 (fengchi –) ....dispels pathogens from the head

Du.14 (dazhui –)................these points dispel external pathogens and clear heat
LI.11 (quchi –)
LI.4 (hegu –)

SJ.5 (waiguan –).................clears heat and facilitates qi flow through the triple burner

PC.3 (quze ↓)....................sea point of the Pericardium and Urinary Bladder
Bl.40 (weizhong ↓)   respectively, these points are used together to cool the blood and clear heat

* with nausea and vomiting add PC.6 (neiguan)
* with diarrhea add Sp.9 (yinlingquan –) and St.25 (tianshu –)
* Ear points: lungs, large intestine, zero point

Gua Sha

See p.426.

Clinical notes

* Summerheat headaches may be diagnosed as acute gastroenteritis, food poisoning, gastric flu, influenza, acute colitis or heatstroke.
* When heat exposure is the cause of the headache, ice packs at critical points such as the axillae, neck and groin can help cool the patient quickly.
* Acute summerheat patterns respond well to early treatment, but can drag on or become recurrent if neglected.
* Fluid and electrolyte replacement is important and dehydration can occur due to the volume of sweat lost. This is especially so in infants and children, who can become dehydrated quickly. Oral isotonic fluid replacement solution should be given in small amounts frequently. Isotonic solution can be made by adding 3.5 grams of ordinary salt (NaCl), 2.5 grams of sodium bicarbonate, 1.5 grams of potassium chloride (KCl) and 20 grams of sugar to one liter of water.

肝气郁滞 9.2. LIVER QI CONSTRAINT

- with heat
- with blood deficiency

Liver qi constraint is a common type of headache, typically associated with stress and emotional tension. Liver qi constraint is at the basis of numerous other conditions commonly implicated in headaches, such as Liver fire, ascendant Liver yang and Liver wind. The Liver patterns form a continuum, and in chronic cases, patients may display aspects of all simultaneously. Liver qi constraint can also contribute to Spleen weakness, qi, blood and yin deficiency and/or the development of phlegm damp and blood stasis (Fig 9.1, p.411).

The Liver qi constraint headache often manifests as the classical tension headache, however depending on complicating factors, it may be migrainous in nature, with a premonition or aura. The more heat there is the more tendency to migraine type headaches, the more blood deficiency, the more tendency to dull and persistent headaches.

Clinical features
- Recurrent frontal or temporal headache. The headache is a dull ache, likened to a tight band around the head, and is constant rather than throbbing. It often starts in the occiput, then radiates to the front and behind the eyes. It may be one sided or bilateral.
- The headache often starts soon after rising from bed and gets worse during the day. It may also occur after emotional upset, with a sudden release of stress (at weekends or during holiday), or before a menstrual period. The scalp is tender to touch and painful spots are found in the neck and upper back.
- The headache is preceded by characteristic symptoms which can vary from patient to patient, but include digestive upset, sudden and increasing tiredness or sleepiness, yawning, visual disturbances, sore eyes, photophobia, a sense of heat in the head and increasing irritability.
- stiff, tight neck and shoulders; frowning; general muscular tension
- grinding of the teeth (bruxism); sighing
- depression, moodiness, irritability
- hypochondriac and abdominal discomfort and ache
- maybe nausea or vomiting
- premenstrual syndrome
- **with constrained heat**: red, sore eyes, acid reflux and heartburn, facial flushing, severe irritability, bitter taste, waking in the middle of the night with headache
- **with blood deficiency**: vertex and temples affected, postural dizziness, headaches before and after a menstrual period, light periods or long menstrual cycle, spots in the visual field

T normal or mauve, with a thin, white or yellow coat; with constrained heat, red edges; with blood deficiency, pale or orangey edges

P wiry; rapid with heat; fine with blood deficiency

Treatment principle
Dredge the Liver and regulate Liver qi
Supplement the Spleen, qi and blood

Prescription

XIAO YAO SAN 逍遥散
Rambling Powder

This prescription is a good basis for all Liver qi constraint patterns, and is particularly good when there are elements of blood and Spleen deficiency, a complication commonly seen in women. It can be used for acute headache when suitably modified, and to regulate qi and prevent headaches occurring. When used to regulate qi, the headache relieving modifications are unnecessary and pills are usually adequate.

chai hu (Bupleuri Radix) 柴胡 9–12g
dang gui (Angelicae sinensis Radix) 当归 9–12g
bai shao (Paeoniae Radix alba) 白芍 12–18g
bai zhu (Atractylodes macrocephalae Rhizoma) 白术 9–12g
fu ling (Poria) 茯苓 12–15g
wei jiang (roasted Zingiberis Rhizoma recens) 煨姜 3–6g
bo he (Mentha haplocalycis Herba) 薄荷 3–6g
zhi gan cao (Glycyrrhizae Radix preparata) 炙甘草 3–6g
Method: Decoction, powder or pills. **Bo he** is added a few minutes before the end of cooking a decoction. **Chai hu** dredges the Liver and regulates qi; **dang gui** and **bai shao** nourish Liver blood and soften the Liver; **bai zhu** and **fu ling** strengthen the Spleen and dry damp; **zhi gan cao** supplements qi and, with **bai shao**, eases muscle spasm; **wei jiang** warms and harmonizes the Stomach; **bo he** assists **chai hu** in moving Liver qi. (Source: *Shi Yong Zhong Yi Nei Ke Xue* [*He Ji Ju Fang*])

Modifications

- During a headache or in anticipation of a headache, add **chuan xiong** (Chuanxiong Rhizoma) 川芎 9–30g (see also p.421) and **man jing zi** (Viticis Fructus) 蔓荆子 9–12g.
- With constrained heat, add **mu dan pi** (Moutan Cortex) 牡丹皮 6–9g and **shan zhi zi** (Gardeniae Fructus) 山栀子 6–9g.
- With heartburn or acid reflux, add **wu zhu yu** (Evodiae Fructus) 吴茱萸 1–3g and **huang lian** (Coptidis Rhizoma) 黄连 3–6g.
- With constipation or sluggish bowel movements (without hard or dry stools) from reduced peristalsis, add **wu yao** (Linderae Radix) 乌药 6–9g and **bing lang** (Arecae Semen) 槟榔 6–9g or **zhi shi** (Aurantii Fructus immaturus) 枳实 6–9g.
- For constipation with dry stools, add **tao ren** (Persicae Semen) 桃仁 9–12g.
- With chest oppression, difficulty getting a deep and satisfying breath or fullness and discomfort in the hypochondrium, add **zhi xiang fu** (Cyperi Rhizoma preparata) 制香附 6–9g, **yu jin** (Curcumae Radix) 郁金 9–12g and **zhi ke** (Aurantii Fructus) 枳壳 6–9g.
- With belching, add **chen pi** (Citri reticulatae Pericarpium) 陈皮 9–12g and **chen xiang** (Aquilariae Lignum resinatum) 沉香 3–6g.

- With premenstrual headaches, breast tenderness and edema, add **chuan xiong** (Chuanxiong Rhizoma) 川芎 6–12g, **mei gui hua** (Rosae rugosae Flos) 玫瑰 花 6–9g and **yi mu cao** (Leonurus Herba) 益母草 12–15g.

Variations and additional prescriptions
Qi constraint without deficiency
In relatively acute patterns, or in young or otherwise robust patients, the qi constraint may be uncomplicated by any deficiency or other significant pathology. The treatment is to regulate qi and dredge the Liver with CHAI HU SHU GAN SAN (Bupleurum Powder to Dredge the Liver 柴胡疏肝散, p.790).

Prepared medicines
Concentrated powder
Xiao Yao San (Bupleurum & Tangkuei Formula)
Jia Wei Xiao Yao San (Bupleurum & Peony Formula)
Chai Hu Shu Gan San (Bupleurum & Cyperus Combination)

Pills
Xiao Yao Wan (Free and Easy Wanderer Teapills, Hsiao Yao Wan)
Jia Wei Xiao Yao Wan (Free and Easy Wanderer Plus Teapills, Dan Zhi Xiao Yao Wan)
Chai Hu Shu Gan Wan (Bupleurum Soothe Liver Teapills)

Acupuncture (select from)
The points below are used in addition to points selected on the basis of the location of the headache (Boxes 9.5–9.8, pp.415–418)

Du.20 (baihui) ....these points alleviate headache, and have a shen
taiyang (M–HN–9)   calming effect
yintang (M–HN–3)

GB.20 (fengchi) ....regulates Liver qi, subdues Liver yang and alleviates
headache

Liv.3 (taichong –)..............source point of the Liver, dredges the Liver and
regulates qi; for all types of Liver headache

LI.4 (hegu).......................combined with Liv.3 to form the 'four gates', a
combination for pain and muscle spasm

GB.41 (zulinqi –)..............these points cool the Liver and regulate qi; for
SJ.5 (waiguan)   temporal headaches and premenstrual headaches

GB.34 (yanglingquan –)......sea point of the Gallbladder, regulates qi and
subdues ascendant Liver yang; especially good [with
GB.21 (jianjing –)] when there is tension in the
neck

GB.21 (jianjing –)..............releases tension in the neck and subdues ascendant
yang

ahshi points ....tender points on the upper back and neck (sternocleidomastoid, trapezius); usually trigger points

Lu.7 (lieque).......................used to restrain Liver wood by strengthening the
Lung metal via the controlling (ke 克) cycle; best
when there is evidence of Lung weakness

- with heat, add Liv.2 (xingjian –)
- with blood or yin deficiency, add Sp.6 (sanyinjiao +), St.36 (zusanli +), Bl.18 (ganshu +) and Bl.23 (shenshu +)
- Ear points: liver, spleen, zero point, sympathetic, shenmen

Clinical notes

- Liver qi constraint type headaches may be diagnosed as tension headaches, migraine headaches, referred pain from myofascial trigger points, hypertension, premenstrual syndrome, postural headache or headache originating from the cervical spine.
- Liver qi constraint is a common type of stress induced headache, and the precursor to a variety of other more severe and persistent headaches. The best treatment is prevention by instituting appropriate stress relieving measures.
- Increasing exercise levels (see p.103), neck mobilization and massage and deactivation of latent or active trigger points can assist significantly. There is often a myofascial component, so detailed examination of the suboccipital muscles, trapezius, sternocleidomastoid, levator scapulae, splenius, semispinalis and scalene muscles may uncover trigger points.
- Hot spot therapy is strongly indicated, p.923.
- A qi mobilizing diet is recommended. See Clinical Handbook, Vol.2 p.878.

肝
火
头
痛

9.3 LIVER FIRE

Liver fire headaches are usually a complication of prolonged qi constraint, in combination with alcohol, coffee, or other heating and stimulating substances. Liver fire headaches usually occur as an acute exacerbation of a more persistent or background headache of a qi constraint type. When recurrent or persistent, the heat depletes Liver yin and can evolve into yin deficiency with ascendant Liver yang.

Clinical features

- Acute severe, pounding or splitting, hot headache, typically initiated by over-indulgence in alcohol, emotional outburst or sudden increase in stress levels. The headache often affects the forehead or temporal area, and may concentrate behind or over one eye. There may be nausea and vomiting, which can alleviate the headache. The headache is alleviated by a cold compress on the neck and forehead.
- red, flushed face
- sore, distended, red eyes
- bitter taste in the mouth
- constipation
- maybe scleral hemorrhage or epistaxis
- severe irritability, restlessness, anger, violent temper outburst
- heavy menstrual bleeding, menorrhagia

T red or with red edges and a thick, yellow, dry coat (during headaches)
P wiry, strong, rapid (during headaches)

Prescription

LONG DAN XIE GAN TANG 龙胆泻肝汤
Gentian Decoction to Purge the Liver

jiu long dan cao (wine fried Gentianae Radix) 酒龙胆草 3–9g
huang qin (Scutellariae Radix) 黄芩.. 6–12g
shan zhi zi (Gardeniae Fructus) 山栀子 6–12g
ze xie (Alismatis Rhizoma) 泽泻 6–12g
mu tong (Akebiae Caulis) 木通 3–6g
che qian zi (Plantaginis Semen) 车前子 9–15g
sheng di (Rehmanniae Radix) 生地.. 9–15g
dang gui (Angelicae sinensis Radix) 当归 6–12g
chai hu (Bupleuri Radix) 柴胡 3–9g
gan cao (Glycyrrhizae Radix) 甘草 3–6g
Method: Decoction. **Che qian zi** is usually cooked in a cloth bag. **Jiu long dan cao**, very bitter and cold, cools the Liver and clears heat; **shan zhi zi** and **huang qin** clear heat from all three burners; the relatively small dose of **chai hu** assists in clearing heat, dredging the Liver and relieving qi constraint; **ze xie**, **che qian zi** and **mu tong** promote urination to provide an escape route for the heat; **sheng di** cools the blood; **dang gui** nourishes and protects blood; **gan cao** protects the Stomach. (Source: *Zhong Yi Nei Ke Xue* [*Yi Fang Ji Jie*])

Modifications

- During headaches, a few herbs to specifically address the pain can be added,

such as **gou teng** (Uncariae Ramulus cum Uncis) 钩藤 9–12g, **bai ji li** (Tribuli Fructus) 白蒺藜 9–12g, **xia ku cao** (Prunellae Spica) 夏枯草 12–15g, **chuan niu xi** (Cyathulae Radix) 川牛膝 12–15g or **jue ming zi** (Cassiae Semen) 决明子 9–12g.
- With constipation, add **da huang** (Rhei Radix et Rhizoma) 大黄 6–9g and **mang xiao** (Natrii Sulfas) 芒硝 6g, or use DANG GUI LONG HUI WAN (Tang-kuei, Gentian and Aloe Pill 当归龙会丸 p.117).
- With concentrated or painful urination, add **bai mao gen** (Imperatae Rhizoma) 白茅根 12–18g and **hua shi** (Talcum) 滑石 9–12g.

Prepared medicines
Concentrated powders
Long Dan Xie Gan Tang (Gentiana Combination)
Dang Gui Long Hui Wan (Tangkuei, Gentiana & Aloe Formula)
Pills
Long Dan Xie Gan Wan (Snake and Dragon Teapills)
Ming Mu Shang Qing Pian (Ming Mu Shang Ching Pien)

Acupuncture (select from)
The points below are used in addition to points selected on the basis of the location of the headache (Boxes 9.5–9.8, pp.415–418)
GB.20 (fengchi) ....regulates Liver qi, clears heat and subdues Liver yang
Liv.2 (xingjian –)................clears heat and drains fire
GB.41 (zulinqi –)...............these points open daimai, cool the Liver, regulate
SJ.5 (waiguan –)   qi and direct fire away from the head
GB.34 (yanglingquan –).....cools the Liver, stops pain and eases muscles spasm
ah shi points ....tender points on the upper back and neck (sterno-
                                cleidomastoid, trapezius); usually trigger points
- points on the head are avoided in this pattern as they can aggravate headache
- Ear points: liver, gallbladder, sympathetic, shenmen, lowering blood pressure groove (↓ to reduce blood pressure)

Clinical notes
- Headaches of Liver fire type may be diagnosed as migraine, cluster headache, alcohol or substance abuse headache, cholecystitis, hypertension or referred pain from myofascial trigger points.
- Alcohol can play a significant part in the creation of a Liver fire headache. A cooling diet can be helpful. Avoidance of known dietary triggers is essential. For dietary recommendations, see Clinical Handbook, Vol.2 p.882.
- The myofascial component can be significant, especially suboccipital muscles, trapezius, sternocleidomastoid, levator scapulae, splenius, semispinalis and scalenus.
- Hot spot therapy is strongly indicated, p.923.
- Activities to regulate Liver qi are essential for long term resolution. See Clinical notes, p.437.

肝 9.4 ASCENDANT LIVER YANG, WITH YIN DEFICIENCY
阳
头
痛

Headaches from ascendant Liver yang are caused by an imbalance in the distribution of yin and yang. Too much yang qi ends up in the head. This can happen as the result of a sudden explosion of pent up qi, or more commonly because yin and/or blood are insufficient to anchor yang and provide a counterweight to its active and rising nature. When the anchoring yin reaches a critical point of deficiency, the yang loses its moorings, becomes excessively mobile and rises to the head. When ascendant yang reaches a certain level of chaotic intensity, it is redefined as wind. The greater the deficiency of yin the more likely and more vigorously the yang is to slip its moorings and ascend to the head. For ascendant yang from blood deficiency see p.464–465.

There are two phases of treatment, during a headache and in between headaches. Treatment during a headache aims to subdue the ascendant yang. Treatment in between episodes aims to rebuild yin and blood and regulate qi to prevent headaches from occurring.

Clinical features
• Recurrent headaches, usually severe, splitting or pounding, with a sense of distension and pressure in the head. The headache may be bilateral or one sided, and focused in the temples, vertex, the orbital ridge or behind the eyes. Pain may radiate down the back of the neck to the shoulder. The headache is better for sitting up and with a cold compress, and worse for lying down. Headaches may be initiated by emotional stress or occur when stress is released (the 'weekend headache').
• During or preceding headaches there may be dizziness, visual disturbances such as blurring, flashing lights and photophobia, nausea and vomiting, increasing tiredness and yawning, and pain, stiffness and tightness of the neck and upper back.
• red complexion, facial flushing or malar flush; red eyes and ears
• night sweats
• tinnitus or hearing loss
• anger, irritability
• insomnia; waking between 1–3am, may wake with a headache
• aching and weakness of the lower back and legs
• sensation of heat in the chest, palms and soles
• weakness, fatigue
• muscles spasms, tics or tremors
• numbness in the extremities
T red, with little or no coat
P wiry, fine, rapid; during headaches strong and rapid

Treatment principle
Calm the Liver and subdue ascendant yang
Clear heat and stop pain
Nourish Liver and Kidney yin

Prescription

TIAN MA GOU TENG YIN 天麻钩藤饮
Gastrodia and Uncaria Drink

This formula is selected when ascendant yang and Liver heat are the main features and there is relatively little underlying deficiency. It is best used during periods of frequent headaches. Once the headaches are reduced, a more general qi regulating and cooling strategy can be adopted.

tian ma (Gastrodiae Rhizoma) 天麻...6–9g
gou teng (Ramulus Uncariae cum Uncis) 钩藤 9–12g
shi jue ming (Haliotidis Concha) 石决明 15–30g
shan zhi zi (Gardeniae Fructus) 山栀子..6–9g
huang qin (Scutellariae Radix) 黄芩...6–9g
chuan niu xi (Cyathulae Radix) 川牛膝...9–15g
du zhong (Eucommiae Cortex) 杜仲 9–12g
sang ji sheng (Taxilli Herba) 桑寄生..9–12g
yi mu cao (Leonurus Herba) 益母草...9–12g
fu shen (Poria Sclerotium pararadicis) 茯神.....................................9–12g
ye jiao teng (Polygoni multiflori Caulis) 夜交藤 15–30g

Method: Decoction. **Shi jue ming** is cooked for 30 minutes prior to the other herbs, **gou teng** is added 5 minutes before the end of cooking. **Tian ma** and **gou teng** calm the Liver and extinguish wind; **shi jue ming** cools the Liver subdues ascendant Liver yang; **shan zhi zi** and **huang qin** clear heat; **yi mu cao** activates blood and promotes urination to provide an outlet for the heat; **sang ji sheng** and **chuan niu xi** supplement the Liver and Kidneys, and assist in leading qi and blood downwards; **ye jiao teng** and **fu shen** calm the Heart and shen. (Source: *Zhong Yi Nei Ke Xue [Za Bing Zheng Zhi Xin Yi]*)

Modifications (to Tian Ma Gou Teng Yin)

- For a severe or resistant headache, a large dose of **chuan xiong** (Chuanxiong Rhizoma) 川芎 15–30g can be added for a day or two. To alleviate any negative consequences of its qi and blood dispersing at this dose, increase the dose of **chuan niu xi** to 18g, and add **bai shao** (Paeoniae Radix alba) 白芍 9–12g and **gou qi zi** (Lycii Fructus) 枸杞子 9–12g.
- With Liver qi constraint, add **chai hu** (Bupleuri Radix) 柴胡 6–9g.
- With fire, add **xia ku cao** (Prunellae Spica) 夏枯草 12–15g and **mu dan pi** (Moutan Cortex) 牡丹皮 9–12g.

ZHEN GAN XI FENG TANG 镇肝熄风汤
Sedate the Liver and Extinguish Wind Decoction

This formula is selected when ascendant yang is severe and clearly the result of Liver and Kidney yin deficiency. The prescription is not suitable for long term use, and the big doses of herbs should be reduced as the pain is alleviated. A more specific Liver and Kidney yin supplement can be phased in as the yang is stabilized and brought under control.

huai niu xi (Achyranthis bidentatae Radix) 怀牛膝................................15–30g
dai zhe shi (Haematitum) 代赭石 15–30g

long gu (Fossilia Ossis Mastodi) 龙骨 9–15g
mu li (Ostreae Concha) 牡蛎 9–15g
gui ban (Testudinis Plastrum) 龟板 9–15g
bai shao (Paeoniae Radix alba) 白芍 9–15g
xuan shen (Scrophulariae Radix) 玄参 9–15g
tian dong (Asparagi Radix) 天冬 9–15g
chuan lian zi (Toosendan Fructus) 川楝子 6–9g
mai ya (Hordei Fructus germinantus) 麦芽 6–9g
yin chen (Artemisiae scopariae Herba) 茵陈 6–9g
gan cao (Glycyrrhizae Radix) 甘草 3–6g

Method: Decoction. The mineral and shell ingredients are decocted for 30 minutes prior to the other herbs. **Huai niu xi** directs yang qi and blood downwards and away from the head, while supplementing the Liver and Kidneys to anchor yang; **dai zhe shi** pacifies the Liver, subdues yang and extinguishes wind; **long gu**, **mu li** and **gui ban** subdue yang and calm the Liver; **xuan shen**, **tian dong** and **bai shao** enrich the yin, nourish blood and soften the Liver; **yin chen**, **chuan lian zi** and **mai ya** cool the Liver and regulate Liver qi; **mai ya** and **gan cao** protect and harmonize the Stomach. (Source: *Zhong Yi Nei Ke Xue* [*Yi Xue Zhong Zhong Can Xi Lu*])

Modifications (to Zhen Gan Xi Feng Tang)

- For a severe or resistant headache, a large dose of **chuan xiong** (Chuanxiong Rhizoma) 川芎 15–30g can be added for a day or two. To alleviate any negative consequences of its qi and blood dispersing at this dose, use **huai niu xi** at the upper end of the dosage range, and add **gou qi zi** (Lycii Fructus) 枸杞子 9–12g.
- If the shells and mineral cause digestive upset, combine with a small dose of the prepared medicine Sɪ Jᴜɴ Zɪ Wᴀɴ (Four Gentlemen Teapills) or Jɪᴀɴ Pɪ Wᴀɴ (Ginseng Stomachic Pills, Spleen Digest Aid Pill).
- With marked yin deficiency, add **sheng di** (Rehmanniae Radix) 生地 9–12g **bie jia** (Trionycis Carapax) 鳖甲 9–12g [cooked first], **zhi mu** (Anemarrhenae Rhizoma) 知母 9–12g and **huang bai** (Phellodendri Cortex) 黄柏 9–12g.
- With severe wind, causing unsteady gait, tremor or numbness of the extremities, add **shan yang jiao** (Naemorhedi Cornu) 山羊角 9–12g [powdered or shaved and cooked first].
- With constipation, add **quan gua lou** (Trichosanthis Fructus) 全栝楼 18–24g and **zhi shi** (Aurantii Fructus immaturus) 枳实 6–9g.
- With loose stools, delete **dai zhe shi** and **gui ban**, and add **chi shi zhi** (Halloysitum rubrum) 赤石脂 15–24g.
- With blood stasis, add **dan shen** (Salviae miltiorrhizae Radix) 丹参 12–15g and **tao ren** (Persicae Semen) 桃仁 9–12g.
- With persistent hypertension, add **xia ku cao** (Prunellae Spica) 夏枯草 15–18g, **gou teng** (Uncariae Ramulus cum Uncis) 钩藤 9–12g, **ju hua** (Chrysanthemi Flos) 菊花 9–12g and **di long** (Pheretima) 地龙 6–9g.
- With phlegm heat, add **dan nan xing** (Arisaemae cum Bile) 胆南星 6–9g.

Variations and additional prescriptions
Treatment of underlying imbalance
Both the formulas above are designed for use during periods of ascendant yang

and are not recommended for continuous use. The headaches and other symptoms should clearly improve within a few weeks. If the headaches continue, reappraisal of the diagnosis is warranted. ZHEN GAN XI FENG TANG in particular can weaken the Spleen and cause iatrogenic complications if overused. Once the headaches have been alleviated or reduced to a manageable level, the treatment strategy should aim at rectifying the underlying imbalance that allows yang to get out of control. In the case of Liver qi constraint and Liver heat, a formula such as JIA WEI XIAO YAO SAN (Augmented Rambling Powder 加味逍遥散, p.713) can be used in conjunction with modification of the contributing lifestyle factors. When yin deficiency is the main contributor, a suitable yin supplement such as QI JU DI HUANG WAN (Lycium Fruit, Chrysanthemum and Rehmannia Pill 杞菊 地黄丸, p.467) can be used.

Prepared medicines
Concentrated powders
Tian Ma Gou Teng Yin (Gastrodia & Gambir Combination)
Zhen Gan Xi Feng Tang (Hematite & Scrophularia Combination)
Qi Ju Di Huang Wan (Lycium, Chrysanthemum & Rehamannia Formula)
– for long term rebuilding of Liver and Kidney yin during remission

Pills
Tian Ma Gou Teng Wan (Tian Ma Gou Teng Teapills)
Zhen Gan Xi Feng Wan (Zhen Gan Xi Feng Teapills)
Yang Yin Jiang Ya Wan (Pill to Nourish Yin and Relieve Hypertension)
Hu Po Bao Long Wan (Po Lung Yuen Medical Pills)
Long Dan Xie Gan Wan (Snake and Dragon Teapills)
– with Liver fire

Acupuncture (select from)
The points below are used in addition to points selected on the basis of the location of the headache (Boxes 9.5–9.8, pp.415–418)
Du.20 (baihui –) ....subdues ascendant yang and extinguishes wind, clears the mind and calms the shen
GB.20 (fengchi –) ....extinguishes wind, calms the Liver and subdues ascendant yang, alleviates headache
Liv.3 (taichong –)...............source point of the Liver, subdues Liver yang, extinguishes wind and alleviates spasm
SJ.5 (waiguan –).................these points cool the Liver and sedate yang;
GB.39 (xuanzhong –)   indicated for temporal headache and when insomnia is an accompanying problem
GB.34 (yanglingquan –)......sea point of the Gallbladder, regulates qi and subdues ascendant Liver yang; especially good [with GB.21 (jianjing –)] when there is muscular tension in the neck
GB.21 (jianjing –)..............releases tension in the neck and subdues ascendant yang

Bl.18 (ganshu).....................transport points of the Liver and Kidneys, nourish
Bl.23 (shenshu +)   Liver and Kidney yin to restrain yang
- with heat, add Liv.2 (xingjian –)
- with nausea or belching, add PC.6 (neiguan –)
- Ear points: liver, kidney, ear apex ↓, lowering blood pressure groove ↓

Clinical notes

- Headaches of an ascendant Liver yang type may be associated with hypertension, migraine or cluster headaches, temporal arteritis, transient ischemic attacks, arteriosclerosis or referred pain from myofascial trigger points.
- Persistent or severe headaches of an ascendant yang type can represent a potentially dangerous condition or an impending catastrophe. Acupuncture with relatively strong stimulation can be effective in the case of dangerously high blood pressure or impending stroke. Persistently high blood pressure that does not respond to Chinese medical treatment quickly, should be thoroughly investigated and treated with other modalities.
- Liver yang headaches usually have a significant myofascial component. The muscles of the neck and upper back should be examined for tender or reactive points, which when deactivated can assist in quickly alleviating the headache. Both yin and blood deficiency lead to increased irritability of the muscles of the upper back and neck, and patients may find that massage aggravates the headaches.
- Headaches from ascendant Liver yang are often complicated by phlegm and blood stasis, especially in the middle aged and elderly, and can be challenging to treat successfully. In such cases there may be complicating cardiovascular and cerebrovascular disease. For these patients, experience suggests that focusing initially on the blood stasis can be helpful. Activating blood can allowing yin and yang to find a balance, without forcing yang downwards. See blood stasis, p.451, for more.
- Hot spot therapy is strongly indicated, p.923.
- Diet, regular exercise and stress reduction are important components of management.
- A yin nourishing diet is recommended, see Clinical Handbook, Vol.2, p.876.

寒
邪
侵
犯
厥
阴

9.5 COLD AFFECTING THE LIVER AND STOMACH

The headache associated with cold in the Liver and Stomach is due to pathological rebellion of yang qi through the jueyin channels brought about by blockage of the middle burner qi dynamic by cold. The cold is the product of disharmony between the Liver and Stomach and a cold diet which weakens Spleen yang qi. The cold accumulates in the middle burner and blocks the qi dynamic. The obstructed qi ascends to the head through the Liver channel ending at the vertex. This pattern is also known as cold encroaching on the jueyin channels.

Clinical features

- Recurrent headaches affecting the vertex or temporal region. The headache can be intense, and is accompanied by nausea, vomiting or dry retching and neck stiffness. During episodes the patient is cold and weak, with cold extremities but may appear flushed. They may have diarrhea. Headaches are worse or more frequent premenstrually or when the patient is upset, stressed or hungry.
- facial pallor (in between headaches)
- acid reflux, heartburn
- epigastric pain and distension
- hyper salivation
- reduced sense of taste
- fatigue with restlessness and irritability

T pale, with a greasy, white coat
P slow and fine, or wiry (during pain episodes)

Treatment principle

Warm the Liver and Stomach and dispel cold
Downbear counterflow qi and stop pain

Prescription

WU ZHU YU TANG 吴茱萸汤
Evodia Decoction

wu zhu yu (Evodiae Fructus) 吴茱萸 3–6g
ren shen (Ginseng Radix) 人参 9–12g
sheng jiang (Zingiberis Rhizoma recens) 生姜 15–20g
da zao (Jujubae Fructus) 大枣 ....4 fruit

Method: Decoction. **Wu zhu yu** warms the Stomach and Liver, dispels cold, downbears counterflow qi and stops vomiting; **sheng jiang** warms the Spleen and Stomach, dispels cold and assists the **wu zhu yu** in stopping vomiting; **ren shen** strengthens the Spleen and protects Stomach qi and yin from the effects of vomiting; **da zao** moderates the dispersing and drying nature of **wu zhu yu**. (Source: *Shi Yong Zhong Yi Nei Ke Xue* [*Shang Han Lun*])

Modifications

- For severe headache, add **chuan xiong** (Chuanxiong Rhizoma) 川芎 9–15g and **gao ben** (Ligustici Rhizoma) 藁本 6–9g.
- With persistent acid reflux, add **duan mu li** (calcined Ostreae Concha) 煅牡蛎 15–30g and **duan wa leng zi** (calcined Arcae Concha) 煅瓦楞子 12–15g.

- With marked vomiting, add **zhi ban xia** (Pinelliae Rhizoma preparatum) 制半夏 6–9g and **sha ren** (Amomi Fructus) 砂仁 6–9g.

Prepared medicines
Concentrated powders
Wu Zhu Yu Tang (Evodia Combination)

Acupuncture (select from)
The points below are used in addition to points selected on the basis of the location of the headache (Boxes 9.5–9.8, pp.415–418)

Du.20 (baihui −)................directs qi downward and stops pain
Liv.3 (taichong +▲)..........source point of the Liver, dredges the Liver and directs jueyin qi downward
PC.6 (neiguan −)................directs qi in the jueyin and yangming channels downwards, stops nausea and vomiting
St.36 (zusanli +▲) ....warms the Stomach and dispels cold
- Ear points: liver, stomach, zero point, shenmen

Clinical notes
- Headaches of a Liver and Stomach cold type may be diagnosed as migraine, neurogenic or hormonal headache.
- This is not a very common type of headache, but when encountered is quite distinctive and amenable to treatment.
- Diet is an important part of treatment. Food should be warming, well cooked and easily digested. A yang warming diet is recommended. See Clinical Handbook, Vol.2, p.873.
- Hot spot therapy in the region of T7–T10 can be helpful, p.923.

痰
湿
头
痛

9.6 PHLEGM DAMP

Headache and head distension associated with phlegm damp is a chronic and recurrent problem. Phlegm damp headaches can be severe and may be episodic, with headaches occurring in clusters interspersed with variable periods of remission. The sporadic nature of the headaches is due to the alternate congealing and dispersal of phlegm damp in response to changes in the diet and emotions, or exposure to strong dispersing substances like perfume and gasoline.

Phlegm damp headaches are often complicated by Spleen qi deficiency, and occasionally by ascendant Liver yang or wind. Phlegm damp headaches can appear similar to those due to wind damp (9.1.3, p.429). See also clinical notes.

Clinical features

- Dull, aching, distending headache, as if the head is 'wrapped in a wet sack' or being 'squeezed in a vice'. The forehead or the entire head may be affected. There may be superficial insensitivity or numbness on the scalp. Headaches may be triggered by phlegm inducing or Spleen weakening food, increase in emotional turmoil and stress or strong smells.
- dizziness or vertigo
- poor concentration, foggy head, or a feeling of a 'veil over the senses'
- fatigue, lethargy, heaviness
- nausea or vomiting; nausea may precede or accompany headaches and the headache may be alleviated after vomiting
- abdominal distension and chest oppression

T swollen, may be pale, with a thick, greasy, white coat
P slippery and wiry or soft and soggy

Treatment principle

Transform phlegm damp and stop pain
Strengthen the Spleen and supplement qi

Prescription

BAN XIA BAI ZHU TIAN MA TANG 半夏白术天麻汤
Pinellia, White Atractylodes, and Gastrodia Decoction

zhi ban xia (Pinelliae Rhizoma preparatum) 制半夏 9–12g
bai zhu (Atractylodes macrocephalae Rhizoma) 白术 12–15g
tian ma (Gastrodiae Rhizoma) 天麻 9–12g
chen pi (Citri reticulatae Pericarpium) 陈皮 6–9g
fu ling (Poria) 茯苓 9–15g
gan cao (Glycyrrhizae Radix) 甘草 3–6g
sheng jiang (Zingiberis Rhizoma recens) 生姜 9–12g
da zao (Jujubae Fructus) 大枣 .... 3 fruit

Method: Decoction. **Zhi ban xia** transforms phlegm, dries damp, downbears counterflow Stomach qi and stops nausea and vomiting; **tian ma** calms the Liver and extinguishes wind; **bai zhu** and **fu ling** strengthen the Spleen and dry phlegm damp; **chen pi** transforms phlegm damp, regulates middle burner qi and corrects the qi dynamic; **sheng jiang** transforms phlegm and assists the other herbs in stopping nausea and vomiting; **da zao** and **gan cao** strengthen the Spleen and harmonize the Stomach. (Source: *Zhong Yi Nei Ke Xue* [*Yi Xue Xin Wu*])

Modifications

- For frontal headache, add **bai zhi** (Angelicae dahuricae Radix) 白芷 6–9g and **cang er zi** (Xanthii Fructus) 苍耳子 6–9g.
- For temporal or vertex headache, add **bai ji li** (Tribuli Fructus) 白蒺藜 9–12g and **man jing zi** (Viticis Fructus) 蔓荆子 9–12g.
- For occipital headache and stiff neck, add **qiang huo** (Notopterygii Rhizoma seu Radix) 羌活 6–9g and **ge gen** (Puerariae Radix) 葛根 9–12g.
- With Spleen qi deficiency, add **dang shen** (Codonopsis Radix) 党参 12–15g and **huang qi** (Astragali Radix) 黄芪 12–15g.
- With ascendant Liver yang and hypertension, add **gou teng** (Uncariae Ramulus cum Uncis) 钩藤 12–15g [added at the end of cooking] and **shi jue ming** (Haliotidis Concha) 石决明 15–30g [cooked first].
- With foggy head, confusion or muddled thinking, add **cang zhu** (Atractylodis Rhizoma) 苍术 9–12g, **shi chang pu** (Acori tatarinowii Rhizoma) 石菖蒲 6–9g and **yuan zhi** (Polygalae Radix) 远志 6–9g.
- With edema, combine with Wu Ling San (Five Ingredient Powder with Poria 五苓散, p.219–220).
- With hiccup or belching, add **dai zhe shi** (Haematitum) 代赭石 12–18g and **xuan fu hua** (Inulae Flos) 旋复花 9–15g.
- With Liver qi constraint, add **zi su ye** (Perillae Folium) 紫苏叶 9–12g, **zhi shi** (Aurantii Fructus immaturus) 枳实 6–9g and **hou po** (Magnoliae officinalis Cortex) 厚朴 9–12g.
- With heat, add **zhu ru** (Bambusae Caulis in taeniam) 竹茹 6–9g and **huang lian** (Coptidis Rhizoma) 苍术 3–6g, or combine with Wen Dan Tang (Warm Gallbladder Decoction 温胆汤, p.87).
- With cold, add **gan jiang** (Zingiberis Rhizoma) 干姜 6–9g and **gui zhi** (Cinnamomi Ramulus) 桂枝 6–9g.
- With severe vertigo and nausea, increase the dose of **tian ma** (Gastrodiae Rhizoma) 天麻 to 15g, and add one or two of the following herbs: **dai zhe shi** (Haematitum) 代赭石 12–18g, **xuan fu hua** (Inulae Flos) 旋复花 9–15g, **bai jiang can** (Bombyx Batryticatus) 白僵蚕 9–12g or **dan nan xing** (Arisaemae cum Bile) 胆南星 6–9g.
- With epigastric distension and loss of appetite, add **hou po** (Magnoliae officinalis Cortex) 厚朴 9–12g and **sha ren** (Amomi Fructus) 砂仁 6–9g.

Variations and additional prescriptions
When wind and ascendant yang predominate

Patients with phlegm damp and qi constraint or ascendant yang may occasionally experience episodes of wind phlegm. The pressure of the qi constraint is suddenly released causing a sudden severe pounding or distending headache, accompanied by a red complexion, vertigo and vomiting. The tongue has a thick greasy, mostly yellow coat. The treatment is to quickly subdue yang, extinguish wind and transform phlegm with a prescription such as Zhen Gan Xi Feng Tang (Sedate the Liver and Extinguish Wind Decoction 镇肝熄风汤, p.441), suitably modified.

In between episodes to strengthen the Spleen

Ensuring the Spleen and Liver are working as efficiently as possible will help to prevent phlegm damp from being created. This can be achieved with any of the Spleen strengthening prescriptions, usually given in prepared form for long term supplementation. One of the best for Spleen deficiency with phlegm damp and qi stagnation is XIANG SHA LIU JUN ZI TANG (Six Gentlemen Decoction with Aucklandia and Amomum 香砂六君子汤, p.618).

Prepared medicines

Concentrated powders

Ban Xia Bai Zhu Tian Ma Tang (Pinellia & Gastrodia Combination)
Xiang Sha Liu Jun Zi Tang (Vladmiria & Amomum Combination)

Pills

Ban Xia Bai Zhu Tian Ma Wan (Head Clear Pill)
Xiang Sha Liu Jun Zi Wan (Aplotaxis–Ammomum Pills, Six Gentlemen Tea Pills)
Wen Dan Wan (Rising Courage Teapills)
    – phlegm heat

Acupuncture (select from)

The points below are used in addition to points selected on the basis of the location of the headache (Boxes 9.5–9.8, pp.415–418)

Du.20 (baihui) ....alleviates headache and clears the mind
St.8 (touwei) ....dispels phlegm from the head
GB.20 (fengchi) ....clears the head, extinguishes wind, soothes the Liver and subdues ascendant Liver yang
Ren.12 (zhongwan) ....alarm point of the Stomach, strengthens Stomach and Spleen to assist in transforming phlegm
St.40 (fenglong –) ....connecting point of the Stomach, transforms phlegm, calms the shen
St.41 (jiexi –).....................strengthens the Spleen and Stomach to transform phlegm damp
PC.5 (jianshi –) ....river point of the Pericardium, transforms phlegm
Bl.20 (pishu) ....transport point of the Spleen, strengthens the Spleen and supplements qi to transform phlegm damp

- with Spleen deficiency add St.36 (zusanli +)
- with Liver qi constraint, add GB.34 (yanglingquan –) and Liv.3 (taichong –)
- with foggy head and poor concentration, add Bl.62 (shenmai)
- with muscle aches, add Sp.21 (dabao)
- with edema, add Sp.9 (yinlingquan –) and Sp.6 (sanyinjiao)
- with somnolence, add Kid.6 (zhaohai) and Bl.62 (shenmai)
- with heat, add St.44 (neiting –)
- with cold, apply moxa cones to Bl.20 (pishu ▲) and Bl.21 (weishu ▲)
- with marked abdominal distension, add St.25 (tianshu –) and Sp.15 (daheng –)
- Ear points: spleen, liver, zero point, subcortex, sympathetic, shenmen

Clinical notes

- Headaches of a phlegm damp type may be diagnosed as chronic headache, cerebral atherosclerosis, hypoglycemia, Meniere's disease or hypertension.
- Phlegm damp headaches can appear similar to those due to wind damp (9.1.3, p.429). Wind damp headaches have a more significant environmental component and are associated with more generalized muscle aching and stiffness. Wind damp is less disruptive to the senses than phlegm, and lacks the dizziness, vertigo and cognitive disturbance that is so characteristic of phlegm.
- Phlegm damp can respond well to correct treatment and dietary modification, although treatment usually needs to be quite lengthy for a sustained result.
- Diet, weight loss, regular exercise and stress management are important components of long term successful treatment. A phlegm damp transforming diet is recommended. See Clinical Handbook, Vol.2, p.880.
- Hot spot therapy can be helpful, p.923.

血
瘀
头
痛

9.7 BLOOD STASIS

Headaches due to blood stasis may be acute or chronic. When acute, there will be a history of head trauma or concussion; when chronic, there is often a long history of constrained Liver qi, chronic heat or cold, or various deficiency states. Stasis of the blood obstructs the free movement of qi and blood in the network vessels of the head, causing rather intense focal pain.

Blood stasis is a common type of headache, and depending on the etiology, may not always display the classic signs and symptoms of blood stasis. It was noted by the author of the two prescriptions below, Wang Qing–Ren (Corrections of Errors among Physicians, *Yi Lin Gai Cuo* 1830) that the diagnosis of blood stagnation should be considered when other approaches have failed, or when there are chronic headaches without indications of other pathology, i.e. no clear diagnosis.

Clinical features
- Recurrent focal headaches. The headache tends to occur in the same spot, resolving to a small area that the patient is able to point to with a finger, often in the region of the taiyang acupoint, behind the eyes or above the orbital ridge. An acute focal headache of a similar nature may follow head trauma. The pain is usually described as sharp, stabbing, drilling, boring, or words to that effect. Depending on the degree of qi constraint there may occasionally be an emotional component. Blood stasis headaches may also occur before a menstrual period, in which case there may be dysmenorrhea, clotted menstrual flow and irregular menses.
- purplish lips, sclera, conjunctiva and nail beds; dark rings around the eyes
- congested vessels or spider nevi on the face, trunk, inner knee and ankle
- irritability, short temper, depression, mood swings
- dry, scaly skin
- left iliac fossa pressure pain (p.925–926)

T in acute cases the tongue body may be unremarkable; in chronic cases dark or red purple with brown or purple stasis spots and a thin, white coat; sublingual veins are distended and dark

P deep, fine, choppy or wiry, or irregular and intermittent

Treatment principle
Activate blood and dispel blood stasis
Regulate qi, free circulation in the network vessels of the head and stop pain

Prescription

TONG QIAO HUO XUE TANG 通窍活血汤
Unblock the Orifices and Activate the Blood Decoction

tao ren (Semen Persicae) 桃仁	9–12g
hong hua (Flos Carthami Tinctorii) 红花	9–12g
chi shao (Paeoniae Radix rubra) 赤芍	9–12g
chuan xiong (Radix Ligustici Chuanxiong) 川芎	9–15g
sheng jiang (Zingiberis Rhizoma recens) 生姜	9–12g

da zao (Jujubae Fructus) 大枣 .... 4 fruit
cong bai (Allii fistulosi Bulbus) 葱白 .... 3 stalks
ren gong she xiang (synthetic muscone) 人工麝香 0.1g
Method: Decoction. **Tao ren, hong hua, chi shao** and **chuan xiong** activate blood and disperse stagnant blood; **chuan xiong** activates qi and blood stasis and alleviates headache; **ren gong she xiang** opens the orifices, activates blood and frees up circulation through the channels and network vessels; **sheng jiang** and **da zao** protect the Spleen and Stomach; **cong bai** promotes the flow of yang qi through the upper body and diffuses the lungs to promote normal descent of Lung qi. **Ren gong she xiang** is used instead of **she xiang** (Moschus) 麝香 which appeared in the original prescription, and which is not used today due to the endangered status of the musk deer. Synthetic muscone is a good substitute and appears in many prepared medicines. When used in decoction, **ren gong she xiang** can be substituted with **bai zhi** (Angelicae dahuricae Radix) 白芷 9–12g. When used, the pungent warmth of **bai zhi** disperses stagnation and alleviates facial, sinus and frontal pain. (Source: *Shi Yong Zhong Yi Nei Ke Xue* [*Yi Lin Gai Cuo*])

XUE FU ZHU YU TANG 血府逐瘀汤
Drive Out Stasis in the Mansion of Blood Decoction

This is an excellent prescription for both acute and chronic blood stasis headaches, as it takes account of the most common etiology, qi constraint.
chuan xiong (Chuanxiong Rhizoma) 川芎 9–30g
dang gui (Angelicae sinensis Radix) 当归 9–12g
sheng di (Rehmanniae Radix) 生地 9–12g
chi shao (Paeoniae Radix rubrae) 赤芍 9–15g
tao ren (Persicae Semen) 桃仁 9–12g
hong hua (Carthami Flos) 红花 6–9g
chai hu (Bupleuri Radix) 柴胡 6–9g
zhi ke (Aurantii Fructus) 枳壳 6–9g
gan cao (Glycyrrhizae Radix) 甘草 3–6g
chuan niu xi (Cyathulae Radix) 川牛膝 9–15g
jie geng (Platycodi Radix) 桔梗 3–6g
Method: Decoction. **Chuan xiong, dang gui, sheng di, chi shao, tao ren** and **hong hua** nourish, regulate and gently activate blood; the large dose of **chuan xiong** activates blood and stops pain; **chai hu, zhi ke, gan cao** and **chi shao** soothe the Liver and regulate qi; **jie geng** frees the movement of qi through the chest and diaphragm, and can raise qi to the upper body; **chuan niu xi** leads blood downwards–together **jie geng** and **chuan niu xi** re–establish the correct ascent and descent of qi and blood. (Source: *Zhong Yi Nei Ke Xue* [*Yi Lin Gai Cuo*])

Modifications (to both prescriptions)
- With severe headache, **chuan xiong** can be used in doses of up to 50 grams per packet for short periods of time. When **chuan xiong** is used in large doses, increase the dose of **dang gui** to 15g and **chuan niu xi** to 25g to balance **chuan xiong's** strong dispersing action and mitigate any iatrogenic effects. (see also Table 9.2, p.421).
- With neuralgic pain, add **quan xie** (Scorpio) 全蝎 1–3g, **wu gong** (Scolopendra) 蜈蚣 1–3g [both powdered and added to the strained decoction], and **di long** (Pheretima) 地龙 6–9g.
- If the headache occurs premenstrually, add **yi mu cao** (Leonurus Herba) 益母草 12–15g, **ze lan** (Lycopi Herba) 泽兰 9–12g and **gui zhi** (Cinnamomi

Ramulus) 桂枝 6–9g.

- With heat, delete **jie geng** and **zhi ke** (from Xᴜᴇ Fᴜ Zʜᴜ Yᴜ Tᴀɴɢ), increase the dose of **sheng di** to 18g, and add **mu dan pi** (Moutan Cortex) 牡丹皮 9–12g, **zhi mu** (Anemarrhenae Rhizoma) 知母 9–12g and **huang bai** (Phellodendri Cortex) 黄柏 9–12g.
- With nausea or vomiting, add **zhi ban xia** (Pinelliae Rhizoma preparatum) 制 半夏 9–12g and **chen pi** (Citri reticulatae Pericarpium) 陈皮 6–9g.
- With dizziness, add **gou teng** (Ramulus Uncariae cum Uncis) 钩藤 9–12g and **tian ma** (Gastrodiae Rhizoma) 天麻 6–9g.
- With qi deficiency, add **huang qi** (Astragali Radix) 黄芪 30–60g.
- With cold, add **xi xin** (Asari Herba) 细辛 3–6g and **gui zhi** (Cinnamomi Ramulus) 桂枝 9–12g.
- With phlegm, add **bai jie zi** (Sinapsis Semen) 白芥子 6–9g, **shi chang pu** (Acori tatarinowii Rhizoma) 石菖蒲 6–9g and **zhi ban xia** (Pinelliae Rhizoma preparatum) 制半夏 9–12g.

Variations and additional prescriptions
Headache following head trauma
Headaches or focal pain following head trauma can be treated with one of the primary prescriptions above. In cases of recent trauma with relatively severe pain and extensive bruising however, a more specific formula for trauma can be employed. The treatment strategy is to transform and expel blood stasis with Fᴜ Yᴜᴀɴ Hᴜᴏ Xᴜᴇ Tᴀɴɢ (Revive Health by Activating the Blood Decoction 复元活血汤). This prescription is usually only used for a couple of weeks or less, depending on how acute the trauma is. If there is extensive bruising the patient should experience loose stools or diarrhea as the bruising and pain resolve.

jiu da huang (wine fried Rhei Radix et Rhizoma) 酒大黄 9–12g
dang gui (Angelicae sinensis Radix) 当归 9–12g
tian hua fen (Trichosanthes Radix) 天花粉 9–12g
tao ren (Persicae Semen) 桃仁 6–9g
hong hua (Carthami Flos) 红花 6–9g
chai hu (Bupleuri Radix) 柴胡 6–9g
gan cao (Glycyrrhizae Radix) 甘草 3–6g
wang bu liu xing (Vaccariae Semen) 王不留行 9–12g

Method: Decoction, taken with a little yellow wine or vodka. **Jiu da huang** breaks up and moves stagnant blood, stimulates metabolism of old blood and provides an outlet for it through the bile and the bowel; **dang gui**, **tao ren**, **hong hua** and **wang bu liu xing** activate blood, reduce swelling, disperse static blood and stop pain; **wang bu liu xing** frees the channels and network vessels; **chai hu** dredges the Liver and regulates qi to lead blood; **tian hua fen** reduces swelling and stimulates healing; **gan cao** protects the Stomach and eases spasms. **Wang bu liu xing** is substituted for **chuan shan jia** (Squama Manitis) 穿山甲, the scales of the endangered pangolin that appeared in the original prescription. (Source: *Zhong Yi Nei Ke Xue* [*Yi Xue Fa Ming*])

Headache following wind stroke
Persistent headache is relatively common in the aftermath of a wind stroke, and usually has components of blood stasis and qi deficiency. As long as there is no residual ascendant yang, Bᴜ Yᴀɴɢ Hᴜᴀɴ Wᴜ Tᴀɴɢ (Supplement Yang to Restore

Five Tenths Decoction 补阳还五汤) modified, can be used to supplement qi to move blood and unblock the network vessels.

huang qi (Astragali Radix) 黄芪 30–120g
dang gui wei (rootlets of Angelicae sinensis Radix) 当归尾 6–12g
chi shao (Paeoniae Radix rubra) 赤芍 6–9g
chuan xiong (Chuanxiong Rhizoma) 川芎..6–9g
tao ren (Persicae Semen) 桃仁..6–9g
hong hua (Carthami Flos) 红花 6–9g
di long (Pheretima) 地龙..6–12g
ju hua (Chrysanthemi Flos) 菊花 6–9g
man jing zi (Viticis Fructus) 蔓荆子...6–9g

Method: Powder or Decoction. **Huang qi** supplements and activates the distribution of Spleen and Lung qi to the extremities, and thus leads blood to the periphery; **dang gui wei** supplements and activates the blood; **chi shao**, **chuan xiong**, **tao ren** and **hong hua** activate blood and dispel blood stasis; **di long** 'drills through' blockages in the channels and network vessels, opening them up and allowing free flow of qi and blood. **Ju hua** and **man jing zi** alleviate headache. **Chuan xiong** is used in a modest dose here, as support to the main strategy of promoting qi movement to move the blood. (Source: *Zhong Yi Nei Ke Xue* [*Yi Lin Gai Cuo*])

Prepared medicines
Concentrated powders
Tong Qiao Huo Xue Tang (Persica & Ligusticum Combination)
Xue Fu Zhu Yu Tang (Persica & Carthamus Combination)
Fu Yuan Huo Xue Tang (Tangkuei & Persica Combination)
Bu Yang Huan Wu Tang (Astragalus & Peony Combination)
Tao Hong Si Wu Tang (Tangkuei Four, Persica & Carthamus Combination)
– blood stasis with blood deficiency

Pills
Tong Qiao Huo Xue Wan (Tong Qiao Huo Xue Teapills)
Xue Fu Zhu Yu Wan (Stasis in the Mansion of Blood Teapills)
Tao Hong Si Wu Wan (Tao Hong Si Wu Tang Teapills)
Sheng Tian Qi Pian 生田七片 (Raw Tian Qi Ginseng Tablets)

Acupuncture (select from)
The points below are used in addition to points selected on the basis of the location of the headache (Boxes 9.5–9.8, pp.415–418)

Du.20 (baihui) ....these points are useful for treating the location of the
taiyang (M–HN–9)   headache, calming the shen and clearing stagnation
yintang (M–HN–3)   from the head
GB.20 (fengchi) ....moves qi and blood in the head
ahshi points ....tender points on the head, upper back and neck (splenius, suboccipital muscles, sternocleidomastoid, trapezius, scalene muscles); usually trigger points
Bl.17 (geshu –)..................meeting point for blood, dispels static blood
Sp.6 (sanyinjiao –)..............these points activate blood and dispel static blood
Sp.10 (xuehai –)
LI.4 (hegu –)

Liv.3 (taichong –) ....dredges the Liver, regulates qi and activates Liver
blood
SI.3 (houxi –) ....the master and couple points of the dumai, these
Bl.62 (shenmai)   points open up the circulation of dumai qi to assist
in moving blood through the head
- with dysmenorrhea or premenstrual headaches, add St.28 (guilai)
- Bleeding the congested vessels that may be found around taiyang (M–HN–9)
and at the back of the neck can be helpful. The veins are pierced with a surgical
lancet and a few drops of blood extracted. Stagnation is being cleared when the
blood runs black at first, then fresh red. This technique can be performed weekly for a few sessions, then intermittently thereafter. See also Appendix 4, p.929.
- Ear points: liver, heart, head, brain, sympathetic, shen men

Clinical notes
- Headache of a blood stasis type may be associated with head injury, post traumatic stress disorder, post concussion syndrome, tumors, chronic depression,
cluster headaches, chronic migraines or referred pain from myofascial trigger
points. Acute blood stasis headaches from trauma respond well to correct treatment. Chronic blood stasis type headaches can also respond quite well depending on the biomedical etiology. Headaches associated with masses and tumors
should be managed with a combination of Western and Chinese medicine.
- During a headache, or in anticipation of a headache, the dose of **chuan xiong**
required is usually quite large, up to 50 grams in severe cases. The high doses
should only be used for the duration of the headache before being scaled back
as pain is alleviated. See also Table 9.2, p.421.
- Caution when using high doses of **chuan xiong** premenstrually, and for patients with bleeding, or for those taking anticoagulant agents such as coumarin,
aspirin and fish oils.
- On occasion, the diagnosis of blood stasis is made by default, when other approaches that seemed more appropriate have failed, or when persistent blood
stasis like headaches occur without clear features of systemic pathology.
- Hot spot therapy can be helpful, p.923.

胃热头痛 9.8 STOMACH HEAT

Stomach heat headaches have a strong relationship to diet, and are triggered by foods such as chocolate, cheese, chillies, coffee, shellfish and red wine, or simply overeating. Most patients subject to headaches of this type have evidence of low grade heat in the Stomach in between headaches, causing chronic indigestion and heartburn. Prolonged Stomach heat can lead to damage of Stomach and Liver yin.

A Stomach heat headache may also be associated with an invasion of external heat into the qi level, but in this case the headache will be secondary to high fever, thirst and profuse sweating. This is a type of yangming syndrome (see p.321). Occasionally, headaches can persist in the aftermath of an acute qi level fever.

Clinical features
- Frontal headache (occasionally temporal), that are set off by ingestion of specific foods (see above). The headache can be intense, may feel hot or burning and is alleviated by a cold compress over the forehead.
- nagging epigastric discomfort or burning pain; indeterminate gnawing hunger
- acid reflux, heartburn, indigestion
- sore, red, bleeding gums
- halitosis
- thirst
- dry stools or constipation

T red, especially in the center, with a dry yellow or centrally peeled coat (with Stomach yin damage)

P slippery, strong, especially in the middle positions

Treatment principle
Clear heat from the Stomach
Activate the qi dynamic

Prescription

QING WEI SAN 清胃散
Clear the Stomach Powder

sheng di (Rehmanniae Radix preparata) 生地	9–15g
huang lian (Coptidis Rhizoma) 黄连	3–6g
sheng ma (Cimicifugae Rhizoma) 升麻	3–6g
mu dan pi (Moutan Cortex) 牡丹皮	6–9g
dang gui (Angelicae sinensis Radix) 当归	6–12g

Method: Decoction. **Huang lian** clears heat from the Stomach; **sheng ma** assists in clearing and dispersing heat, its ascending nature counterbalancing the descending nature of **huang lian** to drive the qi dynamic, uncover heat and facilitate its dispersal; **mu dan pi** cools the blood and clears deeply hidden heat; **sheng di** cools the blood and nourishes yin; **dang gui** nourishes and activates blood, and stops pain. (Source: *Lan Shi Mi Cang*)

Modifications
- With pronounced heat, a red face, thirst and dryness and red gums, add **shi gao** (Gypsum fibrosum) 石膏 15–30g [cooked first].

- With constipation, add **da huang** (Rhei Radix et Rhizoma) 大黄 6–9g [added towards the end of cooking] and **mang xiao** (Natrii Sulfas) 芒硝 6–9g [dissolved into the strained decoction].
- With yin deficiency, add **xuan shen** (Scrophulariae Radix) 玄参 12–15g.
- For headaches, dryness and damage to Stomach fluids that persist in the aftermath of an unresolved qi level fever, use ZHU YE SHI GAO TANG (Lophatherus and Gypsum Decoction 竹叶石膏汤 p.370).

Prepared medicines
Concentrated powders
Qing Wei San (Coptis & Rehmannia Formula)
Yu Nu Jian (Rehmannia & Gypsum Combination)

Pills
Huang Lian Shang Qing Pian (Huang Lien Shang Ching Pien)
Qing Wei San Wan (Qing Wei San Teapills)

Acupuncture (select from)
The points below are used in addition to points selected on the basis of the location of the headache (Boxes 9.5–9.8, pp.415–418)

yintang (M–HN–3) ....these points alleviate frontal headache
Du.23 (shangxing)
GB.14 (yangbai)
Ren.12 (zhongwan) ....alarm point of the Stomach, clears heat from the Stomach and corrects the qi dynamic
St.44 (neiting –) ....water point of the Stomach, clears heat from the Stomach and Stomach channel
PC.8 (laogong –) ....fire point of the Pericardium, clears heat from the Stomach channel
LI.4 (hegu –) ....source point of the Large Intestine, clears heat and alleviates frontal headache
LI.11 (quchi –) ....sea point of the Large Intestine, clears heat from yangming
- with severe heat, add St.45 (lidui ↓) and SJ.2 (yemen –)
- with constipation, add SJ.6 (zhigou –) and St.25 (tianshu –)
- with nausea, add PC.6 (neiguan)
- Ear points: stomach, zero point, sympathetic, shenmen

Clinical notes
- Headaches of a Stomach heat type may be diagnosed as food related headache or migraine, food allergy, food intolerance or trigeminal neuralgia.
- Modifying the diet to exclude known triggers is an essential part of treatment. Pharmaceutical analgesics can aggravate damage to Stomach yin and should be reduced as much as possible. A cooling diet is recommended, see Clinical Handbook, Vol.2, p.882.
- Hot spot therapy can be helpful, p.923.

胆
胃
不
和

9.9 STOMACH AND GALLBLADDER DISHARMONY

Stomach and Gallbladder disharmony is a pattern associated with persistent low grade heat and/or phlegm in the Gallbladder, usually from the diet or prolonged qi constraint. The irritated Gallbladder, when inflamed by stress or fatty foods, invades the Stomach via the controlling cycle, and causes Stomach and Gallbladder qi to counterflow upwards to the head.

Clinical features
- Temporal and frontal headache that may radiate behind the eyes, to the jaw and temporomandibular joint. The pain is intense and throbbing, and patients may be woken from sleep with a headache. Headaches are accompanied by nausea and vomiting of bitter or bile stained fluid, and sometimes sinus congestion, maxillary pain and muscle spasm in the neck and upper back. Headaches are aggravated by stress and/or foods such as alcohol and fats, and may be alleviated by vomiting.
- bitter taste in the mouth; belching; flatulence
- grey or green complexion during headaches
- abdominal and hypochondriac distension and discomfort or pain
- indeterminate gnawing hunger
- acid reflux, heartburn; aversion to fats and oils
- sluggish stools, constipation; stools may be pale
- may be mild jaundice

T greasy white or yellow coat
P slippery or wiry pulse, maybe rapid

Treatment principle
Harmonize the Gallbladder and Stomach
Clear heat and downbear counterflow Stomach qi

Prescription

HUANG LIAN WEN DAN TANG 黄连温胆汤
Warm Gallbladder Decoction with Coptis, modified

huang lian (Coptidis Rhizoma) 黄连 3–6g
zhu ru (Bambusae Caulis in taeniam) 竹茹 9–12g
zhi ban xia (Pinelliae Rhizoma preparatum) 制半夏 9–12g
zhi ke (Aurantii Fructus) 枳壳 6–9g
chen pi (Citri reticulatae Pericarpium) 陈皮 6–9g
fu ling (Poria) 茯苓 9–12g
sheng jiang (Zingiberis Rhizoma recens) 生姜 6–9g
huang qin (Scutellariae Radix) 黄芩 6–9g
chai hu (Bupleuri Radix) 柴胡 6–9g
wu zhu yu (Evodiae Fructus) 吴茱萸 1–2g

Method: Decoction. **Huang lian** and **zhu ru** clear heat and alleviate irritability, harmonize the Stomach and stop vomiting; **zhi ban xia** downbears counterflow Stomach qi, dries damp and transforms phlegm; **chen pi**, **fu ling** and **zhi ke** strengthen the Spleen, harmonize the Stomach, transform phlegm and regulate qi; **chai hu** and **huang qin** dredge the Liver and Gallbladder, alleviate constraint and clear heat; **sheng jiang** and **wu zhu yu** stop vomiting and pain. (Source: *Zhong Yi Nei Ke Xue* [*Wen Re Jing Wei*])

Modifications

- During a headache, herbs to specifically address the pain, such as **bai ji li** (Tribuli Fructus) 白蒺藜 9–12g, **xia ku cao** (Prunellae Spica) 夏枯草 12–15g and **jue ming zi** (Cassiae Semen) 决明子 9–12g, can be added.
- With jaundice, add **yin chen** (Artemisiae scopariae Herba) 茵陈 12–18g.
- With marked heat, add **shan zhi zi** (Gardeniae Fructus) 山栀子 9–12g and **pu gong ying** (Taraxaci Herba) 蒲公英 18–30g.
- With constipation, add **da huang** (Rhei Radix et Rhizoma) 大黄 6–9g [added towards the end of cooking].
- With severe vomiting, add **xuan fu hua** (Inulae Flos) 旋复花 9–12g and **dai zhe shi** (Haematitum) 代赭石 9–12g.
- With gall stones or gallbladder sludge, add **yu jin** (Curcumae Radix) 郁金 9–12g, **jin qian cao** (Lysimachiae Herba) 金钱草 30–60g, **hai jin sha** (Lygodii Spora) 海金沙 15g [decocted in a cloth bag] and **ji nei jin fen** (powdered Gigeriae galli Endothelium corneum) 鸡内金粉 5g [added to strained decoction].
- With colicky or spasmodic abdominal pain, add **bai shao** (Paeoniae Radix alba) 白芍 9–12g, and **gan cao** (Glycyrrhizae Radix) 甘草 3–6g.
- With insomnia and waking with headaches, add **mu li** (Ostrea Concha) 牡蛎 15–30g and **long gu** (Fossilia Ossis Mastodi) 龙骨 15–30g.
- With food stagnation, add **lian qiao** (Forsythiae Fructus) 连翘 9–12g and **shan zha** (Crataegi Fructus) 山楂 12–15g.

Prepared medicines
Concentrated powders
Zhu Ru Wen Dan Tang (Bamboo & Ginseng Combination)
Xiao Chai Hu Tang (Minor Bupleurum Combination)
Xuan Fu Dai Zhe Shi Tang (Inula & Hematite Combination)
   – with severe vomiting

Pills
Wen Dan Wan (Rising Courage Teapills)
Xiao Chai Hu Wan (Minor Bupleurum Teapills)
Qing Gan Li Dan Pian (Qing Gan Li Dan Tablets)
Li Dan Pian (Lidan Tablets)

Acupuncture (select from)
The points below are used in addition to points selected on the basis of the location of the headache (Boxes 9.5–9.8, pp.415–418).
yintang (M–HN–3) ....these points alleviate frontal and temporal headache
taiyang (M–HN–9)
GB.14 (yangbai)
GB.24 (riyue –).................alarm point of the Gallbladder, dredges the Liver and promotes Gallbladder function
PC.6 (neiguan –)................connecting point of the Pericardium, directs Stom-

ach qi downwards

Ren.12 (zhongwan –) ....alarm point of the Stomach, directs Stomach qi
downwards

Bl.18 (ganshu)....................transporting point of the Liver and Gallbladder

Bl.19 (danshu)   respectively, these points dredge the Liver and
Gallbladder

dannangxue (M–LE–23) ....extra point for the Gallbladder, use if tender

GB.40 (qiuxu)....................source point of the Gallbladder, dredges the Gallbladder and regulates qi

GB.34 (yanglingquan –).....sea point of the Gallbladder, dredges the Liver and
Gallbladder and stops pain

St.36 (zusanli –) ....sea point of the Stomach, supplements qi and corrects the qi dynamic

- with marked heat, add St.44 (neiting –)
- with constipation, add SJ.6 (zhigou –) and St.25 (tianshu –)
- with jaundice, add Du.9 (zhiyang –)
- with severe insomnia, use SJ.5 (waiguan –) and GB.39 (xuanzhong –)
- Ear points: liver, gallbladder, spleen, zero point, sympathetic, shenmen

Clinical notes

- Headaches of a Stomach and Gallbladder disharmony type may be diagnosed as migraine, cholecystitis or gallstones.
- Modifying the diet and excluding known triggers is an essential part of treatment. A cooling, phlegm transforming diet is recommended, see Clinical Handbook, Vol.2, p.882.
- Hot spot therapy can be helpful, p.923.

气
虚
头
痛

9.10 QI DEFICIENCY

Headache associated with qi deficiency is due to a failure of qi (and blood not being lead) to reach the head. The deficiency may affect the Spleen and Stomach, Lungs and/or Heart, and can be complicated by blood deficiency, blood stasis or yang deficiency. Qi and blood deficiency are often seen together, but each causes a distinct type of headache, with predictable complications, and can be distinguished when independent.

Clinical features

- Dull, intermittent background headaches that are worse when tired, following exertion, at the end of the day and with exposure to cold. Headache may also start soon after rising from bed and moving around. The pain is poorly localized, although may be frontal in some patients. The head feels cold and vulnerable and patients feel the need to keep the head covered in a scarf or hat. Muscle weakness lack of tone can cause the patients head to slump forward, increasing stress on the posterior neck.
- mental and physical fatigue; lack of vitality; poor muscle tone
- poor immunity; frequent colds and flu
- waxy, pale complexion
- breathlessness, weak, low voice
- spontaneous sweating
- poor appetite
- loose stools

T pale, swollen and scalloped with a thin, white coat
P weak and fine

Treatment principle

Strengthen the Lungs and Spleen
Supplement qi and raise yang qi to the head

Prescription

BU ZHONG YI QI TANG 补中益气汤
Supplement the Middle to Augment the Qi Decoction

huang qi (Astragali Radix) 黄芪 15–24g
ren shen (Ginseng Radix) 人参 9–12g
bai zhu (Atractylodes macrocephalae Rhizoma) 白术 9–12g
dang gui (Angelicae sinensis Radix) 当归 6–9g
chen pi (Citri reticulatae Pericarpium) 陈皮 6–9g
zhi gan cao (Glycyrrhizae Radix preparata) 炙甘草 3–6g
sheng ma (Cimicifugae Rhizoma) 升麻 3–6g
chai hu (Bupleuri Radix) 柴胡 3–6g

Method: Decoction. **Huang qi**, **ren shen** and **bai zhu** strengthen the Spleen, supplement qi and assist the Spleen in holding blood in the vessels; **huang qi** supplements and secures wei qi and raises yang qi; **chai hu** and **sheng ma** raise **yang qi**; **dang gui** supplements blood and prevents excessive dispersal by the pungent herbs; **chen pi** and **zhi gan cao** regulate qi and harmonize the middle burner. (Source: *Shi Yong Zhong Yi Nei Ke Xue* [*Pi Wei Lun*])

Modifications

- Treatment in between headaches focuses on supplementing qi. During a headache, specific herbs can be added to address the pain. Small doses are recommended, bearing in mind the fact that analgesic herbs can disperse zheng qi and may ultimately aggravate the condition if overused.
- With generalized headache, add **man jing zi** (Viticis Fructus) 蔓荆子 3–6g.
- With frontal headache, maxillary pain or chronic sinus congestion, add **bai zhi** (Angelicae dahuricae Radix) 白芷 3–6g.
- With frontal headache and chronic rhinitis, add **du zhong** (Eucommiae Cortex) 杜仲 9–12g and **bu gu zhi** (Psoraleae Fructus) 补骨脂 9–12g.
- With vertex headache or pain inside the head, add **gao ben** (Ligustici Rhizoma) 藁本 3–6g.
- With temporal headache or dull facial pain, add **chuan xiong** (Chuanxiong Rhizoma) 川芎 3–6g.
- With blood stasis, add **ji xue teng** (Spatholobi Caulis) 鸡血藤 15–30g and **chuan xiong** (Chuanxiong Rhizoma) 川芎 6–9g, or use BU YANG HUAN WU TANG (Supplement Yang to Restore Five Tenths Decoction 补阳还五汤, p.600) as guiding prescription.
- With yang deficiency, add **gan jiang** (Zingiberis Rhizoma) 干姜 6–9g.

Variations and additional prescriptions

Common qi deficiency variations

Qi deficiency can evolve in numerous ways and there are many variants of the basic pattern of qi deficiency. If Spleen yang is compromised the patient may develop more severe digestive weakness, diarrhea with undigested food, headaches after ingestion of cold or raw food and cold sensitivity. The strategy is to warm Spleen yang with FU ZI LI ZHONG WAN (Prepared Aconite Pill to Regulate the Middle 附子理中丸 p.624). When Spleen qi and Heart blood are deficient, chronic headaches are accompanied by anxiety, palpitations and insomnia, and GUI PI TANG (Restore the Spleen Decoction 归脾汤 p.387) is recommended. When there is a sense of emptiness in the head and lower abdominal distension from qi sinking downwards, SHENG XIAN TANG (Raise the Sunken Decoction 升陷汤 p.273) is appropriate. Qi deficiency is frequently complicated by generalized blood deficiency, in which case one of the many qi and blood supplements will help, REN SHEN YANG YING TANG (Ginseng Decoction to Nourish the Nutritive Qi 人参养营汤 p.384) being a popular example.

Prepared medicines

Concentrated powders

Bu Zhong Yi Qi Tang (Ginseng & Astragalus Combination)
Gui Pi Tang (Ginseng & Longan Combination)
Ren Shen Yang Ying Tang (Ginseng & Rehmannia Combination)
 – qi and blood deficiency

Pills

Bu Zhong Yi Qi Wan (Central Chi Teapills)

Gui Pi Wan (Kwei Be Wan, Gui Pi Teapills)

Acupuncture (select from)

The points below are used in addition to points selected on the basis of the location of the headache (Boxes 9.5–9.8, pp.415–418)

Du.20 (baihui ▲) ....raises yang qi to the head

Ren.4 (guanyuan +▲).......strengthens yuan qi and supports qi systemically

Lu.9 (taiyuan +) ....source point of the Lungs, strengthens the Lungs and supplements qi deficiency

Bl.13 (feishu +▲)..............transport point of the Lungs, strengthens the Lungs and supplements qi

Bl.20 (pishu +▲) ....transport point of the Spleen, warms and strengthens the Spleen and supplements qi

St.36 (zusanli +) ....sea point of the Stomach, strengthens the Spleen and Stomach and supplements qi

Sp.6 (sanyinjiao +▲).........strengthens the Spleen and supplements qi

• Ear points: lung, spleen, zero point, shenmen, adrenal

Clinical notes

• Qi deficiency headaches may be diagnosed as hypoglycemic episodes, diabetes, mental and physical exhaustion, burn out, poor muscle tone and postural weakness.

• A qi supplementing diet is an essential component of treatment. See Clinical Handbook, Vol.2 p.870.

• Regular rest balanced with graded exercise, built up over a period of time, is an essential component to the rebuilding of Lung and Spleen qi. Breathing exercises and swimming are particularly helpful. Some people find singing in a structured fashion, such as joining a choir to be beneficial.

血虚头痛

9.11 BLOOD DEFICIENCY

Blood deficiency headaches are common, and due to failure of blood to reach the head, or failure of the weakened blood to anchor yang securely. These headaches are more frequent in women of reproductive age, and in general are more severe than those associated with qi deficiency. Blood deficiency headaches are often complicated by Liver qi constraint and may be sporadically compounded by ascendant yang.

Clinical features

- Dull background headaches, that are initiated or aggravated by blood loss, menstruation, childbirth or during breast feeding. The vertex, the region behind the eyes or whole head can be affected. Headaches can be brought on by exertion, prolonged use of the eyes and may be worse at the end of the day. The patient may wake from sleep with a headache (as blood returns to the Liver) or may start upon rising (as blood drains from the head).
- The background headache may occasionally and suddenly get a lot worse and become pounding or splitting, affecting the temples. This is caused by ascendant yang not being anchored by blood. Acute exacerbations are associated with increasing stress, emotional upset or blood loss.
- sore and tender neck and shoulders
- creaking or crackles in the neck with rotation; creaky joints
- pale complexion, conjunctivae and nails
- dry hair and skin; dry stools
- postural dizziness
- insomnia, dream disturbed sleep
- palpitations
- scanty menses, irregular menses
- fatigue, low energy reserves

T pale and thin, or with orangy edges
P fine

Treatment principle

Supplement blood

Prescription

JIA WEI SI WU TANG 加味四物汤
Augmented Four Substance Decoction

dang gui (Angelicae sinensis Radix) 当归 6–12g
shu di (Rehmanniae Radix preparata) 熟地 9–15g
bai shao (Paeoniae Radix alba) 白芍 9–12g
chuan xiong (Chuanxiong Rhizoma) 川芎 6–9g
ju hua (Chrysanthemi Flos) 菊花 6–9g
man jing zi (Viticis Fructus) 蔓荆子 3–6g
gan cao (Glycyrrhizae Radix) 甘草 3–6g

Method: Decoction. **Dang gui**, **shu di** and **bai shao** nourish blood and yin; **bai shao** softens the

Liver; **chuan xiong**, **man jing zi** and **ju hua** clear the head and eyes and stop pain; **gan cao** harmonizes the formula and protects the Spleen. (Source: *Shi Yong Zhong Yi Nei Ke Xue* [*He Ji Ju Fang*])

Modifications

- With qi deficiency, add **huang qi** (Astragali Radix) 黄芪 12–18g, **ren shen** (Ginseng Radix) 人参 6–9g and **bai zhu** (Atractylodes macrocephalae Rhizoma) 白术 9–12g, or use **Ren Shen Yang Ying Tang** (Ginseng Decoction to Nourish the Nutritive Qi 人参养营汤 p.384).
- With marked palpitations, anxiety and insomnia add **suan zao ren** (Ziziphi spinosae Semen) 酸枣仁 12–15g and **yuan zhi** (Polygalae Radix) 远志 6–9g or use **Gui Pi Tang** (Restore the Spleen Decoction 归脾汤 p.387).
- With ascendant yang and sudden onset of increasing pounding headache, dizziness and muscle spasms, add **shi jue ming** (Haliotidis Concha) 石决明 15–30g, **mu li** (Ostreae Concha) 牡蛎 15–30g [both cooked first], **nu zhen zi** (Ligustri Fructus) 女贞子 9–12g and **gou teng** (Uncariae Ramulus cum Uncis) 钩藤 9–12g [added at the end of cooking].
- With Liver qi constraint, tension headaches, premenstrual headaches, muscle tension and a pale tongue, consider **Xiao Yao San** (Rambling Powder 逍遥散 p.435) as guiding prescription.

Prepared medicines
Concentrated powders
Gui Pi Tang (Ginseng & Longan Combination)
– Spleen qi and Heart blood deficiency
Ba Zhen Tang (Tangkuei & Ginseng Eight Combination)
– qi and blood deficiency
Shi Quan Da Bu Tang (Ginseng & Dang Gui Ten Combination)
– qi and blood deficiency with cold
Ren Shen Yang Ying Tang (Ginseng & Rehmannia Combination)
– qi and blood deficiency with cold
Xiao Yao San (Bupleurum & Tangkuei Formula)
– blood deficiency with Liver qi constraint

Pills
Gui Pi Wan (Kwei Be Wan, Gui Pi Teapills)
Bai Zi Yang Xin Wan (Pai Tzu Yang Hsin Wan)
– Heart blood deficiency
Shi Quan Da Bu Wan (Ten Flavour Teapills)
Dang Gui Ji Jing (Tang Kuei Essence of Chicken)
– excellent for postpartum blood deficiency
Xiao Yao Wan (Free and Easy Wanderer Teapills, Hsiao Yao Wan)

Acupuncture
The points below are used in addition to points selected on the basis of the location of the headache (Boxes 9.5–9.8, pp.415–418)
Du.20 (baihui +)................helps to raise yang qi and blood to the head
Bl.18 (ganshu +▲)............transport point of the Liver, nourishes Liver blood

Bl.20 (pishu +▲) ....transport point of the Spleen, strengthens the Spleen and supplements qi and blood

Bl.21 (weishu +▲) ....transport point of the Stomach, strengthens the Stomach and supplements qi and blood

Bl.25 (shenshu +▲) ....transport point of the Kidney, strengthens the Kidneys to support the Spleen and supplement qi and blood

Ren.4 (guanyuan +▲) ....strengthens yuan qi and supports qi systemically

St.36 (zusanli +) ....sea point of the Stomach, strengthens the Spleen and Stomach and supplements qi to produce blood

Sp.6 (sanyinjiao +▲) ....strengthens the Spleen and supplements qi

Liv.3 (taichong –) ....source point of the Liver, nourishes Liver blood and restrains ascendant yang

• Ear points: liver, heart, spleen, zero point, shenmen

Clinical notes

• Headaches due to blood deficiency may be diagnosed as anemia from nutritional deficiency, low iron stores, chronic blood loss, menstrual or hormonal headaches, myofascial trigger points or tension headaches.

• Blood and yin deficiency can lead to increased irritability of the muscles of the upper back and neck and an increased likelihood of harbouring trigger points. Deep massage can further irritate the already sensitive muscles and may aggravate the headache.

• These headaches are responsive to treatment, but depending on the patients diet and duration of the deficiency, can take some time to resolve.

• A blood nourishing diet is an essential component of treatment. See Clinical Handbook, Vol.2, p.874.

肾
虚
头
痛

9.12 KIDNEY DEFICIENCY

1. Yin deficiency
2. Yang deficiency

Kidney deficiency headaches can be divided into two main types, yin and yang deficiency. Various combinations of yin and yang deficiency also occur. The mechanism of each is different. In the yin deficiency pattern the headache is due to two factors; deficiency of the 'sea of Marrow', i.e. the brain, and the rising of heat and ascendant yang that is created by the deficiency. Yang deficiency headache is due to a failure of yang qi to reach the head and the constricting effects of cold on the circulation of qi and blood.

阴
虚

9.12.1 KIDNEY YIN DEFICIENCY

Kidney yin deficiency is responsible for two types of headache. The first is the dull persistent background pain, which is occasionally superseded by the second, the more intense splitting headache characteristic of ascendant yang (see Ascendant Liver yang, p.440).

Clinical features
- Chronic background headache with a dull empty feeling in the head or occiput; the head may feel slightly warm. Patients sometimes describe this sensation as the 'head feels inflamed'. Headaches are worse in the evening, aggravated by exertion and after sex.
- dryness of the skin, hair, eyes, vagina, mouth and throat; warm, dry palms
- facial flushing, night sweats, low grade fever in the evening
- insomnia, nightmares, vivid exhausting dreams
- tiredness and exhaustion, yet irritable and easily angered
- lower back and legs aching and weak
- dizziness, tinnitus, forgetfulness
- visual weakness, blurring vision
- muscle spasms, calf cramps
- dry stools or constipation
- infertility, menstrual disorders, amenorrhea

T red, thin and dry with little or no coat
P fine and rapid

Treatment principle
Nourish and supplement Kidney yin
Clear deficiency heat

Prescription

QI JU DI HUANG WAN 杞菊地黄丸
Lycium Fruit, Chrysanthemum and Rehmannia Pill

shu di (Rehmanniae Radix preparata) 熟地 24g
shan yao (Dioscoreae Rhizoma) 山药 12g

shan zhu yu (Corni Fructus) 山茱萸 12g
mu dan pi (Moutan Cortex) 牡丹皮 9g
fu ling (Poria) 茯苓 9g
ze xie (Alismatis Rhizoma) 泽泻 9g
ju hua (Chrysanthemi Flos) 菊花 9g
gou qi zi (Lycii Fructus) 枸杞子 12g
Method: Pills or powder. Can also be decocted with the doses as shown. **Shu di** supplements Kidney yin and blood; **shan zhu yu** warms and supplements the Liver and Kidneys and preserves yin; **shan yao** strengthens the Spleen; **ze xie** clears heat and fire from the Kidneys through the urine; **mu dan pi** cools and activates the blood, and clears heat from the Liver; **fu ling** strengthens the Spleen and leaches damp out through the urine; **ju hua** calms the Liver and alleviates headaches; **gou qi zi** nourishes Liver yin and blood. (Source: *Shi Yong Zhong Yi Nei Ke Xue* [*Yi Ji Bao Jian*])

Prepared medicines
Concentrated powders
Qi Ju Di Huang Wan (Lycium, Chrysanthemum & Rehamannia Formula)
Pills
Qi Ju Di Huang Wan (Lycium Rehmannia Teapills)
Ming Mu Di Huang Wan (Ming Mu Di Huang Teapills)

Acupuncture (select from)
The points below are used in addition to points selected on the basis of the location of the headache (Boxes 9.5–9.8, pp.415–418)
Ren.4 (guanyuan +)............these points supplement Kidney yin and yuan qi
Ren.6 (qihai +)
Kid.3 (taixi +)....................source point of the Kidneys, supplements Kidney
                                yin
Liv.3 (taichong +)...............source point of the Liver, supplements Liver yin and
                                blood, pacifies ascendant Liver yang
Lu.7 (lieque).......................master and couple points of renmai, these points
Kid.6 (zhaohai)   open up circulation of renmai qi and supplement
                                Kidney yin
Sp.6 (sanyinjiao)................nourishes Kidney, Liver and Spleen yin
Bl.23 (shenshu +) ....transport point of the Kidneys, supplements Kidney
                                yin
Bl.52 (zhishi +)...................supplements the Kidneys
- with insomnia, add Ht.7 (shenmen) and PC.6 (neiguan –)
- with night sweats, add Ht.6 (yinxi –)
- with anxiety, add yintang (M–HN–3) and Du.20 (baihui)
- with forgetfulness, add Du.20 (baihui)
- with palpitations or arrhythmias add Ht.5 (tongli)
- Ear points: kidney, liver, shenmen, adrenal, subcortex, endocrine

Clinical notes
- Kidney yin deficiency headaches may be diagnosed as migraine or cluster headache, temporal arteritis or hormonal headache.
- A yin nourishing diet is recommended. See Clinical Handbook, Vol.2, p.876.

阳
虚

9.12.2 KIDNEY YANG DEFICIENCY

Clinical features
- Chronic, dull, persistent background headache with a dull empty or cold feeling in the head or occipital region; during headaches the patient feels cold or even shivers.
- cold intolerance, cold extremities
- lower back ache, coldness and weakness
- frequent urination, nocturia; copious thin watery leukorrhea
- low energy, low motivation, low libido

T pale, swollen and scalloped with a moist white coat
P deep, slow, weak

Treatment principle
Warm and supplement Kidney yang

Prescription

YOU GUI WAN 右归丸
Restore the Right [Kidney] Pill

shu di (Rehmanniae Radix preparata) 熟地 24g
shan yao (Dioscoreae Rhizoma) 山药 12g
gou qi zi (Lycii Fructus) 枸杞子 12g
lu jiao jiao (Cervi Cornus Colla) 鹿角胶 12g
du zhong (Eucommiae Cortex) 杜仲 12g
tu si zi (Cuscutae Semen) 菟丝子 12g
dang gui (Angelicae sinensis Radix) 当归 9g
shan zhu yu (Corni Fructus) 山茱萸 9g
zhi fu zi (Aconiti Radix lateralis preparata) 制附子 6–18g
rou gui (Cinnamomi Cortex) 肉桂 6–12g

Method: Pills or powder. The herbs are ground to a fine powder and formed into 9 gram pills with honey. The dose is one pill twice daily. Can also be decocted, in which case **zhi fu zi** is cooked for 30 minutes before the other herbs and **lu jiao jiao** is melted into the strained decoction. **Shu di**, **gou qi zi** and **dang gui** nourish Kidney yin and blood; **shan zhu yu** supplements the Liver; **shan yao** strengthens the Spleen and Kidneys; **tu si zi** and **du zhong** supplement Kidney yang; **zhi fu zi** and **rou gui** warm yang; **lu jiao jiao** benefits yang and jing. (Source: *Zhong Yi Nei Ke Xue* ([*Jing Yue Quan Shu*])

Modification
- With stubborn and persistent headaches, add 'meaty' substances that deeply enrich the jing to support the creation of yin and yang, such as **gui ban** (Testudinis Plastrum) 龟板, **bie jia** (Trionycis Carapax) 鳖甲, **ge jie** (Gecko) 蛤蚧 and **lu rong** (Cervi Cornu pantotrichum) 鹿茸. Add herbs to temper the richness of these substances, such as **sha ren** (Amomi Fructus) 砂仁 and **chen pi** (Citri reticulatae Pericarpium) 陈皮.
- With nocturia or copious leucorrhea, add **qian shi** (Euryales Semen) 芡实 9–12g, **sang piao xiao** (Mantidis Ootheca) 桑螵蛸 6–9g, **fu pen zi** (Rubi Fructus) 覆盆子 9–12g and **sha yuan ji li** (Astragali complanati Semen) 沙苑

蒺藜 6–9g.

- With early morning diarrhea, add **bu gu zhi** (Psoraleae Fructus) 补骨脂 12g and **wu wei zi** (Schizandrae Fructus) 五味子 6g, or combine with **SI SHEN WAN** (Four Miracle Pill 四神丸 p.920).
- With Spleen yang deficiency, poor appetite and abdominal distension, combine with **LI ZHONG WAN** (Regulate the Middle Pill 理中丸, p.732).
- With indigestion or nausea, add **gan jiang** (Zingiberis Rhizoma) 干姜 9g.

Prepared medicines
Concentrated powder
You Gui Wan (Eucommia & Rehmannia Formula)
Ba Wei Di Huang Wan (Rehmannia Eight Formula)
Pills
You Gui Wan (Right Side Replenishing Teapills)
Jin Kui Shen Qi Wan (Fu Gui Ba Wei Wan, Golden Book Teapills)

Acupuncture (select from)
The points below are used in addition to points selected on the basis of the location of the headache (Boxes 9.5–9.8, pp.415–418)

Du.20 (baihui ▲) ....raises yang qi to the head
Ren.6 (qihai +▲) ....these points warm Kidney yang
Ren.4 (guanyuan +▲)
Ren.8 (shenque ▲) ....warms yang when treated with moxa on salt; place a piece of thin cloth over the navel and fill it with salt; burn large cones of moxa on the salt. The cloth enables quick removal of the salt and prevents excessive burning.
Kid.3 (taixi +).....................source point of the Kidneys, supplements Kidney yang
St.36 (zusanli +▲) ....sea point of the Stomach, strengthens the Spleen and Stomach and supplements yang qi
Sp.6 (sanyinjiao +▲).........strengthens the Spleen and Kidneys
Bl.23 (shenshu +▲) ....transport point of the Kidneys, warms yang
Du.4 (mingmen +▲) ....warms and supports Kidney yang
- with abdominal distension, add Sp.1 (yinbai)
- with edema, add Kid.7 (fuliu –), Ren.9 (shuifen ▲) and Sp.9 (yinlingquan –)
- Ear points: kidney, adrenal, subcortex, sympathetic, zero point, shenmen

Clinical notes
- Kidney yang deficiency headache may be diagnosed as hypothyroidism, Addison's disease, hormonal headache, cervical osteoarthritis or uremia.
- A diet to warm yang is recommended. See Clinical Handbook, Vol.2, p.873.

Table 9.3 Summary of headache patterns

Pattern		Features	Prescription
External pathogens	wind cold	Occipital headache with stiff neck; aversion to wind & cold, chills & fever, no sweating, muscle aches, nasal obstruction or a runny nose, thin white tongue coat, floating, or floating & tight pulse	Chuan Xiong Cha Tiao San
	wind heat	Frontal headache, fever, red face & eyes, thirst, dry cough or cough with sticky yellow sputum, sore throat, red tipped tongue with a yellow coat, floating, rapid pulse	Xiong Zhi Shi Gao Tang
	wind damp	Occipital or frontal headache, heavy head, neck stiffness, chills with mild fever, muscle & joint pain, loss of appetite, nausea & vomiting, loose stools, thick greasy white coat, floating, soft, soggy pulse	Qiang Huo Sheng Shi Tang
	summerheat	Frontal headache with high fever, sweating or hot dry flushed skin, dryness & thirst, scanty, concentrated urine, vomiting & diarrhea, dry, yellow tongue coat, rapid & strong, or rapid & fine pulse	Xin Jia Xiang Ru Yin
Liver qi constraint		Recurrent occipital or temporal headaches worse with stress, stiff neck & shoulders, muscular tension, depression, premenstrual syndrome; **with constrained heat:** flushing, red sore eyes, heartburn, bitter taste, waking in the middle of the night with headaches, normal or mauve tongue, or with red edges, wiry and rapid	Xiao Yao San Jia Wei Xiao Yao San
Liver fire		Severe, pounding or splitting temporal headache, worse with alcohol, and stress, flushed face, sore red eyes, bitter taste, constipation, scleral hemorrhage, bad temper, red tongue with a thick yellow dry coat (during headaches), wiry, strong, rapid pulse (during headaches)	Long Dan Xie Gan Tang
Ascendant Liver yang; Liver wind		Splitting temporal or vertex headache, dizziness, visual disturbances, nausea & vomiting, red complexion, anger, insomnia, lower backache, heat in the chest, palms & soles, night sweats; muscle spasms and tremors, numbness, red tongue with little coat, or a peeled coat, wiry, strong, rapid pulse	Zhen Gan Xi Feng Tang Tian Ma Gou Teng Tang
Cold affecting the Liver and Stomach		Vertex or temporal headache with vomiting, cold intolerance and cold extremities, hyper salivation, pale tongue with a white coat, slow wiry pulse	Wu Zhu Yu Tang

Table 9.3 Summary of headache patterns (cont.)

Pattern		Features	Prescription
Phlegm damp		Dull heavy aching headache, vertigo, poor concentration, foggy head, nausea or vomiting, chest oppression, swollen tongue with a thick greasy tongue coat, slippery pulse	Ban Xia Bai Zhu Tian Ma Tang
Blood stasis		Intense focal stabbing headache, purple lips, sclera, conjunctiva and nail beds, vascular congestion, depression, left iliac fossa pressure pain, purple tongue, choppy pulse	Tong Qiao Huo Xue Tang Xue Fu Zhu Yu Tang Fu Yuan Huo Xue Tang
Stomach heat		Frontal headache associated with specific foods, epigastric pain; indeterminate gnawing hunger, heartburn, halitosis, sore gums, thirst, constipation, thick yellow tongue coat, slippery strong pulse	Qing Wei San
Stomach and Gallbladder disharmony		Pounding frontal and temporal headache with nausea and vomiting, bitter taste, belching and flatulence, abdominal and hypochondriac pain, greasy white or yellow tongue, slippery wiry pulse	Huang Lian Wen Dan Tang
Qi deficiency		Dull headache worse in the morning, when tired and after exposure to cold, fatigue, poor immunity, pale complexion, breathlessness, weak voice, spontaneous sweating, poor appetite, pale tongue, weak pulse	Bu Zhong Yi Qi Tang
Blood deficiency		Dull headaches, worse after blood loss, menstruation, with eyestrain and at the end of the day. Pale complexion, conjunctivae and nail beds, dry hair, skin and eyes, postural dizziness, insomnia, palpitations, scanty or irregular menses, low energy reserve, pale thin tongue, fine pulse	Jia Wei Si Wu Tang
Kidney deficiency	yin	Chronic dull headache, worse in the evening, after exertion and sex. Dryness of the skin, hair, eyes, vagina, mouth and throat; warm dry palms, flushing, night sweats, lower back and leg pain, dizziness, tinnitus, muscle spasms and calf cramps, insomnia, dry stools or constipation, red dry tongue with little or no coat, fine rapid pulse	Qi Ju Di Huang Wan
	yang	Chronic dull headache with a dull empty or cold feeling in the head; cold intolerance, cold extremities, lower back ache, nocturia; copious thin watery leukorrhea, pale swollen and scalloped tongue, deep, slow weak pulse	You Gui Wan

HU HUO DISEASE
A model for chronic inflammation

The disease described as *hú huò bing*[1] (狐惑病) was first recorded during the Han dynasty by Zhang Zhong–Jing, in his classic Jin Gui Yao Lüe (Synopsis of Prescription of the Golden Chamber). Zhang states that 'the signs and symptoms of hu huo disease are similar to those of exogenous febrile disease; the pathogenic ulcerations attack the throat or external genitals. When ulcers develop, the patient loses appetite and feels nauseated with food....'

The main features of hu huo disease are ulceration of the mouth, throat, anus and external genitals, inflammation of the eyes, joint pains and digestive disturbance (Table 10.1, p.474). Modern commentators consider hu huo disease to be synonymous with Behçet's disease, an autoimmune disease that attacks veins and arteries. Hu huo bing translates enigmatically as 'puzzled fox disease', but according to the source text (clause 3–10), hu 狐 refers to ulceration of the external genitals and huo 惑 is ulceration of the throat.

Hu huo disease is rare in Europe, the United States and Australia, but is relatively common in a band running from China westwards to Turkey, hence its first modern description by a Turkish dermatologist Hulusi Behçet, and its other name, the silk road disease. Although practitioners are unlikely to encounter patients with hu huo disease, it serves as a model for understanding the pathology of more common chronic inflammatory diseases (p.478).

In Zhang's description of hu huo disease, he recommended the formula GAN CAO XIE XIN TANG (Licorice Decoction to Drain the Epigastrium 甘草泻心汤) as the main treatment. This formula is one of the harmonizing group. The harmonizing group of formulae have two main areas of therapeutic activity. The first is their use in treating lingering pathogenic invasion. Here, harmonizing refers to a gentle balancing method that closes the space available to the pathogen and so encourages it to leave. This technique is considered harmonizing because it is quite different to the harsh techniques usually employed to forcibly expel pathogens, such as purgation, diaphoresis or emesis. Harmonizing formulae also treat complex disorders by balancing the function and relationships of the internal organ systems, in particular the Liver, Spleen and Intestines, while clearing heat, supplementing qi and transforming dampness. Although not made explicit in the original text, the selection of Gan Cao Xie Xin Tang reveals that Zhang recognized the etiology of the heat in hu huo disease to be disharmony of the internal organs. This has implications for the

---

1 Practical Dictionary of Chinese Medicine (1998) – 'fox creeper disease'

473

way we look at chronic inflammatory conditions, including autoimmune diseases such as Systemic Lupus Erythematosus, rheumatoid arthritis and Grave's disease, and other inflammatory disorders such as ulcerative colitis and Crohn's disease.

Table 10.1 Main features of hu huo disease

Symptom	Interpretation
Oral ulceration	heat in the Heart (tongue) and Spleen (buccal cavity)
Genital ulceration	heat in the Liver
Inflammation of the eyes	heat in the Liver
Vasculitis, thrombosis	heat in the Heart, blood stasis
Arthritis, usually knees and large joints	damp heat sinking downwards
Psychiatric disorders, personality changes	heat disturbing the shen
Skin lesions, nodular lesions	damp heat, heat affecting the blood, blood stasis
Abdominal pain, diarrhea, loss of appetite, nausea, fatigue	damp heat, Spleen deficiency
Low grade fever, night sweats	damp heat; yin deficiency

ETIOLOGY

Heat

The main pathology of hu huo disease is heat, typically damp heat, affecting the Liver, Spleen and Heart. The source of the heat is the primary pathological triad. The primary pathological triad (PPT) is so called because it is comprised of three patterns of pathology that are seen frequently together, are tightly interlinked and mutually engendering.

The triad comprises Liver qi stagnation, Spleen qi deficiency, and the heat that is created as a result of the Liver and Spleen imbalance. The type and intensity of heat created can vary, and may be in the form of constrained heat, damp heat, phlegm heat, toxic heat or fire. In hu huo disease the heat is concentrated in the Spleen, Liver and Heart organ systems. In terms of intensity, constrained heat is the mildest, toxic heat and fire the most severe. Constrained heat is usually the first form of heat generated and the precursor to the other more severe forms. Toxic heat and fire are highly concentrated types of heat and create suppurative and ulcerated lesions. Damp heat is seen in cases with swelling and inflammatory exudate.

In addition to the basic triad of pathology, there are usually complicating factors such as blood and yin deficiency, blood stasis and shen disturbances (Fig. 10.1, p.476). The development of the PPT is promoted by the usual etiological factors that disrupt the Liver and Spleen. Chronic stress and worry, poor diet and eating habits and increasingly sedentary habits and occupations all contribute.

A strong emotional component has been observed in hu huo disease, with onset or aggravation of the disease frequently preceded by periods of increasing stress and emotional turmoil. The primary pathological triad is the main pathology in the early to mid stages of hu huo disease, after which the complications – qi and yin deficiency, and blood stasis – start to become more prominent.

Deficiency

One of the features of heat is that it waxes and wanes. Heat is a yang pathogen and will dissipate over time, either of its own accord or as the result of treatment. In clinical practice a progression is observed in chronic inflammatory conditions from states with abundant heat at the onset of the illness or during a flare–up of a chronic pattern, to gradually decreasing heat and eventual weakening or loss of function.

TREATMENT

As huo huo disease is rare, our specific clinical experience is limited. The patterns of hu huo disease from p.482 can be used as general models for analyzing inflammatory conditions, with less emphasis made on the ulceration which is typical of Behçet's disease. The following statements are applicable to chronic inflammatory disease in general.

The majority of patients diagnosed with a chronic inflammatory disease (of an autoimmune type) will be medicated with various combinations of pharmaceuticals such as anti–inflammatory, corticosteroid, immunosuppressant, and/or anti–coagulant agents. These drugs provide relief from symptoms, but complicate Chinese medical diagnosis and treatment. Patients who are well managed do not present to Chinese medicine practitioners. Those who do seek Chinese medical treatment do so because the drugs are not working very well, or they are unhappy with the side effects. Even though the pharmaceuticals alleviate most symptoms, in practice we find that in such patients there are usually sufficient features, albeit somewhat muted, to be able to make a rational Chinese medicine diagnosis.

The Chinese medical treatment depends on what medication the patient is taking. The ultimate aim of treatment is to enable the patient to reduce the amount of all medications required to the minimum necessary to remain functional and comfortable. As a general rule, if patients are already taking numerous medications, or large doses of medication, we avoid prescribing more. When the existing medication load is small (one or two drugs in low or maintenance doses), herbs can be judiciously added. For those using multiple or high dose medications, frequent acupuncture (at least 2–3 times per week is needed to gain momentum), given in several courses, is the recommended approach. Over time (usually several months), and in keeping with the patients improvement, the medication load can be reviewed and adjusted as appropriate, by their specialist.

Large doses of gan cao (Glycyrrhizae Radix) 甘草

Most of the prescription recommended for hu huo disease use quite large doses of gan cao. It is used primarily for its heat clearing, toxin resolving action. Large doses of **gan cao** over a prolonged period can lead to fluid retention, aggravation of edema and hypertension in some patients. This is not an issue in the first weeks of treatment, but needs to be monitored in long term therapy. As patients improve, in particular as the ulcerations resolve, the dose of **gan cao** should be reduced.

Figure 10.1 The primary pathological triad and hu huo disease

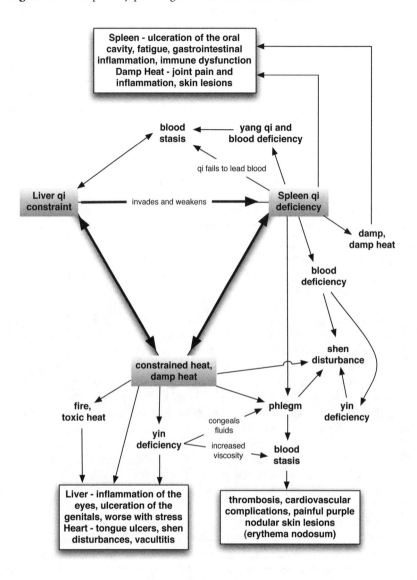

Figure 10.2 Harmonizing formulae can be mapped according to therapeutic bias

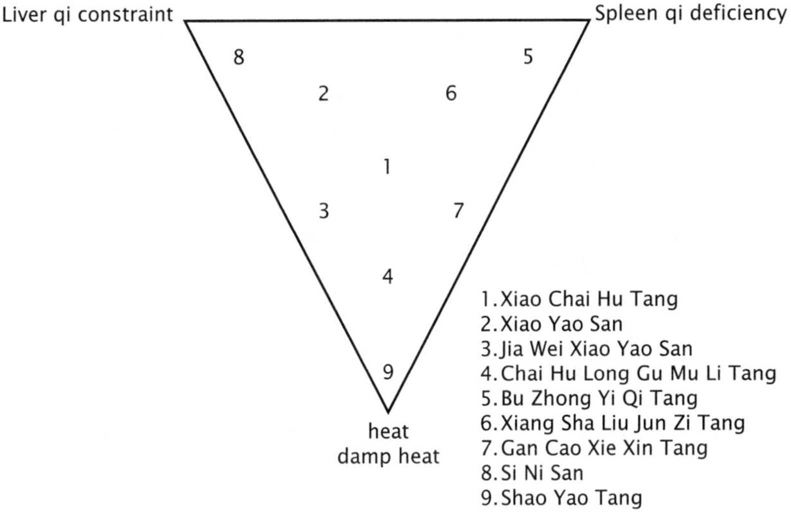

Liver qi constraint

8

2   6

5

Spleen qi deficiency

1

3   7

4

9

heat
damp heat

1. Xiao Chai Hu Tang
2. Xiao Yao San
3. Jia Wei Xiao Yao San
4. Chai Hu Long Gu Mu Li Tang
5. Bu Zhong Yi Qi Tang
6. Xiang Sha Liu Jun Zi Tang
7. Gan Cao Xie Xin Tang
8. Si Ni San
9. Shao Yao Tang

Biomedical treatment

Corticosteroids and immunosuppressant agents (Imuran, Cyclosporin) and Thalidomide are the usual therapies for hu huo disease, and while they are effective in calming down a flare–up or controlling severe symptoms, the side effects make their prolonged use undesirable. The aim of therapy is always to reduce the dose to the minimum possible to maintain a satisfactory result.

Long term use of corticosteroids may cause pathological change that can be described in Chinese medical terms. Steroids are pungent and very dispersing to qi and yin, and work by mobilizing the body's yang to dissipate any obstruction or accumulation. By continually activating yang however, they deplete yin and disperse yang qi. Qi and yin deficiency is the most common early effect of prolonged steroid use. Because yin and yang are interdependent, ultimately yang is dispersed as well, and patients become both yin and yang deficient.

CHINESE MEDICINE AND CHRONIC INFLAMMATION

Chronic inflammation is the primary disease process in a variety of conditions (Box 10.2). The unifying factor that links these conditions is heat of some type, at least during the significant and active portion of their natural history. The heat can occur in numerous forms, from fire and toxic heat, damp heat, constrained heat to heat associated with yin deficiency. To start to address these conditions effectively and in the long term, we need to know where the heat has come from.

We propose a preliminary model to explain the presence of the heat in diseases characterized by chronic inflammation, based on our observations in the clinic.

There are two broad types of prolonged heat observed in chronic inflammatory diseases

1. Heat derived from internal organ system dysfunction

There are two variants that give rise to prolonged heat:

- The first is associated with chronic stress and emotional turmoil, usually in combination with a less than optimal diet. The stress is usually relatively low grade, but persistent, with periodic exacerbation. The combined effects of the stress and diet disrupt the Liver and Spleen axis, which in turn creates heat and damp. This is the primary pathological triad (PPT), and is commonly observed in a wide range of diseases with chronic inflammation, including Behçet's disease (Fig. 10.1, p.476), ulcerative colitis, rheumatoid arthritis, allergies (skin, respiratory and gastrointestinal) and hyperthyroidism.

- The second is associated with a sudden severe shock or emotional trauma. This is usually a significant life event, such as a major motor vehicle accident, death of a loved one, period of extreme fear, combat trauma or environmental catastrophe. The traumatic event disrupts the Heart Kidney axis, one of the fundamental relationships of the body. This upsets the balance between water and fire, with the result that fire flares out of control. This has been observed in cases of type 1 diabetes, Grave's disease (hyperthyroidism) and Hashimoto's thyroiditis, where onset of the illness is preceded by a traumatic event, usually around 6–9 months before. The shaoyin disruption also renders patients vulnerable to subsequent pathogenic invasion and development of a lingering pathogen. Hashimoto's thyroiditis is a special case where the inflammatory phase is short, and the patient quickly progresses to yang deficiency (see shaoyin level disorder, pp.522–523).

2. Heat derived from a lingering pathogen

Heat and damp heat can enter the body from outside, and once inside linger in different locations in the body for prolonged periods of time. Depending on the nature and location of the pathogen, quite a diverse range of clinical pictures can emerge, but the features that link them are those that are frequently seen in chronic inflammatory conditions – fever, sweating, swollen lymph glands, fatigue and painful joint or muscle pathology. A discussion of Lingering pathogens can be found in Chapter 11.

Although many patients will show clear signs of one source of heat, some patients will exhibit elements of both internal and external causes in their pathology.

An inherited or acquired predisposition is common

Patients who develop a chronic inflammatory disease often have a predisposition to this particular type of illness. It is the combination of the heat creating factors or the pathogenic influence with the underlying weakness, that enables the full blown condition to arise. The common predisposition is a weakness of the shaoyin (Heart and Kidneys), and it can be inherited or acquired. When in-

> **BOX 10.2 EXAMPLES OF CHRONIC INFLAMMATORY DISEASE**
>
> Autoimmunity
> – Behçet's disease
> – Systemic lupus erythematosus
> – Rheumatoid arthritis
> – Grave's disease
> – Hashimoto's thyroiditis
> – Polymyositis
> Inflammatory bowel disease
> – Ulcerative colitis
> – Crohn's disease
> Allergies

herited, we find other members of the family with the same or a related condition. A predisposition can also be acquired with ageing and the relative Kidney deficiency that accompanies age, by harmful life habits, poor diet, drug use and sudden shock as noted above.

Identifying the source of the heat is critical

The important point to appreciate is that even though the superficial features may appear somewhat similar (they are all due to heat), the treatments are quite different, so identifying the source of the heat is critical to success. For disorder of the PPT, treatments that harmonize, as well as exercise and stress management are important. For disruption of the Heart Kidney axis, supplementation of Heart and Kidney yin and/or yang, along with rejuvenating rest are indicated. For a lingering pathogen, the pathogen must be vented towards the surface or an exit point and expelled from the body.

There are a few simple clues that help distinguish between the two types. Those associated with the PPT are distinctly worse with, or initiated by, stress and can be alleviated when relaxed or on holiday. Those associated with a lingering pathogen do not show the relationship to the emotional state, and instead display signs of pathogenic involvement, such as a specific history ('never well since....'), swollen glands, cyclical fever patterns and other traits described in Chapter 11.

Stages of inflammatory disease

Once heat is being created, or is trapped in the body, it can exist in different states. Most chronic inflammatory diseases pass through various stages, from periods of intense inflammation, to low grade illness, and in some cases to remission. Broadly speaking, these periods can be divided into three.

1. The acute flare up, where inflammation is intense. This corresponds to toxic heat or fire. Intense heat quickly damages yin and fluids, and congeals blood, and so must be cleared with priority, with minimal regard to the origin of the heat. The representative formula given here (for hu huo disease, Long Dan

Figure 10.3 The sources of heat in chronic inflammatory diseases

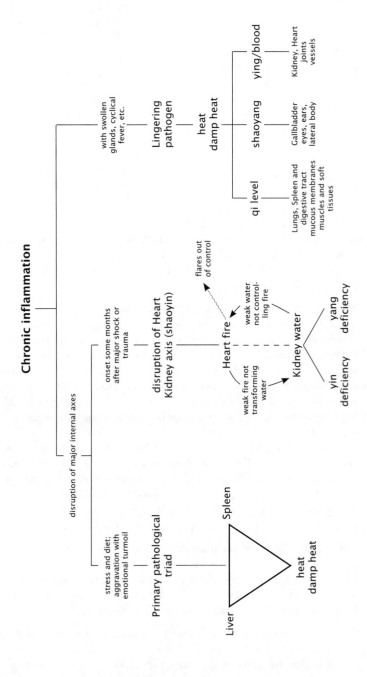

Xie Gan Tang) specifically clears fire and toxic heat from the Liver and Spleen. Depending on the precise location of the inflammation, other formulae could be selected to quickly cleat heat (Huang Lian Jie Di Tang, Qing Wen Bai Du Tang, Gan Lu Xiao Du Yin are examples). This phase of treatment should not last longer than several weeks.

2. The low grade illness, where inflammation is still obvious, but muted or manageable. This corresponds to heat or damp heat affecting various organ systems, or heat or damp heat located in the qi, shaoyang, ying or blood levels, and is the most prolonged phase. This phase is the one in which the underlying cause of the heat can be most efficiently addressed. In the case of hu huo disease, this is achieved by Gan Cao Xie Xin Tang (or other suitable harmonizing formula, depending on precisely where the patients symptom pattern falls on the map in Fig. 10.2, p.477.

3. The late stage where the damage done by the inflammatory process becomes more prominent than the inflammation. In Chinese medicine terms, this is when pathology such as yin or yang deficiency, Spleen deficiency and blood stasis come to the fore. At this stage, the heat has usually diminished, and repairing the damage and any remaining underlying vulnerability, is the priority of treatment.

Table 10.2 Comparison of features of some chronic inflammatory diseases. Main features are in bold.

Behcets disease (hu huo)	Systemic Lupus Erythematosus	Rheumatoid arthritis	Ulcerative colitis
wide spread ulceration	mouth ulcers		**ulcers in the large intestine**
arthritis (knees, non destructive)	**arthritis** (hands and feet, non destructive)	**arthritis (symmetrical, destructive)**	may be arthritis
inflammation of the eyes	inflammation of the eyes	inflammation of the eyes	inflammation of the eyes
vasculitis, erythema nodosum	**rashes, vasculitis, photosensitivity**	vasculitis	erythema nodosum
fever, malaise, fatigue, weight loss	fever, malaise, fatigue, weight loss	fever, malaise, fatigue, weight loss	fever, malaise, fatigue, weight loss
anorexia, diarrhea	abdominal pain	anorexia	**frequent bloody diarrhea**, tenesmus, anorexia
	lymphadenopathy	lymphadenopathy	
PPT the common etiology	Lingering pathogen a common etiology	Lingering pathogen a common etiology	PPT the common etiology

肝脾毒热 10.1 TOXIC HEAT IN THE LIVER AND SPLEEN

Toxic heat is seen in the early stages of hu huo disease, or during a flare–up of a chronic pattern. This pattern is in fact a mixture of toxic heat and damp heat. Damp heat becomes toxic when highly concentrated and destructive. The toxic heat is seen in tissue damage, ulceration, suppuration and pain; the damp heat in the systemic nature of the heat, inflammatory exudate and red swollen joints.

Clinical features
- Painful ulceration and suppuration of the mouth, throat and/or external genitals and anus. The lesions are red with raised margins and may exude pus.
- painful, red, burning eyes, severe photophobia
- low grade fever (occasionally high) that tends to be worse in the afternoon and evening; night sweats
- joint pain and stiffness, warm swollen joints, usually knees, but other joints may be affected
- erythematous nodules on the lower limbs
- vasculitis, painful congested veins on the legs
- general malaise – aversion to food, nausea, desire to sleep
- concentrated urine
- dry stools, constipation or sluggish stools
- thick, yellow, malodorous leucorrhea

T red with a thick, greasy, yellow coat
P slippery and rapid

Treatment principle
Clear toxic heat and damp heat from the Liver and Spleen

Prescription

LONG DAN XIE GAN TANG 龙胆泻肝汤
Gentian Decoction to Purge the Liver, plus
XIE HUANG SAN 泻黄散
Drain the Yellow Powder, modified

jiu long dan cao (wine fried Gentianae Radix) 酒龙胆草	3–9g
huang qin (Scutellariae Radix) 黄芩	6–12g
shan zhi zi (Gardeniae Fructus) 山栀子	6–12g
ze xie (Alismatis Rhizoma) 泽泻	6–12g
mu tong (Akebiae Caulis) 木通	3–6g
che qian zi (Plantaginis Semen) 车前子	9–15g
sheng di (Rehmanniae Radix) 生地	9–15g
chai hu (Bupleuri Radix) 柴胡	3–6g
gan cao (Glycyrrhizae Radix) 甘草	15–30g
shi gao (Gypsum fibrosum) 石膏	15–30g
huo xiang (Pogostemonis Herba) 藿香	9–15g
fang feng (Saposhnikoviae Radix) 防风	9–12g
huang lian (Coptidis Rhizoma) 黄连	3–6g

pei lan (Eupatorii Herba) 佩兰 9–12g
Method: Decoction. **Shi gao** is cooked for 30 minutes prior to the other herbs. **Jiu long dan cao**, **shan zhi zi**, **huang lian**, **huang qin** and **shi gao** clear heat and damp heat from both the Liver and Spleen; **chai hu** and **fang feng** disperse constrained heat in the Liver and Spleen; **che qian zi**, **mu tong** and **ze xie** promote urination to drain dampness and heat; **sheng di** cools the blood and protects yin; **huo xiang** and **pei lan** fragrantly dissipate dampness; **gan cao** clear heat and toxin. (Source: *Shi Yong Zhong Yi Nei Ke Xue* [*Yi Fang Jin Jie* / *Xiao Er Yao Zheng Zhi Jue*).

Modifications

- With severe heat and inflammation, add two or three of the following herbs: **pu gong ying** (Taraxaci Herba) 蒲公英 18–30g, **jin yin hua** (Lonicerae Flos) 金银花 15–30g, **xuan shen** (Scrophulariae Radix) 玄参 12–15g, **ban lan gen** (Isatidis/Baphicacanthis Radix) 板蓝根 15–24g and **bai hua she she cao** (Hedyotis diffusae Herba) 白花蛇舌草 18–30g, or consider Dang Gui Long Hui Wan (Tangkuei, Gentian and Aloe Pill 当归龙会丸, p.117) as guiding prescription.
- With very painful, red eyes, add **jue ming zi** (Cassiae Semen) 决明子 9–12g.
- With painful genital ulcerations and sores, add **tu fu ling** (Smilacis glabrae Rhizoma) 土茯苓 15–30g.
- With painful, red or nodular skin lesions and vasculitis, add **mu dan pi** (Moutan Cortex) 牡丹皮 9–12g and **chi shao** (Paeoniae Radix rubra) 赤芍 9–12g.
- With joint pain, add **qin jiao** (Gentianae macrophyllae Radix) 秦艽 9–15g, **ren dong teng** (Lonicerae Caulis) 忍冬藤 15–30g and **tou gu cao** (Herba Speranskia) 透骨草 12–15g.
- With constipation, add **da huang** (Rhei Radix et Rhizoma) 大黄 6–9g, or consider Dang Gui Long Hui Wan (Tangkuei, Gentian and Aloe Pill 当归龙会丸, p.117) as guiding prescription..

Variations and additional prescriptions

With severe joint pain

When joint pains are severe, with swelling, heat and stiffness, the treatment should focus on unblocking yang, activating qi and blood, dispelling wind and eliminating damp with a formula such as Gui Zhi Shao Yao Zhi Mu Tang (Cinnamon Twig, Peony and Anemarrhena Decoction 桂枝芍药知母汤 p.659).

With concerns about yin damage

The primary prescription is excellent for clearing toxic heat and fire from the Liver and Spleen. However, the intense bitterness of the main herbs can damage yin and Spleen yang in some patients. This is more likely in patients with underlying yin deficiency or Spleen weakness, in older people, and in those experiencing a flare up of a recurrent problem. A milder, yet still powerful alternative in such cases is Qing Xin Tang (Cool the Heart Decoction 清心汤).

jin yin hua (Lonicerae Flos) 金银花 60g
gan cao (Glycyrrhizae Radix) 甘草 30g
xuan shen (Scrophulariae Radix) 玄参 15g
ban lan gen (Isatidis/Baphicacanthis Radix) 板蓝根 15g
mu dan pi (Moutan Cortex) 牡丹皮 4.5g
chi fu ling (Poria Rubra) 赤茯苓 15g

shi chang pu (Acori tatarinowii Rhizoma) 石菖蒲 3g
Method: Decoction. **Jin yin hua** clears toxic heat without drying or damaging yin; **gan cao** alleviates toxicity and supports the Spleen; **xuan shen** and **mu dan pi** cool the blood; **xuan shen** also nourishes yin; **ban lan gen** clears toxic heat; **chi fu ling** promotes urination to clear heat; **shi chang pu** guides the formula to the Heart. (Source: *Zhong Yi Zhi Liao Nin Nan Za Bing Mi Yao* [*Jing Yan Fang*]).

External wash (for genitals)

KU SHEN TANG 苦参汤
Sophora Decoction

These herbs are used for the itch and inflammation of genital ulcers.
ku shen (Sophorae flavescentis Radix) 苦参 30g
she chuang zi (Cnidii Fructus) 蛇床子 12g
Method: Boil the herbs in three liters of water for 20 minutes and strain off the dregs. The remaining liquid can be used as a sitzbath or applied with a cloth. (Source: *Zhong Yi Zhi Liao Nin Nan Za Bing Mi Yao*)

Prepared medicines
Concentrated powders
Long Dan Xie Gan Tang (Gentiana Combination) plus Xie Huang San (Siler & Licorice Formula)

Pills
Long Dan Xie Gan Wan (Snake and Dragon Teapill)
San Jin Xi Gua Shuang (Watermelon Frost)
Shuang Liao Hou Feng San (Superior Sore Throat Powder)
 – the latter two topically for painful mouth ulcers
Ling Zhi (Reishi Mushroom)

Acupuncture (select from)
Ren.12 (zhongwan –) ....clears heat from the Spleen and Stomach
LI.11 (quchi –) ....clear heat from yangming and have a beneficial effect
LI.4 (hegu –)   on the mouth and eyes
St.44 (neiting –)
Sp.9 (yinlingquan –) ....water and metal points of the Spleen, these points
Sp.5 (shangqiu –)   cool fire and promote urination to clear damp heat
Liv.2 (xingjian –) ....fire point of the Liver, drains fire and clears damp heat
GB.34 (yanglingquan –)......sea point of the Gallbladder, regulates qi, clears damp heat and calms hyperactive Liver yang
• with eye pain and blurring vision, add GB.41 (zulinqi) and SJ.3 (zhongzhu –)
• with severe genital ulceration, add Liv.5 (ligou –)
• with painful mouth ulcers, add PC.8 (laogong –), Ren.24 (chengjiang), St.6 (jiache) or St.4 (dicang)
• with nausea, add PC.6 (neiguan)
• with constipation, add St.25 (tianshu –) and St.37 (shangjuxu –)
• with diarrhea, add zhixie (N–CA–3) and Bl.25 (tianshu)
• Ear points: mouth, liver, spleen, zero point, sympathetic, shenmen

Clinical notes

• The large number of bitter cold herbs is aimed at quickly reducing the heat, and should not be used for too long to avoid iatrogenic damage to Spleen yang qi and yin. Once the obvious inflammation has settled and the ulcers are less painful and beginning to heal, the treatment strategy should adopt a more harmonizing approach, to balance the Liver and Spleen and correct the underlying pathological triad.

• A cooling diet is recommended. See Clinical Handbook, Vol. 2, p.882.

湿
重
于
热

10.2 DAMP HEAT

This is the classic presentation of hu huo disease, with the inflammatory stage calming down and sticky dampness the predominant feature. The damp heat is concentrated in the Liver and Spleen, and there will be some degree of Spleen qi deficiency and Liver qi constraint. The latter is seen in the relationship between increasing stress levels and the aggravation or onset of symptoms.

Clinical features

- Ulceration of the mouth and throat, external genitals and anus. The lesions are moderately painful, slightly red, moist or crusting. The gums may be swollen and painful.
- sore, irritated eyes, visual blurring, photophobia
- low grade afternoon fever, contained fever (see p.367); occasional night sweats
- erythematous nodules on the lower limbs
- vasculitis, painful congested veins on the legs
- joint pain and swelling, especially knees
- anorexia, nausea and vomiting; epigastric distension and discomfort
- fatigue, weakness, but restlessness and difficulty sleeping
- diarrhea or sluggish stools

T slightly red, with a greasy, white or yellow coat
P soggy or soft and slightly rapid

Treatment principle

Clear damp heat from the Liver and Spleen
Harmonize the middle burner

Prescription

GAN CAO XIE XIN TANG 甘草泻心汤
Licorice Decoction to Drain the Epigastrium

---

gan cao (Glycyrrhizae Radix) 甘草 30g
huang qin (Scutellariae Radix) 黄芩 9–12g
huang lian (Coptidis Rhizoma) 黄连 3–6g
zhi ban xia (Pinelliae Rhizoma preparata) 制半夏 6–9g
gan jiang (Zingiberis Rhizoma) 干姜 3–6g
ren shen (Ginseng Radix) 人参 6–9g
da zao (Jujubae Fructus) 大枣 .... 4 fruit

Method: Decoction. **Gan cao** clears heat, alleviates toxin and strengthens the Spleen; **huang qin** and **huang lian** clear damp heat from the upper burner, Stomach and Heart; **zhi ban xia** transforms phlegm; **ren shen** supplements qi and strengthens the Spleen; the ascending pungent heat of **gan jiang** protects the Stomach and combines with the bitter cold descent of **huang qin** and **huang lian** to activate the qi dynamic; **da zao** protects the Stomach. (Source: *Zhong Yi Zhi Liao Yi Nan Za Bing Mi Yao* [*Jin Gui Yao Lüe*])

Modifications

- With painful, red eyes, add **jue ming zi** (Cassiae Semen) 决明子 9–12g.
- With painful genital ulcerations and sores, add **tu fu ling** (Smilacis glabrae

Rhizoma) 土茯苓 15–30g.
- With painful, red or nodular skin lesions and vasculitis, add **mu dan pi** (Moutan Cortex) 牡丹皮 9–12g and **chi shao** (Paeoniae Radix rubra) 赤芍 9–12g.
- With joint pain, add **qin jiao** (Gentianae macrophyllae Radix) 秦艽 9–15g, **ren dong teng** (Lonicerae Caulis) 忍冬藤 15–30g and **cang zhu** (Atractylodis Rhizoma) 苍术 12–15g.
- With constipation, add **da huang** (Rhei Radix et Rhizoma) 大黄 6–9g.

External wash (for genitals)
See Ku Shen Tang p.484.

Prepared medicines
Concentrated powders
Gan Cao Xie Xin Tang (Pinellia & Licorice Combination)

Pills
Tong Xuan Li Fei Pian (Tung Hsuan Li Fei Pien)
San Jin Xi Gua Shuang (Watermelon Frost)
Shuang Liao Hou Feng San (Superior Sore Throat Powder)
 – the latter two topically for painful mouth ulcers
Ling Zhi (Reishi Mushroom)

Acupuncture (select from)
Ren.12 (zhongwan –) ....clears damp heat from the Spleen and Stomach
Sp.9 (yinlingquan –)...........water and metal points of the Spleen, these points
Sp.5 (shangqiu –)   cool fire and promote urination to clear damp heat
LI.11 (quchi –)...................clear heat from yangming and have a beneficial effect
LI.4 (hegu –)   on the mouth and eyes
St.44 (neiting –)
- with eye pain and blurring vision, add GB.41 (zulinqi) and SJ.3 (zhongzhu –)
- with genital ulceration, add Liv.5 (ligou –)
- with painful mouth ulcers, add PC.8 (laogong –), Ren.24 (chengjiang), St.6 (jiache) or St.4 (dicang)
- with nausea, add PC.6 (neiguan)
- with constipation, add St.25 (tianshu –) and St.37 (shangjuxu –)
- with diarrhea, add zhixie (N–CA–3) and Bl.25 (tianshu)
- Ear points: mouth, liver, spleen, zero point, sympathetic, shenmen

Clinical notes
- This is the classic harmonizing approach advocated by Zhang Zhong–Jing. The prescription can also be helpful, in between flare ups, to balance the pathological triad, in which case a reduced dose of **gan cao** is used. See note on p.475.
- A damp heat clearing diet is recommended. See Clinical Handbook, Vol. 2, p.884.

脾
虚
来
湿

10.3 SPLEEN DEFICIENCY WITH DAMP

This pattern is seen in patients with a constitutional tendency to yang qi deficiency, and during the remission phase of the heat patterns. It can also be the result of excessive heat clearing during the acute phase.

Clinical features
- Chronic non–healing ulceration of the mouth, genitals, anus. The ulcers are pale pink and flat or indented, and not especially painful.
- blurring vision, irritated eyes
- fatigue, lethargy, weakness
- heavy aching legs, nodular rash, painful congested veins
- aching, slightly swollen joints, especially knees
- poor appetite or anorexia; abdominal distension; diarrhea
- pale complexion, may be puffy around the eyes
- heavy, foggy head

T pale, swollen and scalloped with a thin, white or greasy coat
P deep, fine, or wiry

Treatment principle
Strengthen the Spleen and supplement qi
Raise yang qi and eliminate dampness

Prescription

BU ZHONG YI QI TANG 补中益气汤
Supplement the Middle to Augment the Qi Decoction, modified

huang qi (Astragali Radix) 黄芪	12–18g
ren shen (Ginseng Radix) 人参	6–9g
bai zhu (Atractylodes macrocephalae Rhizoma) 白术	9–12g
dang gui (Angelicae sinensis Radix) 当归	6–9g
chen pi (Citri reticulatae Pericarpium) 陈皮	6–9g
gan cao (Glycyrrhizae Radix) 甘草	9–12g
zhi gan cao (Glycyrrhizae Radix preparata) 炙甘草	9–12g
sheng ma (Cimicifugae Rhizoma) 升麻	3–6g
chai hu (Bupleuri Radix) 柴胡	3–6g

Method: Decoction. **Huang qi**, **ren shen** and **bai zhu** strengthen the Spleen and supplement qi; **huang qi** supplements and fortifies wei qi and elevates yang; **chai hu** and **sheng ma** elevate yang qi; **dang gui** supplements blood; **chen pi** and **zhi gan cao** regulate qi and harmonize the middle burner; the large dose of raw **gan cao** alleviates toxin. (Source: *Zhong Yi Nei Ke Xue* [*Pi Wei Lun*])

Modifications
- With pronounced damp, weeping or crusting lesions, aching joints and thick tongue coat, add **yi ren** (Coicis Semen) 苡仁 15–30g, **fu ling** (Poria) 茯苓 9–12g and **cang zhu** (Atractylodis Rhizoma) 苍术 9–15g.
- With food stagnation, abdominal distension and pain, bad breath and foul stools, add **ji nei jin** (Gigeriae galli Endothelium corneum) 鸡内金 3–6g [as powder added to the strained decoction], **mai ya** (Hordei Fructus germinan-

tus) 麦芽 15–30g and **gu ya** (Setariae Fructus germinatus) 谷芽 15–30g.
• For ulcers that refuse to heal, add **mu hu die** (Oroxyli Semen) 木蝴蝶 6–9g.

External wash (for genitals)
See She Chuang Zi Tang, p.497.

Prepared medicines
Concentrated powders
Bu Zhong Yi Qi Tang (Ginseng & Astragalus Combination)
Xiang Sha Liu Jun Zi Tang (Vladmiria & Amomum Combination)
– with more damp

Pills
Bu Zhong Yi Qi Wan (Central Chi Teapills)
San Jin Xi Gua Shuang (Watermelon Frost)
Shuang Liao Hou Feng San (Superior Sore Throat Powder)
– the latter two topically for painful mouth ulcers
Ling Zhi (Reishi Mushroom)

Acupuncture (select from)
Ren.12 (zhongwan) ....alarm point of the Stomach, fortifies Stomach and
Spleen function to assist in transforming phlegm
St.36 (zusanli +) ....sea point of the Stomach, strengthens the Spleen
and Stomach, supplements qi and activates the qi
dynamic
Sp.9 (yinlingquan –)...........sea point of the Spleen, promotes urination to
drain damp; also good for pain and swelling in the
external genitals
Sp.6 (sanyinjiao +)..............strengthens the Spleen, supplements qi and assists
Sp.9 in draining damp
Bl.20 (pishu +▲) ....transport point of the Spleen, strengthens the Spleen
and supplements qi
• with abdominal distension, add Sp.3 (taibai –) and St.25 (tianshu –)
• with muscle heaviness, add Sp.21 (dabao)
• with blurred vision, add St.8 (touwei), Bl.2 (zanzhu) and GB.37 (guanming)
• with foggy head, add Bl.62 (shenmai)
• Ear points: mouth, lung, spleen, adrenal, sympathetic, point zero, shenmen

Clinical notes
• Treatment will be more prolonged than those employed on the previous patterns, so the issue of large doses of **gan cao** may become relevant. See treatment
on p.475.
• A diet to strengthen the Spleen and qi is recommended. See Clinical Handbook, Vol. 2, p.870.

阴
虚
内
热

10.4 YIN DEFICIENCY

Yin deficiency is a mid to late stage pattern seen in chronic hu huo disease, and in older patients with hu huo disease. There will be varying grades of heat created by the deficiency. Yin deficiency is usually a progression from a toxic heat or damp heat pattern, but may be the result of excessive or prolonged use of bitter cold medicines or high doses of corticosteroids in the acute phase.

Clinical features
• Ulceration of the mouth, throat, genitals and anus. The lesions are dark red and moderately painful.
• sore, dry, scratchy eyes, photophobia, blurring or weakening vision
• low grade fever rising in the afternoon or evening; night sweats; heat in the palms and soles
• pale face with red cheeks, malar flush
• lower back ache and weakness, knee pain
• irritability, restlessness, insomnia
• tiredness and fatigue with an inability to rest
• dizziness and tinnitus
• dry stools or constipation; concentrated urine
T red and dry with little or no coat, or a mirror tongue
P wiry, fine, rapid

Treatment principle
Nourish and supplement Liver and Kidney yin, clear deficiency heat

Prescription

QI JU DI HUANG WAN 杞菊地黄丸
Lycium Fruit, Chrysanthemum and Rehmannia, plus
ZENG YE TANG 增液汤
Increase the Fluids Decoction, modified

sheng di (Rehmanniae Radix preparata) 生地 12–18g
shu di (Rehmanniae Radix preparata) 熟地 12–18g
shan zhu yu (Corni Fructus) 山茱萸 9–12g
shan yao (Dioscoreae Rhizoma) 山药 9–12g
mu dan pi (Moutan Cortex) 牡丹皮 9–12g
fu ling (Poria) 茯苓 9–12g
ze xie (Alismatis Rhizoma) 泽泻 9–12g
gou qi zi (Lycii Fructus) 枸杞子 9–15g
xuan shen (Scrophulariae Radix) 玄参 15–24g
mai dong (Ophiopogonis Radix) 麦冬 9–12g
gan cao (Glycyrrhizae Radix) 甘草 12–15g

Method: Decoction or powder. **Sheng di**, **shu di**, **xuan shen**, **gou qi zi** and **shan zhu yu**, nourish Liver and Kidney yin; **mai dong**, **xuan shen** and **sheng di** moisten dryness, clear heat and nourish yin; **mu dan pi**, **fu ling** and **ze xie** regulate blood and drain damp without damaging yin; **gan cao** and **xuan shen** alleviates toxin and eases ulceration. (Source: *Zhong Yi Nei Ke Shou Ce* [*Ma Zhen Quan Shu* / *Wen Bing Tiao Bian*]).

Modifications

- With painful ulcerations, add **lian qiao** (Forsythiae Fructus) 连翘 9–12g and **jin yin hua** (Lonicerae Flos) 金银花 15–30g.
- With joint pain, add **qin jiao** (Gentianae macrophyllae Radix) 秦艽 9–15g, **ren dong teng** (Lonicerae Caulis) 忍冬藤 30g and **hai feng teng** (Piperis kadsurae Caulis) 海风藤 9–12g.
- With very dry, sore eyes and photophobia, add **chong wei zi** (Leonuri Fructus) 茺蔚子 9–12g.
- With nodular or purple skin lesions, add **dan shen** (Salviae miltiorrhizae Radix) 丹参 9–12g and **ji xue teng** (Spatholobi Caulis) 鸡血藤 15–30g.
- With relatively severe deficient heat, add **di gu pi** (Lycii Cortex) 地骨皮 12–15g, or **zhi mu** (Anemarrhenae Rhizoma) 知母 9–12g and **huang bai** (Phellodendri Cortex) 黄柏 9–12g, or combine with Dᴀ Bᴜ Yɪɴ Wᴀɴ (Great Supplement the Yin Pill 大补阴丸, p.914).
- With fever or bone steaming, add **qing hao** (Artemisiae annuae Herba) 青蒿 9–15g.
- With severe dry mouth and irritability, combine with Zʜᴜ Yᴇ Sʜɪ Gᴀᴏ Tᴀɴɢ (Lophatherus and Gypsum Decoction 竹叶石膏汤, p.370).
- With dampness and weeping genital lesions, add **tu fu ling** (Smilacis glabrae Rhizoma) 土茯苓 12–15g, **yi ren** (Coicis Semen) 苡仁 15–30g and **bi xie** (Dioscoreae hypoglaucae Rhizoma) 萆薢 9–12g.
- With poor appetite, add **chen pi** (Citri reticulatae Pericarpium) 陈皮 6–9g and **shan zha** (Crataegi Fructus) 山楂 12–15g.
- With insomnia, add **suan zao ren** (Ziziphi spinosae Semen) 酸枣仁 12–15g and **ye jiao teng** (Polygoni multiflori Caulis) 夜胶藤 15–30g.
- With concentrated urine, add **huai niu xi** (Achyranthis bidentatae Radix) 怀牛膝 9–12g and **che qian zi** (Plantaginis Semen) 车前子 9–12g [decocted in a cloth bag].

External wash (for genitals)

See Ku Shen Tang p.484.

Prepared medicines

Concentrated powders

Qi Ju Di Huang Wan (Lycium, Chrysanthemum & Rehamannia Formula) plus Yi Guan Jian (Linking Combination) and Er Zhi Wan (Ligustrum & Eclipta Combination)

Zhi Bai Di Huang Wan (Anemarrhena, Phellodendron & Rehmannia Formula)

Pills

Qi Ju Di Huang Wan (Lycium–Rehmannia Pills) plus Yi Guan Jian Wan (Linking Decoction Teapills)

Zhi Bai Ba Wei Wan (Eight Flavor Rehmannia Teapills)

San Jin Xi Gua Shuang (Watermelon Frost)

Shuang Liao Hou Feng San (Superior Sore Throat Powder)
 – the latter two used topically for painful mouth ulcers

Ling Zhi (Reishi Mushroom)

Acupuncture (select from)

Ren.4 (guanyuan +)............these points supplement Kidney yin and yuan qi and
Ren.6 (qihai +)   influence the genital region
Kid.3 (taixi +).....................source point of the Kidneys, nourishes Kidney yin
Liv.3 (taichong +)...............source point of the Liver, supplements Liver yin and
                             blood
Lu.7 (lieque).....................master and couple points of renmai, these points
Kid.6 (zhaohai)   open up circulation of renmai qi, nourish Kidney
                             yin
Sp.6 (sanyinjiao)................nourishes Kidney, Liver and Spleen yin
Bl.23 (shenshu +)..............transport point of the Kidneys, nourishes Kidney yin
Bl.52 (zhishi +)..................supplements the Kidneys
- for painful mouth ulcers, add Ren.24 (chengjiang), St.6 (jiache) or St.4 (dicang)
- with genital ulceration, add Liv.5 (ligou –)
- with blurred or weakening vision, sore eyes or cataracts, add GB.37 (guan-ming) and SI.6 (yanglao)
- with dizziness or vertigo, add GB.20 (fengchi–) and Du.20 (baihui)
- with painful nodules, add Bl.40 (weizhong –) and Du.10 (lingtai –)
- With joint pains, add LI.11 (quchi –) and St.36 (zusanli +)
- With fever, add Kid.2 (rangu –)
- Ear points: mouth, liver, kidney, sympathetic, shenmen

Clinical notes
- See note on p.475 regarding large doses of **gan cao**.
- Yin can be replenished, but the course of treatment is likely to be long. The most distressing symptoms can be relieved to some extent after some weeks, but 6–12 months of treatment, or even longer, will usually be required for a sustained result.
- A yin nourishing diet is recommended. See Clinical Handbook, Vol. 2, p.876.

气
血
瘀
滞

10.5 QI AND BLOOD STAGNATION

This is a late stage pattern, where the heat has congealed blood. There may be some residual heat, but the heat may have dissipated by the time blood stasis is the primary pathology. Blood stasis will usually be complicated by secondary pathology, such as yin or yang qi deficiency, and/or blood deficiency.

Clinical features

- Chronic non–healing ulcerations of the mouth, throat and external genitals. The ulcers may be painful, have a dark margin and coalesce into larger lesions with a mottled or purple base. The gums may be purple or mottled and receding.
- pale, darkish or mottled complexion; purple lips
- painful, purple or brown congested veins and nodular skin lesions on the legs
- purpura, or purple or brown discoloration of the skin
- weak blurring vision; dark rings around the eyes
- abdominal or chest pain
- left iliac fossa pressure pain (p.925–926)
- stiff, painful joints
- may be rectal or urinary bleeding

T purple or mauve or with purple or brown patches or stasis spots; congested sublingual veins

P choppy, fine, wiry

Treatment principle

Activate blood and dispel blood stasis
Dredge the Liver and regulate qi

Prescription

XUE FU ZHU YU TANG 血府逐瘀汤
Drive Out Stasis in the Mansion of Blood Decoction, modified

tao ren (Persicae Semen) 桃仁	9–12g
hong hua (Carthami Flos) 红花	6–9g
dang gui (Angelicae sinensis Radix) 当归	9–12g
sheng di (Rehmanniae Radix) 生地	9–12g
chi shao (Paeoniae Radix rubra) 赤芍	6–9g
chuan xiong (Chuanxiong Rhizoma) 川芎	6–9g
chai hu (Radix Bupleuri) 柴胡	6–9g
zhi ke (Aurantii Fructus) 枳壳	6–9g
gan cao (Glycyrrhizae Radix) 甘草	12–15g
chuan niu xi (Cyathulae Radix) 川牛膝	9–12g
jie geng (Platycodi Radix) 桔梗	3–6g

Method: Decoction. **Dang gui, sheng di, chuan xiong, chi shao, tao ren** and **hong hua** nourish and activate blood; **chai hu, zhi ke** and **chi shao** dredge the Liver and regulate qi; **jie geng** frees qi in the chest and diaphragm, and raises qi; **chuan niu xi** leads blood downwards–together, the last two herbs seek to re–establish the correct elevation and descent of qi and blood; the large dose of **gan cao** alleviates toxin and protects the Stomach. (Source: *Yi Lin Gai Cuo*)

Modifications

- With joint pain, add **qin jiao** (Gentianae macrophyllae Radix) 秦艽 9–15g, **ren dong teng** (Lonicerae Caulis) 忍冬藤 15–30g and **tou gu cao** (Herba Speranskia) 透骨草 12–15g.
- With declining vision or irritated eyes, add **gou qi zi** (Lycii Fructus) 枸杞子 9–12g and **nu zhen zi** (Ligustri Fructus) 女贞子 9–12g.
- With focal headache or migraine, increase the dose of **chuan xiong** up to 24g.
- With colicky or spasmodic abdominal pain, **bai shao** (Paeoniae Radix alba) 白芍 can be used instead of **chi shao**.
- With masses in the upper abdomen, add **dan shen** (Salviae miltiorrhizae Radix) 丹参 9–12g, **yu jin** (Curcumae Radix) 郁金 9–12g, **san leng** (Sparganii Rhizoma) 三棱 6–9g and **e zhu** (Curcumae Rhizoma) 莪术 6–9g.
- With depression, add **he huan pi** (Albizziae Cortex) 合欢皮 12–15g.
- With severe insomnia, add **he huan pi** (Albizziae Cortex) 合欢皮 12–15g and **ye jiao teng** (Polygoni multiflori Caulis) 夜交藤 15–30g.
- With qi deficiency and for very weak patients, add **huang qi** (Astragali Radix) 黄芪 12–15g and **ren shen** (Ginseng Radix) 人参 6–9g.
- With yang deficiency, add **zhi fu zi** (Aconiti Radix lateralis preparata) 制附子 6–12g.
- With yin deficiency, add **bie jia** (Trionycis Carapax) 鳖甲 9–12g.
- With bleeding, purpura or bruising, add **san qi fen** (powdered Notoginseng Radix) 三七粉 3–6g [added to the strained decoction].
- With significant blood deficiency, replace **sheng di** with **shu di** (Rehmanniae Radix preparata) 熟地.
- With marked qi and blood deficiency, pale tongue with stasis spots and dizziness, combine with Ba Zhen Tang (Eight Treasure Decoction 八珍汤, p.275).

External wash (for genitals)

Boil **da huang** (Rhei Radix et Rhizoma) 大黄 15g and **bai ji** (Bletillae Rhizoma) 白芨 15g in 2 liters of water for 25 minutes and when cool, use the resulting liquid to wash the genital area. A paste made from finely powdered **ru xiang** (Olibanum) 乳香 and **mo yao** (Myrrha) 没药 mixed in vaseline or sorbolene can also be helpful.

Prepared medicines

Concentrated powders

Xue Fu Zhu Yu Tang (Persica & Carthamus Combination)
Ba Zhen Tang (Tangkuei & Ginseng Eight Combination)
  – add for qi and blood deficiency

Pills

Xue Fu Zhu Yu Wan (Stasis in the Mansion of Blood Teapills)
San Shen Jian Kang Wan (Sunho Multi Ginseng Tablets)
San Jin Xi Gua Shuang (Watermelon Frost)
Shuang Liao Hou Feng San (Superior Sore Throat Powder)
  – the latter two topically for painful mouth ulcers
Ling Zhi (Reishi Mushroom)

Acupuncture (select from)

LI.11 (quchi –)...................these points together have a special effect on blood
Sp.10 (xuehai –)   stasis in general, and on the mouth and genital
LI.4 (hegu –)   region
Sp.6 (sanyinjiao)
Liv.5 (ligou –)....................connecting point of the Liver, activates blood and
                         clears heat from the lower burner
Bl.15 (xinshu +) ....transport point of the Heart, strengthens the Heart
                         and stimulates circulation of qi and blood
Bl.17 (geshu –)..................transport point for the diaphragm, meeting point for
                         blood, dispels static blood
Bl.18 (ganshu –).................transport point of the Liver, dredges the Liver and
                         regulates qi, activates blood
Bl.20 (pishu –) ....transport point of the Spleen, promotes manufacture
                         of new blood and supplements qi
Liv.14 (qimen –) ....alarm point of the Liver, soothes the Liver and
                         regulates qi, dispels static blood
Liv.13 (zhangmen –) ....alarm point of the Spleen and meeting point of the
                         internal organs, strengthens the Spleen and pro-
                         motes Liver function

- Bleeding the congested vessels that may be found over the thoracic region, lower back and around the knee and ankle can be helpful. The veins are pierced with a surgical lancet and a few drops of blood extracted. Ideally the blood should run black at first, then fresh red. Those on the back can be cupped if the patient is strong enough. This technique can be performed weekly for a few sessions, then intermittently thereafter. See also p.929.
- with focal abdominal pain, add Sp.8 (diji –) and St.34 (liangqiu –)
- with spasmodic or cramping pain, add Du.8 (jinsuo –)
- for painful mouth ulcers, add Ren.24 (chengjiang), St.6 (jiache) or St.4 (dicang)
- with Spleen deficiency, add Ren.12 (zhongwan), St.36 (zusanli)
- Ear points: liver, heart, shenmen, adrenal, endocrine

Clinical notes

- See note on p.475 regarding large doses of **gan cao**.
- Prolonged treatment will usually be necessary to make significant impact in this pattern, although the most distressing symptoms can often be alleviated to some extent within some weeks. Treatment courses of 6–12 months are not uncommon. Be aware of the potential of strong blood activation to damage the zheng qi and blood, and watch for signs of increasing deficiency. A good rule of thumb is to break from the main prescription every few months, and use a qi and blood supplement for 2–3 weeks.
- A qi and blood mobilizing diet is recommended. See Clinical Handbook, Vol. 2, p.878 and 886.

脾
肾
两
虚

10.6 SPLEEN AND KIDNEY DEFICIENCY

This pattern is a mixture of yin and yang deficiency. Usually yang deficiency is prominent, but depending on the prevailing circumstances the pattern can oscillate between one or the other. The common way for a mixed pattern of yin and yang deficiency to present is with signs of heat in the upper body and cold below. Yin and yang deficiency is a common side effect of prolonged corticosteroid use.

Clinical features
- Chronic non–healing ulceration of the mouth and external genitals. The ulcers are pale, flat, not especially painful and may coalesce into a large ulcerated area. The ulcers may be aggravated or initiated by cold weather or changes of season.
- in warm weather heat in the palms and soles; in cooler weather cold extremities and cold intolerance
- flushed face, malar flush
- spontaneous sweating, mild night sweats or bone steaming fever
- slightly painful eyes with blurring or double vision
- abdominal pain, better for warmth
- aching, stiff joints
- lower back, knees and legs aching and weak
- edema of the ankles
- frequent urination or nocturia
- poor appetite, diarrhea

T pale or pink, swollen, dry and slightly scalloped
P deep, fine and weak

Treatment principle
Strengthen and supplement the Spleen and Kidneys
Support yin and yang and alleviate toxicity

Prescription

ER XIAN TANG 二仙汤
Two Immortal Decoction, modified

xian mao (Curculiginis Rhizoma) 仙茅	9–12g
xian ling pi (Epimedii Herba) 仙灵脾	12–15g
dang gui (Radix Angelicae Sinensis) 当归	9–12g
ba ji tian (Morindae officinalis Radix) 巴戟天	9–12g
huang bai (Phellodendri Cortex) 黄柏	9–12g
zhi mu (Anemarrhenae Rhizoma) 知母	9–12g
gan cao (Glycyrrhizae Radix) 甘草	9–15g
zhi gan cao (Glycyrrhizae Radix preparata) 炙甘草	9–15g
jiao bai zhu (baked Atractylodis macrocephalae Rhizoma) 焦白术	12–15g

Method: Decoction. **Xian mao** and **xian ling pi** warm Kidney yang and support jing; **ba ji tian** warms Kidney yang and strengthens the tendons and bones; **dang gui** nourishes and protects Blood and yin, softens the Liver, and, combined with **xian mao** and **xian ling pi**, regulates and supplements the chongmai and renmai; **zhi mu** and **huang bai** nourish Kidney yin, clear deficiency heat, and moderate the pungent hot dispersing nature of **xian mao** and **xian ling pi**; **gan cao** alleviates toxicity, and with **jiao bai zhu**, strengthens the Spleen. (Source: *Zhong Yi Zhi Liao Ning Nan Za Bing Mi Yao [Shanghai Shu Guang Yi Yuan Jing Yan Fang]*)

Modifications

- If the yang deficiency is predominant, combine with Jɪɴ Gᴜɪ Sʜᴇɴ Qɪ Wᴀɴ (Kidney Qi Pill from the Golden Cabinet 金匮肾气丸 p.826).
- If the yin deficiency is predominant, delete **xian mao** and add **sheng di** (Rehmanniae Radix) 生地 12–15g and **xuan shen** (Scrophulariae Radix) 玄参 9–12g.
- With weak vision or pain in the eyes, add **sha yuan ji li** (Astragali complanati Semen) 沙苑蒺藜 9–12g and **nu zhen zi** (Ligustri Fructus) 女贞子 9–12g.
- When edema is pronounced or there is hypertension, decrease the dose of **gan cao** and **zhi gan cao** by 50%.

External wash (for the genitals)

SHE CHUANG ZI TANG 蛇床子汤
Cnidium Fruit Decoction

she chuang zi (Cnidii Fructus) 蛇床子 15g
cang zhu (Atractylodis Rhizoma) 苍术 15g
Method: Boil the herbs in 2–3 liters of water for 20 minutes and strain off the dregs. When cool, wash the genital area or soak in a sitzbath. (Source: *Shi Yong Zhong Yao Xue*)

Prepared medicines

Concentrated powders
Er Xian Tang (Curculigo & Epimedium Combination)
Ba Wei Di Huang Wan (Rehmannia Eight Formula) plus Gan Cao Xie Xin Tang (Pinellia & Licorice Combination)

Pills
Er Xian Wan (Two Immortals Teapills)
San Jin Xi Gua Shuang (Watermelon Frost)
Shuang Liao Hou Feng San (Superior Sore Throat Powder)
  – the latter two topically for painful mouth ulcers
Ling Zhi (Reishi Mushroom)

Acupuncture (select from)

LI.11 (quchi)	these points clear heat from the upper body and
LI.4 (hegu)	stimulate the flow of yang qi through the yangming channels and mouth; moxa can be used when there is no heat
Ren.4 (guanyuan +▲)	these points warm Kidney and Spleen yang
Ren.6 (qihai +▲)	
Sp.6 (sanyinjiao)	strengthens the Spleen and Kidney, regulates qi and activates blood
Kid.3 (taixi –)	source point of the Kidneys, benefits yin and yang
St.36 (zusanli +▲)	sea point of the Stomach, strengthens the Spleen and Stomach and supplements qi, activates the qi dynamic

Bl.20 (pishu +▲) ....transport points of the Spleen and Kidney, these
Bl.23 (shenshu +▲)   points warm Spleen and Kidney yang
- with severe mouth ulcers, add Kid.9 (zhubin –), Ren.24 (chengjiang) and St.6 (jiache)
- with painful genital ulcers, add Liv.8 (ququan)
- with double vision, add Kid.7 (fuliu)
- with edema, add Kid.7 (fuliu) and Sp.9 (yinlingquan –)
- Ear points: mouth, spleen, kidney, heart, shenmen, adrenal, endocrine

Clinical notes

- The large dose of **gan cao**, see p.475, is more likely to cause problems in patients with Spleen and Kidney deficiency because of their propensity to fluid metabolism problems. A smaller dose than that recommended here may be better for patients with hypertension or significant edema.
- Yang qi can be restored, but the course of treatment will be lengthy. The most distressing symptoms can be relieved to some extent after some weeks, but 3–6 months of treatment, or even longer, will usually be required for a sustained result.
- A yang warming diet is recommended. See Clinical Handbook, Vol. 2, p.873.

Table 10.3 Summary of hu huo disease patterns

Pattern	Features	Prescription
Toxic heat affecting the Liver and Spleen	Ulceration and suppuration of the mouth and genitals, painful eyes, photo-phobia, fever, night sweats, nodules on the lower limbs, vasculitis, joint pain, malaise, concentrated urine, constipation, red tongue with a thick greasy yellow coat, slippery, rapid pulse	Long Dan Xie Gan Tang + Xie Huang San
Damp heat	Moderately painful ulceration of the mouth and genitals, sore eyes and blurring vision, low grade fever, nodules on the lower limbs, vasculitis, occasional night sweats, nausea and vomiting, anorexia, diarrhea, slightly red tongue with a greasy yellow coat, soggy or soft, slightly rapid pulse	Gan Cao Xie Xin Tang
Spleen qi deficiency with damp	Chronic non-healing ulceration of the mouth and genitals, blurring vision, fa-tigue, heavy aching legs; nodular rash; poor appetite, pale complexion, diarrhea, pale, swollen, scalloped tongue with a thin white coat, deep, fine, weak pulse	Bu Zhong Yi Qi Tang
Yin deficiency with heat	Ulceration of the mouth and genitals, dry sore eyes, blurring or weakening vi-sion, low grade fever, night sweats, heat in the palms and soles, malar flush, insomnia, fatigue and agitation, tinnitus, constipation, concentrated urine, lower back ache, red, dry tongue with little or no coat, fine rapid pulse	Qi Ju Di Huang Wan + Zeng Ye Tang
Qi and blood stagnation	Chronic non-healing ulcerations with dark margins and a mottled or purple base. Purple receding gums, purple lips, vascular congestion, nodular skin lesions, joint pain, purpura, purple or mauve tongue with stasis spots, choppy pulse	Xue Fu Zhu Yu Tang
Spleen and Kidney deficiency (yin and yang deficiency)	Chronic non-healing ulceration that are pale, flat, not especially painful and may coalesce into a large ulcerated area; flushed face, sweating, painful eyes with double vision, abdominal pain, aching joints, lower back and knee pain, edema, frequent urination or nocturia, pale or pink tongue, deep, weak pulse	Er Xian Tang

LINGERING PATHOGENS

Descriptions of lingering pathogens are scattered through some of the great classics of Chinese medicine, however a comprehensive framework for their analysis is lacking in modern clinical reference books. The approach taken in this chapter therefore departs somewhat from the concise and clearly summarized formats we have used for the rest of the diseases described in the Clinical Handbook series. In this chapter we describe a hybrid model for analyzing and understanding a common subset of lingering pathogen problems, based on our clinical experience. This subset of lingering pathogen pathology is defined by an objectively verifiable abnormal immune response, and a small group of specific identifying features (Box 11.3).

Lingering pathogens are pathogenic influences that remain in the body and provoke a persistent immune response

that produces characteristic signs and symptoms. Pathogenic influences in this context include living organisms (viruses, bacteria, fungi and parasites) as well as allergens, chemicals, drugs and environmental toxins.

Lingering pathogens manifest in a number of ways. An infection from the past may still be making its presence felt with recurrent symptoms (often arising when the patient is stressed or run down), or is perhaps detectable as persistent antibodies or other markers, in blood tests. Examples include glandular fever (Epstein Barr virus), cytomegalovirus, toxoplasmosis, brucellosis, aspergillus, malaria, viral hepatitis, and the active factors in immunizations. Some normal fauna, such as Candida albicans, can also manifest as a lingering pathogen if they are not maintained in a proper balance.

In clinic we often suspect a lingering pathogen when the patient presents with a history that begins 'I have never been well since...'. They are usually referring to an acute infection they suffered some time ago, and occasionally an immunization. Alternatively, the initial insult which has left the patient with chronic or recurrent symptoms may have been exposure to environmental toxins such as volatile gases, or fumes or heavy metals, or in some cases drugs or substances causing an allergic reaction.

500

> **BOX 11.2 BIOMEDICAL DISEASES THAT MAY BE ASSOCIATED WITH A LINGERING PATHOGEN (AS DEFINED IN THIS MODEL)**
>
> - chronic viral infections such as influenza, glandular fever, cytomegalovirus, hepatitis, HIV, Ross River fever and herpes
> - chronic bacterial, protozoal and fungal infections such as malaria, giardia, Lyme disease, toxoplasmosis, brucellosis, aspergillus and candida
> - chronic fatigue syndrome; post viral syndrome
> - reaction to immunization
> - allergies and food intolerance
> - reaction to environmental toxins and chemicals; post chemotherapy fever
> - chronic inflammatory and autoimmune diseases such as systemic lupus erythematosus, rheumatoid arthritis, ulcerative colitis, polymyositis, Graves disease and Hashimoto's thyroiditis

In some cases, the initial infection or injury is not recalled or apparent, however the pattern of recurrent symptoms fits the picture of a lingering pathogen and will be treated as such.

Historical background

The concept of a pathogen that can penetrate the body's defenses and then persist, causing chronic illness without necessarily killing the host is ancient, with roots stretching back to the Shang dynasty, some 4000 years ago. From the Han dynasty (206 BCE–220 CE), the reference to lurking pathogens from the Huang Di Nei Jing Su Wen[1] is well known:

Su Wen, Chapter 3

> *'If during spring one is affected by wind that is not expelled, it will attack the Spleen causing diarrhea, indigestion and food retention. If during the summer one is invaded by summerheat, malaria may occur in the autumn. During the autumn, if one is affected by dampness and the damp accumulates in the Lung it will cause cold and flaccid limbs, cough and emaciation. Cold invading in winter will incubate and manifest as a febrile disease in spring.....'*

In addition to this passage, there are references scattered throughout the classical literature to persistent pathogenic phenomena, including the gu worms of antiquity, sections of the Shang Han Lun and Wen Re Lun, and more recently Qing dynasty developments by Lei Feng[2] and Liu Bao–Yi[3].

Those that have generated the most interest in recent years, are gu toxins and lurking pathogens, because they resemble, in certain respects, some of the more difficult and intractable conditions encountered in modern clinical practice. Lurking pathogens (*fú xié* 伏邪, also known as hidden, deep lying or residual pathogenic factor), are characterized by a period of latency before onset of symptoms.

---

1 Translation by Maoshing Ni (1995)
2 Discussion of Seasonal Diseases (*Shi Bing Lun* 时病论)
3 Encountering the Source of Warm–Heat Pathogenic Diseases (*Wen Re Feng Yuan* 温热逢原)

This looks much like infectious conditions with an incubation period. The other attribute of a lurking pathogen is the sudden onset of a full blown internal pattern, with the characteristics of an external invasion, but without the classic progression from the surface through the various levels. The illness appears to spring directly from the interior. The timing of onset and emergence of the pathogen is variable, but often coincides with a change of season, a secondary external invasion, a build up of yang qi internally or ascendant yang that pushes the pathogen towards the surface.

Even older is the concept of gu toxin (or gu worms), from the Shang dynasty. The original connotation of gu was of a hidden evil, a form of black magic used by those in possession of gu, to kill and confuse their enemies. Gu toxins were thought responsible for many of the illnesses of the time, in which victims would fall ill and slowly expire. The character *gǔ* 蛊 (old character 蠱), reflects the idea of worms in a vessel, hinting at rottenness and decay, with the suggestion of the body being consumed from within. Over the centuries various antidotes were developed (herbal, mineral, ground up gu worms) and entire villages were turned over to their production.

Gradually, the malevolent worm spirit was replaced by a more rational world view, where the relationship between humans and the environment, rather than unseen spirits evolved. Medical texts began to describe a situation where the vessel of the human body was inhabited by parasites and influences from the environment. Ultimately the concept evolved into the understanding that gu involved the relationship between the body and one or more parasitic inhabitants.

While fascinating, these ideas lack detail and precision, and as a result are difficult to translate effectively into clinical practice. The offending pathogens are not clearly described, nor is their location. The necessary details to make a clear diagnosis are lacking and thus a precise treatment plan is difficult to formulate.

Even in China a formal framework for clearly understanding the many varieties of lingering pathogens has been lacking, prompting Liu Bao–Yi (1842–1901) to declare:

> 'Nowadays people all put Ye Tian–Shi [author of the Discussion of Warm–Heat Pathogen Disorders, Wen Re Lun] on a pedestal and just shelve the idea of a lurking pathogen and never mention it....W they run into a warm pathogen, no matter whether it is a sudden exposure or lurking, they simply use Ye's light cooling method and Yin Qiao or San Ju just flow off their brush.....there is no–one to put forward the theory of deep lying pathogens, they even see it as some weird theory. What a pity! It is such a common illness, especially in the South (of China). It is recorded in the Nei Jing, Nan Jing and Shang Han Lun, and thus not some weird theory'

11.1 HOW TO IDENTIFY A LINGERING PATHOGEN

There are a number of signs and symptoms that point to the presence of a lingering pathogen. Not all will be present in any particular individual, and their appearance can vary depending on any complicating pathology or deficiency, the duration of the condition, the age of the patient and any medications the patient may be taking.

> **BOX 11.3 KEY SIGNS OF A LINGERING PATHOGEN**
>
> - fever / abnormal heat in the body
> - abnormal sweating
> - dryness; damage to fluids
> - swollen lymph nodes &/or tonsils

A thorough physical examination is essential in the discovery of lingering pathogens, as signs like abnormal heat distribution or isolated sweating may be quite subtle and not obvious to the patient. The golden rule is that while patients are often unreliable witnesses, the body never lies. A physical examination, in the context of a lingering pathogen, requires systematic assessment of the neck for lymphadenopathy, observation of the tonsils for swelling, and palpation of the skin of the arms and hands, chest, head and feet for abnormal temperature sensations and moisture.

History

A positive history of infection or other event (immunization, chemotherapy) from which the patient has never completely recovered, or following which has been 'never well since' is the strongest indicator that a lingering pathogen is in situ. In such cases, the lingering pathogen may present as a persistent illness after the initial episode has passed, or as an 'echo' of the initial illness that appears from time to time, recurring in much the same fashion as the first episode, although generally less severe, and usually when the patient is run down or stressed.

The sudden onset of an uncharacteristic symptom, in the absence of any clear etiology, may also suggest a possible pathogenic influence. This is seen most commonly in middle aged people who suddenly develop an uncharacteristic problem, such as insomnia, headaches, asthma or allergies, with no identifiable changes in diet, habits, environment, routine or relationships to explain it. In such cases, a lingering pathogen should be part of the differential diagnosis.

Low grade fever and abnormal heat sensations

A fever is an abnormal elevation, or the perception of an elevation in body temperature, that may be either systemic or localized. The fever type most typical of a lingering pathogen is a low grade fever (p.367), but depending on the duration of the condition, the degree of dampness and any complicating deficiency, the heat sensation can vary considerably. Abnormal heat sensations in the body may also point to the possibility of a lingering pathogen, and these may be subjective or objective. When subjective, the patient feels hot or heat intolerant in one part of the body – the hands and feet, head or chest are common. The heat may be suggested by symptoms such as night sweats, flushing, light or inadequate dressing for the weather, or throwing the bedclothes off the feet at night. When objective, the patient is generally unaware of any heat, and it is detected by the practitioner during the course of the physical examination, usually as a region of the body (commonly the chest, upper back, upper abdomen, hands and feet or head) that is distinctly warmer than the surrounding area.

The more heat, or heat relative to damp, the more distinct the heat sensation or fever is likely to be. In cases with relatively little heat, with damp predominance or significant complicating deficiency, heat sensations may be muted or absent. In this case a 'contained fever' (p.367) may be detected. Low grade fevers are cyclical, appearing daily at specific times. Periods of fever may come and go, occurring for a few weeks, then abating for a variable time before beginning again. Low grade fevers are typical of qi level and ying and blood level pathogens.

A common variant is alternating fever and chills. These are characterized by distinct episodes of fever alternating with distinct chills, shivering, cold intolerance or goose bumps. In acute cases the fever and chill pattern is clear and unmistakable, but when prolonged and in patients with underlying deficiency, the fever and chill episodes can be muted to point that they may only appear sporadically when the patient is run down, and are then often described vaguely as 'flu like feelings' or 'getting hot and cold'. In some patterns, the fever and chills episodes may appear every few days for a few hours, or just in the afternoon. Alternating fever and chills are typical of shaoyang level pathogens.

Swollen lymph nodes and tonsils

Palpable lymph nodes in the neck are a common finding, and often the initial clue that points towards a lingering pathogen diagnosis. The nodes have a very specific feel. Lymph nodes suggestive of a lingering pathogen are non tender or slightly tender, well defined, round, soft or slightly rubbery and yielding. They feel just like small peas under the skin, and are able to be moved slightly over the subcutaneous tissues. Lymph node swelling can come and go during to course of a prolonged lingering pathogenic illness. The more swollen the glands are, the more tender they can be.

Careful and systematic palpation of the jawline and neck is necessary to detect swollen nodes, as they are spread over a relatively wide area and are easy to miss (Fig. 11.1). The discovery of a single positive node is sufficient to arouse suspicion. Be aware of false positives, such as tight or contracted bands in muscles, old scars, the edges of the hyoid bone and very hard fibrous nodes. Very hard and unyielding nodes may suggest malignancy or a 'shotty' node. A shotty node is so called because it feels hard and small like buckshot. These nodes have been damaged to such an extent that the lymphoid tissue has died and been replaced with fibrous scar tissue. Shotty nodes are constant, do not fluctuate in size, and are usually the remnants of an old lingering pathogen that has long since dissipated.

Chronically swollen tonsils are another important indicator, especially in children, and are obvious with oral examination. The tonsils are enlarged, but not red or inflamed. There is rarely any pain, but the enlarged tonsils may cause some irritation or difficulty swallowing. If the tonsils have been removed the back of the hard palate may appear duskier than normal.

Figure 11.1 Cervical lymph nodes

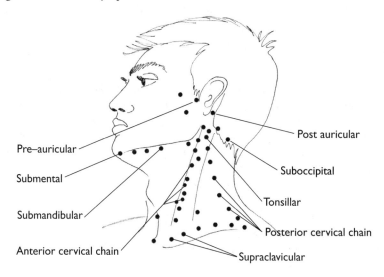

Pre–auricular

Submental

Submandibular

Anterior cervical chain

Post auricular

Suboccipital

Tonsillar

Posterior cervical chain

Supraclavicular

Abnormal sweating

Abnormal sweating is a common finding in patients with a lingering pathogen, and one that is easy to overlook. Troublesome, debilitating or embarrassing sweating (usually night sweats or sweaty palms) will be reported, but patients are often insensible to sweating, or it is considered normal and thus disregarded. A thorough physical examination is essential in assessing the presence or absence of moisture on the skin. Particular attention should be paid to the hands and feet, forearms and shins, back of the neck and chest and upper abdomen. Be aware, however, of the influences of anxiety, the warmth of the environment, and whether or not the patient has rushed to the appointment.

Night sweats

Night sweats are a common feature of lingering pathogens, and particularly characteristic of a pathogen in the qi and shaoyang levels. They are less common in the ying and blood levels, due to the degree of fluid and yin damage that complicates these patterns. Night sweats can occur with both heat and damp heat pathogens, and should be distinguished from the night sweats due to yin deficiency. Night sweats due to a lingering pathogen usually occur once or twice per night, whereas the sweats of yin deficiency can occur many times at more or less regular intervals. The more damp heat, the stickier, and potentially more odorous, the sweat.

Spontaneous sweating

Spontaneous sweating is the appearance of sweat on the skin during the daytime without exertion or environmental heat to justify it. The sweat can be systemic or isolated to one part of the body, continuous or intermittent. Spontaneous sweating, in the context of a lingering pathogen, suggests heat or damp heat in the qi level. When heat is the primary pathogen, the sweat tends to be continuous. The more damp heat, the more intermittent the appearance of the sweat. The intermittent nature of damp heat sweat occurs as sweating clears some heat and as the heat diminishes, the sweating stops. However, the obstructing damp soon leads to a buildup of heat and the sweating starts again.

Sweating on parts of the body

Sweating may be localized to parts of the body, or distinctly more prominent on parts of the body. This is most commonly seen on the hands and feet, chest, head and neck, upper abdomen, armpits or genitals. Localized sweating, in the context of a lingering pathogen, is always due to a pathogen in the qi or shaoyang levels. Sweating on the head is suggestive of a damp heat pathogen, as damp blocks the expression of heat on the trunk and acts to funnel the heat upwards as if through a chimney, to appear as heat and sweat on the head and neck. Abnormal sweating only on the chest suggests heat in the qi level, while clammy hands and feet points to heat or damp heat in the qi level. Abnormal, or sudden onset of, sweating from the armpits and genital region is suggestive of a shaoyang pathogen.

Sour, strong or otherwise unusual smelling sweat

Strong smelling sweat, or sweat that stains the clothes is due to damp heat in the qi level or shaoyang.

Nature of the sweat

Sweat can be watery or sticky and viscous. When watery, it runs down the body in rivulets; when viscous it accumulates in droplets (often seen on the forehead and top lip) that feel somewhat oily between the fingers. The more heat, the more watery the sweat; the more damp heat the more viscous.

Dryness; damage to body fluids

Body fluids are inevitably damaged by a lingering pathogen. The fluid damage is due to the heat itself which dries and scorches fluids, and the sweating that is part of the bodies response to the presence of a lingering pathogen. This can manifest in numerous ways, including thirst, dry skin, hair eyes and mucous membranes, constipation, dryness of the linings of the respiratory and gastrointestinal systems and the thickening of fluids and bodily secretions. In very chronic or severe cases, damage to fluids may eventually drain the deeper true yin of the Liver and Kidneys.

Energy levels

Poor energy is often the presenting complaint of a patient with a lingering pathogen. The fatigue associated with a lingering pathogen can be debilitating, and its depth is due to two factors – the presence of the pathogen itself which obstructs the circulation of qi and blood, and the amount of qi required to contain the pathogen and prevent it from doing more damage. Persistent fatigue since a previous illness, or a sudden and otherwise inexplicable drop in energy lasting from a few hours to days or longer, may suggest a lingering pathogen, when accompanied by abnormal heat, sweating or lymph node swelling.

Tongue

Certain features of the tongue, in particular the prominent red protrusions (thorns) that appear anteriorly, around the edges of the tongue and on the root of the tongue, are suggestive of a lingering pathogen. The distribution of thorns can give clues as to the depth of the pathogen (Fig.11.2). The other main benefit of the tongue is as a prognostic indicator and a measure of how well a treatment is progressing, especially in the deeper patterns of ying and blood. When lingering heat occurs at the ying and blood level, progress of treatment can sometimes be slow, but an early indicator that treatment is progressing is a return of the previously absent tongue coat. Conversely, if the tongue coat becomes further denuded during the course of a qi level or shaoyang treatment, something is going wrong and the pathogen moving deeper.

The color of the tongue is variable. When a heat pathogen is in the qi level, fluids, qi and yin are damaged. The tongue will be dry and red, or redder than normal with a thin or peeled coat and anterior thorns. When qi damage is significant, however, the tongue may appear pale and possibly swollen, even though there is still heat in situ. When damp or damp heat are in the qi level, the drying qualities of heat are muted and a thick white or yellow coat is seen.

Shaoyang patterns usually do not produce characteristic tongue signs unless there is damp heat, in which case a thick tongue coat will be seen. Depending on the degree of heat and deficiency, the edges of the tongue may be red or have red spots or thorns, or be pale and slightly swollen.

As the pathogen moves deeper into the ying and blood levels, the tongue becomes redder and the fluid damage more profound. The tongue coat begins to diminish until it is completely absent and the tongue a deep red or scarlet. Thorns appear further back on the tongue body. In the absence of a scarlet tongue there is little likelihood of a pathogen in the ying or blood, although overlapping qi and ying or blood level pathogens can modify the color somewhat. Be aware

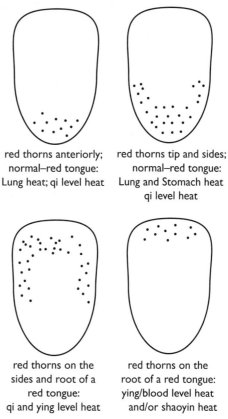

red thorns anteriorly; normal–red tongue: Lung heat; qi level heat

red thorns tip and sides; normal–red tongue: Lung and Stomach heat qi level heat

red thorns on the sides and root of a red tongue: qi and ying level heat

red thorns on the root of a red tongue: ying/blood level heat and/or shaoyin heat

Figure 11.2 Thorns are suggestive of a lingering pathogen

that some patients are fond of brushing their tongues, especially when the coating is thick.

Skin lesions and rashes

Skin lesions and rashes characteristic of lingering pathogens include macules, papules and vesicles. Macules and papules often appear together as a maculopapular rash. They can appear in qi, ying and blood level pathology, but their primary clinical significance is in prognosis and determination of the progress of treatment. Depending on their nature and when they appear, their appearance can be encouraging, or a sign that something is going wrong. In general however, if other symptoms are improving when a rash appears, it is a good sign. Ye Tian–Shi[4] noted that when treating pathogens:

'It is favorable for macules and papules to appear, but not in great numbers'.

Macules

Macules are flat, dull red, brown or purple, contiguous with the skin, and may appear on the trunk and extremities. They cannot be felt and do not blanch with pressure. Macules are an indication of a pathogen at the blood level. Macules appearing during the course of a blood or ying level treatment are generally considered favorable and an expression of the pathogen coming out. Macules appearing during the treatment of a qi level pathogen, on the other hand, may mean that the pathogen is heading deeper into the body.

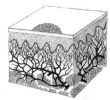

Figure 11.3 Macule

Papules

Papules are raised lesions like small pale pimples, appearing mostly on the trunk. They can be easily felt, blanch with pressure, and are an indication of a pathogen in the ying and qi levels. Papules appearing when attempting to vent a ying level pathogen are a sign that the treatment is working, and the pathogen emerging. On the other hand, the appearance of a papular or maculopapular rash during the course of a qi level treatment indicates that something is going wrong and the pathogen heading deeper.

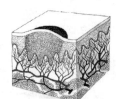

Figure 11.4 Papule

Vesicles

Vesicles are small fluid filled blisters which can appear anywhere on the body, but tend to affect the lips and fingers (qi level), trunk, genitals (shaoyang) and lower body. They always indicate damp of some type. They tend to be intensely itchy and may appear repeatedly during treatment, as damp is gradually cleared from the body.

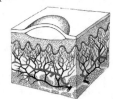

Figure 11.5 Vesicle

---

4 Discussion of Warm Heat Pathogen Disorders (*Wen Re Lun*) 1792

11.2 ETIOLOGY

Weakness of anti–pathogenic qi, weakness of Lung, Spleen and Kidney qi, weak constitution

Any pre–existing constitutional or acquired weakness can predispose patients to a pathogenic invasion, which they cannot repel. Weakness of Lung and Spleen qi can enable a pathogen to penetrate into the qi level. Weakness of the Kidneys can enable deeper penetration in the ying, blood and shaoyin levels. Patients presenting with ying and blood level heat pathogens are often found to have a constitutional predisposition to Kidney weakness, and a family history of related conditions may be seen.

Overwork

One of the most common contributing factors is failure to rest and look after oneself during an acute illness. Patients who try to 'sweat it out' and soldier on, or simply ignore the illness and continue to work through it, are especially likely to end up with a lingering pathogen. The diversion of resources away from the fight leads to an incomplete response from the anti–pathogenic qi.

Overwork in general, both physical and mental, drains the basic reserves of yuan qi and weakens the Kidneys. This weakness enables a pathogen to easily enter, and once in to linger, especially at the deep levels, ying, blood and shaoyin. The anti–pathogenic qi is unable to mount a robust defense. Prolonged 'burning the candle at both ends' is a common finding in patients who go on to develop chronic fatigue syndrome and other persistent fatigue patterns. Shift workers and those working long hours in stressful situations are particularly vulnerable. These patients tend to develop very prolonged illnesses because the acquired weakness of yuan qi and jing essence complicates removal of the pathogen and restoration of normal function and recovery.

Immunization

Immunizations may cause a lingering pathogen in some circumstances. Patients who are weak to start with, or who are vaccinated during an acute illness, are especially vulnerable. The use of antipyretic drugs such as paracetamol and aspirin, directly after an immunization, in an attempt to allay the resulting fever can short circuit or inhibit the immune response, causing the pathogen to get trapped. Immunization can transmit a pathogen directly into the qi, shaoyang, ying or blood levels.

Antibiotics during acute viral illness

Antibiotics are bitter and cold, and can weaken Spleen yang qi. They act like a bitter cold purge, often causing diarrhea. They effectively clear heat, but are unable to completely disperse the pathogen, so a residue, often in the form of damp, is left behind, creating a medium for repeated infection. The weakened Spleen yang leads to poor resistance and enables pathogens to gain easy access deep into the qi level.

Wrong treatment

Wrong or poorly administered treatment for the type and location of a pathogen can weaken anti–pathogenic qi, trap a pathogen or drag it deeper into the body. Wrong treatments include diaphoresis when a pathogen is already beyond the surface, excessive purging, and prescriptions of bitter cold herbs or antibiotics when a pathogen is still on the surface. Supplementing inappropriately (as can occur when mistaking fatigue for deficiency) with qi and yin supplements is another common trap, which can lock the pathogen in rather than disperse it. Repeated use of antipyretic drugs during mild childhood fevers is also implicated.

Environmental exposure

Repeated exposure to certain climates, chemicals or toxins can lead to a lingering pathogen pattern. The climactic factors are the most common, with prolonged exposure to hot humid weather, a damp house or frequent contact with water, especially when tired or vulnerable, enabling dampness and damp heat to seep into the body.

Exposure to farm and industrial chemicals, pesticides, volatile fumes and pollutants can induce a lingering pathogen reaction in some people, especially those already weakened or vulnerable due to constitution, age or pre–existing illness. This may be seen in rural workers, the residents of badly polluted cities, in the inhabitants of new and hermetically sealed buildings ('sick building syndrome') and in those working with volatile substances, such as perfumes, paints, varnishes, solvents and gasoline.

Strong pathogen

A strong or epidemic pathogen can overwhelm even the most robust of defenses, deplete qi and damage yin, and become persistent. This is seen in certain new strains of flu and other viral and bacterial illnesses that sweep through populations affecting many regardless of health. A strong pathogen may also be something other than an infectious agent, such as a chemical, poison or radiation, that is able to create a persistent immune response regardless of how robust the patient.

Drugs (pharmaceutical, recreational)

Some drugs weaken the Spleen and can damage qi, for example, laxatives and antibiotics. Some drugs deplete yin, weaken the Kidneys and open the shaoyin to invasion. These include stimulants such as amphetamines and cocaine, antidepressants, steroids and cytotoxic agents.

Emotional factors

Any emotional factor that leads to depletion of Spleen, Lung or Kidney qi can enable a pathogen to get past the body's defences and into the deeper levels where the weak qi is unable to adequately expel it. Chronic Liver qi constraint will eventually weaken Spleen qi, whereas a sudden or severe fright or shock can damage Kidney qi, or disrupt the Heart Kidney axis and leave the ying and blood levels vulnerable.

11.3 A SIMPLIFIED MODEL

A model for analyzing lingering pathogens exists in the Shang Han Lun and the Wen Re Lun, but this model has been obscured by an over emphasis on the role of these texts in the treatment of acute illness. In addition, the conceptual division between them (different number of levels, different pathogenic emphasis – Shang Han Lun for cold, Wen Re Lun for heat) has caused confusion amongst teachers and students, and leads to misunderstanding about how to use them effectively. It has not helped that the text is often opaque, the clauses difficult to understand and relate to the modern world, and are sometimes contradictory. A clearer framework, derived from observations in clinical practice in combination with a simplified way of looking at the classic texts, is warranted and will be presented here.

Definition

A lingering pathogen, according to this model, is a pathogenic influence, either heat or damp heat (with varying degrees of heat), that is located in a specific region of the body as described in the Shang Han Lun and Wen Re Lun. Regardless of the initial pathogen, once it has breached the body's defenses and is inside, it is transformed into heat or damp heat, and can persist for long periods of time in the qi/shaoyang level and/or the ying/blood level.

The classic texts are maps of the immune response

The Shang Han Lun and Wen Re Lun provide two descriptions of the immune response. They can be seen as maps describing the same terrain, although they focus on different surface features. They describe the territory of the body and the immune response under different conditions and from different perspectives. Although they appear superficially dissimilar, they can be hybridized to provide a simplified, yet more comprehensive and user friendly model of host pathogen interactions. The ten levels they jointly describe can be resolved into three (Fig. 11.3). The multiplicity of pathogens they describe are heat or damp heat once inside the body.

Although simplistic, this model has two advantages. First, it provides a clear framework for understanding the nature and location of lingering pathogens with some precision, enabling a precisely targeted response and a way of assessing the

Figure 11.3 Ten levels resolve into three

Wei	Taiyang
Qi	Shaoyang Yangming Taiyin
Ying Blood	Shaoyin Jueyin

responses to treatment. Secondly, the model reflects clinical reality and is not simply theoretical. In the authors experience, many commonly seen disorders associated with a persistent immune response can be effectively analysed in this way.

This model, however, does not attempt to, nor can it, explain all host pathogen interactions. The model excludes some conditions which may be the result of a pathogenic agent, but nevertheless do not exhibit the characteristic features of a lingering pathogen. For example, some viral infections, such as some hepatitis cases and post herpetic neuralgia, can present with organ system dysfunction or disorder of qi, blood and fluids, and diagnoses of Liver qi constraint, various deficiency states, and qi and blood stasis, etc., are more appropriate. No single model can incorporate all possible variations and different problems need different ways of thinking. From here on the term lingering pathogen is used according to the definition outlined on page 511.

11.3.1 THE MAIN PATHOGENS ARE HEAT AND DAMP HEAT

There are numerous types of pathogens[5] described in the Shang Han Lun and Wen Re Lun that can invade the body, but once they have penetrated the defensive layer and are internal they are transformed into two main types[6], heat and damp heat.

Heat

Heat is created when a pathogen, regardless of its original nature, breaches the defensive layers of the body and comes into conflict with the anti–pathogenic qi. The physical presence of a pathogen also obstructs qi and blood which can in turn generate heat, and also prevents efficient dispersal of surplus physiological heat.

Heat is a yang and expansive pathogen, can move and change rapidly, tends to sit more superficially within a level due to its rising nature, and can be vented and expelled with relative ease. Persistent heat always damages body fluids and yin.

When heat lingers in the body, it can exist in various degrees, from relatively pronounced to quite muted (Fig. 11.4). There are several factors that influence the degree and expression of heat:

- The nature of heat itself. Heat is yang, and as such tends to dissipate naturally over time. The longer a heat pathogen is present the more it tends to disperse and the less heat may be apparent.

- The interaction between the patients qi and the pathogen. The degree and presentation of heat can be muted in patients with concurrent or pre–existing yang qi deficiency or internal cold. When yang qi is weak, the anti–pathogenic response is unable to put up much of a fight, and cold can 'freeze' the heat pathogen in situ. Conversely a patient with robust anti–pathogenic qi or a hot constitution confronted with a trapped or lingering pathogen is likely to show a good deal more heat.

---

5 wind warmth, damp warmth, spring warmth, autumn dryness, warm toxin, summerheat, wind, cold, damp, heat
6 Their presence can however, occasionally give rise to pathology that ultimately presents as cold or yang deficient. See shaoyin cold transformation, p.522–523.

Figure 11.4 Typical range of lingering pathogenic heat. The degree of heat observed in most cases of lingering pathogens is mild to moderate.

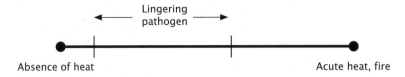

- Certain treatments can reduce heat, without dispelling the pathogen. This occurs with antibiotic treatment, when applied inappropriately for a viral illness, for example. The same iatrogenic potential exists for toxic heat clearing herbs. The coldness of the drugs cools the heat, but the contracting bitterness prevents dispersal of the pathogen, may injure the Spleen and further compromise qi.
- The pathological effects of heat on the patient. Persistent pathogenic heat damages fluid and yin, and uses up a great deal of the patients qi in the effort to expel or contain the pathogen. Symptoms of a lingering pathogen include not only those caused by the remnant pathogen itself, but also those caused by the damage its presence has wrought. Qi deficiency and fluid damage will be apparent if the lingering pathogen is at the qi level, but if a persistent lingering pathogen has penetrated deeper, yin and yang deficiency with blood stasis will develop. The deficiency not only makes it more difficult to expel the pathogen, but mutes the expression of the heat as well.

Damp heat

Damp heat is the result of an invasion of a damp or damp heat pathogen, or the interaction between a patient with pre–existing damp and any other pathogen that transforms into heat once inside the body. Pre–existing damp and damp heat are common in the Western world due to the abundance of food available, the relatively fat rich and sweet diet, and high alcohol consumption.

Damp heat is sticky, viscous, obstructing and heavy, and tends to sink into the deeper layers of the qi and shaoyang levels. Like pure heat, damp heat can have varying degrees of heat associated with it. In practice we see the full spectrum from almost pure dampness with very little heat to a moderate degree of damp with predominant heat. The clinical features can help discriminate the relative proportions of heat and damp (Table 11.1, p.514).

In combination, yin damp and yang heat moderate each others expression. Damp 'wraps' and contains the heat, preventing its full expression. Heat congeals the damp further making it more sticky and difficult to shift. In general, the longer a damp heat pathogen persists, the more the heat tends to dissipate. The sticky obstructive nature of damp, however, easily blocks qi and blood circulation which in turn creates more heat, leading to a cyclical increase of damp heat. Damp heat conditions are typically characterized by exacerbations and remissions.

The relative degrees of dampness and heat are also dependent on the constitu-

Table 11.1 Comparison of damp and heat predominance

	Damp > Heat	Heat > Damp
Fever	low grade fever that rises in the afternoon; may be contained fever, or heat only on the head or hands and feet	higher, more obvious and more persistent fever that results in an oozy sweat; fever does not break with sweating
Sweating	clamminess; can be isolated to the hands and feet or head	with fever as above, night sweats common
Muscles	generalized aching prominent, commonly the thigh and upper arms, with heaviness and easy fatigue with use; soggy or pudgy feel to the muscles	muscle weakness and mild aching; sense of heat in the muscles; can concentrate in joints (esp. knees); may be swelling with redness and pain
Bowels	loose stools or diarrhea, may be with mucus	urgent foul explosive diarrhea with tenesmus or a sense of incomplete bowel emptying; sluggish stools that are hard to shift but not dry and hard
Urination	cloudy or frothy	yellow, concentrated, scanty, maybe turbid
Head, cognition	foggy head, heavy head, poor concentration, dull headache; dizziness	more profound headache, foggy head, unclear thinking or confusion; sore throat
Digestion	no appetite, nausea	vomiting
Thirst, mouth	no thirst; sticky sensation in the mouth	thirst with dry mouth and throat, or a sticky unpleasant sensation in the mouth, but little actual drinking
Demeanor	lethargic, listless, sleepiness, heavy sleeping and waking feeling tired	agitation, restlessness; insomnia and broken sleep
Tongue	greasy, white or mixed white and yellow coat	greasy, yellow coat
Pulse	soggy	slippery, rapid

tion of the patient, as well as the effects of treatment and concurrent pathology. The more robust the patients anti–pathogenic qi, the more likely the pathogen will be contained, with the resulting battle creating greater heat. If the Spleen is weak however, and damp is being created internally, damp will tend to predominate. Similarly, weak yang qi will favor more damp and less heat, whereas a hot constitution, heating diet or yin deficiency will promote heat over damp.

The sticky viscosity of yin damp, with or without heat, impedes the circulation of qi and blood and disrupts the qi dynamic, which has an impact on the function of the Spleen.

11.3.2 PATHOGENS LINGER IN SPECIFIC LOCATIONS

The Shang Han Lun and Wen Re Lun together describe a total of 10 locations[7] that a pathogen can access. In practice, these multiple layers can be resolved into three – the surface, the region between the surface and the deep yin organ systems, and the deep interior of the 'yin yin' organ systems. Pathogens can persist in all three, but by far the most common and important, in the authors experience, is the qi level.

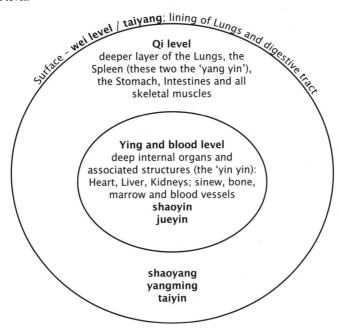

Figure 11.5 The levels of the body, according to the Shang Han Lun and Wen Re Lun

The surface

The surface, the wei/taiyang level, is the most superficial part of the body and includes the surface of the skin, the pores, and mucous membranes of the Lungs and respiratory tract, and the lining of the digestive tract. Wei qi circulates on these surfaces and protects them from pathogenic invasion. Pathogens can occasionally persist on the surface when wei qi is weak, or the yin yang (ying and wei) balance of the skin is disturbed. Being the exterior of the body, the pathogen has not yet met with major resistance and thus transformed into heat or damp heat, and can still be in its original form of wind, heat, cold and so on. In general, lingering pathogens on the surface are minor disorders and are dealt with in the section on persistent colds, p.73.

---

7 taiyang, shaoyang, yangming, taiyin, shaoyin, jueyin, wei, qi ying, blood

The qi level

Most lingering pathogens end up in the qi level. The qi level is associated function-ally and structurally with the Lungs, Spleen, Stomach and Large Intestine. The qi level is where the body mounts its most robust defense against external invasion, to prevent pathogens from getting into the deepest and most vulnerable organs. Acute qi level pathology is therefore characterized by symptoms of a strong fight, the classic identifying features of the qi level, the 'four bigs' – high fever, profuse sweat, large thirst and surging pulse. When a qi level pathogen persists, these key features remain, but they change in nature and intensity[8].

The Lungs and Spleen are the 'yang yin' organs, because they are yin organs with a connection to the exterior, directly in the case of the Lungs, indirectly via the Stomach in the case of the Spleen. The qi level lies between the surface wei level and the deepest level of the body, where the 'yin yin' organ systems, the Heart, Liver and Kidneys are found. The qi level includes the deeper layer of the Lungs and its associated subcutaneous tissues, the Stomach and the deeper tissues of the digestive tract, and the Spleen and its associated tissues, the skeletal muscles, lips and extremities.

Qi level pathology can be diverse, but is characterized by a specific group of key identifying features (Table 11.2), with the addition of varying proportions of respiratory and gastrointestinal symptoms, disorder of energy production, and pathology of the skeletal muscles, mucous membranes and skin. The persistent presence of a pathogen in the qi level always leads to fluid damage and various degrees of qi deficiency, both of which compound the body's inability to eject the pathogen.

The qi level has various depths within it (Fig. 11.6). Different pathogens inhabit different levels, influence different systems, and produce distinct clinical pictures.

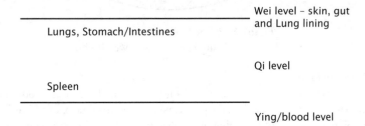

Figure 11.6 Depths of the qi level

Heat, being a yang, expansive pathogen, tends to sit high up in the qi level and thus affects the superficial tissues of the Lungs, Stomach and mucous membranes. Damp heat, on the other hand, is heavy and sinks deeper in the qi level, impacting

---

8 Not all lingering qi level pathology follows acute qi level disorder. Lingering qi level pathology can occur gradually and may lack a specific history. The end result is the same however, with the core group of identifying features, and varying proportions of associated features as per Table 11.2.

Table 11.2 Identifying features of acute and lingering qi level patterns.

	Acute	Lingering heat	Lingering damp heat
Key features	continuous high fever	low grade fever, cyclical fever, heat in one part of the body	afternoon fever, contained fever unrelieved by sweating
	large thirst	dryness, moderate thirst; dry skin and hair	dryness with little or no desire to drink
	profuse sweat	night sweats, spontaneous sweating, abnormal sweating on one part of the body	night sweats, sticky sweat in the afternoon, abnormal sweating on one part of the body
	surging, rapid pulse	fine, rapid pulse	slippery, wiry, soft pulse
	red tongue	red dry tongue	thick greasy tongue coat
	malaise	fatigue	fatigue, heaviness
	tender swollen glands	non tender swollen glands and tonsils	rubbery non tender swollen glands and tonsils
Primary focus		Lungs and upper gastrointestinal tract; cough, nausea, vomiting	Spleen, lower digestive tract, lips, extremities and muscles
muscles		muscle weakness, mild aches	muscle and joint aches and heaviness; poor tone
skin		dry itchy skin lesions	vesicular skin lesions
shen, demeanor		insomnia, irritability, restlessness; behavioral problems	lethargy, sleepiness, listlessness
bowels		tendency to constipation or dry stools	loose stools or diarrhea
mucous membranes		hypersensitivity of mucous membranes – allergies, food intolerances	mucus congestion, sticky serous discharges; post nasal drip, sinus congestion, glue ear, vaginal discharge
other		pathology is peripheral and central; peripheral affecting the muscles and limbs; central, affecting digestive tract, Lungs, sinuses and lips	

more on the Spleen and the skeletal muscles.

There are eight distinct qi level patterns that the authors encounter (Table 11.8, p.541) but they all share the key identifying features which locate the pathogen in the qi level. In general, qi level pathogens respond reliably to the correct treatment. Heat is easy to vent, and conditions of even considerable duration can be resolved within a few weeks at most. Damp heat is stickier and deeper, and so takes longer to resolve, but still responds in a reliable manner.

The qi level and shaoyang level inhabit the same space between the surface and deep interior, and in fact can be seen as different poles within the same level (Fig.

Figure 11.7 Shaoyang and qi level share the same space

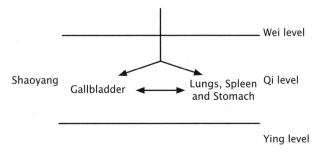

11.7). The difference between them is simply that the pathology of the qi level is skewed towards the Lungs, Spleen and Stomach, the centre of the body and limbs, whereas the shaoyang is skewed towards the Gallbladder and lateral parts of the body. The clinical picture oscillates sometimes between qi level and shaoyang pathology.

Key features
- Low grade fever, or abnormal heat sensations
- Sweating
- Dryness and thirst
- Swollen glands and/or tonsils
- Increasing levels of fatigue

Secondary features
- Respiratory and digestive tract symptoms such as cough, sinus congestion, nausea, vomiting and diarrhea. These are associated with dryness and irritation of the linings of these systems.
- Increasing fatigue and lethargy. Fatigue, both physical and mental, is one of the main features of a lingering pathogen, and a frequent presenting complaint.
- Sleep disturbances, insomnia, irritability or behavioral changes may occur as heat disturbs the Heart and shen. Patients with behavioral problems from qi level heat may be diagnosed with conditions such as attention deficit hyperactivity disorder (ADHD).
- Hypersensitivity of the superficial tissues lining the respiratory and gastrointestinal tracts, causing allergic[9] or intolerance type symptoms, skin rashes, serous discharges and excessive mucus production. The heat located beneath the surface influences the mucous membranes and skin, making them more irritable and reactive to stimuli.
- Dry itchy skin lesions such as eczema and dermatitis, or vesicular lesions like herpes when damp heat is the pathogen.

---

9 Clinical experience suggests that the increase in allergies in the developed world can, at least partly, be linked to the rise in lingering pathogens resulting from immunization and subsequent use of anti-phlogistic drugs to allay the resulting fever (see p. 509–510).

Table 11.3 Identifying features of acute and lingering shaoyang patterns.

Acute (1-2 weeks)	Lingering heat	Lingering damp heat
distinct alternating fever and chills	sporadic periods of fever and chilliness; hot and cold sensations; 'flu like' feelings	alternating fever and chills starting in the afternoon
fatigue	increasing fatigue	increasing fatigue, foggy head, heaviness
dizziness, giddiness	dizziness, giddiness, balance problems	vertigo, balance problems
bitter taste in the mouth	bitter or odd taste in the mouth; food tastes bad	bitter, odd taste or cloying sensation in the mouth, food tastes bad; bad breath
irritability	irritability	irritability, sleepiness
loss of appetite	loss of appetite	loss of appetite
nausea	nausea, worse in the morning	nausea, vomiting
hypochondriac ache	hypochondriac ache	hypochondriac ache, muscle aches, chest oppression
wiry pulse	fine, wiry pulse	slippery, soggy, wiry pulse
unremarkable tongue, or coated on one side only	red edges or slightly pale tongue	thick greasy tongue coat
tender swollen glands	non tender swollen glands and tonsils	non tender swollen glands and tonsils; white spots on the tonsils

- Dampness in the qi level leads to muscle and joint aching and weakness, cognitive changes, increasing lower gastrointestinal dysfunction and discharge from mucous membranes.

The shaoyang level

In this model, the shaoyang is a subset of the qi level. They both exist in the intermediate zone between the surface and the interior, but while the qi level is aligned with the Lungs, Spleen, Stomach and Intestines, the shaoyang is aligned with the Gallbladder. The shaoyang level is distinct from the qi level pathologically and symptomatically, but because they inhabit the same relative space, we sometimes see patients oscillating between qi level and shaoyang type disorders.

The shaoyang level has various depths, and the deeper a pathogen lies within the shaoyang, the harder it can be to resolve. The deepest level is known as the 'membrane source' (*mó yuán* 膜原), a conceptual area thought to be located between the diaphragm and pleura. This is where malarial pathogens (i.e. pathogens which may, or may not be, true plasmodium malaria but which produce malaria like intermittent fever symptoms), are thought to hide. The depth is responsible for the relative difficulty in thoroughly evicting them.

The shaoyang is one of the commonest presentations of a lingering pathogen, but is often missed because of the variability and diversity of its identifying features. The classical acute features of shaoyang syndrome, noted in Table 11.3, persist when the pathogen lingers, but can be muted to such an extent that they may be difficult to recognize.

Area of influence

Shaoyang disorders affect those parts of the body associated with the Gallbladder and shaoyang channel pathways. In addition to the basic identifying features, we can see a diverse range of lateral and genital pathology, including temporal headaches, temporomandibular, shoulder and hip pain, tightness and spasm of lateral structures like the sternocleidomastoid and the iliotibial band, ear problems, and eczematous and vesicular lesions on the sides of the body and genitals.

The ying and blood levels

The ying and blood levels are the deepest levels of the body. They exist on a continuum, with the ying level shallower than the blood level. The difference in depth has implications for therapy, specifically that pathogens in the ying level can still

Table 11.4 Identifying features of lingering ying and blood level patterns

	Lingering heat in the ying	Lingering heat in the blood
Common features	persistent low grade fever, worse at night	
	may or may not be night sweats	
	deep red or scarlet tongue with thorns and no coat	
	dryness – skin, hair, mucous membranes, stools	
	fine, rapid pulse	
	fatigue and exhaustion	
	insomnia, restlessness	
	lymphadenopathy	
	joint pain and inflammation	
	vasculitis	
	weight loss, emaciation	
	mouth ulcers	
Specific features	mild, indistinct erythematous or papular skin rashes; rashes worse or increasingly itchy at night	distinct erythematous, dark red or purple skin rashes and macules on the face, trunk and shins; worse at night
	irrational behavior, personality change, incoherent speech	severe irritability, confusion, personality change, mania
		bleeding, mild and persistent – menorrhagia, abnormal uterine bleeding, purpura, rectal
		numbness, tics, tremor, spasms

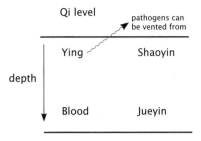

Figure 11.8 Depth of ying and blood

be vented towards the exterior, while pathogens in the blood cannot (Fig. 11.8). In general, only heat is seen at these levels. Pathogenic heat in the ying and blood levels is characterized by a group of common features and a few specific features related to the increasing depth (Table 11.4). The ying and blood levels are aligned with the most yin of the internal organs, the Kidneys and Heart (shaoyin organs) and Liver (jueyin), thus pathogenic influences in the ying and blood influence the behavior and activity of these organs. By the time a pathogen is in the ying and blood levels, significant damage to yin and blood has occurred. A heat pathogen damages Kidney and Liver yin, depletes the fluid portion of blood and causes blood stasis. In some patients with pre–existing yang weakness, Kidney yang is depleted as well, giving rise to a paradoxical yang deficiency (see shaoyin level, p.522). Kidney deficiency, either inherited or acquired, predisposes an individual to invasion and persistence of pathogens in the ying and blood levels.

These patterns are always complex, and can be difficult to manage successfully. In practice, mixtures of qi, ying and blood level pathogens are seen simultaneously. The difficulty in resolving these patterns is due not only to the depth of the pathogen and degree of concurrent damage done by it, but also the fact that many patients with these problems are medicated with strong drugs that can block the effects of herbs and acupuncture. Heat in the ying and blood often corresponds to chronic inflammatory disorders or autoimmune disease – rheumatoid arthritis, Systemic Lupus Erythematosus and Graves disease for example – and patients are frequently medicated with drugs such as corticosteroids, immunosuppressants

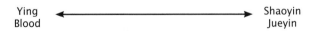

Ying Blood		Shaoyin Jueyin
• Clear features of lingering pathogen • More systemic, less organ specific • Main principal is to eliminate excess		• Clear features of organ system deficiency • No specific evidence of pathogen • Main principal is to replenish deficiency

Figure 11.9 Difference between ying/blood, and shaoyin/jueyin pathology

and anticoagulants.

Although the ying and blood occupy the same region of the body (Fig. 11.8, p.521), there are differences between them.

Ying level

A pathogen in the ying level is always due to an external invasion. Heat in the ying can be vented back towards the qi level. In practice, the fact that ying level heat can be vented presents both challenges and opportunities. If a pathogen moves from the ying level into the qi level, features of the qi level may appear. Gastrointestinal symptoms such as nausea, thirst or constipation, an increasing fever and muscle aches may be seen. This is a good sign and presents the practitioner with an opportunity to expedite elimination of the pathogen, as venting pathogens from the qi level is easier than from the ying. To the patient and unaware practitioner, however, this can look like an aggravation, or wrong treatment, and the temptation is to abandon the course of treatment. In our experience, if patients are informed that this may happen, they will put up with a temporary aggravation gladly, as it is a positive sign of advancement. If qi level symptoms do occur and are treated appropriately (with qi level treatment), they should resolve within a few weeks, after which the patient feels considerably better.

Blood level

A pathogen in the blood level can be the result of an external invasion, or be due to internal dysfunction. Internally generated heat usually arises as a result of Liver dysfunction. The heat is transferred to the blood when the blood returns to the Liver at night. Once a pathogen is predominantly in the blood, it cannot be vented and must cooled in situ.

The shaoyin level

The shaoyin organs, the Heart and Kidneys, are located within the ying and blood levels. Shaoyin pathology represents the end result of an external pathogenic invasion. The main difference between the ying and blood level pathology and shaoyin pathology, is the relative balance of the excess (the pathogen) and the resulting deficiency (Fig. 11.9, p.521). Shaoyin pathology is organ specific and characterized by deficiency of the shaoyin organs, with little or no sign of a remnant pathogen. The pathogen may have diminished into insignificance, or the depleted host may be too weak to mount an adequate defense and thus produce the characteristic symptoms of a lingering pathogen. As treatment progresses, the deficiency is replenished, the patient grows stronger and is more able to evict any remnant pathogen. Specific signs of a lingering pathogen (swollen glands, changing fever pattern) may begin to emerge. Because damage to organ systems is the defining character of a shaoyin pattern, the pathology can lean towards either yin or yang deficiency, depending on the initial conditions, the constitution of the patient, diet and treatment. Most commonly, chronic lingering heat damages the yin, leading to heat transformation, but occasionally in those with a pre–existing Kidney yang qi deficiency, an invading pathogen, rather than generating a heat response, can be 'frozen' in place. The containment of the pathogen also saps more and more yang qi (Fig. 11.10, p.524). These factors can lead to a cold transforma-

Table 11.5 Features of shaoyin level patterns

Heat transformation	Cold transformation
low grade fever, rising in the afternoon and evening	cold intolerance, feels cold to the touch especially the extremities and abdomen
heat in the palms and soles; palmar erythema	cold extremities
facial flushing	bluish discoloration of the lips; pale puffy face and eyes
insomnia	somnolence
anxiety, panic attacks, restlessness, irritability	depression, withdrawal, lack of motivation
palpitations, tachycardia	bradycardia, arrythmia, poor circulation
dizziness, tinnitus	loss of hearing
night sweats	coarse dry skin
dry mouth and throat	no thirst
fatigue, exhaustion, yet with an inability to settle and rest	severe tiredness, exhaustion; breathlessness or wheezing with exertion
poor concentration and memory	poor concentration and memory
lower back and legs aching and weak	lower back and legs aching and cold
frequent concentrated urine, dysuria	frequent copious urination; nocturia
	pitting edema, especially ankles
dry stools, constipation	diarrhoea with undigested food or constipation
mouth or tongue ulcers	pale and painless oral ulcers
joint pain and inflammation	cold, stiff, aching joints
vasculitis, erythema	
red, dry, cracked tongue with no coat	pale, wet, swollen, scalloped tongue
fine rapid pulse	deep, weak, slow, irregular or imperceptible pulse

tion of what was initially a heat pattern.

The features of shaoyin pathology (Table 11.5) reflect the standard yin and yang deficiency patterns, but the onset may be more acute. These conditions are rarely diagnosed as a lingering pathogen until the pathogen begins to emerge and make its presence felt. Diagnosis of a lingering pathogen in such cases is made in retrospect. Patients presenting with these patterns, especially the cold transformation, rarely relate a relevant history, as the pre–existing deficiency leaves them open to swift invasion directly into shaoyin. A surface pathogen may encounter such feeble resistance as to be unopposed and unnoticed before slipping in deeper, and as the shaoyin level is related to the taiyang level (Heart – Small Intestine, Kidneys – Urinary Bladder), a pathogen can bypass the taiyang level altogether and directly

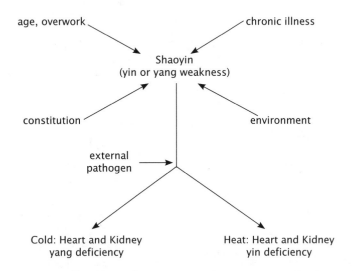

Figure 11.10 Cold and heat transformation of a shaoyin disorder

enter the shaoyin when the Kidneys are weak (Fig.11.11, p.526). Conversely a pathogen in shaoyin may express itself through taiyang, causing skin rashes and inflammation of superficial tissues. Shaoyin pathology also manifests in the tissues associated with the Heart and Kidneys, the vessels and joints. Chronic shaoyin pathology often involves joint swelling, inflammation and pain, and vasculitis. This is seen in some connective tissue diseases, such as lupus and Behçets disease.

The jueyin level

The jueyin level is aligned with the Liver and Pericardium, and closely associated with the blood. Jueyin pathology is rare in the Chinese medicine clinic (in the authors clinical experience), and represents a potentially fatal deterioration of a shaoyin pathology, in which both yin and yang are seriously depleted. An example of jueyin deterioration is seen in the fatal outcome of untreated type 1 diabetes mellitus (p.162). The pathology of jueyin syndrome is associated with a disruption of the fundamental yin and yang of the body, specifically the relationship between the Kidney water and Heart fire. The heat differential that exists between Kidney water and Heart fire creates a natural current that flows through the wood element, the jueyin. This current is a form of physiological wind that assists in elevating those aspects of normal physiological activity that ascend, such as Spleen qi. The jueyin relies on the correct temperature differential for normal functioning. When the differential is too small or too large pathology results.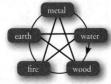

When the differential is too great, that is, Heart fire is in excess or Kidney water (yin) is deficient, too much current is generated and the wind becomes gusty, chaotic and pathological. The result is an imbalance between heat and cold, with

Table 11.6 Features of jueyin patterns

cold below, heat above	cold congealing
consumptive thirst[1]	no thirst
painful heat in the chest	icy cold blue or purple extremities
sense of heat rushing upwards	numbness in the extremities
irritability and restlessness; confusion, delirium, irrational behavior, loss of consciousness	
muscle spasms, tremors, convulsions	
vertigo, balance problems	
abdominal pain, vomiting	abdominal pain
frequent urination, nocturia	dysmenorrhea
chronic diarrhoea with undigested food	coldness and pain in the testicles
lower back and legs cold and aching	
pale swollen tongue with a red tip	pale tongue
	imperceptible pulse

1 Consumptive thirst is thirst with copious drinking, the volume of which is not reflected in the urinary output. Volume of urine is less that fluid ingested.

too much heat above the diaphragm and too much cold below. The pathological wind created by this differential can be quite intense, leading to muscles spasms, involuntary movement, balance problems, vertigo or in severe cases, convulsions. The involvement of the Pericardium and heat above the diaphragm can give rise to mental symptoms such as incoherence, confusion, irrational behavior and loss of consciousness.

When the differential is too small, that is Heart fire is weak or Kidney water is in excess, not enough current is generated and flow of qi and blood is slowed and stalled. This is equivalent to a pattern such as Heart and Kidney yang deficiency. The blood becomes cold and frozen and its distribution to the extremities is compromised. The main features are icy cold, pale or blue extremities.

11.4 MODE OF PENETRATION

The mode of transmission depends on the nature of the initial pathogen, the constitution of the patient and other factors such as treatment and behaviour during the acute phase. Pathogens can penetrate in an orderly fashion, from the surface through the various layers to the interior. This is seen when a cold or flu is not resolved in the acute phase and symptoms reflecting penetration of the deeper levels begin. When wei qi is weak or compromised, the surface can be bypassed altogether and a pathogen may get straight into the qi or shaoyang. In patients with Spleen and/or Kidney yin or yang deficiency the pathogen may get deep into ying and blood or shaoyin. Immunizations inject pathogens directly in the qi, shaoyang and deep levels.

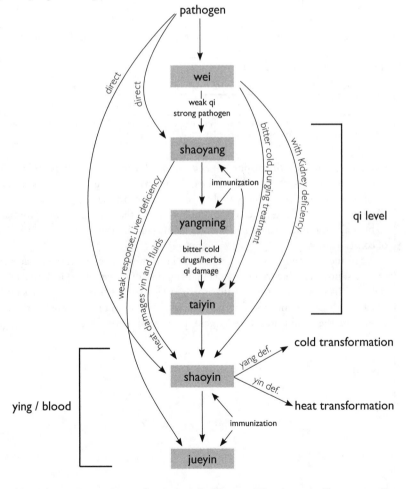

Figure 11.11 Penetration of an external pathogen. This diagram illustrates some of the many ways pathogens can enter the body.

Figure 11.12 Diagnostic flowchart for the analysis of lingering pathogens

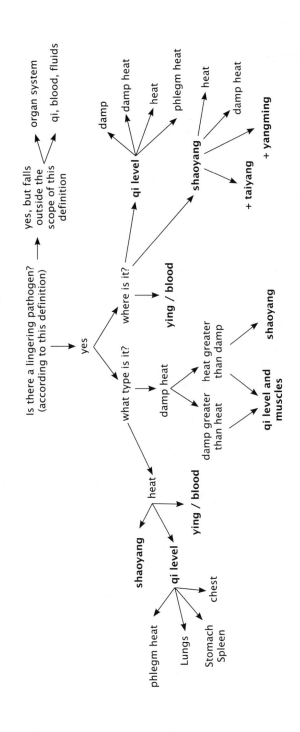

11.5 HOW TO EXPEL LINGERING PATHOGENS

The key points
- Keep all pathways of elimination open
  - keep the surface free
  - keep the bowels open and Lung and Stomach qi descending
  - actively encourage the qi dynamic
  - promote normal urination
- Encourage the natural tendency of heat pathogens to expand
- Close off the space available to a pathogen
- Exploit the sinking nature of damp to guide it towards the natural drainage conduits
- Clear heat with salty, pungent, sweet herbs
- Protect and restore anti–pathogenic qi, yin, fluids and blood

11.5.1 VENTING

Venting is the fundamental technique for evicting pathogens from the body. Venting works by gently encouraging a pathogen at one level of the body to move toward the surface or towards a yang organ, where it can then be eliminated. It does this by taking advantage of the spreading and expanding tendency that is inherent in yang pathogens. The aim is to encourage them to expand right out of the body. The Chinese word for venting is *tou* 透, which means to pass through or move outwards.

Which pathogens can be vented?

Venting is used in the treatment of insubstantial pathogens in the qi and ying levels. It is mostly used for heat, but can also be applied to damp heat that is relatively superficial. When used for damp heat, venting is used in conjunction with other specific damp draining techniques.

Insubstantial pathogens

Insubstantial pathogens lack concentrated form, are generally diffuse in nature, and may be distributed throughout various tissues. Insubstantial pathogens include wind, heat, dampness and damp heat. Insubstantial pathogens must be guided out of the body by light lifting that encourages the natural expansion of the yang pathogens, wind and heat, or that provides a lift to the relatively more yin pathogens, dampness and damp heat.

Substantial pathogens

Substantial pathogens are those with physical form, blood stasis and phlegm. Substantial pathogens cannot be vented. They must be broken up and expelled through one of the organs of elimination. Substantial pathogens require a strong 'attacking' type of treatment that can damage qi and yin if improperly used. Substantial pathogens, especially blood stasis, frequently complicate deep lying lingering pathogens in the ying and blood levels, and can be a significant impediment to treatment. Herbal treatments for pathogens in the ying and blood take this complication into account in their design.

Characteristics of the herbs used to vent lingering pathogens

Venting emphasizes the use of light natured, pungent, cool herbs (Table 11.7, pp.532–533). The pungency is the essential attribute, as it lifts upwards and outwards and reinforces the natural spreading tendency of the pathogen. Pungency not only encourages the pathogen to move up and out, it also keeps the pores open to allow the pathogen to escape. The aim however, is not to induce sweating, although this may occur. If a sweat is induced it must be very slight so as not to exacerbate any fluid damage that may already have occurred.

In general, light natured herbs are usually leaves, flowers and other aerial parts. The herbs are used in smaller than typical doses, in the range of one half to three quarters the standard dose. The small dose maintains the lightness of touch necessary to nudge the pathogen up and out, whereas larger doses can encourage too much movement and cause excessive sweating. Herbs are briefly decocted in a pot with a tight fitting lid, for no more than 10 minutes. Short cooking maintains the pungency and light lifting quality of the herbs, and the lid stops the essential oils from escaping.

Characteristics of venting acupuncture points

Acupuncture points that have a venting effect are primarily those that stimulate the diffusing action of the Lungs, and activate the movement of yang qi. The Lung organ system is yin and internal, yet opens directly to the exterior. It is therefore a convenient portal between the interior and exterior. Stimulating the Lungs diffusing action encourages movement towards the surface. Activating the quality and activity of yang qi has a similar effect, as the nature of yang is to expand and rise. Encouraging expansive movement in the body can assist in dislodging and wafting a pathogen towards the surface, or from a deep level towards and yang organ and an exit point.

Pathogens can be vented from the qi and ying levels

Venting a heat pathogen from the qi level is usually quite straightforward, with a reliable and predictable outcome. In addition to venting herbs, formulae for qi level heat pathogens use sweet or pungent cold herbs to clear heat. Bitter cold herbs are generally not used, or are used judiciously in quite small doses when heat is severe, or when constipation is a major issue and purging is required. Bitter cold herbs have a descending and contracting nature, that stands in opposition to the aims of venting so care is needed when they are used. They may also damage the Spleen and create a relative emptiness in the middle burner that sucks the pathogen further inward.

The basic treatment to vent heat from the qi level usually uses one or two mild diuretic herbs to maintain urinary flow and so maintain another outlet for pathogens. Excessive diuresis with too many or overly strong herbs, however, can further damage fluids. Good choices of herbs are those that promote urination while protecting fluids (Table 11.7, pp.532–533).

A lingering heat pathogen in the ying level is usually more complex, and is always accompanied by yin damage and blood stasis, both of which complicate things further. Both yin deficiency and blood stasis need to be addressed if progress is to be made. Bitter cold herbs are avoided because they can congeal heat and blood further. One regularly encountered difficulty in treating ying and blood level lingering heat is that patients are often taking strong pharmaceuticals, such as steroids, immunosuppressants and anticoagulants. The strong pungency of corticosteroids disperses heat and allays the worst of the inflammation, but inhibits the effects of treatment with both acupuncture and herbs, and may gradually aggravate both yin and yang deficiency when used long term or in high doses. Patients on anticoagulant therapy cannot use some important herbs and formulas, as clotting can be compromised. In patients taking numerous strong medications, adding more medicine to their load can overtax the liver and lead to unwanted interactions. In such cases, acupuncture can form the basis of treatment until the medication load is reduced sufficiently so as to be able to include appropriate herbs.

Pathogens can be vented from the ying back towards the qi level, but the course of treatment and prognosis is less predictable. Pathogens generally cannot be vented from the blood and must be cleared in situ. In practice when a patient presents with heat in the deepest levels there are usually aspects of both ying and blood level involvement. Trying to assess how much heat lies in each level can assist in weighting the treatment appropriately.

Pathogens are expelled in unpredictable ways

What happens as a lingering pathogen is vented? Do they retrace their inward journey in reverse? The classics describe an orderly exit fashion through the associated channel pathways, for example from shaoyin to taiyang, jueyin to shaoyang and taiyin to yangming. However, this is not commonly observed, and Lei Shou–Yi, writing in the Discussion of Seasonal Diseases, noted

> '*The outward expression of a lingering pathogen must follow the weak spots in channel qi: there is no certain route out of the body*'

When treating a lingering pathogen successfully, the pathogen is vented and the condition just resolves, but it may follow a more circuitous course as the pathogen changes location. As the pathogen changes location the symptom picture also changes. Sometimes, symptoms may appear to get worse. An increase in fever or fever and chills, sweating, restlessness, constipation, nausea or vomiting may be seen. These changes can indicate that the pathogen is coming up out of the ying level through the qi or shaoyang level. Although this may appear to be an aggravation, it presents a valuable opportunity to more efficiently expel the pathogen. Patients may be alarmed, but courage and a good understanding of possible pathogen progression can avoid premature abandonment of a treatment strategy. Patients will generally accept any perceived aggravation if alerted to the possibility and likely course, and in fact will usually welcome it as a sign of improvement. The tongue and appearance of skin rashes are important indicators as to which direction the pathogen is heading, and to the likely outcome of the treatment (see pp.526–527).

11.5.2 TECHNICAL ASPECTS OF VENTING

1. Encouraging the natural spreading tendency of the pathogen

This is the key feature of the technique and is applicable to heat at any level. Light, pungent, lifting herbs, used in small doses and briefly decocted provide the venting stimulus to the pathogen to dislodge it and nudge it towards an exit point. Qi level and shaoyang heat pathogens are easy to vent, usually with a predictable outcome. Heat in the ying level is more complicated and less predictable. Venting is also be used for damp heat, with additional techniques aimed at promoting healthy fluid metabolism, but the course of treatment is longer.

2. Freeing the surface (keeping the pores open)

Freeing the surface means encouraging the pores to remain open. This is achieved with light pungent herbs, used in doses insufficient to cause diaphoresis, but enough to have an expansive effect on the pores. The aim is to keep the pores open to enable the pathogen to escape. Causing more sweating is contraindicated, as it can exacerbate damage to qi, fluids and yin which may already have occurred due to the heat. Freeing the surface is quite different to the sweat inducing [diaphoretic; *fā hàn* 发汗] method used to expel wind cold from the surface.

3. Promoting Lung function

An essential feature of venting pathogens from the qi level is maintenance of good Lung function. This means encouraging both the diffusion and descent of Lung qi. When we diffuse the Lungs we assist the natural venting of the Lungs, sending fluids and wei qi to the surface. By encouraging the natural descent of Lung qi we maintain the Lungs control over the 'water passages' and urinary flow, and assist the descent of Large Intestine qi and proper elimination through the bowel. These are important exit points for lingering pathogens.

4. Venting with fragrant herbs

Fragrant herbs are a subset of light pungent herbs that have an extra dissipating effect on dampness. The herbs work at the level of the Lungs, Spleen and Stomach, and are used when there is damp heat in the qi level. In addition to breaking up and venting dampness towards the surface and yang organs, they have a stimulating effect on the qi dynamic, thus maintaining elimination through the Intestines.

11.5.2 HARMONIZING

Harmonizing is the method used to expel pathogens from the shaoyang level. In the context of a lingering pathogen, harmonizing has two different connotations. In the first it can be seen as a type of venting, in that it dislodges and lifts pathogens towards the surface, while closing the space available to the pathogen. This aspect is considered to be harmonizing because it gets rid of pathogens without resorting to the relatively harsh pathogen expelling methods such as diaphoresis, purgation or emesis. Harmonizing, in this sense, is a strong pathogen expelling technique, yet unlike the others, is mild enough to be suitable for prolonged use.

The second connotation of harmonizing refers to the technique of balancing the various organ systems and processes responsible for homeostasis, in particular

Table 11.7 Venting herbs

Qi level		
light venting, heat clearing	**Lian Qiao** Forsythiae Fructus 连翘	Forsythia fruit; pungent, cool, bitter; Heart, Lung, Gallbladder, Small Intestine. Cools and vents heat from the qi and ying levels, cools the blood; has the ability to penetrate deeply, hence its use for nodules and heat in the blood.
	Jin Yin Hua Lonicerae Flos 金银花	Honeysuckle flower; sweet, cold; Lung, Stomach, Large Intestine. Vents and clears heat from the qi and ying levels.
	Zhu Ye Phyllostachys Folium 竹叶	Bamboo leaves; sweet, cold, bland; Heart, Stomach, Lung, Small Intestine. Clears heat from the qi level, Lungs and chest; promotes urination to drain damp heat.
	Dan Dou Chi Sojae Semen preparatum 淡豆豉	Prepared soybean; pungent, sweet, cool; Lung, Stomach. Vents heat and diffuses the Lungs to clear heat from the chest. Frequently combined with **xuan shen** or **sheng di** to vent ying level pathogens.
	Bo He Menth haplocalycis Herba 薄荷	Mint; pungent, aromatic, cool; Lung, Liver. Vents heat and rashes from the qi level.
	Ju Hua Chrysanthemi Flos 菊花	Chrysanthemum flower; sweet, bitter, cool; Lung, Liver. Vents heat from the qi level.
	Chai Hu Bupleuri Radix 柴胡	Bupleurum root; pungent, bitter, cool. Liver, Gallbladder, Small Intestine. Vents heat from shaoyang, the qi level and muscle layer.
	Sheng Ma Cimicifugae Rhizoma 升麻	Black cohosh rhizome; pungent, sweet, cool; Lung, Large Intestine, Spleen, Stomach. Vents heat and rashes from the qi level.
	Niu Bang Zi Arctii Fructus 牛蒡子	Burdock seed; pungent, bitter, cold; Lung, Stomach. Vents heat from the qi level and brings rashes to the surface. Also keeps bowels moving to provide another outlet for heat.
strong heat clearing	**Shi Gao** Gypsum fibrosum 石膏	Gypsum; pungent, sweet, very cold; Lung, Stomach. Clears heat from the qi level and vents to the exterior; protects fluids.

Table 11.7 Venting herbs (cont.)

Qi level

diffusing the Lungs	**Xing Ren** Armeniacae Semen 杏仁	Apricot kernel; bitter, warm; Lung, Large Intestine. Diffuses the Lungs and encourages descent of Lung qi; vents pathogens from the qi level and assists Lungs regulation of the water passages.
	Lu Gen Phragmitis Rhizoma 芦根	Phragmites reed; sweet, cold; Lung, Stomach. Clears heat and generates fluids; vents heat from the qi level and promotes urination.
	Jie Geng Platycodi Radix 桔梗	Balloon flower root; pungent, bitter; Lung. Diffuses the Lungs and opens up the flow of Lung qi.
fragrant venting	**Huo Xiang** Pogostemonis/ Agastaches Herba 藿香	Patchouli; pungent, warm; Lung, Spleen, Stomach. Vents pathogens from the exterior, qi level and muscles; diffuses Lung qi and stimulates the qi dynamic.
	Pei Lan Eupatorii Herba 佩兰	Eupatorium; pungent; Spleen, Stomach. Vents pathogens from the exterior, qi level and muscles; diffuses Lung qi and stimulates the qi dynamic.
	Bai Dou Kou Amomi Fructus rotundus 白豆蔻	Round cardamon; pungent, warm, aromatic; Lung, Spleen, Stomach. Diffuses Lung qi, stimulates the Spleen and qi dynamic, lifts and disperses damp.
	Shi Chang Pu Acori tatarinowii Rhizoma 石菖蒲	Acorus; pungent, bitter, warm, aromatic; Stomach, Heart. Rouses the Spleen and disperses dampness and phlegm from the qi level, especially the muscles and head.

Ying level

deep venting, heat clearing	**Qing Hao** Artemisiae annuae Herba 青蒿	Sweet wormwood; bitter, cold, aromatic; Liver, Gallbladder, Kidney. Major herb for venting deep lying pathogens in all levels, qi, ying and shaoyang. Unparalleled ability to dredge and uproot persistent and deeply hidden pathogens.
	Qin Jiao Gentianae macrophyllae Radix 秦艽	Large gentian root; pungent, bitter, cool; Stomach, Liver, Gallbladder. Vents heat from the ying level. An important herb for heat in the ying and blood especially when there is joint pain.

the Liver and Spleen and the qi dynamic. Harmonizing in this sense is aimed at restoring homeostasis, and improving the function of the organ systems involved in defense and general qi regulation, thereby creating a hostile environment and promoting anti–pathogenic qi. The process of maintaining a pathogen in the shaoyang is energetically expensive. The longer a pathogen is held in the shaoyang level, the more the Spleen is drained, and qi deficiency complicates the pathology, so supporting qi production is an essential feature of treatment. The treatment of lingering pathogens in the shaoyang employs both these aspects of harmonizing.

11.5.3 CLEARING DAMP AND DAMP HEAT

In addition to venting, there are additional methods of clearing damp and damp heat. The combined pathology of yin dampness and yang heat produces a more resistant pathogen and complicates treatment. The damp wraps the heat and prevents it escaping, while the heat congeals and thickens the damp, and makes it harder to eliminate. The longer a damp heat pathogen persists the more complex it becomes and the more damage to the Spleen, qi and yin ensues.

General principles

There are two main components to the treatment of damp heat lingering pathogens; venting towards the surface or a drainage channel, and maximizing the efficiency of fluid metabolism. In general, we focus on eliminating the dampness, because by so doing, heat is liberated and more easily vented.

The treatment of damp heat involves venting with light, cool and fragrant herbs, and promotion of healthy function of the organs of fluid metabolism, the Lungs, Spleen and Kidneys.

There are four techniques, and the proportion of each technique used in any particular treatment will vary depending on the relative balance of damp and heat, and the depth and location of the pathogen. In the common formulae for qi level damp heat, all four methods are represented.

1. Promote Lung function

This method is the same one employed in general venting. The aim is to stimulate the Lung diffusion (*xuān* 宣) to the surface and promote normal descent of Lung qi and maintenance of the 'water passages'. Diffusing the Lungs pushes damp heat towards the surface. Promoting descent of Lung qi and governance of the water passages, assists in maintaining adequate urinary flow and stimulating the bowels to provide additional outlets for the damp.

2. Dry damp in the middle burner and rectify the qi dynamic

This method employs pungent warm herbs and, sparingly, bitter cold herbs to dry damp and clear heat from the middle burner and keep things moving through the Intestines. The pungent warmth of the herbs disperses and lifts damp off the Spleen and frees up the natural ascent of Spleen qi, while the bitterness dries the damp and assists the descent of Stomach qi. The sum total of these effects is to free and stimulate the qi dynamic, and encourage its proper operation. A healthy qi dynamic further assists transformation and elimination of damp.

Figure 11.16 Summary of venting techniques

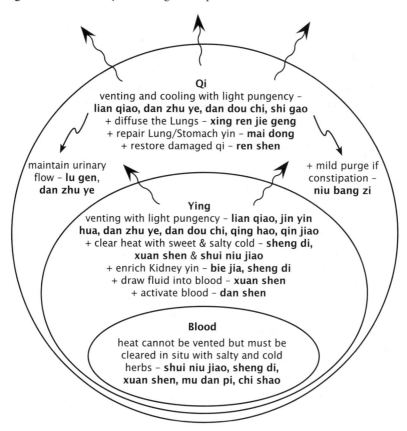

Freeing the qi dynamic, the pivot for triple burner qi movement, has ramifications beyond the middle burner and elimination through the Intestines. By encouraging normal qi movement it promotes good organ function in all three burners. This is the main treatment method when digestive symptoms and signs of disruption to the qi dynamic are prominent.

3. Provide an outlet for the damp by promoting urinary flow

Bland diuretic herbs are included to ensure the water passages remain open and clear. Gentle herbs with a mild damp leaching action are preferred. Herbs that combine a venting and damp draining effect are particularly useful (see Table 11.7, pp.532–533). This technique is included to one degree or another in all damp heat treatments. Care must be used when using diuretic herbs, however, to avoid excessive diuresis and damage to yin. This is especially the case when there is concurrent yin deficiency.

4. Drain heat with bitter cold herbs

The more heat, the more bitter cold herbs can be employed, although always in relatively small amounts. This is especially appropriate when heat is significantly disturbing the shen. These herbs must be used with caution, however, and practitioners should be mindful of the fact that bitter contracts, pulls inward and descends, while cold freezes and constricts, all actions that are in opposition to the expansive opening intended with venting. Therefore, while bitter cold herbs are sometimes required, small quantities, around ¼ – ⅓ of a normal dose, should be used to avoid the potential problem of locking the pathogen in place.

11.5.4 CLEARING HEAT FROM THE YING AND BLOOD

In addition to venting pathogens from the ying level towards the surface, heat must be cooled, the yin replenished and fluid drawn back into the blood so it can flow. Once heat has reached the blood it generally cannot be vented and must be cleared in situ. Bitter cold heat clearing herbs are generally not used, or are used only in small amounts, in combination with herbs that promote expulsion of heat.

The best heat clearing herbs for ying and blood level heat are those that are salty and cold, or sweet and cold. The saltiness goes to the Kidneys and has a softening and yin protecting effect while strongly cooling heat. The sweetness protects and generates fluids and yin. Cooling herbs that activate and draw fluid back into the blood are always included, as blood is invariably dried out, thickened, and stagnant. Salty herbs are required to replenish the fluid portion of blood sufficiently to enable blood to flow again.

11.5.5 RESTORING QI AND YIN

The restoration of fluids, yin and qi is necessary when they have been damaged. Fluid and qi damage always occurs in lingering qi level heat patterns, and the prescriptions for venting qi level pathogens takes this damage into account in their construction. Damaged fluids and superficial yin (Lung and Stomach surfaces) are replenished with the mild, shallow acting and fluid moistening yin supplements.

Damage to the deeper yin of the Kidneys and Liver is most likely in prolonged patterns when heat and sweating have been quite severe, or when a heat pathogen affects the ying and blood. In all cases of ying and blood heat, the yin will require replenishment. This is necessary not only to rebuild the yin but also to fortify it sufficiently to be able to expel the pathogen and throw it off, with the help of the venting herbs. Formulae for treating ying and blood level heat always include Kidney yin enriching herbs, which must be used at the same time as the heat venting and blood cooling herbs.

In the shaoyang level, it is usually the qi that is damaged due to the energy required to contain the pathogen. Harmonizing formulae always include qi supplements and Spleen strengthening herbs.

After a pathogen has been expelled, patients are often left with residual qi and yin damage. Getting rid of the pathogen usually leads to a significant improvement in symptoms, but treatment often needs to continue for a period of time to repair the damage done by the pathogen.

Figure 11.17 Main principles of damp and damp heat treatment

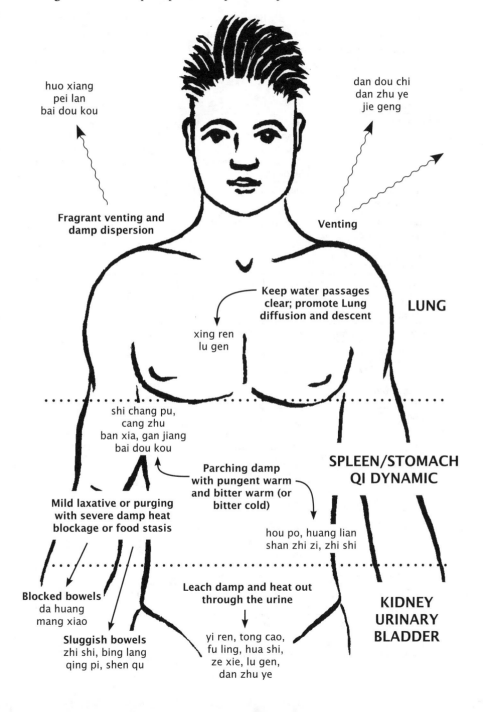

11.6 ACUPUNCTURE PROTOCOLS

Although herbs have historically been the primary modality for treating lingering pathogens, venting pathogens from the qi and shaoyang levels with acupuncture can also be effective. Treatment of ying and blood level pathogens is difficult and less reliable when using acupuncture alone.

Qi level

Heat

Lu.7 lieque	the main point to vent pathogens from the qi and shaoyang levels; diffuses the Lungs and directs Lung qi downwards thereby encouraging movement from inside to out, and up to down and out (via the Urinary Bladder)
LI.11 quchi St.44 neiting	clear heat from the qi level and yangming
Du.14 dazhui Du.13 taodao Du.12 shenzhu	clear lingering heat from the yang portion of the body
with fluid damage	+ Kid.6 zhaohai
with cough	+ Lu.5 chize or Lu.6 kongzui and Ren.17 shanzhong
with nausea and vomiting	+ PC.6 neiguan
with constipation	+ St.25 tianshu and St.37 shangjuxu
with muscle weakness and aches	+ Sp.21 dabao and GB.34 yanglingquan

Damp heat

Lu.7 lieque	the main point to vent pathogens from the qi level; diffuses the Lungs and directs Lung qi downwards thereby encouraging movement from inside to out, and up to down and out (via the Urinary Bladder)
Ren.12 zhongwan	stimulates the qi dynamic
Sp.9 yinlingquan	promotes urination and drains damp
St.36 zusanli	strengthens the Spleen and stimulates the qi dynamic
Bl.39 weiyang	keeps the Urinary Bladder water passage open
Kid.7 fuliu	promotes urination and vents pathogens
LI.11 quchi	clears damp heat
Du.14 dazhui	vents heat from the qi level
with muscle aches and joint pain	+ Sp.21 dabao, GB.34 yanglingquan and Bl.11 dazhu
with nausea and vomiting	+ PC.6 neiguan
with diarrhea or sluggish stools	+ St.25 tianshu and St.37 shangjuxu

Shaoyang

Lu.7 lieque	the main point to vent pathogens from the qi and shaoyang levels due to its ability to encourage movement in general from the inside to the outside
SJ.5 waiguan GB.41 zulinqi	vents pathogens from, and closes off, the shaoyang level
SJ.5 waiguan GB.39 xuanzhong	vents pathogens from the shaoyang level; used instead of the above points when sleep disturbances are a feature
GB.34 yanglingquan SJ.6 zhigou	used when there is lateral pain, headaches, rib pain and sluggish stools
Sp.9 yinlingquan St.36 zusanli Bl.39 weiyang LI.11 quchi Bl.22 sanjiaoshu	for damp heat; these points clear heat, drain damp, strengthen the Spleen, stimulate the qi dynamic and maintains urinary flow

Ying

Kid.7 fuliu	vents pathogens from the ying level and shaoyin and promotes urination
Kid.3 taixi	replenishes damaged yin
Bl.23 shenshu Bl.15 xinshu Bl.18 ganshu	clear heat from the organ systems at the deepest level; improve organ function
SI.3 houxi Bl.62 shenmai Lu.7 lieque Kid.6 zhaohai	Master and couple points of dumai and renmai, used together to activate the central dynamo of the body and mobilize yang qi. By activating yang qi systemically, deep lying pathogens can be encouraged towards the surface or an exit point. Can be connected across the body with ion pumping cords to create a figure eight pattern (i.e. left SI.3 connected to right Bl.62; right Lu.7 connected to left Kid.6) for 10–15 minutes. If the patient feels odd or agitated change the polarity.

Blood

PC.3 quze Bl.40 weizhong	these points cool the blood when bled or needled with vigor
LI.11 quchi Sp.10 xuehai Liv.2 xingjian Sp.6 sanyinjiao	cool the blood, cool the Liver and nourish yin and fluids
Kid.3 taixi Kid.6 zhaohai	to help preserve yin
SI.3 houxi Bl.62 shenmai Lu.7 lieque Kid.6 zhaohai	Master and couple points of dumai and renmai. See ying level treatment above.

Table 11.8 Patterns of lingering pathogens seen in the authors practices.

Location	Key features	Pattern	Other symptoms	Prescription
Wei level (taiyang)	• floating pulse • swollen glands	Wind in the skin; ying wei disharmony	clammy skin, itchy skin lesions that are worse for cold weather and changes of weather	Gui Zhi Tang p.76
		Cold in the surface with qi deficiency[1]	persistent runny or congested nose in clammy, listless children	Shen Su Yin p.79
Qi level[2]	• low grade fever • dryness, thirst • sweating • fatigue • swollen glands • muscle weakness or aching • insomnia • restlessness, irritability • dry or peeled tongue coat	Heat in the Lungs, with qi and fluid damage[3]	dry hacking cough that is worse at night; respiratory allergies	Zhu Ye Shi Gao Tang p.370
		Heat in the Stomach, with qi and fluid damage[4]	nausea, vomiting, dry retching, indeterminate gnawing hunger; food intolerances or allergies	Zhu Ye Shi Gao Tang p.370
		Heat in the chest[5]	restlessness and fitful sleep, marked irritability, depression, burning sensation and sweating on the chest	Zhi Zi Chi Tang p.371
		Heat and cold in the qi level and middle burner; qi dynamic disruption[6]	epigastric fullness, acid, reflux, nausea, belching, diarrhea	Ban Xia Xie Xin Tang, p.914
		Heat and phlegm accumulating in the tonsils[7]	chronically swollen tonsils, chronic sore throat, dysphagia	Add Xiao Luo Wan p.921 to appropriate prescription

1 Seen in those who catch cold while weak or run down.
2 The more heat, the more dryness and hypersensitivity of tissues and mucous membranes, and the more influence on the shen.
3 Qi level heat concentrated in the Lungs usually follows an upper respiratory or vaccination. Can last months.
4 Qi level heat concentrated in the Stomach follows gastrointestinal infection or ingestion of toxic substances like chemotherapy. Can last months.
5 Qi level heat concentrated in the chest follows an inappropriate purge or enema given for a surface pattern. Can last months.
6 Can follow an acute surface pattern that was treated by purgation or enema, or a disorder characterized by severe vomiting. This type of disruption can occur for reasons other than an external pathogen, but will then lack the swollen glands, fever and sweating.
7 May display features of a qi or shaoyang level disorder. Most common in adolescents, who have had multiple courses of antibiotics.

Table 11.8 Patterns of lingering pathogens seen in the authors practices (cont).

Location	Key features	Pattern		Other symptoms	Prescription
Qi level	• low grade fever • tiredness, fatigue • sweating • muscle and joint aches • swollen glands • vesicular skin lesions • mucus congestion, serous discharge • thick tongue coat	Damp heat[1]	damp > heat	heaviness, pronounced muscle aches, white tongue coat	Huo Po Xia Ling Tang p.84
			damp = heat	fatigue, heaviness and muscle aches, contained fever, mixed white/yellow tongue coat	San Ren Tang p.375
			heat > damp	afternoon fever, night sweats or sweating on the head, yellow tongue coat	Lian Po Yin p.377
		Phlegm heat[2]		fatigue, anxiety, palpitations, insomnia, dizziness, nausea	Wen Dan Tang p.87
Shaoyang	• alternating fever and chills • swollen glands • fatigue • dizziness • nausea • loss of appetite • lateral pathology (temporal headache, TMJ pain, lesions on the sides of the body etc.)	Heat[3]		fever > chills, food tastes bad, hypochondriac pain	Xiao Chai Hu Tang p.373
		Damp heat[4]		muscle aches, chills and fever starting in the afternoon, sticky sweat, greasy yellow tongue coat	Hao Qin Qing Dan Tang p.373
		plus Taiyang[5]		chills > fever, joint and muscle aches (neck, upper and lower back), creaking joints	Chai Hu Gui Zhi Tang p.90
		plus Yangming		constipation or clay like stools, frequent vomiting, fever > chills, abdominal pain	Da Chai Hu Tang p.91

1 Generally more common in hot humid climates, but often seen in societies with an overabundance of food, a sweet, rich diet, and high level of alcohol consumption. Can persist for years. Repeated antibiotics are common, and decrease heat but promote damp.
2 Follows in the aftermath of a high fever, the heat of which is required to quickly congeal normal fluids into phlegm.
3 The fatigue is often the main complaint, and when particularly tired, patients may complain of feeling 'fluey' or hot and cold. The more prolonged the pattern, the more qi deficiency and Spleen weakness intervene. Can last months or years.
4 More common in the tropics, unusual in temperate climates. Can last months or years.
5 Can look as if there is no heat due to the residual pathogen on the surface, especially when chills or cold intolerance are prominent. This is a common pattern in children.

Table 11.8 Patterns of lingering pathogens seen in the authors practices (cont).

Location	Key features	Pattern	Other symptoms	Prescription
Ying	• recurrent low grade fever at night • dryness	joint pain and inflammation, vasculitis, mouth ulcers, insomnia, weight loss, transitory skin rashes that flare at night		Qing Ying Tang p.349 Qing Hao Bie Jia Tang p.381
Blood	• fatigue and exhaustion • swollen glands • red or crimson, dry tongue with no coat	bleeding, distinct purple skin rashes, disturbances of consciousness, irrational behavior, personality change, joint pain, vasculitis, tics, tremors and spasms		Shui Niu Jiao Di Huang Tang p.351
Shaoyin[1]	• lower back ache • urinary disfunction • tinnitus, hearing loss	Heat transformation	facial flushing, night sweats, dysuria, insomnia, anxiety, palpitations, joint inflammation, red dry tongue	Tian Wang Bu Xin Dan p.147
		Cold transformation	cold intolerance, urinary frequency and nocturia or edema and oliguria, stiff swollen aching joints, pale swollen tongue	Jin Gui Shen Qi Wan p.826 Zhen Wu Tang p.249
Jueyin[2]	• cold below, heat above	thirst, flushing, restlessness and confusion, muscle spasms and tremor, vertigo, frequent urination and diarrhea, cold legs and feet		Wu Mei Wan p.921

1 Can be due to factors other than pathogen invasion, and rarely diagnosed as a lingering pathogenic problem, except in hindsight, as the pathogen emerges during the course of treatment.
2 An rare presentation, and in clinic one that should ring alarm bells.

MUSCLE WEAKNESS AND ATROPHY

Muscle weakness and atrophy is based on the Chinese disease of *wěi zhèng*[1] 痿证. Wei zheng represents a group of disorders characterized by muscular weakness, loss of motor control, wasting and paralysis. The onset of muscular weakness can be sudden or gradual. If atrophy occurs, it happens gradually, slowly complicating the weakness. Sudden onset of weakness may occur in the aftermath of an infectious illness, with weakness and eventual atrophy developing over a period of weeks. In the majority of cases, however, the symptoms develop progressively, starting with minor weakness and loss of function or sensory change, tingling, numbness, loss of tendon reflexes or foot drop. Finally, paralysis and atrophy may intervene.

> **BOX 12.1 PATTERNS OF MUSCLE WEAKNESS AND ATROPHY**
>
> Lung and Stomach heat
> Damp heat
> Phlegm damp
> Spleen and Stomach qi deficiency
> Qi and blood deficiency
> Blood stasis
> Liver and Kidney yin deficiency
> Spleen and Kidney yang deficiency

Muscle weakness and atrophy is caused by pathology of the muscle tissue or of the motor nerves that supply the muscles. In general, with muscle pathology, tendon reflexes are still present, despite weakness. Weakness is principal feature, with wasting minimal or absent, and there are no sensory changes or fasciculation. When the lesion is neurological, reflexes are diminished or absent, wasting is greater than weakness, and there are sensory changes, numbness, fasciculation and tremors.

The disorders described in the chapter are often serious and debilitating conditions for which orthodox medicine has few effective treatments. Depending on the condition, Chinese medicine can be an effective management tool, and while rarely curative, can often assist physical function and arrest further deterioration.

The Chinese medical viewpoint

The first description of muscle weakness and atrophy appears in the Huang Di Nei Jing Su Wen (Simple Questions, Chapter 44), where five types are described.

1. **Vessel** (*mài wěi* 脉痿) : atrophy and weakness of the lower limbs caused by heat affecting the Heart and blood vessels.
2. **Flesh** (*ròu wěi* 肉痿): numbness in the skin, atrophy, flaccidity and weakness of the muscles, caused by dampness and damp heat invading the muscles and Spleen, and damaging fluids and yin.
3. **Bone** (*gǔ wěi* 骨痿) : atrophy of the lower limbs and weakness of the waist and spine making sitting up difficult, caused by exhaustion of Kidney yin and jing, with deficient fire that dries out the tissues
4. **Sinew** (*jīn wěi* 筋痿) : muscle contraction, spasm and loss of sensation, caused by deficiency of Liver blood

---

1 Practical Dictionary of Chinese Medicine (1998) – 'wilting patterns'

5. **Skin** (*pí wěi* 皮痿): cracked and brittle skin with weakness in the extremities caused by heat affecting the Lungs

The common thread of these ancient descriptions is heat drying fluids leading to failure of nourishment of the various tissues, with consequent weakness and withering. Today our analysis is broader, and incorporates other pathogens observed in atrophy and weakness patterns, in particular phlegm damp and blood stasis.

The main organ systems involved in the acute onset of weakness and atrophy are the Lungs, Stomach and Spleen. In the chronic or slowly progressive patterns, pathology of the Spleen, Liver and Kidney is responsible. The Spleen is in charge of maintaining the tone, bulk and strength of skeletal muscles. The Liver presides over the sinews, and is responsible for maintenance of smooth and coordinated movement of the limbs and joints. The Kidney rules the bones and articulations, and the integrity of the musculoskeletal system as a whole. Spleen pathology leads to weakness and wasting of the muscles, while Liver pathology leads to dryness and tightness of the sinews, causing stiffness and loss of function and mobility. All chronic pathology drains the Kidneys, which leads to an increased loss of yin structure (and atrophy of all involved tissues) and yang function, with more serious wasting and weakness, to the point of immobility.

ETIOLOGY

External pathogens

Invasion by external pathogens is seen in both acute onset and slowly progressive cases of muscular weakness and atrophy. A strong wind heat or warm disease (*wēn*

BOX 12.2 KEY DIAGNOSTIC POINTS

Weakness
- without wasting – damp heat, phlegm damp, early stages of Spleen qi deficiency, acute onset of qi and blood deficiency

Atrophy
- more pronounced than weakness – Liver and Kidney yin deficiency, Spleen and Kidney yang deficiency

Muscle tone
- flaccid – Spleen yang qi deficiency
- spastic, cramping – qi and blood deficiency
- weak yet without major loss of tone – damp heat, phlegm damp

Onset
- acute – Lung and Stomach heat, damp heat, blood stasis, qi and blood deficiency
- gradual – damp heat, Spleen qi deficiency, qi and blood deficiency, Liver and Kidney yin deficiency, Spleen and Kidney yang deficiency

Worse for
- heat – damp heat
- activity – Spleen qi deficiency, qi and blood deficiency, yin and yang deficiency
- prolonged inactivity – damp heat, phlegm damp

bìng) pathogen was historically the most frequent cause of the paralysis and muscle wasting we now associate with poliomyelitis. While less common in the West than it once was, thanks to public health measures and vaccination, it still occurs in some parts of Asia, Africa and South America. The wind heat or warm pathogen invades the qi level, the Lungs and Stomach. Heat in the qi level directly damages fluids and yin, depletes zheng qi, and ultimately plunders Kidney yin. The damaged yin and fluids are unable to nourish and maintain the muscles and sinews. The typical pattern of onset is muscular weakness in the lower limbs a week or so after the onset of a wind heat pattern.

BOX 12.3 BIOMEDICAL CAUSES OF WEAKNESS AND ATROPHY

- acute inflammatory polyneuritis (Guillain–Barré syndrome)
- acute myelitis, poliomyelitis
- weakness following an infection of the central nervous system, such as encephalitis and meningitis
- myasthenia gravis
- muscular dystrophy
- motor neurone disease
- progressive myopathy
- amyotrophic lateral sclerosis
- multiple sclerosis
- sequelae of stroke
- periodic paralysis
- peripheral neuropathy
  – drug related
  – diabetes
  – vitamin deficiency

External dampness and damp heat are the other pathogens responsible for muscle weakness and atrophy. Dampness generally doesn't cause an acute illness, but seeps into the tissues gradually, slowly compromising the circulation of qi and blood and the strength and function of the peripheral muscles. The damp in the muscles blocks qi and blood movement creating heat and damp heat. The damp can be contracted by chronic exposure to damp or humid conditions, such as living in a damp house, prolonged habitation in damp climates or by frequent exposure to water.

Damp heat is usually the product of chronic damp in the muscles, and is thus associated with the gradual development of weakness and atrophy. It can occasionally be more acute, when a seasonal damp heat pathogen invades the qi level.

Diet

The most common dietary habits that contribute to weakness and atrophy are those that weaken the Spleen, lead to qi and blood deficiency, or generate dampness and damp heat.

Restrictive or fad diets are a common cause of Spleen qi and yang deficiency. Diets low in protein lead to blood deficiency. Prolonged starvation or digestive insult seriously damages Spleen yang qi. Overuse of slimming aids that suppress the appetite has the same potential to damage Spleen qi. A diet too biased towards cold natured or raw food weakens Spleen qi and yang. Some herbs and drugs weaken the Spleen and deplete Spleen qi and yang or create dampness. These include heat clearing herbs, hypoglycemic agents (Box 4.2, p.167) and antihypertensive drugs, purgative laxatives and antibiotics. Eating irregularly, missing meals, eating at odd hours or late at night weakens the Spleen and Stomach.

Figure 12.1 Etiology and pathology of atrophy and weakness

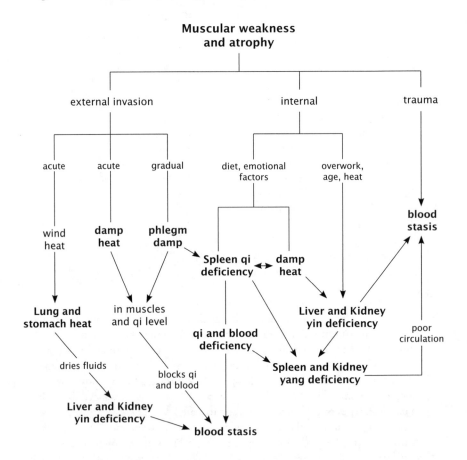

Overconsumption in general, and excessive consumption of alcohol or rich, heating or supplementing foods and herbs in particular, contribute to dampness and damp heat. An excess of heating foods, such as chilies, coffee, spirits, spices, fats and meat can introduce heat and damage yin. The inappropriate or excessive use of supplementing or hot herbs, such as aconite or red ginseng can easily contribute to internal heat and yin damage.

Emotional factors

The emotional factors that impact upon the Spleen, Kidney and Liver are significant in contributing to the development of weakness and atrophy. The Liver is affected by anger, frustration and repressed emotion, while worry, rumination, obsessive thinking, sadness and prolonged concentration, in combination with

BOX 12.4 POINTS TO ACTIVATE QI AND BLOOD, FOR ALL PATTERNS OF WEAKNESS AND ATROPHY

As a general principle, body points to influence weakness and wasting on the limbs are selected from the yangming channels as they are the repository of qi and blood. These points can be treated with electroacupuncture for patients with excess patterns. Moxibustion should be used for yang qi and blood deficiency patterns. Scalp acupuncture is also helpful (Box 12.5, p.550).

Face
- GB.14 (yangbai) → yuyao (M–HN–6)
- St.2 (sibai) → St.4 (dicang)
- St.4 (dicang) → St.6 (jiache)
- St.6 (jiache) → St.7 (xiaguan)

Arm
- LI.15 (jianyu)
- LI.11 (quchi)
- LI.10 (shousanli)
- LI.4 (hegu)
- SJ.5 (waiguan)
- SI.3 (houxi)
- Du.14 (dazhui)
- Huatuo Jiaji points from T1–T5

Leg
- St.31 (biguan)
- St.32 (futu)
- St.36 (zusanli)
- St.38 (tiaokou)
- St.40 (fenglong)
- St.41 (jiexi)
- GB.30 (huantiao)
- GB.34 (yanglingquan)
- GB.39 (xuanzhong)
- GB.40 (qiuxu)
- Du.3 (yaoyangguan)
- Du.4 (mingmen)
- Huatuo Jiaji points from L2–L5

a sedentary life–style and poor diet, weaken the Spleen. Any of these emotional factors, if prolonged or extreme, can disrupt the function of the Liver and Spleen, or cause the Liver to invade the Spleen. This then leads to deficiency of qi and blood, creation of dampness and a failure of the Spleen to nourish the muscles. Chronic Liver qi constraint may also lead to blood stasis, phlegm accumulation or heat which can deplete yin.

Sudden shock, extreme fear or terror, or a major life upheaval, as may occur in an accident, following the death of a loved one, or as the result of a profound physical or emotional trauma, can damage the Kidneys and shaoyin, drain them of vitality and damage yang qi and yin.

Trauma
A significant trauma to a limb, the spine or the head can lead to weakness and atrophy, due to blood stasis in the channels.

Constitution
A constitutional weakness of the Kidneys or Spleen may predispose a patient to more easily develop weakness and atrophy in response to other factors such as diet and external pathogenic invasion.

PATHOLOGY
The weakness and atrophy described in this chapter affects the skeletal muscles

Figure 12.2 Degrees of severity of muscular weakness and atrophy

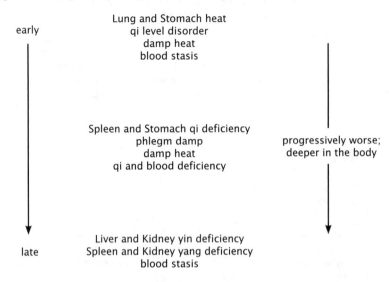

and sinews. It may be confined to the muscle layer with little internal organ system involvement, but more commonly there is a mixture of muscle and organ pathology. By the time symptoms of weakness or wasting have developed the functions of the Spleen, Liver or Kidneys are likely to be compromised. In clinical practice, patients with muscular weakness and atrophy usually present with a composite of different patterns. The natural history usually follows a progression from an excess condition in the early stages, to a mixed excess and deficiency condition in the mid to late stages. The pathology of the early stages contributes to the pathology of the latter stages. For example, heat in the Lungs and Stomach or damp heat will damage yin and can lead to Liver and Kidney yin deficiency. Dampness in the muscles will gradually weaken the Spleen and lead to Spleen qi deficiency, qi and blood deficiency or Spleen and Kidney yang deficiency.

Although an excess pattern is most commonly seen in the early stages of weakness and atrophy, this is not always the case. Sometimes deficiency patterns can occur suddenly or develop quickly, and may be seen in muscle weakness of recent onset. An example is a major hemorrhage that causes sudden onset of qi and blood deficiency. Similarly, the late stages of a weakness and wasting condition are most commonly associated with profound deficiency, however, there are cases where an excess of some type is the principal feature, such as the blood stasis that frequently complicates yin and yang deficiency.

DIFFERENTIAL DIAGNOSIS

Painful obstruction syndrome (*bì zhèng* 痹证): Both painful obstruction and muscular weakness and atrophy may exhibit numbness, heaviness and atrophy, but painful obstruction syndrome is focused on pain, which is usually absent or minimal in atrophy and weakness patterns.

Hemiplegia (*piān kū* 偏枯): Atrophy and weakness of the limbs on one side of the body are symptoms of hemiplegia. The upper and/or lower limb may be affected and there may be facial paralysis and slurring speech. Hemiplegia follows a wind–stroke, and although considered distinct (usually analyzed within the Chinese medical disease diagnosis of wind–stroke), there are obvious overlaps, so some of the patterns in this section can apply to hemiplegia.

Hysteria (*yì bìng* 癔病): A neurotic disorder characterized by periodic paralysis and loss of function, but without residual symptoms once the episode has passed.

TREATMENT

Muscular weakness and atrophy can be continuous and progressive, or intermittent, with periods of active disease and remission. During the active phase, treatment needs to be frequent and persistent, with a minimum of two acupuncture treatments per week, in combination with herbs, to stabilize the condition and try and prevent further deterioration. During periods of remission appropriate constitutional treatment is vigorously pursued to correct the underlying imbalance. As the maintenance phase begins, treatments can be spaced out to weekly, fortnightly or monthly, depending on how the patient holds up in between. Maintenance of the immune system and swift intervention in any acute viral or other external pathogenic invasion are important factors that can help prevent relapse.

Duration of treatment is usually long, with a minimum of 3–6 months required to make a significant impact in long standing cases. Six to eight weeks at a minimum is needed to assess whether the treatment is working, and as change in weakness and atrophy cases is likely to be slow, persistence is the key to success.

In addition to acupuncture and herbal treatment, physical activities such as taijiquan and qigong can be helpful in improving muscle control and balance and calming the shen.

Muscular weakness and wasting patterns can often be difficult depending on the biomedical disease involved. When nerves and muscles are seriously damaged, cure is unlikely. Many patients, however, can receive significant benefit in terms of improvement in wellbeing and function, a slowing of the progress of the condition and better quality of life. Depending on the condition, treatment and appropriate lifestyle changes need to be ongoing to maintain any benefits attained, and the earlier treatment commences, the better the outcome.

BOX 12.5 SCALP ACUPUNCTURE

Scalp acupuncture is a simple and convenient technique for weakness and atrophy. It is particularly useful when patients are immobile, have significant spasticity or twitching of the limbs, or it is simply difficult to do a systemic treatment. Treatment can be done with the patient sitting comfortably. Points can be selected from the relevant areas on the scalp and needled obliquely along the line being treated.

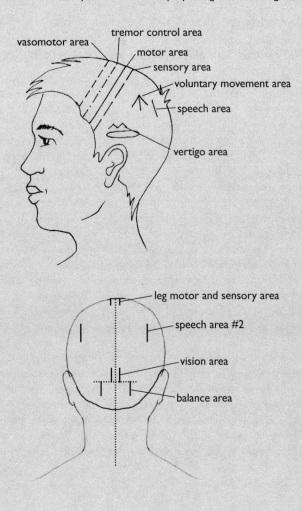

肺胃热津伤 12.1 LUNG AND STOMACH HEAT WITH FLUID DAMAGE

Lung and Stomach heat is due to invasion of wind heat or a warm disease pathogen (*wēn bìng* 温病). It is an acute pattern, most common in children and young people, in which paralysis or loss of motor function follows an upper respiratory tract infection. Heat invades the Lungs, Stomach and qi level, consumes qi, and damages yin and fluids. The qi level is aligned with the muscles, and thus the damaged yin and fluids fail to moisten and nourish the muscles and sinews, resulting in weakness, dryness, loss of function and gradual atrophy.

Clinical features

- Gradual and progressive weakness and flaccidity of the limbs, usually the legs, a week or so following the onset of an acute episode of high fever. Atrophy may develop gradually over weeks to months.
- headache, stiff neck, photophobia, cough
- thirst, dry mouth, throat and mucous membranes
- dry, cracked skin
- dry, unproductive cough
- concentrated urine
- constipation
- cervical lymphadenopathy

T red or red tip with a thin, dry, yellow coat
P thready, rapid

Treatment Principle

Clear heat from the Lungs and Stomach
Moisten dryness and generate fluids

Prescription

QING ZAO JIU FEI TANG 清燥救肺汤
Eliminate Dryness and Rescue the Lungs Decoction

This prescription is suitable when the condition is still relatively acute.

shi gao (Gypsum fibrosum) 石膏 18–30g
sang ye (Mori Folium) 桑叶 6–9g
mai dong (Ophiopogonis Radix) 麦冬 6–9g
hei zhi ma (Sesame Semen nigrum) 黑芝麻 6–9g
zhi pi pa ye (honey fried Eriobotryae Folium) 炙枇杷叶 6–9g
e jiao (Asini Corii Colla) 阿胶 6–9g
xing ren (Armeniacae Semen) 杏仁 6–9g
ren shen (Ginseng Radix) 人参 3–6g
gan cao (Glycyrrhizae Radix) 甘草 3–6g

Method: Decoction. **Shi gao** is decocted for 30 minutes prior to the other herbs, **e jiao** is melted into the strained decoction. The sweet coldness of **shi gao** and **mai dong** cools and moistens the Lungs; **sang ye**, **xing ren** and **zhi pi pa ye** diffuse the Lungs and direct Lung qi downward to stop cough; **e jiao** and **hei zhi ma** nourish Lung yin; **ren shen** and **gan cao** supplement and support Lung qi; **ren shen** generates fluids and with **mai dong** assist in moistening the Lungs. (Source: *Zhong Yi Nei Ke Xue* [*Yi Men Fa Lu*])

Modifications

- With persistent high fever and profuse sweating, use 60–90 grams of **shi gao** and add **jin yin hua** (Lonicerae Flos) 金银花 15–30g and **lian qiao** (Forsythiae Fructus) 连翘 9–12g.

- With persistent dry cough, add **gua lou** (Trichosanthis Fructus) 栝楼 15–24g, **chuan bei mu** (Fritillariae cirrhosae Bulbus) 川贝母 9–12g and **sang bai pi** (Mori Cortex) 桑白皮 9–12g.

- With severe thirst and dryness, add **tian hua fen** (Trichosanthes Radix) 天花粉 15–30g, **sha shen** (Glehniae/Adenophorae Radix) 沙参 9–12g and **lu gen** (Phragmitis Rhizoma) 芦根 60g.

- With toxic heat, malaise, stiff neck and vomiting add **da qing ye** (Isatidis Folium) 大青叶 15–30g and **ban lan gen** (Isatidis/Baphicacanthis Radix) 板蓝根 30g.

Variations and additional prescriptions

Stomach yin deficiency

A few weeks after the initial wind heat, the damage to Stomach yin and fluids becomes more apparent. At this stage the fever has receded, but the thirst and dryness are severe, the patient has no appetite or is nauseous and dry retches, and the tongue is peeled in the center. The treatment is to replenish Stomach yin and fluids, and protect the source of qi and blood, with YI WEI TANG (Benefit the Stomach Decoction 益胃汤), modified.

bei sha shen (Glehniae Radix) 北沙参	9–12g
mai dong (Ophiopogonis Radix) 麦冬	12–15g
sheng di (Rehmanniae Radix) 生地	12–15g
yu zhu (Polygonati odorati Rhizoma) 玉竹	12–15g
bing tang (rock sugar) 冰糖	6g
yi ren (Coicis Semen) 苡仁	15–30g
shan yao (Dioscoreae Rhizoma) 山药	12–15g
gu ya (Setariae Fructus germinatus) 谷芽	15–30g

Method: Decoction. **Bei sha shen**, **mai dong** and **yu zhu** nourish Stomach yin and fluids; **sheng di** nourishes yin and cools the blood; **yi ren** strengthens the Spleen and clears damp heat; **shan yao** strengthens the Spleen, supplements qi and benefits Stomach yin; **gu ya** benefits digestion and improves the appetite; **bing tang** harmonizes the Spleen and Stomach. (Source: *Zhong Yi Nei Ke Xue* [*Wen Bing Tiao Bian*])

Phlegm and blood stasis

As the result of a high fever, fluids can be quickly congealed into phlegm and the blood dried and damaged. The patient has recovered from the fever, but weakness and flaccidity of the limbs remains. In addition, qi deficiency, blood stasis and phlegm are apparent in the fatigue, pallor, mottling and numbness of the hands and feet, confusion, weak choppy pulse and pale tongue with purple stasis spots. The treatment at this stage is to activate qi and blood, transform phlegm and open up the channels and network vessels with BU YANG HUAN WU TANG (Supplement Yang to Restore Five Tenths Decoction 补阳还五汤, p.600), plus **shi chang pu** (Acori tatarinowii Rhizoma) 石菖蒲 and **yu jin** (Curcumae Radix) 郁金.

Prepared medicines

Concentrated powders

Qing Zao Jiu Fei Tang (Eriobotrya & Ophiopogon Combination)

Zhu Ye Shi Gao Tang (Bamboo Leaves & Gypsum Combination)

   – post acute residual heat and dryness with qi and fluid damage

Sha Shen Mai Men Dong Tang (Glehnia & Ophiopogon Combination)

   – Stomach yin deficiency

Bu Yang Huan Wu Tang (Astragalus & Peony Combination)

Pills

Yang Yin Qing Fei Wan (Pills to Nourish Yin and Cool the Lungs)

Sha Shen Mai Men Dong Wan (Autumn Rain Teapills)

Bu Yang Huan Wu Wan (Great Yang Restoration Teapills)

Acupuncture (select from)

In addition to points chosen according to the affected limbs (Box 12.4, p.547) select from the following:

Lu.7 (lieque).....................vents heat from the qi level

Du.14 (dazhui –)...............meeting point of the yang channels, clears heat from the qi level, Lungs and Stomach

LI.11 (quchi –)...................sea point of the Large Intestine, dispels wind and clears heat from the qi level, Lungs and Stomach

LI.4 (hegu –).....................source point of the Large Intestine, clears heat, dispels wind heat and diffuses the Lungs

SJ.5 (waiguan –) ....connecting point of the triple burner, dispels wind and clears heat

Bl.13 (feishu – Ω) ....back transport point of the Lungs, diffuses the Lungs, clears heat and directs Lung qi downward

St.34 (liangqiu –) ....cleft point of the Stomach, clears heats from the Stomach and activates qi and blood in the legs

Sp.6 (sanyinjiao +)..............nourishes yin and fluids

Kid.6 (zhaohai +) ....nourishes Kidney yin and benefits fluids

- with marked heat, add Lu.10 (yuji)
- with headache, add Bl.60 (kunlun –) and SI.3 (houxi –)
- with cough, add Lu.5 (chize –)
- with sore, swollen throat, add Lu.11 (shaoshang ↓)
- Ear points: lung, large intestine, tonsils

Clinical notes

- Weakness and atrophy of a Lung and Stomach heat type may be diagnosed as acute myelitis, poliomyelitis or muscular impairment in the aftermath of a febrile illness such as meningitis or encephalitis.

湿
热
浸
淫

12.2 DAMP HEAT

Damp heat can be acute or insidious in onset. The acute pattern is associated with an invasion of external damp heat into the qi level. The gradual onset pattern is caused by damp heat accumulating internally as a result of poor diet or prolonged exposure to hot humid or damp conditions. Damp or damp heat seeps into the superficial muscle layer, obstructs qi and blood flow, weakens the Spleen and interrupts the supply of nutrition to the muscles. Damp heat, being heavy, sinks downwards and mainly affects the lower body.

If the external damp heat is severe, it can quickly damage yin and fluids. Gradual onset of damp heat is usually complicated by varying degrees of Spleen qi and yin deficiency. In the early stage of a damp heat pattern of muscular weakness, atrophy is minimal or absent, but as underlying qi and yin damage become more prominent, wasting starts to occur.

Clinical features
- Muscle weakness, primarily of the lower limbs, accompanied by mild edema. The limbs are heavy, aching and numb, and feel warm to the touch. Numbness or a burning sensation may begin in the soles of the feet and gradually progress up the leg. The weakness and other symptoms are worse in hot weather and after a hot bath. In general, at this stage there is little or no muscle wasting.
- heat intolerance, feels generally warm to the touch
- flushed complexion; greasy skin
- low grade fever, afternoon fever or contained fever (p.367); night sweats
- heaviness and lethargy
- itchy or weeping skin lesions; suppurative sores
- chest oppression and abdominal distension
- concentrated or uncomfortable urination
- may be swollen lymph glands

T red with a greasy, yellow coat
P slippery, rapid

Treatment Principle
Clear damp heat from the muscles and sinews

Prescription

JIA WEI ER MIAO SAN 加味二妙散
Augmented Two Marvel Powder, modified

This prescription is selected for damp heat of gradual onset.

huang bai (Phellodendri Cortex) 黄柏 9–12g
cang zhu (Atractylodis Rhizoma) 苍术 9–12g
bi xie (Dioscoreae hypoglaucae Rhizoma) 萆薢 9–12g
chuan niu xi (Cyathulae Radix) 川牛膝 12–15g
han fang ji (Stephaniae tetrandrae Radix) 汉防己 9–12g
mu tong (Akebiae Caulis) 木通 6–9g

yi ren (Coicis Semen) 苡仁 30–60g
mu gua (Chaenomelis Fructus) 木瓜 9–12g
can sha (Bombycis Faeces) 蚕沙 6–9g
gan cao (Glycyrrhizae Radix) 甘草 3–6g

Method: Decoction. **Huang bai** clears damp heat, **cang zhu** and **yi ren** dry damp and strengthen the Spleen, and support **huang bai** in clearing damp heat; **bi xie**, **mu tong** and **han fang ji** promote urination to clear damp heat through the urine; **can sha**, **chuan niu xi** and **mu gua** ease the sinews and activate the flow of qi and blood through the legs; **gan cao** harmonizes the formula. (Source: *Zhong Yi Nei Ke Xue [Dan Xi Xin Fa]*)

Modifications

- With aching and numbness in the legs, add **xi xian cao** (Siegesbeckia Herba) 豨莶草 9–15g and **luo shi teng** (Trachelospermi Caulis) 络石藤 15–30g.
- With chest oppression, heavy limbs and edema, add **fu ling** (Poria) 茯苓 12–15g, **ze xie** (Alismatis Rhizoma) 泽泻 9–12g and **hou po** (Magnoliae officinalis Cortex) 厚朴 9–12g.
- With weeping, itchy skin lesions, add **tu fu ling** (Smilacis glabrae Rhizoma) 土茯苓 12–15g and **bai xian pi** (Dictamni Cortex) 白藓皮 9–12g.
- With yin damage, burning in the soles of the feet, and a peeled tongue coat on the back of the tongue, add **sheng di** (Rehmanniae Radix) 生地 12–15g and **mai dong** (Ophiopogonis Radix) 麦冬 9–12g.
- With blood stasis, add **chi shao** (Paeoniae Radix rubra) 赤芍 9–12g, **tao ren** (Persicae Semen) 桃仁 9–12g and **hong hua** (Carthami Flos) 红花 6–9g.

Variations and additional prescriptions

Sudden onset

Damp heat muscle weakness can follow some days or weeks after an acute damp warm disease. There are still signs of a pathogen in the qi level, such as a relatively high fever, sore throat, lymphadenopathy, nausea and vomiting, muscle aches, muscular flaccidity and weakness and a thick, greasy, yellow tongue coat. The treatment is to clear damp heat from the qi level with GAN LU XIAO DU DAN (Sweet Dew Special Pill to Eliminate Toxin 甘露消毒丹, p.325).

Chronic damp heat with Kidney yin deficiency

Chronic damp heat depletes Kidney yin, and as the features of yin deficiency become more apparent, atrophy may be seen. The features of yin deficiency and damp heat are often segregated into the upper and lower body, with the damp heat apparent in the lower burner and legs (weakness and wasting, urinary dysfunction and pain), and the yin deficiency in the upper body (flushing, red dry tongue, tinnitus). The treatment is to nourish Kidney yin and clear damp heat with a mixture of ZHI BAI DI HUANG WAN (Anemarrhena, Phellodendron and Rehmannia Pill 知柏地黄丸, p.922) plus SI MIAO SAN (Four Marvel Powder 四妙散, p.595).

Prepared medicines

Concentrated powders

Dang Gui Nian Tong San (Tangkuei & Anemarrhena Combination)
  – damp heat in the legs

San Miao San (Atractylodes & Phellodendron Formula)
Gan Lu Xiao Du Dan (Forsythia & Acorus Formula)
Zhi Bai Di Huang Wan (Anemarrhena, Phellodendron & Rehmannia Formula)
Pills
Bi Xie Sheng Shi Wan (Subdue the Dampness Teapills)
Zhi Bai Ba Wei Wan (Eight Flavor Rehmannia Teapills)

Acupuncture (select from)
In addition to points chosen according to the affected limbs (Box 12.4, p.547) select from the following:

Du.14 (dazhui –)................meeting point of the yang channels, clears heat and pathogens from the Lungs and qi level

LI.11 (quchi –)...................these points clear damp heat from the qi level
St.44 (neiting –)

Sp.9 (yinlingquan –)...........water and metal points of the Spleen, together these
Sp.5 (shangqiu –)   points promote urination and clear damp heat

St.32 (futu –) ....these points clear damp heat and from the lower
St.36 (zusanli –)   limbs, activate qi and blood flow through the legs
St.38 (tiaokou –)   and are specifically indicated for muscular weakness
St.41 (jiexi –)   and atrophy

SI.4 (wangu –) ....source point of the Small Intestine, clears damp heat
Ren.5 (shimen –)................alarm point of the triple burner, clears damp heat
Bl.20 (pishu) ....transport point of the Spleen, strengthens the Spleen to dry damp

- for acute external damp heat, add Lu.7 (lieque –) and SJ.6 (zhigou –)
- with nausea add PC.6 (neiguan)
- with diarrhea add zhixie (N–CA–3) and Bl.25 (tianshu)
- with myalgia add Sp.21 (dabao)
- Ear points: zero, spleen, stomach, lung, shenmen, sympathetic

Clinical notes
- Damp heat type muscular weakness may be diagnosed as weakness following an infection of the central nervous system, encephalitis, meningitis, acute myelitis, polyneuritis, Guillain–Barré syndrome, acute inflammatory polyneuritis, glandular fever, multiple sclerosis or periodic paralysis.
- This can be a difficult condition, but an aggressive approach with frequent acupuncture and decocted herbs can help arrest progress of the illness. Rapidly progressive weakness should be managed in hospital. In slowly progressive cases, treatment should persist for a minimum of 6–8 weeks before a judgement is made about its effectiveness.
- A damp heat clearing diet is recommended. See Clinical Handbook, Vol.2, pp.880–884.
- Damp heat is often complicated by qi and yin deficiency, so caution must be observed when prescribing the bitter cold and pungent drying herbs, which themselves can contribute to yin damage if excessively or improperly used.

痰
湿
阻
络

12.3 PHLEGM DAMP BLOCKING THE NETWORK VESSELS

Phlegm damp can accumulate in the muscles and network vessels as a result of Spleen deficiency, or prolonged damp stagnation in the muscles. The damp congeals and thickens further into phlegm. There is usually cold associated with this pattern, but heat may sporadically be generated by the stagnation. This is predominantly an excess pattern, but will gradually be complicated by more and more qi deficiency.

Clinical features

- Gradual and progressive weakness, heaviness, numbness and tingling of the arms, legs, hands or feet, and eventually, difficulty walking. The weakness may follow an intermittent course, with exacerbations and remissions. The muscles may feel firm or flaccid, but in general there is no muscle wasting.
- cold, pale extremities
- dizziness and vertigo
- blurred vision or double vision
- hoarse voice, throat congestion or difficulty swallowing
- foggy and heavy head, difficulty concentrating
- chest oppression
- symptoms worse in damp and humid weather
- even though the condition may be chronic, the patient still appears relatively robust

T normal color, or slightly pale and swollen with thick, white, greasy coat
P deep and slippery

Treatment Principle

Transform phlegm and dry damp
Strengthen the Spleen and unblock the network vessels

Prescription

ER ZHU TANG 二术汤
Dual Atractylodes Decoction

cang zhu (Atractylodis Rhizoma) 苍术	12–15g
bai zhu (Atractylodis macrocephalae Rhizoma) 白术	12–15g
zhi ban xia (Pinelliae Rhizoma preparatum) 制半夏	9–12g
chen pi (Citri reticulatae Pericarpium) 陈皮	9–12g
fu ling (Poria) 茯苓	9–12g
xiang fu (Cyperi Rhizoma) 香附	9–12g
dan nan xing (Arisaema cum Bile) 胆南星	6–9g
wei ling xian (Clematidis Radix) 威灵仙	6–9g
qiang huo (Notopterygii Rhizoma seu Radix) 羌活	6–9g
huang qin (Scutellariae Radix) 黄芩	6–9g
sheng jiang (Zingiberis Rhizoma recens) 生姜	6–9g
gan cao (Glycyrrhizae Radix) 甘草	3–6g

Method: Decoction. **Cang zhu** and **bai zhu** dry phlegm damp and strengthen the Spleen; **zhi ban xia** and **chen pi** dry dampness and transform phlegm; **fu ling** strengthens the Spleen and promotes urination to drain damp; **xiang fu** regulates qi; **dan nan xing** scours out phlegm; **wei ling xian** and **qiang huo** promote movement of qi through the channels and network vessels and disperse phlegm damp; **huang qin** clears heat and dries damp; **sheng jiang** harmonizes the Stomach; **gan cao** protects the Spleen and Stomach. (Source: *Wan Bing Hui Chun*)

Modifications

- If the legs are most affected, add **chuan niu xi** (Cyathulae Radix) 川牛膝 12–15g and **mu gua** (Chaenomelis Fructus) 木瓜 9–12g.
- If the arms are most affected, add **gui zhi** (Cinnamomi Ramulus) 桂枝 6–9g and **jiang huang** (Curcumae longae Rhizoma) 姜黄 6–9g.
- With cold extremities or blanching fingers, delete **huang qin**, replace **sheng jiang** with **gan jiang** (Zingiberis Rhizoma) 干姜 6–9g, and add **xi xin** (Asari Herba) 细辛 3–6g.
- With poor concentration and foggy head, add **shi chang pu** (Acori tatarinowii Rhizoma) 石菖蒲 6–9g and **yuan zhi** (Polygalae Radix) 远志 6–9g.
- With marked qi deficiency, add **ren shen** (Ginseng Radix) 人参 3–6g.
- With ptosis, add **chai hu** (Bupleuri Radix) 柴胡 6–9g and **sheng ma** (Cimicifugae Rhizoma) 升麻 3–6g.
- With blood stasis, add **chuan xiong** (Chuanxiong Rhizoma) 川芎 6–9g, **hong hua** (Carthami Flos) 红花 6–9g and **ji xue teng** (Spatholobi Caulis) 鸡血藤 12–18g.

Variations and additional prescriptions

In the remission phase

If the patient does well and the symptoms improve, it is a good idea to continue the treatment with a gentler, more balanced prescription. The aim of treatment is to strengthen the Spleen, improve fluid metabolism and prevent phlegm formation with a formula such as XIANG SHA LIU JUN ZI TANG (Six Gentlemen Decoction with Aucklandia and Amomum 香砂六君子汤 p.618) or SHEN LING BAI ZHU SAN (Ginseng, Poria and White Atractylodes Powder 参苓白术散, p.621).

Prepared medicines

Concentrated powders

Er Zhu Tang (Atractylodes & Arisaema Combination)

Ding Xian Wan (Gastrodia and Amber Combination)

Zhu Ru Wen Dan Tang (Bamboo & Ginseng Combination)
  – phlegm heat

Xiao Huo Luo Dan (Myrrh & Aconite Formula)
  – cold phlegm and blood stasis and no sign of heat; this is a strong formula with the potential for side effects, so is best used in a small dose, 10–25% by weight, added to an appropriate constitutional formula, such as one of those noted in Variations above

Pills

Wen Dan Wan (Rising Courage Teapills)

Xiao Huo Luo Dan (Xiao Huo Luo Dan Teapills)

Niu Huang Qing Xin Wan (Tong Ren Niu Huang Qing Xin Wan)
– phlegm heat

Acupuncture (select from)

In addition to points chosen according to the affected limbs (Box 12.4, p.547) select from the following:

St.40 (fenglong –) ....connecting and source points of the Stomach
Sp.3 (taibai +)   and Spleen, these points resolve and transform phlegm, strengthen the Spleen and are effective for heaviness and weakness in the limbs
PC.5 (jianshi –)..................river point of the Pericardium, transforms phlegm
Ren.12 (zhongwan)............alarm point of the Stomach, strengthens Stomach and Spleen function to assist in transforming phlegm
Bl.20 (pishu) ....transport point of the Spleen, strengthens and supplements Spleen qi and yang to promote transformation and resolution of phlegm
Liv.3 (taichong –)...............regulates the Liver and resolves qi constraint, an essential feature of all phlegm treatments
• with muscle heaviness, add Sp.21 (dabao)
• with vertigo, add GB.43 (xiaxi –) and Du.20 (baihui)
• with blurred vision, add St.8 (touwei), Bl.2 (zanzhu) and GB.37 (guanming)
• with foggy or heavy head, add Bl.62 (shenmai)
• with aphasia, add Ht.5 (tongli –)
• with Spleen deficiency add St.36 (zusanli +)
• with cold, apply moxa to Bl.20 (pishu ▲) and Bl.21 (weishu ▲)
• with heat, add St.44 (neiting –)
• Ear points: stomach, spleen, liver, zero point, sympathetic, shenmen

Clinical notes

• Weakness and wasting of a phlegm damp type may be diagnosed as multiple sclerosis, polyneuropathy or myasthenia gravis.
• If the onset of this type of weakness is recent, the patient can respond reasonably well to persistent treatment, or at least the progression of the weakness may be slowed. This pattern tends to have an intermittent course, reflecting the gathering and dispersal of phlegm in response to diet, qi constraint and invasion of pathogens into the qi level. If a patient has had an episode that has responded to treatment or gone into spontaneous remission and is symptom free, continued treatment with Chinese medicine to maintain healthy Spleen and Lung function, fluid metabolism, and plentiful qi and blood, is of great value in preventing recurrence.
• A phlegm damp drying diet is an essential part of treatment. See Clinical Handbook, Vol.2, pp.880–881.

脾
胃
虚
弱 | 12.4 SPLEEN AND STOMACH QI DEFICIENCY

The Spleen maintains the strength, tone and bulk of the muscles. The Stomach, being associated with yangming, is replete with qi and blood. Weakness or dysfunction of these organs has a significant impact on muscle strength and bulk. All muscles can be affected, but the muscles along the yangming and taiyin channel pathways are most affected. Spleen qi deficiency is often complicated by accumulation of dampness and phlegm, Kidney qi deficiency or yin and blood deficiency. Conversely, Spleen qi deficiency may develop as a result of chronic dampness, damp heat and phlegm.

Clinical features

- Progressive muscular weakness and atrophy. The peripheral muscles are affected first, with gradual involvement of the respiratory and swallowing muscles in severe cases. The first sign may be ptosis, or weakness along the taiyin channels, for example, weakness of brachioradialis, with difficulty turning door handles or opening jars, or the yangming channels with difficulty standing, walking and holding the head up. The weakness is worse following activity and when tired. Muscle atrophy occurs gradually and is usually worse in the lower limbs. Muscles feel soft and flaccid.
- fatigue, tiredness, listlessness
- loss of appetite, early satiety
- abdominal distension
- loose stools, or sluggish bowel habits with no urge
- breathlessness, weak voice
- frequent urination
- cold intolerance, cold extremities
- pale, sallow or translucent complexion
- facial or orbital edema, fingers may be puffy in the mornings

T pale, swollen and scalloped with a thin, white, maybe greasy coat
P deep, thready , weak

Treatment Principle

Strengthen the Spleen, Stomach and Lungs and supplement qi
Elevate yang qi

Prescription

BU ZHONG YI QI TANG 补中益气汤
Supplement the Middle to Augment the Qi Decoction

huang qi (Astragali Radix) 黄芪	15–24g
ren shen (Ginseng Radix) 人参	9–12g
bai zhu (Atractylodes macrocephalae Rhizoma) 白术	9–12g
dang gui (Angelicae sinensis Radix) 当归	6–9g
chen pi (Citri reticulatae Pericarpium) 陈皮	6–9g
zhi gan cao (Glycyrrhizae Radix preparata) 炙甘草	3–6g
sheng ma (Cimicifugae Rhizoma) 升麻	3–6g

chai hu (Bupleuri Radix) 柴胡 3–6g
Method: Decoction. **Huang qi**, **ren shen** and **bai zhu** strengthen the Spleen, supplement qi and promote qi movement to the extremities; **huang qi** fortifies and secures wei qi and raises yang qi; **chai hu** and **sheng ma** raise yang qi; **dang gui** supplements blood; **chen pi** and **zhi gan cao** regulate qi and harmonize the middle burner. (Source: *Zhong Yi Nei Ke Xue* [*Pi Wei Lun*])

Modifications

- In severe cases, the doses of **huang qi** and **ren shen** can be increased by 100%.
- If the lower limbs are most affected, add **wu jia pi** (Acanthopanacis Cortex) 五加皮 12–15g, **ji xue teng** (Spatholobi Caulis) 鸡血藤 15–30g, **du zhong** (Eucommiae Cortex) 杜仲 9–12g and **chuan niu xi** (Cyathulae Radix) 川牛膝 9–12g.
- If the upper limbs are most affected, add **gui zhi** (Cinnamomi Ramulus) 桂枝 6–9g, **ji xue teng** (Spatholobi Caulis) 鸡血藤 15–30g and **jiang huang** (Curcumae longae Rhizoma) 姜黄 9–12g.
- With weakness of the low back and waist, add **du zhong** (Eucommiae Cortex) 杜仲 9–12g and **xu duan** (Dipsaci Radix) 续断 9–12g.
- With numbness, add **wei ling xian** (Clematidis Radix) 威灵仙 6–9g.
- With dampness, add **cang zhu** (Atractylodis Rhizoma) 苍术 9–12g and **hou po** (Magnoliae officinalis Cortex) 厚朴 9–12g.
- With cold, add **gan jiang** (Zingiberis Rhizoma) 干姜 6–9g and **zhi fu zi** (Aconiti Radix lateralis preparata) 制附子 6–9g [cooked first].
- With blood deficiency, add **gou qi zi** (Lycii Fructus) 枸杞子 9–12g and **long yan rou** (Longan Arillus) 龙眼肉 9–12g.
- With yin deficiency, wheezing or a dry cough, add **wu wei zi** (Schizandrae Fructus) 五味子 6–9g and **mai dong** (Ophiopogonis Radix) 麦冬 9–12g.
- With foggy head and poor concentration, add **shi chang pu** (Acori tatarinowii Rhizoma) 石菖蒲 6–9g and **yuan zhi** (Polygalae Radix) 远志 6–9g.
- A poor appetite can be a big impediment to recovery and can be addressed with herbs such as **shan zha** (Crataegi Fructus) 山楂 12–15g, **gu ya** (Setariae Fructus germinatus) 谷芽 15–30g and **sha ren** (Amomi Fructus) 砂仁 6–9g.
- With loose stools or diarrhea, add **yi ren** (Coicis Semen) 苡仁 15–30g, **shan yao** (Dioscoreae Rhizoma) 山药 12–15g and **lian zi** (Nelumbinis Semen) 莲子 6–9g.
- With sluggish bowels and no urge to defecate, increase the dose of **bai zhu** to 30g and add **mu xiang** (Aucklandiae Radix) 木香 9–12g.
- With breathlessness and spontaneous sweating, increase the dose of **huang qi** up to 45g.
- With palpitations, add **yuan zhi** (Polygalae Radix) 远志 6–9g and **long yan rou** (Longan Arillus) 龙眼肉 9–12g.
- The more prolonged the Spleen qi deficiency, the more the Kidneys will be drained, giving rise to dual Spleen and Kidney qi deficiency. In addition to the Spleen deficiency symptoms, the patient will start to display urinary symptoms or incontinence, worse weakness or wasting in the legs, difficulty walking and back ache. Combine the primary prescription with LIU WEI DI HUANG WAN (Six Ingredient Pill with Rehmannia 六味地黄丸, p.192).

Prepared medicines
Concentrated powders
Bu Zhong Yi Qi Tang (Ginseng & Astragalus Combination)
Xiang Sha Liu Jun Zi Tang (Vladmiria & Amomum Combination)
– with damp and phlegm
Pills
Bu Zhong Yi Qi Wan (Central Chi Teapills)
Xiang Sha Liu Jun Zi Wan (Aplotaxis–Ammomum Pills, Six Gentlemen Tea Pills)

Acupuncture (select from)
In addition to points chosen according to the affected limbs (Box 12.4, p.547) select from the following:

Bl.13 (feishu +▲)...............transport point of the Lungs, strengthens the Lungs and supplements qi
Bl.20 (pishu +▲) ....transport point of the Spleen, warms and strengthens the Spleen and supplements qi
Bl.23 (shenshu +▲) ....transport point of the Kidney, warms and strengthens the Kidney to support the Spleen
Ren.4 (guanyuan +▲)........strengthens yuan qi and supports qi systemically
Ren.12 (zhongwan)...........alarm point of the Stomach, strengthens Stomach and Spleen function to supplement qi
St.36 (zusanli +) ....sea point of the Stomach, warms and strengthens the Spleen and Stomach and supplements qi
Sp.6 (sanyinjiao +▲)..........strengthens the Spleen and supplements qi
Lu.9 (taiyuan +) ....source point of the Lung channel, strengthens the Lungs and supplements qi deficiency
• with damp and edema, add Sp.3 (taibai –) and Sp.9 (yinlingquan –)
• with phlegm, add St.40 (fenglong –) and Sp.3 (taibai –)
• with muscle heaviness, add Sp.21 (dabao)
• with vertigo, add GB.43 (xiaxi –) and Du.20 (baihui)
• with blurred vision, add St.8 (touwei), Bl.2 (zanzhu) and GB.37 (guanming)
• with foggy or heavy head, add Bl.62 (shenmai)
• Ear points: lung, spleen, adrenal, sympathetic, zero point, shenmen

Clinical notes
• Weakness and wasting of a Spleen and Stomach qi deficiency type may be diagnosed as polyneuropathy, myasthenia gravis, muscular dystrophy, periodic paralysis, multiple sclerosis or syringomyelia.
• Maintaining a strong Spleen and Lung, and immune system is especially important both during and in between episodes. This can have a significant preventative effect and reduce the likelihood of relapse.
• A Spleen strengthening diet is essential. See Clinical Handbook, Vol.2, pp.870–871.

气
血
两
虚

12.5 QI AND BLOOD DEFICIENCY

This pattern of weakness and atrophy is associated with Liver blood deficiency, due to the relationship of Liver blood to integrity and function of the sinews. It is often complicated by wind. In general it is gradual in onset, but may on occasion follow a sudden or catastrophic blood loss, surgery or pregnancy.

Clinical features

- Muscle weakness with stiffness, cramping and spasticity which is worse following exertion. Numbness and tingling of the extremities. There may be a mild tremor, tics or fasciculation. Muscle wasting may gradually intervene.
- pale sallow complexion; pale nails and conjunctivae
- blurring or weakening vision
- postural dizziness, light–headedness
- dry skin and hair
- insomnia, dream disturbed sleep
- scanty menstruation, amenorrhea

T pale, thin and dry
P thready and weak or choppy

Treatment Principle

Nourish Liver blood, strengthen the Spleen and supplement qi

Prescription

SHENG YU TANG 圣愈汤
Sage–like Healing Decoction, modified

dang gui (Angelicae sinensis Radix) 当归 6–12g
shu di (Rehmanniae Radix preparata) 熟地 9–15g
bai shao (Paeoniae Radix alba) 白芍 9–12g
chuan xiong (Chuanxiong Rhizoma) 川芎 6–9g
ren shen (Ginseng Radix) 人参 6–9g
huang qi (Astragali Radix) 黄芪 12–18g
ji xue teng (Spatholobi Caulis) 鸡血藤 12–15g
gou qi zi (Lycii Fructus) 枸杞子 9–12g
he shou wu (Polygoni multiflori Radix) 何首乌 9–12g

Method: Decoction. **Shu di** nourishes yin and blood; **dang gui** and **ji xue teng** supplement and activate the blood; **bai shao** nourishes blood and softens the Liver; **ren shen** and **huang qi** strengthen the Spleen to produce blood; **gou qi zi** nourishes blood and supports Kidney jing; **chuan xiong** activates blood and moves qi; **he shou wu** supplements and strengthens blood, the Liver and Kidneys, and supports jing. (Source: *Zhong Yi Nei Ke Xue* [*Lan Shi Mi Cang*])

Modifications

- With visual weakness or blurring vision, add **jue ming zi** (Cassiae Semen) 决明子 9–15g and **chu shi zi** (Broussonetiae Fructus) 楮实子 6–9g.
- With wind, muscle spasms, fasciculation, tremors or numbness, add **mu gua** (Chaenomelis Fructus) 木瓜 6–9g, **tian ma** (Gastrodiae Rhizoma) 天麻 6–9g and **bai jiang can** (Bombyx Batryticatus) 白僵蚕 6–9g.

- With postural dizziness, add **nu zhen zi** (Ligustri Fructus) 女贞子 9–12g and **ci shi** (Magnetitum) 磁石 15–30g.
- With insomnia or dream disturbed sleep, add **he huan pi** (Albizziae Cortex) 合欢皮 12–15g and **ye jiao teng** (Polygoni multiflori Caulis) 夜交藤 15–30g.
- With Liver qi constraint, add **xiang fu** (Cyperi Rhizoma) 香附 9–12g.
- With anxiety and palpitations, add **yuan zhi** (Polygalae Radix) 远志 6–9g.
- With dampness or weak digestion, add **bai zhu** (Atractylodis macrocephalae Rhizoma) 白术 9–12g and **chen pi** (Citri reticulatae Pericarpium) 陈皮 6–9g.
- With blood stasis, add **tao ren** (Persicae Semen) 桃仁 9–12g, **hong hua** (Carthami Flos) 红花 6–9g and **dan shen** (Salviae miltiorrhizae Radix) 丹参 9–12g.

Prepared medicines
Concentrated powder
Ba Zhen Tang (Tangkuei & Ginseng Eight Combination)
Shi Quan Da Bu Tang (Ginseng & Dang Gui Ten Combination)
Pills
Ba Zhen Wan (Women's Precious Pills, Nu Ke Ba Zhen Wan)
Shi Quan Da Bu Wan (Ten Flavour Teapills)
Dang Gui Ji Jing (Tang Kuei Essence of Chicken)

Acupuncture (select from)
In addition to points selected according to the affected limbs (Box 12.4, p.547) select from the following:
Ren.12 (zhongwan +▲).......alarm point of the Stomach, strengthens the Spleen and Stomach and supplements qi and blood
Ren.4 (guanyuan +▲)........supplements yuan qi to build blood
Bl.18 (ganshu +).................transport point of the Liver, nourishes and supplements Liver blood
Bl.20 (pishu +▲) ....transport point of the Spleen, warms and strengthens the Spleen and supplements qi and blood
Sp.6 (sanyinjiao +▲)..........strengthens the Spleen, nourishes and activates qi and blood and calms the shen
St.36 (zusanli +▲) ....sea point of the Stomach, warms and strengthens the Spleen and Stomach and supplements qi and blood
Liv.3 (taichong –)...............nourishes and activates Liver blood
- with muscle spasms, add GB.34 (yanglingquan) and Du.8 (jinsuo)
- with visual weakness or spots before the eyes, add GB.37 (guanming +)
- with postural dizziness, add Du.20 (baihui ▲)
- Ear points: liver, spleen, zero point, shenmen, sympathetic

Clinical notes
- Weakness and wasting of a qi and blood deficiency type may be diagnosed as polyneuritis, motor neuron disease, myasthenia gravis, muscular dystrophy, periodic paralysis or multiple sclerosis.
- A qi and blood supplementing diet is recommended. See Clinical Handbook, Vol.2, pp.870–875.

瘀
阻
络
脉

12.6 BLOOD STASIS IN THE CHANNELS AND NETWORK VESSELS

Blood stasis type weakness and atrophy can be acute or chronic. When chronic, it is usually a complication of another pattern such as Liver and Kidney yin deficiency, Spleen and Kidney yang deficiency or phlegm damp. If the blood stasis continues unabated, it gradually becomes more and more prominent, until it becomes the primary pathology. When acute, blood stasis type weakness and atrophy may follow a wind stroke or an incompletely resolved physical trauma. When blood stasis is the primary diagnosis it usually complicated by cold, heat or deficiency.

Clinical features

- Weakness and atrophy of the limbs, with numbness or paresthesia. The affected limb or limbs may be sensitive to pressure, with pain upon palpation. There may be stiffness and pain with movement of the limbs.
- venous congestion on the limbs, or darkening and discoloration of the skin on the affected limb or limbs
- dry scaly skin on the extremities
- purplish lips, sclera, conjunctiva and nail beds
- left iliac fossa pressure pain, p.925–926

T in acute cases the tongue body may be unremarkable; in chronic cases it will be purple or mauve with brown or purple stasis spots and a thin white coat; sublingual veins are distended and dark

P deep, choppy, wiry, thready , or irregular and intermittent

Treatment Principle

Activate blood and dispel blood stasis
Supplement qi and blood

Prescription

TAO HONG SI WU TANG 桃红四物汤
Four Substance Decoction with Safflower and Peach Pit, modified

tao ren (Persicae Semen) 桃仁 9–12g
hong hua (Carthami Flos) 红花 6–9g
dang gui (Angelicae sinensis Radix) 当归 9–12g
shu di (Rehmanniae Radix preparata) 熟地 12–15g
bai shao (Paeoniae Radix alba) 白芍 9–15g
chuan xiong (Chuanxiong Rhizoma) 川芎 6–9g
chuan niu xi (Cyathulae Radix) 川牛膝 9–12g
zhi huang qi (honey fried Astragali Radix) 炙黄芪 18–30g
dang shen (Codonopsis Radix) 党参 12–18g
gan cao (Glycyrrhizae Radix) 甘草 6–9g

Method: Decoction. **Dang gui** supplements and activates blood; **shu di** and **bai shao** nourish and supplement blood; **bai shao** softens the Liver and alleviates spasmodic pain; **tao ren** and **hong hua** activate blood; **chuan xiong** activates qi and blood, and stops pain; **chuan niu xi** activates blood and leads the action of the formula to the lower body; **zhi huang qi** moves qi to lead blood and supplements qi; **dang shen**, **zhi huang qi** and **gan cao** strengthen the Spleen and supplement qi.
(Source: *Zhong Yi Nei Ke Xue* [*Yi Zong Jin Jian*])

Modifications

- With atrophy of the lower limbs, add **suo yang** (Cynomorii Herba) 锁阳 12–15g, **rou cong rong** (Cistanches Herba) 肉苁蓉 15–24g and **ba ji tian** (Morindae officinalis Radix) 巴戟天 9–12g.
- With numbness, use **chi shao** (Paeoniae Radix rubra) 赤芍 9–12g instead of **bai shao**, and add **ji xue teng** (Spatholobi Caulis) 鸡血藤 18–30g, **san qi fen** (powdered Notoginseng Radix) 三七粉 3–6g, **di long** (Pheretima) 地龙 6–9g and **mu tong** (Akebiae Caulis) 木通 6–9g.
- With cold extremities, add **gui zhi** (Cinnamomi Ramulus) 桂枝 6–9g.
- With heat, substitute **chi shao** (Paeoniae Radix rubra) 赤芍 9–12g for **bai shao** and **sheng di** (Rehmanniae Radix) 生地 12–15g for **shu di**; with relatively severe heat add **mu dan pi** (Moutan Cortex) 牡丹皮 6–9g and **shan zhi zi** (Gardeniae Fructus) 山栀子 6–9g.
- With severe blood stasis, add **shui zhi** (Hirudo) 水蛭 3–6g and **di long** (Pheretima) 地龙 6–9g, or **wu gong** (Scolopendra) 蜈蚣 1–3g and **quan xie** (Scorpio) 全蝎 1–3g [as powder taken separately].
- For loss of function, pain or bruising following a traumatic injury, add **ji xue teng** (Spatholobi Caulis) 鸡血藤 18–30g, **ru xiang** (Olibanum) 乳香 6–9g and **mo yao** (Myrrha) 没药 6–9g.

Variations and additional prescriptions

Qi deficiency with blood stasis post wind–stroke atrophy

Following recovery from the acute phase of a wind–stroke, patients are often left with residual hemiplegia. This is frequently associated with a combination of blood stasis and qi deficiency. In addition to the weakness or atrophy, which can also involve the face, the patient is pale, easily fatigued and breathless. The treatment is to supplement qi to move blood and unblock the network vessels with a prescription such as the excellent BU YANG HUAN WU TANG (Supplement Yang to Restore Five Tenths Decoction 补阳还五汤, p.600).

Weakness and loss of function in a robust patient with blood stasis

Muscle weakness and loss of function soon after a trauma in a patient with minimal underlying deficiency can be treated with a more powerful blood activating formula, as long as there is no residual bleeding. XUE FU ZHU YU TANG (Drive Out Stasis in the Mansion of Blood Decoction 血府逐瘀汤, p.402) or FU YUAN HUO XUE TANG (Revive Health by Activating the Blood Decoction 复元活血汤, p.403) can be considered.

Prepared medicines

Concentrated powders

Tao Hong Si Wu Tang (Tangkuei Four, Persica & Carthamus Combination)
Bu Yang Huan Wu Tang (Astragalus & Peony Combination)
    – with qi deficiency
Xue Fu Zhu Yu Tang (Persica & Carthamus Combination)
Fu Yuan Huo Xue Tang (Tangkuei & Persica Combination)

Dang Gui Si Ni Tang (Tangkuei & Jujube Combination)
– with cold

Pills
Tao Hong Si Wu Wan (Tao Hong Si Wu Tang Teapills)
Bu Yang Huan Wu Wan (Great Yang Restoration Teapills)
Xue Fu Zhu Yu Wan (Stasis in the Mansion of Blood Teapills)
Sheng Tian Qi Pian (Raw Tian Qi Ginseng Tablets)
San Shen Jian Kang Wan (Sunho Multi Ginseng Tablets)

Acupuncture (select from)

In addition to points chosen according to the affected limbs (Box 12.4, p.547) select from the following:

Bl.17 (geshu –)...................meeting point for blood, dispels static blood
Sp.6 (sanyinjiao –)..............these points activate blood and dispel static blood
Sp.10 (xuehai –)
LI.4 (hegu –)
Bl.18 (ganshu –)................transport point of the Liver, dredges the Liver and
regulates qi, activates blood
Liv.14 (qimen –) ....alarm point of the Liver, dredges the Liver and
regulates qi, dispels static blood

- Bleeding the congested vessels that are often found around the knee and ankle can be helpful. The veins are pierced with a surgical lancet and a few drops of blood extracted. If stagnation is released, the blood should run black at first, then fresh red. This technique can be performed weekly for a few sessions, then intermittently thereafter. See also Appendix 4, p.929.
- Ear points: liver, heart, sympathetic, zero point, shenmen

Clinical notes

- Blood stasis muscular weakness and atrophy may be diagnosed as post traumatic brain or spinal cord injury, myasthenia gravis, late stage of poliomyelitis or motor neuron disease.
- Depending on the etiology and the extent of any damage to the spinal cord, blood stasis weakness can respond reasonably well to treatment. Weakness following a brain injury generally has a better outcome. Paralysis and loss of function following a wind–stroke has a good prognosis if it is treated soon after the event and no longer than six months after.

肝
肾
亏
损

12.7 LIVER AND KIDNEY YIN DEFICIENCY

Liver and Kidney yin deficiency is often the end result of other heat patterns, such as Lung heat or, more commonly, damp heat. It can also represent a deterioration of the deficiency patterns, especially blood deficiency.

Clinical features
- Gradual onset of weakness, loss of function, stiffness and wasting. Difficulty walking or standing. Obvious wasting of the large proximal muscles of the legs. In severe cases the patient is completely disabled and wheelchair bound.
- weak, aching, lower back and spine with an inability to sit for very long
- fatigue, weakness, exhaustion
- blurring vision or weakening vision, cataracts
- dizziness and tinnitus
- hair loss, premature greying of the hair
- dry mouth and throat
- weight loss, emaciation
- may be a tremor
- frequent urgent urination or incontinence of urine
- irregular menses, scanty menstruation, amenorrhea

T red and dry with little or no coat
P thready and rapid

Treatment Principle
Supplement and strengthen the Liver and Kidneys
Support the sinews and bones

Prescription

ZHUANG GU WAN 壮骨丸
Pill to Strengthen the Bones

shu di (Rehmanniae Radix preparata) 熟地 120g
gui ban (Testudinis Plastrum) 龟板 120g
huai niu xi (Achyranthis bidentatae Radix) 怀牛膝 90g
dang gui (Angelicae sinensis Radix) 当归 60g
bai shao (Paeoniae Radix alba) 白芍 60g
huang bai (Phellodendri Cortex) 黄柏 60g
zhi mu (Anemarrhenae Rhizoma) 知母 60g
chen pi (Citri reticulatae Pericarpium) 陈皮 60g
suo yang (Cynomorii Herba) 锁阳 45g
gou gu (Canis Os) 狗骨 30g
zhi gan cao (Glycyrrhizae Radix preparata) 炙甘草 30g
gan jiang (Zingiberis Rhizoma) 干姜 15g

Method: Pills. Grind all substances to a thready powder and form into 9 gram pills with honey. The dose is one pill 2–3 times daily with salty water. The main herbs, **shu di** and **gui ban** supplement the Liver and Kidneys, yin and blood; **gou gu** and **huai niu xi** strengthen the sinews and bones and support the Liver and Kidneys; **dang gui** and **bai shao** nourish blood and ease the sinews; **huang bai** and **zhi mu** clear heat from deficiency and support yin; **suo yang** supports yang and jing; **chen**

pi and **gan jiang** regulate qi, warm the middle burner and strengthen the Spleen to alleviate any difficulty with digestion of the formula; **gan jiang** protects the stomach from the bitter cold of **huang bai**; **zhi gan cao** harmonizes the formula. (Source: *Zhong Yi Nei Ke Xue*)

Modifications

- With marked heat, omit **suo yang** and **gan jiang**.
- With qi deficiency, add **huang qi** (Astragali Radix) 黄芪 60g and **dang shen** (Codonopsis Radix) 党参 60g.
- With yang deficiency, delete **huang bai** and **zhi mu**, and add **lu jiao jiao** (Cervi Cornus Colla) 鹿角胶 90g and **gou ji** (Cibotii Rhizoma) 狗脊 60g.
- With weakness and aching in the lower back and spine, add **gou ji** (Cibotii Rhizoma) 狗脊 60g, **xu duan** (Dipsaci Radix) 续断 90g and **bu gu zhi** (Psoraleae Fructus) 补骨脂 60g.
- With dizziness, add **gou qi zi** (Lycii Fructus) 枸杞子 60g and **ju hua** (Chrysanthemi Flos) 菊花 60g.
- With incontinence of urine, add **sang piao xiao** (Mantidis Ootheca) 桑螵蛸 60g and **fu pen zi** (Rubi Fructus) 覆盆子 60g.

Prepared medicines

Concentrated powders

Hu Qian Wan (Phellodendron & Testudinis Formula)
Zhi Bai Di Huang Wan (Anemarrhena, Phellodendron & Rehmannia Formula) – yin deficiency with residual damp heat

Pills

Jian Bu Qiang Sheng Wan (Aches and Pains Relief Pill)
Jian Bu Zhuang Gu Wan (Tong Ren Tang Jian Bu Zhuang Gu Wan)
Zhi Bai Ba Wei Wan (Eight Flavor Rehmannia Teapills)

Acupuncture (select from)

In addition to points chosen according to the affected limbs (Box 12.4, p.547) select from the following:

Ren.4 (guanyuan +)............these points supplement Kidney yin and yuan qi
Ren.6 (qihai +)
Kid.3 (taixi +).....................source point of the Kidneys, supplements Kidney yin
Liv.3 (taichong +)...............source, transport and earth point of the Liver, supplements Liver yin and blood
Lu.7 (lieque).....................master and couple points of renmai, these points
Kid.6 (zhaohai)   open up circulation of renmai qi, supplement Kidney yin
Sp.6 (sanyinjiao)................nourishes Kidney, Liver and Spleen yin
Bl.23 (shenshu +)..............transport point of the Kidneys, supplements Kidney yin
Bl.52 (zhishi +)..................supplements the Kidneys
- with dizziness or vertigo, add GB.20 (fengchi–) and Du.20 (baihui)
- with slurred speech, add Ht.5 (tongli)

- with blurred or weakening vision, or cataracts, add GB.37 (guanming) and SI.6 (yanglao)
- with urinary incontinence, add Bl.28 (pangguangshu) and Ren.3 (zhongji)
- Ear points: liver, kidney, zero point, adrenal, sympathetic, shenmen

Clinical notes

- Atrophy syndrome of a Liver and Kidney yin deficiency type may be diagnosed as motor neuron disease, syringomyelia, Guillain–Barré syndrome, the sequelae of poliomyelitis or other inflammatory conditions of the central nervous system.
- The prognosis is variable. In advanced cases the prognosis for the atrophy is poor, although many quality of life indicators can be improved with persistent treatment. Regardless of the stage, for treatment to be successful at all, acupuncture must be frequent, and both herbs and acupuncture should continue for at least six months.
- A yin supplementing diet is recommended. See Clinical Handbook, Vol.2, pp.876–877.

脾
肾
阳
虚

12.8 SPLEEN AND KIDNEY YANG DEFICIENCY

Spleen and Kidney yang deficiency represents a profound and late stage of weakness with significant atrophy.

Clinical features

- Weakness, loss of function, flaccidity and wasting, mostly in the legs but may affect the arms and neck as well. Difficulty walking and standing, lifting or using the arms or holding the head up. Obvious wasting of the large proximal muscles of the limbs. In severe cases the patient is completely disabled and wheelchair bound. There may be ankle edema.
- weak aching, cold lower back and spine with an inability to sit for very long
- disabling physical and mental exhaustion; little energy reserve
- cold intolerance, cold extremities
- frequency or incontinence of urine, nocturia; or scanty urine with edema
- fecal incontinence
- breathlessness, wheezing, rattle in the chest
- poor appetite
- dysphagia
- hearing loss, tinnitus

T pale or mauve, swollen and scalloped with a thin, white, greasy coat
P deep, weak or imperceptible

Treatment Principle

Vigorously warm and supplement Spleen and Kidney yang

Prescription

YOU GUI WAN 右归丸
Restore the Right [Kidney] Pill

shu di (Rehmanniae Radix preparata) 熟地	24g
shan yao (Dioscoreae Rhizoma) 山药	12g
gou qi zi (Lycii Fructus) 枸杞子	12g
tu si zi (Cuscutae Semen) 菟丝子	12g
du zhong (Eucommiae Cortex) 杜仲	12g
lu jiao jiao (Cervi Cornus Colla) 鹿角胶	12g
shan zhu yu (Corni Fructus) 山茱萸	9g
dang gui (Angelicae sinensis Radix) 当归	9g
zhi fu zi (Aconiti Radix lateralis preparata) 制附子	6–12g
rou gui (Cinnamomi Cortex) 肉桂	6–12g

Method: Pills or powder. Grind the herbs to a fine powder and form into 9 gram pills with honey. The dose is one pill twice daily. Can also be decocted with the doses as shown, in which case **zhi fu zi** is cooked for 30 minutes before the other herbs and **lu jiao jiao** is melted into the strained decoction. **Shu di, gou qi zi** and **dang gui** nourish Kidney yin and blood; **shan zhu yu** supplements the Liver; **shan yao** strengthens the Spleen and Kidneys; **tu si zi** and **du zhong** supplement Kidney yang; **zhi fu zi** and **rou gui** warm yang; **lu jiao jiao** benefits yang and jing. (Source: *Zhong Yi Nei Ke Xue* ([*Jing Yue Quan Shu*]))

Modifications

- With fecal incontinence, add **bu gu zhi** (Psoraleae Fructus) 补骨脂 9–12g, **wu wei zi** (Schizandrae Fructus) 五味子 6–9g, **rou dou kou** (Myristicae Semen) 肉豆蔻 3–6g and **wu zhu yu** (Evodiae Fructus) 吴茱萸 2–3g.
- With frequent urination or nocturia, add **sang piao xiao** (Mantidis Ootheca) 桑螵蛸 6–9g, **qian shi** (Euryales Semen) 芡实 9–12g, **jin ying zi** (Rosae laevigatae Fructus) 金樱子 9–12g and **yi zhi ren** (Alpiniae oxyphyllae Fructus) 益智仁 6–9g.
- With poor appetite and digestion, add **chao bai zhu** (stir fried Atractylodes macrocephalae Rhizoma) 炒白术 9–12g and **gan jiang** (Zingiberis Rhizoma) 干姜 6–9g.
- With wheezing and breathing difficulty, add **bu gu zhi** (Psoraleae Fructus) 补骨脂 9–12g and **wu wei zi** (Schizandrae Fructus) 五味子 6–9g.
- With severe weakness and aching in the low back and spine, add **gou ji** (Cibotii Rhizoma) 狗脊 9–12g, **xu duan** (Dipsaci Radix) 续断 9–12g and **bu gu zhi** (Psoraleae Fructus) 补骨脂 9–12g.
- With qi deficiency and fading yang, add **hong ren shen** (Ginseng Radix) 红人参 15–30g.

Variations and additional prescriptions

With edema

If edema is severe, and this can include peripheral edema and fluid accumulating in the Lungs, fluids must be quickly mobilized by warming and supporting Heart yang to transform and process fluids. For Kidney and Heart yang deficiency with significant edema, breathlessness and a pale bluish cast to the face and tongue, the treatment is to support Heart and Kidney yang with ZHEN WU TANG (True Warrior Decoction 真武汤, p.249).

Prepared medicines

Concentrated powder

You Gui Wan (Eucommia & Rehmannia Formula)
Ba Wei Di Huang Wan (Rehmannia Eight Formula)
Fu Zi Li Zhong Tang (Aconite, Ginseng and Ginger Combination)
  – add with Spleen yang deficiency
Jin Suo Gu Jing Wan (Lotus Stamen Formula)
  – add when there is frequent urination and nocturia

Pills

You Gui Wan (Right Side Replenishing Teapills)
Jin Kui Shen Qi Wan (Fu Gui Ba Wei Wan, Golden Book Teapills)
Da Huo Luo Dan (Tong Ren Tang Da Huo Luo Dan)

Acupuncture (select from)

In addition to points chosen according to the affected limbs (Box 12.4, p.547) select from the following:

Ren.6 (qihai +▲) ....regulates qi and supports Kidney yang
Ren.4 (guanyuan +▲) ....supplements yuan qi, warms yang and regulates qi

Ren.8 (shenque ▲) ....treated with moxa on salt; place a piece of thin cloth over the navel and fill it with salt; burn cones of moxa on the salt; strongly warms Kidney yang

Kid.3 (taixi +).....................source point of the Kidneys, supplements and supports Kidney yang

St.36 (zusanli +▲) ....sea point of the Stomach, strengthens the Spleen and Stomach and supplements yang qi

Sp.6 (sanyinjiao +▲)..........strengthens the Spleen and Kidneys

Bl.23 (shenshu +▲) ....transport point of the Kidneys, warms and supports yang

Du.4 (mingmen +▲)........warms and supports Kidney yang

- with edema, add Kid.7 (fuliu –), Ren.9 (shuifen ▲) and Sp.9 (yinlingquan –)
- with urinary incontinence, add Bl.28 (pangguangshu) and Ren.3 (zhongji)
- with dysphagia, add PC.5 (jianshi)
- Ear points: kidney, spleen, zero point, shenmen, adrenal, subcortex

Clinical notes

- Muscular weakness and atrophy of a Spleen and Kidney yang deficiency type is a late stage pattern, and the patient is debilitated. The prognosis is generally poor, but treatment can improve some functions. Atrophy is unlikely to change, but the progression of the illness can sometimes be slowed down, and the energy, appetite and digestive function, and quality of life can often be improved. For any result, treatment needs to continue for at least some months. Depending on the duration and severity of the initial condition, 6–12 months of treatment may be required to rebuild and sustain Kidney yang.
- A yang warming diet is recommended. See Clinical Handbook, Vol.2, p.873.

Table 12.1 Summary of muscular weakness and atrophy patterns

Pattern	Features	Prescription
Lung and Stomach heat with fluid damage	Gradual and progressive weakness and flaccidity of the legs, following an acute upper respiratory tract infection with fever, sore throat, cough and generalized dryness.	Qing Zao Jiu Fei Tang Yi Wei Tang
Damp heat	Muscle weakness of the legs with mild edema, heaviness, numbness, low grade fever, night sweats, lymphadenopathy, red tongue with a greasy yellow coat, slippery rapid pulse.	Jia Wei Er Miao San Gan Lu Xiao Du Dan
Phlegm damp	Weakness, heaviness, numbness and tingling of the limbs. The muscles feel firm or flaccid, with no wasting. Vertigo, foggy head, chest oppression, swollen tongue with a thick greasy coat, deep slippery pulse	Er Zhu Tang
Spleen qi deficiency	Weakness and atrophy, worse with activity and when tired. Muscles soft and flaccid. Fatigue, poor appetite, loose stools, breathlessness, weak voice, pale swollen scalloped tongue, deep weak pulse.	Bu Zhong Yi Qi Tang
Qi and blood deficiency	Muscle weakness with stiffness and spasticity, worse with exertion. Numbness and tingling of the extremities, mild tremor or fasciculation. Pale face, nails and conjunctivae, blurring vision, postural dizziness, scanty menstruation, pale thin tongue, thready weak pulse.	Sheng Yu Tang
Qi and blood stasis	Weakness and atrophy with numbness or paresthesia. Stiffness and pain with movement of the limbs; venous congestion, skin discoloration, purple or mauve tongue with stasis spots and congested sublingual veins, choppy, wiry pulse.	Tao Hong Si Wu Tang Bu Yang Huan Wu Tang
Liver and Kidney yin deficiency	Weakness, stiffness and wasting. Difficulty walking or standing. Weak aching lower back, exhaustion, blurring vision, dizziness, weight loss, tremor, amenorrhea, red dry tongue with little or no coat, thready rapid pulse.	Zhuang Gu Wan
Spleen and Kidney yang deficiency	Profound weakness flaccidity and wasting; difficulty walking and using the arms; ankle edema, weak low back, exhaustion, cold intolerance incontinence of urine and feces, breathlessness, dysphagia, hearing loss, tinnitus, pale or mauve, swollen and scalloped tongue with a white coat, deep weak or imperceptible pulse.	You Gui Wan

NUMBNESS AND PARESTHESIA

Numbness is diminished or loss of sensation in the skin. Paresthesia is abnormal sensation in the skin, such as tingling and pins and needles. In Chinese medicine, these sensory disturbances are known collectively as *má mù*[1] 麻木. Má 麻 is abnormal sensation, tingling and pins and needles, and mù 木 is reduced sensation or numbness.

Numbness and paresthesia, as defined in this chapter, occur without significant pain or weakness. Numbness may be observed as a part of painful obstruction syndrome (Chap.15) and muscular weakness and atrophy (Chap.12), but in both those conditions, the sensory component is overshadowed by pain and weakness respectively.

> **BOX 13.1 PATTERNS OF NUMBNESS AND PARESTHESIA**
>
> Ying wei disharmony
> Cold in the channels
> Phlegm in the network vessels
> Qi and blood stasis
> Phlegm and blood stasis
> Wind damp
> Damp heat
> Qi deficiency
> Qi deficiency with blood stasis
> Blood deficiency
> Liver and Kidney yin deficiency

In Chinese medicine, numbness and paresthesia are due to failure of blood to reach and nourish the skin. The skin relies on a steady supply of blood to maintain its elasticity and sensitivity. If blood is inadequate, poorly distributed or blocked by a pathogen, numbness and paresthesia can result. As a general rule, deficiency gives rise to tingling and pins and needles, whereas the blocking presence of a pathogen gives rise to numbness. In practice, various degrees of numbness and tingling are often seen together.

In biomedical terms, there are two broad causes of numbness and paresthesia; mechanical compression and traumatic damage to a sensory nerve, or nerve damage from metabolic disturbance, ischemia, autoimmunity, infection or nutritional deficiency.

ETIOLOGY
External pathogens
External pathogens such as wind damp and damp heat can infiltrate the surface and block the distribution of qi and blood through the superficial tissues. This can occur if wei qi is systemically weak, or if a patch of skin is temporarily undefended. When pathogenic wind is strong, it can disperse wei qi from the area exposed to the wind. Numbness and paresthesia may then be seen in discrete patches of skin. When wind is predominant it gives rise to tingling and pins and needles, often seen on the trunk and proximal limbs. When damp is predominant, the congealing nature of the damp leads to more sensory loss and a heavy wooden feeling in the tissues, most commonly the lower limbs. Numbness and paresthesia of this type tend to be

---

1 Practical Dictionary of Chinese Medicine (1998) – 'numbness and tingling'

relatively acute.

Dampness can also seep gradually into the tissues and create numbness. This is seen in patients exposed to prolonged damp climactic or environmental conditions. The distal extremities are usually the first part affected.

Qi and blood deficiency

Factors which weaken qi and blood can lead to numbness and paresthesia. An inadequate diet, or any factor that weakens the Spleen, can lead to reduced supply of qi and blood to the skin. When qi is weak, it may be unable to lead the blood up to the most superficial layers of the skin. Weak qi will also lead to a failure of protective wei qi, enabling external pathogens to gain access. Qi and blood deficiency can also be caused by factors such as overwork, prolonged breast feeding or loss of qi and blood from hemorrhage during childbirth.

Yin deficiency

There are two mechanisms whereby yin deficiency can cause numbness and paresthesia; failure of yin to nourish the tissues, and failure of yin to restrain yang leading to creation of internal wind. Both are associated

---

13.2 BIOMEDICAL CAUSES OF NUMBNESS AND PARESTHESIA

Nerve impingement
- scalene and pectoralis minor – ulnar and median nerve affected with tingling in the middle, ring and little fingers
- carpal tunnel – median nerve
- spinal nerve root compression
- sciatica, piriformis syndrome
- post surgical or traumatic nerve damage
- compression from tumors

Autoimmune
- scleroderma
- rheumatoid arthritis
- Raynaud's syndrome
- polyarteritis nodosa
- polyneuritis
- multiple sclerosis

Other
- beri–beri, nutritional deficiency
- leprosy
- diabetes, peripheral neuropathy
- hypothyroidism
- acromegaly
- acute and chronic infections, myelitis
- thrombophlebitis
- vascular claudication
- herpes zoster
- frostbite

---

with a decline in yin from ageing, depletion of yin by fever or chronic disease, or damage to yin by a heating diet, chronic damp heat, drug use or deterioration of qi and blood deficiency.

Yin and blood share the role of nourishing, moistening and maintaining the elasticity of skin, hair, joints and sinews. Weak yin can lead to dryness and thinning of the skin, with loss of sensitivity. When yin deficiency is the main pathology the numbness is usually part of a deeper pattern of disharmony involving the sinews and bones, with general weakness, stiffness and possibly pain and atrophy.

In the second mechanism, yin deficiency can lead to ascendant yang and the development of internal wind. The numbness in this case is usually relatively acute, affecting the extremities, upper body and face. It is usually accompanied by vertigo, tinnitus and headaches, and may be a sign of an impending wind–stroke.

Phlegm

Phlegm causes numbness and paresthesia by congealing in the tissues, obstructing the network vessels and impeding the circulation of qi and blood. The phlegm can be the result of congealing of normal physiological fluids or dampness, a constitutional predisposition to phlegm, or can be introduced in the diet. Fluids can be congealed into phlegm by being slowed down, congested or cooked. Fluids are slowed and congested by constrained qi that fails to lead them, or by poor fluid metabolism from weakness of the Lungs, Spleen and Kidneys. Fluids and dampness can be cooked and thickened into phlegm by heat from yin deficiency, damp heat or constrained heat. Chronic damp in the tissues, from the diet or an external invasion, can gradually thicken into phlegm. Phlegm can be introduced in the diet with rich, fatty, sweet foods, persistent overeating, or with cold raw foods that weaken the Spleen and cause damp accumulation.

Blood stasis

Numbness and paresthesia from blood stasis can be acute and chronic. When acute it is usually the result of physical trauma or surgery. When chronic it is the end result of other pathology that slows or impedes blood flow, such as Liver qi constraint, cold, phlegm, damp heat or deficiency of yang qi, blood or yin. Blood stasis that contributes to numbness can also result from prolonged inactivity, an awkward sleeping position, sitting in one position for long periods of time, heavy cigarette smoking and dehydration. In general, blood stasis causes complete loss of sensation and a wooden feeling in tissues.

Nerve compression

Interference with sensory nerves as they exit the spinal cord, or at some point along the nerve pathway can cause numbness and paresthesia. This can be caused by a narrowing of the gap between vertebrae due to thinning of the intervertebral disc, growth of osteophytes or muscle spasm. When specific nerves are compressed the numbness and paresthesia are seen in the relevant dermatome (Fig.13.1, p.575).

A number of common types of numbness and paresthesia are due to temporary nerve compression. Numbness in the hands and fingers, for example, often wakes people from sleep, and can be caused by constriction of the brachial plexus by an awkward sleeping position. The plexus can be squeezed as it passes through the scalene muscles in the neck, or under the attachment of pectoralis minor in the anterior shoulder. The ulnar nerve can be compressed where it navigates the elbow joint. Numbness or tingling in the middle three fingers can be due to compression of the median nerve as it passes through the carpal tunnel.

Numbness of this type can be the result of simple mechanical factors, such as an awkward sleeping position or a pillow that is too low or high. It may also be part of a systemic pathology. Muscular shortening and tension due to Liver qi constraint, for example, can squeeze the sensory nerves as they pass through. Spleen qi deficiency can lead to edema, dampness and phlegm accumulation in tissues; this may be seen in the wrist and can contribute to carpal tunnel. Qi and blood deficiency can make nerves more sensitive to interference and more likely to react to trivial stimuli.

Figure 13.1 Dermatomes

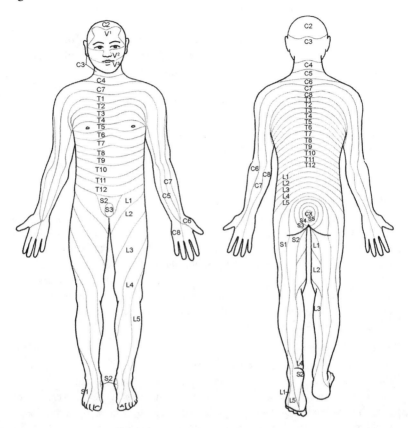

PATHOLOGY OF THE NETWORK VESSELS

The network vessels are fine vessels that branch off from the main channels. They are widely distributed through the surface tissues of the body, and enable distribution of qi and blood to the surface beyond the main channel pathways. They reinforce the links between the yin and yang pairs of channels. They also connect the main channels to the surrounding tissues. The network vessels serve to maintain a balance in the ebb and flow of yin and yang through the channels system. They also connect the surface of the body to the internal organ systems, via the intermediary of the main channels.

When numbness is the main complaint, the disease is usually located in the network vessels. Because the network vessels are so fine and diffuse, obstruction within them is insufficiently concentrated to produce pain, the classic feature of qi and blood blockage. When a pathogen is restricted to the network vessels, numbness and paresthesia are the main symptoms. As the disease progresses and moves deeper into the channel system, the blockage becomes more focused and intense, and pain, weakness and wasting start to develop.

TREATMENT

There are two needling methods that are of particular use in treating numbness and paresthesia; hair needling and plum blossom.

Hair needling (*máo cì* 毛刺)

This is a special needling technique for numbness and paresthesia, and is one of the nine ancient needling methods. The method involves using fine needles (0.16–0.20mm) inserted obliquely, almost parallel to the skin from the edge of the numb area towards its center. The needles should lie between the surface and the muscle layer, but not penetrate the muscle layer. With blood and/or phlegm stasis a slightly greater angle of insertion, between 30–45°, is required. The needles are placed at regular intervals around the numb area when presenting as a discrete patch, or around the upper limits of the numbness on a limb. The needles are placed about every 1–2 cm. Hair needling is best for relatively small areas of numbness.

Plum blossom needle (*méi huā zhēn* 梅花针)

Plum blossom needling is a technique used to dispel pathogens from, and activate the circulation of qi and blood in, the network vessels. It can be applied in both deficiency and excess conditions, with a variation of technique. Plum blossom needling is suited to relatively large areas of numbness, and can be combined with hair needling. It is not suited for use in the damp heat pattern or where there is edema.

The technique is simple but requires some practice to perform efficiently. The main aim is to keep the needle tips parallel with the skin while maintaining a constant rhythm and even pressure. This keeps the point of contact as wide as possible, preventing undue discomfort while stimulating the skin evenly. The skin to be treated should be stretched between the fingers to tension it. For very large areas, the stimulation can focus on the channel pathways that pass through it. For deficient patterns and for weak patients a light touch is required, with mild tapping until the skin reddens or very slight bleeding seems imminent. With excess conditions, a more robust approach is necessary, with firm tapping maintained until obvious pinpoints of blood appear. The treatment can be repeated twice a week.

Nerve compression

The main treatment for numbness and paresthesia from nerve compression is primarily local, aimed at the site of the compression. Acupuncture, massage and mobilization are the treatments of choice. Herbal medicine is supportive and aimed at correcting any systemic imbalances that may be present. In many cases of cervical, thoracic or lumbar spondylosis, deep acupuncture to the level of the tissues surrounding the vertebral outlet can be very effective in relieving numbness. When significant physical obstruction is present, such as osteophytes, stenosis or vertebral lipping, surgery may be required to relieve the compression.

DIFFERENTIAL DIAGNOSIS

Numbness can be due to wind–stroke (Clinical Handbook, Vol.1), and be seen in painful obstruction (Ch.15) and muscular weakness and atrophy (Ch.13).

营
卫
失
调

13.1 YING WEI DISHARMONY

Ying wei disharmony occurs when weak yang qi is unable to prevent the penetration of wind or damp into the superficial tissues. The location of the invasion is very shallow, affecting only the network vessels. Impediment to the circulation of qi and blood is mild, hence the absence of pain. The pathogenic invasion usually occurs when the patient is sweating heavily with exertion. Numbness of this type may also be caused by disruption of the ying wei from local trauma, surgery or following blood loss.

Clinical features
- Numbness and a feeling of thickness or woodenness in discrete areas. The numbness can occur anywhere, and typically appears in patches on the trunk or large muscles of the thighs and upper arm.
- mild fever and chills, hot and cold sensations
- aversion to wind and sudden change of temperature
- sweating and clamminess with mild exertion
- dry, mildly itchy skin, worse during cold dry weather

P choppy, floating or weak

T thin, white tongue coat

Treatment principle
Dispel wind from the exterior
Balance the relationship between ying qi and wei qi
Supplement qi, activate blood and warm the network vessels

Prescription

HUANG QI GUI ZHI WU WU TANG 黄芪桂枝五物汤
Astragalus and Cinnamon Twig Five Substance Decoction

huang qi (Astragali Radix) 黄芪 15–30g
bai shao (Paeoniae Radix alba) 白芍 9–12g
gui zhi (Cinnamomi Ramulus) 桂枝 9–12g
sheng jiang (Zingiberis Rhizoma recens) 生姜 12–15g
da zao (Jujubae Fructus) 大枣 .... 6 fruit

Method: Decoction. **Huang qi** supplements qi and secures the exterior; **bai shao** nourishes yin and blood; **gui zhi** warms and opens up qi and blood flow through the network vessels and supports **huang qi** in moving qi and blood; the large dose of pungent warm **sheng jiang** assists in moving qi and blood; **da zao** supports the Spleen and with **sheng jiang** harmonizes ying and wei qi. (Source: *Shi Yong Zhong Yi Nei Ke Xue* [*Jin Gui Yao Lüe*])

Modifications
- With blood stasis, use **chi shao** (Paeoniae Radix rubra) 赤芍 9–12g instead of **bai shao**.
- If the numbness moves from place to place and is accompanied by mild itching, add **fang feng** (Saposhnikovae Radix) 防风 9–12g and **bai ji li** (Tribuli Fructus) 白蒺藜 6–9g.
- For numbness following childbirth, menstrual period or hemorrhage, add **ch-**

uan xiong (Chuanxiong Rhizoma) 川芎 6–9g, **dang gui** (Angelicae sinensis Radix) 当归 9–12g, **ji xue teng** (Spatholobi Caulis) 鸡血藤 15–30g.
• With numbness of the lower body, add **huai niu xi** (Achyranthis bidentatae Radix) 怀牛膝 9–12g.

Prepared medicines
Concentrated powders
Huang Qi Wu Wu Tang (Astragalus & Cinnamon Five Herb Combination)
Pills
Gui Zhi Tang Wan (Gui Zhi Tang Teapills)

Acupuncture
Plum blossom needle over the affected area, until the skin is red. Distal points are selected according to the affected area. Discrete patches of numbness on the skin can be treated with the hair needle technique (p.579). Points to harmonize ying and wei qi can be selected from those below

Lu.9 (taiyuan) ....source point of the Lungs, strengthens the Lungs, wei qi, and fortifies the surface

Sp.6 (sanyinjiao)................strengthens the Spleen and Kidney, supplements ying qi and regulates the Liver

Du.14 (dazhui)..................meeting point of the yang channels, secures the exterior

LI.4 (hegu –) ....source point of the Large Intestine, dispels wind and diffuses the Lungs (with Lu.7 [lieque])

Lu.7 (lieque –)..................connecting point of the Lungs, diffuses the Lungs and directs Lung qi downward, dispels wind

St.36 (zusanli +▲) ....sea point of the Stomach, strengthens the Spleen and Stomach, and supplements qi to assist in dispelling pathogenic invasion; fortifies and secures wei qi

• Ear points: points related to the affected area, lung, spleen, large intestine, zero point, shenmen

Clinical notes
• Numbness of a yang wei disharmony type may be diagnosed as terminal neuritis, the sequelae of stroke, dermatitis, post traumatic or surgical nerve damage, postpartum numbness or numbness associated with malnutrition.
• A qi and blood supplementing diet is recommended. See Clinical Handbook, Vol.2, p.870 and 874.

寒 入 经 络

13.2 COLD IN THE CHANNELS

Cold in the channels is a localized phenomenon, where the cold has permeated the channels and network vessels of the extremities, constricted the vessels and diminished the flow of yang qi and blood.

Clinical features
- Numbness and cold in the hands and feet (to the wrist and ankle), aggravated or initiated by exposure to cold. Fingers and toes may blanch white or purple when exposed to cold. The affected limb or limbs may be pale or purplish and discolored, and feel icy cold, rough and dry to the touch. Once cold, the hands and feet are slow to warm up even when covered in gloves or socks or exposed to a heat source.

T pale or bluish with a white coat
P deep or imperceptible in the affected limb or limbs

Treatment Principle
Warm the channels and network vessels and disperse cold
Nourish blood and unblock blood vessels

Prescription

DANG GUI SI NI TANG 当归四逆汤
Tangkuei Decoction for Frigid Extremities

dang gui (Angelicae sinensis Radix) 当归 9–12g
bai shao (Paeoniae Radix alba) 白芍 9–12g
gui zhi (Cinnamomi Ramulus) 桂枝 6–9g
tong cao (Tetrapanacis Medulla) 通草 6–9g
zhi gan cao (Glycyrrhizae Radix preparata) 炙甘草 3–6g
xi xin (Asari Herba) 细辛 2–3g
da zao (Jujubae Fructus) 大枣 .... 8 fruit

Method: Decoction. **Dang gui** and **bai shao** supplement and nourish yin and blood; **dang gui** gently activates blood; **xi xin** and **gui zhi** warm the channels, dispel cold and encourage the circulation of yang qi to the extremities; **da zao** supports **dang gui** in nourishing blood; **zhi gan cao** and **bai shao** alleviate vasospasm, muscle spasm and pain; **tong cao** assists in opening up the peripheral channels and network vessels. (Source: *Shang Han Lun*)

Modifications
- With marked cold, add **zhi fu zi** (Aconiti Radix lateralis preparata) 制附子 6–9g and **gan jiang** (Zingiberis Rhizoma) 干姜 6–9g.
- With qi deficiency, add **huang qi** (Astragali Radix) 黄芪 12–18g, **bai zhu** (Atractylodes macrocephalae Rhizoma) 白术 9–12g and **ji xue teng** (Spatholobi Caulis) 鸡血藤 15–30g.

Prepared medicines
Concentrated powder
Dang Gui Si Ni Tang (Tangkiei & Jujube Combination)

Pills
Dang Gui Si Ni Wan (Dang Gui Si Ni Teapills)

Acupuncture (select from)
LI.11 (quchi +▲) ....sea point of the Large Intestine, warms and dispels
cold and promotes circulation of qi and blood
through the arm

LI.4 (hegu +▲) ....local point for the hand and fingers

Lu.9 (taiyuan) ....meeting point for the vessels

PC.4 (ximen) ....these points stimulate qi and blood circulation to

PC.6 (neiguan)   the hand

St.36 (zusanli +▲)..............sea point of the Stomach, promotes circulation of qi
and blood through the legs and systemically (with
LI.11)

Sp.6 (sanyinjiao +▲) ....warms the channels and activates qi and blood
circulation to the feet

Ren.4 (guanyuan ▲) ....warms Kidney yang and promotes distribution of
yang qi to the extremities

• Ear points: points related to the affected area, heart, liver, sympathetic, adrenal

Clinical notes
• Numbness from cold in the channels may be diagnosed as Raynaud's syndrome, Buerger's disease, frostbite, intermittent claudication or peripheral vascular disease.
• The cold in this pattern is confined to the extremities, thus this pattern differs from that in which yang is systemically weak and unable to reach the limbs. In systemic yang deficiency, the whole limb is cold and there are systemic signs of yang deficiency.
• A warming diet is recommended. See Clinical Handbook, Vol.2, p.873.

痰
湿
阻
络

13.3 PHLEGM BLOCKING THE NETWORK VESSELS

Phlegm can infiltrate the tissues and network vessels as a result of chronic constrained qi that causes congealing of fluids, from chronic damp or damp heat in the tissues or qi deficiency. When phlegm has congealed in the tissues and network vessels, it produces a particularly viscous obstruction to qi and blood flow, and a persistent and progressive, or recurrent type of numbness.

Clinical features

- Gradually progressive or recurrent numbness, tingling and heaviness in the arms, legs, hands and feet. The numbness may start at the tips of the extremities, gradually progressing to a 'stocking and glove' distribution. When severe the numbness can make walking and using the hands difficult. The muscles of the limbs may feel firm and cold to the touch.
- dizziness or vertigo
- foggy or heavy head, difficulty concentrating
- chest oppression
- may be blurred vision or double vision
- symptoms often worse in damp or humid weather

T normal color, or slightly pale and swollen with thick, white, greasy coat
P deep and slippery

Treatment Principle

Transform phlegm damp
Promote qi movement and disperse stubborn phlegm accumulation
Supplement qi and unblock the network vessels

Prescription

DI TAN TANG 涤痰汤
Scour Phlegm Decoction, modified

zhi ban xia (Pinelliae Rhizoma preparatum) 制半夏	9–12g
zhu ru (Bambusae Caulis in taeniam) 竹茹	9–12g
fu ling (Poria) 茯苓	9–12g
dan nan xing (Arisaema cum Bile) 胆南星	6–9g
chen pi (Citri reticulatae Pericarpium) 陈皮	6–9g
zhi shi (Aurantii Fructus immaturus) 枳实	6–9g
shi chang pu (Acori tatarinowii Rhizoma) 石菖蒲	6–9g
ren shen (Ginseng Radix) 人参	3–6g
gan cao (Glycyrrhizae Radix) 甘草	3–6g
sheng jiang (Zingiberis Rhizoma recens) 生姜	6–9g
da zao (Jujubae Fructus) 大枣	4 fruit
wei ling xian (Clematidis Radix) 威灵仙	6–9g

Method: Decoction. **Zhi ban xia, zhu ru** and **chen pi** dry dampness and phlegm; **fu ling** strengthens the Spleen and promotes urination to drain damp; **zhi shi** regulates qi and assist descent of Stomach qi; **dan nan xing** and **shi chang pu** dispel and vaporize phlegm; **ren shen, da zao** and **gan cao** supplement qi and protects the Spleen and Stomach; **sheng jiang** assists **zhi ban xia** and **chen pi** in transforming phlegm damp; **wei ling xian** breaks through obstruction in the channels and network vessels and disperses phlegm. (Source: *Zhong Yi Zhi Liao Yi Nan Za Bing Mi Yao* [*Ji Sheng Fang*])

Modifications

- If the legs are most affected, add **chuan niu xi** (Cyathulae Radix) 川牛膝 12–15g and **mu gua** (Chaenomelis Fructus) 木瓜 9–12g.
- If the arms are most affected, add **gui zhi** (Cinnamomi Ramulus) 桂枝 6–9g and **jiang huang** (Curcumae longae Rhizoma) 姜黄 6–9g.
- With cold extremities, replace **sheng jiang** with **gan jiang** (Zingiberis Rhizoma) 干姜 6–9g, and add **xi xin** (Asari Herba) 细辛 3–6g.
- With heat, delete **sheng jiang**, and add **ren dong teng** (Lonicerae Caulis) 忍冬藤 15–30g and **shan zhi zi** (Gardeniae Fructus) 山栀子 9–12g.
- With chest oppression, add **gua lou** (Trichosanthis Fructus) 栝楼 18–30g.
- With marked Spleen qi deficiency, add **bai zhu** (Atractylodis macrocephalae Rhizoma) 白术 9–12g.
- With blood stasis, add **chuan xiong** (Chuanxiong Rhizoma) 川芎 6–9g, **hong hua** (Carthami Flos) 红花 6–9g and **ji xue teng** (Spatholobi Caulis) 鸡血藤 12–18g.

Variations and additional prescriptions

In the remission phase

If the patient does well and the symptoms improve, it is a good idea to continue the treatment with a milder phlegm transforming prescription. The treatment at this point is to strengthen the Spleen, improve fluid metabolism and prevent phlegm formation. Formulae to consider include XIANG SHA LIU JUN ZI TANG (Six Gentlemen Decoction with Aucklandia and Amomum 香砂六君子汤 p.618) or SHEN LING BAI ZHU SAN (Ginseng, Poria and White Atractylodes Powder 参苓白术散, p.621).

Prepared medicines

Concentrated powders

Er Zhu Tang (Atractylodes & Arisaema Combination)
Ding Xian Wan (Gastrodia and Amber Combination)
Zhu Ru Wen Dan Tang (Bamboo & Ginseng Combination)
 – with phlegm heat

Pills

Wen Dan Wan (Rising Courage Teapills) plus Ping Wei San (Calm Stomach Teapills, Tabellae Pingwei)
Qing Qi Hua Tan Wan (Clean Air Teapills, Pinellia Expectorant Pills)
 – phlegm heat

Acupuncture

Define the limits of the numb region with a surgical marker and use the hair needle technique (p.579) towards the numbness. If the points listed below fall in the numb region, they can be needled obliquely with shallow insertion, not penetrating the muscle layer. Those outside the numb region can be needled in the standard fashion.

Ren.12 (zhongwan) ....alarm point of the Stomach, strengthens the Spleen
and Stomach to assist in transforming phlegm

St.40 (fenglong –) ....connecting and source points of the Stomach

Sp.3 (taibai +)   and Spleen, these points strengthen the Spleen and
resolve phlegm, and are effective for heaviness and
weakness in the limbs

PC.5 (jianshi –)..................river point of the Pericardium, transforms phlegm

Bl.20 (pishu) ....transport point of the Spleen, strengthens the Spleen
and supplements qi to promote transformation and
resolution of phlegm

Liv.3 (taichong –)...............regulates the Liver and resolves qi constraint, an
essential consideration for all phlegm treatments

- with muscle heaviness, add Sp.21 (dabao)
- with vertigo, add GB.43 (xiaxi –) and Du.20 (baihui)
- with blurred vision, add St.8 (touwei), Bl.2 (zanzhu) and GB.37 (guanming)
- with foggy or heavy head, add Bl.62 (shenmai)
- with Spleen deficiency add St.36 (zusanli +)
- with cold, apply moxa to Bl.20 (pishu ▲) and Bl.21 (weishu ▲)
- with heat, add St.44 (neiting –)
- Ear points: points related to the affected area, zero point, stomach, spleen, liver, zero point, sympathetic, shenmen

Clinical notes

- Numbness of a phlegm type may be diagnosed as multiple sclerosis, peripheral neuropathy or polyneuropathy.
- Numbness of recent onset associated with phlegm can respond quite well to persistent treatment. This pattern usually has an intermittent course, reflecting the congealing and dispersal of phlegm in response to diet, qi constraint and invasion of pathogens into the qi level. A patient who has responded to treatment or has had a spontaneous remission and is symptom free, should be advised that continued treatment is still of great value in preventing recurrence. Treatment to maintain healthy Spleen and Lung function, support fluid metabolism, and build plentiful qi and blood is important.
- A phlegm transforming diet and one that supports Spleen function is an essential part of treatment. See Clinical Handbook, Vol.2, p.880.

气血瘀滞 13.4 QI AND BLOOD STASIS

Numbness from qi and blood stasis can be acute or chronic. When acute it follows a traumatic injury or surgery. When chronic the stasis can be the result of chronic Liver qi constraint, prolonged cold, damp heat or phlegm blocking the channels, or qi and blood deficiency. It can also result from heavy cigarette smoking and disorders that congeal the blood or lead to increased viscosity of blood, such as high fever or chronic dehydration.

Clinical features
- Numbness, insensitivity and a wooden feeling in a limb that is discolored and with thickened dry scaly skin. There may be purple congested veins, varicosities, or spider nevi in the affected area. The limbs are generally cold, and may ache.
- vascular congestion or venous ulceration
- left iliac fossa pressure pain (p.925–926)

T mauve or purple with stasis spots; dark, congested, sublingual veins
P deep, choppy, fine; diminished or absent in the affected limb or limbs

Treatment Principle
Activate blood and disperse stagnant blood
Open up the channels and network vessels
Warm and dispel cold

Prescription

TONG MAI TANG 通脉汤
Unblock the Vessels Decoction

huang qi (Astragali Radix) 黄芪	15–30g
ji xue teng (Spatholobi Caulis) 鸡血藤	15–30g
dang gui (Angelicae sinensis Radix) 当归	12–15g
chi shao (Paeoniae Radix rubra) 赤芍	12–15g
huai niu xi (Achyranthis bidentatae Radix) 怀牛膝	12–15g
chuan xiong (Chuanxiong Rhizoma) 川芎	9–12g
tao ren (Persicae Semen) 桃仁	9–12g
hong hua (Carthami Flos) 红花	9–12g
si gua luo (Luffae Fructus) 丝瓜络	9–12g
liu ji nu (Artemesiae anomalae Herba) 刘寄奴	9–12g
zhi ru xiang (Olibanum preparata) 炙乳香	9–12g
gui zhi (Cinnamomi Ramulus) 桂枝	9–12g

Method: Decoction. **Huang qi, ji xue teng** and **si gua luo** promote circulation of qi and blood to the extremities; **dang gui** nourishes blood; **chi shao, huai niu xi, chuan xiong, tao ren, hong hua, liu ji nu** and **zhi ru xiang** activate blood and disperse blood stasis; **gui zhi** warms the blood and promotes flow of yang qi to the extremities. (Source: *Shi Yong Zhong Yi Wai Ke Xue* [*Xi An Yi Xue Yuan*])

Modifications
- With cold, add **zhi fu zi** (Aconiti Radix lateralis preparata) 制附子 6–9g.

Prepared medicines

Concentrated powder

Tao Hong Si Wu Tang (Tangkuei Four, Persica & Carthamus Combination)

Xue Fu Zhu Yu Tang (Persica & Carthamus Combination)

Pills

Tao Hong Si Wu Wan (Tao Hong Si Wu Tang Teapills)

Xue Fu Zhu Yu Wan (Stasis in the Mansion of Blood Teapills)

Sheng Tian Qi Pian (Raw Tian Qi Ginseng Tablets)

Acupuncture

Plum blossom needle with some vigor over the affected area, until mild bleeding occurs. Bloodletting on congested veins to draw a few drops of dark blood may be helpful. Local points are selected according to the affected area. Discrete patches of numbness on the skin can be treated with the hair needle technique (p.579), inserted at 30–45⁰, at intervals of a few centimeters, towards the numb area. In addition points can be selected from those below to activate blood. Points within the numb area are avoided and the plum blossom technique is preferred.

Bl.17 (geshu −)..................meeting point for blood, disperses stagnant blood

Bl.18 (ganshu +)................transport point of the Liver, activates Liver qi and blood

Bl.20 (pishu +) ....transport point of the Spleen, strengthens the Spleen to manufacture new blood

Sp.6 (sanyinjiao −)..............these points activate blood and disperse stagnant

Sp.10 (xuehai −)   blood

LI.4 (hegu −)

Sp.8 (diji −).......................cleft point of the Spleen, rectifies qi and activates blood

Liv.3 (taichong −)..............source point of the Liver, regulates qi and activates blood, frees the channels and network vessels and stops pain

St.36 (zusanli) ....sea point of the Stomach, strengthens the Spleen, supplements qi and activates qi and blood flow

- Ear points: points related to the affected area, liver, spleen, zero point, sympathetic, shenmen

Clinical notes

- Qi and blood stasis type numbness may be diagnosed as intermittent claudication, peripheral vascular disease, peripheral atherosclerosis, fibromyalgia, deep venous thrombosis, vascular scarring or Buerger's disease.
- Watch for signs of bleeding in patients using anticoagulant drugs such as Warfarin.

痰
瘀
阻
滞

13.5 PHLEGM AND BLOOD STASIS

Phlegm and blood stasis is a chronic and recalcitrant pattern of numbness. Both phlegm and blood stasis alone can give rise to numbness, but when combined, they cause complete deadening and loss of sensation.

Clinical features

- Chronic numbness with complete loss of sensation. The numbness may be anywhere in the body, although the extremities are the most common location. When the legs and feet are affected, walking is difficult or impossible.
- weakness in the extremities; cold extremities
- dark skin discoloration or congested veins and spider nevi over or near the affected area

T mauve or purple, or with brown or purple stasis spots; may be a thick or greasy coat; sublingual veins congested and dark
P deep and choppy or deep and slippery

Treatment principle

Activate blood and disperse blood stasis
Transform and eliminate phlegm

Prescription

XIAO HUO LUO DAN 小活络丹
Minor Activate the Network Vessels Special Pill

This formula is only used in prepared form. It contains powerful heating and dispersing herbs that are toxic when used improperly.

zhi cao wu (Aconiti kusnezoffii Radix preparata) 制草乌 20g
zhi chuan wu (Aconiti Radix preparata) 制川乌 20g
zhi tian nan xing (Arisaematis Rhizoma preparatum) 制天南星 20g
di long (Pheretima) 地龙 20g
mo yao (Myrrha) 没药 10g
ru xiang (Olibanum) 乳香 10g

Method: Pills or powder. Available in small pills and powdered extract. These formats enable reliable and precise dose management. Always start with a small dose to assess the patients response before increasing to a therapeutic dose, and do not exceed the manufacturers recommended dose. Not suitable for very weak patients, those with underlying yin deficiency and prolonged use. **Zhi chuan wu** and **zhi cao wu** dispel cold, warm the channels and network vessels and break through stubborn blockages; **zhi tian nan xing** transforms phlegm and disperses phlegm from the channels and network vessels; **ru xiang** and **mo yao** activate blood and disperse blood stasis; **di long** 'burrows' through obstructions and clears the channel system of obstruction. (Source: *He Ji Ju Fang*)

Modifications.

- With severe blood stasis, add **wu gong** (Scolopendra) 蜈蚣 1–3g, **quan xie** (Scorpio) 全蝎 1–3g and **di bie chong** (Eupolyphaga/Steleophaga) 地鳖虫 3–6g [all powdered and taken separately].
- With numbness in the face, combine with **QIAN ZHENG SAN** (Lead to Symmetry Powder 牵正散, p.917).
- With Liver and Kidney deficiency, combine with **DU HUO JI SHENG TANG**

(Pubescent Angelica and Taxillus Decoction 独活寄生汤, p.690).

Variations and additional prescriptions

For weak patients

Phlegm and blood stasis will usually be complicated by some degree of qi and blood deficiency. When there is significant deficiency the primary prescription above is too dispersing and not recommended. A milder compromise prescription that is slower in action but better tolerated can be constructed from a mixture of mild blood activating and phlegm dispersing prescriptions such as TAO HONG SI WU TANG (Four Substance Decoction with Safflower and Peach Pit 桃红四物汤, p.921) and DI TAN TANG (Scour Phlegm Decoction 涤痰汤, p.584).

Prepared medicines

Concentrated powder

Xiao Huo Luo Dan (Myrrh & Aconite Formula)
Tao Hong Si Wu Tang (Tangkuei Four, Persica & Carthamus Combination) plus Er Zhu Tang (Atractylodes & Arisaema Combination)
– for phlegm and blood stasis with qi and blood deficiency

Pills

Xiao Huo Luo Dan (Xiao Huo Luo Dan Teapills)
Tao Hong Si Wu Wan (Tao Hong Si Wu Tang Teapills) plus Er Chen Wan (Pinellia Pachyma Pills, Erh Chen Wan)
– for phlegm and blood stasis with qi and blood deficiency

Acupuncture

Plum blossom needle with some vigor over the affected area, until mild bleeding occurs. Bloodletting on congested veins to draw a few drops of dark blood may be helpful. Local points are selected according to the affected area. Discrete patches of numbness on the skin can be treated with the hair needle technique (p.579), inserted at 30–45^0, at intervals of a few centimeters, towards the numb area. In addition points can be selected from those below to activate blood and transform phlegm. Points within the numb area are avoided and the plum blossom technique is preferred.

Bl.17 (geshu –).................meeting point for blood, disperses stagnant blood
Bl.18 (ganshu +).................transport point of the Liver, activates Liver qi and blood
Bl.20 (pishu +) ....transport point of the Spleen, strengthens the Spleen to manufacture new blood and transform phlegm
Bl.23 (shenshu +) ....transport point of the Kidneys, strengthens the Kidneys to support the Spleen
Sp.6 (sanyinjiao –)..............these points activate blood and disperse stagnant
Sp.10 (xuehai –)   blood
LI.4 (hegu –)
Sp.8 (diji –) ....cleft point of the Spleen, rectifies qi and activates blood
Liv.3 (taichong –)...............source point of the Liver, regulates qi and activates

blood, frees the channels and network vessels and
stops pain

St.40 (fenglong –) ....connecting point of the Stomach, transforms
phlegm and clears heat and phlegm from the
Stomach, calms the shen

St.36 (zusanli) ....sea point of the Stomach, strengthens the Spleen and
supplements qi to transform phlegm and activate
blood

• Ear points: points related to the affected area, liver, spleen, zero point, sympathetic, shenmen

Clinical notes

• Phlegm and blood stasis type numbness is difficult to treat effectively, but is worth trying if only to relieve discomfort and help mobility. Some patients can respond reasonably well.

• In all cases where relatively high doses of **fu zi** and its more powerful relatives are being used, it is wise to begin with a small dose and work up to a therapeutic dose over a week or two, and carefully assess the patients response. Patients with subclinical yin deficiency or hidden heat can become overheated quickly, causing symptoms such as increasing insomnia and restlessness, flushing and thirst to become apparent. In such cases, the dose of medicine should be reduced, or the prescription taken with a decoction of counterbalancing herbs such as **zhi mu** (Anemarrhenae Rhizoma) 知母, **bai shao** (Paeoniae Radix alba) 白芍 and **xuan shen** (Scrophulariae Radix) 玄参.

风
湿
痹
阻

13.6 WIND DAMP

Wind damp obstructs the circulation of qi and blood and prevents blood from reaching the skin. There are two types of wind damp numbness, one chronic and other acute. Chronic wind damp numbness has parallels to wind damp painful obstruction (p.651), with the pain component minimal or absent. An acute episode of wind damp numbness occurs as a result of invasion of the network vessels and often involves the face and upper body.

Clinical features

• Gradual and progressive, or acute onset of, numbness in the extremities or head, accompanied by aching and stiffness of muscles and joints. The numbness is worse during, or preceding cold or wet weather or increasing humidity. Numbness and aching may be relieved by warmth.

T normal or pale, with a thin, white or greasy coat
P deep, moderate, slow

Treatment principle

Dispel wind damp
Open up flow of qi and blood through the channels and network vessels

Prescription

CHENG SHI JUAN BI TANG 程氏蠲痹汤
Remove Painful Obstruction Decoction (from the Cheng Clan), modified

qiang huo (Notopterygii Rhizoma seu Radix) 羌活 6–9g
du huo (Angelicae pubescentis Radix) 独活 6–9g
qin jiao (Gentianae macrophyllae Radix) 秦艽 6–9g
dang gui (Angelicae sinensis Radix) 当归 6–9g
chuan xiong (Chuanxiong Rhizoma) 川芎 6–9g
mu xiang (Aucklandiae Radix) 木香 3–6g
zhi gan cao (Glycyrrhizae Radix preparata) 炙甘草 3–6g
sang zhi (Mori Ramulus) 桑枝 15–30g
hai feng teng (Piperis kadsurae Caulis) 海风藤 15–30g
gui zhi (Cinnamomi Ramulus) 桂枝 6–9g
ji xue teng (Spatholobi Caulis) 鸡血藤 15–30g

Method: Decoction. **Qiang huo**, **du huo**, **qin jiao**, **hai feng teng** and **sang zhi** dispel wind damp; **dang gui**, **chuan xiong** and **mu xiang** activate qi and blood; **gui zhi** and **ji xue teng** open up qi and blood flow through the network vessels; **zhi gan cao** harmonizes the formula and protects the Stomach. (Source: *Shi Yong Zhong Yi Nei Ke Xue* [*Yi Xue Xin Wu*])

Modifications

• With wind predominant, add **fang feng** (Saposhnikovae Radix) 防风 9–12g.
• With damp predominant, add **han fang ji** (Stephaniae tetrandrae Radix) 汉防己 9–12g, **cang zhu** (Atractylodis Rhizoma) 苍术 9–12g, **yi ren** (Coicis Semen) 苡仁 15–30g and **can sha** (Bombycis Faeces) 蚕沙 6–9g.
• With cold predominant, add **ma huang** (Ephedra Herba) 麻黄 6–9g and **zhi fu zi** (Aconiti Radix lateralis preparata) 制附子 6–12g.

- If the primary location of the numbness is the upper body, add **wei ling xian** (Clematidis Radix) 威灵仙 9–12g and **jiang huang** (Curcumae longae Rhizoma) 姜黄 9–12g.
- If the legs are affected, add **huai niu xi** (Achyranthis bidentatae Radix) 怀牛膝 9–12g, **mu gua** (Chaenomelis Fructus) 木瓜 6–9g and **xu duan** (Dipsaci Radix) 续断 9–12g.
- In very chronic or resistant cases, a small dose of XIAO HUO LUO DAN (Minor Activate the Network Vessels Special Pill 小活络丹, p.589) in concentrated powder or pill form can be helpful to break through stubborn blockages.

Variations and additional prescriptions
Acute onset of wind damp
Acute wind damp invasion into the network vessels can cause numbness and loss of motor function. This is a type of wind–stroke, in which a preexisting deficiency allows wind damp to gain access to the exposed channels and network vessels. The onset is sudden, with numbness in the extremities or face. There will usually be symptoms of an external pathogen, such as fever and chills, myalgia and malaise and a floating pulse, a week or two before the numbness sets in. The treatment is to dispel wind damp and activate blood with a prescription such as **DA QIN JIAO TANG** (Major Large Gentian Decoction 大秦艽汤, p.914).

Wind damp with Liver and Kidney deficiency
A chronic wind damp condition often becomes complicated by weakness of the Liver and Kidneys, and thus a deeper pathology of the sinews and bones develops. This is especially so in older patients. The deficiency aspects can be diverse, with mixtures of qi, blood, yin and yang deficiency underlying the superficial wind damp. In addition to the numbness, stiffness and dull aches of the legs and waist, the patient exhibits the classic features of deficiency such as fatigue, pallor, dizziness, breathlessness, pale tongue and weak pulse. The treatment is to supplement the Liver and Kidneys and dispel wind damp with a prescription such as **DU HUO JI SHENG TANG** (Pubescent Angelica and Taxillus Decoction 独活寄生汤, p.690) or **SAN BI TANG** (Three Painful Obstruction Decoction 三痹汤, p.680).

Prepared medicines
Concentrated powder
Juan Bi Tang (Notopterygium & Turmeric Combination)
Da Qin Jiao Tang (Major Gentiana Macrophylla Root Combination)
   – acute wind damp numbness or facial paralysis
Du Huo Ji Sheng Tang (Tuhuo and Loranthus Combination)
   – with Liver and Kidney deficiency

Pills
Juan Bi Wan (Clear Channel Teapills)
Xuan Bi Tang Wan (Xuan Bi Teapills)
   – damp heat
Du Huo Ji Sheng Wan (Solitary Hermit Teapills)
   – with Liver and Kidney deficiency

Acupuncture

Local points are selected according to the affected area. Points proximal to, or surrounding, the region of sensory loss are chosen. Discrete patches of numbness on the skin can be treated with the hair needle technique (p.579). Plum blossom needle is also suitable (p.579). In addition, points can be selected from those below to expel wind damp. If any of these points are located in the numb area, they can be needled obliquely and superficially, otherwise they are needled in the standard fashion.

LI.4 (hegu –).....................source point of the Large Intestine, dispels wind and clears the channels, good for numbness in the face

LI.11 (quchi –)...................sea point of the Large Intestine, expels wind and damp, regulates qi and blood

Sp.9 (yinlingquan –)...........sea point of the Spleen, transforms damp stagnation

GB.31 (fengshi –)...............dispels wind and relaxes the sinews

GB.33 (xiyangguan –)........for numbness in the legs

GB.34 (yanglingquan –).....sea point of the Gallbladder and meeting point for the sinews, strengthens sinews and bones

St.36 (zusanli) ....sea point of the Stomach, regulates qi and blood and eliminates damp

- with cold, use plenty of moxa and warm needle technique
- with heat, add St.43 (xianggu –)
- Ear points: points related to the affected area, spleen, kidney, zero point, shen-men, sympathetic

Clinical notes

- Wind damp numbness may be diagnosed as rheumatoid arthritis or osteoarthritis, atypical autoimmune disease, diabetic peripheral neuropathy, early stage of scleroderma or polyneuritis from poisoning.

湿
热
浸
淫

13.7 DAMP HEAT

Numbness and paresthesia caused by damp heat is usually a chronic problem of insidious onset, although may occasionally be acute and rapidly progressive. The damp heat can be environmental, seeping slowly into the body with prolonged exposure to hot humid or damp conditions, or can invade the qi level quickly during unseasonal weather. Damp heat can also be generated internally, as a result of diet and alcohol, or Spleen weakness. Any pre–existing internal damp heat or Liver and Kidney deficiency renders one more vulnerable to external damp heat invasion. Damp heat is heavy and tends to sink down towards the lower body. It is mainly deposited in the superficial muscle layer and network vessels of the legs. Persistent damp heat will gradually damage yin and further weaken the Liver and Kidneys.

Clinical features
- Numbness, heaviness, tingling and paresthesia of the feet and lower legs, with mild edema. The limbs feel warm to the touch. The numbness or a burning sensation may begin in the soles of the feet and gradually progress up the leg. The symptoms may develop gradually or quickly. There may be mild edema of the feet, muscle aches or weakness.
- heat intolerance, may feel worse in warm weather or with hot baths
- low grade fever, afternoon fever or contained fever (p.367); night sweats
- heaviness, lethargy
- flushed complexion; greasy skin
- chest oppression
- abdominal distension
- may be lymphadenopathy

T red with a greasy, yellow coat
P slippery, rapid

Treatment Principle
Clear damp heat from network vessels and muscles
Activate circulation of qi and blood

Prescription

SI MIAO SAN 四妙散
Four Marvel Powder

---

cang zhu (Atractylodis Rhizoma) 苍术 12–15g
huang bai (Phellodendri Cortex) 黄柏 12–15g
yi ren (Coicis Semen) 苡仁 30–60g
chuan niu xi (Cyathulae Radix) 川牛膝 12–15g

Method: Decoction. **Huang bai** clears damp heat, **cang zhu** and **yi ren** dry and leach out dampness and strengthen the Spleen and thus support **huang bai** in clearing damp heat; **chuan niu xi** activates the flow of qi and blood through the legs. (Source: *Shi Yong Zhong Yi Nei Ke Xue* [*Cheng Fang Bian Du*])

Modifications

- The formula above is usually augmented with herbs to open up flow in the network vessels, clear heat and treat numbness, such as **lao guan cao** (Erodii/ Geranii Herba) 老鹳草 15–30g, **ren dong teng** (Lonicerae Caulis) 忍冬藤 15–30g, **xi xian cao** (Siegesbeckia Herba) 豨莶草 9–15g and **ji xue teng** (Spatholobi Caulis) 鸡血藤 15–30g.

- A couple of blood activating herbs are useful to promote flow in the channels and network vessels. Select from **dan shen** (Salviae miltiorrhizae Radix) 丹参 9–12g, **chi shao** (Paeoniae Radix rubra) 赤芍 9–12g, **lu lu tong** (Liquidambaris Fructus) 路路通 6–12g, **di long** (Pheretima) 地龙 9–12g and **si gua luo** (Luffae Fructus) 丝瓜络 9–12g.

- With marked heat, burning feet, a yellow tongue coat, afternoon fever and sweats, use **huang bai** at the top of the dosage range, and add **shan zhi zi** (Gardeniae Fructus) 山栀子 9–12g and **shi gao** (Gypsum fibrosum) 石膏 15–30g [cooked first].

- With damp greater than heat, edema, lethargy and a thick greasy tongue coat, use **cang zhu** at the top of the dosage range, and add **han fang ji** (Stephaniae tetrandrae Radix) 汉防己 9–12g, **chi fu ling** (Poria Rubra) 赤茯苓 12–15g and **bi xie** (Dioscoreae hypoglaucae Rhizoma) 萆薢 9–12g.

- With painful or concentrated urination, add **dan zhu ye** (Lophatheri Herba) 淡竹叶 6–9g and **che qian zi** (Plantaginis Semen) 车前子 9–12g [cooked in a cloth bag].

- With weeping, itchy skin lesions, add **tu fu ling** (Smilacis glabrae Rhizoma) 土茯苓 12–15g and **bai xian pi** (Dictamni Cortex) 白藓皮 9–12g.

- With yin damage, burning in the soles of the feet and peeled tongue coat on the root of the tongue, add **sheng di** (Rehmanniae Radix) 生地 12–15g and **mai dong** (Ophiopogonis Radix) 麦冬 9–12g.

- For peripheral neuropathy associated with diabetes, see modifications, p.182.

Variations and additional prescriptions

Sudden onset
See p.555.

Chronic damp heat with Kidney yin deficiency
See p.555.

Prepared medicines

Concentrated powders
San Miao San (Atractylodes & Phellodendron Formula)
Dang Gui Nian Tong San (Tangkuei & Anemarrhena Combination)
Gan Lu Xiao Du Dan (Forsythia & Acorus Formula)
   – sudden onset of damp heat with exterior signs and symptoms
Zhi Bai Di Huang Wan (Anemarrhena, Phellodendron & Rehmannia Formula)
   – with Kidney yin damage

Pills
Bi Xie Sheng Shi Wan (Subdue the Dampness Teapills)

– damp greater than heat
Long Dan Xie Gan Wan (Snake and Dragon Teapills)
– heat greater than damp
Zhi Bai Ba Wei Wan (Eight Flavor Rehmannia Teapills)

Acupuncture (select from)

Local points are selected according to the affected area. Points proximal to the region of sensory loss are chosen. Discrete patches of numbness on the skin can be treated with the hair needle technique (p.579). In addition points can be selected from those below to systemically strengthen Lung and Spleen qi. Plum blossom is not suitable.

Sp.9 (yinlingquan –)...........sea and river points of the Spleen these points
Sp.5 (shangqiu –)   promote urination and clear damp heat
Sp.3 (taibai).....................source and connecting points of the Spleen and
St.40 (fenglong –)   Stomach, strengthen the Spleen and transform damp
                              and phlegm
LI.11 (quchi –)..................these points clear damp heat from the qi level
St.44 (neiting –)
SJ.6 (zhigou –) ....river point of the triple burner, promotes movement
                              through the triple burner to dispel damp heat
Bl.20 (pishu) ....transport point of the Spleen, strengthens the Spleen
                              to dry dampness
- for acute damp heat, add Lu.6 (kongzui)
- with nausea, add PC.6 (neiguan)
- with diarrhea, add zhixie (N–CA–3) and Bl.25 (tianshu)
- with myalgia, add Sp.21 (dabao)
- Ear points: points related to the affected area, spleen, stomach, zero point, shenmen, sympathetic, endocrine

Clinical notes

- Damp heat numbness may be diagnosed as peripheral neuropathy associated with diabetes, Guillain–Barré syndrome, polyneuritis, alcoholic poisoning or infection of the central nervous system.
- Diet is an essential part of treatment. See Clinical Handbook, Vol.2, p.884 for suggestions.
- Damp heat is often complicated by yin deficiency, so be careful with the bitter cold and pungent drying herbs, which can contribute to yin damage if overused.

气虚失运 | 13.8 QI DEFICIENCY

The qi deficiency here is associated with the Lung, Heart and Spleen. The Lungs govern the qi and the overall movement of qi, the Heart governs blood circulation, and the Spleen is responsible for distribution of qi to the limbs and muscles. The combined weakness of these organ systems is unable to propel blood to the furthest points of the body, here the far extremities.

Clinical features

- Numbness and paresthesia, mostly in the hands and feet. There may be heaviness, a feeling as if walking on cotton wool, and mild edema.
- waxy, pale complexion
- fatigue, weakness
- spontaneous sweating
- breathlessness with exertion; weak voice
- frequent colds and flu
- loss of appetite, abdominal distension, loose stools

T pale, swollen and scalloped with a thin, white coat
P weak, fine, especially in the distal position

Treatment principle

Supplement qi to lead the blood
Secure and consolidate wei qi

Prescription

BU ZHONG YI QI TANG 补中益气汤
Supplement the Middle to Augment the Qi Decoction

huang qi (Astragali Radix) 黄芪 18–45g
ren shen (Ginseng Radix) 人参 9–12g
bai zhu (Atractylodis macrocephalae Rhizoma) 白术..............................9–12g
dang gui (Angelicae sinensis Radix) 当归 6–9g
chen pi (Citri reticulatae Pericarpium) 陈皮 6–9g
sheng ma (Cimicifugae Rhizoma) 升麻..3–6g
chai hu (Bupleuri Radix) 柴胡 3–6g
zhi gan cao (Glycyrrhizae Radix preparata) 炙甘草..................................3–6g

Method: Decoction. **Huang qi** strengthens the Lungs and Spleen and elevates qi; **ren shen**, **bai zhu** and **zhi gan cao** supplement qi; **chai hu** and **sheng ma** support the principal herbs in elevating qi and by doing so assist in correcting the qi dynamic and the distribution of yang qi; **dang gui** nourishes and activates blood; **chen pi** regulates qi and stimulates the qi dynamic. (Source: *Shi Yong Zhong Yi Nei Ke Xue* [*Pi Wei Lun*])

Modifications

- The channel opening effect of the prescription can be augmented by herbs such as **ji xue teng** (Spatholobi Caulis) 鸡血藤 15–30g, **qing feng teng** (Sinomenium Caulis) 清风藤 9–15g and **shen jin cao** (Lycopodii Herba) 伸筋草 9–15g.
- With cold extremities and cold intolerance, add **gui zhi** (Cinnamomi Ramulus) 桂枝 6–9g.

- With phlegm, add one or two of the following herbs: **bai jie zi** (Sinapsis Semen) 白芥子 3–6g, **zhi ban xia** (Pinelliae Rhizoma preparatum) 制半夏 6–9g, **zhe bei mu** (Fritillariae thunbergii Bulbus) 浙贝母 9–12g and **gua lou** (Trichosanthis Fructus) 栝楼 18–30g.
- With edema and heaviness, add **cang zhu** (Atractylodis Rhizoma) 苍术 9–12g.
- For peripheral neuropathy associated with diabetes of a qi deficiency type, add **shan yao** (Dioscoreae Rhizoma) 山药 12–18g, **tian hua fen** (Trichosanthes Radix) 天花粉 9–12g and **ge gen** (Puerariae Radix) 葛根 9–12g. See also p.175.

Prepared medicines
Concentrated powders
Bu Zhong Yi Qi Tang (Ginseng & Astragalus Combination)
Er Chen Tang (Citrus & Pinellia Combination)
　　– add with phlegm or damp

Pills
Bu Zhong Yi Qi Wan (Central Chi Teapills)

Acupuncture (select from)
Local points are selected according to the affected area, generally drawn from the yangming and taiyin channels. Points proximal to the region of sensory loss are chosen. Discrete patches of numbness on the skin can be treated with the hair needle technique (p.579). In addition points can be selected from those below to systemically strengthen Lung and Spleen qi.

Bl.13 (feishu +▲)...............transport point of the Lungs, strengthens the Lungs
　　　　　　　　　　　　and supplements qi
Bl.20 (pishu +▲) ....transport point of the Spleen, strengthens the Spleen
　　　　　　　　　　　　and supplements qi
Bl.23 (shenshu +▲) ....transport point of the Kidneys, strengthen the
　　　　　　　　　　　　Kidneys to support the Lungs and Spleen
Ren.4 (guanyuan +▲)........these points strengthen yuan qi to support qi
Ren.6 (qihai +)　　　　　　systemically
Ren.12 (zhongwan)............alarm point of the Stomach, supplements qi
St.36 (zusanli + ▲) ....sea point of the Stomach, strengthens the Spleen and
　　　　　　　　　　　　Stomach and supplements qi
Sp.6 (sanyinjiao +▲)..........strengthens the Spleen and supplements qi
Lu.9 (taiyuan +) ....source point of the Lungs, strengthens the Lungs
　　　　　　　　　　　　and supplements qi
- with damp, add Sp.3 (taibai –) and Sp.9 (yinlingquan –)
- with phlegm, add St.40 (fenglong –)
- Ear points: points related to the affected area, lung, spleen, zero point, adrenal

Clinical notes
- Numbness of a qi deficiency type may be diagnosed as numbness from malnutrition, diabetic neuropathy, post–stroke numbness or post surgical numbness.
- A qi supplementing diet is recommended, modified appropriately for diabetics. See Clinical Handbook, Vol.2, p.870.

气
虚
血
瘀

13.9 QI DEFICIENCY AND BLOOD STASIS

Qi deficiency with blood stasis is commonly seen pattern in patients with numbness and weakness following a wind–stroke. The treatment is focused on motivating the qi to lead the blood, with gentle blood stasis activation secondary.

Clinical features
- Numbness or complete loss of sensation, with weakness and loss of function. There may be facial paralysis or hemiplegia, with mild vascular congestion or discoloration over the affected region. Usually one side of the body or the face is affected.
- fatigue, weakness
- breathlessness with exertion
- palpitations
- loss of appetite
- waxy pale complexion, puffy face and eyes
- frequent urination or incontinence of urine

T mauve, pale or purplish body with a white coat
P moderate, weak, fine or choppy

Treatment principle
Supplement qi and activate blood
Open the channels and free the network vessels

Prescription

BU YANG HUAN WU TANG 补阳还五汤
Supplement Yang to Restore Five Tenths Decoction

huang qi (Astragali Radix) 黄芪 30–120g
dang gui wei (rootlets of Angelicae sinensis Radix) 当归尾 6–12g
chi shao (Paeoniae Radix rubra) 赤芍...6–9g
chuan xiong (Chuanxiong Rhizoma) 川芎.....................................6–9g
tao ren (Persicae Semen) 桃仁 6–9g
hong hua (Carthami Flos) 红花 6–9g
di long (Pheretima) 地龙...6–12g

Method: Decoction. **Huang qi**, supplements qi and stimulating circulation of qi and blood to the extremities; **dang gui wei** supplements and activates the blood; **chi shao**, **chuan xiong**, **tao ren** and **hong hua** activate blood and dispel blood stasis; **di long** 'drills through' blockages in the channels and network vessels, opening them up and allowing free flow of qi and blood. (Source: *Shi Yong Zhong Yi Nei Ke Xue* [*Yi Lin Gai Cuo*])

Modifications
- The addition of herbs with specific effects in opening up the channels and network vessels can improve the overall effectiveness of the formula. These include **ji xue teng** (Spatholobi Caulis) 鸡血藤 18–30g, **wu gong** (Scolopendra) 蜈蚣 2–3g [as powder taken separately], and **dan shen** (Salviae miltiorrhizae Radix) 丹参 9–12g.
- In cases with yang deficiency, and when the pattern is more than a few months

old, **zhi fu zi** (Aconiti Radix lateralis preparata) 制附子 6–9g [cooked first] can be added to activate the distribution of yang qi into the periphery.
- If the upper limbs are affected, add **sang zhi** (Mori Ramulus) 桑枝 15–30g.
- If the lower limbs are affected, add **chuan niu xi** (Cyathulae Radix) 川牛膝 9–12g and **du zhong** (Eucommiae Cortex) 杜仲 9–12g.
- With constipation, increase the dose of **tao ren** to 12g.
- With numbness in the face, add **zhi bai fu zi** (Typhonii Rhizoma preparatum) 制白附子 3–6g, **bai jiang can** (Bombyx Batryticatus) 白僵蚕 3–6g and **quan xie** (Scorpio) 全蝎 2–3g [as powder taken separately].
- With incontinence of urine, add **yi zhi ren** (Alpiniae oxyphyllae Fructus) 益智仁 6–9g.

Prepared medicines
Concentrated powders
Bu Yang Huan Wu Tang (Astragalus & Peony Combination)
Pills
Bu Yang Huan Wu Wan (Great Yang Restoration Teapills)

Acupuncture (select from)
Local points are selected according to the affected area, typically drawn from the yangming and taiyin channels. Points proximal to the region of sensory loss are chosen. Discrete patches of numbness on the skin can be treated with the hair needle technique (p.579), inserted obliquely at intervals of a few centimeters, towards the numb area. In addition points can be selected from those below to supplement qi and activate blood.

Bl.17 (geshu –) ....meeting point for blood, dispels stagnant blood
Bl.20 (pishu +▲) ....transport point of the Spleen, warms and strengthens the Spleen and supplements qi
Bl.23 (shenshu +▲) ....transport point of the Kidneys, strengthens the Kidneys to support the Spleen
Ren.4 (guanyuan +▲)........strengthens yuan qi and supports qi systemically
Ren.12 (zhongwan)...........alarm point of the Stomach, supplements qi
St.36 (zusanli + ▲) ....sea point of the Stomach, strengthens the Spleen and Stomach and supplements qi
Sp.10 (xuehai –) ....activates blood and dispels static blood
Sp.6 (sanyinjiao +▲)..........strengthens the Spleen and supplements qi
- Ear points: points related to the affected area, zero point, adrenal

Clinical notes
- This pattern responds well when not too chronic. If the numbness has persisted longer than six months, the prognosis is poor. Combining acupuncture and herbs with physiotherapy, tuina or massage gives better results.
- A qi and blood nourishing diet is recommended. See Clinical Handbook, Vol.2, pp.870–874.

血
虚
不
荣

13.10 BLOOD DEFICIENCY

Blood deficiency is a common cause of sensory loss, as blood is responsible for nourishment and sensitivity of the skin, and its overall health. Lack of blood in the skin and network vessels can be from deficiency of blood in general, as here, or from blockage to a specific area by a pathogenic entity such as static blood, phlegm or damp heat.

Clinical features
- Numbness of the hands and feet, fingertips and toes, or patches of skin anywhere on the body. The skin in general may be pale, thin, dry, cracked or scaly. The numbness is often worse at night and may contribute to sleep loss.
- pale, sallow complexion; pale, lusterless lips, nails and conjunctivae
- postural dizziness
- insomnia, difficulty falling asleep
- palpitations
- fatigue, tiredness worse at the end of the day
- dry stools or constipation
- dry eyes and visual weakness or spots before eyes
- weight loss, emaciation

T pale, thin and dry
P fine

Treatment principle
Nourish and supplement blood
Gently activate blood and open up flow in the network vessels

Prescription

SI WU TANG 四物汤
Four Substance Decoction, modified

dang gui (Angelicae sinensis Radix) 当归 6–12g
shu di (Rehmanniae Radix preparata) 熟地 9–15g
bai shao (Paeoniae Radix alba) 白芍 9–12g
chuan xiong (Chuanxiong Rhizoma) 川芎 6–9g
dan shen (Salviae miltiorrhizae Radix) 丹参 9–12g
qin jiao (Gentianae macrophyllae Radix) 秦艽 9–12g
hong hua (Carthami Flos) 红花 6–9g
ji xue teng (Spatholobi Caulis) 鸡血藤 15–30g

Method: Decoction. **Dang gui** supplements and gently activates blood; **shu di** nourishes yin and supplements blood; **bai shao** supplements blood, softens the Liver and preserves yin; **chuan xiong** activates blood and moves qi; **dan shen**, **hong hua** and **ji xue teng** gently activate blood and disperse blood stasis; **qin jiao** dispels wind damp and with **ji xue teng** and **dan shen**, opens up qi and blood flow in the channels and network vessels. (Source: *Shi Yong Zhong Yi Nei Ke Xue* [*He Ji Ju Fang*])

Modifications
- With numbness in the hands and fingers, add **sang zhi** (Mori Ramulus) 桑枝 15–30g and **bai ji li** (Tribuli Fructus) 白蒺藜 9–12g.

- With numbness in the lower limbs, add **huai niu xi** (Achyranthis bidentatae Radix) 怀牛膝 9–15g and **mu gua** (Chaenomelis Fructus) 木瓜 9–12g.
- With Liver wind, fasciculation, tics, tremors or muscle twitching, add **bai ji li** (Tribuli Fructus) 白蒺藜 9–12g, **tian ma** (Gastrodiae Rhizoma) 天麻 9–12g and **sha yuan ji li** (Astragali complanati Semen) 沙苑蒺藜 9–12g.
- With heat, substitute **sheng di** (Rehmanniae Radix) 生地 for **shu di** and **chi shao** (Paeoniae Radix rubra) 赤芍 9–12g for **bai shao**, and add **mu dan pi** (Moutan Cortex) 牡丹皮 6–9g and **huang qin** (Scutellariae Radix) 黄芩 6–9g.
- With qi deficiency, add **ren shen** (Ginseng Radix) 人参 6–9g and **huang qi** (Astragali Radix) 黄芪 15–24g.
- With blood stasis, use **dang gui wei** (rootlets of Angelicae sinensis Radix) 当归尾 instead of **dang gui**, substitute **chi shao** (Paeoniae Radix rubra) 赤芍 9–12g for **bai shao**, and add **tao ren** (Persicae Semen) 桃仁 9–12g.
- With cold, add **rou gui** (Cinnamomi Cortex) 肉桂 3–6g and **gan jiang** (Zingiberis Rhizoma) 干姜 6–9g.
- With Liver qi constraint, add **xiang fu** (Cyperi Rhizoma) 香附 6–9g.
- With digestive upset, loose stools and bloating, add **sha ren** (Amomi Fructus) 砂仁 3–6g and **chen pi** (Citri reticulatae Pericarpium) 陈皮 6–9g.
- For severe numbness and joint stiffness, add herbs such as **wei ling xian** (Clematidis Radix) 威灵仙 9–12g, **xi xian cao** (Siegesbeckia Herba) 豨莶草 9–12g, **sang zhi** (Mori Ramulus) 桑枝 15–30g, **fang feng** (Saposhnikovae Radix) 防风 9–12g or **jiang huang** (Curcumae longae Rhizoma) 姜黄 9–12g.

Prepared medicines
Concentrated powder
Tao Hong Si Wu Tang (Tangkuei Four, Persica & Carthamus Combination)
Dang Gui Si Ni Tang (Tangkiei & Jujube Combination)

Pills
Tao Hong Si Wu Wan (Tao Hong Si Wu Tang Teapills)
Dang Gui Si Ni Wan (Dang Gui Si Ni Teapills)

Acupuncture (select from)
Local points are selected according to the affected area. Points proximal to the region of sensory loss are chosen. Discrete patches of numbness on the skin can be treated with the hair needle technique (p.579), inserted obliquely at intervals of a few centimeters, towards the numb area. Light plum blossom needling over the affected area until the skin is red can be used. In addition points can be selected from those below to supplement qi and blood.

Ren.12 (zhongwan +▲) ....alarm point of the Stomach, strengthens the Spleen and Stomach and supplements qi and blood
Ren.4 (guanyuan +▲) ....strengthens the Kidneys, supplements yuan qi to build blood
Bl.17 (geshu +) ....meeting point for the blood
Bl.18 (ganshu +) ....transport point of the Liver, nourishes and supplements Liver blood

Bl.20 (pishu +▲)................transport point of the Spleen, strengthens the Spleen
and supplements qi and blood
Sp.10 (xuehai) ....activates blood
Sp.6 (sanyinjiao +▲) ....strengthens the Spleen, nourishes and activates qi
and blood
GB.39 (xuanzhong)............meeting point of the marrow and the three leg yang
channels
St.36 (zusanli +▲)...............sea point of the Stomach, strengthens the Spleen and
Stomach and supplements qi and blood
Liv.3 (taichong –) ....source point of the Liver, nourishes and activates
Liver blood
• with tics, tremors or spasms, add GB.34 (yanglingquan), Liv.8 (ququan +) and
Du.8 (jinsuo)
• with visual weakness or spots before the eyes, add GB.37 (guanming +)
• with postural dizziness, add Du.20 (baihui ▲)
• Ear points: points related to the affected area, liver, spleen, zero point, shen-
men, adrenal

Clinical notes
• Numbness and paresthesia of a blood deficiency type may be diagnosed as malnutrition, anemia, chronic skin disease or peripheral neuropathy.
• A blood nourishing diet is an essential part of treatment. See Clinical Handbook, Vol.2, p.874.

肝
肾
亏
损

13.11 LIVER AND KIDNEY YIN DEFICIENCY

Liver and Kidney yin deficiency is often the end result of a heat pattern such as damp heat. It can also represent a deterioration of other deficiency patterns, in particular blood deficiency. There are two types of Liver and Kidney deficiency that can cause numbness. The first is a progressive depletion of the Liver and Kidneys and their ability to maintain the integrity of the sinews, bones and related tissues. This type is usually associated sensory disturbances and weakness in the lower body, and is related to muscular weakness and atrophy (Chapter 12). The second type of Liver and Kidney yin deficiency numbness is associated with the ascendant yang and internal wind, and is a precursor to wind–stroke.

Clinical features

- Numbness in the limbs. When the lower limbs are affected there may also be weakness or wasting of the limbs. In the upper limbs, there may be muscle spasms, tics or tremors. The skin may be pale or have a purplish hue.
- weak, aching lower back and spine with an inability to sit for very long
- facial flushing, low grade fever, night sweats
- fatigue, weakness, exhaustion
- blurring vision or weakening vision, cataracts
- insomnia, with repeated waking feeling hot or anxious
- dizziness and tinnitus
- hair loss, premature graying of the hair
- dry mouth and throat
- weight loss, emaciation
- may be a tremor
- irregular menses, scanty menstruation, amenorrhea

T red and dry with little or no coat
P fine and rapid

Treatment Principle

Supplement and strengthen the Liver and Kidneys
Support the sinews and bones

Prescription

HU QIAN WAN 虎潜丸
Hidden Tiger Pill, modified

This prescription is used when numbness is accompanied by weakness, muscle wasting or loss of function.

jiu huang bai (wine fried Phellodendri Cortex) 酒黄柏 240g
zhi gui ban (honey fried Testudinis Plastrum) 炙龟板 120g
shu di (Rehmanniae Radix preparata) 熟地 60g
jiu zhi mu (wine fried Anemarrhenae Rhizoma) 酒知母 60g
bai shao (Paeoniae Radix alba) 白芍 60g
chen pi (Citri reticulatae Pericarpium) 陈皮 60g
chuan niu xi (Cyathulae Radix) 川牛膝 60g

dang gui (Angelicae sinensis Radix) 当归 60g
suo yang (Cynomorii Herba) 锁阳 45g
gan jiang (Zingiberis Rhizoma) 干姜 15g
mu li* (Ostreae Concha) 牡蛎 120g
Method: Pills. Grind the herbs to a fine powder and form into 9 gram pills with honey. The dose is
one pill 2–3 times daily with salty water. **Jiu huang bai** and **jiu zhi mu** clear heat from deficiency
and support yin; **shu di** and **zhi gui ban** supplement the Liver and Kidneys and deeply enrich yin
and blood; **chuan niu xi** strengthens the sinews and bones and supports the Liver and Kidneys;
dang gui and **bai shao** nourish blood and ease the sinews; **suo yang** supports yang and jing; **chen
pi** and **gan jiang** regulate qi, warm the middle burner and strengthen the Spleen to alleviate any
difficulty with digestion of the herbs; **gan jiang** protects the stomach from the bitter cold of **huang
bai**. *The **hu gu** (Os Tigris) 虎骨 that appeared in the original prescription is substituted by **mu li**
(Ostreae Concha) 牡蛎. (Source: *Shi Yong Zhong Yi Nei Ke Xue* [*Yi Fang Ji Jie*])

Modifications

- Herbs to open up flow through the network vessels, such as **ji xue teng**
  (Spatholobi Caulis) 鸡血藤 60g and **ren dong teng** (Lonicerae Caulis) 忍冬
  藤 60g can be added.
- With marked heat, omit **suo yang** and **gan jiang**, and substitute **sheng di**
  (Rehmanniae Radix) 生地 for **shu di**.
- With blood stasis, add **dan shen** (Salviae miltiorrhizae Radix) 丹参 60g and
  chi shao (Paeoniae Radix rubra) 赤芍 60g.
- With qi deficiency, add **huang qi** (Astragali Radix) 黄芪 60g and **ren shen**
  (Ginseng Radix) 人参 30g.
- With weakness and aching in the lower back and spine, add **gou ji** (Cibotii
  Rhizoma) 狗脊 60g, **xu duan** (Dipsaci Radix) 续断 90g and **bu gu zhi** (Pso-
  raleae Fructus) 补骨脂 60g.
- With dizziness, add **gou qi zi** (Lycii Fructus) 枸杞子 60g and **ju hua** (Chry-
  santhemi Flos) 菊花 60g.
- With incontinence of urine, add **sang piao xiao** (Mantidis Ootheca) 桑螵蛸
  60g and **fu pen zi** (Rubi Fructus) 覆盆子 60g.

Variations and additional prescriptions

Yin deficiency with ascendant yang

Liver and Kidney yin deficiency is frequently complicated by ascendant yang. As
yin becomes progressively more depleted, the inability of the yin to anchor the
yang becomes more and more apparent. As the unanchored yang becomes more
chaotic it can transform into wind. When wind is being created, numbness and
tingling in the extremities gets worse, and is accompanied by visual disturbances,
blurring vision, dizzy spells, tinnitus and tremors. This may be a precursor to a
wind–stoke. The treatment is to sedate Liver yang, extinguish wind, and nourish Liver and Kidney yin to anchor yang with a prescription such as ZHEN GAN
XI FENG TANG (Sedate the Liver and Extinguish Wind Decoction 镇肝熄风汤,
p.441) or TIAN MA GOU TENG YIN (Gastrodia and Uncaria Drink 天麻钩藤饮,
p.441). See also Headache, p.440, Dizziness (Vol.1) and Wind–stroke (Vol.1)

Prepared medicines

Concentrated powders

Hu Qian Wan (Phellodendron & Testudinis Formula)

Tian Ma Gou Teng Yin (Gastodia & Gambir Combination)

Zhen Gan Xi Feng Tang (Hematite & Scrophularia Combination)

Qi Ju Di Huang Wan (Lycium, Chrysanthemum & Rehamannia Formula)
– for long term rebuilding of Liver and Kidney yin during remission

Pills

Da Bu Yin Wan (Abundant Yin Teapills)

Zhi Bai Ba Wei Wan (Eight Flavor Rehmannia Teapills)

Tian Ma Gou Teng Wan (Tian Ma Gou Teng Teapills)

Zhen Gan Xi Feng Wan (Zhen Gan Xi Feng Teapills)

Acupuncture (select from)

Local points are selected according to the affected area. Points proximal to the region of sensory loss are chosen. Discrete patches of numbness on the skin can be treated with the hair needle technique (p.579), inserted obliquely at intervals of a few centimeters, towards the numb area. In addition points can be selected from those below to supplement Liver and Kidney yin. Points within the numb area are needled obliquely and shallowly.

Ren.4 (guanyuan +)............these points supplement Kidney yin and yuan qi

Ren.6 (qihai +)

Kid.3 (taixi +)....................source points of the Kidneys and Liver, supplement

Liv.3 (taichong +)   Kidney and Liver yin

St.36 (zusanli +) ....sea point of the Stomach, strengthens the Spleen to
supplement qi and yin

Liv.8 (ququan +)................sea point of the Liver, nourishes Liver yin

Sp.6 (sanyinjiao)................nourishes Kidney, Liver and Spleen yin

Bl.18 (ganshu +)................transport points of the Liver and Kidneys,

Bl.23 (shenshu +)   supplement Liver and Kidney yin and restrain yang

Bl.52 (zhishi +)..................supplements the Kidneys

• with wind, add GB.20 (fengchi –), LI.11 (quchi –) and LI.4 (hegu –)

• Ear points: points related to the affected area, liver, kidney, adrenal, sympathetic, shenmen

Clinical notes

• Numbness of a Liver and Kidney deficiency type may be diagnosed as multiple sclerosis, diabetic peripheral neuropathy, the sequelae of poliomyelitis or other inflammatory condition of the central or peripheral nervous system, hypertension and an impending sign of a potential cerebrovascular accident.

• The prognosis is variable. In advanced cases the prognosis is poor, although quality of life indicators can be improved with persistent treatment.

• A yin nourishing diet is recommended. See Clinical Handbook, Vol.2, p.876.

Table 13.1 Summary of numbness and paresthesia patterns

Pattern	Features	Prescription
Ying wei disharmony	Numbness and a feeling of thickness or woodenness in patches on the skin, mild fever and chills, aversion to wind, sweating, dry skin, floating, weak pulse; thin, white tongue coat	Huang Qi Gui Zhi Wu Wu Tang
Cold in the channels	Numb cold fingers or toes worse with exposure to cold; extremities may blanch white or purple, deep or imperceptible pulse	Dang Gui Si Ni Tang
Phlegm	Progressive numbness, tingling and heaviness of the arms, legs, hands or feet. The numbness gradually progresses in a 'stocking and glove' distribution. Vertigo, foggy head, blurred vision, swollen tongue with a thick coat; deep, slippery pulse	Di Tan Tang
Qi and blood stasis	Numbness and a wooden feeling in a limb that is discolored and with thickened dry scaly skin. Purple congested veins, varicosities, or spider nevi in the affected area. The limbs are cold and may ache, purple tongue; choppy, fine, wiry pulse	Tong Mai Tang
Phlegm and blood stasis	Chronic, intractable numbness with complete loss of sensation, skin discoloration, spider nevi, mauve or purple tongue with a thick or greasy coat; congested sublingual veins; choppy or deep and slippery pulse	Xiao Huo Luo Dan
Wind damp	Numbness in the extremities accompanied by aching and stiffness of muscles and joints, worse during, or preceding cold or wet weather or increasing humidity, normal or pale tongue, with a thin, white or greasy coat, deep, slow pulse	Cheng Shi Juan Bi Tang Da Qin Jiao Tang
Damp Heat	Numbness, heaviness and tingling of the feet and lower legs with mild edema; heat intolerance, low grade fever, night sweats, lethargy, flushed complexion, red tongue with a greasy yellow coat; slippery, rapid pulse	San Miao San
Qi deficiency	Numbness and tingling in the hands and feet, pale complexion, spontaneous sweating, sensitivity to wind and temperature changes, fatigue, weakness, breathlessness, frequent colds and flu, loss of appetite, loose stools, pale, swollen, scalloped tongue with a thin white coat; weak, fine pulse	Bu Zhong Yi Qi Tang
Qi deficiency with blood stasis	Numbness and loss of motor control of one limb or one side of the body, facial numbness and paralysis, fatigue, weakness, dry scaly skin, pale or mauve tongue; weak, fine pulse	Bu Yang Huan Wu Tang

Table 13.1 Summary of numbness and paresthesia patterns (cont.)

Pattern	Features	Prescription
Blood deficiency	Numbness of the hands, feet, fingertips and toes, or patches of skin anywhere on the body, worse at night. Pale, thin, dry, cracked or scaly skin, postural dizziness, insomnia, palpitations, fatigue, dry stools, dry eyes, spots before eyes, pale, thin, dry tongue; fine pulse	Si Wu Tang
Liver and Kidney yin deficiency	Numbness in the limbs with weakness or wasting or spasms or tremors, lower back ache, facial flushing, low grade fever, night sweats, exhaustion, blurring vision, dizziness and tinnitus, dry mouth and throat, weight loss, red, dry tongue with no coat; fine, rapid pulse	Hu Qian Wan Tian Ma Gou Teng Yin Zhen Gan Xi Feng Tang

OBESITY

Obesity (*féi pàng* 肥胖) is on the rise worldwide and is the most common nutrition related disorder in the developed world. Most commonly it is associated with an increase in the energy value and quantity of food consumed, coupled with a decrease in activity. There are however, some diseases that can contribute to increased weight (Box 14.2, p.612).

While there are no quick fixes, and no substitute for the basic therapeutic principle of eating less and exercising more, Chinese medicine can play a valuable supportive role, and can improve some of the physiological components that contribute to obesity, specifically slow metabolism, digestive inefficiency, problems with insulin metabolism and the fatigue that prevents activity.

The line between a healthy weight and obesity is usually clear but there are standard parameters that can be useful in determining the progress of treatment. These are based on the body mass index (BMI), and the waist to hip circumference ratio (W/H ratio). The body mass index is calculated by dividing the weight (kg) by the square of the height (m²).

$$BMI = \frac{weight\ (kg)}{height\ (m^2)}$$

The waist to hip circumference ratio is derived by dividing the waist measurement by the hip measurement, for which a health range is less than 0.9.

BOX 14.1 PATTERNS OF OBESITY

Stomach heat and food stagnation
Phlegm damp
Spleen qi deficiency with damp
Spleen and Kidney yang deficiency
Liver and Kidney yin deficiency
Qi and blood stagnation

Table 14.1 Classification of obesity and BMI

BMI	Grade
<18.5	underweight
18.5 – 25	considered a healthy range
25 – 30	overweight
30 – 35	Grade 1 obesity
35 – 40	Grade 2 obesity
>40	Grade 3 morbid obesity

In terms of the general health of obese individuals, the standard classification can be too rigidly applied, and the BMI should always be considered in the context of the individual concerned. There are many people with a BMI outside the consensus healthy range who are perfectly well. However, the risk levels for some chronic illnesses can increase significantly with increasing BMI. These include diabetes and metabolic syndrome, cardiovascular and gall bladder disease, osteoarthritis and infertility.

Obesity and insulin resistance

Rising in tandem with increasing frequency of obesity are disorders of sugar metabolism, specifically insulin resistance and diabetes mellitus (see Chapter 4). Insulin resistance is a condition which occurs when somatic cells do not respond appropriately to insulin. Obesity and insulin resistance are clearly linked. The glucose that should be taken up by cells and consumed to power their metabolic activity, with the assistance of insulin, is instead routed into fat storage. Insulin resistance and diabetes are increasing because the makeup of the diet, availability of food and modern lifestyles have evolved too rapidly for our bodies to keep pace. We are still genetically programmed to live like our ancestors, whose diet, as far as we can tell, was low in refined carbohydrates and volume of food, and who sustained greater levels of movement and exercise. The insulin system evolved to deal with slowly digested food stuffs and periods of food scarcity. During periods of food abundance, the extra energy was stored as fat as insurance against the lean times. Obesity associated with insulin resistance tends to be central (abdominal) in its distribution. The more weight gained, the greater the insulin resistance and higher the compensatory insulin production, which leads to even more weight gain.

ETIOLOGY

The main cause of obesity is taking in more energy than is used by activity. Weakness and inefficiency in harvesting, transforming, distributing and utilizing the qi derived from food resulting from poor organ system function, can further compound weight gain.

Spleen and Stomach

Weakness of the Spleen and Stomach leads to inefficient digestion, causing a buildup of damp and phlegm in the form of fat and fluid in the tissues. The weakness and tendency to phlegm damp accumulation may be inherited, or acquired through poor eating habits. Patients with a real or perceived weight problem are often drawn to slimming diets of various types, many of which use bitter cold purgatives, diuretics and appetite suppressants as their main therapy. All of these can damage the Spleen; the patient loses appetite, some weight and fluid, but once dieting stops the weight usually returns worse than before. This 'yo yo' pattern of weight loss and weight gain can deplete Spleen and Kidney yang. Inactivity is another factor which weakens the Spleen. It was noted in the Simple Questions (Huang Di Nei Jing Su Wen), Chapter 23, that 'too much lying down damages the qi and too much sitting damages the flesh'.

Habitual overeating overloads the Spleen and Stomach and exceeds their processing capacity. Instead of being efficiently processed and moved quickly through the Intestines, unprocessed food accumulates, stagnates and produces heat. The heat causes an increase in appetite, and a vicious cycle occurs in which Spleen and Stomach are further weakened and digestion becomes increasingly inefficient. Damp is produced which combines with the heat to produce damp heat, or is further congealed into phlegm.

The damp, damp heat and phlegm so produced can accumulate in the tissues and internal organs, and have further ramifications for the health. For example, phlegm can accumulate in the cardiovascular and cerebrovascular systems causing chest pain, obstruction of blood vessels and peripheral circulation, wind–stroke, tremors, anxiety states and vertigo. Chronic heat or damp heat in the yangming system can injure Intestinal yin and damage the Intestinal lining. The local circulation of qi and blood is weakened, phlegm and blood stasis can accumulate and polyps, nodules and tumors may form.

Liver

Chronic Liver qi constraint can weaken the Spleen, retard fluid movement and lead to accumulation of damp and phlegm. Prolonged or severe Liver qi constraint can also generate heat, which may then combine with any damp present to form damp heat or phlegm, or may injure fluids and yin. Qi constraint also has an impact on the Gallbladder and the distribution of bile, and in combination with damp readily forms gallstones. Gallstones can further impair digestive efficiency and lead to the accumulation of more damp.

Kidneys

As we age and our Kidney yang declines, the metabolic fire that underpins the yang functions of the other organ systems diminishes. Spleen yang, the basis of efficient digestion is weakened, and damp, phlegm and blood stasis occur more readily. A decline in Kidney yin reduces yin fluids and leads to deficient heat, which causes thickening of fluids, accumulation of phlegm and blood stasis. In addition, the general decline of yang qi often leads to a decrease in overall activity and more sedentary habits.

There is a constitutional component to weight gain, with a tendency to obesity running through some families, however, whether this is learned behavior and poor eating habits imprinted from an early age, or part of an inherited template can be difficult to determine.

BOX 14.2 BIOMEDICAL CAUSES OF WEIGHT GAIN

Endocrine
- hypothyroidism
- Cushing's syndrome
- acromegaly
- hypogonadism
- hyperprolactinoma
- insulin secreting tumors
- polycystic ovarian syndrome

Other
- cardiac failure
- liver failure
- nephrotic syndrome
- hypothalamic tumors
- premenstrual syndrome
- early pregnancy
- depression

Drugs
- tricyclic antidepressants
- oral contraceptive pill, hormone replacement therapy
- corticosteroids

TREATMENT

The treatment of obesity can be challenging. In many cases the reasons for overeating are complex, and intertwined with social and emotional factors. For sustained success, treatment requires a substantial commitment from both patient and practitioner, and is usually prolonged. Initial weight loss is often dramatic, but this is largely fluid. Real weight loss, i.e. decrease in fat deposits, should be gradual and ideally no more than 0.25kg per week. In this way, the metabolic changes necessary to keep the weight off can be embedded. During this process, regular support and encouragement, reinforcement of goals and monitoring of progress are the keys to success. The Chinese medicine clinic is an ideal environment to provide such a framework. Regular appointments for acupuncture treatments provide a good forum for encouraging motivation and reviewing progress, as well as improving physiological function. A typical treatment course will run over 3–12 months, during which time acupuncture is given weekly.

Food and activity diary
A food and activity diary is a useful way of assessing the nature and volume of food consumed and the relative energy expenditure. This can help not only in tailoring a rational plan, but creates an awareness in the patient of what is being ingested and what is being used. People generally underestimate, unintentionally or otherwise, the amount of food they eat. Be aware, however, that for patients with Spleen deficiency, a food diary may become a source of obsession and encourage a counterproductive preoccupation with food and diet.

Diet
A diet that reflects the pathology being treated should be advised and introduced gradually. Radical or sudden changes in diet are not advised since they generally do not to last. See Clinical Handbook, Vol.2, p.862, for diets tailored to specific pathology.

Some simple dietary guidelines can apply to all people wishing to lose weight.
1. Cut down volume of food by 30%. Having small meals which include some protein at regular times through out the day will regulate blood sugar levels and reduce appetite.
2. Avoid fatty or fried foods. Eat more fresh fruits and vegetables.
3. Avoid soft drinks and fruit juices.
4. High protein (or low GI) meals are often recommended because they are relatively low calorie, don't raise blood sugar or produce so much insulin and they manage hunger better. However any diet which reduces calories will help reduce weight.
5. Breakfast and lunch are the more important meals as their energy value will be consumed in daily activity, while the calories from a large evening meal will tend to be stored as fat. The old saying 'eat like a king at breakfast, a prince at lunch and a pauper at dinner' is excellent advice. Chinese medicine with its understanding of the flow of qi in the 12 channels has long recognized that it

is in the early part of the day that the digestive organs are at their peak. The time of maximal energy available for digestion is between 7–11am (Stomach and Spleen time).

6. Snacking between meals should be avoided.

7. Good digestion and regular bowel movements are also an important part of weight control.

8. A disciplined and persistent approach is essential, but rigidity is counterproductive, especially so for those with Spleen deficiency.

9. The 80/20 rule could be applied here – do the right thing 80% of the time and 20% of the time you can get away with small indiscretions.

Exercise

A realistic and regular program of exercise is an essential part of any weight loss plan. Exercise consumes calories, but more importantly it makes muscle tissue more insulin sensitive, so the pancreas can reduce its output, and less sugar is shunted to fat deposits.

The goal should be for a minimum of 30–40 minutes of sustained aerobic activity every day, or at least several times a week. This means getting the heart rate up to about 50% above the resting rate (i.e. to 120 beats per minute if the resting rate is 80) and keeping it there for 30–40 minutes. Walking is ideal. The benefits of regular aerobic activity are cumulative and become self sustaining over time.

胃
热
脾
滞

14.1 STOMACH HEAT WITH FOOD STAGNATION

Stomach heat with food stagnation is seen primarily in younger people and in men. The results of overeating lead to accumulation of food in the middle burner, causing food stagnation, damp heat or phlegm heat. It is an excess pattern without too much damage to the organ systems involved. There are numerous variations depending on the individual concerned (see Variations), but the basic principles are the same: keeping all pathways of elimination open and clear, removing any blockages to elimination and supporting healthy digestive function. Treatment has to proceed carefully, as the herbs, in the process of clearing heat and stagnation, can damage Spleen yang. In the short term this is useful as it suppresses the appetite, but it has to be managed carefully to avoid pushing the patient into Spleen deficiency.

Clinical features
- Obesity associated with a high intake of food. The weight is predominantly upper body and abdominal, giving the patient the classic apple shape.
- red, glossy or oily complexion
- constipation or alternating constipation and diarrhea; foul smelling stools
- abdominal distension; the abdomen feels firm
- bitter taste, thirst, dry mouth
- bad breath, heartburn, acid reflux, foul belching
- sweating, clearly seen on the forehead and around the lips
- fatigue, often related to sleep apnoea
- poor sleep; sleep apnea

T red with a thick, greasy, white or yellow coat
P deep, slippery, strong

Treatment Principle
Keep all pathways of elimination open
Clear heat, eliminate food stagnation

Prescription

ZHI SHI DAO ZHI WAN 枳实导滞丸
Unripe Bitter Orange Pill to Guide Out Stagnation

da huang (Rhei Radix et Rhizoma) 大黄........................30g
zhi shi (Aurantii Fructus immaturus) 枳实........................15g
shen qu (Massa medicata fermentata) 神曲........................15g
huang qin (Scutellariae Radix) 黄芩........................9g
huang lian (Coptidis Rhizoma) 黄连........................9g
fu ling (Poria) 茯苓........................9g
bai zhu (Atractylodis macrocephalae Rhizoma) 白术........................9g
ze xie (Alismatis Rhizoma) 泽泻........................6g

Method: Grind the herbs to powder and form into 9 gram pills with water. The dose is one pill 2–3 times daily. **Da huang** clears heat and purges accumulation from the Stomach and Intestines; it is assisted in this by **zhi shi** which also regulates qi and alleviates epigastric distension; **shen qu** alleviates food stagnation; **huang qin** and **huang lian** clear damp heat; **fu ling** and **ze xie** promote urination to clear damp heat; **bai zhu** and **fu ling** strengthen the Spleen and dry damp. (Source: *Nei Wai Shang Bian Huo Lun*])

Variations and additional prescriptions
Damp heat in the qi level
Damp heat can be diffusely spread through the qi level, concentrated in the Liver or Gallbladder, or may congeal further into phlegm heat. The symptoms are similar to the Stomach heat pattern but are more concentrated in the muscles. The additional influence of the damp is seen in the urgent loose stools or diarrhea, foggy head, night sweats and muscle aches and weakness. The patient feels warm to the touch. The treatment is to clear damp heat from the qi level with LIAN PO YIN (Coptis and Magnolia Bark Drink 连朴饮, p.377).

Damp heat in the Liver and Stomach
Damp heat can concentrate in the Liver, especially when alcohol and stress are involved, in addition to the dietary factors. In addition to the symptoms of Stomach heat, there are specific Liver symptoms such as red, sore eyes, anger, irritability and hypochondriac pain. The treatment can initially focus on clearing damp heat with a prescription such as LONG DAN XIE GAN TANG (Gentian Decoction to Purge the Liver 龙胆泻肝汤, p.438).

With damp heat and Gallbladder qi constraint
A common complication of obesity and damp heat is disruption to Gallbladder function and the formation of stones. This pattern is characterized by right hypochondriac pain, dark urine, pale, sticky or clay like stools and possibly jaundice. The treatment is to clear damp heat from the Gallbladder and regulate Liver and Gallbladder qi with a formula such as DA CHAI HU TANG (Major Bupleurum Decoction 大柴胡汤, p.330).

Prepared medicines
Concentrated powders
Fang Feng Tong Sheng San (Siler & Platycodon Formula)
San Ren Tang (Triple Nut Combination)
   – damp heat in the qi level
Long Dan Xie Gan Tang (Gentiana Combination)
Da Chai Hu Tang (Major Bupleurum Combination)
Pills
Fang Feng Tong Sheng Wan (Ledebouriella Sagely Unblocks Teapills)
Long Dan Xie Gan Wan (Snake and Dragon Teapills)
Da Chai Hu Wan (Major Bupleurum Teapills)
Da Huang Jiang Zhi Wan (Rhubarb Teapills)
   – with constipation and high triglycerides

Acupuncture (select from)
Ren.12 (zhongwan –).........these points clear heat from the Spleen and Stomach,
St.25 (tianshu)   regulate Intestinal function and promote bowel
Sp.15 (daheng)   movement

St.44 (neiting –) ....these points clear heat from the Stomach and
LI.11 (quchi –)   Intestines
LI.4 (hegu –)
SJ.6 (zhigou –) ....fire point of the triple burner, spreads qi, disperses
                              accumulation from the Intestines and promotes
                              bowel movement to maintain elimination
GB.34 (yanglingquan –).....dredges the Liver and encourages qi movement
                              through the Intestine to promote bowel movement
St.36 (zusanli –) ....sea point of the Stomach, regulates Stomach and
                              Intestine function, strengthens the Spleen and
                              Stomach and supplements qi
St.37 (shangjuxu –) ....lower sea point of the Large Intestine, clears heat
                              and regulates the Intestines

- with nausea, add PC.6 (neiguan –)
- with phlegm, add St.40 (fenglong –)
- with heat in the Liver, add Liv.2 (xingjian –)
- with damp heat, add St.45 (lidui ↓) and St.40 (fenglong –)
- with Spleen deficiency, add Sp.6 (sanyinjiao)
- with abdominal pain, add Sp.8 (diji –) and Sp.4 (gongsun –)
- Ear points: mouth, spleen, stomach, zero point, large intestine, shenmen, endocrine

Clinical notes

- This is one of the common patterns of obesity in the modern era, when too much energy rich food is consumed relative to the amount of physical activity. The unused surplus goes into fat storage and creates heat. Eventually the Spleen and Stomach are weakened, and one of the deficiency patterns develops. This is also the stage that patients are likely to begin radical weight loss programs or use bitter cold diuretic and purgative slimming aids that further weaken Spleen yang qi.
- The prescriptions recommended above are not suitable for long term use, generally no longer than 4–6 weeks, as their bitter coldness will damage Spleen yang. They can be used as long as the heat remains obvious. Once the heat has dissipated, elimination is proceeding regularly and the patient is getting used to a new diet, a more Spleen strengthening strategy can be phased in. Loose bowel movements are expected and desirable in the early stages of treatment but persistent loose bowels suggest that the Spleen is being weakened and it is time to ease off on the bitter cold herbs.
- Basic dietary advice as per p.613. A specific diet aimed at reducing heat and damp heat should be adopted. See Clinical Handbook, Vol. 2, p.884.

痰湿壅阻 | 14.2 PHLEGM DAMP

Phlegm damp type obesity can be the result of overeating, but can be constitutional. Patients with phlegm damp will often note they were overweight from an early age. Phlegm damp is often complicated by constrained Liver qi, and the longer it persists, the more Spleen deficiency will develop. The guiding principle of treatment is not to simply resolve phlegm damp, but to maintain all passageways of elimination and ensure the Spleen and Stomach are working as efficiently as possible.

Clinical features
- Obesity, with the weight distributed in the lower body, lower abdomen, hips and thighs resulting in the classic pear shape
- Puffy face; thick fingers; muscles feel firm
- tiredness, heaviness, somnolence
- abdominal bloating, acid reflux, belching
- sweet cravings
- heavy feelings in the limbs
- alternating loose and sluggish stools; or constipation (but stools not dry); after elimination the patient feels more energetic and lighter
- tendency to mucus congestion and throat clearing
- dizziness, vertigo
- yellow or brown xanthoma

T swollen with a thin or thick greasy, white coat
P deep, wiry, slippery

Treatment Principle
Transform phlegm damp and assist the qi dynamic
Strengthen the Spleen and Stomach and supplement qi

Prescription

XIANG SHA LIU JUN ZI TANG 香砂六君子汤
Six Gentlemen Decoction with Aucklandia and Amomum

ren shen (Ginseng Radix) 人参	6–9g
chao bai zhu (stir fried Atractylodis macrocephalae Rhizoma) 炒白术	12–15g
fu ling (Poria) 茯苓	12–15g
zhi ban xia (Pinelliae Rhizoma preparatum) 制半夏	9–12g
chen pi (Citri reticulatae Pericarpium) 陈皮	9–12g
mu xiang (Aucklandiae Radix) 木香	6–9g
sha ren (Fructus Amomi) 砂仁	6–9g
zhi gan cao (Glycyrrhizae Radix preparata) 炙甘草	3–6g

Method: Decoction. **Sha ren** is added towards the end of cooking. **Ren shen** supplements qi and strengthens the Spleen; **chao bai zhu** strengthens the Spleen, supplements qi and dries damp; **fu ling** strengthens the Spleen and leaches out damp; **zhi ban xia** transforms phlegm damp and down-bears counterflow Stomach qi; **chen pi** transforms phlegm, regulates middle burner qi and corrects the qi dynamic; **zhi gan cao** strengthens the Spleen and harmonizes the Stomach; **sha ren** and **mu xiang** regulate qi and correct the qi dynamic. (Source: *Zhong Yi Nei Ke Xue* [*He Ji Ju Fang*])

Modifications

- The addition of mild diuretic herbs, such as **yi ren** (Coicis Semen) 苡仁 15–30g, **ze xie** (Alismatis Rhizoma) 泽泻 9–12g and **chi xiao dou** (Phaseoli Semen) 赤小豆 15–30g can be helpful in maintaining a good urinary flow and ensuring an escape route for the phlegm damp. Take care not to overdo the diuresis, to avoid damage to yin.
- With food stagnation, add **shan zha** (Crataegi Fructus) 山楂 12–15g, **chao shen qu** (stir fried Massa medicata fermentata) 炒神曲 12–15g and **chao lai fu zi** (stir fried Raphani Semen) 炒莱菔子 6–9g. The addition of a couple of these herbs in the early stages of treatment is good practice to assist with digestion and gentle elimination.
- With sluggish bowels, add **jue ming zi** (Cassiae Semen) 决明子 9–12g and **he shou wu** (Polygoni multiflori Radix) 何首乌 9–12g.
- With Liver qi constraint, add **chai hu** (Bupleuri Radix) 柴胡 6–9g, **bai shao** (Paeoniae Radix alba) 白芍 9–12g and **bing lang** (Arecae Semen) 槟榔 9–12g.
- With abdominal and epigastric bloating and a thick tongue coat, add **cang zhu** (Atractylodis Rhizoma) 苍术 9–12g and **hou po** (Magnoliae officinalis Cortex) 厚朴 9–12g.
- With foggy or heavy head, add **shi chang pu** (Acori tatarinowii Rhizoma) 石菖蒲 6–9g and **yuan zhi** (Polygalae Radix) 远志 6–9g.
- With mucus congestion, throat clearing or productive cough, add **chao lai fu zi** (stir fried Raphani Semen) 炒莱菔子 6–9g, **su zi** (Perillae Fructus) 苏子 6–9g and **bai jie zi** (Sinapsis Semen) 白芥子 6–9g.

Variations and additional prescriptions
Phlegm heat
Prolonged obstruction by phlegm damp can produce heat. Heat may also occur in response to stress, qi constraint or overindulgence on heating food and alcohol. Phlegm heat has a propensity to affect the Heart and shen, so when phlegm heat is created (it can also be a constitutional tendency), there are shen symptoms in addition to the weight problem. In fact overeating itself may be related to psychological states caused by the phlegm heat, such as anxiety, nervousness and lack of self–confidence. It is further compounded by gnawing hunger that leads to frequent snacking. The tongue may be red with a greasy yellow coat, the pulse slippery and rapid. The treatment is to clear heat, transform phlegm and calm the shen with a prescription such as HUANG LIAN WEN DAN TANG (Warm Gallbladder Decoction with Coptis 黄连温胆汤 p.915).

Prepared medicines
Concentrated powders
Xiang Sha Liu Jun Zi Tang (Vladmiria & Amomum Combination)
Xiang Sha Ping Wei San (Cyperus, Amomum & Atractylodes Formula)
  – with food stagnation, sluggish stools and disruption to the qi dynamic
Xiang Sha Yang Wei Tang (Cyperus & Cardamon Combination)
  – phlegm damp with indigestion and heartburn

Zhu Ru Wen Dan Tang (Bamboo & Ginseng Combination)
– phlegm heat

Pills

Bojenmi Chinese Tea (Bao Jian Mei Cha 保健美茶)
Mu Xiang Shun Qi Wan (Aplotaxis Carminative Pills, Shun Qi Wan)
– with Liver qi constraint
Ping Wei San (Calm Stomach Teapills, Tabellae Pingwei)
Xiang Sha Yang Wei Wan (Appetite and Digestion Pill, Hsiang Sha Yang Wei Pien)
– with abdominal bloating and reflux

Acupuncture (select from)

Ren.12 (zhongwan –) ....alarm point of the Stomach, strengthens the Spleen and Stomach, supplements qi to transform phlegm damp

Sp.3 (taibai).....................source and connecting points of the Spleen and
St.40 (fenglong –)   Stomach, these points transform phlegm damp, strengthen the Spleen and correct the qi dynamic

St.36 (zusanli +▲) ....sea point of the Stomach, strengthens the Spleen and Stomach and corrects the qi dynamic

Sp.5 (shangqiu –) ....river point of the Spleen, transforms damp

PC.5 (jianshi)....................river point of the Pericardium, transforms phlegm, harmonizes the Stomach

- with foggy head, add GB.20 (fengchi)
- with sluggish stools or constipation, add SJ.6 (zhigou –), St.37 (shangjuxu –) and St.41 (jiexi –)
- with phlegm heat, add St.41 (jiexi –) and PC.7 (daling –)
- with cold, apply moxa cones to Bl.20 (pishu ▲) and Bl.21 (weishu ▲)
- Ear points: mouth, spleen, stomach, zero point, shenmen, endocrine

Clinical notes

- When constitutional, phlegm damp obesity can be difficult to resolve to the satisfaction of the patient. Some weight can be lost, but patients often reach a point beyond which no more weight loss can be achieved regardless of dietary restrictions and amount of exercise. Their natural weight sits at the upper end of the bell curve, and the problem becomes one of perception rather than of health.
- Women with phlegm damp weight problems may be found to have polycystic ovarian syndrome.
- The heaviness and lethargy typical of phlegm damp can be impediments to getting started with exercise, but graded exercise in groups has a motivating effect and can achieve good results.
- A specific diet designed for phlegm damp should be adopted. See Clinical Handbook, Vol. 2, p.880.

脾
虚
不
运

14.3 SPLEEN QI DEFICIENCY

Spleen qi deficiency is a common cause of weight problems, and can lead to both weight loss or weight gain. When weight is gained, it is due to the inefficient processing of food which leaves a residue of damp, phlegm and fluid that settles in the flesh.

Clinical features

- Obesity, with flabby, flaccid muscles and superficial edema. The edema can be seen most clearly around the eyes and in the fingers and hands.
- muscles are weak and easily fatigued
- Fatigue, tiredness and sleepiness, worse after eating and especially after lunch. The fatigue of qi deficiency is one of the main impediment to exercise and losing weight and patients are usually quite sedentary.
- A tendency to obsess about food; an overly rigid or exclusive eating plan or multiple food sensitivities.
- pale complexion
- abdominal distension
- sweet cravings
- loose or sluggish stools
- breathlessness, spontaneous sweating
- copious white, or egg white like, vaginal discharge

T pale, swollen and scalloped with a thin, white or greasy coat
P deep, weak, moderate, soft

Treatment Principle

Strengthen the Spleen and Stomach and supplement qi

Prescription

SHEN LING BAI ZHU SAN 参苓白术散
Ginseng, Poria and White Atractylodes Powder

ren shen (Ginseng Radix) 人参	100g
bai zhu (Atractylodes macrocephalae Rhizoma) 白术	100g
fu ling (Poria) 茯苓	100g
shan yao (Dioscoreae Rhizoma) 山药	100g
zhi gan cao (Glycyrrhizae Radix preparata) 炙甘草	100g
bai bian dou (Dolichos Semen) 白扁豆	75g
yi ren (Coicis Semen) 苡仁	50g
lian zi (Nelumbinis Semen) 莲子	50g
jie geng (Platycodi Radix) 桔梗	50g
sha ren (Amomi Fructus) 砂仁	50g

Method: Powder or pills. Grind the herbs to a fine powder and take in 6–9 gram doses, two or three times daily with warm water. Can also be decocted with an 80–90% reduction is dose. **Ren shen**, **bai zhu**, **yi ren**, **fu ling**, **bian dou**, **shan yao** and **zhi gan cao** strengthen the Spleen and supplement qi; **bai zhu** dries damp; **yi ren**, **fu ling** and **bai bian dou** leach out damp by promoting urination; **lian zi** astringes the Intestines and stops diarrhea; **jie geng** diffuses the Lungs, raises yang qi and collaborates with the descending bitterness of **bai zhu** to correct the qi dynamic; **sha ren** transforms damp and regulates qi. (Source: *Zhong Yi Nei Shou Ce* [*He Ji Ju Fang*])

Modifications

- With insulin resistance or type 2 diabetes of a Spleen qi deficiency type, add **huang qi** (Astragali Radix) 黄芪 15–30g, **tian hua fen** (Trichosanthes Radix) 天花粉 12–15g and **ge gen** (Puerariae Radix) 葛根 12–15g.
- With puffy eyes and edema, increase the dose of **fu ling**, and add **ze xie** (Alismatis Rhizoma) 泽泻 9–12g and **che qian zi** (Plantaginis Semen) 车前子 9–12g.
- With a pale tongue with a thick greasy tongue coat, belching and heartburn, add **cang zhu** (Atractylodis Rhizoma) 苍术 9–12g and **hou po** (Magnoliae officinalis Cortex) 厚朴 9–12g.
- With mucus congestion, add **zhi ban xia** (Pinelliae Rhizoma preparatum) 制半夏 6–9g and **chen pi** (Citri reticulatae Pericarpium) 陈皮 6–9g.
- With Liver qi constraint, add **chai hu** (Bupleuri Radix) 柴胡 6–9g and **bai shao** (Paeoniae Radix alba) 白芍 9–12g.
- With food stagnation, add **shan zha** (Crataegi Fructus) 山楂 12–15g, **chao mai ya** (stir fried Hordei Fructus germinantus) 炒麦芽 15–30g and **chao shen qu** (stir fried Massa medicata fermentata) 炒神曲 12–15g.
- With wei qi deficiency, add **zhi huang qi** (honey fried Astragali Radix) 炙黄芪 15–30g and **wu wei zi** (Schizandrae Fructus) 五味子 6–9g.
- With yang deficiency, add **zhi fu zi** (Aconiti Radix lateralis preparata) 制附子 6–12g [decocted for 30 minutes before the other herbs] and **pao jiang** (Zingiberis Rhizoma preparatum) 炮姜 6–9g.

Variations and additional prescriptions
With significant edema, sweating and knee pain
A commonly seen variation occurs primarily in women over 35, and is characterized by the patient being overweight, puffy, pale, fatigued and clammy, with marked swelling and pain in the knees. The initial treatment is to strengthen the Spleen and move fluids with FANG JI HUANG QI TANG (Stephania and Astragalus Decoction 防己黄芪汤, p.653). After the fluids are moving, swelling and pain reduced, a more balanced Spleen strengthening prescription, such as the primary prescription above, can be phased in.

Prepared medicines
Concentrated powders
Shen Ling Bai Zhu San (Ginseng & Atractylodes Formula)
Ping Wei San (Magnolia & Ginger Formula)
    – add with damp
Fang Ji Huang Qi Tang (Stephania & Astragalus Combination)
Pills
Shen Ling Bai Zhu Wan (Absorption and Digestion Pill, Shen Ling Bai Zhu Pian)
Ping Wei San (Calm Stomach Teapills, Tabellae Pingwei)
Zi Sheng Wan (Zi Sheng Stomachic Pills)
Jian Pi Wan (Ginseng Stomachic Pills, Spleen Digest Aid Pill)

Acupuncture (select from)

Ren.12 (zhongwan +▲) ....alarm point of the Stomach, strengthens the Spleen
and Stomach and supplements qi

St.36 (zusanli +▲) ....sea point of the Stomach, strengthens the Spleen and
Stomach, supplements qi to transform damp

Sp.3 (taibai).....................source and connecting points of the Spleen and

St.40 (fenglong –)   Stomach, these points transform phlegm damp,
strengthen the Spleen and correct the qi dynamic

Du.20 (baihui ▲) ....clears the head and elevates qi

Bl.20 (pishu +▲) ....transport points of the Spleen and Stomach, warm

Bl.21 (weishu +▲)   and strengthen middle burner qi

- with foggy head, add Bl.62 (shenmai)
- with edema, add Sp.9 (yinlingquan –) and Sp.6 (sanyinjiao)
- with somnolence, add Kid.6 (zhaohai) and Bl.62 (shenmai –)
- with abdominal pain, add Sp.4 (gongsun –)
- with diarrhea, moxa can be applied with a moxa stick to Du.20 (baihui)
- with marked abdominal distension, add St.25 (tianshu –)
- Ear points: mouth, spleen, stomach, zero point, shenmen, endocrine

Clinical notes

- Treatment to strengthen Spleen function and clear damp can result in rapid initial weight loss as urinary output increases and edema resolves. Patients may lose several kilos per week for the first few weeks. While the initial results are often dramatic and welcome, the real work of burning fat deposits is a much slower process and patients should be counselled to expect losses of no more than 1–2 kilograms per month. Gradual weight loss combined with strengthening of Spleen function results in a much better long term outcome and sustained healthy weight.
- Exercise is essential, and is best performed in the morning, between 7 and 11am, when qi is at its daily peak. It may be best to begin with some type of mild activity, such as gentle walking, yoga or taijiquan, before gradually building up to a more aerobic regime.
- A specific diet suitable for Spleen qi deficiency should be adopted. See Clinical Handbook, Vol. 2, p.870.

脾
肾
阳
虚

14.4 SPLEEN AND KIDNEY YANG DEFICIENCY

This pattern is associated with weight gain from both fluid and fat due to reduced metabolic rate. Some patients with this type of obesity may be diagnosed with hypothyroidism. The weight is accompanied by marked lack of energy and motivation. Damage to Spleen and Kidney yang is often the result of repeated crash or restrictive diets, or the use of slimming aids in an attempt to treat phlegm damp or damp heat weight problems.

In general the treatment initially focuses on restoring Spleen yang to improve digestive efficiency. If necessary, treatment addressing Kidney yang can follow.

Clinical features
- Obesity, puffiness of the face and eyes. Patients complain that they hardly eat anything and still do not lose weight.
- waxy, pale complexion
- edema, worse in the lower limbs
- exhaustion, low energy reserves, somnolence
- severe abdominal bloating; the abdomen feels flaccid and cool to touch
- chronic diarrhea with undigested food, or chronic atonic constipation
- breathlessness, panting with exertion
- cold intolerance, cold extremities
- frequent urination, nocturia
- lower back and legs aching and weak

T pale, swollen and scalloped and a thin, white or greasy coat
P deep, weak or slippery, slow

Treatment Principle
Warm and supplement Spleen and Kidney yang

Prescription

FU ZI LI ZHONG WAN 附子理中丸
Prepared Aconite Pill to Regulate the Middle

---

zhi fu zi (Aconiti Radix lateralis preparata) 制附子 9–15g
ren shen (Ginseng Radix) 人参 6–12g
bai zhu (Atractylodes macrocephalae Rhizoma) 白术 6–12g
gan jiang (Zingiberis Rhizoma) 干姜 6–9g
zhi gan cao (Glycyrrhizae Radix preparata) 炙甘草 3–6g

Method: Decoction. **Zhi fu zi** is cooked for 30 minutes before the other herbs. **Zhi fu zi** and **gan jiang** warm the middle burner, dispel cold and restore Spleen yang; a large dose of **zhi fu zi** is usually required in the early stages to provide sufficient yang to get fluids moving and digestion working at all; **ren shen** strengthens the Spleen and supplements qi; **bai zhu** strengthens the Spleen and dries damp; **zhi gan cao** strengthens the Spleen and harmonizes the middle burner. (Source: *Zhong Yi Nei Ke Xue* [*He Ji Ju Fang*])

Modifications
- With marked edema, add **fu ling** (Poria) 茯苓 9–12g and **ze xie** (Alismatis Rhizoma) 泽泻 6–9g.

- With marked qi deficiency, increase the dose of **ren shen** to 15g.
- With damp, substitute **cang zhu** (Atractylodis Rhizoma) 苍术 for **bai zhu**.
- With acid reflux, belching or persistent hiccups from counterflow Stomach qi, add **ding xiang** (Caryophylli Flos) 丁香 1.5g and **bai dou kou** (Amomi Fructus rotundus) 白豆蔻 6g [added at the end of cooking].
- With colicky abdominal pain, add **mu xiang** (Aucklandiae Radix) 木香 6–9g and **chao bai shao** (stir fried Paeoniae Radix alba) 炒白芍 9–12g.

Variations and additional prescriptions
With significant edema
When there is significant edema, it should be quickly mobilized and eliminated before employing the primary prescription above. The treatment is to warm Spleen and Kidney yang and stimulate fluid metabolism with a prescription such as ZHEN WU TANG (True Warrior Decoction 真武汤, p.249).

As weight is reducing and the Spleen is stronger
After a month or two, Spleen yang is usually strong enough to handle the richness of Kidney supplements. At this point, combining a Kidney yang supplement in pill form, such as JIN GUI SHEN QI WAN (Kidney Qi Pill from the Golden Cabinet 金匮肾气丸, p.826) with the primary prescription above, is recommended for long term rebuilding of Spleen and Kidney yang. Start with a small dose to see how the patient's Spleen reacts, then, if all goes well, build up to a therapeutic dose over a week or two.

Prepared medicines
Concentrated powders
Fu Zi Li Zhong Tang (Aconite, Ginseng and Ginger Combination)
Zhen Wu Tang (Ginger, Aconite, Poria & Peony Combination)
   – with pronounced edema
Ji Sheng Shen Qi Wan (Cyathula & Plantago Formula)
   – for long term Kidney supplementation with persistent tendency to fluid problems
Ba Wei Di Huang Wan (Rehmannia Eight Form.)
   – Kidney yang deficiency

Pills
Fu Zi Li Zhong Wan (Fu Tzu Li Chung Wan, Li Chung Yuen Medical Pills)
Zhen Wu Tang Wan (True Warrior Teapills)
Jin Kui Shen Qi Wan (Fu Gui Ba Wei Wan, Golden Book Teapills)
   – Kidney yang deficiency

Acupuncture (select from)
Ren.12 (zhongwan +▲) .....alarm point of the Stomach, warms and strengthens the Spleen and Stomach and supplements qi

St.25 (tianshu +▲) ....alarm point of the Large Intestine, regulates Intestinal function and directs qi downwards to promote elimination

Ren.4 (guanyuan +▲) ....alarm point of the Small Intestine, supplements yuan qi, warms yang and regulates qi

St.36 (zusanli +▲)...............sea point of the Stomach, strengthens the Spleen and Stomach, supplements qi and corrects the qi dynamic

Sp.6 (sanyinjiao +▲) ....strengthens the Spleen and Kidneys, and supplements qi

Bl.20 (pishu +▲)................transport point of the Spleen, warms Spleen yang

Bl.21 (weishu +▲) ....transport point of the Stomach, warms the Stomach and regulates the qi dynamic

Bl.23 (shenshu +▲)............transport point of the Kidneys, warms Kidney yang to support Spleen yang

Du.4 (mingmen +▲) ....warms Kidney yang to support Spleen yang

- a moxa box over the upper abdomen is very helpful
- with edema, add Ren.9 (shuifen ▲) and Sp.9 (yinlingquan –)
- Ear points: mouth, spleen, kidney, zero point, shenmen, adrenal, endocrine

Clinical notes

- Spleen and Kidney yang deficiency type obesity may be the result of digestive damage from weight loss programs, or prolonged use of cold medications or herbs. Patients may be diagnosed with hyperthyroidism or polycystic ovaries.
- A diet aimed at warming Spleen yang is an essential component of treatment. See Clinical Handbook, Vol. 2, p.873.
- The low energy levels of patients with yang deficiency is a major impediment to increasing activity levels. In many cases, it is best to wait until the patients yang qi is returning before embarking on any program. Once exercise is possible, it should be introduced gradually and in a graded fashion, starting with some type of mild and well supported activity, such as aquaerobics in a heated pool. This is especially useful where there is lower back pain. As Spleen and Kidney yang recover, a more aerobic regime can be phased in.

肝
肾
阴
虚

14.5 LIVER AND KIDNEY YIN DEFICIENCY

Liver and Kidney yin deficiency is a common pattern in overweight people, and is most commonly seen in women after menopause. It can also be the result of a chronic damp heat pattern that depletes yin, or excessive dieting and the use of bitter purgative and appetite suppressant slimming aids.

Although the most characteristic feature of yin deficiency is weight loss and thinning of tissues, the deficiency can affect certain tissues preferentially, for example the tissues lining the genitourinary tract, leaving muscle and fat tissue unaffected. The weight loss is slower than in the Spleen deficiency and heat patterns, with none of the initial loss from improved fluid metabolism.

Clinical features
- Obesity, usually in older patients, most commonly seen in women over 50 years, although men may also be affected.
- dryness of the skin, hair, vagina and mucous membranes; thirst
- multiple xanthoma and skin tags
- lower back, leg and knee pain
- facial flushing, malar flush
- low grade afternoon fever, night sweats
- visual weakness, blurring vision; dry, irritated eyes
- headaches, irritability, dizziness and tinnitus
- insomnia and palpitations

T red and dry with little or no coat
P deep, fine and rapid

Treatment Principle
Nourish and supplement Liver and Kidney yin

Prescription

YI GUAN JIAN 一贯煎
Linking Decoction, modified

sheng di (Rehmanniae Radix preparata) 生地	24–45g
gou qi zi (Lycii Fructus) 枸杞子	9–18g
sha shen (Glehniae/Adenophorae Radix) 沙参	9–12g
mai dong (Ophiopogonis Radix) 麦冬	9–12g
dang gui (Angelicae sinensis Radix) 当归	9–12g
chuan lian zi (Toosendan Fructus) 川楝子	3–6g
he shou wu (Polygoni multiflori Radix) 何首乌	9–12g
han lian cao (Ecliptae Herba) 旱莲草	9–12g
nu zhen zi (Ligustri Fructus) 女贞子	9–12g

Method: Decoction. **Sheng di** and **gou qi zi** enrich Liver and Kidney yin and blood; **sha shen** and **mai dong** nourish and supplement Stomach yin; **dang gui** supplements and activates Liver blood and softens the Liver; the small dose of **chuan lian zi** regulates qi without damaging yin; **he shou wu, han lian cao** and **nu zhen zi** support **sheng di** in nourishing Liver and Kidney yin. (Source: *Zhong Yi Nei Ke Xue [Xu Ming Yi Lei An]*)

Modifications
- With marked deficient heat, add **mu dan pi** (Moutan Cortex) 牡丹皮 9–12g, and **zhi mu** (Anemarrhenae Rhizoma) 知母 9–12g.
- With Stomach yin deficiency and a peeled or mirror tongue, add **yu zhu** (Polygonati odorati Rhizoma) 玉竹 12–15g.
- With constipation, add **huo ma ren** (Cannabis Semen) 火麻仁 9–12g or **gua lou ren** (Trichosanthis Semen) 栝楼仁 9–12g.
- With abdominal pain, add **bai shao** (Paeoniae Radix alba) 白芍 9–12g and **gan cao** (Glycyrrhizae Radix) 甘草 3–6g.
- With food stagnation, add **mai ya** (Hordei Fructus germinantus) 麦芽 15–30g and **gu ya** (Setariae Fructus germinatus) 谷芽 15–30g.
- With acid reflux, add **hai piao xiao** (Sepiae Endoconcha) 海螵蛸 9–12g [as powder added to the strained decoction].

Prepared medicines
Concentrated powders
Yi Guan Jian (Linking Combination) plus Er Zhi Wan (Ligustrum & Eclipta Combination)

Tian Wang Bu Xin Dan (Ginseng & Zizyphus Formula)
  – with sleep and shen disturbances

Pills
Yi Guan Jian Wan (Linking Decoction Teapills)

Tian Wang Bu Xin Dan (Emperor's Teapills, Tian Wang Pu Hsin Tan)

Acupuncture (select from)
Ren.4 (guanyuan +)............these points supplement Liver and Kidney yin
Ren.6 (qihai +)

St.36 (zusanli +) ....sea point of the Stomach, strengthens the Spleen and Stomach and improves digestive function

Kid.3 (taixi +)......................source point of the Kidneys, supplements Kidney yin and clears heat from deficiency

Liv.3 (taichong +)................source point of the Liver, supplements Liver yin

Sp.6 (sanyinjiao +)..............nourishes Kidney, Liver and Spleen yin

Bl.18 (ganshu +).................transport points of the Liver and Kidney,
Bl.23 (shenshu +)   supplement Liver and Kidney yin

- with insomnia, add Ht.7 (shenmen) and PC.6 (neiguan –)
- with night sweats, add Ht.6 (yinxi –)
- with anxiety, add yintang (M–HN–3) and Du.20 (baihui)
- with palpitations or arrhythmias add Ht.5 (tongli)
- Ear points: mouth, liver, kidney, zero point, spleen, shenmen, endocrine

Clinical notes.
- Even though building yin to treat weight gain may seem counter intuitive, improving the quality of the body's yin will restore homeostasis and assist in trimming down.
- A yin nourishing diet is recommended. See Clinical Handbook, Vol. 2, p.876.

气
滞
血
瘀

14.6 QI AND BLOOD STAGNATION

Qi and blood stasis is the result of chronic obesity, and represents obesity with significant cardiovascular complications. Stagnation will gradually complicate all other patterns, and so this pattern will have features of phlegm, heat or deficiency.

Clinical features

- obesity, usually with predominance of abdominal fat and the classic apple shape
- chest pain or oppression, breathlessness with exertion
- pains in the legs worse with walking; hip, knee and ankle pain and stiffness
- purple or dark discoloration of the lower legs with dry, scaly skin
- dark or mottled complexion, purple lips
- varicose veins, spider veins, spider nevi
- multiple xanthoma and dark skin tags
- left iliac fossa pressure pain (p.925–926)

T purple or mauve, or with purple or brown patches or stasis spots; congested, dark sublingual veins

P deep, choppy or imperceptible, or irregular

Treatment Principle

Activate blood and dispel blood stasis
Dredge the Liver and regulate qi

Prescription

XUE FU ZHU YU TANG 血府逐瘀汤
Drive Out Stasis in the Mansion of Blood Decoction

tao ren (Persicae Semen) 桃仁	9–12g
hong hua (Carthami Flos) 红花	6–9g
dang gui (Angelicae sinensis Radix) 当归	9–12g
sheng di (Rehmanniae Radix) 生地	9–12g
chi shao (Paeoniae Radix rubra) 赤芍	6–9g
chuan xiong (Chuanxiong Rhizoma) 川芎	6–9g
chai hu (Radix Bupleuri) 柴胡	6–9g
zhi ke (Aurantii Fructus) 枳壳	6–9g
gan cao (Glycyrrhizae Radix) 甘草	3–6g
chuan niu xi (Cyathulae Radix) 川牛膝	9–12g
jie geng (Platycodi Radix) 桔梗	3–6g

Method: Decoction. **Tao ren** and **hong hua** activate blood and disperse blood stasis; **dang gui**, **chuan xiong** and **chi shao** nourish blood and activate blood; **sheng di** and **chi shao** cool the blood; **sheng di** and **dang gui** nourish and protect yin and blood; **chai hu** and **zhi ke** dredge the Liver and regulate qi to lead the blood; **chuan niu xi** activates blood and leads it downwards; **jie geng** frees qi in the chest and diaphragm, and its ascending nature collaborates with the descending actions of **chuan niu xi** and **zhi ke**, to stimulate the qi dynamic; **gan cao** harmonizes the other herbs and protects the Spleen. (Source: *Zhong Yi Nei Ke Xue* [*Yi Lin Gai Cuo*])

Modifications

- With constipation, add **da huang** (Rhei Radix et Rhizoma) 大黄 9–12g [added at the end of cooking] until the bowels are moving, then reduce the dose or cook for the same time as the rest of the herbs.

- With severe stasis, add **shui zhi** (Hirudo) 水蛭 1–1.5g and **san qi fen** (powdered Notoginseng Radix) 三七粉 3–6g [both powdered and taken separately].
- With abdominal pain, add **zhi mo yao** (Myrrha preparata) 炙没药 6–9g and **zhi ru xiang** (Olibanum preparata) 炙乳香 6–9g.
- With masses, add **dan shen** (Salviae miltiorrhizae Radix) 丹参 9–12g, **yu jin** (Curcumae Radix)郁金 9–12g, **san leng** (Sparganii Rhizoma) 三棱 6–9g and **e zhu** (Curcumae Rhizoma) 莪术 6–9g.
- With depression, add **he huan pi** (Albizziae Cortex) 合欢皮 12–15g.
- With insomnia, add **he huan pi** (Albizziae Cortex) 合欢皮 12–15g and **ye jiao teng** (Polygoni multiflori Caulis) 夜交藤 15–30g.

Variations and additional prescriptions

With blood deficiency

Patients with chronic blood stasis often have significant deficiency as well. When there is qi and blood deficiency, a milder blood activating strategy may be best to begin with. Prescriptions such as **TAO HONG SI WU TANG** (Four Substance Decoction with Safflower and Peach Pit 桃红四物汤, p.921) for blood deficiency with stasis, or **BU YANG HUAN WU TANG** (Supplement Yang to Restore Five Tenths Decoction 补阳还五汤, p.600) for qi deficiency with stasis may be more acceptable.

Prepared medicines

Concentrated powders

Xue Fu Zhu Yu Tang (Persica & Carthamus Combination)
Tao Hong Si Wu Tang (Tangkuei Four, Persica & Carthamus Combination)
 – with blood deficiency
Bu Yang Huan Wu Tang (Astragalus & Peony Combination)
 – with qi deficiency

Pills

Xue Fu Zhu Yu Wan (Stasis in the Mansion of Blood Teapills)
Sheng Tian Qi Pian (Raw Tian Qi Ginseng Tablets)
 – thought to help with hyperlipidemia as well as activating blood
Tao Hong Si Wu Wan (Tao Hong Si Wu Tang Teapills)
Bu Yang Huan Wu Wan (Great Yang Restoration Teapills)

Acupuncture (select from)

Ren.12 (zhongwan +▲).....alarm point of the Stomach, strengthens the Spleen and Stomach and supplements qi
Ren.4 (guanyuan +▲)........supplements yuan qi to build new blood
Bl.17 (geshu –)...................meeting point for blood, dispels stagnant blood
Bl.18 (ganshu)....................transport point of the Liver, nourishes and activates Liver blood
Bl.20 (pishu +▲)..............transport point of the Spleen, strengthens the Spleen and supplements qi and blood
Sp.10 (xuehai –).................activates blood and dispels stasis

Sp.6 (sanyinjiao +▲).........strengthens the Spleen and nourishes and activates qi
and blood

Sp.4 (gongsun –)...............connecting point of the Spleen and master point of
chongmai, regulates the Spleen and Stomach and
activates blood

St.36 (zusanli +▲) ....sea point of the Stomach, strengthens the Spleen and
Stomach and supplements qi and blood

Liv.3 (taichong –)...............source point of the Liver, activates Liver blood

• moxa can be used unless there is heat
• Ear points: mouth, liver, spleen, stomach, zero point, shenmen, endocrine

Clinical notes

• The prognosis is relative to the degree of the blood stasis. If the patient is able
to take part in more physical activity and aerobic exercise, even relatively severe
blood stasis can be improved.
• A diet suitable for blood stasis should be adopted. See Clinical Handbook, Vol.
2, p.886

Table 14.1 Summary of common patterns of obesity

Pattern	Features	Prescription
Stomach heat with food stagnation	Obesity with a red plethoric complexion, constipation or loose foul smelling stools, distended abdomen, bad breath, heartburn, sleep apnea, red tongue with a thick, greasy, white or yellow coat, deep, slippery, strong pulse	Zhi Shi Dao Zhi Wan Lian Po Yin Long Dan Xie Gan Tang Da Chai Hu Tang
Phlegm damp	Obesity, pear shape; puffy face; firm muscles, somnolence, reflux, sweet cravings, mucus congestion, dizziness, swollen tongue with a thin or thick, greasy, white coat, deep, wiry, slippery pulse	Xiang Sha Liu Jun Zi Tang
Spleen qi deficiency	Obesity with poor muscle tone and edema; weak muscles, tiredness pallor, sweet cravings, loose stools, copious leucorrhea, pale, swollen and scalloped tongue with a thin white or greasy coat, deep, weak, moderate, soft pulse	Shen Ling Bai Zhu San
Spleen and Kidney yang deficiency	Similar to the Spleen qi deficiency pattern above with cold intolerance, marked edema and digestive weakness, urinary frequency and nocturia	Fu Zi Li Zhong Wan
Liver and Kidney yin deficiency	Obesity, facial flushing, afternoon fever, night sweats, visual weakness headaches, irritability, dizziness and tinnitus, insomnia, palpitations, red, dry tongue with little or no coat, deep, fine, rapid pulse	Yi Guan Jian
Qi and blood stasis	Obesity, chest pain and breathlessness, leg pain with walking; purple legs with dry scaly skin, mottled complexion, purple lips, varicose and spider veins, purple or mauve tongue, dark sublingual veins, deep, rough, imperceptible or irregular pulse	Xue Fu Zhu Yu Tang

PAINFUL OBSTRUCTION SYNDROME

Painful obstruction syndrome, or bi syndrome, (*bì zhèng*[1] 痹证), is acute or chronic pain and stiffness in the musculoskeletal system. There may also be swelling, numbness, paresthesia and decreased range of motion. These symptoms primarily affect joints and their related soft tissues. Traditionally, the painful obstruction syndrome model has focused on the bones and joints, in a manner similar to the western orthopedic model, and is primarily concerned with what would be diagnosed biomedically as inflammatory and degenerative joint disease. Because painful obstruction syndrome is concerned with pain, however, there has been a tendency to use it to analyze and treat all kinds of musculoskeletal pain, often with less than satisfactory results. Clinical experience has demonstrated that a significant proportion of musculoskeletal pain presenting to the average Chinese medical practice is of muscular and myofascial origin, and falls outside the painful obstruction model. All musculoskeletal pain can technically be classified as painful obstruction, but it does not follow that the painful obstruction model can be used to effectively analyze and manage all musculoskeletal pain.

> **BOX 15.1 PAINFUL OBSTRUCTION SYNDROME**
>
> Wind damp
> Cold damp
> Localized heat in a joint
> Damp heat
> Lingering heat in the ying level
> Toxic heat
> Blood stasis
> Phlegm
> Phlegm and blood stasis
> Qi and blood deficiency
> Qi and yin deficiency
> Liver and Kidney deficiency
> – yin deficiency
> – yang deficiency
> – yin and yang deficiency

Two models for understanding and managing pain

There are two ways of seeing musculoskeletal pain, the anatomical (Western) model and the constitutional (Chinese) model. Both have strengths and weaknesses.

The Chinese model is concerned with the relationship between pathogenic invasion, organ system function and local pathology of joints and soft tissues, and understands how the interior and exterior, and distant parts of the body are linked through the channel system. With its attention on the functional and structural unity of the whole organism, Chinese medicine is more concerned with systemic dysfunction, at the expense of local precision. Areas are treated, rather than the specific tissues involved.

The anatomical model is based on an understanding of the structure, function and biomechanics of the components of the musculoskeletal system. Its advantages are the precision with which it is possible to identify and treat a pain causing structure. Its weakness is in missing the relationship between the function of the organism as a whole and pathology of a specific part. Constitutional and systemic factors

---

1 Practical Dictionary of Chinese Medicine (1998) – 'impediment pattern'

are generally not considered in the treatment plan. While this approach is often effective in swiftly improving pain, the condition may recur.

When used together, the anatomical and the constitutional models complement each other, compensating for each others weaknesses and capitalizing on their strengths. A broader understanding of diagnosis and prognosis can be achieved and more effective treatment plans designed. The combined approach leads to:–

- a better understanding of exactly where the pain is coming from, and a more focused response as a result
- the ability to improve the functional characteristics of the affected tissues by treating the systemic pattern or patterns that contribute to the problem in the first place
- better use of the tools of Chinese medicine; acupuncture, moxibustion, cupping, guasha and tuina are rendered more powerful when applied with the precision of the anatomical model
- a reduced incidence of relapse when constitutional or systemic factors are addressed (often with herbal medicine)

A detailed discussion of the myofascial model of pain management is beyond the scope of this chapter, but the system is laid out with clarity by Janet Travell and David Simons (1983) in their seminal work on the topic. See also Legge (2010) for a Chinese medical approach to myofascial pain.

PATHOLOGY
Qi and blood stasis is at the root of all pain
The main features of painful obstruction syndrome, pain and stiffness, are caused by disruption to the normal distribution of qi and blood. This disruption may be due to a number of different factors, including physical blockage from scarring, trauma or other structural phenomena, the presence of an obstructing pathogen, poor or sluggish flow of qi and blood from weak Heart and Lungs qi, increased blood viscosity from yin deficiency or internal heat, or a general lack of circulatory momentum from yang deficiency. Regardless of the cause, the result is localized stagnation and accumulation of qi and blood, which at a certain level of stasis causes pain. Treatment of painful obstruction syndrome always involves therapeutic strategies and techniques to remove obstruction and stimulate the local circulation of qi and blood.

Different pathogens can influence the flow of qi and blood in different ways. For example, wind and damp tend to obstruct the qi, and so their characteristic pain is dull, aching and diffuse. Cold on the other hand is particularly good at constricting the vessels and slowing blood circulation, resulting in the characteristic intense and localized pain.

The diagnosis of qi and blood stagnation at the basis of all pain reveals one of the weaknesses of the Chinese model. The symptoms of qi and blood stagnation can be described accurately, but the precise location of the stasis, in terms of anatomy, cannot. Working out precisely where the stasis is located and the tissues involved leads to a much finer focus and better treatment outcomes.

BOX 15.2 BIOMEDICAL CAUSES OF MUSCULOSKELETAL PAIN

Most common
- myofascial pain syndromes
- osteoarthritis
- tendonitis
- bursitis
- trauma
- nerve compression disorders such as carpal tunnel and sciatica
- degenerative joint disease
- biomechanical strain

Viral and infectious arthralgia/myalgia
- Rheumatic fever
- Dengue fever
- influenza
- gonococcal, staphylococcal
- toxoplasma
- herpes zoster

Drug induced
- cholesterol lowering statins
- amoxycillin
- methyldopa
- carbimazole

Connective tissue disease, autoimmune
- rheumatoid arthritis
- systemic lupus erythematosus
- scleroderma
- mixed connective tissue disease
- Behçet's syndrome
- Reiter's syndrome
- myositis
- dermatomyositis
- polymyositis
- ankylosing spondylitis
- psoriatic arthritis

Metabolic disorders
- gout
- hypocalcaemia

Other
- tumors
- vasculitis
- thrombophlebitis
- fibromyalgia

Painful obstruction syndrome is primarily located in the musculoskeletal system

Painful obstruction syndrome is primarily an external disorder, with the main pathology located in the musculoskeletal system. The musculoskeletal system is considered yang and external, relative to the organ systems. Although the external layers of the body are contiguous with the internal organ systems and linked through the channels network, they are distinct. Pathology in the musculoskeletal system, even when severe, may have no adverse effect on systemic circulation of qi and blood or function of the internal organs.

The integrity of qi and blood flow through the channel network and the musculoskeletal system, however, is influenced by the function of the internal organ systems. Weakness or dysfunction of one or more organ systems can predispose to, or exacerbate, painful obstruction syndrome. Any organ system, especially those with a direct effect on the manufacture and distribution of qi and blood, can influence the volume and quality of qi and blood in the channels and its ability to circulate freely. Lack of adequate qi and blood to nourish and protect the superficial tissues can predispose them to injury from pathogenic invasion, overuse and trauma.

Imbalance in any organ system can also affect the integrity of qi and blood dis-

Figure 15.1 Progression of external pathogens

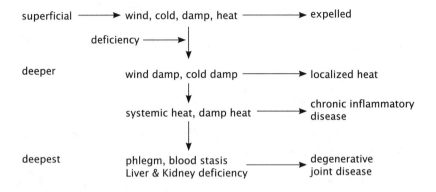

tribution through the related channel network and the tissues under its control. For example, pathology of the Large Intestine organ, such as heat, can predispose a patient to pathology along the pathway of the related channel. In the case of the Large Intestine, pathology of the elbow and shoulder, such as inflammation of the lateral tendons, epicondylitis and supraspinatus tendonitis, may result.

Painful obstruction syndrome involves the exterior, interior or both

There are three ways that internal and external conditions influence the development of painful obstruction syndrome, and the strategies appropriate to their resolution.

Purely external

Purely external pathology is confined to the musculoskeletal system, and is the result of trauma or pathogenic invasion. The local qi and blood circulation has been compromised, but the internal organ systems remain unaffected. Treatment is predominantly local, aimed at removing the obstruction and correcting qi and blood flow through the local channels and tissues.

External conditions with internal organ dysfunction

This is a common finding in chronic pain problems, and is the most common presentation of patients with painful obstruction syndrome as described in this chapter. The main symptoms are external, but there is an organ system imbalance or weakness that contributes to the pathology. This situation can occur in two ways. Firstly, an unresolved external pathogen may linger in the tissues, eventually impacting on the internal organ systems. For example, a persistent damp pathogen will gradually deplete the Spleen, chronic cold will drain Kidney yang and unresolved heat will damage Liver and Kidney yin. Secondly, an internal organ system dysfunction can predispose the tissues and regions of the body controlled by it to invasion by an external pathogen or to damage from overuse. Treatment is both local and systemic, and herbs play an important role.

Internal organ system dysfunction with symptoms externally
In this case, the main problem is in an internal organ system, but the symptoms are reflected in the external pathways and tissues related to the affected system. Examples include the dull lower back pain and aching weak knees of Kidney deficiency, or hip, shoulder and temporomandibular joint pain from Gallbladder dysfunction. Treatment is aimed at the organ system, with herbs as the primary modality, and improvement or resolution often occurs with little attention paid to the local manifestations.

Deficiency and excess
By definition, the primary pathology of painful obstruction syndrome, stagnation of qi and blood, is an excess condition, even though the underlying cause of the stasis may be from weakness of an organ system or localized deficiency. In general, the status of qi and blood at a particular locus can be assessed by the symptoms. If there is too much qi and blood at a particular locus due to the damming effects of trauma or spasm, the symptoms reflect localized obstruction and tend to be acute, quite painful, with swelling, redness and reactive spasm of the overlying tissues.

Pain can also arise when qi and blood fails to reach an area, either because of a deficiency of the relevant internal organs or because an obstruction prevents qi and blood from getting in to the area. This is seen in conditions that are chronic, with pain that tends to be mild to moderate, aching and dull, with the affected area appearing atrophic, pale or cool.

ETIOLOGY
Trauma
Trauma in a variety of forms can contribute to painful obstruction syndrome. Physical trauma involves not only the obvious injury to tissues that follows a fall or contusion, but also damage that slowly accretes from poor posture or overuse.

In most cases of simple trauma, the lesion is confined to the superficial tissues. Once damaged however, the area may be weakened and predisposed to later invasion by pathogens or further traumatic injury.

Severe or prolonged stress and emotional trauma may also play a part in chronic pain by inhibiting systemic circulation in general and localized circulation of qi and blood in particular. Stress and emotional factors can cause muscle spasm, increase the mechanical traction on joints, reduce qi and blood flow, and predispose the affected tissues to pathological invasion and mechanical damage.

Ergonomics, overuse, under use
Bad posture held for prolonged periods can contribute to painful obstruction syndrome. Poor furniture design, awkward placement of computer screens and keyboards and working long hours under stress can all lead to pain in the back, neck or arms.

The right amount of physical activity and exercise is essential to health. Excessive and repetitive use of any body part, however, can wear it out and weaken it, enabling penetration by external pathogens or predisposition it to mechanical damage. Similarly, insufficient physical activity can weaken both muscles and the qi required to maintain their tone and integrity. It was noted in the Simple Questions (*Huang Di Nei Jing Su Wen*), chapter 23, that 'excessive running damages the sinews and Liver blood, excessive standing damages the bones and Kidneys, excessive sitting damages the Spleen and muscles and excessive lying down damages the Lungs and qi'.

Pathogens

The pathogens primarily responsible for painful obstruction syndrome are wind, cold, damp and heat. External pathogens can gain access to the body (of a vulnerable individual) when the individual is in contact with specific environmental conditions, for example, prolonged exposure to a humid or cold climates, or a damp or wet work or living environment, that allows damp to seep into the body.

A diagnosis of wind, heat, cold or damp can also be made on the basis of an individuals physiological response to pathology of the superficial tissues. A history of exposure to an environmental pathogen in unnecessary. For example, pain that is the result of chronic overuse, repetitive strain or accumulated micro–trauma may exhibit the hallmark signs and symptoms of a cold or damp pathogen (focal pain, heaviness, swelling etc.), and will be diagnosed and treated as such.

Wind

Wind enables other pathogens to gain access to the body by dispersing wei qi and carrying other pathogens into the superficial tissues. Wind relies on a relative blood deficiency to maintain a foothold in the tissues, so systemic or localized blood deficiency can render tissues vulnerable to wind invasion.

The nature of wind is light, active, airy and changeable and these qualities are reflected in the symptoms. Wind is often seen in the early stages of a pain pattern, when the pain is not localized and appears in different parts of the body at different times. Being light and airy by nature, wind tends to affect the upper body, and the pain varies in intensity. The pain pattern typical of wind can be clearly seen in the migratory pain of early rheumatic disease and some viral arthralgias.

Cold

Cold 'freezes and constricts'. Its presence significantly inhibits the local circulation of qi and blood. It tends to have an affinity for joints, especially the peripheral joints of the hands and feet. Its effects are usually quite localized, producing relatively severe pain that is improved with topical warmth. A cold pattern may arise as a result of pathogenic cold lodged in a joint or tissue, or as an absence of the warming action of yang qi and blood flow if there is blockage or inadequate circulation. Cold type pain is accompanied by significant stiffness, and the affected area may feel cooler than the surrounding tissues. Heat gives significant relief. Patients with yang deficiency are predisposed to cold patterns.

Damp

Damp is sticky, congesting, heavy and congealing, and a major impediment to qi and blood flow. Damp causes a sense of deep or dull aching or heaviness, usually

Figure. 15.2 Types of musculoskeletal pain

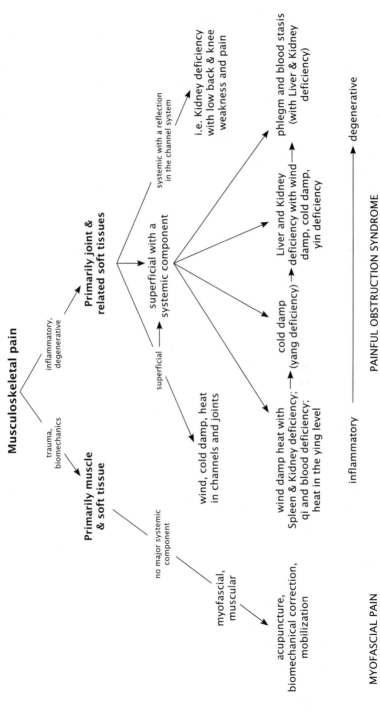

with swelling and edema of the affected tissues. Tissues feel boggy when palpated. Being a heavy pathogen it tends to sink downwards and often affects the lower body. Damp pain is worse with changes of weather, especially increasing humidity. The stickiness of damp causes it to adhere to the host tissues more readily and it is usually slow to resolve. Patients with Spleen weakness or pre–existing damp are prone to damp type painful obstruction syndrome.

Heat
Heat results in pain with redness and swelling of joints or soft tissues. The heat can result from an external invasion, in which case it is usually acute and systemic. It can also be the product of transformation of a pre–existing cold or damp pathogen into heat. Heat can be created internally by internal organ system dysfunction, and chronic heat is a common component of pathology such as the primary pathological triad (p.780).

Internal organ system dysfunction
Dysfunction of the internal organ systems can predispose patients to the development of musculoskeletal pain. The production, quality and distribution of qi and blood through the associated channel network and tissues may be compromised and leave the superficial tissues vulnerable to trauma or invasion.

Lung/Large Intestine
Lung and/or Large Intestine disorders can influence the anterior aspects of the shoulder, lateral elbow, radial aspect of the wrist, thumb and index finger. Heat disorders of the Large Intestine may contribute to inflammatory conditions along the pathway of the yangming (Large Intestine and Stomach) channels.

Lung weakness tends to cause people to slump forward with the shoulders internally rotated. This puts mechanical stress on the upper thorax and neck which can lead to chronic pain.

Spleen/Stomach
Disorders of the Spleen and Stomach can influence the jaw, knees and ankles. Spleen qi deficiency can lead to general qi and blood deficiency and poor muscle tone, leaving tissues prone to injury and hyperextension. Spleen deficiency also contributes to damp and a tendency to damp painful obstruction syndrome.

Liver/Gallbladder
Disorders of the Liver and Gallbladder can influence the suboccipital area, posterior shoulder, hip, groin, lateral aspects of the trunk, thigh, ankle and big toe.

Liver qi constraint is a major contributor to neck, upper back and shoulder pain. Liver blood has a special effect on lubricating, nourishing and maintaining the integrity of sinews. Dryness, loss of elasticity, stiffness and creaking of joints can be seen when Liver blood is deficient.

Kidney/Urinary Bladder
Pathology of the Kidney and Urinary Bladder can influence the entire spine and its many joints, the sacrum, coccyx, posterior leg, knee, heel and sole.

The Kidney has specific control over the bones. Pathology of the Kidney can contribute to bone and joint pathology and degeneration.

Qi and blood

Insufficiency of qi and blood inhibits the body's ability to repel pathogens and repair damage. External pathogens can invade more easily, and once in, are harder to evict. Musculoskeletal tissues are subject to wear and tear from normal activity, and maintenance and repair is a continual process requiring a steady and reliable supply of qi and blood. Qi and blood deficiency, either systemic or localized, reduce the ability of the body to efficiently repair itself, leading to the gradual accumulation of multiple areas of weakness that expose the tissues to invasion and encourage the processes of degeneration.

Phlegm

Phlegm is seen in chronic degenerative changes in joints. The phlegm congeals into dense nodules, such as rheumatoid nodules. Phlegm is often associated with numbness rather than pain, and usually occurs with blood stasis.

TREATMENT

The aim of treatment is to expel any pathogen affecting the tissues, restore the circulation of qi and blood and correct any underlying organ system imbalance or deficiency. A clearly formulated diagnosis will determine the mode and level of treatment. Treatment of painful obstruction syndrome can be prolonged, more so when there is underlying Liver and Kidney deficiency, phlegm or blood stasis. In chronic patterns, patients often get some temporary relief following a treatment, but sustained results may not become apparent for some weeks or even longer. It is important to persevere for a reasonable time before deciding whether the treatment is working or not.

When the painful obstruction is related to an external pathogen, without organ system involvement or deficiency complication, the treatment is focused on the affected area, with the use of local acupuncture and ahshi points, with internal medicine to assist in expelling the pathogen if necessary.

When there is external pathology with internal organ system complications, treatment is a more even mixture of local therapy and internal medicine. Appropriate local and distal acupuncture or other topical therapy is combined with herbal formulae aimed at dispelling pathogens and correcting organ system imbalance. Biomechanical correction, mobilization and exercises will be recommended as appropriate.

When the primary pathology is an internal organ imbalance which is reflected in the channel system, treatment is directed at the internal pathology, usually with herbs, although acupuncture is also effective. The greater the deficiency, the more herbs are necessary to replenish it. On the whole, little or no specific attention is paid to the musculoskeletal component.

Pharmaceutical medications

Many patients presenting with painful obstruction syndrome will be taking a pharmaceutical medication of some kind. It is quite appropriate for patients to use some form of analgesia, as necessary, while treatment with Chinese medicine proceeds. Some medications, however, appear to block the effects of Chinese

BOX 15.3 OTHER TREATMENTS

Topical treatment for cold
- Hot plasters to dispel cold and activate qi and blood, such as chilli and mustard plasters
- Anything with capsacin, the hot component of chilli; a simple version can be made by adding a teaspoon of tabasco sauce to a small amount of a neutral oil
- Hot packs and infrared heat lamps

Heat (inflammation)
- Heat clearing poultices can be made from herbs such as **pu gong ying** (Taraxaci Herba) 蒲公英, **da huang** (Rhei Radix et Rhizoma) 大黄, **huang qin** (Scutellariae Radix) 黄芩 and **huang lian** (Coptidis Rhizoma) 黄连

Massage
- Can activate the local circulation of qi and blood, reduce swelling and spasm
- Excellent when done with warming and dispersing liniments, such as Po Sum On oil (*bǎo xīn ān yóu* 保心安油) or similar
- Not suitable for heat and inflammation

Bloodletting
- Useful technique for blood stasis. See Appendix 4, p.929

Cupping
- Disperses qi and blood stasis; for congestion and spasm, often used with blood letting for blood stasis

Mobilization
- Essential to keep joints and tissues as mobile as possible. Painful areas should be mobilized passively or actively through as full a range of motion as possible, without causing undue pain
- Not for acute trauma

medicine treatment and prolong the course of treatment. Corticosteroids and immunosuppressant medications used for chronic inflammatory disease are notable for this. These drugs must not be stopped suddenly, and should only be modified in consultation with the patient's specialist. In many cases we can expect a slow and steady withdrawal of, or decreased need for, pharmaceutical medications as the treatment progresses.

Some patients with chronic pain related to inflammatory disease are also treated with anticoagulants such as coumarin (Warfarin) and aspirin, a recognition of the critical role blood stasis plays. Blood activating herbs must be used with extra caution in patients taking such medicines, and **dan shen** (Salviae miltiorrhizae Radix) 丹参 is contraindicated. These patients must be monitored carefully for signs of bleeding or purpura.

Table 15.1 Herbs that treat painful obstruction syndrome

Region	Herb	Action
	The regional designation does not restrict the use of the herbs to that location alone, but that they have been found to be most effective for pain in these areas.	
upper body	**Qiang Huo** Notopterygii Rhizoma seu Radix 羌活	Notopterygium root; pungent, bitter, warm; Urinary Bladder, Liver, Kidney. Disperses wind cold damp and stops pain. For wind cold damp pain of the neck and upper back, especially along the pathway of the upper half of the Urinary Bladder channel. 3-9 grams in decoction.
	Gui Zhi Cinnamomi Ramulus 桂枝	Cinnamon twigs; pungent, sweet, warm; Lung, Heart, Spleen, Stomach, Liver, Kidney, Urinary Bladder. Warms the channels and stops pain. An important herb for wind cold damp pain, especially in the neck, upper back, shoulders and arms. Can also be used for damp heat with suitable cooling herbs. 3-9 grams in decoction.
	Sang Zhi Mori Ramulus 桑枝	Mulberry twigs; bitter, neutral; Liver. Dispels wind and opens up flow in the channels. Especially good for shoulder, hand, finger and arm pain. Can be used for both cold and hot patterns. 15-30 grams in decoction.
	Jiang Huang Curcumae longae Rhizoma 姜黄	Curcuma root; bitter, pungent, warm; Spleen, Liver. Activates blood, opens up flow in the channels and stops pain. For wind damp shoulder and upper arm pain. 3-9 grams in decoction.
	Tou Gu Cao Herba Speranskia 透骨草	Speranskia; pungent, warm; Liver, Kidney. Dispels wind damp, activates blood and stops pain. For acute and chronic wind damp pain, especially when there is bony deformity or stubborn pain. Best for the shoulder and neck. 9-15 grams in decoction.
	Qing Feng Teng Sinomenium Caulis 清风藤	Sinomenium vine; pungent, bitter, warm; Liver, Kidney. Dispels wind damp and nourishes blood. For wind damp with blood deficiency in the shoulders, neck and upper body. 9-15 grams in decoction.
	Qin Jiao* Gentianae macrophyllae Radix 秦艽	Gentiana macrophylla root; bitter, pungent; Stomach, Large Intestine, Liver, Gallbladder. Dispels wind and stops pain. For wind damp pain in general, but best for pain in the extremities and neck. Can be used for cold or hot patterns. Especially good when there is inflammation and pain from a deep lying heat pathogen in the qi and ying levels. 6-12 grams in decoction.
	Ge Gen Pueraria Radix 葛根	Kudzu root; sweet, pungent, cool; Spleen, Stomach. For neck and upper back pain and stiffness from a variety of causes, including wind cold, wind damp and damp heat. 9-20 grams in decoction.

Table 15.1 Herbs that treat painful obstruction syndrome (cont.)

Region	Herb	Action
lower body and spine	**Han Fang Ji*** Stephaniae tetrandrae Radix 汉防己	Strephania root; very bitter, pungent, cold; Urinary Bladder, Spleen, Lung. Expels wind and stops pain. For wind damp and damp heat pain and swelling in the legs and knees. 6–9 grams in decoction.
	Yi Ren* Coicis Semen 苡仁	Job's tears; sweet, bland, cool; Spleen, Lung, Kidney. Drains damp and relieves obstruction. For damp heat pain and swelling, especially in the knees and ankles. 15–30 grams in decoction.
	Xi Xian Cao* Siegesbeckia Herba 豨莶草	Siegesbeckia; pungent, bitter, cold, slightly toxic; Liver, Kidney. Dispels wind damp. For wind damp or damp heat pain and numbness in the extremities. 9–15 grams in decoction.
	Du Huo Angelicae Pubescentis Radix 独活	Angelica pubescens root; pungent, bitter, slightly warm; Kidney, Liver. Dispels wind damp and stops pain. For wind damp pain along the lower half of the Urinary Bladder channel. 3–9 grams in decoction.
	Xu Chang Qing Cynanchi paniculati Radix 徐长卿	Cynanchum root; pungent, warm; Lung, Stomach, Liver, Kidney. Dispels wind, opens up flow in the channels and promotes urination. For wind damp pain, swelling and edema in the lower back and legs. 9–15 grams in decoction.
	Lu Xian Cao Pyrolae Herba 鹿衔草	Pyrola; sweet, warm; Lung, Liver, Kidney. Supplements the Liver and Kidneys and dispels wind damp. For pain, weakness and bony deformity in the joints. Also used for neurological pain. 9–30 grams in decoction.
	Lao Guan Cao* Erodii/Geranii Herba 老鹳草	Geranium; bitter, slightly pungent, neutral; Liver, Kidney. Dispels wind damp and opens up flow in the channels. For wind damp or damp heat pain and numbness. Also used for neurological pain like sciatica and nerve impingement. 15–30 grams in decoction.
	Hai Tong Pi Erythrinae Cortex 海桐皮	Flame tree bark; bitter, neutral; Liver, Kidney. Dispels wind and opens up flow in the channels. For wind damp lower back and leg pain. 6–12 grams in decoction
	Huai Niu Xi Achyranthis bidentatae Radix 怀牛膝	Achyranthes root; bitter, sour, neutral; Liver, Kidney. Supplements the Liver and Kidneys, strengthens the sinews and bones. For lower back, leg and knee pain from Liver and Kidney deficiency. 9–30 grams in decoction.
	Chuan Niu Xi Cyathulae Radix 川牛膝	Cyathula root; bitter, sour, neutral; Liver, Kidney. Activates blood, opens up flow in the channels and stops pain. For wind damp pain in the legs. Can be used for both heat and cold patterns. 9–30 grams in decoction.

Table 15.1 Herbs that treat painful obstruction syndrome (cont.)

Region	Herb	Action
lower body and spine	**Mu Gua** Chaenomelis Fructus 木瓜	Chinese quince; sour, warm; Liver, Spleen. Expels damp and eases sinews. For lower back and knee pain and swelling. 6-15 grams in decoction.
	Du Zhong Eucommiae Cortex 杜仲	Eucommia bark; sweet, slightly pungent, warm; Liver, Kidney. Supplement Liver and Kidney yin and yang and strengthens sinews and bones. An important herb for lower back and leg pain and weakness from Kidney deficiency. 9-15 grams in decoction, although up to 60 grams can be used in severe cases. Usually combined with xu duan.
	Xu Duan Dipsaci Radix 续断	Dipscus root; bitter, pungent, sweet, warm; Liver, Kidney. Supplements the Liver and Kidneys, activates the channels and stops pain. For lower back and leg pain and weakness from wind damp or Liver and Kidney yin or yang deficiency. 9-15 grams in decoction. Usually combined with du zhong.
	Sang Ji Sheng Taxilli Herba 桑寄生	Mistletoe; bitter, sweet, neutral; Liver, Kidney. Dispels wind and opens up flow in the channels. For lower back, leg and knee pain, stiffness and weakness from wind damp, Kidney yin and blood deficiency 15-30 grams in decoction.
	Xian Ling Pi Epimedii Herba 仙灵脾	Epimedium leaf; pungent, sweet, warm; Liver, Kidney. Dispels wind damp and warms Kidney yang. For pain, weakness and numbness in the lower back and legs from wind cold damp or Kidney yang deficiency. 9-15 grams in decoction.
	Gou Ji Cibotii Rhizoma 狗脊	Cibotium root; bitter, sweet, warm; Liver, Kidney. Dispels wind damp and strengthens the low back and spine. For back and spine pain and weakness from wind cold damp or Kidney yang deficiency. 3-9 grams in decoction.
	Wu Jia Pi Acanthopanacis Cortex 五加皮	Acanthopanax bark; pungent, sweet, warm; Liver, Kidney. Dispels wind damp and strengthens the sinews and bones. For lower back and leg pain and swelling from wind cold damp with damp predominant, or Liver and Kidney deficiency. 6-12 grams in decoction.

*cooling herbs for inflammatory conditions with obvious heat

Table 15.1 Herbs that treat painful obstruction syndrome (cont.)

Region	Herb	Action
four limbs, fingers, toes	**Ren Dong Teng*** Lonicerae Caulis 忍冬藤	Lonicera vine; sweet, cold; Lung, Heart, Stomach. Clears heat and opens up flow in the channels. An important herb for heat and damp heat in the joints. 15-30 grams in decoction.
	Luo Shi Teng* Trachelospermi Caulis 络石藤	Trachelospermum vine; bitter, cool; Heart, Liver. Dispels wind and opens up flow in the channels. For wind damp or damp heat in the joints of the extremities with stiffness and pain. 15-30 grams in decoction.
	Wei Ling Xian Clematidis Radix 威灵仙	Clematis root; pungent, salty, warm; influences all twelve channels. Dispels wind damp, opens up flow in the channels and stops pain. For wind cold damp pain and numbness. A very dispersing herb, also used for phlegm and blood stasis with joint deformity. 3-9 grams in decoction.
	Ji Xue Teng Spatholobi Caulis 鸡血藤	Milletia vine; bitter, slightly sweet, warm, Liver, Kidney. Activates and supplements blood, opens up the channels. For wind damp pain, paresthesia, weakness and numbness with underlying blood deficiency and stasis. 15-60 grams in decoction.
	Hai Feng Teng Piperis kadsurae Caulis 海风藤	Kadsura vine; pungent, bitter, warm; Liver, Spleen. Dispels wind damp and opens up flow in the channels. For wind damp in the joints of the extremities with stiffness and pain. 9-15 grams in decoction.
	Shen Jin Cao Lycopodii Herba 伸筋草	Lycopodium; pungent, bitter, warm; Liver, Kidney. Dispels wind and opens up flow in the channels. For pain, stiffness and numbness in the joints of the extremities. 9-15 grams in decoction.
*cooling herbs for inflammatory conditions with obvious heat		

Table 15.2 Acupuncture points for painful obstruction syndrome. Points with major effects on specific regions. TPs are trigger points in muscles that can refer pain to the area.

NECK	
local	• GB.20 (fengchi): dispels wind, affects upper neck, suboccipital region and entire head • BI.10 (tianzhi): dispels wind and affects the deep muscles of the neck • GB.21 (jianjing): tightness and stiffness; major point for qi stagnation; affects neck, shoulder and upper back
distal	• luozhen (M-UE-24): located proximal to the heads of the 2nd and 3rd metacarpals; used for acute pain and restricted rotation, needled strongly while the patient rotates the head • SI.3 (houxi): master point of the dumai, for pain and stiffness along the spine and posterior neck; combined with UB.62 (shenmai) for spinal pathology • GB.39 (xuanzhong) + SJ.5 (waiguan): for lateral neck pain and stiffness • BI.60 (kunlun): dispels wind and relaxes sinews and muscles; for posterior neck pain and stiffness
TPs	• suboccipital muscles • semispinalis • splenius • trapezius • levator scapulae
SHOULDER	
local	• LI.15 (jianyu) + SJ.14 (jianliao): dispel wind; main points for the lateral shoulder, glenohumeral joint and supraspinatus tendon • jianneiling (M-UE-48): midway between the shoulder tip and anterior axilliary fold, for anterior should pain • SI.9 (jianzhen), SI.10 (naoshu), SI.11 (tianzong): posterior shoulder and scapula pain
distal	• LI.4 (hegu), LI.11 (quchi): lateral shoulder pain • SI.6 (yanglao): cleft point of the Small Intestine; posterior shoulder and scapula pain • Lu.7 (lieque): anterior shoulder pain • St.38 (tiaokou): for acute pain, stiffness and restricted rotation; needled strongly while mobilizing joint
TPs	• infraspinatus (anterior pain) • supraspinatus (lateral pain) • subscapularis (posterior pain) • teres major (posterior pain) • deltoids

Table 15.2 Acupuncture points for painful obstruction syndrome (cont.)

ELBOW	
local	• LI.11 (quchi) • LI.10 (shousanli) • Lu.5 (chize) • PC.3 (quze) • SJ.10 (tianjing)
distal	• Lu.6 (kongzui): cleft point of the Lung channel, for anteromedial pain • LI.4 (hegu): lateral pain • Ht.7 (shenmen): medial pain
TPs	• supinator • triceps • supraspinatus
WRIST, HAND, FINGERS	
local	• SJ.4 (yangchi) • SI.5 (yanggu) • Lu.9 (taiyuan) • LI.5 (yangxi) • PC.7 (daling) • LI.4 (hegu) • SI.3 (houxi) • baxie (M–UE–9): just proximal to the metacarpophalangeal joints on the dorsum of the hand, four on each hand; for pain and stiffness in the fingers
proximal	• Lu.7 (lieque) • SJ.5 (waiguan) • LI.11 (quchi)
TPs	• subscapularis (wrist) • infraspinatus (radial aspect of the hand) • interosseous muscles
SPINE	
local	• Huatuo Jiaji points at the relevant segment • Urinary bladder points at the relevant segment • Du.3 (yaoyangguan) • Du.4 (mingmen) • Du.8 (jinsuo) • Du.14 (dazhui)
distal	• SI.3 (houxi) + Bl.62 (shenmai): used together for spinal pain and stiffness
TPs	• multifidis

Table 15.2 Acupuncture points for painful obstruction syndrome (cont.)

SACRUM	
local	• Bl.31 (shangliao) • Bl.32 (ciliao) • Bl.33 (zhongliao) • Bl.34 (xialiao)
distal	• Bl.58 (feiyang), Bl.62 (shenmai)
TPs	• quadratus lumborum • iliocostalis lumborum • gluteus maximus • longissimus
HIPS, GROIN, BUTTOCKS	
local	• GB.30 (huantiao): an important point for pain in the hips and legs • GB.29 (juliao)
distal	• GB.41 (zulinqi) • GB.39 (xuanzhong) • GB.31 (fengshi) • Bl.62 (shenmai) + SI.3 (houxi) and Kid.6 (zhaohai) + Lu.7 (lieque): to balance the yinqiaomai and yangqiaomai for tightness in the lateral muscles and laxness in the medial adductor muscles
TPs	• quadratus lumborum • gluteus minimus • gluteus medius • piriformis
KNEES	
local	• xiyan (M-LE-5): located on either side of the inferior margin of the patella when the knee is flexed, for pain inside the knee • St.36 (zusanli), GB.34 (yanglingquan), St.34 (liangqiu): lateral knee pain; influences the lateral collateral ligament • Sp.9 (yinlingquan), Sp.10 (xuehai), Kid.10 (yingu), Liv.8 (ququan): medial and posteromedial pain; influences the medial collateral ligament • Bl.40 (weizhong, Bl.39 (weiyang): posterior and popliteal fossa pain
distal	• Sp.5 (shangqiu), Sp.6 (sanyinjiao), Kid.3 (taixi): medial pain • St.41 (jiexi), GB.40 (qiuxu): lateral pain
TPs	• rectus femoris • medial head of quadriceps femoris
ANKLES	
local	• GB.40 (qiuxu): lateral pain, influences the coronary ligament • St.41 (jiexi): lateral pain, transforms damp • Bl.60 (kunlun): posterior ankle pain
distal and proximal	• GB.34 (yanglingquan), GB.39 (xuanzhong): lateral pain • Sp.6 (sanyinjiao), Sp.8 (diji): medial pain • Liv.3 (taichong): dorsal pain
TPs	• soleus • gastrocnemius

Table 15.2 Acupuncture points for painful obstruction syndrome (cont.)

TOES	
local	• bafeng (M-LE-10): just proximal to the metatarsopalangeal joints on the dorsum of the foot, for pain and stiffness in the toes • Sp.3 (taibai): also resolves damp • Liv.3 (taichong) • St..43 (xianggu) • GB.42 (diwuhui)
proximal	• St.36 (zusanli), GB.34 (yanglingquan), GB.39 (xuanzhong): lateral toes • Liv.5 (ligou), Sp.5 (shangqiu), Sp.6 (sanyinjiao), Kid.3 (taixi): medial toes
TPs	• tibialis anterior (big toe) • lumbricals and interosseous muscles

Table 15.3 Metal water points for inflammation

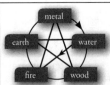 Metal and water points are used together for inflammation and pain at locations along the relevant channel pathway. Their use is based on the principle of cooling fire by manipulating the controlling and generating cycles. Metal is the mother of water; plentiful water can restrain fire.

Metal water pair	Area of influence
LI.1 (shangyang) + LI.2 (erjian)	radial aspect of the wrist, lateral elbow and lateral shoulder
Lu.8 (jingqu) + Lu.5 (chize)	radial aspect of the wrist, anterolateral aspect of the elbow and anterior shoulder
SI.1 (shaoze) + S.I.2 (qiangu)	ulnar aspect of wrist, medial elbow, posterior shoulder, scapula, posterior neck
SJ.1 (guanchong) + SJ.2 (yemen)	lateral fingers, lateral aspect of elbow, shoulder and neck
GB.44 (zuqiaoyin) + GB.43 (xiaxi)	lateral ankle, knee, hip and neck
Bl.67 (zhiyin) + Bl.65 (tonggu)	posterior ankle, achilles tendon, posterior knee, sacrum, spine, neck
St.45 (lidui) + St.44 (neiting)	anterolateral aspect of ankle, knee, anterior hip, clavicle
Kid.7 (fuliu) + Kid.10 (yingu)	posteromedial aspect of ankle, knee and costosternal junction

风
湿
痹
阻

15.1 WIND DAMP

Wind damp is a common presentation of both acute and chronic painful obstruction syndrome. The symptom picture depends on the balance of wind and damp. In the early stages (the first weeks), wind symptoms tends to predominate. If the condition persists, damp symptoms start to dominate the clinical picture, and the pain settles into a joint or joints, or muscle. Patients with pre–existing damp or Spleen qi deficiency are more susceptible. Chronic wind damp in joints can easily transform into heat (see damp heat, p.659 and 662).

Clinical features

- Joint and muscle pain, soreness, aching, with heaviness or numbness. The pain most commonly affects the large joints, but may be localized in muscles. The pain may be worse during or prior to the onset of humid or wet weather.
- swelling, a boggy feel or edema of the affected area
- stiffness, decreased range of motion
- in the early stages there may be fever and aversion to wind, and the pain may be migratory

T greasy, white coat; pale body (with Spleen deficiency)
P wiry, slippery, soft, soggy, moderate

Treatment principle

Dispel wind and damp
Mobilize qi and blood in the channels and network vessels

Prescription

CHENG SHI JUAN BI TANG 程氏蠲痹汤
Remove Painful Obstruction Decoction (from the Cheng Clan)

This is a versatile formula that can be adapted according to the location of the pain and the balance of pathogens.

qiang huo (Notopterygii Rhizoma seu Radix) 羌活 6–9g
du huo (Angelicae pubescentis Radix) 独活 6–9g
qin jiao (Gentianae macrophyllae Radix) 秦艽 6–9g
dang gui (Angelicae sinensis Radix) 当归 6–9g
chuan xiong (Chuanxiong Rhizoma) 川芎 6–9g
mu xiang (Aucklandiae Radix) 木香 3–6g
ru xiang (Olibanum) 乳香 3–6g
zhi gan cao (Glycyrrhizae Radix preparata) 炙甘草 3–6g
sang zhi (Mori Ramulus) 桑枝 15–30g
hai feng teng (Piperis kadsurae Caulis) 海风藤 15–30g
rou gui (Cinnamomi Cortex) 肉桂 1.5–3g

Method: Decoction. **Qiang huo, du huo, qin jiao, hai feng teng** and **sang zhi** dispel wind damp; **dang gui, chuan xiong, mu xiang** and **ru xiang** activate qi and blood and stop pain; **rou gui** scatters cold and warms the channels; **zhi gan cao** harmonizes the formula and protects the Stomach. (Source: *Zhong Yi Nei Ke Xue [Yi Xue Xin Wu]*)

Modifications

- With wind predominant, add **fang feng** (Saposhnikovae Radix) 防风 9–12g.
- With damp predominant, add **cang zhu** (Atractylodis Rhizoma) 苍术 9–12g, **yi ren** (Coicis Semen) 苡仁 24–30g and **han fang ji** (Stephaniae tetrandrae Radix) 汉防己 9–12g.
- With cold, add **ma huang** (Ephedra Herba) 麻黄 6–9g and **zhi fu zi** (Aconiti Radix lateralis preparata) 制附子 6–9g.
- With heat, add **jin yin hua** (Lonicerae Flos) 金银花 15–30g and **lian qiao** (Forsythiae Fructus) 连翘 9–12g.
- When the upper body is affected, add **wei ling xian** (Clematidis Radix) 威灵仙 6–9g, **jiang huang** (Curcumae longae Rhizoma) 姜黄 9–12g and **tou gu cao** (Herba Speranskia) 透骨草 9–12g.
- When the lower body is affected, add **chuan niu xi** (Cyathulae Radix) 川牛膝 12–15g, **mu gua** (Chaenomelis Fructus) 木瓜 9–12g and **xu duan** (Dipsaci Radix) 续断 12–15g.
- With numbness or tingling, add **ji xue teng** (Spatholobi Caulis) 鸡血藤 15–30g.

Variations and additional prescriptions

With wind predominant and migratory pain

Joint pain without swelling that moves from place to place is a sign that wind is the main pathogen. This is sometimes seen in the early stages of a rheumatic condition or viral arthralgia. There will be signs and symptoms reflecting the acute nature of the exterior invasion, such as fever and chills, sore throat and a floating pulse. The treatment is to dispel wind and activate qi in the superficial tissues with FANG FENG TANG (Saposhnikova Decoction 防风汤).

fang feng (Saposhnikovae Radix) 防风 9–12g
dang gui (Angelicae sinensis Radix) 当归 9–12g
xing ren (Armeniacae Semen) 杏仁 9–12g
fu ling (Poria) 茯苓 9–12g
qin jiao (Gentianae macrophyllae Radix) 秦艽 9–12g
ge gen (Puerariae Radix) 葛根 9–12g
gui zhi (Cinnamomi Ramulus) 桂枝 6–9g
ma huang (Ephedra Herba) 麻黄 6–9g
qiang huo (Notopterygii Rhizoma seu Radix) 羌活 6–9g
huang qin (Scutellariae Radix) 黄芩 3–6g
gan cao (Glycyrrhizae Radix) 甘草 3–6g
sheng jiang (Zingiberis Rhizoma recens) 生姜 3–6g
da zao (Jujubae Fructus) 大枣 .... 5 fruit

Method: Decoction. **Fang feng** and **qin jiao** dispel wind from the surface and stop pain; **fu ling** leaches damp out through the urine; **qiang huo, gui zhi, ma huang** and **ge gen** dispel wind cold from the surface and release pathogens from the muscle layer; **dang gui** nourishes and activates blood; **xing ren** diffuses the Lungs and mobilizes Lung qi and wei qi; the bitter coldness of **huang qin** balances the pungent warmth of the other herbs and prevents the pathogen from transforming into heat. **Sheng jiang, gan cao** and **da zao** harmonize the ying and wei, and assist in shoring up the surface against invasion. (Source: *Zhong Yi Nei Ke Shou Ce* [*Xuan Ming Fang Lun*])

Acute wind damp pain with exterior symptoms

In the acute phase of an external wind damp attack, the pathogen penetrates the superficial tissues through open pores when the individual is sweating and thus sits superficially in the muscles and joints. The symptoms are acute muscle and joint aching, stiffness and heaviness especially in the upper body, neck and upper back. In addition there is fever and mild chills, with the fever worse in the afternoon and unrelieved by sweating, headache or foggy head, nausea and vomiting, a thick greasy white tongue coat and a floating, soft or soggy pulse. The treatment is to dispel wind damp with **QIANG HUO SHENG SHI TANG** (Notopterygium Decoction to Overcome Dampness 羌活胜湿汤).

qiang huo (Notopterygii Rhizoma seu Radix) 羌活 9–12g
du huo (Angelicae pubescentis Radix) 独活 6–9g
gao ben (Ligustici Rhizoma) 藁本 6–9g
fang feng (Saposhnikoviae Radix) 防风 9–12g
chuan xiong (Chuanxiong Rhizoma) 川芎 6–9g
man jing zi (Fructus Viticis) 蔓荆子 6–9g
zhi gan cao (Glycyrrhizae Radix preparata) 炙甘草 3–6g

Method: Decoction. **Qiang huo** and **du huo** dispel wind damp and stop pain; as a pair they are especially effective for pain along the path of the taiyang channels. **Gao ben** and **fang feng** reinforce the action of **qiang huo** and **du huo** in dispelling pathogens from taiyang. **Chuan xiong** and **man jing zi** alleviate headache. **Zhi gan cao** harmonizes the formula and assists in preventing excessive dispersal of qi and yin by the pungent herbs. (Source: *Zhong Yi Nei Ke Xue* [*Nei Wai Shang Bian Huo Lun*])

Knee pain and swelling in overweight individuals with Spleen deficiency

A common pattern of wind damp pain manifests as chronic or recurrent pain and swelling of the knees. There is usually a significant degree of Spleen deficiency which predisposes the patient to edema. The main features are knee pain and swelling in clammy, tired, overweight individuals, most commonly women. In addition there may be frequent colds and flu, a pale complexion, a pale tongue and a weak soggy pulse. The treatment is to strengthen the Spleen and supplement qi, dispel wind and drain damp, and stop pain with **FANG JI HUANG QI TANG** (Stephania and Astragalus Decoction 防己黄芪汤).

han fang ji (Stephaniae tetrandrae Radix) 汉防己 9–12g
huang qi (Astragali Radix) 黄芪 15–30g
bai zhu (Atractylodes macrocephalae Rhizoma) 白术 9–12g
zhi gan cao (Glycyrrhizae Radix preparata) 炙甘草 3–6g
sheng jiang (Zingiberis Rhizoma recens) 生姜 6–9g
da zao (Jujubae Fructus) 大枣 6pce

Method: Decoction. **Han fang ji** dispels wind and damp, promotes urination and alleviates edema; **huang qi** fortifies wei qi and secures the exterior, mobilizes fluids and stops sweating; **bai zhu** and **gan cao** strengthen the Spleen and supplement qi and; **sheng jiang** and **da zao** harmonize and protect the Stomach. (Source: *Zhong Yi Nei Ke Xue* [*Shang Han Lun*])

Prepared medicines
Concentrated powders

Juan Bi Tang (Notopterygium & Turmeric Combination)

Shang Zhong Xia Tong Yong Tong Feng Wan (Cinnamon & Angelica Formula)
– with wind predominant
Yi Yi Ren Tang (Coix Combination)
Qiang Huo Sheng Shi Tang (Notopterygium & Tuhuo Combination)
Fang Ji Huang Qi Tang (Stephania & Astragalus Combination)

Pills
Juan Bi Wan (Clear Channel Teapills)
Qu Feng Zhen Tong Wan (Qu Feng Zhen Tong Capsule)

Acupuncture
Primary treatment is based on the location of the pain (Table 15.2, p.647–650)
with the addition of systemic points below, depending on the pathogen:

Damp

Sp.5 (shangqiu –) ....river and metal point of the Spleen, transforms
damp stagnation and alleviates painful obstruction

Sp.9 (yinlingquan –)...........sea point of the Spleen, transforms damp stagnation
and clears damp and heat

Sp.6 (sanyinjiao –)...............strengthens the Spleen and transforms damp
(especially when used with Sp.9), activates qi and
blood and removes obstructions from the channels
and network vessels

St.36 (zusanli +) ....sea point of the Stomach, strengthens the Spleen and
supplements qi, transforms damp

Wind

Du.14 (dazhui –)................dispels wind
Bl.11 (dazhu) ....dispels wind
Bl.12 (fengmen) ....dispels wind
Sp.10 (xuehai –) ....nourishes and activates blood to dispel wind
GB.39 (xuanzhong –).........these points dispel wind and damp
SJ.5 (waiguan –)
LI.4 (hegu –) ....these points dispel wind and clear obstruction from
LI.11 (quchi –)   the channels

• Ear points: points relating to affected area, lung, spleen, shenmen

Clinical notes
• This is one of the most common presentations of painful obstruction syndrome,
with mild to moderate pain and stiffness in joints and muscles. When chronic,
wind damp painful obstruction syndrome may be diagnosed as osteoarthritis,
rheumatoid arthritis, fibromyalgia or chronic soft tissue lesions and myofascial
pain. It may also reflect an infectious process, such as rheumatic fever, influenza
or viral arthritis.
• Wind cold damp painful obstruction often goes through periodic change into
wind damp heat, with increasing redness, swelling and pain of the affected area.
See. p.659.

寒 | 15.2 COLD DAMP
湿
痹
阻

Cold damp is the designation of a pain pattern that is predominantly cold, and is most often seen as a progression of wind damp in a patient with pre–existing yang deficiency. The damp component is seen in any swelling that is present. The freezing and constricting nature of cold causes significant impediment to blood flow and relatively severe and localized pain. Chronic cold lodged in a joint is usually complicated by blood stasis and phlegm accumulation, and bony deformity.

Clinical features
- Joint, muscle or neuralgic pain that is fixed and intense. Range of motion is decreased and there is marked stiffness. When joints are involved, cold tends to affect the small joints of the hands and feet. The pain is worse at night and with exposure to cold. Stiffness and pain are worse following prolonged inactivity and are significantly improved by heat.
- the affected area may appear pale and cool to the touch (unless topical heat packs have been applied)
- there may or may not be swelling, depending on the degree of damp

T pale with a white coat
P tight, wiry

Treatment principle
Warm and dispel cold and dry damp
Activate qi and blood movement in the channels and network vessels

Prescription

FU ZI TANG 附子汤
Prepared Aconite Decoction

Most texts recommend the formula Wu Tou Tang (next page) for this pattern. Its toxicity, however, makes it impractical for use outside China. Fu Zi Tang is the preferred option as it is quite safe when used correctly and is effective for most cold pain patterns.

zhi fu zi (Aconiti Radix lateralis preparata) 制附子 12–15g
bai zhu (Atractylodis macrocephalae Rhizoma) 白术 9–12g
fu ling (Poria) 茯苓 9–12g
bai shao (Paeoniae Radix alba) 白芍 9–12g
ren shen (Ginseng Radix) 人参 6–9g

Method: Decoction. **Zhi fu zi** is decocted for 30–60 minutes prior to the other herbs. It warms Spleen and Kidney yang, dispels cold, dries damp and stops pain; **ren shen** supplements yuan qi and augments the ability of **zhi fu zi** to support yang qi; **bai zhu** and **fu ling** strengthen the Spleen, dry and drain damp, and assist **zhi fu zi** in transforming damp; **bai shao** nourishes and protects yin and blood against the drying effects of the principle herbs and assists **zhi fu zi** in alleviating pain. (Source: *Zhong Yi Nei Ke Xue* [*Shang Han Lun*])

Modifications
- With severe cold and pain, **zhi fu zi** can be used in doses of up to 30g for short periods of time, 1–2 weeks maximum, until the pain is controlled. At

this dose, it should be boiled for at least two hours before the other herbs to ensure conversion of the toxic principle.

- With pain in the upper body, fingers, wrist and elbow, add **gui zhi** (Cinnamomi Ramulus) 桂枝 9–12g and **sang zhi** (Mori Ramulus) 桑枝 15–30g.
- For pain in the lower limbs, add **du huo** (Angelicae Pubescentis Radix) 独活 6–9g and **chuan niu xi** (Cyathulae Radix) 川牛膝 9–12g.
- For numbness or a wooden feeling in the limbs, add **xi xian cao** (Siegesbeckia Herba) 豨莶草 9–12g and **lu lu tong** (Liquidambaris Fructus) 路路通 6–9g.
- For facial pain, add **xi xin** (Asari Herba) 细辛 3–6g.
- With dampness, joint swelling, heaviness and aching, add **yi ren** (Coicis Semen) 苡仁 24g and increase the dose of **bai zhu** to 30–60g.
- With qi deficiency, sweating and fatigue, add **huang qi** (Astragali Radix) 黄芪 12–18g.
- With blood stasis, sharp pain and vascular congestion, add **ru xiang** (Olibanum) 乳香 6–9g and **mo yao** (Myrrha) 没药 6–9g.

WU TOU TANG 乌头汤
Aconite Decoction

This is the classical prescription for severe cold damp pain. It is rarely used outside of China due to the toxicity of the principle ingredient.

zhi chuan wu (Aconiti Radix preparata) 制川乌 9–15g
ma huang (Ephedra Herba) 麻黄 6–9g
chao bai shao (stir fried Paeoniae Radix alba) 炒白芍 6–9g
huang qi (Astragali Radix) 黄芪 12–18g
zhi gan cao (Glycyrrhizae Radix preparata) 炙甘草.............................6–9g
feng mi (honey) 蜂蜜 60g

Method: Decoction. To be rendered safe, **zhi chuan wu** must be decocted for a minimum of 45–60 minutes, and preferably 2 hours with **feng mi** prior to the addition of the other herbs. Start with a small dose, 30–50 mls of the decoction, and increase as required until a therapeutic effect is achieved. **Zhi chuan wu** warms yang, dispels cold and alleviates severe pain; **ma huang** dispels cold and stimulates qi flow through the surface tissues; **huang qi** and **chao bai shao** protect qi and blood from excessive dispersal; **zhi gan cao** and **feng mi** moderate the toxicity of **zhi chuan wu** and assist in alleviating spasmodic pain. (Source: *Zhong Yi Nei Ke Xue* [*Jin Gui Yao Lüe*])

XIAO HUO LUO DAN 小活络丹
Minor Activate the Network Vessels Special Pill

This formula is only used in prepared form. Even though it contains the same toxic ingredients as the prescription above, it is available in small pills and powdered extract. These formats enable reliable and precise dose management.

zhi cao wu (Aconiti kusnezoffii Radix preparata) 制草乌 20g
zhi chuan wu (Aconiti Radix preparata) 制川乌 20g
zhi tian nan xing (Arisaematis Rhizoma preparatum) 制天南星............20g
di long (Pheretima) 地龙...20g
mo yao (Myrrha) 没药 10g
ru xiang (Olibanum) 乳香 10g

Method: Pills or powder. A commonly available prepared medicine. **Zhi chuan wu** and **zhi cao wu** dispel cold damp, warm the channels and network vessels and stop pain; **zhi tian nan xing** transforms phlegm and dries damp, and has a particular effect on clearing phlegm damp from the channels and network vessels; **ru xiang** and **mo yao** activate blood, disperse blood stasis and stop pain; **di long** 'burrows' through obstructions and clears the channel system of obstruction. (Source: *He Ji Ju Fang*)

Prepared medicines
Concentrated powder
Zhen Wu Tang (Ginger, Aconite, Poria & Peony Combination)
Xiao Huo Luo Dan (Myrrh & Aconite Formula)
Pills
Zhen Wu Tang Wan (True Warrior Teapills)
Xiao Huo Luo Dan (Xiao Huo Luo Dan Teapills)
– The big advantage of using these pills is the ability to carefully monitor the dose. A small dose, usually ¼ to ½ the recommended dose, is given initially to assess the patients response, then gradually increased to the therapeutic dose over a week or two.

Topical treatment
La Jiao Gao (Porous Capsicum Plaster)
Gou Pi Gao (Gou Pi Gao)
– this is the classic 'dog skin' plaster, infused with chuan wu and cao wu and thus very hot and stimulating
Mustard plasters
Hot stimulating liniments with capsaicin, the hot component of chillies
Tabasco sauce added to a suitable carrier oil in about 1:10 proportion

Acupuncture
Select points on the basis of the location of the pain (Table 15.2, p.647–650) and use plenty of local moxa. Warm needle technique is preferred. Be careful when starting treatment with moxa, as patients with severe cold pathology may not feel the heat before they start to burn. Do not rely on their subjective perception of heat. This applies especially to the elderly. Systemic points to warm yang and dispel cold can be selected from the following:

St.36 (zusanli ▲)................sea points of the Stomach and Large Intestine, warm
LI.11 (quchi ▲)   yang and activate the circulation of qi and blood
Ren.6 (qihai ▲) ....these points supplement the Kidneys and warm yang
Ren.4 (guanyuan ▲)   systemically
Du.4 (mingmen ▲)
Bl.23 (shenshu ▲)..............transport point of the Kidneys, warms yang and
                               dispels cold
• Ear points: kidney, spleen, adrenal, shenmen, points relating to affected area

Clinical notes
• Cold damp painful obstruction syndrome may be diagnosed as chronic osteoarthritis or rheumatoid arthritis, post traumatic or post surgical pain, trigeminal neuralgia, post–herpetic neuralgia or sciatica.

- Wu tou is toxic and rarely used outside China, where it is sometimes still used for severe or unresponsive cases, due to its unparalleled analgesic effects. When it is used it must be cooked for a minimum of 1–2 hours, the larger the dose the longer the cooking. Signs of toxicity include numbness and tingling of the lips and tongue, slurred speech, dizziness and arrhythmia. Being so hot it easily causes overheating and can damage yin. Zhi fu zi is weaker but still quite effective and much easier to use safely. The dose of zhi fu zi can be as high as 30 grams for short periods, but the cooking time must be increased proportionately.

- In all cases where relatively high doses of fu zi and its more powerful relatives are being used, it is wise to begin with a small dose and work up to a therapeutic dose over a week or two, to assess the patients response. Patients with subclinical yin deficiency or hidden heat can become overheated quite quickly, with symptoms such as increasing insomnia and restlessness, flushing and thirst. In such cases, the dose of medicine can be reduced or the prescription modified with appropriate counterbalancing herbs, such as **zhi mu** (Anemarrhenae Rhizoma) 知母, **bai shao** (Paeoniae Radix alba) 白芍 and **xuan shen** (Scrophulariae Radix) 玄參.

寒
热
错
杂

15.3 LOCALIZED HEAT IN A JOINT OR JOINTS

Localized heat in a joint is usually an acute exacerbation of a chronic cold damp or wind damp joint pain. The knees, ankles, sacroiliac joint and spine are particularly prone to heat transformation of this type. Cold and damp can lodge in a joint for prolonged periods of time, blocking qi and blood movement and inhibiting the dispersal of physiological heat. The local constraint and heat accumulation combine with the pre–existing pathogen. The main feature of this pathology is the localized nature of the heat, being confined to the joint or joints in question, with little or no systemic heat.

The transformation of an existing cold damp pathogen into heat is encouraged in patients with a hot or yang constitution and in those with pre–existing yin deficiency. Trauma or periods of overuse are also contributing factors.

Clinical features
- Gradual or sudden onset of increasing pain, redness, stiffness and swelling, usually of a single joint. Pain is worse at night. The skin overlying the affected joint may be mottled red, and the patient may get some relief with the topical application of moderate heat. The knees, ankles, sacroiliac joint and spine are the joints most commonly affected, but any joint may be involved.
- unaffected regions, limbs and extremities, may be cold
- no fever, thirst, sweating or other signs of systemic heat

T white coat
P wiry, tight

Treatment principle
Dispel wind damp and clear heat
Promote movement of yang qi, unblock the channels and stop pain

Prescription

GUI ZHI SHAO YAO ZHI MU TANG 桂枝芍药知母汤
Cinnamon Twig, Peony and Anemarrhena Decoction

The balance of heat and cold can vary considerably and the prescription can be adjusted to address this. In the very early stages, heat may be only just apparent, and cold or damp still dominant, so the warming herbs are emphasized. As the heat develops and becomes more intense, the dose of the cooling herbs can be increased, and more cooling herbs added.

gui zhi (Cinnamomi Ramulus) 桂枝 9–12g
bai shao (Paeoniae Radix alba) 白芍 6–9g
sheng jiang (Zingiberis Rhizoma recens) 生姜 9–15g
zhi gan cao (Glycyrrhizae Radix preparata) 炙甘草 3–6g
ma huang (Ephedra Herba) 麻黄 3–6g
bai zhu (Atractylodis macrocephalae Rhizoma) 白术 12–15g
zhi mu (Anemarrhenae Rhizoma) 知母 9–12g
fang feng (Saposhnikovae Radix) 防风 9–12g
zhi fu zi (Aconiti Radix lateralis preparata) 制附子 6–9g

Method: Decoction. The pungent warmth of **gui zhi**, **ma huang** and **fang feng** unblocks the channels and network vessels; **sheng jiang** supports the dispersing action of these herbs; **bai zhu** dries damp and supports the Spleen; **zhi fu zi** and **gui zhi** warm, open and unblock the channels to enable dispersal of the pathogenic damp and heat; **zhi fu zi** stops pain; **bai shao** and **zhi mu** clear heat and protect yin and fluids from damage by the pungent dispersing herbs; **zhi gan cao** and **sheng jiang** balance and harmonize the diverse elements of the formula and protect the Spleen and Stomach. (Source: *Zhong Yi Nei Ke Xue* [*Jin Gui Yao Lüe*]).

Modifications

- With stiff painful joints that are slightly warm, but are alleviated somewhat by heat, use **gui zhi**, **ma huang** and **zhi fu zi** at the upper end of the dosage range.
- With marked damp, causing swelling, heaviness, aching and numbness in the joints that is worse in humid or wet weather, use **zhi fu zi** and **bai zhu** at the upper end of the dosage range, and add **han fang ji** (Stephaniae tetrandrae Radix) 汉防己 9–12g, **bi xie** (Dioscoreae hypoglaucae Rhizoma) 萆薢 9–12g and **yi ren** (Coicis Semen) 苡仁 15–30g.
- With marked heat, manifesting in quite hot and obviously red joint or joints that are worse at night, use **zhi mu** and **gan cao** at the upper end of the dosage range, **chi shao** (Paeoniae Radix rubra) 赤芍 9–12g instead of **bai shao**, and add **sheng di** (Rehmanniae Radix) 生地 9–12g, **luo shi teng** (Trachelospermi Caulis) 络石藤 15–30g and **ren dong teng** (Lonicerae Caulis) 忍冬藤 15–30g.
- With joint deformity or osteophytes, add **tou gu cao** (Herba Speranskia) 透骨草 9–15g.
- With yin deficiency, a red uncoated tongue, dryness and tendency for joints to become inflamed with use, delete **zhi fu zi**, and add **sheng di** (Rehmanniae Radix) 生地 9–12g, **di gu pi** (Lycii Cortex) 地骨皮 12–15g, **qin jiao** (Gentianae macrophyllae Radix) 秦艽 9–12g and **bai wei** (Cynanchi atrati Radix) 白薇 9–12g.

Prepared medicines

Concentrated powders

Gui Zhi Shao Yao Zhi Mu Tang (Cinnamon & Anemarrhena Combination)

Pills

Guan Jie Yan Wan (Joint Inflammation Teapills)

Xuan Bi Tang Wan (Xuan Bi Teapills)

Acupuncture

Select points on the basis of the location of the pain (Table 15.2, p.647–650). Heat clearing points along the relevant channel pathways can be selected. These include the Metal Water pairs which have the ability to cool and control fire (Table 15.3, p.650). Systemic points to clear heat can be selected from:

LI.11 (quchi –)...................these points clear heat, clear obstruction from the
LI.4 (hegu –)   channels, and stop pain
St.43 (xianggu –)
GB.39 (xuanzhong –).........dispels wind damp heat

Du.14 (dazhui –)................meeting point of the yang channels, clears heat
- Ear points: points relating to affected area, spleen, kidney, sympathetic, shen-men

Clinical notes
- Localized heat in a joint may be diagnosed as an acute inflammatory exacerbation of an existing osteoarthritic or rheumatoid condition, joint pain in connective tissue disease, gout or infectious arthritis.
- A diet that is cooling and anti–inflammatory can be helpful. See Clinical Handbook, Vol.2, p.882. Fish oils are beneficial. Juice fasting can help some patients with acute inflammatory pain and rheumatoid arthritis.

湿
热
痹
阻

15.4 DAMP HEAT

The damp heat in this pattern is both local and systemic, with joint and/or soft tissue inflammation, swelling and pain. The pattern can be acute or chronic. When acute, the damp heat is the result of an external invasion into the qi level, and the onset of pain and swelling are abrupt. When chronic, the damp heat can be due to heat transformation of a pre–existing condition, or the gradual accumulation of damp heat derived from the diet. The pain and swelling are gradual in onset and the pain and systemic symptoms less intense.

Clinical features
- Pain, stiffness, redness and swelling of joints and soft tissues; the painful areas are warm to the touch, and stiff with reduced range of motion. The pain is a deep, heavy ache with morning stiffness; there may be difficulty walking and getting started in the morning; the pain is exacerbated by hot humid weather. Single or multiple joints and/or tissues may be affected.
- fever, afternoon fever or contained fever (p.367)
- night sweats
- scanty, concentrated urine
- thirst, or dry mouth and throat
- chest oppression
- may be lymphadenopathy

T greasy, yellow tongue coat
P slippery or soggy, possibly rapid pulse

Treatment principle
Clear damp heat from the joints and muscles
Unblock the channels and network vessels

Prescription

XUAN BI TANG 宣痹汤
Disband Painful Obstruction Decoction

han fang ji (Stephaniae tetrandrae Radix) 汉防己	12–15g
xing ren (Armeniacae Semen) 杏仁	12–15g
hua shi (Talcum) 滑石	12–15g
lian qiao (Forsythiae Fructus) 连翘	9–12g
shan zhi zi (Gardeniae Fructus) 山栀子	9–12g
zhi ban xia (Pinelliae Rhizoma preparatum) 制半夏	9–12g
can sha (Bombycis Faeces) 蚕沙	9–12g
yi ren (Coicis Semen) 苡仁	15–30g
chi xiao dou (Phaseoli Semen) 赤小豆	15–30g

Method: Decoction. **Hua shi** and **can sha** are decocted in a cloth bag. The bitter cold of **han fang ji** clears damp heat and promotes urination to provide an escape route, while its pungency dispels wind, unblocks the channels and stops pain. **Xing ren** diffuses the Lungs and directs Lung qi downwards to assist in regulation of the water passages and the drainage of damp heat; **yi ren** strengthens the Spleen, drains damp and unblocks the channels; **can sha** expels wind and dries damp; **zhi ban xia** dries damp; **lian qiao, shan zhi zi, hua shi** and **chi xiao dou** clear damp heat and promote urination to enable the damp heat to escape. (Source: *Zhong Yi Nei Ke Xue* [*Wen Bing Tiao Bian*])

Modifications

- With severe stiffness and pain, add two or three of the following herbs: **luo shi teng** (Trachelospermi Caulis) 络石藤 15–30g, **hai tong pi** (Erythrinae Cortex) 海桐皮 6–9g, **ren dong teng** (Lonicerae Caulis) 忍冬藤 15–30g, **xi xian cao** (Siegesbeckia Herba) 豨莶草 10–15g or **wei ling xian** (Clematidis Radix) 威灵仙 6–9g.

- With marked redness and erythema, add **sheng di** (Rehmanniae Radix) 生地 9–15g, **chi shao** (Paeoniae Radix rubra) 赤芍 9–12g, **mu dan pi** (Moutan Cortex) 牡丹皮 9–12g and **dan shen** (Salviae miltiorrhizae Radix) 丹参 9–12g.

- With relatively high fever and thirst, add **han shui shi** (Glauberitum) 寒水石 15–30g [decocted first] and **sheng di** (Rehmanniae Radix) 生地 9–15g.

- With marked swelling in the joints, add **cang zhu** (Atractylodis Rhizoma) 苍术 9–12g, **ze xie** (Alismatis Rhizoma) 泽泻 9–12g and **bi xie** (Dioscoreae hypoglaucae Rhizoma) 萆薢 9–12g.

- If the lower limbs are affected, add **cang zhu** (Atractylodis Rhizoma) 苍术 9–12g, **huang bai** (Phellodendri Cortex) 黄柏 9–12g and **chuan niu xi** (Cyathulae Radix) 川牛膝 12–15g.

- With constipation, add **da huang** (Rhei Radix et Rhizoma) 大黄 6–9g and **mang xiao** (Natrii Sulfas) 芒硝 6–9g [dissolved in the strained decoction].

Variations and additional prescriptions

With sudden onset and migratory pain

Wind damp heat joint and muscle pain can appear suddenly as part of an external invasion into the qi level. The initial illness is characterized by fever and chills, sore throat, cough, arthralgia and myalgia. The treatment is to dispel wind and clear heat with a prescription based on **MA XING SHI GAN TANG** (Ephedra, Apricot Kernel, Gypsum and Licorice Decoction 麻杏石甘汤), modified.

zhi ma huang (honey fried Ephedra Herba) 炙麻黄 6–9g
xing ren (Armeniacae Semen) 杏仁 9–12g
shi gao (Gypsum fibrosum) 石膏 15–30g
zhi gan cao (Glycyrrhizae Radix preparata) 炙甘草 3–6g
ren dong teng (Lonicerae Caulis) 忍冬藤 15–30g
qin jiao (Gentianae macrophyllae Radix) 秦艽 9–12g
sang zhi (Mori Ramulus) 桑枝 15–30g
jin yin hua (Lonicerae Flos) 金银花 15–30g
lian qiao (Forsythiae Fructus) 连翘 9–12g
niu bang zi (Arctii Fructus) 牛蒡子 9–12g
dan dou chi (Sojae Semen preparatum) 淡豆豉 9–12g

Method: Decoction. **Zhi ma huang** directs Lung qi downward and dispels any remaining pathogen from the surface. Its pungent warmth is balanced by the large dose of the pungent cold **shi gao**. When used together, the diaphoretic nature of **zhi ma huang** is restrained by the **shi gao**, but the pores are kept open to allow the pathogen an escape route. **Xing ren** diffuses and directs Lung qi downward, while moistening the Lungs; **shi gao** clears heat from the Lungs and generates fluids; **zhi gan cao** protects the Stomach and harmonizes the action of the other herbs; **ren dong teng**, **qin jiao** and **sang zhi** clear heat and stop pain; **jin yin hua**, **lian qiao** and **niu bang zi** clear wind heat and toxic heat; **dan dou chi** vents heat to the surface. (Source: *Shi Yong Zhong Yi Nei Ke Xue* [*Shang Han Lun*])

Prepared medicines
Concentrated powders
Dang Gui Nian Tong Tang (Dang Gui & Anemarrhena Combination)
Shang Zhong Xia Tong Yong Tong Feng Wan (Cinnamon & Angelica Formula)
Pills
Xuan Bi Tang Wan (Xuan Bi Teapills)
Guan Jie Yan Wan (Joint Inflammation Teapills)

Acupuncture
Select points on the basis of the location of the pain (Table 15.2, p.647–650). Heat clearing points along the relevant channel pathways should be selected. These include the Metal Water pairs which have the ability to cool and control fire (Table 15.3, p.650). Systemic points to clear heat can be selected from:

Lu.7 (lieque –)....................diffuses the Lungs and vents pathogens from the qi level
LI.11 (quchi –)..................these points clear heat from yangming, clear the
LI.4 (hegu –)   channels and stop pain
St.43 (xianggu –)
Du.14 (dazhui –)...............meeting point of the yang channels, clears heat
Sp.9 (yinlingquan –)...........water and metal points of the Spleen, these points
Sp.5 (shangqiu –)   clear heat and promote urination to drain damp heat
• Ear points: spleen, stomach, sympathetic, shenmen, points relating to affected area

Clinical notes
• Damp heat painful obstruction may be diagnosed as Ross River fever, rheumatic fever, Lyme disease, Dengue fever, acute rheumatoid arthritis, connective tissue disease such as systemic lupus erythematosus or Behçet's disease, infectious arthritis, bursitis or gout.
• A diet that is anti–inflammatory can be helpful for chronic patterns. See Clinical Handbook, Vol.2, p.882. Fish oils are of benefit. Juice fasting can help some patients with acute inflammatory pain and rheumatoid arthritis.

热
留
营
分

15.5 LINGERING HEAT IN THE YING LEVEL

Heat can get into the ying level in patients with a pre–existing shaoyin (Kidney) weakness. The weakness may be inherited, in which case there will be a positive family history, or can be acquired by aging, a severe shock or trauma, overwork, drug use and life habits. In both cases, the pathogen bypasses the exterior altogether and penetrates directly into the ying, where it may remain quietly for some time. A suitable trigger event, such as an intervening infection, change of season, or period of increased stress sufficient to dampen the zheng qi, can then induce the pathogen to emerge and cause symptoms.

Clinical features
• Joint pain and stiffness. The pain is usually moderate, worse at night, with increased stiffness in the morning. The joints may be warm to touch, but are usually not swollen. Pain is worse with prolonged activity.
• low grade fever, worse at night; the heat at night may be followed by coldness in the early hours of the morning
• thirst, or dryness of mucous membranes without thirst
• insomnia or fitful dream disturbed sleep; irritability and restlessness
• may be night sweats
• malaise and weight loss
• faint erythema, purpura or maculopapular rash; vasculitis
• mouth ulcers
• swollen lymph nodes
T dry, deep red or scarlet with thorns, and little or no coat
P fine and rapid

Treatment principle
Clear and vent heat from the ying level
Nourish yin and moisten dryness

Prescription

QING YING TANG 清营汤
Clear the Nutritive Level Decoction, modified

shui niu jiao (Cornu Bubali) 水牛角 30–60g
sheng di (Rehmanniae Radix) 生地.. 15–30g
xuan shen (Scrophulariae Radix) 玄参 9–18g
mai dong (Ophiopogonis Radix) 麦冬 6–12g
jin yin hua (Lonicerae Flos) 金银花.. 9–15g
lian qiao (Forsythiae Fructus) 连翘 6–15g
dan zhu ye (Lophatheri Herba) 淡竹叶... 3–6g
huang lian (Coptidis Rhizoma) 黄连 3–6g
dan shen (Salviae miltiorrhizae Radix) 丹参 6–15g
qin jiao (Gentianae macrophyllae Radix) 秦艽.............................. 9–15g
Method: Decoction. **Shui niu jiao** is shaved into fine strips and cooked for 30 minutes prior to the other herbs. **Shui niu jiao** clears heat from the ying level and cools the blood; **xuan shen** and **sheng**

di cool the blood and protect yin; **mai dong** clears heat, nourishes yin and moistens dryness; **jin yin hua, lian qiao, dan zhu ye** vent heat from the qi and ying levels; **huang lian** clears heat from the Heart and Stomach; **dan shen** clears heat, activates the blood, and helps prevent the blood stasis that may complicate both heat and the use of cold herbs; **qin jiao** vents heat from the ying and alleviates joint pain. **Shui niu jiao** is used instead of **xi jiao** (Rhinocerotis Cornu) 犀角, the horn of the critically endangered rhinoceros. (Source: *Wen Bing Tiao Bian*)

Modifications
* With marked pain, add **hai tong pi** (Erythrinae Cortex) 海桐皮 6–9g and **ji xue teng** (Spatholobi Caulis) 鸡血藤 15–30g.
* With fever and sweating, add **qing hao** (Artemisiae annuae Herba) 青蒿 12-15g, **yin chai hu** (Stellariae Radix) 银柴胡 9–12g and **di gu pi** (Lycii Cortex) 地骨皮 12–15g.

Prepared medicines
Concentrated powders
Qin Jiao Bie Jia San (Gentiana Macrophylla Root & Turtle Shell Formula)
Pills
Xuan Bi Tang Wan (Xuan Bi Teapills)
Guan Jie Yan Wan (Joint Inflammation Teapills)

Acupuncture (select from)
Select points on the basis of the location of the pain (Table 15.2, p.647–650). Heat clearing points along the relevant channel pathways should be selected. These include the Metal Water pairs which have the ability to cool and control fire (Table 15.3, p.650). Systemic points to clear heat can be selected from:

Kid.7 (fuliu –)....................vents pathogens from the ying level
PC.3 (quze –).....................together these points clear heat from the ying and
Bl.40 (weizhong –)   blood, and activate the blood
Sp.10 (xuehai –)
Kid.3 (taixi +).....................replenishes damaged yin
Bl.23 (shenshu +) ....these points clear heat and replenish damaged yin
Bl.18 (ganshu +)   and fluids
* Ear points: liver, kidney, heart, subcortex, endocrine, shenmen

Clinical notes
* Lingering heat in the ying level may be diagnosed as rheumatoid arthritis, systemic lupus erythematosus, and other connective tissue diseases.
* Heat in the ying level can respond to treatment or be difficult, depending on the associated biomedical disease process. Patients may be medicated with drugs such as steroids or immunosuppressants, which complicate treatment.

热
毒
痹
阻

15.6 TOXIC HEAT

Toxic heat is a pattern of severe heat that is localized in a single joint, or multiple joints, with marked systemic heat symptoms. It is an acute pattern that may follow joint trauma or be associated with an intensification of a damp heat pattern.

Clinical features
• Acute heat, redness, swelling and pain in one or more joints. The pain is continuous and cannot bear palpation; affected joints are hot to the touch and better with cold. Stiffness and immobility are marked. When isolated in one joint, the heat and pain symptoms are severe; if the toxic heat is part of a systemic pattern, the pain tends to affect multiple joints and has less severe localized symptoms and more systemic heat.
• high fever and red complexion
• intense thirst
• profuse sweating
• general malaise; nausea and vomiting, lethargy
• concentrated urine
• may be constipation
• in severe cases, confusion or mild delirium, erythema, purpura or bleeding
T scarlet or red, with a dry, yellow or greasy, yellow
P slippery, wiry or surging and rapid

Treatment principle
Clear toxic heat and cool the blood
Unblock the channels and network vessels and stop pain

Prescription
BAI HU TANG 白虎汤
White Tiger Decoction, plus
HUANG LIAN JIE DU TANG 黄连解毒汤
Coptis Decoction to Resolve Toxicity, modified

shi gao (Gypsum fibrosum) 石膏 30–90g
zhi mu (Anemarrhenae Rhizoma) 知母 9–15g
gan cao (Glycyrrhizae Radix) 甘草 3–6g
huang bai (Phellodendri Cortex) 黄柏 9–12g
huang qin (Scutellariae Radix) 黄芩 9–12g
huang lian (Coptidis Rhizoma) 黄连 3–9g
shan zhi zi (Gardeniae Fructus) 山栀子 9–12g
hu zhang (Polygoni cuspidati Rhizoma) 虎杖 9–12g
Method: Decoction. **Shi gao** is cooked for 30 minutes prior to the other herbs. **Shi gao** clears heat from the Lungs, Stomach and Intestines, generates fluids and alleviate thirst; **zhi mu** clears heat and protects yin; **gan cao** protects the Stomach; **huang qin, huang bai, huang lian** and **shan zhi zi** clear toxic heat and cool the blood; **hu zhang** clears heat, activates blood and stops pain. (Source: *Shi Yong Zhong Yi Ne Ke Xue [Qian Jin Yao Fang]*)

Modifications
- With constipation, add **da huang** (Rhei Radix et Rhizoma) 大黄 6–12g and **mang xiao** (Natrii Sulfas) 芒硝 6–9g [dissolved in the strained decoction].
- With fluid damage, a peeled tongue and thirst, add **xuan shen** (Scrophulariae Radix) 玄参 18–30g and **yu zhu** (Polygonati odorati Rhizoma) 玉竹 12–15g.
- With purpura or a maculopapular rash, add **da qing ye** (Isatidis Folium) 大青叶 15–30g and **mu dan pi** (Moutan Cortex) 牡丹皮 9–12g.
- With severe pain, add **zhi mo yao** (Myrrha preparata) 炙没药 6–9g and **zhi ru xiang** (Olibanum preparata) 炙乳香 6–9g.

Prepared medicines
Concentrated powders
Bai Hu Tang (Gypsum Combination) plus Huang Lian Jie Du Tang (Coptis & Scute Combination)
Pu Ji Xiao Du Yin (Scute & Cimicifuga Combination)

Pills
Huang Lian Jie Du Wan (Huang Lian Jie Du Teapills) plus Wu Wei Xiao Du Wan (Five Flavor Teapills)

Acupuncture
Select points on the basis of the location of the pain (Table 15.2, p.647–650). Heat clearing points along the relevant channel pathways should be selected. These include the Metal Water pairs which have the ability to cool and control fire (Table 15.3, p.650). Systemic points to clear heat can be selected from:

PC.3 (quze ↓) ....sea points of the Pericardium and Urinary Bladder
Bl.40 (weizhong ↓)   respectively, these points cool the blood, clear toxic heat and reduce fever
Du.14 (dazhui −)................meeting point of the yang channels, clears heat and drains fire
shixuan ↓ (M–UE–1)..........clear heat from the blood when bled; used when there is disturbance of consciousness
LI.11 (quchi −)...................these points clear heat systemically
St.44 (neiting −)
LI.4 (hegu −)
- treatment can be given every 6–8 hours
- Ear points: liver, sympathetic, shenmen, points relating to affected area

Clinical notes
- Toxic heat type painful obstruction represents a serious inflammatory or infectious disorder. Infectious arthritis can quickly lead to joint destruction and should be managed promptly with intravenous antibiotics in hospital.
- Toxic heat painful obstruction syndrome may be diagnosed as infectious arthritis, an acute exacerbation of a connective tissue disorder such as Systemic Lupus erythematosus, Behçet's syndrome, polyarteritis nodosa, or acute rheumatoid arthritis.

瘀
血
痹
阻

15.7 BLOOD STASIS

Blood stasis occurs as a complication of other pathogenic processes, or as the result of physical trauma. Physical trauma can include direct injury, surgery or accumulation of micro traumata from chronic postural and biomechanical stress.

Blood stasis often follows years of qi stagnation, especially when it appears in the neck and upper back. In such cases there will usually be a long history of neck pain, headaches and tightness and knots in the muscles of the upper back.

Although this is a common pattern of musculoskeletal pain, the diagnosis may not always be immediately apparent. Because the location of the blood stasis is in the exterior, the internal organ systems are not necessarily affected, and the classical systemic blood stasis signs are not always present. It can be easy to confuse blood stasis pain with that of cold damp, especially when both pathologies are present. A blood stasis diagnosis may occasionally be one of exclusion or default when other treatments fail to produce a result. This is a type of stubborn painful obstruction syndrome (*wán bì* 顽痹).

Clinical features
- Chronic joint and musculoskeletal pain, stiffness, paresthesia; the pain is focal, fixed, stabbing, sharp, or boring, and aggravated by inactivity, sleep and pressure. The pain may be intermittent, but will recur repeatedly in the same location. The pain can be quite intense, but is not influenced by weather change or emotional states. Joints may exhibit bony deformity, hypertrophy, osteophytes and other structural change.
- The tissues overlying the affected region may be discolored, dry and scaly, or have vascular congestion, spider vessels or nevi. The affected area may feel hard or lumpy.

The following may only occur when blood stasis is systemic:
- purple discoloration of face, lips, conjunctivae, nails
- spider naevi and congested vessels on the lower limbs
- chronic depression and insomnia
- left iliac fossa pressure pain (p.925–926)

T purple, or with brown or purple stasis spots, dark, congested, sublingual veins
P choppy, wiry or fine pulse

Treatment principle
Activate blood and move qi, break up and dispel blood stasis
Unblock the channels and network vessels, and stop pain

Prescription
SHEN TONG ZHU YU TANG 身痛逐瘀汤
Drive Out Blood Stasis from a Painful Body Decoction

qin jiao (Gentianae macrophyllae Radix) 秦艽 6–9g
chuan xiong (Chuanxiong Rhizoma) 川芎 3–6g
tao ren (Persicae Semen) 桃仁 6–9g
hong hua (Carthami Flos) 红花 3–6g

gan cao (Glycyrrhizae Radix) 甘草 3–6g
qiang huo (Notopterygii Rhizoma seu Radix) 羌活................................ 3–9g
mo yao (Myrrha) 没药 3–6g
dang gui (Angelicae sinensis Radix) 当归 6–9g
chao wu ling zhi (stir fried Trogopterori Faeces) 炒五灵脂 3–6g
xiang fu (Cyperi Rhizoma) 香附 3–6g
chuan niu xi (Cyathulae Radix) 川牛膝... 6–9g
di long (Pheretima) 地龙... 6–9g

Method: Decoction. **Tao ren, hong hua, chuan xiong, dang gui** and **mo yao** activate the blood and dispels static blood, **chuan niu xi, chao wu ling zhi** and **di long** free the channels and network vessels and stop pain; **qiang huo** and **qin jiao** dispel wind damp and stop pain; **xiang fu** mobilizes qi to lead the blood; **gan cao** protects the Stomach and supplemens qi. (Source: *Zhong Yi Nei Ke Xue* [*Yi Lin Gai Cuo*])

Modifications

- With cold and intense pain, add **zhi fu zi** (Aconiti Radix lateralis preparata) 制附子 6–12g [cooked first] and **gui zhi** (Cinnamomi Ramulus) 桂枝 6–9g.
- With severe focal, piercing, stabbing or neuropathic pain, add **shui zhi** (Hirudo) 水蛭 3–6g, **wu gong** (Scolopendra) 蜈蚣 3g and **quan xie** (Scorpio) 全蝎3g [the last two powdered and taken separately].
- With heat or inflammation, add **huang bai** (Phellodendri Cortex) 黄柏 9–12g, **ren dong teng** (Lonicerae Caulis) 忍冬藤 15–30g and **cang zhu** (Atractylodis Rhizoma) 苍术 9–12g.
- With marked stiffness, rigidity or deformity of the joint, add **lu xian cao** (Pyrolae Herba) 鹿衔草 15–30g, **tou gu cao** (Herba Speranskia) 透骨草 12–15g and **ji xue teng** (Spatholobi Caulis) 鸡血藤 18–30g.
- With qi deficiency, sweating and breathlessness, add **zhi huang qi** (honey fried Astragali Radix) 炙黄芪 15–30g and **ren shen** (Ginseng Radix) 人参 6–9g.
- With yin deficiency, add **sheng di** (Rehmanniae Radix) 生地 9–12g, **xuan shen** (Scrophulariae Radix) 玄参 12–15g and **zhi mu** (Anemarrhenae Rhizoma) 知母 9–12g.

Topical treatments

Die Da Gao (Trauma Plaster)
Yunnan Baiyao Gao (Yunnan White Herb Plasters)
Die Da Zhi Tong Gao (Plaster for Analgesic and Bruise)
Die Da Feng Shi Gao (Die Da Feng Shi Plaster)
Zheng Gu Shui (Mend Bone Water)

Prepared medicines

Concentrated powders

Shen Tong Zhu Yu Tang (Ligusticum & Notopterygium Combination)
Xiao Huo Luo Dan (Myrrh & Aconite Formula)
　 – with cold and severe pain
Shu Jing Huo Xue Tang (Clematis & Stephania Combination)

Pills

Shen Tong Zhu Yu Wan (Great Invigorator Teapills)

Xiao Huo Luo Dan (Xiao Huo Luo Dan Teapills)
Huo Luo Xiao Ling Dan (Red Vessel Teapills)
Shu Jin Huo Xue Wan (Ease Sinew and Activate Blood Pill)
Kang Gu Zeng Sheng Pian (Inhibit Bony Proliferation Pill)
– for bony deformity and osteophytes

Acupuncture

Points are selected on the basis of the location of the pain (Table 15.2, p.647–650), and treated with a strong reducing technique to vigorously move qi and blood locally. Moxa can be used as long as there is no obvious heat. Blood letting with a surgical lancet on any local congested vessels is helpful; vigorous plum blossom needle can be used for the robust patient. The area can be cupped to encourage flow. When blood is let, it should be allowed to run until fresh red. This may require a reasonable volume of old dark blood to be let, so don't be too quick to staunch it. Blood letting can be applied on any vascular congestion along the relevant channel pathway. Local treatment is the most effective, but points that influence blood stasis systemically may be selected from the following:

Bl.11 (dazhu –) ....meeting point for bones, for pain with deformity
Bl.17 (geshu –) ....meeting point for blood, disperses static blood
Liv.3 (taichong –) ....source point of the Liver, regulates qi and activates
                                   blood, supplements Liver blood, frees the channels
                                   and network vessels and stops pain
Sp.6 (sanyinjiao –)..............these points activate blood and disperse static blood
Sp.10 (xuehai –)
LI.4 (hegu –)
Sp.8 (diji –) ....cleft point of the Spleen, rectifies qi and activates
                                   blood
• Ear points: points relating to affected area, liver, sympathetic, shenmen

Clinical notes

• Blood stasis painful obstruction syndrome may be diagnosed as chronic osteoarthritis, chronic rheumatoid arthritis, chronic tendonitis, traumatic arthritis, frozen shoulder, rotator cuff injury, osteophytes, heel spurs or post–herpetic neuralgia.
• For such a chronic pathology, blood stasis pain often responds surprisingly well to local and systemic treatment.
• Caution must be observed in those patients taking anticoagulant medications or supplements, including warfarin, coumarin, fish oils, Vitamin E and aspirin. Watch for bruising and increased bleeding tendency.
• Long term use of blood activating herbs can damage zheng qi and blood. Watch for signs of blood deficiency and change to a blood supplementing strategy for a few weeks if necessary.

痰
浊
痹
阻

15.8 PHLEGM

The hallmark of phlegm painful obstruction syndrome is paresthesia which is more pronounced than pain, and nodules in the affected area. Phlegm in the tissues is usually a consequence of chronic wind cold damp that blocks distribution of fluids. The obstructed fluids and damp gradually congeal into phlegm. This is a type of stubborn painful obstruction syndrome (*wán bì* 顽痹).

Clinical features

- Mild to moderate joint ache, heaviness, pain and distension, with numbness, woodenness, tingling and stiffness. Numbness may be the main feature. The fingers, elbow, hips, knees and ankles are most commonly affected. The affected area may be swollen, and feel soft or rubbery, lumpy or nodular when palpated. There is no significant aggravation with changes of weather, but symptoms may be aggravated by ingestion of phlegm inducing foods such as sugar, wheat and dairy products.
- dizziness, vertigo
- heavy head, foggy head
- chest oppression, abdominal distension
- nausea, poor appetite
- may be overweight
- even after years of suffering from painful obstruction syndrome, the patient may still appear quite robust

T swollen, with a greasy, white coat
P deep, wiry, slippery

Treatment principle

Transform and disperse phlegm and mobilize qi
Free the channels and network vessels and stop pain and paresthesia

Prescription

BAN XIA BAI ZHU TIAN MA TANG 半夏白术天麻汤
Pinellia, White Atractylodes, and Gastrodia Decoction, plus
YANG HE TANG 阳和汤
Yang Heartening Decoction

---

zhi ban xia (Pinelliae Rhizoma preparatum) 制半夏 9–12g
fu ling (Poria) 茯苓 12–15g
chao bai zhu (stir fried Atractylodes macrocephalae Rhizoma) 炒白术 ... 12–15g
ju hong (Citri reticulatae Exocarpium rubrum) 橘红 6–9g
bai jie zi (Sinapsis Semen) 白芥子 6–9g
ma huang (Ephedra Herba) 麻黄 1.5–3g
lu jiao jiao (Cervi Cornus Colla) 鹿角胶 9–12g
shu di (Rehmanniae Radix preparata) 熟地 12–15g
pao jiang (Zingiberis Rhizoma preparatum) 炮姜 3–6g
gan cao (Glycyrrhizae Radix) 甘草 3–6g
da zao (Jujubae Fructus) 大枣 .... 3 fruit

Method: **Zhi ban xia** dries damps and transforms phlegm; **ju hong** transforms phlegm, rectifies qi and corrects the qi dynamic; **chao bai zhu, fu ling** and **gan cao** strengthen the Spleen and supplement qi; **chao bai zhu** and **fu ling** strengthen the Spleen and dry damp; **da zao** harmonizes the Spleen and Stomach; **shu di** supplements yin and blood; **lu jiao jiao** nourishes blood and supports yang qi and assists **shu di** in nourishing jing and blood and strengthening the bones; **pao jiang** warms yang qi, dispels cold and unblocks the blood vessels; **bai jie zi** disperses phlegm; **ma huang** and **bai jie zi** assist **pao jiang** in warming the channels and removing blockages. (Source: *Zhong Yi Nei Ke Xue* [*Yi Xue Xin Wu* / *Wai Ke Zheng Zhi Quan Sheng Ji*])

Modifications

- The doses of **shu di** and **lu jiao jiao** should not be increased, as aggravation of the phlegm may occur.
- With subcutaneous nodules or lumpiness, increase the dose of **bai jie zi** to 15g and add **dan nan xing** (Arisaema cum Bile) 胆南星 6–9g, **wei ling xian** (Clematidis Radix) 威灵仙 6–9g and **zao jiao ci** (Gleditsiae Spina) 皂角刺 3–6g.
- If the knees and ankles are affected, add **chuan niu xi** (Cyathulae Radix) 川牛膝 12–15g.
- If the fingers, elbows and toes are affected, add **wei ling xian** (Clematidis Radix) 威灵仙 6–9g.
- If the shoulder and neck are affected, add **jiang huang** (Curcumae longae Rhizoma) 姜黄 9–12g and **sang zhi** (Mori Ramulus) 桑枝 15–30g.
- With joint swelling and distension, add **cang zhu** (Atractylodis Rhizoma) 苍术 9–12g, **yi ren** (Coicis Semen) 苡仁 15–30g and **bi xie** (Dioscoreae hypoglaucae Rhizoma) 萆薢 9–12g.
- With chest oppression, add **gua lou** (Trichosanthis Fructus) 栝楼 15–24g and **gui zhi** (Cinnamomi Ramulus) 桂枝 6–9g.
- With tiredness and sweating add **huang qi** (Astragali Radix) 黄芪 15–30g.
- With poor appetite, add **mu xiang** (Aucklandiae Radix) 木香 9–12g.

Prepared medicines

Concentrated powders
Er Zhu Tang (Atractylodes & Arisaema Combination)
Ding Xian Wan (Gastrodia and Amber Combination)
 – a formula for seizures, but can also be used for phlegm in the tissues

Pills
Kang Gu Zeng Sheng Pian (Inhibit Bony Proliferation Pill)
 – for bony deformity and osteophytes
Xiao Huo Luo Dan (Xiao Huo Luo Dan Teapills)
 – for severe numbness and stiffness; only used when there is no trace of heat

Acupuncture
Points are selected according to the affected area (Table 15.2, p.647–650). Additional points can be added from the following to systemically transform phlegm. Moxa can be used with caution, as excessive use can congeal phlegm further.
Bl.11 (dazhu –) ....meeting point for bones, for pain with deformity
Ren.12 (zhongwan)............alarm point of the Stomach, strengthens the Spleen and Stomach to transform phlegm

St.40 (fenglong −) ....connecting point of the Stomach, transforms phlegm

Sp.5 (shangqiu −) ....metal point of the Spleen, transforms damp

St.41 (jiexi −)......................fire point of the Stomach, strengthens Spleen and Stomach qi and transforms phlegm

PC.5 (jianshi −)..................river point of the Pericardium, transforms phlegm

Bl.20 (pishu) ....transport point of the Spleen, strengthens the Spleen and supplements qi to promote transformation of damp and phlegm

- with Spleen deficiency, add St.36 (zusanli +)
- with Liver qi constraint, add GB.34 (yanglingquan −) and Liv.3 (taichong −)
- with cold, apply moxa cones to Bl.20 (pishu ▲) and Bl.21 (weishu ▲)
- with muscle aches and heaviness, add Sp.21 (dabao)
- with edema, add Sp.9 (yinlingquan −) and Sp.6 (sanyinjiao)
- Ear points: spleen, kidney, zero point, shenmen, points relating to affected area

Clinical notes

- Phlegm type painful obstruction syndrome may be diagnosed as chronic rheumatoid arthritis, osteoarthritis, cystic swelling in joints, bunions or ganglia.
- This is a difficult pattern to treat successfully, and will require long term persistent treatment.
- A phlegm transforming diet is recommended. See Clinical Handbook, Vol.2, p.880.

痰
瘀
痹
阻

15.9 PHLEGM AND BLOOD STASIS

This is very chronic joint pathology. The proportion of blood stasis and phlegm can vary. The greater the blood stasis component, the more pain and vascular congestion. The more phlegm, the greater the numbness, paresthesia and nodularity of the joint and surrounding tissues. In addition to the stasis, there may be heat or cold, and patients usually have varying degrees of qi, blood or Kidney deficiency. The primary prescription recommended below is quite powerful and dispersing, and aimed at providing some relief from pain and stiffness relatively quickly. Care must be taken not to further damage the patient's qi and blood. A form of stubborn painful obstruction syndrome (*wán bì* 顽痹).

Clinical features
* Recurrent or persistent joint pain, with stiffness, rigidity and joint deformity. There may be palpable nodules, lipping or osteophytes around the joint margin. The skin overlying the joint may be discolored or show signs of vascular congestion. The pain can be variable, either relatively severe, or with less pain and more numbness and stiffness. The joints may occasionally be warm and swollen. There is little relationship between pain and stiffness and changes in the weather.
T purple tongue, or brown or purple spots on the tongue, dark and distended sublingual veins; may be swollen
P choppy, wiry, slippery or fine pulse

Treatment principle
Activate blood and disperse phlegm and blood stasis
Free the channels and network vessels
Support qi, blood and the Kidneys as necessary

Prescription

SHEN TONG ZHU YU TANG 身痛逐瘀汤
Drive Out Blood Stasis from a Painful Body Decoction, modified

This is a strong prescription suitable for robust patients. It should provide some pain and stiffness relief within a few weeks and can then be used for a few months before a break is needed. For less robust patients see p.676.

tao ren (Persicae Semen) 桃仁	9–12g
hong hua (Carthami Flos) 红花	9–12g
chi shao (Paeoniae Radix rubra) 赤芍	9–12g
chuan xiong (Chuanxiong Rhizoma) 川芎	6–9g
dang gui (Angelicae sinensis Radix) 当归	6–9g
chuan niu xi (Cyathulae Radix) 川牛膝	9–12g
bai jie zi (Sinapsis Semen) 白芥子	6–9g
qiang huo (Notopterygii Rhizoma seu Radix) 羌活	9–12g
di long (Pheretima) 地龙	9–12g
dan nan xing (Arisaema cum Bile) 胆南星	6–9g
zao jiao ci (Gleditsiae Spina) 皂角刺	3–6g

Method: Decoction. **Tao ren, hong hua, chuan xiong, dang gui** and **chi shao** activate the blood and dispel static blood, **chuan niu xi** and **di long** free the channels and network vessels and stop pain; **qiang huo** dispels wind and eliminates damp; **bai jie zi, dan nan xing** and **zao jiao ci** transform and disperse phlegm. (Source: *Zhong Yi Nei Ke Shou Ce* [*Yi Lin Gai Cuo*])

Modifications

- With severe pain, add **zhi mo yao** (Myrrha preparata) 炙没药 3–6g and **zhi ru xiang** (Olibanum preparata) 炙乳香 3–6g.
- For neuropathic pain, add **wu gong** (Scolopendra) 蜈蚣 3g and **quan xie** (Scorpio) 全蝎 3g [both powdered and taken separately], and **wu shao she** (Zaocys) 乌梢蛇 6–9g.
- With joint swelling, add **cang zhu** (Atractylodis Rhizoma) 苍术 9–12g and **yi ren** (Coicis Semen) 苡仁 15–30g.
- With severe stiffness, rigidity or deformity of the joint, add **lu xian cao** (Pyrolae Herba) 鹿衔草 15–30g, **tou gu cao** (Herba Speranskia) 透骨草 12–15g, **bu gu zhi** (Psoraleae Fructus) 补骨脂 9–12g and **ba ji tian** (Morindae officinalis Radix) 巴戟天 9–12g and **ji xue teng** (Spatholobi Caulis) 鸡血藤 18–30g.
- With qi deficiency, add **huang qi** (Astragali Radix) 黄芪 18–30g and **ren shen** (Ginseng Radix) 人参 6–9g.
- With heat, add r**en dong teng** (Lonicerae Caulis) 忍冬藤 15–30g, **mu dan pi** (Moutan Cortex) 牡丹皮 9–12g and **lian qiao** (Forsythiae Fructus) 连翘 9–12g.
- With cold, add **gui zhi** (Cinnamomi Ramulus) 桂枝 9–12g and **xi xin** (Asari Herba) 细辛 3–6g.

Variations and additional prescriptions

Weak and deficient patients

The powerful dispersing action of the primary prescription can be detrimental to patients with significant deficiency, and a gentler but more prolonged strategy is better tolerated. In addition to the joint symptoms, patients will be fatigued, dizzy, pale and run down. The treatment is to gently activate and protect blood and transform phlegm with a formula such as **SHUANG HE TANG** (Dual Combination Decoction 双合汤). This prescription is suited to long term use without breaks.

tao ren (Persicae Semen) 桃仁	6–9g
hong hua (Carthami Flos) 红花	6–9g
bai shao (Paeoniae Radix alba) 白芍	9–12g
chuan xiong (Chuanxiong Rhizoma) 川芎	6–9g
dang gui (Angelicae sinensis Radix) 当归	6–9g
shu di (Rehmanniae Radix preparata) 熟地	9–12g
zhi ban xia (Pinelliae Rhizoma preparatum) 制半夏	6–9g
chen pi (Citri reticulatae Pericarpium) 陈皮	6–9g
bai jie zi (Sinapis Semen) 白芥子	6–9g
fu ling (Poria) 茯苓	9–15g
zhu li (Bambusae Succus) 竹沥	6–9g
sheng jiang (Zingiberis Rhizoma recens) 生姜	6–9g
gan cao (Glycyrrhizae Radix) 甘草	3–6g

Method: Decoction. **Tao ren, hong hua, chuan xiong, dang gui, shu di** and **bai shao** activate, nourish and protect the blood, while gently dispelling static blood; **zhi ban xia**, **chen pi**, **bai jie zi** and **zhu li** transform phlegm and open up the network vessels; **fu ling** supplements the Spleen and leaches out damp and assists in transforming phlegm; **sheng jiang** assists in phlegm transformation and, with **gan cao**, protects the Stomach. (Source: *Zhong Yi Nei Ke Xue*[*Za Bing Yuan Liu Xi Zhu*])

With severe joint deformity

In many chronic cases of phlegm and blood stasis in the joints, the joint deformity is the main problem leading to stiffness and loss of function. Pain is a secondary consideration. An experimental formula, Gu Zhi Zeng Sheng Wan (Bony Proliferation Pills 骨质增生丸) from the Jilin Fourth Clinical Teaching Hospital Orthopedic Department, is aimed at supplementing the Liver and Kidneys, activating blood and transforming phlegm to address some of the worst restriction and improve mobility.

shu di (Rehmanniae Radix preparata) 熟地 150g
rou cong rong (Cistanches Herba) 肉苁蓉 100g
lu xian cao (Pyrolae Herba) 鹿衔草 100g
xian ling pi (Epimedii Herba) 仙灵脾 100g
gu sui bu (Drynariae Rhizoma) 骨碎补 100g
ji xue teng (Spatholobi Caulis) 鸡血藤 100g
lai fu zi (Raphani Semen) 莱菔子 50g

Method: Boil the last five herbs in sufficient water to cover the herbs by 2–3cm for 90 minutes, strain off and conserve the remaining liquid. Add fresh water to cover the dregs and boil again for 90 minutes, then strain off and conserve the liquid and discard the dregs. Combine the two liquid portions and mix with powdered **shu di** and **rou cong rong**, and sufficient honey to form 3 gram pills. The dose is 2–3 pills per day. **Shu di** enriches Kidney yin and blood; **xian ling pi** warms Kidney yang; **rou cong rong** benefits jing; **gu sui bu** and **lu xian cao** supplement the Kidneys and transform bony growths; **ji xue teng** promotes movement through the channels and supplements blood; **lai fu zi** transforms phlegm and helps digestion of the principal herbs. With digestive upsets or diarrhea, add **shan yao** (Dioscoreae Rhizoma) 山药 100g and **bai dou kou** (Amomi Fructus rotundus) 白豆蔻 60g. (Source: *Ji Lin Di Si Lin Chuang Xue Yuan Gu Ke Jing Yan Fang*)

Prepared medicines
Concentrated powders
Shen Tong Zhu Yu Tang (Ligusticum & Notopterygium Combination) plus Er
    Zhu Tang (Atractylodes & Arisaema Combination)
    – the proportions of these two formulae above can be altered to reflect the
    proportions of phlegm and blood stasis
Shu Jin Li An San (Clematis & Carthamus Combination)
Xiao Huo Luo Dan (Myrrh & Aconite Formula)
    – for robust patients without heat or yin deficiency
Pills
Shen Tong Zhu Yu Wan (Great Invigorator Teapills)
Xiao Huo Luo Dan (Xiao Huo Luo Dan Teapills)
Kang Gu Zeng Sheng Pian (Inhibit Bony Proliferation Pill)

Acupuncture
Points are selected on the basis of the location of the pain (Table 15.2, p.647–650), and treated vigorously to move qi and blood locally. Moxa can be used

cautiously as long as there is no obvious heat. Blood letting with a surgical lancet on any local congested vessels is helpful (see p.929). Local treatment is the most effective, but points that influence blood stasis and phlegm systemically may be selected from the following:

Bl.11 (dazhu –) ....meeting point for bones, for pain with deformity

Bl.17 (geshu –).................meeting point for blood, disperses stagnant blood

Liv.3 (taichong –)...............source point of the Liver, regulates qi and activates blood, frees the channels and network vessels and stops pain

St.40 (fenglong –) ....connecting point of the Stomach, transforms phlegm

St.36 (zusanli) ....sea point of the Stomach, strengthens the Spleen and supplements qi to transform phlegm and move blood stasis

Sp.6 (sanyinjiao –)..............these points activate blood and disperse stagnant

Sp.10 (xuehai –)   blood

LI.4 (hegu –)

Sp.8 (diji –) ....cleft point of the Spleen, rectifies qi and activates blood

• Ear points: points relating to affected area, liver, kidney, zero point, sympathetic, shenmen

Clinical notes

• Phlegm and blood stasis may be diagnosed as chronic rheumatoid or osteoarthritis, ankylosing spondylitis, bunions and degenerative joint disease.

• This is a difficult pattern to treat successfully, but some symptomatic relief can be achieved.

• A phlegm transforming diet is recommended. See Clinical Handbook, Vol.2, p.880.

气
血
虚
弱

15.10 QI AND BLOOD DEFICIENCY

Plentiful blood is required to maintain elasticity of tissues and lubricate the joints. Blood deficiency is a component of all chronic joint pathology, while lack of qi leads to weakness and loss of tone in the supporting soft tissues. Qi and blood deficiency painful obstruction syndrome is a chronic pain pattern that occurs after the inflammatory phase of a joint or soft tissue pathology has subsided, or when the bony and soft tissues are chronically starved of qi and blood. The main symptom is usually stiff, dry, creaky joints from the failure of blood to nourish and lubricate the joint, muscles and sinews, along with atrophy of the soft tissues around the affected joint or joints. There may be joint deformity, but the deficiency aspects are primary. The relative lack of qi and blood in the superficial tissues also enables wind and damp to gain access and linger.

In practice, qi and blood deficiency often overlaps with yin deficiency, and the predominance of either yin or blood deficiency depends on the age and constitution of the patient, and the medications used. A tendency to yin deficiency is more common in those over 40 and in those who have taken a lot of pungent, dispersing medications, such as cortisone and strong analgesics (including Chinese herbs). Blood deficiency tends to affect a younger age group, in particular women of reproductive age, and also appears in patients with inadequate diets.

Clinical features
- Dull persistent or intermittent stiffness, pain, paresthesia or numbness. Stiffness is often the main complaint. Pain is alleviated by rest and is worse with use and flexion, and during cold weather. The affected tissues may be atrophic and feel lax and without tone. Muscle weakness is pronounced, and there may be muscle fasciculation and spasm. Mild nodulation or vascular congestion around the affected area may be observed, and there may be stiffness of the back and spine.
- pale complexion, nails, conjunctivae
- weakness and fatigue
- dry skin and hair
- poor appetite, loose stools
- low grade fever
- postural dizziness
- palpitations and insomnia
- weight loss, emaciation

T pale with a thin, white coat
P deep, weak, fine

Treatment principle
Supplement qi and blood
Nourish and ease the sinews and bones
Free the channels and network vessels and stop pain

Prescription

SAN BI TANG 三痹汤
Three Painful Obstruction Decoction

ren shen (Ginseng Radix) 人参 6–9g
huang qi (Astragali Radix) 黄芪 12–15g
fu ling (Poria) 茯苓 9–12g
zhi gan cao (Glycyrrhizae Radix preparata) 炙甘草 3–6g
dang gui (Angelicae sinensis Radix) 当归 9–12g
sheng di (Rehmanniae Radix) 生地 12–18g
bai shao (Paeoniae Radix alba) 白芍 9–12g
chuan xiong (Chuanxiong Rhizoma) 川芎 6–9g
sheng jiang (Zingiberis Rhizoma recens) 生姜 6–9g
fang feng (Saposhnikovae Radix) 防风 9–12g
qin jiao (Gentianae macrophyllae Radix) 秦艽 9–12g
xi xin (Asari Herba) 细辛 3–6g
du huo (Angelicae pubescentis Radix) 独活 9–12g
xu duan (Dipsaci Radix) 续断 9–12g
du zhong (Eucommiae Cortex) 杜仲 9–12g
huai niu xi (Achyranthis bidentatae Radix) 怀牛膝 9–12g
rou gui (Cinnamomi Cortex) 肉桂 3–6g

Method: Powder or decoction. **Huang qi**, **ren shen**, **fu ling** and **zhi gan cao** supplement qi and assist in the transformation of damp; **sheng di**, **dang gui**, **bai shao** and **chuan xiong** supplement and activate blood; **sheng jiang** warms the Spleen and assists in the digestion of the rich supplements; **du huo**, **xi xin**, **fang feng** and **qin jiao** dispel wind damp and stop pain; **xu duan**, **du zhong** and **huai niu xi** supplement the Kidneys, strengthen the back, spine and knees, warm yang qi and support sinews and bones; **rou gui** supports yang qi, dispels cold and assists in stimulating the movement of qi and blood; (Source: *Zhong Yi Nei Ke Xue* [*Fu Ren Liang Fang*])

Variations and additional prescriptions

With predominant qi deficiency
When qi deficiency is the predominant feature, muscle tone is poor and the tissues feel lax and weak. The treatment is to focus on rebuilding Spleen qi and improving qi and blood flow to the affected region. A modified version of **Bu Zhong Yi Qi Tang** (Supplement the Middle to Augment the Qi Decoction 补中益气汤 p.598) can be used with the addition of **zhi fu zi** (Aconiti Radix lateralis preparata) 制附子 and two or three wind damp dispelling herbs, as necessary. Consider **wei ling xian** (Clematidis Radix) 威灵仙, **qin jiao** (Gentianae macrophyllae Radix) 秦艽, **xi xian cao** (Siegesbeckia Herba) 豨莶草, **sang zhi** (Mori Ramulus) 桑枝, **fang feng** (Saposhnikovae Radix) 防风 or **jiang huang** (Curcumae longae Rhizoma) 姜黄.

With predominant blood deficiency
When blood deficiency is the main feature, dryness of the soft tissues, stiffness and creaking joints, tics, tremors and muscle fasciculation are seen. The treatment is to build the blood and alleviate stiffness and pain with a formula such as **Si Wu Tang** (Four Substance Decoction 四物汤 p.920), with the same additions as for

qi deficiency above.

Prepared medicines
Concentrated powders
San Bi Tang (Tuhuo & Astragalus Combination)
Pills
San Bi Tang Wan (San Bi Tang Teapills)

Acupuncture
Points are chosen based on the location of the pain (Table 15.2, p.647–650), with the addition of moxa and use of points to supplement qi and blood systemically, as follows:

Ren.12 (zhongwan +▲) ....alarm point of the Stomach, strengthens the Spleen and supplements qi and blood

St.36 (zusanli +▲) ....sea point of the Stomach, strengthens the Spleen and Stomach, and supplements qi and blood

Sp.6 (sanyinjiao +)..............strengthens the Spleen and Kidneys, supplements qi and blood

LI.11 (quchi +▲)...............sea point of the Large Intestine, stimulates movement of qi and blood by activating yangming (which is rich in qi and blood)

Bl.20 (pishu +▲) ....transport point of the Spleen, strengthens the Spleen and supplements qi and blood

Bl.21 (shenshu +▲) ....transport point of the Kidneys, warms and supplements the Kidneys to support qi and blood

• Ear points: points relating to affected area, spleen, liver, zero point, shenmen

Clinical notes
• Qi and blood deficiency is a common form of chronic pain and stiffness, and can respond quite well to prolonged treatment.
• Painful obstruction syndrome of a qi and blood deficiency type may be diagnosed as age related degenerative changes of articular cartilage and soft tissue, and tendinopathy such as rotator cuff syndrome.
• Diet is an essential feature in the treatment of qi and blood deficiency. Adequate protein must be consumed to build blood. See Clinical Handbook, Vol.2, p.870 and 874. There are some tasty traditional dishes that are considered effective for qi and blood deficiency patterns with pain. A slow cooked stew of lamb shanks, beef tendons or other gelatinous cut of meat with dang gui, ginger, bai shao and gui zhi is popular in some parts of China, particularly the cold north west.

15.11 QI AND YIN DEFICIENCY

气
阴
两
虚

Qi and yin deficiency painful obstruction syndrome is characterized by dryness of joints and tissues, with inflammation and heat. The etiology can be varied, with the qi and yin damaged by age and use, a persistent heat pattern in a joint or tissue, or a long history of pungent dispersing medications such as cortisone and strong analgesics, including Chinese herbs for pain of an excess type. The dispersing qualities of these medicines effectively removes blockages, but can also disperse qi and damage yin.

This pattern is more common in an older age group, over 50 years, but is also seen in younger patients who have used a lot of medication, or depleted their qi and yin through overwork, poor sleep and eating habits or illicit drug use.

Clinical features
- Joint stiffness, dull pain, paresthesia and numbness. The pain is alleviated by rest, and is worse with use and massage. The tissues feel dry and stiff. Joints crackle and creak with movement and feel dry subjectively. Stiffness and rigidity can be severe. Joints and affected tissues may feel slightly warm, and are easily aggravated and inflamed with use.
- dry, scaly skin, dry hair
- weight loss, emaciation
- weakness and fatigue
- facial flushing, malar flush
- insomnia, palpitations
- red conjunctivae
- low grade fever, night sweats, patient easily overheated
- acupuncture and massage may leave large red marks

T slightly swollen, pink or red with multiple surface cracks and little or no coat
P fine, weak, rapid

Treatment principle
Supplement qi and yin
Nourish and ease the sinews and bones
Free the network vessels and stop pain

Prescription
SHENG MAI SAN 生脉散
Generate the Pulse Powder, plus
HUANG QI GUI ZHI WU WU TANG 黄芪桂枝五物汤
Astragalus and Cinnamon Twig Five Substance Decoction

ren shen (Ginseng Radix) 人参 6–9g
huang qi (Astragali Radix) 黄芪 30–60g
gui zhi (Cinnamomi Ramulus) 桂枝 6–9g
bai shao (Paeoniae Radix alba) 白芍 9–12g
dang gui (Angelicae sinensis Radix) 当归 9–12g
mai dong (Ophiopogonis Radix) 麦冬 9–12g

wu wei zi (Schizandrae Fructus) 五味子 3–6g
sheng jiang (Zingiberis Rhizoma recens) 生姜 12–15g
da zao (Jujubae Fructus) 大枣 .... 6 fruit
zhi gan cao (Glycyrrhizae Radix preparata) 炙甘草 3–6g

Method: Powder or decoction. **Ren shen** and **huang qi** supplement qi; **bai shao** and **dang gui** nourish blood and yin; **mai dong** nourishes Lung and Stomach yin; **gui zhi** opens up qi flow through the superficial tissues, and, with **bai shao**, harmonizes ying and wei qi to secure the surface; **wu wei zi** supplements the Kidneys, astringes the Lungs and secures wei qi; **sheng jiang**, **da zao** and **zhi gan cao** support the Spleen and Stomach. (Source: *Zhong Yi Nei Ke Xue* [*Nei Wai Shang Bian Huo Lun* / *Jin Gui Yao Lüe*])

Modifications

- With blood deficiency, add **sheng di** (Rehmanniae Radix) 生地 9–12g, **shu di** (Rehmanniae Radix preparata) 熟地 9–12g and **ji xue teng** (Spatholobi Caulis) 鸡血藤 15–30g.
- With marked yin deficiency, add **xuan shen** (Scrophulariae Radix) 玄参 9–12g, **shan zhu yu** (Corni Fructus) 山茱萸 9–12g and **yu zhu** (Polygonati odorati Rhizoma) 玉竹 12–15g.
- With marked deficiency heat, sweats and flushing, delete **gui zhi**, and add **sang zhi** (Mori Ramulus) 桑枝 15–30g, **di gu pi** (Lycii Cortex) 地骨皮 12–15g and **qin jiao** (Gentianae macrophyllae Radix) 秦艽 9–12g.
- With loose stools, delete **mai dong**, and add **cang zhu** (Atractylodis Rhizoma) 苍术 6–9g and **bai zhu** (Atractylodis macrocephalae Rhizoma) 白术 6–9g.
- With blood stasis, add **tao ren** (Persicae Semen) 桃仁 9–12g and **hong hua** (Carthami Flos) 红花 6–9g.
- With muscle spasms or numbness, add **ji xue teng** (Spatholobi Caulis) 鸡血藤 15–30g and **tian ma** (Gastrodiae Rhizoma) 天麻 6–9g.
- With poor appetite and abdominal distension, add **mu xiang** (Aucklandiae Radix) 木香 9–12g and **chen pi** (Citri reticulatae Pericarpium) 陈皮 6–9g.

Prepared medicines

Concentrated powders

Sheng Mai San (Ginseng & Ophiopogon Formula) plus Huang Qi Wu Wu Tang (Astragalus & Cinnamon Five Herb Combination)

Pills

Sheng Mai Wan (Great Pulse Teapills) plus Gui Zhi Tang Wan (Gui Zhi Tang Teapills)

Acupuncture

Points are chosen based on the location of the pain or stiffness (Table 15.2, p.647–650), with systemic points added to supplement qi and yin as follows:

Ren.4 (guanyuan +) ....supplements Kidney yin to support yin systemically
Kid.3 (taixi) ....source point of the Kidneys, supplements yin
St.36 (zusanli +) ....sea point of the Stomach, strengthens the Spleen and Stomach and supplements qi
Sp.6 (sanyinjiao +) ....strengthens the Spleen and Kidneys, supplements qi and yin

Bl.20 (pishu +) ....transport point of the Spleen, supplements Spleen qi
                                to build blood and yin
Bl.23 (shenshu +) ....transport point of the Kidneys, supplements the
                                Kidneys to build yin, qi and blood
Lu.7 (lieque).....................master points of renmai and yinqiaomai, used
Kid.6 (zhaohai)   together to supplement Kidney yin and Lung qi
- Ear points: points relating to affected area, kidney, liver, spleen, zero point, shenmen

Clinical notes

- Qi and yin deficiency is a relatively common type of chronic pain and stiffness and can respond reasonably well to prolonged treatment. This type of painful obstruction syndrome may be diagnosed as chronic inflammatory and degenerative changes in soft tissues, age related degeneration of articular cartilage and joint capsules, chronic tendinopathy (rotator cuff, lateral epicondyle, Achilles tendonitis etc.) and myopathy.
- A qi and yin nourishing diet is recommended. See Clinical Handbook, Vol.2, p.870 and 876.

肝
肾
两
虚

15.12 LIVER AND KIDNEY DEFICIENCY

1. Yang deficiency
2. Yin deficiency
3. Yin and yang deficiency

Liver and Kidney deficiency is a chronic degenerative pathology. The main difference between Liver and Kidney deficiency type painful obstruction syndrome and the other deficiency patterns is the depth of the pathology. Liver and Kidney deficiency represents a deterioration of joint structures and soft tissues, with increasing systemic weakness.

The pattern can veer towards either yin or yang deficiency, or have aspects of both. How the pattern develops depends on the constitution of the patient, the nature of the original pathogen, work and rest habits, and the medication history. Patients tend to be older, mostly over 50 years.

Common clinical features
• Chronic, persistent or intermittent joint ache, pain and stiffness. On the whole, the pain is mild to moderate and may be secondary to weakness or stiffness and inflexibility of joints. The lower back, spine, sacrum, legs and knees are most commonly affected. There may be difficulty in walking and severe restriction of movement. Bony deformity and osteophytes are common.

阳
虚

15.12.1 YANG DEFICIENCY
Kidney yang deficiency is a common pattern of chronic joint pain and stiffness. Pain and stiffness may go through cycles of exacerbation and remission, depending on factors such as the activity levels of the patient and the weather.

The treatment strategy depends on the degree of pain and debility. When the pain is mild or absent, often during summer and warm weather, the strategy focuses on strengthening Kidney yang to prevent deterioration during the winter. When the pain is more intense or unmanageable, a more specific cold dispelling strategy can be adopted until control is maintained and pain relieved.

Specific features
• Pain and stiffness, worse during cold weather and winter, when the patient is chilled, overworked or fatigued, or with wind cold invasion. Tissue tone in the affected area and, in general, tends to be lax.
• joints may be swollen and edematous
• cold intolerance, cold extremities
• increased desire to sleep
• fatigue, mental and physical exhaustion
• waxy pale complexion
• urinary frequency or nocturia
T pale, swollen and scalloped with a white coat
P deep, weak, slow pulse

Treatment principle
Warm and supplement yang
Dispel cold and promote circulation of qi and blood

Prescription

JIN GUI SHEN QI WAN 金匮肾气丸
Kidney Qi Pill from the Golden Cabinet p.826

This is an excellent prescription for all Kidney yang deficiency problems, and one well suited to strengthen the Kidneys to support, and prevent deterioration of, a yang deficiency pain pattern. It is best used when pain is mild or in remission.

Modifications
- With swelling and edema, add **cang zhu** (Atractylodis Rhizoma) 苍术 9–12g, **bai zhu** (Atractylodis macrocephalae Rhizoma) 白术 12–15g, **yi ren** (Coicis Semen) 苡仁 15–30g and **che qian zi** (Plantaginis Semen) 车前子 9–12g.
- If the lower body is affected, add **huai niu xi** (Achyranthis bidentatae Radix) 怀牛膝 12–15g.
- With stiffness of the spine and lower back ache, add **xu duan** (Dipsaci Radix) 续断 12–15g, **gou ji** (Cibotii Rhizoma) 狗脊 9–12g and **du zhong** (Eucommiae Cortex) 杜仲 12–15g.
- With joint deformity and nodularity, combine with YANG HE TANG (Yang Heartening Decoction 阳和汤 p.792).
- With Liver blood deficiency, add **dang gui** (Angelicae sinensis Radix) 当归 9–12g and **bai shao** (Paeoniae Radix alba) 白芍 12–15g.
- With blood stasis, add **ji xue teng** (Spatholobi Caulis) 鸡血藤 30g and **wei ling xian** (Clematidis Radix) 威灵仙 12–15g.

FU ZI TANG 附子汤
Prepared Aconite Decoction, p.655

This prescription is selected for exacerbations of pain and stiffness that may periodically occur during cold spells and with over exertion. It is used for a week or two until the pain is managed, after which the constitutional treatment can be resumed.

Prepared medicines
Concentrated powders
Ba Wei Di Huang Wan (Rehmannia Eight Formula)
You Gui Wan (Eucommia & Rehmannia Formula)
Zhen Wu Tang (Ginger, Aconite, Poria & Peony Combination)
   – for periods of exacerbation of pain

Pills
Jin Kui Shen Qi Wan (Fu Gui Ba Wei Wan, Golden Book Teapills)
You Gui Wan (Right Side Replenishing Teapills)
Zhen Wu Tang Wan (True Warrior Teapills)

Acupuncture

Points are chosen based on the location of the pain or stiffness (Table 15.2, p.647–650), with the addition of moxa, and systemic points to warm and supplement Kidney yang, as follows:

Ren.6 (qihai +▲) .... these points warms and strengthen Kidney yang and
Ren.4 (guanyuan +▲)   stimulate circulation of yang qi to the extremities
Kid.3 (taixi +).................... source point of the Kidneys, supplements Kidney
                            yang
St.36 (zusanli +▲) .... sea point of the Stomach, strengthens the Spleen and
                            Stomach and supplements yang qi
SI.3 (houxi)....................... master and couple points of dumai, stimulate the
Bl.62 (shenmai)   circulation of yang qi through the dumai
Bl.23 (shenshu +▲) .... transport point of the Kidneys, warms and supple-
                            ments Kidney yang
Du.4 (mingmen +▲) .... warms and supplements Kidney yang

• Ear points: points relating to affected area, kidney, adrenal, shenmen

Clinical notes

• Kidney yang deficiency painful obstruction syndrome may be diagnosed as chronic rheumatoid arthritis, osteoarthritis, chronic lumbago, sciatica or prolapsed lumbar intervertebral disc.
• Kidney yang deficiency pain can respond well to prolonged treatment.
• A warming diet is recommended. See Clinical Handbook, Vol.2, p.873.

15.12.2 YIN DEFICIENCY

Kidney and Liver yin deficiency, with joint pathology and pain, may follow an acute or prolonged episode of excess heat in the joints, such as damp heat or toxic heat. This pattern is also seen around menopause and in those with a history of stimulant drug use, or large amounts of steroids and other pungent dispersing medications. This is one of those situations in which herbs are essential.

Specific features

• Joints may be slightly warm or feel warm to the touch, relative to surrounding tissues. The pain is worse at night and during hot weather, and is aggravated by moxa, warming liniments and plasters. The soft tissues surrounding the joints may be atrophic, tight or contracted. Joints and soft tissues become inflamed and irritated easily when over used. Stiffness and inflexibility is often a main component, and tissues feel tight and contracted, or dry.
• lower back weak and aching, hot aching feet
• muscle spasms and cramps, calf cramps, restless legs
• heat intolerance, easily over heated; heat in the hands and feet
• generalized dryness–skin, mouth, hair, vagina, joints
• constipation
• night sweats
• facial flushing
• insomnia

- dizziness
- irritability
- fatigue, with difficulty resting and jitteriness

T red with little or no coat
P fine and rapid

Treatment principle

Nourish and supplement Liver and Kidney yin
Nourish and activate blood

Prescription

LIU WEI DI HUANG WAN 六味地黄丸
Six Ingredient Pill with Rehmannia, plus
SI WU TANG 四物汤
Four Substance Decoction

This prescription is most effective when used long term, and is suitable when aches, pains and stiffness are relatively mild and manageable. It can be used as a base for modification during exacerbations of pain with inflammation.

shu di (Rehmanniae Radix preparata) 熟地 12–24g
shan yao (Dioscoreae Rhizoma) 山药 12–15g
shan zhu yu (Corni Fructus) 山茱萸 12–15g
mu dan pi (Moutan Cortex) 牡丹皮 9–12g
fu ling (Poria) 茯苓 9–12g
ze xie (Alismatis Rhizoma) 泽泻 9–12g
dang gui (Angelicae sinensis Radix) 当归 9–12g
bai shao (Paeoniae Radix alba) 白芍 9–12g
chuan xiong (Chuanxiong Rhizoma) 川芎 6–9g

Method: Powder is the best form for long term use, while decoction can be used to settle pain down during exacerbations. **Shu di** is the main herb to nourish and supplement Kidney yin, and, with **dang gui**, supplements blood; **shan zhu yu** warms and supplements the Liver and Kidneys, its astringency helping to preserve yin and retain leakage of fluids; **shan yao** strengthens the Spleen, secures jing and, with **shan zhu yu**, restrains excessive urination. **Ze xie** clears heat and fire from the Kidneys through the urine; **mu dan pi** cools and activates the blood, and clears heat from the Liver; **fu ling** strengthens the Spleen and leaches damp out through the urine. **Dang gui** supplements and gently activates blood; **bai shao** supplements blood, softens the Liver and preserves yin; **chuan xiong** activates blood and moves qi. (Source: *Shi Yong Zhong Yi Nei Ke* [*Xiao Er Yao Zheng Zhi Jue* / *He Ji Ju Fang*])

Modifications

- With mild to moderate pain and stiffness in the upper body, add **sang zhi** (Mori Ramulus) 桑枝 15–30g, **ji xue teng** (Spatholobi Caulis) 鸡血藤 30g and **qing feng teng** (Sinomenium Caulis) 清风藤 9–15g.
- With mild to moderate pain and stiffness in the legs, add **sang ji sheng** (Taxilli Herba) 桑寄生 12–15g, **huai niu xi** (Achyranthis bidentatae Radix) 怀牛膝 12–15g, **mu gua** (Chaenomelis Fructus) 木瓜 9–12g and **luo shi teng** (Trachelospermi Caulis) 络石藤 15–30g.
- With pain in the fingers or toes, add **xi xian cao** (Siegesbeckia Herba) 豨莶草 9–12g, **ji xue teng** (Spatholobi Caulis) 鸡血藤 30g, **dan shen** (Salviae miltior-

rhizae Radix) 丹参 9–12g and **shen jin cao** (Lycopodii Herba) 伸筋草 9–15g.

- With lower back weakness and aching, add **tu si zi** (Cuscutae Semen) 菟丝子 9–12g, **xu duan** (Dipsaci Radix) 续断 9–12g, **gou qi zi** (Lycii Fructus) 枸杞子 9–12g and **du zhong** (Eucommiae Cortex) 杜仲 12–15g.
- With relatively severe pain, add **chi shao** (Paeoniae Radix rubra) 赤芍 9–12g, **tao ren** (Persicae Semen) 桃仁 9–12g, **hong hua** (Carthami Flos) 红花 6–9g and **dan shen** (Salviae miltiorrhizae Radix) 丹参 9–12g.
- With ascendant Liver yang, add **shi jue ming** (Haliotidis Concha) 石决明 15–30g, **gou teng** (Uncariae Ramulus cum Uncis) 钩藤 9–12g and **mu li** (Ostreae Concha) 牡蛎 15–30g.
- With muscle spasms and cramps, add **sha yuan ji li** (Astragali complanati Semen) 沙苑蒺藜 9–12g, **mu gua** (Chaenomelis Fructus) 木瓜 9–12g and **tian ma** (Gastrodiae Rhizoma) 天麻 9–12g, or combine with Sʜᴀᴏ Yᴀᴏ Gᴀɴ Cᴀᴏ Tᴀɴɢ (Peony and Licorice Decoction 芍药甘草汤 p.919).
- With marked systemic heat, add **zhi mu** (Anemarrhenae Rhizoma) 知母 9–12g and **huang bai** (Phellodendri Cortex) 黄柏 9–12g.
- With marked local heat in the affected area, add **di long** (Pheretima) 地龙 9–12g, **cang zhu** (Atractylodis Rhizoma) 苍术 9–12g, **huang bai** (Phellodendri Cortex) 黄柏 12–15g, **bi xie** (Dioscoreae hypoglaucae Rhizoma) 萆薢 9–12g and **yi ren** (Coicis Semen) 苡仁 15–30g.

Prepared medicines

Concentrated powders

Liu Wei Di Huang Wan (Rehmannia Six Formula) plus Si Wu Tang (Tangkuei Four Combination)

Pills

Liu Wei Di Huang Wan (Six Flavor Teapills) plus Si Wu Wan (Four Substances for Women Teapills)

Zhuang Yao Jian Shen Pian 壮腰健身片 (Zhuang Yao Jian Shen Tablet)

Acupuncture

Points are chosen based on the location of the pain or stiffness (Table 15.2, p.647–650), with systemic points added to supplement Liver and Kidney yin as follows:

Ren.4 (guanyuan +)............these points supplement Kidney yin and yuan qi
Ren.6 (qihai +)

Kid.3 (taixi +)....................source point of the Kidneys, supplements Kidney yin and clears heat

Kid.7 (fuliu –)....................connecting point of the Kidneys, supplements Kidney yin and clears heat

Lu.7 (lieque)......................master and couple points of renmai, these points
Kid.6 (zhaohai)   open up circulation of renmai qi, and supplement Kidney yin

Sp.6 (sanyinjiao).................nourishes Kidney, Liver and Spleen yin

Bl.23 (shenshu +)...............transport point of the Kidneys, supplements Kidney yin

Bl.52 (zhishi +).................supplements the Kidneys
- with insomnia, add Ht.7 (shenmen) and PC.6 (neiguan –)
- with night sweats, add Ht.6 (yinxi –)
- with anxiety, add yintang (M–HN–3) and Du.20 (baihui)
- with palpitations or arrhythmias add Ht.5 (tongli)
- with dizziness, add Du.20 (baihui)
- Ear points: points relating to affected area, kidneys, adrenal, shenmen

Clinical notes
- Liver and Kidney deficiency painful obstruction may be diagnosed as chronic rheumatoid arthritis, osteoarthritis, chronic lumbago, sciatica or prolapsed lumbar intervertebral disc.
- The pain and stiffness of Liver and Kidney yin deficiency painful obstruction syndrome can respond reasonably well to prolonged treatment.
- Take care not to use too many sour, cold or bitter, cold herbs when clearing heat, to avoid aggravating stagnation.

阴
阳
两
虚

15.12.3 YIN AND YANG DEFICIENCY
This pattern is characterized by chronic stiffness and pain without a specific bias towards heat or cold. The clinical features are those described in the Liver and Kidney and qi and blood deficiency patterns above, and include lower back ache, fatigue, nocturia and urinary frequency and tinnitus, with chronic or recurrent joint and muscle aches, pain, stiffness, numbness and paresthesia.

Treatment principle
Supplement the Liver, Kidneys, qi and blood
Dispel wind damp and stop pain

Prescription

DU HUO JI SHENG TANG 独活寄生汤
Pubescent Angelica and Taxillus Decoction

du huo (Angelicae pubescentis Radix) 独活	9–12g
sang ji sheng (Taxilli Herba) 桑寄生	15–30g
qin jiao (Gentianae macrophyllae Radix) 秦艽	9–12g
fang feng (Saposhnikovae Radix) 防风	9–12g
xi xin (Asari Herba) 细辛	3–6g
du zhong (Eucommiae Cortex) 杜仲	9–12g
huai niu xi (Achyranthis bidentatae Radix) 怀牛膝	9–12g
dang gui (Angelicae sinensis Radix) 当归	9–12g
bai shao (Paeoniae Radix alba) 白芍	9–12g
chuan xiong (Chuanxiong Rhizoma) 川芎	6–9g
shu di (Rehmanniae Radix preparata) 熟地	12–18g
fu ling (Poria) 茯苓	9–12g
ren shen (Ginseng Radix) 人参	6–9g
rou gui (Cinnamomi Cortex) 肉桂	3–6g

zhi gan cao (Glycyrrhizae Radix preparata) 炙甘草................................ 3–6g

Method: Powder or decoction. **Du huo, xi xin, fang feng** and **qin jiao** dispel wind damp and stop pain; **ren shen, fu ling** and **zhi gan cao** supplement qi and assist in the transformation of damp; **shu di, dang gui, bai shao** and **chuan xiong** supplement and activate blood; **rou gui** supports yang qi and dispels cold and assists in stimulating the movement of qi and blood; **du zhong, huai niu xi** and **sang ji sheng** assist **shu di** in supplementing the Liver and Kidneys, as well as strengthening the lower back and knees and supporting the sinews and bones. (Source: *Zhong Yi Nei Ke Xue* [*Qian Jin Yao Fang*])

Modifications

- With cold, add **zhi fu zi** (Aconiti Radix lateralis preparata) 制附子 6–12g.
- With a moderate degree of heat, delete **rou gui**, use **sheng di** (Rehmanniae Radix) 生地 and **chi shao** (Paeoniae Radix rubra) 赤芍 rather than **shu di** and **bai shao**, and add **ren dong teng** (Lonicerae Caulis) 忍冬藤 15–30g and **sang zhi** (Mori Ramulus) 桑枝 15–30g.
- With Spleen deficiency and diarrhea or loose stools, delete **shu di** and add **cang zhu** (Atractylodis Rhizoma) 苍术 9–12g and **yi ren** (Coicis Semen) 苡仁 15–30g.
- With blood stasis, add **tao ren** (Persicae Semen) 桃仁 9–12g and **hong hua** (Carthami Flos) 红花 6–9g.
- For atrophy and weakness of the limbs, add **wu jia pi** (Acanthopanacis Cortex) 五加皮 6–12g, **ji xue teng** (Spatholobi Caulis) 鸡血藤 15–30g and **shen jin cao** (Lycopodii Herba) 伸筋草 9–15g.

Prepared medicines

Concentrated powder

Du Huo Ji Sheng Tang (Tuhuo and Loranthus Combination)
San Bi Tang (Tuhuo & Astragalus Combination)

Pills

Du Huo Ji Sheng Wan (Solitary Hermit Teapills)
San Bi Tang Wan (San Bi Tang Teapills)
Jian Bu Qiang Shen Wan (Aches and Pains Relief Pill)
Da Huo Luo Dan (Tong Ren Da Huo Luo Wan)

Acupuncture

Points are chosen based on the location of the pain or stiffness (Table 15.2, p.647–650), with systemic points added to supplement the Liver and Kidneys drawn from yin deficiency and yang deficiency sections above (pp.687 and 689).

Clinical notes

- Liver and Kidney deficiency painful obstruction may be diagnosed as chronic rheumatoid arthritis, osteoarthritis, chronic lumbago, sciatica or prolapsed lumbar intervertebral disc.
- Treatment of Liver and Kidney deficiency painful obstruction syndrome can be relatively successful, but takes a long time to achieve results.

Table 15.2 Summary of common patterns of painful obstruction syndrome

Pattern	Pain	Other Features	Prescription
Wind damp	joint aches, pain, stiffness and heaviness	pain is diffuse and aching, with swelling and puffiness, a boggy feel to the tissues; worse in humid or overcast weather; mostly affects large joints; greasy white tongue coat, soggy pulse	Juan Bi Tang Qiang Huo Sheng Shi Tang Fang Ji Huang Qi Tang
Cold damp		severe focal pain, worse for cold and significantly better for heat; local tissues may feel cooler than those surrounding; tends to affect the small joints of the hands and feet; pale tongue with a white coat, wiry, tight pulse	Fu Zi Tang Wu Tou Tang Xiao Huo Luo Dan
Heat localized in a joint	red, swollen, painful joint or joints with severely restricted movement	usually a single joint affected; no signs of systemic heat	Gui Zhi Shao Yao Zhi Mu Tang
Damp heat		deep aching pain; single or multiple joints affected; signs of systemic heat; low grade fever, sweats; red tongue with a greasy yellow coat, slippery pulse	Xuan Bi Tang Ma Xing Shi Gan Tang
Toxic heat		high fever, malaise, subcutaneous hemorrhage or other bleeding, disturbances of consciousness; scarlet red tongue with a dry or peeled coat, slippery, surging, wiry, rapid pulse	Bai Hu Tang + Huang Lian Jie Du Tang
Lingering heat in the ying level	joint pain and stiffness, worse at night; may be warm	low grade fever, swollen glands, night sweats; deep red or scarlet tongue with thorns and no coat, fine rapid pulse	Qing Ying Tang
Blood stasis	chronic, intense, focal stabbing pain	joint deformity, hypertrophy, osteophytes; congested vessels and skin discoloration over the affected area; purple tongue with dark congested sublingual veins, rough, wiry, fine pulse	Shen Tong Zhu Yu Tang
Phlegm	mild dull pain, numbness, tingling, paresthesia	joints feel lumpy and nodular, swollen tongue with a greasy white coat, slippery pulse	Ban Xia Bai Zhu Tian Ma Tang + Yang He Tang

Table 15.2 Summary of common patterns of painful obstruction syndrome (cont.)

Pattern	Pain	Other Features	Prescription
Phlegm & blood stasis	focal pain and paresthesia	severe joint deformity, with a mix of phlegm and blood stasis systemic symptoms	Shen Tong Zhu Yu Tang Shuang He Tang Gu Zheng Zeng Sheng Wan
Qi and blood deficiency	dull, intermittent pain, stiffness, weakness and paresthesia	pain better with rest and worse with activity, weak, lax or atrophic tissues; muscle fasciculation; pallor, fatigue, pale tongue, deep, weak pulse	San Bi Tang
Qi and yin deficiency		creaking dry joints with relatively severe stiffness; pain better for rest, worse with use and massage, joints easily inflamed and irritated; dryness, weight loss, pink fat tongue with surface cracks, fine, rapid, weak pulse	Sheng Mai San + Huang Qi Gui Zhi Wu Wu Tang
Liver & Kidney deficiency		yang deficiency: low back and knees mostly affected; edema, cold intolerance, pale, swollen, scalloped tongue	Jin Gui Shen Qi Wan Fu Zi Tang
		yin deficiency: low back, ankles and feet; heat intolerance, sweats, flushing, weight loss; red, dry tongue with no coat	Liu Wei Di Huang Wan + Si Wu Tang
		yin and yang deficiency: no major heat or cold signs; general signs of Liver and Kidney weakness; fatigue and exhaustion, urinary frequency, dizziness, tinnitus; pale tongue	Du Huo Ji Sheng Tang

SWEATING

Sweating occurs constantly and is essential to the body as a means of temperature regulation and as a pathway of elimination. Sweat increases in response to elevated environmental and internal temperatures and serves to assist the body in shedding heat by way of evaporative cooling. As external and internal temperature decreases sweating stops to prevent heat loss. Sweat glands are under the control of the autonomic nervous system. Increasing sympathetic nervous system activity in response to stress and arousal can lead to increased sweating. There are two types of glands that produce secretions on the skin, eccrine and apocrine. Eccrine glands are distributed all over the body, open directly onto the skin, and release a dilute sodium chloride solution. Their primary function is thermoregulation. Apocrine glands release their secretions into hair follicles and are concentrated in the armpits, groin and scalp. They secrete a more viscous, oily sweat that is thought to be associated with mammalian pheromones.

> **BOX 16.1 ABNORMAL SWEATING**
>
> Night sweats, p.702
> Spontaneous, p.726
> Hands and feet, p.739
> Underarm, p.743
> Head and chest, p.751
> Unilateral, p.758
> Genitals, p.762
> Yellow, p.766

Sweating is not perceived as a problem until it impacts on daily life. The most likely type of abnormal sweating to present in the Chinese medicine clinic is night sweats, as these are distinctly uncomfortable and can be a significant disruption to sleep and wellbeing. Patients with excessively sweaty palms can also present as clammy hands are considered a liability in business and social situations. Spontaneous sweating, on the other hand, is a rare presentation unless severe, but a common finding, and one that is important in Chinese medical diagnosis.

VARIETIES OF ABNORMAL SWEATING

Night sweats (*dào hàn* 盗汗)
Literally 'thief sweats', a night sweat is sweating that occurs while the patient is asleep, and stops upon waking. Patients wake suddenly, hot and sweaty, dry off and fall asleep again, at which time the sweating may begin again.

Spontaneous sweating (*zì hàn* 自汗)
Sweating with little or no exertion, which increases significantly with exertion and is not the result of hot weather, overdressing, exercise or consumption of diaphoretic foods or herbs. Spontaneous sweating should be clearly differentiated from the sweating that accompanies acute fever. Spontaneous sweating can be general or localized on the hands and feet, head, chest, armpits or genitals.

Unilateral sweat (*bàn shēn hàn* 半身汗)
Also known as hemihydrosis, this is sweating on one side of the body only. The problem is actually on the side that doesn't sweat. This is usually related to some

type of neurological condition, such as a stroke.

Yellow sweating (*huáng hàn* 黄汗)
Sweat which stains the clothing yellow.

PHYSIOLOGY OF SWEAT

Sweating is an important mechanism by which the body maintains the balance of yin and yang. Sweat is derived from body fluids, which in turn are derived from ingested food and fluids. Sweating is closely associated with the function of the Heart, Lungs and Spleen, and is a function of the relationship between yin fluids and yang qi, in particular the yang qi that inhabits the surface, the wei or protective qi. The wei qi functions as a gatekeeper, allowing the escape of excess physiological heat as sweat, while preventing incursion by external pathogens. Similarly when heat needs to be retained the wei qi shuts down the exits and prevents excessive cooling.

Heart

Sweat is the fluid of the Heart. The Heart governs the blood, and both blood and sweat are derived from the essence of food and fluid. Excessive sweating can deplete the blood and damage the Heart. What these statements refers to is the sensitivity of the Heart to excessive sweating, which when severe, can lead to cardiovascular collapse. Similarly, Heart yang deficiency is observed to cause profuse sweating. In less dramatic circumstances, sweating disorders can be associated with deficiency of Heart qi and disturbances of the shen. Sweating associated with the Heart and shen has an emotional component, and occurs when the patient is nervous or anxious.

Lungs

Wei qi is contiguous with Lung qi, and controls the closing of the pores. Any factor that weakens the Lungs will weaken wei qi and the control of the surface.

Spleen and Stomach

The Spleen and Stomach are the root of acquired qi and thus the qi of all other organ systems. Weakness of the Spleen in gathering sufficient qi is a common contributor to weakness of wei qi. The Spleen and Stomach control the limbs, and pathology of the Spleen and Stomach is often implicated in sweating on the hands and feet.

Liver

The Liver plays a secondary role in sweating. The Livers main influence is through the generation of internal heat from constrained qi, and the weakening of the Spleen and qi that results when the Liver and Spleen axis is disrupted. Prolonged Liver qi constraint can generate heat, which in turn scorches the yin, eventually leading to unrestrained and ascendant yang. The expansive nature of heat and ascendant yang, in concert with the body's attempts to shed the heat, result in sweating. The Liver can also indirectly influence the Lungs, and the Lungs control of wei qi and the pores, by invading the Lungs via the reverse controlling cycle. This accounts for some types of excessive sweating seen in stressful situations.

PATHOLOGY

There are two broad types of abnormal sweating, excess and deficiency. The excess types are due to the presence of a pathogen, typically heat or damp heat, that the body is trying to eliminate. These pathogens may be the result of an external invasion, or can be created by internal imbalances. When generated internally, heat and damp heat are due to prolonged qi constraint, yin deficiency or are introduced with the diet.

Heat and damp heat give rise to different types of pathological sweating. A heat pathogen with its yang, expansive nature, is already forcing fluids towards the surface, and when combined with the efforts of the body's anti–pathogenic qi to eject the pathogen, a vigorous sweat is created. A damp heat pathogen on the other hand, combines the yin stickiness of damp with the yang expansiveness of heat. The damp tends to wrap up the heat and mute it, with the result that the sweat tends to be less pronounced, and concentrated in the afternoon, at night, or on specific regions of the body.

The deficiency types of sweating are associated with weakness of the surface and inability of wei qi to keep the pores properly closed, or creation of internal heat and the expansive force of unrestrained yang. The weakness of wei qi deficiency, and its inability to keep the pores closed, causes fluids to simply leak out. Yang qi deficiency type sweat mostly occurs during the day because wei qi should be most active on the surface during daylight hours.

Creation of internal heat and the expansive force of unrestrained yang are associated with yin and blood deficiency. Yin and blood deficiency sweating mostly occurs at night because the yin yang imbalance, with the relative excess of yang, is most apparent in the yin phase (night) of the daily cycle. It is compounded by the absence of wei qi from the surface as it retreats to the interior during sleep.

ETIOLOGY

External pathogens

Sweating is a feature of any acute febrile illness, but the sweating is secondary to the other symptoms of fever, cough, diarrhea and so on. Persistent sweating as a presenting symptom is more common in the aftermath of an acute febrile illness, and may persist for some time after the initial illness has passed. This is because the pathogen responsible for the initial episode has not been completely cleared, or because its presence has damaged qi and yin.

There are two general locations in which pathogens can linger and cause excessive sweating, the qi level and ying level. The qi level incorporates the shaoyang level, as they both exist between the surface and the deepest recesses of the body. The difference between the qi level and the shaoyang level is simply that qi level pathology veers towards the Lungs, Spleen and Stomach, whereas shaoyang pathology primarily involves the Gallbladder. In terms of location, pathogens in the qi level lead to sweating on those areas functionally associated with the Lungs, Spleen and Stomach – the whole body, or just the chest, head and face, or hands and feet. Shaoyang sweating can be systemic or just on those areas functionally associated with the Gallbladder and Liver systems – the genitals and armpits. The

BOX 16.2 MECHANISM OF SWEATING

1. Heat or ascendant yang

The expansive nature of heat combines with the body's attempts to shed heat and restore the equilibrium of yin and yang. The heat can be generated by deficiency, be the result of an external invasion or be generated by prolonged qi constraint.

- yin deficiency with deficiency heat – night sweats (frequent and severe)
- yin deficiency with ascendant yang – night sweats (mild to moderate)
- qi and blood deficiency – night sweats, spontaneous sweating
- lingering pathogens (heat, damp heat) – night sweats, spontaneous sweating
     (systemic or localized to a specific region)
- Liver qi constraint with heat – night sweats, underarm, head
- Heart and Liver fire – underarms

2. Weak surface and wei qi

Failure of pores to remain closed so fluids simply leak out.

- qi deficiency – spontaneous (systemic or localized to a specific region)
- yang deficiency – spontaneous sweating, head (weak unanchored yang floats away), hands and feet, genitals,
- ying wei disharmony – spontaneous sweating

3. Scattering and constraint of wei qi in response to stress or anxiety

Anxiety can scatter Heart and Lung qi and lead to a weakening of wei qi and a leakage of sweat. Stress can cause Liver qi to rebel backwards through the controlling cycle to damage Lung and wei qi; qi constraint also prevents free movement of wei qi, so control of pores is lost.

- Sweat is the 'fluid of the Heart', so situations that disturb Heart qi and upset the shen (anxiety, public speaking etc.) can lead to sudden onset spontaneous sweat in the areas associated with the Heart organ and channel – palms of the hands, armpits and chest
- Dispersal and constraint of wei qi by pent up Liver qi causes sweating in response to stress, in areas associated with the Liver and Gallbladder – armpits, head, genitals

sweating of shaoyang syndrome is intermittent, appearing as the feverish phase of the cycle occurs.

Emotional factors

Any emotional state that weakens the Lungs, Spleen or Heart can lead to sweating. Worry, brooding, sadness, rumination and isolation can deplete the Lungs and Spleen, and lead to a decrease in production of qi, including wei qi. Repeated invasion of the Spleen by the Liver in response to repressed emotion will also lead to depleted qi. Any situation that disperses Heart qi, such as a sudden or severe shock or prolonged extreme stress, can lead to chronic sweating.

Constitutional factors

Constitutional or inherited weakness of the Lung and Spleen is often associated with poorly controlled sweating. Patients will also experience general weakness and lack of vitality, respiratory problems such as asthma, and poor immunity. A constitutional weakness of Heart qi can also contribute. These patients tend to be anxious and nervous individuals from an early age. The sweating is triggered by stress or anxiety.

Drugs

Some medications can cause excessive sweating. These include pseudoephedrine, antidepressants, aspirin and non steroidal anti–inflammatory drugs (NSAIDs), hypoglycemic agents, caffeine, theophylline and withdrawal from opiates. Excessive alcohol consumption can also contribute to chronic increased sweating.

TREATMENT

Pathological sweating is caused either by an external pathogen or an internal deficiency. These causes must be carefully distinguished, as the treatments applied are very different. Eliminating external pathogens requires all pathways of elimination to remain open and clear to enable the pathogen to escape. The deficiency patterns require supplementation and astringency to consolidate the leakage and prevent escape of vital fluids. The wrong treatment can cause a pathogen to become even more trapped, or can aggravate a deficiency.

Use of astringent herbs

There are numerous herbs that can effectively stop sweating by constricting the surface and tightening the pores (Table 16.1). Astringent herbs provide symptomatic control of sweating while the underlying disease process is being corrected. These herbs must be used judiciously, and only in the right circumstances. When it is certain that no pathogen remains and the pattern is one of deficiency, astringent herbs can be used in addition to whatever supplementing prescription is appropriate. If a pathogen is still in situ, astringents can trap it inside, aggravating the condition.

Table 16.1 Herbs that stop sweat with astringency, for deficient patterns

Herb	Indications
Ma Huang Gen Ephedrae Radix 麻黄	Ephedra root; sweet; Lung. Stops sweat. For all types of deficiency sweating. Quite a strong herb to stop sweating and thus absolutely contraindicated with any residual pathogen. 9-12 grams in decoction.
Fu Xiao Mai Tritici Fructus levis 浮小麦	Wheat; sweet, cool; Heart. Stops sweat. For all types of deficiency sweating, but best when there is a degree of heat, as in yin deficiency. 15-30 grams in decoction.
Wu Wei Zi Schizandrae Fructus 五味子	Schizandra fruit; sour, warm; Lung, Heart, Kidney. Consolidates wei qi and strengthens the Lungs. Treats both yang qi and yin deficient spontaneous sweating and night sweats, but particularly good for weak wei qi. 3-9 grams in decoction.
Wu Bei Zi Galla Chinensis 五倍子	Wasp gall; sour, salty, cold; Lung, Stomach, Large Intestine. For relatively severe night sweats from yin deficiency. 2-5 grams in powder or pills.
Duan Mu Li Ostreae Concha 煅牡蛎	Oyster shell; salty, astringent, cool; Liver, Kidney. Stops sweating by astringing the surface. For all types of deficient sweating, both spontaneous and night. Used in calcined form for sweating, 15-30 grams in decoction, boiled first.
Duan Long Gu Fossilia Ossis Mastodi 煅龙骨	Fossilized bone; sweet, astringent; Heart, Liver, Kidney. Stops sweating by astringing the surface. For all types of deficient sweating. Less astringent than duan mu li, but better at calming the shen. Good for night sweats with sleep and shen disturbances. Used in calcined form for sweating, 15-30 grams in decoction, boiled first.
Suan Zao Ren Ziziphi spinosae Semen 酸枣仁	Zizyphus seed; sweet, sour; Heart, Liver, Gallbladder, Spleen. Augments yin and stops sweating. For night sweats from yin deficiency. Especially good when sleep and shen disturbances are a feature. 12-15 grams in decoction.
Bai Zi Ren Platycladi Semen 柏子仁	Biota seed; sweet, neutral; Heart, Spleen. Augments yin and stops sweating. For night sweats from yin deficiency. 9-12 grams in decoction.
Shan Zhu Yu Corni Fructus 山茱萸	Cornus fruit; sour, astringent; slightly warm, Liver, Kidney. Supplements the Liver and Kidneys and stops sweat. For night sweats from yin deficiency and severe sweating associated with imminent collapse. 6-30 grams in decoction.
Huang Qi Astragali Radix 黄芪	Astragalus root; sweet, warm; Spleen, Lung. Strengthens wei qi to stop sweating. Can be used for both spontaneous and night sweating. Used in the raw state for sweating. 12-30 grams in decoction.

Table 16.2 Acupuncture points with a specific effect on sweating

Point	Indications
Ht.6 yinxi	Cleft point of the Heart, clears heat, nourishes yin and blood fortifies the exterior and constricts the pores. • night sweats with SI.3 houxi • spontaneous sweating with Kid.7 fuliu
Kid.7 fuliu	Strengthens the Kidneys, supplement yin, clears deficiency heat and regulates sweating. • night sweats from yin deficiency with Ht.6 yinxi • spontaneous sweating from qi deficiency with LI.4 hegu and Du.14 dazhui
LI.4 hegu	Source point of the Large Intestine, diffuses the Lungs, strengthens qi and fortifies the exterior. To stop sweating LI.4 is supplemented. • spontaneous sweating with Kid.7 fuliu and Du.14 dazhui
SI.3 houxi	The master point of dumai, activates and consolidates circulation of yang qi through dumai and on the surface, clears heat from the Heart, alleviates qi constraint, dispels wind and vents pathogens. Specifically alleviates night sweats. Can be used for both excess and deficiency patterns. • night sweats with Ht.6 yinxi • night sweats from qi level pathogens with Lu.7 lieque • night sweats from ying level pathogens with Kid.7 fuliu
Du.14 dazhui	Can be used for both deficient types of sweating and lingering pathogens – supplemented or with moxa to fortify the exterior; reduced to vent pathogens • spontaneous sweating with LI.4 hegu and Kid.7 fuliu
Lu.7 lieque	The main point for venting pathogens from the qi level • with LI.4 hegu, Du.14 dazhui and Bl.13 feishu for fortifying the exterior
Bl.15 xinshu	spontaneous sweating from an easily scattered shen and Heart yin deficiency
Bl.13 feishu	spontaneous sweating from weak wei qi; night sweats from Lung yin deficiency
Bl.18 ganshu	spontaneous sweating and night sweats from Liver yin and blood deficiency, and heat in the Liver

Figure 16.1 Common types of sweating

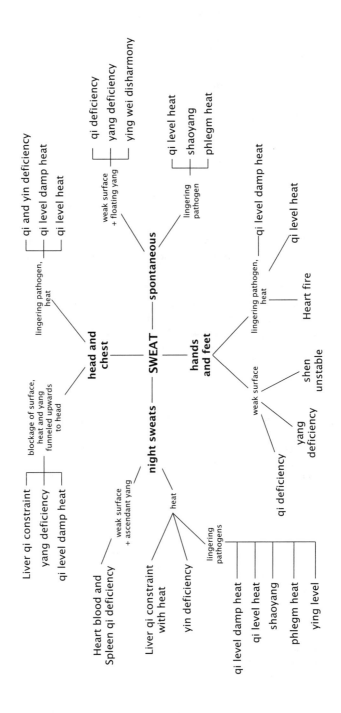

盗汗 16.1 NIGHT SWEATS

1. Yin deficiency with internal heat
2. Heart blood and Spleen qi deficiency
3. Liver qi constraint with heat
4. Lingering pathogens
   • Damp heat in the qi level
   • Heat in the qi level
   • Shaoyang syndrome
   • Phlegm heat
   • Heat in the ying level

A night sweat is characterized by waking from sleep in various degrees of saturation. Once awake, cooling occurs and the sweating ceases. Once dried and with a change of bedclothes, the individual may return to sleep, only for the cycle to repeat itself. In severe cases, sweating can occur many times per night. Night sweats are a common reason to seek treatment, as they can be debilitating, disturbing sleep and leading to chronic tiredness.

Abnormal night sweating should be clearly distinguished from non pathological causes of night sweats related to the environment or food consumed before bed. Causes of non pathological sweats include exercising before bedtime, hot weather or a hot room, too many blankets, heating or rich foods such as red wine, fatty meats, cheese and spices, and sleeping on a full stomach.

BOX 16.3 SOME BIOMEDICAL CAUSES OF NIGHT SWEATS

Infectious
• convalescence from febrile illnesses like pneumonia and influenza
• tuberculosis
• endocarditis
• osteomyelitis
• abscesses (subphrenic, peritoneal, liver, pelvic)
• brucellosis
• histoplasmosis
• chronic malaria
• HIV

Endocrine
• menopause
• carcinoid syndrome
• pheochromocytoma
• hyperthyroidism
• hypoglycemia and diabetes

Malignancy
• lymphoma
• leukemia

Medications
• antidepressants
• niacin
• nitroglycerine
• Viagra
• cortisone, prednisone
• aspirin

Neurological
• syringomyelia
• stroke
• autonomic neuropathy

Other
• sleep apnea
• idiopathic

阴虚火旺
16.1.1 YIN DEFICIENCY WITH INTERNAL HEAT

Yin deficiency with heat or fire is a common cause of night sweats, and can be associated with a gradual loss of yin through ageing, dehydration, drug use and smoking, a sudden loss of yin and blood from hemorrhage or other fluid loss, or yin damage in the aftermath of febrile illness or other heat retained in the body.

The intensity and frequency of the sweats is proportional to the degree of heat, which can range from mild and sporadic to frequent and drenching. The more intense and frequent the sweats, the greater the potential for further damage to yin, through loss of fluids and disturbance to sleep. Even mild degrees of yin deficiency can cause night sweats, and yin deficient sweats often begin gradually, occurring intermittently as yin is damaged by other primary pathology.

The mechanism of the sweating is threefold. First, yin deficiency creates deficiency heat or fire which flares upward and outward, overheating the body, which then attempts to cool itself through sweating. Second, the weakened yin is unable to anchor and restrain yang which floats to the surface, forcing fluids to escape as sweat. Finally, wei qi, which regulates the opening and closing of the pores, retreats internally at night and leaves the surface open to the full effects of the heat and unrestrained yang.

The treatment has two phases. When sweats are severe, the priority is to quickly cool the heat and stop the fluid loss, as continued loss of sweat will aggravate the yin deficiency. In mild to moderate sweats, supplementing yin to cool the heat is the main strategy, with some astringency to secure the exterior as appropriate.

Clinical features
- Night sweats. Multiple sweats may occur each night; sweating occurs at regular intervals and the sweat is watery, non staining and odorless.
- Sweating may be accompanied by a sense of heat emanating from deep within the body ('bone steaming'). Patients may also experience afternoon tidal fever, hot flushes and malar flushing.
- sensation of heat in the palms and soles
- dry mouth, lips, throat and mucous membranes
- scanty, concentrated urine
- dry stools, constipation
- fatigue and exhaustion with an inability to rest or relax
- lower back and legs aching
- thin body type, weight loss
- maybe chronic dry cough
- menstrual irregularity, amenorrhea, perimenopause, menopause

T red and dry with little or no coat
P fine and rapid

Treatment Principle
Clear deficiency heat and supplement yin
Secure the exterior and alleviate sweating

Prescription

DANG GUI LIU HUANG TANG 当归六黄汤
Tangkuei and Six Yellow Decoction

This prescription is focused on clearing heat and cooling the blood, and is used for severe sweating, only until the sweats have been significantly alleviated. This should be no more than a few weeks, after which a more yin supplementing strategy can be adopted. See Clinical notes for more.

dang gui (Angelicae sinensis Radix) 当归 6–9g
shu di (Rehmanniae Radix preparata) 熟地 9–15g
sheng di (Rehmanniae Radix) 生地 9–15g
huang qi (Astragali Radix) 黄芪 9–15g
huang qin (Scutellariae Radix) 黄芩 6–12g
huang bai (Phellodendri Cortex) 黄柏 6–12g
huang lian (Coptidis Rhizoma) 黄连 3–9g

Method: Decoction. **Dang gui**, **sheng di** and **shu di** supplement Liver and Kidney yin and blood, and protect yin and blood from damage by the bitter cold herbs; **sheng di** cools the blood; **huang qin**, **huang lian** and **huang bai** clear heat from all three burners, and cool the blood; **huang qi** fortifies wei qi and secures the exterior to keep the pores closed. (Source: *Zhong Yi Nei Ke Xue* [*Lan Shi Mi Cang*])

Modifications

- Depending on the relative doses of herbs in this prescription, the effect can vary considerably. When heat/fire is predominant, the sweats are frequent and the fluid loss can aggravate the yin deficiency, so clearing heat is a priority. The main herbs in the prescription are sweet cold **sheng di**, and the bitter cold heat clearing **huang qin**, **huang lian** and **huang bai**. Their doses should reflect their status, being towards the upper end of the dosage range. As the heat clears and sweats abate, the possibility of yin damage from the bitterness increases, and the dose of the three bitter cold herbs should decrease and the emphasis placed on supplementing yin. The doses of **shu di** and **sheng di** can be increased, with **huang lian**, **qin** and **bai** towards the low end of the dosage range, or even less.

- For persistent sweating (beyond a week or two), add **shan zhu yu** (Corni Fructus) 山茱萸 12–15g, **ma huang gen** (Ephedrae Radix) 麻黄根 9–12g and **wu wei zi** (Schizandrae Fructus) 五味子 3–6g, or **duan mu li** (calcined Ostreae Concha) 煅牡蛎 18–30g and **duan long gu** (calcined Fossilia Ossis Mastodi) 煅龙骨 18–30g [the last two cooked first].

- For tidal fever and bone steaming, add **yin chai hu** (Stellariae Radix) 银柴胡 9–12g, **zhi mu** (Anemarrhenae Rhizoma) 知母 6–9g and **bie jia** (Trionycis Carapax) 鳖甲 12–15g.

- With dry eyes and visual weakness, add **gou qi zi** (Lycii Fructus) 枸杞子 12–15g and **ju hua** (Chrysanthemi Flos) 菊花 9–12g.

- With dry cough or hemoptysis, add **bai mao gen** (Imperatae Rhizoma) 白茅根 12–15g, **xuan shen** (Scrophulariae Radix) 玄参 12–15g and **chuan bei mu** (Fritillariae cirrhosae Bulbus) 川贝母 6–9g.

- With constipation, add **xuan shen** (Scrophulariae Radix) 玄参 15–18g and **mai dong** (Ophiopogonis Radix) 麦冬 9–12g.

Variations and additional prescriptions

Less fire, moderate or intermittent night sweats, or following alleviation of the worst of the sweats

In situations where the heat and sweats are less severe and therefore less likely to be a contributing factor to swift yin depletion, a more yin supplementing strategy is more suitable. A good choice is ZHI BAI DI HUANG WAN (Anemarrhena, Phellodendron and Rehmannia Pill 知柏地黄丸, p.922), suitable for Kidney yin deficiency patterns with moderate deficiency heat, intermittent night sweats, flushing and heat intolerance. With relatively little heat and intermittent sweats, LIU WEI DI HUANG WAN (Six Ingredient Pill with Rehmannia 六味地黄丸, p.192) can be selected to rebuild the yin in the long term.

Fever or tidal fever, restless sleep with occasional sweats

When the patient has recurrent tidal, afternoon or night fever as the main feature, with intermittent night sweating, the treatment is to clear deficiency heat and alleviate bone steaming with QING GU SAN (Cool the Bones Powder 清骨散, p.391) or DA BU YIN WAN (Great Supplement the Yin Pill 大补阴丸, p.914).

Lung yin deficiency

Lung yin deficiency was a major cause of night sweats in the days when tuberculosis was widespread. Lung yin deficiency can also result from smoking, exposure to respiratory irritants or long term steroid use in the treatment of asthma. When Lung yin deficiency is the main pathology, the features include a chronic, weak, dry cough with small amounts of blood streaked sputum, in addition to frequent night sweats. The treatment is to nourish and moisten Lung and Kidney yin, and clear heat with BAI HE GU JIN TANG (Lily Bulb Decoction to Preserve the Metal 百合固金汤).

bai he (Lilii Bulbus) 百合 9–15g
shu di (Rehmanniae Radix preparata) 熟地 9–12g
sheng di (Rehmanniae Radix) 生地 9–12g
dang gui (Angelicae sinensis Radix) 当归 6–9g
bai shao (Paeoniae Radix alba) 白芍 6–9g
jie geng (Platycodi Radix) 桔梗 3–6g
xuan shen (Scrophulariae Radix) 玄参 6–9g
chuan bei mu (Fritillariae cirrhosae Bulbus) 川贝母 3–6g
mai dong (Ophiopogonis Radix) 麦冬 6–9g
gan cao (Glycyrrhizae Radix) 甘草 3–6g

Method: Decoction or powders. **Bai he** nourishes yin, clears heat, moistens the Lungs and stops cough; **sheng di** and **shu di** supplement yin and blood; **sheng di** and **xuan shen** cool the blood and clear heat; **mai dong** cools and moistens the Lungs; **chuan bei mu** cools the Lungs, transforms phlegm and stops cough; **dang gui** and **bai shao** nourish and harmonize blood; **jie geng** expels phlegm, stops cough and directs the action of the formula to the upper body; **gan cao** harmonizes the other herbs. (Source: *Yi Fang Ji Jie*)

Liver yin deficiency

Liver yin deficiency causes milder and less frequent night sweats than Kidney yin deficiency (although of course they can occur together). One of the reasons that the sweats are relatively infrequent is that insomnia is a major problem, and unless the patient sleeps, night sweats will not occur. The insomnia of Liver yin deficiency is aggravated by worrying about the insomnia itself. Other features include intense or violent dreaming, tooth grinding, talking during sleep, or in severe cases, sleep walking. In addition, these patients tend to be quick tempered and have a dry throat, sore, gritty, dry eyes, visual disturbances and dizziness. The pulse is wiry or fine and rapid. The treatment is to nourish Liver blood, calm the hun and shen and stop sweating with Suan Zao Ren Tang (Sour Jujube Decoction 酸枣仁汤) modified.

suan zao ren (Ziziphi spinosae Semen) 酸枣仁 15–18g
fu ling (Poria) 茯苓 12–15g
zhi mu (Anemarrhenae Rhizoma) 知母 9–12g
chuan xiong (Chuanxiong Rhizoma) 川芎 6–9g
gan cao (Glycyrrhizae Radix) 甘草 3–6g
di gu pi (Lycii Cortex) 地骨皮 9–12g
wu wei zi (Schizandrae Fructus) 五味子 6–9g

Method: Decoction. **Suan zao ren** nourishes yin and blood and calms the shen and hun; **fu ling** strengthens the Spleen and calms the shen; **zhi mu** nourishes yin and clears heat; **chuan xiong** regulates and activates qi and blood to prevent stagnation; **gan cao** supplements Heart qi; **di gu pi** clears heat from the blood; **wu wei zi** stops sweating, calms the shen and secures the hun. (Source: *Jin Gui Yao Lüe*)

Kidney yin and yang deficiency

Yin deficiency can be complicated by yang deficiency. The yin deficiency is most apparent in the deficiency heat and ascendant yang in the upper body, seen in frequent night sweats, hot flushing, irritability, insomnia and dizziness. The yang deficiency is typically concentrated below, seen in urinary frequency, nocturia, and cold legs and feet. Patients are easily overheated, then cold and unable to warm up, or hot at night and cold in the early hours of the morning. When the unanchored yang is particularly frenetic, internal wind may result, causing tics, spasms and muscle fasciculation. The treatment is to warm Kidney yang while nourishing Kidney yin and clearing deficiency heat with Er Xian Tang (Two Immortal Decoction 二仙汤).

xian mao (Curculiginis Rhizoma) 仙茅 6–9g
xian ling pi (Epimedii Herba) 仙灵脾 9–15g
dang gui (Radix Angelicae Sinensis) 当归 9–12g
ba ji tian (Morindae officinalis Radix) 巴戟天 9–12g
huang bai (Phellodendri Cortex) 黄柏 6–9g
zhi mu (Anemarrhenae Rhizoma) 知母 6–9g

Method: Decoction. **Xian mao** and **xian ling pi** warm Kidney yang and support jing; **ba ji tian** warms Kidney yang and strengthens the sinews and bones; **dang gui** nourishes blood, softens the Liver; **zhi mu** and **huang bai** nourish Kidney yin and clear deficiency heat, and moderate the pungent hot dispersing nature of **xian mao** and **xian ling pi**. (Source: *Shanghai Shu Guan Yi Yuan Jing Yan Fang*)

Qi and yin deficiency

Prolonged yin deficiency is often accompanied by qi deficiency, especially when the Lungs have been affected. Qi and yin deficiency can follow a Lung heat pattern or other febrile illness, with high fever and profuse sweating. It can also be the result of a chronic cough and smoking. The main symptoms are night sweats and daytime spontaneous sweating, persistent dry cough, breathlessness, dryness of mucous membranes, thirst and a red dry, or red and swollen tongue. The treatment is to nourish Lung and Kidney qi and yin with a mixture of Liu Wei Di Huang Wan (Six Ingredient Pill with Rehmannia 六味地黄丸, p.192) and Sheng Mai San (Generate the Pulse Powder 生脉散, p.728).

Prepared medicines
Concentrated powders
Dang Gui Liu Huang Tang (Tangkuei and Six Yellow Combination)
 – severe and frequent sweats
Da Bu Yin Wan (Rehmannia & Testudinis Combination)
Zhi Bai Di Huang Wan (Anemarrhena, Phellodendron & Rehmannia Formula)
Er Xian Tang (Curculigo & Epimedium Combination)
 – yin and yang deficiency
Suan Zao Ren Tang (Zizyphus Combination)
 – Liver yin deficiency

Pills
Da Bu Yin Wan (Abundant Yin Teapills)
Zhi Bai Ba Wei Wan (Eight Flavor Rehmannia Teapills)
Er Xian Wan (Two Immortals Teapills)
Kun Bao Wan (Women's Treasure Pills)
 – Liver and Kidney yin deficiency
Xu Han Ting (Stop Deficient Sweat)
 – an astringent formula to stop sweating; can be added to any formula above

Acupuncture (select from)
Ht.6 (yinxi –) ....cleft point of the Heart, clears heat, supplements yin and constricts the pores to stop sweating
Kid.7 (fuliu +) ....metal point of the Kidneys, supplements yin, clears deficiency heat and regulates sweating
SI.3 (houxi –) ....master point of dumai, clears heat, cools the Heart, and constricts the pores to stop sweating
Ren.4 (guanyuan +)...........supplements Kidney yin and yuan qi
Bl.13 (feishu +) ....transport point of the Lungs, strengthens wei qi and the control of closing of the pores
Bl.23 (shenshu +) ....transport point of the Kidneys, supplements Kidney yin
Kid.2 (rangu –) ....fire point of the Kidneys, clears heat and cools the blood
Kid.3 (taixi +)....................source point of the Kidneys, supplements Kidney yin and clears deficiency heat
Sp.6 (sanyinjiao).................nourishes Kidney and Liver yin

- With qi deficiency, add LI.4 (hegu +) and St.36 (zusanli +)
- With Liver yin deficiency, add Bl.18 (ganshu +) and Liv.3 (taichong +)
- with insomnia, add Ht.7 (shenmen) and PC.6 (neiguan –)
- with anxiety, add yintang (M–HN–3) and Du.20 (baihui)
- with forgetfulness, add Du.20 (baihui) and Bl.52 (zhishi)
- with palpitations or arrhythmias add Ht.5 (tongli)
- with dizziness, add Du.20 (baihui)
- Ear points: kidney, lung, liver, subcortex, endocrine, shenmen

Clinical notes
- Night sweats of a yin deficiency type may be associated with conditions such as menopausal syndrome, hyperthyroidism, pulmonary tuberculosis, post–operative fever, postpartum convalescence, lymphoma and the aftermath of chronic infection.
- Night sweats from yin deficiency can respond well to treatment, depending on the length and severity of the deficiency. Night sweats associated with a yin deficiency menopause respond well; similarly those associated with post febrile convalescence. If associated with pulmonary tuberculosis or lymphoma, herbal or acupuncture treatment should be combined with appropriate antibiotic or therapy.
- The primary prescription, DANG GUI LIU HUANG TANG, is aimed at quickly alleviating the night sweats by cooling heat rather than enriching yin. Persistent night sweats can further deplete already damaged yin. Being bitter and cold, however, the formula treads a fine line between clearing the heat and aggravating the yin deficiency, and so must be used carefully.
- A yin nourishing diet is recommended. See Clinical Handbook, Vol.2, p.876.

心
脾
兩
虛

16.1.2 HEART BLOOD AND SPLEEN QI DEFICIENCY

Heart blood and Spleen qi deficiency can be a cause of both night sweats and spontaneous daytime sweating, depending on the balance of qi and blood deficiency. The more qi deficiency, the more spontaneous daytime sweating, the greater the blood deficiency, the more likely night sweats. Many patients will experience both to some extent. Heart and Spleen qi deficiency is also a common cause of sweaty palms.

Blood deficiency is able to generate some deficient heat, and patients may feel quite hot or easily overheat. In addition, blood deficiency can lead to Liver qi constraint which in turn can generate constrained heat, a common complication and one likely to aggravate the night sweats. The heat and symptoms of shen disturbance may resemble those observed in the yin deficiency pattern. The key differentiating feature is the pale tongue.

Clinical features
- Night sweats. Depending on the degree of blood deficiency and the degree of heat present, the sweats may occur intermittently or frequently. There may also be spontaneous sweating during the day, general clamminess and cool clammy palms. The sweat may be systemic, or concentrated on the chest and upper

back, and is watery, non staining and odorless.
- insomnia, fitful sleep broken with sweats, dream disturbed sleep
- palpitations; anxiety, panic attacks
- breathlessness with exertion
- fatigue, listlessness
- pale sallow complexion; cheeks and ears may be red
- poor appetite
- scanty periods, amenorrhea, or persistent uterine bleeding; easy bruising

T pale with a thin, white coat; the edges of the tongue may have an orange tint
P weak and fine, or big, floating and weak

Treatment Principle
Supplement Heart blood and Spleen qi
Calm the shen and stop sweating

Prescription

GUI PI TANG 归脾汤
Restore the Spleen Decoction, modified

zhi huang qi (honey fried Astragali Radix) 炙黄芪 9–12g
fu shen (Poria Sclerotium pararadicis) 茯神 9–12g
bai zhu (Atractylodes macrocephalae Rhizoma) 白术 9–12g
long yan rou (Longan Arillus) 龙眼肉 9–12g
suan zao ren (Ziziphi spinosae Semen) 酸枣仁 9–12g
ren shen (Ginseng Radix) 人参 6–9g
dang gui (Angelicae sinensis Radix) 当归 6–9g
yuan zhi (Polygalae Radix) 远志 3–6g
mu xiang (Aucklandiae Radix) 木香 3–6g
gan cao (Glycyrrhizae Radix) 甘草 3–6g
wu wei zi (Schizandrae Fructus) 五味子 3–6g
fu xiao mai (Semen Tritici Aestivi Levis) 浮小麦 12–15g

Method: Decoction. **Zhi huang qi**, **ren shen**, **bai zhu** and **gan cao** strengthen the Spleen and supplement qi; **dang gui** and **zhi huang qi** together have a special effect on building blood; **fu shen** strengthens the Spleen and calms the shen; **suan zao ren**, **long yan rou** and **yuan zhi** nourish the Heart and calm the shen; **fu ling** strengthens the Spleen and calms the shen; **mu xiang** regulates qi and aids the Spleen in digesting the blood supplementing herbs; **wu wei zi** and **fu xiao mai** astringe and secure the surface to alleviate sweating and calm the shen. (Source: *Shi Yong Zhong Yi Nei Ke Xue* [*Ji Sheng Fang*])

Modifications
- With marked blood deficiency, postural dizziness, a very pale tongue and amenorrhea, add one or two of the following herbs: **shu di** (Rehmanniae Radix preparata) 熟地 12–15g, **bai shao** (Paeoniae Radix alba) 白芍 9–12g, **gou qi zi** (Lycii Fructus) 枸杞子 9–12g or **e jiao** (Asini Corii Colla) 阿胶 9–12g [dissolved in the strained decoction].
- With copious sweating, add **duan mu li** (calcined Ostreae Concha) 煅牡蛎 18–30g [cooked first] and **ma huang gen** (Ephedrae Radix) 麻黄根 9–12g.
- With heat in the Liver, add **shan zhi zi** (Gardeniae Fructus) 山栀子 9–12g

and **chai hu** (Bupleuri Radix) 柴胡 6–9g.

- With cold, add **rou gui** (Cinnamomi Cortex) 肉桂 3–6g.
- With digestive weakness, abdominal distension and a poor appetite, use **chao dang gui** (stir fried Angelicae sinensis Radix) 炒当归, and add **shen qu** (Massa medicata fermentata) 神曲 9–12g and **chen pi** (Pericarpium Citri Reticulatae) 陈皮 9–12g.
- With low grade fever, add **yin chai hu** (Stellariae Radix) 银柴胡 9–12g, **di gu pi** (Lycii Cortex) 地骨皮 12–15g and **mu dan pi** (Moutan Cortex) 牡丹皮 9–12g.
- With loose stools and a thick tongue coat, add **cang zhu** (Rhizoma Atractylodis) 苍术 12–15g.

Variations and additional prescriptions
Qi, blood and yin deficiency
A relatively common pattern of night sweats involves Heart qi, blood and yin deficiency. The symptoms are frequent night sweats and palpitations or tachycardia, in a patient with an irregularly irregular pulse. The more irregular the heartbeat, the greater the deficiency. Stopping the sweating quickly is an essential component of rebuilding Heart qi, blood and yin. Continued loss of fluid in this way further weakens the Heart as sweat is the fluid of the Heart. The treatment is to alleviate sweating, supplement qi and nourish blood and yin, unblock yang qi and restore the pulse with ZHI GAN CAO TANG (Prepared Licorice Decoction 炙甘草汤), modified.

zhi gan cao (Glycyrrhizae Radix preparata) 炙甘草 12–15g
sheng di (Rehmanniae Radix) 生地 24–30g
ren shen (Ginseng Radix) 人参 6–9g
sheng jiang (Zingiberis Rhizoma recens) 生姜 6–9g
gui zhi (Cinnamomi Ramulus) 桂枝 6–9g
e jiao (Asini Corii Colla) 阿胶 6–9g
mai dong (Ophiopogonis Radix) 麦冬 15–24g
da zao (Jujubae Fructus) 大枣 ....4–8 fruit
bai zi ren (Platycladi Semen) 柏子仁 9–12g
suan zao ren (Ziziphi spinosae Semen) 酸枣仁 12–15g
duan long gu (calcined Fossilia Ossis Mastodi) 煅龙骨 15–30g
duan mu li (calcined Ostreae Concha) 煅牡蛎 15–30g

Method: Decoction. **Duan mu li** and **duan long gu** are decocted for 30–60 minutes prior to the other herbs, **e jiao** is melted in hot water or rice wine before being added to the strained decoction. **Zhi gan cao** supplements qi, strengthens the Spleen and Stomach and unblocks the flow of yang qi to the Heart; **ren shen** and **da zao** strengthen the Spleen, boost qi, nourish the Heart and support yuan qi; **sheng di**, **mai dong** and **e jiao** nourish yin, and moisten dryness; the pungent warmth of **sheng jiang**, **gui zhi** and the rice wine promote the movement of yang qi in the chest and assist in restoring the pulse; **bai zi ren** and **suan zao ren** nourish the Heart and stop sweating; **duan long gu** and **duan mu li** astringe sweating, settle the Heart and calm the shen. (Source: *Shi Yong Fang Ji Xue* [*Shang Han Lun*])

Instability of the shen and scattering of Heart qi following shock or trauma
Night sweats (here, the classic cold sweat), nightmares, anxiety and panic attacks

may occur suddenly following a major shock or trauma. These symptoms are typical of post traumatic stress disorder, and are associated with a sudden loss communication between the Heart and Kidneys brought on by shock. In addition to the features noted above, patients experience loss of appetite, depression, lack of motivation and hair loss. When the tongue is pale and the pulse weak, the pattern is one of damage to qi and blood, and the treatment is to support Heart qi and nourish Heart blood, rectify the balance of yin and yang and calm the shen with GUI ZHI JIA LONG GU MU LI TANG (Cinnamon Twig Decoction plus Dragon Bone and Oyster Shell 桂枝加龙骨牡蛎汤).

gui zhi (Cinnamomi Ramulus) 桂枝 6–9g
bai shao (Paeoniae Radix alba) 白芍 6–9g
duan long gu (calcined Fossilia Ossis Mastodi) 煅龙骨 15–30g
duan mu li (calcined Ostreae Concha) 煅牡蛎 15–30g
sheng jiang (Zingiberis Rhizoma recens) 生姜 6–9g
da zao (Jujubae Fructus) 大枣 .... 4 fruit
gan cao (Glycyrrhizae Radix) 甘草 3–6g

Method: Decoction. **Duan mu li** and **duan long gu** are decocted for 30–60 minutes prior to the other herbs. **Gui zhi** warms and mobilizes yang and supports fire, while **bai shao** preserves yin, nourishes blood and maintains water. Together they balance each other in such a way as to harmonize and regulate yin and yang, both in the narrow sense of ying wei imbalance on the surface, and in the broader context of a Heart Kidney imbalance, disconnection between water and fire, the zhi and shen. The heaviness of **duan long gu** and **duan mu li** draws the action of the principal herbs away from the surface and into the body. At the same time they anchor yang, astringe sweating and calm the shen. **Sheng jiang**, **da zao** and **gan cao** support the Spleen and qi production. (Source: *Jin Gui Yao Lüe*)

Prepared medicines
Concentrated powders
Gui Pi Tang (Ginseng & Longan Combination)
Yang Xin Tang (Astragalus & Zizyphus Combination)
Zhi Gan Cao Tang (Licorice Combination)
Gui Zhi Jia Long Gu Mu Li Tang (Cinnamon & Dragon Bone Combination)

Pills
Gui Pi Wan (Kwei Be Wan, Gui Pi Teapills)
Bai Zi Yang Xin Wan (Pai Tzu Yang Hsin Wan)
Dang Gui Ji Jing (Tang Kuei Essence of Chicken)
    – especially good for postpartum sweats
Xu Han Ting (Stop Deficient Sweat)
    – an astringent formula to stop sweating; can be added to any formula above

Acupuncture (select from)
LI.4 (hegu +) ....source point of the Large Intestine, fortifies the surface and supplements qi (with St.36)
Kid.7 (fuliu +) ....metal point of the Kidneys, stops sweating and supplements the Kidneys
Ht.6 (yinxi –) ....cleft point of the Heart, nourishes Heart blood and constricts the pores to stop sweating

Du.14 (dazhui +▲)............meeting point of the yang channels, fortifies the exterior and stops sweating

Ren.12 (zhongwan +▲) .....alarm point of the Stomach, strengthens the Spleen and Stomach to supplement qi and blood

St.36 (zusanli +▲) ....sea point of the Stomach, strengthens the Spleen and Stomach and supplements qi and blood

Sp.6 (sanyinjiao +▲)..........strengthens the Spleen and Kidneys and supplements qi and blood

Bl.15 (xinshu +) ....transport point of the Heart, supplements Heart qi, calms the Heart and shen

Bl.20 (pishu +▲) ....transport point of the Spleen, strengthens the Spleen and supplements qi and blood

- Ear points: heart, spleen, lung, zero point, subcortex, sympathetic, shenmen

Clinical notes
- Qi and blood deficiency is a common cause of night sweats in postpartum women, and may also occur during convalescence from a serious illness or following injury and blood loss.
- Heart and Spleen deficiency can also be a cause of spontaneous daytime sweating and sweating from the hands and feet and chest.
- A qi and blood nourishing diet is recommended. See Clinical Handbook, Vol.2, p.870 and 874.

16.1.3 LIVER QI CONSTRAINT WITH HEAT

气郁化火

Liver qi constraint with heat is a common cause of night sweats in premenstrual and perimenopausal women, and although more common in women, it is seen in men as well. Chronic qi constraint with heat will gradually deplete Liver yin, so there will usually be a component of yin deficiency. If the pattern is allowed to progress, yin will be further depleted and the primary pathology will become one of deficiency.

Clinical features
- Intermittent night sweats that are worse during periods of increased stress, before a menstrual period is due or when upset.
- irritability, anger outbursts, depression
- tension or migraine headaches
- hypochondriac ache, chest oppression
- insomnia or restless dream disturbed sleep
- red complexion; red, sore eyes
- bitter taste in the mouth, dry mouth, thirst
- acid reflux, heartburn, nausea, belching
- constipation with dry stools
- neck and shoulder tightness and pain, elevated shoulders (tight trapezius)
- irregular menstruation, short menstrual cycle, heavy periods or abnormal bleeding; premenstrual syndrome with increased irritability and mood swings, premenstrual breast tenderness with hypersensitive nipples, premenstrual acne

T red or with red edges and a thin, yellow coat
P wiry and rapid

Treatment Principle
Dredge the Liver, regulate qi and relieve qi constraint
Cool the Liver and clear heat

Prescription

JIA WEI XIAO YAO SAN 加味逍遥散
Augmented Rambling Powder

chai hu (Bupleuri Radix) 柴胡 9–12g
bai shao (Paeoniae Radix alba) 白芍 12–18g
dang gui (Angelicae sinensis Radix) 当归 9–12g
fu ling (Poria) 茯苓 12–15g
bai zhu (Atractylodis macrocephalae Rhizoma) 白术 9–12g
shan zhi zi (Gardeniae Fructus) 山栀子 9–12g
mu dan pi (Moutan Cortex) 牡丹皮 9–12g
zhi gan cao (Glycyrrhizae Radix preparata) 炙甘草 3–6g
Method: Decoction. **Chai hu** dredges the Liver, regulates qi and clears heat; **bai shao** softens the Liver and, with **dang gui**, nourishes Liver blood; **fu ling**, **bai zhu** and **zhi gan cao** strengthen the Spleen; **fu ling** promotes urination and drains damp; **bai zhu** dries damp; **shan zhi zi** and **mu dan pi** cool the Liver and clear heat. (Source: *Nei Ke Zhai Yao*)

Modifications
- For persistent sweats, add **ma huang gen** (Ephedrae Radix) 麻黄根 9–12g and **duan mu li** (calcined Ostreae Concha) 煅牡蛎 18–30g [cooked first].
- With yin damage, peeled edges on the tongue, a fine pulse and dry eyes, delete **bai zhu** and **sheng jiang**, and add **sheng di** (Rehmanniae Radix) 生地 12–18g, **mai dong** (Ophiopogonis Radix) 麦冬 9–12g and **shan yao** (Dioscoreae Rhizoma) 山药 9–12g.
- With reflux and heartburn, add **huang lian** (Coptidis Rhizoma) 黄连 6–9g and **wu zhu yu** (Evodiae Fructus) 吴茱萸 2–3g.
- With anger outbursts and headaches add **ju hua** (Chrysanthemi Flos) 菊花 9–12g, **bai ji li** (Tribuli Fructus) 白蒺藜 9–12g and **gou teng** (Uncariae Ramulus cum Uncis) 钩藤 9–12g.

Prepared medicines
Concentrated powders
Jia Wei Xiao Yao San (Bupleurum & Peony Formula)

Pills
Jia Wei Xiao Yao Wan (Free and Easy Wanderer Plus Teapills, Dan Zhi Xiao Yao Wan)

Acupuncture (select from)
Ht.6 (yinxi –) ....cleft point of the Heart, clears heat, supplements Heart yin and constricts the pores to stop sweating
Kid.7 (fuliu +) ....metal point of the Kidneys, supplements the Kidneys and stops sweating

SI.3 (houxi –)......................opens dumai to activate circulation of yang qi and alleviate night sweats

Liv.3 (taichong –)................the 'four gates', these points mobilize qi and blood,
LI.4 (hegu +)   calm the shen and hun; LI.4 (hegu) also works with Ht.6 (yinxi) to control sweating

PC.6 (neiguan)...................opens up qi flow through the chest, dredges the liver and moves constrained qi, calms the Heart and shen, downbears counterflow Stomach qi

Liv.2 (xingjian –)................fire point of the Liver, cools the Liver and alleviates constrained qi

GB.34 (yanglingquan –)......sea point of the Gallbladder, regulates qi and calms hyperactive Liver yang

- Ear points: liver, heart, zero point, subcortex, sympathetic, shenmen

Clinical notes
- Liver qi constraint with heat type night sweats may be diagnosed as premenstrual syndrome, menopause, autonomic nervous system imbalance, sympathetic overload, hyperthyroidism, or a response to chronic stress.
- The sweats of this pattern generally respond well to treatment, as long as the lifestyle factors of exercise and stress management are attended to.
- Exercise and stress management are essential components of short and long term management. See p.103.
- Hot spot therapy can be helpful, p.923.
- A qi mobilizing diet is recommended. See Clinical Handbook, Vol.2, p.878.

留邪

16.1.4 LINGERING PATHOGENS

Lingering pathogens are a common cause of night sweats. The sweats can be of relatively short duration, appearing for a few weeks in the convalescent phase of an acute febrile illness, or be chronic and occur continually or intermittently for years. Many patterns of lingering pathogen can cause night sweats (see Chapter 11), but the sweats are usually sporadic and secondary to symptoms of fatigue and weakness, muscles aches and fever. The patterns in which night sweats can be more intense and the main concern are listed in this section.

湿热在气分

16.1.4.1 DAMP HEAT IN THE QI LEVEL

Damp heat in the qi level is a common cause of night sweating. Damp heat can lodge in different locations, with manifestations specific to the organ system or location involved. There are different grades of heat that occur in damp heat patterns. The more heat there is, the more copious and frequent the sweating. When damp heat affects specific organ systems, night sweats may feature, but will usually be incidental to the main presenting problem, such as jaundice or hypochondriac pain when damp heat affects the Liver, painful urination or urgent diarrhea when damp heat is located in the Urinary Bladder or Large Intestine, and so on. When damp heat is located in the qi level, it is more diffusely spread, and night sweats are often prominent. For damp heat located in specific organ systems see the relevant section in Hypochondriac pain (Vol.1), Painful Urination (Vol.1), Dysenteric disorder and Diarrhea (Vol.2).

Clinical features
- Night sweats. Usually only one or two sweats per night, but sweats may occur every night. The sweat is sticky or oily, may stain the bedclothes, and smell. Sweating may also occur in the afternoon, accompanied by a rising low grade fever. Damp heat in the qi level can also cause sweating just on the head, or hands and feet.
- low grade fever which typically rises or reaches a peak mid afternoon
- dull headache, heavy head as if 'wrapped in a wet towel', foggy head
- muscle aches and muscle weakness
- fatigue, lethargy; increased desire to sleep
- chest oppression and abdominal distension
- loss of appetite, nausea
- loose stools, diarrhea or sticky or difficult to pass stools
- swollen lymph nodes

T thick, greasy, yellow coat
P slippery, wiry or soft; maybe rapid

Treatment Principle
Clear and vent damp heat from the qi level
Diffuse the Lungs and direct Lung qi downward to promote urination
Correct the qi dynamic

Prescription

SAN REN TANG 三仁汤
Three Nut Decoction

---

xing ren (Armeniacae Semen) 杏仁 12–15g
bai dou kou (Amomi Fructus rotundus) 白豆蔻 6–9g
yi ren (Coicis Semen) 苡仁.. 18–30g
zhi ban xia (Pinelliae Rhizoma preparatum) 制半夏 9–12g
hou po (Magnoliae officinalis Cortex) 厚朴... 6–9g
dan zhu ye (Lophateri Herba) 淡竹叶.. 6–9g
hua shi (Talcum) 滑石 12–18g
tong cao (Medulla Tetrapanacis Papyriferi) 通草 6–9g

Method: Decoction. **Bai dou kou** is added towards the end of cooking and **hua shi** is decocted in a cloth bag. **Xing ren** directs Lung qi downward and promotes urination to provide an outlet for the damp heat; **bai dou kou** transforms damp and rectifies the qi dynamic; **yi ren** leaches damp heat from the lower burner via the urine; the ascending pungency of **zhi ban xia** counterbalances the bitter descent of **hou po** to drive the qi dynamic; **dan zhu ye**, **hua shi** and **tong cao** promote urination to clear damp heat. (Source: *Wen Bing Tiao Bian*)

Modifications
- With intense heat, frequent sweats, and a red tongue, add **shan zhi zi** (Gardeniae Fructus) 山栀子 6–9g and **huang qin** (Scutellariae Radix) 黄芩 6–9g. See also **LIAN PO YIN** (Coptis and Magnolia Bark Drink 连朴饮, p.850).

- With more prominent damp, add **cang zhu** (Atractylodis Rhizoma) 苍术 9–12g, **cao guo** (Tsaoko Fructus) 草果 3–6g and **shi chang pu** (Acori tatarinowii Rhizoma) 石菖蒲 6–9g. See also **HUO PO XIA LING TANG** (Agastache, Magnolia Bark, Pinellia and Poria Decoction 藿朴夏苓汤, p.848).
- With nausea and vomiting, add **chen pi** (Citri reticulatae Pericarpium) 陈皮, **sheng jiang** (Zingiberis Rhizoma recens) 生姜 6–9g and **zhu ru** (Bambusae Caulis in taeniam) 竹茹 9–12g.
- With headache or heaviness in the head, add **bai zhi** (Angelicae dahuricae Radix) 白芷 6–9g, **qiang huo** (Notopterygii Rhizoma seu Radix) 羌活 6–9g and **chuan xiong** (Chuanxiong Rhizoma) 川芎 6–9g.
- With sluggish stools, add **chao bai zhu** (stir fried Atractylodes macrocephalae Rhizoma) 炒白术 6–9g and **zhi shi** (Aurantii Fructus immaturus) 枳实 6–9g.
- With epigastric distension and pain, add **chao shan zha** (stir fried Crataegi Fructus) 炒山楂 12–15g, **e zhu** (Curcumae Rhizoma) 莪术 9–12g and **chao bai zhu** (stir fried Atractylodes macrocephalae Rhizoma) 炒白术 6–9g.
- With jaundice, add **yin chen** (Artemisiae scopariae Herba) 茵陈 12–18g and **shan zhi zi** (Gardeniae Fructus) 山栀子 9–12g.

Prepared medicines
Concentrated powder
San Ren Tang (Triple Nut Combination)
Gan Lu Xiao Du Dan (Forsythia & Acorus Formula)
  – with more heat
Xing Jun San 行军散 (Marching Powder, Five Pagodas Brand)
  – with more damp

Pills
Bi Xie Sheng Shi Wan (Subdue the Dampness Teapills)
  – damp greater than heat

Acupuncture (select from)
SI.3 (houxi –).....................vents pathogens to alleviate night sweats
SI.4 (wangu –) ....source point of the Small Intestine, clears damp heat
Lu.7 (lieque –)....................diffuses the Lungs and vents pathogens from the qi level
LI.11 (quchi –)...................these points clear damp heat from the qi level
St.44 (neiting –)
Sp.9 (yinlingquan –)...........water and metal points of the Spleen, these points
Sp.5 (shangqiu –)   promote urination to drain damp heat
Ren.5 (shimen –)................alarm point of the triple burner, clears damp heat
Ren.12 (zhongwan –).........alarm point of the Stomach, activates the qi dynamic
- with nausea, add PC.6 (neiguan)
- with diarrhea, add zhixie (N–CA–3) and Bl.25 (tianshu)
- with muscle aches, add Sp.21 (dabao)
- with headache, add GB.20 (fengchi)
- Ear points: spleen, lung, zero point, subcortex, sympathetic, shenmen

Clinical notes
- Night sweats of a damp heat type may be diagnosed as chronic infection, chronic fatigue syndrome, cytomegalovirus, glandular fever, pelvis or subphrenic abscess, chronic colitis, fever of unknown origin, fibromyalgia or sleep apnea.
- The source of the damp heat should be investigated thoroughly to rule out pathologies better suited to surgical or biomedical intervention, such as abscesses that should be opened and drained.
- Clearing damp heat from the qi level can be a relatively slow process, depending on duration of the pattern. It may take several weeks before any effects are noted, and treatment should continue for a week or two after the symptoms have resolved, to ensure all damp has been cleared. Following resolution of the damp heat and sweats, a strategy to reinforce Spleen function can be adopted.
- Astringent herbs are contraindicated, and all exits should be kept free and clear.
- Damp heat can also cause sweating just on the head, or hands and feet.
- A damp heat clearing diet is recommended. See Clinical Handbook, Vol.2 p.884.

热 16.1.4.2 LINGERING HEAT IN THE QI LEVEL
留
气
分
Lingering heat in the qi level is seen in the aftermath of an upper respiratory tract infection or other febrile disease, when the most pronounced symptoms have subsided and the patient is left with low grade fever, fatigue and sweating. Depending on the location of the initial illness, the other features can vary. When the initial illness affected the Lungs, persistent cough is prominent; when the Stomach and gastrointestinal system was affected, nausea, vomiting and indeterminate gnawing hunger are seen.

Clinical features
- Night sweats. The sweating in this pattern usually occurs once or twice a night and is often drenching. The sweat is watery, non staining and doesn't smell.
- The patient may also experience spontaneous sweating during the day, with the clamminess all over or localized to the hands and feet.
- low grade fever, worse at night
- dry, irritating cough that is worse at night; or nausea, vomiting and indeterminate gnawing hunger
- thirst, dry mouth, lips and throat; may be mouth ulcers
- insomnia, restlessness, fitful sleep
- fatigue, tiredness
- irritability
- swollen lymph nodes

T red and dry with little or no coat, or a patchy geographic coat
P fine, rapid

Treatment principle
Vent heat from the qi level
Supplement qi and replenish fluids

Prescription

ZHU YE SHI GAO TANG 竹叶石膏汤
Lophatherus and Gypsum Decoction

dan zhu ye (Lophateri Herba) 淡竹叶 9–15g
shi gao (Gypsum fibrosum) 石膏 15–30g
zhi ban xia (Pinelliae Rhizoma preparatum) 制半夏 6–9g
mai dong (Ophiopogonis Radix) 麦冬 6–15g
ren shen (Ginseng Radix) 人参 3–9g
zhi gan cao (Glycyrrhizae Radix preparata) 炙甘草 3–9g
jing mi (Oryzae Semen) 粳米 9–15g

Method: Decoction. **Shi gao** is decocted for 30 minutes prior to the other herbs. **Dan zhu ye** and **shi gao** clear heat from the qi level; **ren shen** supplements qi and supports the Spleen, and, with **mai dong**, generates fluids and protects yin; **mai dong** assists in clearing heat; **zhi ban xia** downbears counterflow Stomach qi to stop nausea and vomiting; **zhi gan cao** and **jing mi** assist in strengthening the Spleen and protecting the Stomach. (Source: *Shang Han Lun*)

Modifications
- With significant heat, frequent drenching sweats, a red tongue, rapid pulse and oral ulceration, add **zhi mu** (Anemarrhenae Rhizoma) 知母 9–12g and **tian hua fen** (Trichosanthes Radix) 天花粉 12–15g.
- For Stomach qi and yin damage with sweats and nausea following chemotherapy, add **yu zhu** (Polygonati odorati Rhizoma) 玉竹 12–15g and **xuan fu hua** (Inulae Flos) 旋复花 12–15g.

Prepared medicines
Concentrated powders
Zhu Ye Shi Gao Tang (Bamboo Leaves & Gypsum Combination)

Acupuncture (select from)
Lu.7 (lieque –) .... diffuses the Lungs and vents pathogens from the qi level
SI.3 (houxi –) .... vents pathogens to alleviate night sweats
Du.14 (dazhui –) .... meeting point of the yang channels, an important point for clearing lingering pathogens
LI.11 (quchi –) .... these points clear heat from the qi level
LI.4 (hegu –)
St.44 (neiting –)
- with cough, add Lu.5 (chize –) and Ren.17 (shanzhong)
- with nausea and vomiting, add PC.6 (neiguan –) and Ren.12 (zhongwan)
- with irritability, add PC.7 (daling –) or PC.8 (laogong –)
- with dryness and thirst, add Kid.6 (zhaohai +)
- with sore throat, add Lu.10 (yuji –)
- with constipation, add Kid.6 (zhaohai +) and St.37 (shangjuxu –)
- Ear points: lung, stomach, zero point, sympathetic, subcortex, shenmen

Clinical notes
- Lingering heat in the qi level may be diagnosed as the convalescent phase of an

upper respiratory or gastrointestinal tract infection, post viral syndrome or the side effects of chemotherapy or radiation.

- When correctly identified, residual pathogenic influences in the qi level can be reliably dispelled, and the qi and fluids quickly replenished. Only a few days to a week or so of treatment is usually necessary.
- Even when the sweats are profuse and drenching, the use of astringent herbs is contraindicated, and all the exits should be kept free and clear.

16.1.4.3 SHAOYANG SYNDROME

邪
留
少
阳

Pathogens lingering in the shaoyang level are a moderately common cause of night sweats. The pathogen responsible can vary depending on the location and time of year. Heat is common in drier climates, while damp heat is typical in more humid or tropical latitudes. In general, the more damp heat there is, the more pronounced the night sweats.

The mechanism of the night sweats hinges around the pivotal nature of the shaoyang. The most characteristic feature of shaoyang patterns is the fever pattern–distinct periods of fever alternating with distinct periods of chills. This fever type reflects the waxing and waning in the strength of the pathogen and the anti–pathogenic qi. When the pathogen gains the upper hand, it pushes a little deeper into the body, breaching the yangming; this is when fever and sweating ensues. As the anti–pathogenic qi fights back and pushes the pathogen towards the surface, the pathogen rallies close to the surface and the chills occur. During sleep, wei qi moves off the surface, compounding the tendency to sweat by not securing the pores.

Clinical features

- Night sweats. The sweats usually only occur once or twice per night, but may be more frequent when the condition is of relatively short duration. Once the patient has woken from sleep with a sweat, they feel cold and may shiver for a while before starting to heat up again.
- Patients may also sweat intermittently during the day. The sweating occurs as the fever episode reaches its zenith, and may affect the trunk, or be isolated to the armpits.
- alternating fever and chills
- reduced appetite or anorexia
- nausea
- hypochondriac pain or distension
- chest oppression
- dizziness
- irritability
- bitter taste in the mouth; food tastes bad
- swollen lymph nodes

T unremarkable, or coated only on the left side, or slightly red on the edges
P wiry

Treatment principle
Harmonize and vent pathogens from shaoyang

Prescription

XIAO CHAI HU TANG 小柴胡汤
Minor Bupleurum Decoction

chai hu (Bupleuri Radix) 柴胡	6–12g
huang qin (Scutellariae Radix) 黄芩	6–9g
zhi ban xia (Pinelliae Rhizoma preparatum) 制半夏	6–9g
ren shen (Ginseng Radix) 人参	6–9g
zhi gan cao (Glycyrrhizae Radix preparata) 炙甘草	3–6g
sheng jiang (Zingiberis Rhizoma recens) 生姜	6–9g
da zao (Jujubae Fructus) 大枣	4 fruit

Method: Decoction. **Chai hu** harmonizes and vents pathogens from the shaoyang and regulates qi; **huang qin** clears heat; together these herbs dispel pathogens from the shaoyang level. **Zhi ban xia** and **sheng jiang** harmonize the Stomach, downbear counterflow Stomach qi and stop nausea; **ren shen** and **zhi gan cao** strengthen anti–pathogenic qi and assist in preventing the pathogen from penetrating further; **sheng jiang** and **da zao** support **zhi ban xia** in harmonizing the Stomach and stopping nausea and vomiting. (Source: *Shang Han Lun*)

Modifications
• With damp, sporadic night sweats, anorexia, muscle aches, chills greater than fever and heaviness, add **cang zhu** (Atractylodis Rhizoma) 苍术 12–15g, **hou po** (Magnoliae officinalis Cortex) 厚朴 9–12g and **chen pi** (Citri reticulatae Pericarpium) 陈皮 9–12g.

Variations and additional prescriptions
Damp heat in the shaoyang
In tropical or warm, humid climates, the prevailing pathogen is often damp heat. In addition to the characteristic alternating fever and chill pattern, with fever predominant, the night sweats are more frequent and drenching, and the sweat is sticky or oily. Nausea and vomiting, aching and heaviness in the muscles, heavy and foggy head, thick, greasy, yellow tongue coat and a wiry, rapid and slippery pulse tend to be more pronounced. The aim of treatment is to clear damp heat from shaoyang and harmonize the Stomach with **HAO QIN QING DAN TANG** (Sweet Wormwood and Scutellaria Decoction to Clear the Gallbladder 蒿芩清胆汤, p.373).

Prepared medicines
Concentrated powders
Xiao Chai Hu Tang (Minor Bupleurum Combination)

Pills
Xiao Chai Hu Wan (Minor Bupleurum Teapills)

Acupuncture (select from)
SJ.5 (waiguan –) ....these points harmonize and vent pathogens from
GB.41 (zulinqi –)   shaoyang

SI.3 (houxi –).....................vents pathogens to alleviate night sweats
Bl.19 (danshu –) ....transport point of the Gallbladder, regulates qi
- with marked fever, add Du.14 (dazhui –)
- with damp heat, add Sp.9 (yinlingquan –), Liv.8 (ququan –) and Kid.7 (fuliu –)
- with qi deficiency, add St.36 (zusanli +) and Liv.13 (zhangmen +)
- with nausea, add PC.6 (neiguan –) and Bl.21 (weishu)
- with hypochondriac pain, add Liv.14 (qimen –) and Bl.19 (danshu –)
- with dizziness, add GB.20 (fengchi) and GB.43 (xiaxi –)
- Ear points: liver, gall bladder, zero point, subcortex, sympathetic, shenmen

Clinical notes
- Shaoyang syndrome may be diagnosed as post viral syndrome, influenza, the convalescent phase of an upper respiratory tract infection, postpartum fever or cholecystitis.
- Shaoyang syndrome can also cause intermittent spontaneous sweating and excessive sweating from the armpits.
- When correctly identified, shaoyang patterns respond well to treatment. Patterns of weeks to a few months duration can be resolved within a few days. The more deficiency and the more dampness there is, the slower the resolution, but even pathogens of many months duration can often be resolved in a couple of weeks. Once the pathogen is expelled, the strategy should focus on rebuilding damaged qi and yin.

痰
热
盗
汗

16.1.4.4 PHLEGM HEAT

Phlegm heat night sweats are seen in the aftermath of a substantial fever. Physiological fluids are quickly cooked and congealed into phlegm heat by the heat of the battle between wei qi and the pathogenic invader. Typically, a relatively severe Lung heat pattern is the initial illness, and the sweats can persist for some weeks after the initial illness has abated. The location of the phlegm heat is the qi level, and both the Lungs and Stomach may be involved.

Clinical features
- Night sweats. The sweats may be profuse, are mostly over the chest, upper back and head, and occur several times per night; the sweat may be oily or viscous. Even though they are sweating, patient do not feel especially feverish, or may have a contained fever (p.367). They are not hot to the touch, but are clammy during the day.
- palpitations with anxiety and nervousness; hypersensitivity to noise and smells
- tiredness during the day, with an inability to sleep, or fitful nightmare disturbed sleep at night
- productive cough with sticky yellow or green sputum; sinus congestion
- dizziness and vertigo; heavy or foggy head
- chest oppression; abdominal distension
- poor appetite, belching, acid reflux, bitter taste in the mouth
- nausea, vomiting or indeterminate gnawing hunger
- swollen lymph nodes

T thick, greasy, yellow coat, like a smear of butter
P wiry or slippery

Treatment principle
Clear and transform phlegm heat
Harmonize the Stomach, rectify the qi dynamic and calm the shen

Prescription

WEN DAN TANG 温胆汤
Warm Gallbladder Decoction

zhu ru (Bambusae Caulis in taeniam) 竹茹 12–15g
zhi shi (Citri Fructus immaturus) 枳实 9–12g
zhi ban xia (Pinelliae Rhizoma preparata) 制半夏 9–12g
fu ling (Poria) 茯苓 12–15g
chen pi (Citri reticulatae Pericarpium) 陈皮 9–12g
sheng jiang (Zingiberis Rhizoma recens) 生姜 3–6g
gan cao (Glycyrrhizae Radix) 甘草 3–6g
Method: Decoction. **Zhu ru** clears phlegm heat from the qi level and downbears counterflow Stomach qi; **zhi shi** breaks up stagnant qi, downbears qi and alleviates distension; **zhi ban xia** transforms phlegm, downbears counterflow Stomach qi and stops nausea and cough; **chen pi** transforms phlegm, regulates middle burner qi and corrects the qi dynamic; **fu ling** strengthens the Spleen and leaches out damp; **gan cao** strengthens the Spleen and harmonizes the Stomach; **sheng jiang** assists the other herbs in transforming phlegm. (Source: *San Yin Ji Yi Bing Zheng Fang Lun*)

Modifications
- With sticky, hard to expectorate sputum, add **gua lou** (Trichosanthis Fructus) 栝楼 15–24g and **zhe bei mu** (Fritillariae thunbergii Bulbus) 浙贝母 9–12g.
- With cough, add **xing ren** (Armeniacae Semen) 杏仁 9–12g and **qian hu** (Peucedani Radix) 前胡 9–12g.
- With marked irritability, acid reflux and a deep yellow tongue coat, add **huang lian** (Coptidis Rhizoma) 黄连 3–6g.
- With constipation, add **gua lou ren** (Trichosanthis Semen) 栝楼仁 12–18g.

Prepared medicines
Concentrated powder
Wen Dan Tang (Poria & Bamboo Combination)
Pills
Wen Dan Wan (Rising Courage Teapills)

Acupuncture (select from)
SI.3 (houxi –) .... vents pathogens and alleviates night sweats
PC.5 (jianshi) .... river point of the Pericardium, transforms phlegm and clears heat
PC.6 (neiguan –) .... connecting point of the Pericardium, downbears counterflow Stomach qi and stops vomiting, calms the shen, dredges the Liver and rectifies qi
Ren.12 (zhongwan –) .... alarm point of the Stomach, harmonizes the Stom-

ach and rectifies the qi dynamic

St.40 (fenglong –) ....connecting point of the Stomach, transforms phlegm and clears heat

St.36 (zusanli) ....sea point of the Stomach, strengthens the Spleen and Stomach and corrects the qi dynamic

St.43 (xianggu –)...............wood point of the Stomach, clears heat

- with foggy head, add Du.20 (baihui)
- with marked heat, add PC.8 (laogong –) and St.45 (lidui ↓)
- with Stomach discomfort, add St.34 (liangqiu –)
- with dizziness, add GB.43 (xiaxi –)
- with anxiety, add Du.19 (houding) and Du.24 (shenting)
- Ear points: stomach, gallbladder, zero point, subcortex, sympathetic, shenmen

Clinical notes

- Phlegm heat type night sweats may be diagnosed as the convalescent phase of febrile illnesses such as bronchitis and pneumonia, meningitis, encephalitis and gastroenteritis. The high and sustained fever is usually required to congeal fluids into phlegm.
- Night sweats of a phlegm heat type respond well to treatment. Treatment needs to continue until all signs of phlegm are cleared, in particular, until the tongue coat becomes normal.
- Phlegm heat in the qi level can also cause spontaneous daytime sweating.
- A phlegm resolving diet is recommended. See Clinical Handbook, Vol. 2, p.885.

热
入
营
分

16.1.4.5 LINGERING HEAT IN THE YING LEVEL

Lingering heat in the ying level is due to an unresolved pathogenic invasion. A pathogen can gain access to the ying level when the pathogen is strong, or when the patient has a pre–existing Kidney weakness. A heat pathogen in the ying level can significantly damage yin. This pattern and yin deficiency share features and can appear similar but the differences are important to note because the treatment strategies are quite distinct. The lymphadenopathy, maculopapular and deep scarlet color and thorns on the tongue are important differential signs. Heat in the ying level must be vented to the exterior. Applying predominantly yin enriching or astringent strategies can lead to the pathogen being trapped.

Clinical features

- Night sweats. The sweats can be frequent and drenching with multiple sweats each night, or may occur intermittently. The sweats are accompanied by a low grade fever which recedes in the early hours of the morning, followed by feeling cold and an inability to maintain body temperature.
- may be confusion or mild disturbances of consciousness
- faint erythema, purpura or maculopapular rash
- thirst, or dryness of mucous membranes without thirst
- insomnia or fitful dream and sweat disturbed sleep
- irritability and restlessness

- weight loss, malaise, weakness, fatigue and exhaustion
- mouth ulcers
- may be joint pain, redness and swelling
- swollen lymph nodes

T dry, deep red or scarlet with thorns, and little or no coat
P fine and rapid

Treatment principle

Clear and vent heat from the ying level
Nourish yin and moisten dryness

Prescription

QING YING TANG 清营汤
Clear the Nutritive Level Decoction

shui niu jiao (Cornu Bubali) 水牛角 30–60g
sheng di (Rehmanniae Radix) 生地 15–30g
xuan shen (Scrophulariae Radix) 玄参 9–18g
mai dong (Ophiopogonis Radix) 麦冬 6–12g
jin yin hua (Lonicerae Flos) 金银花 9–15g
lian qiao (Forsythiae Fructus) 连翘 6–15g
dan zhu ye (Lophatheri Herba) 淡竹叶 3–6g
huang lian (Coptidis Rhizoma) 黄连 3–6g
dan shen (Salviae miltiorrhizae Radix) 丹参 6–15g

Method: Decoction. **Shui niu jiao** is shaved into fine strips and cooked for 30 minutes prior to the other herbs. **Shui niu jiao** clears heat from the ying level and cools the blood; **xuan shen** and **sheng di** cool the blood and protect yin; **mai dong** clears heat, nourishes yin and moistens dryness; **jin yin hua, lian qiao, dan zhu ye** vent heat from the qi and ying levels; **huang lian** clears heat from the Heart and Stomach; **dan shen** clears heat, activates the blood, and helps prevent the blood stasis that may complicate both heat and the use of cold herbs. **Shui niu jiao** is used instead of **xi jiao** (Rhinocerotis Cornu) 犀角, the horn of the critically endangered rhinoceros. (Source: *Wen Bing Tiao Bian*)

Modifications

- With persistent fever and sweating, add **qing hao** (Artemisiae annuae Herba) 青蒿 12-15g, **yin chai hu** (Stellariae Radix) 银柴胡 9–12g and **di gu pi** (Lycii Cortex) 地骨皮 12–15g.
- With dry cough, add **sang bai pi** (Mori Cortex) 桑白皮 9–12g and **di gu pi** (Lycii Cortex) 地骨皮 12–15g.
- With joint pain and swelling, add **qin jiao** (Gentianae macrophyllae Radix) 秦艽 9–15g.

Prepared medicines
Concentrated powders
Qing Hao Bie Jia Tang (Artemesia & Turtle Shell Combination)
Qin Jiao Bie Jia San (Gentiana Macrophylla Root & Turtle Shell Formula)
    – with joint pain

Acupuncture (select from)

Kid.7 (fuliu −) .... vents pathogens form the ying level and alleviates
  sweating

Ht.6 (yinxi −) .... cleft point of the Heart, clears heat and alleviates
  sweating

SI.3 (houxi −) .... activates dumai to stimulate yang movement, vent
  pathogens and alleviate night sweats

PC.3 (quze −) .... together these points clear heat from the ying and
Bl.40 (weizhong −)   blood, and activate the blood
Sp.10 (xuehai −)

Kid.3 (taixi +) .... replenishes damaged yin

Bl.23 (shenshu +) .... these points clear heat and replenish damaged yin
Bl.18 (ganshu +)   and fluids

• Ear points: liver, kidney, heart, subcortex, sympathetic, shenmen

Clinical notes

• Lingering heat in the ying level may be diagnosed as infection with Human
  Immunodeficiency Virus (HIV), the residual effects of infections such as bacteremia, meningococcal meningitis and encephalitis, leukemia, systemic lupus
  erythematosus, rheumatoid arthritis and other connective tissue diseases.
• Heat in the ying level can respond to treatment or be difficult, depending on
  the associated biomedical disease process. Patients may be medicated with drugs
  such as steroids or immunosuppressants, which complicate treatment. In general though, the heat and sweats, and thus the patients comfort and well being,
  can be managed reasonably well.

16.2 SPONTANEOUS SWEATING

1. Qi deficiency
2. Yang deficiency
3. Ying and wei disharmony
4. Lingering pathogens
   • Heat in the qi level
   • Shaoyang (see p.719)
   • Phlegm heat (p.721)

Spontaneous sweating occurs without the stimulus of environmental heat or physical exertion. The spontaneous sweating discussed in this section may be continuous or intermittent, but will have been going on for some time, and should be clearly distinguished from the sweating that accompanies an acute fever.

16.2.1 QI DEFICIENCY

肺
脾
气
虚

Spontaneous sweating due to qi deficiency is associated with weakness of the protective wei qi that inhibits the surface and controls the opening and closing of the pores. The Spleen and Lungs are the source of the body's acquired qi, and the Lungs in particular exert a powerful influence over the integrity of the skin and surface, and the distribution of wei qi. When wei qi is weak it is unable to keep the pores tightly shut, pathogens easily penetrate resulting in frequent colds and infection, and fluids leak out as spontaneous sweat.

Clinical features
• Daytime sweating that is worse with exertion, but which may occur while at rest and is fairly continuous. A sheen of moisture will be observed on the upper lip, and the patient feels clammy to touch.
• breathlessness with exertion
• aversion to wind and sudden changes in temperature
• pale complexion
• easy fatigue
• frequent colds and flu, poor immunity
T pale, with a thin, white coat
P fine and weak

Treatment Principle
Supplement and strengthen wei qi
Secure the exterior to stop sweating

Prescription

YU PING FENG SAN 玉屏风散
Jade Windscreen Powder

huang qi (Astragali Radix) 黄芪 18–45g
bai zhu (Atractylodes macrocephalae Rhizoma) 白术 12–15g
fang feng (Saposhnikovae Radix) 防风 6–9g

Method: Grind the herbs into a fine powder and take 6–9 grams as a draft 2–3 times daily. Can also be decocted with the doses as shown. **Huang qi** strengthens the Lungs, fortifies wei qi and secures the exterior; **bai zhu** strengthens the Spleen and supplements qi; **fang feng** dispels any lingering wind from the exterior without dispersing anti–pathogenic qi, and prevents the potential trapping of pathogens under the surface, once the pores are shut. (Source: *Zhong Yi Nei Ke Xue [Dan Xi Xin Fa]*)

Modifications

- With marked sweating, add one or two astringent substances such as **duan long gu** (calcined Fossilia Ossis Mastodi) 煅龙骨 15–30g, **duan mu li** (calcined Ostreae Concha) 煅牡蛎 15–30g, **fu xiao mai** (Tritici Fructus levis) 浮小麦 12–18g, **ma huang gen** (Ephedrae Radix) 麻黄根 9–12g or **wu wei zi** (Schizandrae Fructus) 五味子 6–9g.
- With aversion to wind and sensitivity to sudden temperature change, add **gui zhi** (Cinnamomi Ramulus) 桂枝 6–9g and **bai shao** (Paeoniae Radix alba) 白芍 9–12g.
- With yin deficiency, a dry tongue with surface cracks, dry mouth and thirst and a dry cough that is worse at night, add **mai dong** (Ophiopogonis Radix) 麦冬 9–12g, **wu wei zi** (Schizandrae Fructus) 五味子 6–9g and **sheng di** (Rehmanniae Radix) 生地 9–15g.
- With poor appetite, add **gu ya** (Setariae Fructus germinatus) 谷芽 15–30g and **chen pi** (Citri reticulatae Pericarpium) 陈皮 6–9g.

Variations and additional prescriptions

Relatively severe Spleen and Lung qi deficiency

With more profound Lung and Spleen qi deficiency, manifesting with profound fatigue, breathlessness, respiratory and digestive weakness, a more specific Lung and Spleen strategy is necessary. An excellent formula to strengthen the Lungs and Spleen and build qi while fortifying wei qi and securing the surface, is **BU ZHONG YI QI TANG** (Supplement the Middle to Augment the Qi Decoction 补中益气汤) modified.

zhi huang qi (honey fried Astragali Radix) 炙黄芪 12–30g
ren shen (Ginseng Radix) 人参 6–9g
bai zhu (Atractylodis macrocephalae Rhizoma) 白术 9–12g
dang gui (Angelicae sinensis Radix) 当归 6–9g
chen pi (Citri reticulatae Pericarpium) 陈皮 6–9g
sheng ma (Cimicifugae Rhizoma) 升麻 3–6g
chai hu (Bupleuri Radix) 柴胡 3–6g
zhi gan cao (Glycyrrhizae Radix preparata) 炙甘草 3–6g
ma huang gen (Ephedrae Radix) 麻黄根 9–12g
wu wei zi (Schizandrae Fructus) 五味子 6–9g

Method: Decoction or powdered and taken in doses of 9–grams as a draft. **Zhi huang qi** strengthens the Lungs and Spleen and fortifies wei qi; **ren shen**, **bai zhu** and **zhi gan cao** strengthen the Spleen and supplement qi; **chai hu** and **sheng ma** elevating yang qi, assist in correcting the qi dynamic and the distribution of yang qi; **dang gui** nourishes and activates blood; **chen pi** regulates qi; **ma huang gen** stops sweating; **wu wei zi** strengthens the Lungs and stops sweating. (Source: *Zhong Yi Nei Ke Xue [Pi Wei Lun]*)

Qi and blood deficiency

Qi deficiency is often complicated by blood deficiency. A weak Spleen may not produce sufficient blood in the first place, or the qi may be unable to contain blood in the vessels and so it is lost through bleeding. When blood deficiency complicates qi deficiency, the sweating pattern can vary depending on the degree of either qi or blood deficiency. The greater the blood deficiency the more the tendency to sweat at night. Some patients will experience both daytime spontaneous sweating and night sweats. The treatment is to supplement and nourish qi and blood, strengthen the Spleen and stop sweating with GUI PI TANG (Restore the Spleen Decoction 归脾汤 p.820).

Lung qi and yin deficiency

Lung deficiency patterns frequently overlap. Lung qi and yin deficiency often occur together, as fluids lost as sweat due to qi deficiency can deplete yin. The manifestations are a combination of the patterns – spontaneous sweating and occasional night sweats on the head and chest, persistent cough or wheezing with scant sputum that is hard to expectorate, breathlessness, a dry mouth and tongue, a pale or pink and swollen tongue with surface cracks and little coating, and a weak and fine pulse. Treatment is to supplement Lung qi and yin with SHENG MAI SAN (Generate the Pulse Powder 生脉散).

ren shen (Ginseng Radix) 人参 9–15g
mai dong (Ophiopogonis Radix) 麦冬 15–24g
wu wei zi (Schizandrae Fructus) 五味子 6–9g

Method: Decoction. White ginseng (**bai ren shen** 白人参) is preferred here as it is less heating than the red Korean variety. **Ren shen** strengthens the Spleen and Lungs and supplements qi; **mai dong** nourishes Lung yin; **wu wei zi** strengthens the Lungs and Kidneys, secures wei qi and stops cough. (Source: *Nei Wai Shang Bian Huo Lun*)

Instability of the shen

Instability of the shen (also described as Heart and Gallbladder deficiency) is associated with a congenital or acquired weakness of the shen. When the shen is destabilized, the patient sweats copiously in response to anxiety. The sweat may be all over or isolated to the palms or armpits. When congenital, a lifelong history of anxiety and nervousness is noted. A destabilized shen can be acquired through a serious trauma (p.710–711), by deficiency that fails to anchor it (blood and yin deficiency), or by excess pathology (heat and ascendant yang) that irritates and inflames it. In many cases however, there is no clear pathology and in between episodes of excessive sweating, the patient appears well. Anxiety or anticipation of public speaking, a job interview, etc., destabilize and scatter the shen, and with it the fluid of the Heart, i.e. sweat. Most people will experience this to one degree or another, but in some people it can be severe enough to inhibit their ability to function in pressure situations, and becomes a source of self perpetuating anxiety. The treatment is to stabilize and calm the shen and stop sweating with AN SHEN DING ZHI WAN (Calm the Shen and Settle the Emotions Pill 安神定志丸) modified. The base formula, without modifications, can be used for prolonged periods once the sweating is controlled, in conjunction with acupuncture, to consolidate the Heart and anchor the shen.

ren shen (Ginseng Radix) 人参 90g
fu shen (Poria Sclerotium pararadicis) 茯神 90g
shi chang pu (Acori tatarinowii Rhizoma) 石菖蒲 60g
yuan zhi (Polygalae Radix) 远志 60g
gan cao (Glycyrrhizae Radix) 甘草 60g
da zao (Jujubae Fructus) 大枣 60g
duan mu li (calcined Ostreae Concha) 煅牡蛎 60g
ma huang gen (Ephedrae Radix) 麻黄根 60g
fu xiao mai (Tritici Fructus Levis) 浮小麦 60g

Method: Pills. Grind herbs to a powder and form into 9–gram pills with honey. The dose is 1 pill twice daily. May also be decocted with a 90% reduction in dosage. **Ren shen** and **fu shen** supplement Heart qi; **fu shen** calms the shen; **shi chang pu** and **yuan zhi** calm the shen, and clear and tranquilize the mind; **gan cao**, **da zao** and **fu xiao mai** calm the shen; and support Spleen qi; **duan mu li** tranquilizes the shen and stops sweating; **ma huang gen** and **fu xiao mai** stop sweating. (Source: *Qian Jin Yao Fang*)

Sudden onset of sweating following major shock or trauma

Acute onset of copious spontaneous sweating can follow a sudden shock or trauma. See Gui Zhi Jia Long Gu Mu Li Tang (Cinnamon Twig Decoction plus Dragon Bone and Oyster Shell 桂枝加龙骨牡蛎汤, p.711).

Qi deficiency with wind damp

Patients with qi deficiency are vulnerable to invasion by external pathogens. Patients with pre–existing Spleen deficiency are also more prone to wind damp invasion, with aching and swollen joints the result. This pattern is seen in overweight individuals (mostly women), who are chronically clammy, tired, puffy and pale. The damp sinks down to the knees which are swollen and painful. The treatment is to dispel wind damp, supplement qi and secure the exterior with Fang Ji Huang Qi Tang (Stephania and Astragalus Decoction 防己黄芪汤, p.653).

Prepared medicines
Concentrated powders

Yu Ping Feng San (Astragalus & Siler Formula)
Bu Zhong Yi Qi Tang (Ginseng & Astragalus Combination)
Huang Qi Jian Zhong Tang (Astragalus Combination)
 – especially good for children
Sheng Mai San (Ginseng & Ophiopogon Formula)
Yang Xin Tang (Astragalus & Zizyphus Combination)
 – Heart qi deficiency and instability of the shen
Gui Zhi Jia Long Gu Mu Li Tang (Cinnamon & Dragon Bone Combination)
Fang Ji Huang Qi Tang (Stephania & Astragalus Combination)

Pills

Yu Ping Feng Wan (Jade Screen Teapills)
Bu Zhong Yi Qi Wan (Central Chi Teapills)
Sheng Mai Wan (Great Pulse Teapills)
An Shen Ding Zhi Wan (Calm the Shen and Settle the Zhi Pill)

Fang Ji Huang Qi Wan (Stephania and Astragalus Teapills)
Xu Han Ting (Stop Deficient Sweat)
– an astringent formula that can be added to any formula above

Acupuncture (select from)

Du.14 (dazhui +▲)............meeting point of the yang channels, reinforces yang
qi and fortifies wei qi

LI.4 (hegu +).....................source point of the Large Intestine, and metal

Kid.7 (fuliu +)   point of the Kidneys, these points have a special
effect on stopping sweating from qi deficiency

Lu.9 (taiyuan +) ....source point of the Lungs; strengthens the Lungs
and fortifies wei qi

Ren.12 (zhongwan +)..........alarm point of the Stomach, strengthens the Spleen
and Stomach and supplements qi

Ren.4 (guanyuan +▲)........supplements the Kidneys and yuan qi

St.36 (zusanli +▲) ....sea point of the Stomach, strengthens the Spleen and
Stomach and supplements qi and blood

Bl.13 (feishu +▲)...............transport point of the Lungs, strengthens the Lungs
and fortifies wei qi

Bl.20 (pishu +▲) ....transport point of the Spleen, strengthens the Spleen
and supplements qi

- with anxiety and palpitations, add Ht.6 (yinxi) and Bl.15 (xinshu +)
- with instability of the shen, add Ht.7 (shenmen +) and Kid.7 (dazhong)
- with yin and blood deficiency, add Sp.6 (sanyinjiao +)
- Ear points: spleen, lung, heart, zero point, sympathetic, subcortex, shenmen

Clinical notes

- Spontaneous sweating of a qi deficiency type may be diagnosed as having hyper-hidrosis, hypoglycemia, weak immunity, autonomic nervous system dysfunction or malnutrition, and is seen in patients recovering from serious illness.
- This type of sweating responds reliably well to treatment, with improvement in the patient's immune status and general vitality in a relative short period of time. Those prone to constitutional or acquired Lung weakness can benefit from a course of treatment at change of season to prevent potential problems.
- Proper rest and graded exercises are important for rebuilding qi. Breathing exercises, qigong, taijiquan and swimming are particularly helpful.
- A qi supplementing diet is recommended. See Clinical Handbook, Vol.2, p.870.

阳
虚
汗
出

16.2.2 YANG DEFICIENCY

Spontaneous sweating of yang deficiency due to a failure of yang qi to support wei qi. The mechanism of the sweating is similar to that of qi deficiency, but the deficiency is more profound and the sweating more copious. There are two variants of yang deficiency sweating, based on the location of the primary pathology. The first is associated with severe deficiency of wei qi, to the point where the pores are constantly open and sweat leaks out incessantly. This is depleted Heart and Lung yang qi, a condition that may be relatively acute, following excessive and inappropriately induced sweating in the treatment of an exterior pathogen or excessive sweating during exercise or sunstroke. The second variant is a more chronic pattern, involving the Spleen and Stomach, or Spleen and Kidneys. The sweating is copious and persistent, and affects the head and neck or hands and feet, as the feeble yang simply floats away to the periphery.

Clinical features

• Continuous daytime sweating that is worse with exertion. A sheen of moisture will be observed on the upper lip and forehead and the patient feels cold and clammy to the touch. The sweat can affect the trunk but is often more pronounced on the head and neck.
• cold intolerance, cold extremities
• breathlessness with exertion; weak voice, reluctance to speak
• palpitations, arrhythmia
• aversion to wind and sudden changes in temperature
• poor appetite, abdominal distension, loose stools or diarrhea; diarrhea may occur early in the morning
• frequent urination, nocturia; or scanty urination
• lower back ache, weak legs; may be muscle aches or stiffness in the joints
• waxy, pale complexion
• frequent colds and flu, poor immunity
T pale, wet, swollen and scalloped with a moist white coat
P weak; floating and fine; or floating and weak; or intermittent

Treatment Principle

Supplement and strengthen wei qi
Secure the exterior to stop sweating
Warm and supplement Spleen and Kidney yang

Prescription

GUI ZHI JIA FU ZI TANG 桂枝加附子汤
Cinnamon Twig and Prepared Aconite Decoction

This prescription is selected when the yang deficiency is primarily located in the Lungs, Heart and surface, with severe wei qi deficiency. Profuse and continuous cold sweating, scanty urination, and a sense of vulnerability to temperature change as if constantly being in a draft are seen. The main focus of this formula is to stop sweating by strongly reinforcing the surface and boosting yang qi. Once the sweating has abated somewhat, a more fundamental Lung, Spleen and Kidney supplement, such as the prescription in variations below, should be employed.

gui zhi (Cinnamomi Ramulus) 桂枝 6–9g
zhi fu zi (Aconiti Radix lateralis preparata) 制附子 6–12g
bai shao (Paeoniae Radix alba) 白芍 9–12g
zhi gan cao (Glycyrrhizae Radix preparata) 炙甘草 3–6g
sheng jiang (Zingiberis Rhizoma) 生姜 6–9g
da zao (Jujubae Fructus) 大枣 .... 7 fruit

Method: Decoction. **Zhi fu zi** is cooked for 30–60 minutes before the other herbs. **Gui zhi** mobilizes circulation of qi through the muscle layer; **zhi fu zi** warms and strengthens yang qi; **bai shao**, protects yin and its astringency assists wei qi in closing the pores. **Bai shao** and **gan cao** combine sweet and sour flavours to create and protect yin. **Gui zhi** and **zhi gan cao** combine pungent and sweet flavours to create yang and promote movement of yang qi through the surface tissues; **sheng jiang**, **da zao** and **zhi gan cao** support the Spleen and Stomach, harmonize the formula and protect qi and yin. (Source: *Zhong Yi Nei Ke Xue* [*Shang Han Lun*])

Modifications
• With persistent or profuse sweating, add **huang qi** (Astragali Radix) 黄芪 18–45g, **duan long gu** (calcined Fossilia Ossis Mastodi) 煅龙骨 15–30g and **duan mu li** (calcined Ostreae Concha) 煅牡蛎 15–30g.

Variations and additional prescriptions
Spleen and Stomach yang deficiency
Spleen and Stomach yang deficiency is a chronic pattern associated with a poor or cold diet. The Spleen governs the extremities, so the worst of the sweating may occur on the hands and feet, which are cold and clammy or dripping wet. Other signs of middle burner yang deficiency will be evident – abdominal pain and bloating, loss of appetite, edema of the orbits, fingers and abdomen, loose stools, a pale scalloped tongue and fine, weak, deep pulse. The treatment is to focus on rebuilding middle burner yang with a prescription such as LI ZHONG WAN (Regulate the Middle Pill 里中丸) modified.

ren shen (Ginseng Radix) 人参 6–12g
bai zhu (Atractylodes macrocephalae Rhizoma) 白术 6–12g
gan jiang (Zingiberis Rhizoma) 干姜 6–9g
zhi gan cao (Glycyrrhizae Radix preparata) 炙甘草 3–6g
wu mei (Mume Fructus) 乌梅 9–15g

Method: Decoction. **Gan jiang**, warms the middle burner, dispels cold and restores Spleen yang; **ren shen** strengthens the Spleen and supplements qi; **bai zhu** strengthens the Spleen and dries damp; **zhi gan cao** strengthens the Spleen and harmonizes the middle burner; **wu mei** astringes the Lungs and stops sweating. (Source: *Shang Han Lun*)

Spleen and Kidney yang deficiency
The Spleen and Kidneys are the basis of the body's yang and when weak, all other species of yang qi, including wei qi, are affected. The sweating tends to be relatively mild, but is persistent and cold, and accompanied by signs of digestive weakness and urinary frequency. The aim of treatment is to fortify wei qi and supplement yang qi systemically, to support wei qi, by warming and strengthening Spleen and Kidney yang with a mixture of BU ZHONG YI QI TANG (Supplement the Middle

to Augment the Qi Decoction 补中益气汤 p.727) and Jɪɴ Guɪ Sʜᴇɴ Qɪ Wᴀɴ (Kidney Qi Pill from the Golden Cabinet 金匮肾气丸, p.826).

Prepared medicines
Concentrated powders
Gui Zhi Jia Fu Zi Tang (Cinnamon & Aconite Combination)
Bu Zhong Yi Qi Tang (Ginseng & Astragalus Combination) plus Ba Wei Di
  Huang Wan (Rehmannia Eight Formula)
Pills
Jin Kui Shen Qi Wan (Fu Gui Ba Wei Wan, Golden Book Teapills) plus Bu
  Zhong Yi Qi Wan (Central Chi Teapills)
Xu Han Ting (Stop Deficient Sweat)
  – an astringent formula; can be added to any formula above

Acupuncture (select from)
Du.14 (dazhui +▲)............meeting point of the yang channels, reinforces yang
                             qi and fortifies wei qi
LI.4 (hegu +)....................source point of the Large Intestine and metal point
Kid.7 (fuliu +)   of the Kidneys, these points have a special effect on
                             stopping sweating
Lu.9 (taiyuan +) ....source point of the Lungs; strengthens the Lungs
                             and fortifies wei qi
Ren.12 (zhongwan + ▲) ....alarm point of the Stomach, strengthens the Spleen
                             and supplements yang qi
Ren.4 (guanyuan +▲)........warms and supplements yuan qi
St.36 (zusanli +▲) ....sea point of the Stomach, strengthens the Spleen and
                             Stomach and supplements yang qi
Bl.13 (feishu +▲)...............transport point of the Lungs, strengthens the Lungs
                             and fortifies wei qi
Bl.15 (xinshu +▲) ....transport point of the Heart, warms and supple-
                             ments Heart yang to restrain sweating
Bl.20 (pishu +▲) ....transport point of the Spleen, warms and supple-
                             ments Spleen qi and yang
Bl.23 (shenshu +▲) ....transport point of the Kidneys, warms and supple-
                             ments Kidney qi and yang
- with severe and incessant sweating, apply moxa to Ren.8 (shenque). Place a piece of thin cloth over the navel and fill it with salt; burn cones of moxa on the salt. The cloth enables quick removal of the salt and prevents burning.
- with anxiety and palpitations, add Ht.6 (yinxi) and Bl.15 (xinshu +)
- Ear points: lung, heart, spleen, kidney, heart, sympathetic, adrenal, shenmen

Clinical notes
- Spontaneous sweating of a yang deficiency type may be diagnosed as convalescence from prolonged illness, hypoglycemia, immune deficiency, congestive cardiac failure, hypothyroidism, autonomic nervous system imbalance, hypotension or hyperhidrosis.

- Yang deficiency type sweating can respond reasonably well to treatment, depending on the depth of the deficiency. Treatment to replenish and sustain yang will take some time. After the sweating has abated, treatment should continue for some weeks or longer to adequately restore the depleted yang qi, using an appropriate systemic yang supplement (such as JIN GUI SHEN QI WAN (Kidney Qi Pill from the Golden Cabinet 金匮肾气丸, p.826).
- Proper rest and graded exercises are helpful in rebuilding yang qi. Breathing exercises, qigong, taijiquan and swimming are particularly good.
- A yang warming diet is recommended. See Clinical Handbook, Vol.2, p.873.

营卫不和 16.2.3 YING WEI DISHARMONY

Ying wei disharmony describes a disruption to the relationship between the Spleen and Lungs (earth and metal) at the level of the skin and superficial tissues. Wei qi is an extension of lung qi, while ying qi is harvested and distributed by the Spleen. The imbalance can be skewed in one direction or another. Disruption to wei qi gives rise to sweating and sensitivity to wind. Inadequate ying qi causes dryness of the skin, and skin disorders that are aggravated by exposure to cold.

This pattern is a type of wei qi deficiency, but differs from that in 16.2.1 Qi deficiency (p.726), by the fact that here the deficiency is isolated to the surface and does not necessarily affect the internal organs.

Clinical features
- Intermittent spontaneous sweating or clamminess, which may be provoked or aggravated by exposure to wind or changes of temperature
- aversion to wind and sudden changes of temperature
- muscle aches and joint stiffness
- may be mild fever and chills

T thin white coat
P floating moderate or weak

Treatment Principle
Harmonize ying (nutritive) qi and wei (defensive) qi to stop sweating

Prescription
GUI ZHI TANG 桂枝汤
Cinnamon Twig Decoction

gui zhi (Cinnamomi Ramulus) 桂枝 6–9g
bai shao (Paeoniae Radix alba) 白芍 9–12g
sheng jiang (Zingiberis Rhizoma recens) 生姜 6–9g
zhi gan cao (Glycyrrhizae Radix preparata) 炙甘草 3–6g
da zao (Jujubae Fructus) 大枣 .... 4 fruit

Method: Decoction. **Gui zhi** mobilizes circulation of qi through the muscle layer; **bai shao** protects yin and its astringency assists wei qi in closing the pores; **bai shao** and **gan cao** combine sweet and sour flavours to create and protect yin; **gui zhi** and **gan cao** combine pungent and sweet flavours to create yang and promote movement of yang qi through the surface tissues; **sheng jiang**, **da zao** and **zhi gan cao** support the Spleen and Stomach, harmonize the formula and protect qi and yin. (Source: *Zhong Yi Nei Ke Xue [Shang Han Lun]*)

Variations and additional prescriptions
Sweating and shen disturbance following shock
Spontaneous sweating, and sometimes night sweats, can occur following a major shock or trauma. The onset of symptoms may occur suddenly, following an event such as a motor vehicle accident. This can be seen as a type of ying wei imbalance, but at a deeper level. The sudden shock disrupts the relationship between the Heart and Kidneys (and shen and zhi). In this case, the ying wei imbalance is between water and fire, where the yang wei qi represents fire, while the more yin ying qi represents water. The treatment is to harmonize ying and wei qi. To focus the action of the formula internally, heavy mineral substances, here **duan long gu** (calcined Fossilia Ossis Mastodi) 煅龙骨 and **duan mu li** (calcined Ostreae Concha) 煅牡蛎, are added to GUI ZHI TANG to drag the action of the formula internally. This forms the formula GUI ZHI JIA LONG GU MU LI TANG (Cinnamon Twig Decoction plus Dragon Bone and Oyster Shell 桂枝加龙骨牡蛎汤, p.711). In addition to the sweating, sleeplessness, nightmares, palpitations and flashbacks can occur.

Prepared medicines
Concentrated powders
Gui Zhi Tang (Cinnamon Combination)
Gui Zhi Jia Long Gu Mu Li Tang (Cinnamon & Dragon Bone Combination)
Pills
Gui Zhi Tang Wan (Gui Zhi Tang Teapills)
Xu Han Ting (Stop Deficient Sweat)
   – an astringent formula; can be added to any formula above

Acupuncture (select from)
Du.14 (dazhui +▲)...........meeting point of the yang channels, fortifies wei qi
LI.4 (hegu +).....................source point of the Large Intestine and metal point
Kid.7 (fuliu +)   of the Kidneys, these points stop sweating
Lu.9 (taiyuan +)................source point of the Lungs; strengthens the Lungs
                 and fortifies wei qi
St.36 (zusanli +)................strengthens the Spleen and supplements qi
Sp.6 (sanyinjiao +)............supplements ying qi
• Ear points: shen men, spleen, lung, heart, sympathetic

Clinical notes
• Spontaneous sweating of a ying wei disharmony type may be diagnosed as debility in the aftermath of illness, postpartum weakness, convalescence from infection, weak immunity, post traumatic stress disorder or autonomic nervous system dysfunction.
• Proper rest and graded exercises an important part of balancing ying and wei qi, and restoring homeostasis. Moderate walking, breathing exercises, qigong, taijiquan and swimming are helpful in rebuilding qi.
• A qi supplementing diet is recommended. See Clinical Handbook, Vol.2, p.870.

16.2.4 LINGERING PATHOGENS

热
在
气
分

16.2.4.1 HEAT IN THE QI LEVEL

Spontaneous sweating from heat in the qi level can be due to several factors, whereas night sweats of a qi level heat type is always due to a lingering external pathogen. Spontaneous sweating (which includes sweating localized to specific areas of the body), can be due to the introduction of heat into the qi level through the diet, a constitutional tendency to qi level heat, as well as an unresolved external invasion. When constitutional, excessive sweating is a lifelong problem. When related to the diet, the patient is often overweight, and the heat associated with overeating and an excessively rich or heating diet. Excessive volume of food leads to inefficient digestion, and the unprocessed remnants ferment as a type of 'compost' which generate more heat. The heat evaporates body fluids into a 'steam', which appear on the surface as clamminess and sweat.

Clinical features
- Spontaneous sweating and clamminess which may be generalized, or concentrated on the head, chest, or hands and occasionally feet. The sweating may be intermittent or continuous, and worse after eating.
- red, plethoric complexion
- easy overheating, or low grade fever
- thirst, dry mouth, lips and throat
- abdominal and epigastric distension
- flatulence, belching, nausea
- may be constipation, in which case there may be abdominal pain and tidal fever with sweating, increasing in the afternoon and evening
- maybe persistent, dry, irritating cough
- restlessness, irritability
- insomnia, fitful sleep

T red body with a dry, patchy or greasy, yellow coat
P fine or slippery and rapid

Treatment principle
Clear heat from the qi level
Generate fluids and nourish yin
Open the bowels to clear heat and stagnation, if necessary

Prescription
ZHU YE SHI GAO TANG 竹叶石膏汤
Lophatherus and Gypsum Decoction, modified

This formula is used when the bowels are moving freely. It is not suitable when the stools are dry and hard or when the patient is constipated (see Variations).
dan zhu ye (Lophateri Herba) 淡竹叶..9–15g
shi gao (Gypsum fibrosum) 石膏 15–30g
zhi ban xia (Pinelliae Rhizoma preparatum) 制半夏 6–9g

mai dong (Ophiopogonis Radix) 麦冬 6–15g
zhi gan cao (Glycyrrhizae Radix preparata) 炙甘草 3–9g
jing mi (Oryzae Semen) 粳米 9–15g
sha shen (Glehniae/Adenophorae Radix) 沙参 9–12g
Method: Decoction. **Shi gao** is decocted for 30 minutes prior to the other herbs. **Dan zhu ye** and **shi gao** vent heat from the qi level; **sha shen**, which replaces **ren shen**, and **mai dong** clear heat, generate fluids and protect yin; **zhi ban xia** downbears counterflow Stomach qi to stop nausea and vomiting; **zhi gan cao** and **jing mi** strengthens the Spleen and protect the Stomach. (Source: *Shi Yong Zhong Yi Nei Ke Xue* [*Shang Han Lun*])

Modifications
• With significant fluid damage, a peeled, mirror or geographic tongue, add **yu zhu** (Polygonati odorati Rhizoma) 玉竹 12–15g and **tian hua fen** (Trichosanthes Radix) 天花粉 12–15g.

Variations and additional prescriptions
With food stagnation, heat and constipation
When constipation complicates the qi level heat, the dry stool has to be cleared to alleviate the heat and enable clearance of the stagnation. The treatment is to guide the stagnation down and out, and clear heat with ZHI SHI DAO ZHI WAN (Unripe Bitter Orange Pill to Guide Out Stagnation 枳实导滞丸, p.615).

Summerheat
In hot climates, the middle and late periods of summer bring clusters of disorders known as summerheat, characterized by high fever, nausea and vomiting, diarrhea and profuse sweating. The summerheat pathogen is very yang in nature, and quickly damages fluids and qi, and leads to a lingering pathogen that can persist for a few weeks following the initial episode. The typical features low grade fever with profuse sweating, diarrhea and nausea or anorexia, intense thirst and dryness, swollen glands and a large forceless pulse. The treatment is to clear summerheat, replenish fluids and qi and strengthen the Spleen with WANG SHI QING SHU YI QI TANG (Master Wang's Clear Summerheat and Augment the Qi Decoction 王氏清暑益气汤, p.379).

Prepared medicines
Concentrated powders
Zhu Ye Shi Gao Tang (Bamboo Leaves & Gypsum Combination)
Qing Shu Yi Qi Tang (Astragalus & Atractylodes Combination)
    – summerheat in the qi level
Xiao Cheng Qi Tang (Minor Rhubarb Combination)
Mu Xiang Bing Lang Wan (Vladmiria & Areca Seed Formula)
    – the last two when there is constipation

Acupuncture (select from)
Du.14 (dazhui –Ω) ....meeting point of the yang channels, vents heat and lingering pathogens from the qi level
LI.4 (hegu +).....................source point of the Large Intestine, and metal point
Kid.7 (fuliu +)   of the Kidneys, these points vent pathogens and

regulate sweating

Ren.12 (zhongwan –) ....alarm point of the Stomach and Large Intestine,
St.25 (tianshu –)   these points regulate Intestinal function and activate the qi dynamic

St.36 (zusanli –) ....these points strengthen digestion and activate the qi
LI.10 (shousanli –)   dynamic

St.44 (neiting –) ....clears heat from the Stomach and alleviates food stagnation

- with constipation, add St.37 (shangjuxu –) and SJ.6 (zhigou –)
- with nausea, add PC.6 (neiguan –)
- with Spleen deficiency, add Sp.6 (sanyinjiao)
- with abdominal pain, add Sp.8 (diji –), St.34 (liangqiu –) and Sp.4 (gongsun –)
- with borborygmus, add Sp.5 (shangqiu –)
- Ear points: spleen, stomach, large intestine, lung, shenmen

Clinical notes
- Qi level heat is a relatively common cause of excessive sweating, and the main treatment, when related to the diet, is to regulate the diet and stop fueling the fire. Even though sweating is the main feature, astringent herbs are contraindicated as they can lock the pathogen into the body and make the situation worse, possibly driving it further into the ying or blood levels.

16.2.4.2 SHAOYANG SYNDROME
Shaoyang syndrome can give rise to intermittent daytime sweating. The sweat follows the elevation in temperature that occurs in the fever phase of the fever and chill episodes. The treatment is the same as for shaoyang syndrome night sweats, p.719.

16.2.4.3 PHLEGM HEAT
Phlegm heat can cause both spontaneous sweating and night sweats. The treatment is the same as for phlegm heat night sweats, p.721.

16.3. SWEATING FROM THE HANDS AND FEET

1. Qi deficiency (pp.708–709, 726)
2. Yang deficiency (p.731)
3. Instability of the shen (p.728)
4. Heart fire (p.748)
5. Heat or damp heat in the qi level (pp.736, 714)
6. Spleen and Stomach yin deficiency

The hands and feet are under the control of the Spleen and Stomach, while the palms are influenced by the Heart, Pericardium and Lung channels. Both hands and feet may be affected, or only the palms or only the feet.

气
虚

16.3.1 QI DEFICIENCY

Qi deficiency of the Spleen, Heart and Lungs can all contribute, either singly or in combination, to sweating on the palms. There are two broad variations. In the first, Heart qi is weak and the shen unstable, so the palmar sweating occurs in response to anxiety or a stressful event. In addition to typical signs and symptoms of qi deficiency, the shen is disturbed causing nervousness, insomnia and palpitations. In the second, Lung, Spleen and wei qi deficiency enable fluids to simply leak out, and the hands and feet are constantly clammy. Patients immunity and energy may be poor, with digestive weakness and breathlessness. In both cases, the palms or hands and feet are cool and clammy; in some cases dripping wet. The treatment of Heart qi deficiency is the same as for Heart and Spleen deficiency type night sweats, p.708–709; Lung and Spleen qi deficiency can be treated in the same manner as qi deficiency spontaneous sweating, p.726.

阳
虚

16.3.2 YANG DEFICIENCY

The yang deficiency that contributes to excessive sweating on the hands and feet involves the Spleen, and a failure of the Spleen to support the Lungs. The characteristic feature is the coldness of the hands and feet, which may be dripping wet. The sweat can be continuous and profuse, sufficient to cause difficulty gripping objects firmly. Yang deficiency is less common as a cause of hand and feet sweating than qi deficiency, as the cold that complicates yang deficiency can cause the pores of the periphery to 'freeze shut'. The treatment is the same as for yang deficiency type spontaneous sweating, p.731.

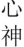
心
神
不
固

16.3.3 INSTABILITY OF THE SHEN

Instability of the shen is associated with a congenital or acquired weakness of the shen. When congenital there is a lifetime history of easy sweating, anxiety and nervousness. A destabilized shen can also be acquired through a serious trauma (p.710–711) or as the result of pathology like qi deficiency (above) or Heart fire (below). In many cases however, there is no clear pathology and in between episodes, the patient appears well. Long term acupuncture and herbs can help to gradually strengthen and stabilize the shen (p.728).

心
火

16.3.4 HEART FIRE

Heart fire, often in association with Liver fire, is the result of chronic pent up Heart and Liver qi in response to ongoing emotional problems or stress. The pent up qi is sporadically exacerbated in anticipation of an event, and fire is generated. The treatment is the same as for Heart and Liver fire type underarm sweating (p.748).

气
分
热

16.3.5 HEAT IN THE QI LEVEL

Both heat or damp heat in the qi level can lead to a steaming of fluids to the furthest points of the extremities, and cause localized sweating on the hands and feet. The more damp there is, the more the feet are affected, and the smellier they tend to become. The features and treatments are the same as for heat in the qi level type spontaneous sweating, p.736, and damp heat in the qi level type night sweats, p.714.

脾
胃
阴
虚

16.3.6 SPLEEN AND STOMACH YIN DEFICIENCY

The sweating of Spleen and Stomach yin deficiency is due to the yin fluids of the Spleen and Stomach being forced peripherally, away from their normal abode in the middle burner to the furthest part of the Spleen and Stomach's sphere of influence, the hands and feet. The upper gastrointestinal tract is dry, while the periphery is clammy.

This pattern can follow a severe gastrointestinal infection with fever that damages middle burner yin, be the result of an overly spicy diet, persistent vomiting, or repeated invasion of the middle burner by pent up Liver qi.

Clinical features

- Clamminess of the hands and feet. The sweat is mild to moderate, but may be continuous, and worse at night. The hands and feet are warm to the touch and may be red (palmar erythema)
- poor digestion; food sits in the stomach for a long time
- abdominal bloating with small amounts of food
- thirst, dry mouth and cracked lips; lack of saliva
- decreased sense of taste
- weakness of the muscles and limbs
- weight loss, or difficulty gaining weight
- easy bruising
- loose stools
- oral ulceration

T slightly red to red and dry, with a peeled coat in the center
P fine and rapid

Treatment Principle

Nourish Spleen and Stomach yin
Encourage normal distribution of fluids

Prescription

SHEN LING BAI ZHU SAN 参苓白术散
Ginseng, Poria and White Atractylodes Powder, modified

tai zi shen (Pseudostellariae Radix) 太子参 9–12g
fu ling (Poria) 茯苓 6–9g
bai zhu (Atractylodes macrocephalae Rhizoma) 白术 6–9g
shan yao (Dioscoreae Rhizoma) 山药 12–15g
lian zi (Nelumbinis Semen) 莲子 6–9g
yi ren (Coicis Semen) 苡仁 12–15g
bai bian dou (Dolichos Semen) 白扁豆 9–12g
jie geng (Platycodi Radix) 桔梗 3–6g
zhi gan cao (Glycyrrhizae Radix preparata) 炙甘草 3–6g
yu zhu (Polygonati odorati Rhizoma) 玉竹 12–15g
ge gen (Puerariae Radix) 葛根 12–15g
Method: Decoction or powder. **Tai zi shen**, used instead of **ren shen**, along with **shan yao**, **bai bian dou** and **yu zhu** moisten and nourish Spleen yin; **fu ling**, **bai zhu** and **yi ren** strengthen the Spleen, supplement qi and drain damp; **lian zi** astringes yin and stops sweating and diarrhea; **jie geng** and **ge gen** assist in elevating Spleen qi; **zhi gan cao** strengthens the spleen and supplements qi. (Source: *He Ji Ju Fang*)

Modifications

• For palmar sweating that occurs postpartum or after hemorrhage, add **dang gui** (Angelicae sinensis Radix) 当归 6–9g and **huang qi** (Astragali Radix) 黄芪 12–15g.
• With incessant loose stools or diarrhea, add **ge gen** (Puerariae Radix) 葛根 12–24g.

Prepared medicines
Concentrated powders
Shen Ling Bai Zhu San (Ginseng & Atractylodes Formula)
Pills
Shen Ling Bai Zhu Wan (Absorption and Digestion Pill, Shen Ling Bai Zhu Pian)

Acupuncture (select from)
Ht.6 (yinxi –) .... cleft point of the Heart, clears heat, supplements yin and constricts the pores to stop sweating
Kid.7 (fuliu +) .... metal point of the Kidneys, supplements the Kidneys, supports yin and stops sweating
Ren.12 (zhongwan +) .... alarm point of the Stomach, supplements middle burner qi and yin
Ren.4 (guanyuan +) .... supplements yin and yuan qi
Bl.20 (pishu +) .... transport point of the Spleen, strengthens Spleen qi and yin
Bl.21 (weishu +) .... transport point of the Stomach, supplements Stomach qi and yin
St.36 (zusanli +) .... sea point of the Stomach, supplements middle

burner qi and yin, and activates the qi dynamic

Sp.6 (sanyinjiao)................nourishes Spleen and Stomach yin

- With qi deficiency, add LI.4 (hegu +)
- with easy bruising, add Sp.10 (xuehai) and Sp.1 (yinbai ▲)
- with insomnia, add Ht.7 (shenmen) and PC.6 (neiguan –)
- with anxiety, add yintang (M–HN–3) and Du.20 (baihui)
- Ear points: spleen, stomach, zero point, subcortex, sympathetic, shenmen

Clinical notes

- Spleen and Stomach yin deficiency type sweating may be part of a picture diagnosed as chronic gastritis or gastroenteritis, the side effects of chemotherapy or radiation therapy, early stage of type 2 diabetes mellitus, malabsorption syndrome or celiac disease.
- A yin nourishing diet is recommended. See Clinical Handbook, Vol.2, p.876.

16.4 SWEATING FROM THE ARMPITS

1. Heart and Liver yin deficiency
2. Liver and Gallbladder damp heat
3. Heart and Liver Fire
4. Shaoyang syndrome (p.719)
5. Instability of the shen (p.728)

Sweating from the armpits is a normal part of the body's thermoregulation. When abnormally profuse, sweat can drip in a continual stream, soaking or staining the clothes. Abnormal underarm sweating occurs with little or no exertion and in a cool environment.

The Liver and Gallbladder organ systems control the sides of the body and the underarm area, and the Heart channel emerges from the axilla. Either the Heart and Liver, or both, may be involved in sweating of this type.

心
肝
阴
虚

16.4.1 HEART AND LIVER YIN DEFICIENCY

This is a chronic type of excessive sweating, more commonly seen in those over 40 years old. It can also be seen in younger individuals who have depleted their yin through drug use and partying, overwork or insufficient sleep and rest.

Clinical features
- Underarm sweating that is profuse and watery, but not especially malodorous or offensive. The sweat can occur at any time, but is more pronounced towards evening and at night, and when the patient is nervous, anxious, or angry and upset.
- facial flushing, malar flush
- heat in the palms and soles
- dry mouth and throat
- **with Liver yin deficiency**: sweating, worse with anger or stress, dizziness, visual weakness, blurred vision, photophobia, tendency to dull headaches or migraines
- **with Heart yin deficiency**: sweating, worse when anxious or nervous, insomnia, fitful sleep, dream disturbed sleep, palpitations, mouth ulcers

T red tongue with little or no coat
P wiry, fine, maybe rapid

Treatment Principle
Supplement Heart and Liver yin and blood
Clear heat and stop sweating

Prescription

QI JU DI HUANG WAN 杞菊地黄丸
Lycium Fruit, Chrysanthemum and Rehmannia Pill, modified

This prescription is selected when Liver yin deficiency is primary.
shu di (Rehmanniae Radix preparata) 熟地 15–24g

shan yao (Dioscoreae Rhizoma) 山药 12–15g
shan zhu yu (Corni Fructus) 山茱萸 12–18g
mu dan pi (Moutan Cortex) 牡丹皮 9–12g
fu ling (Poria) 茯苓 9–12g
ze xie (Alismatis Rhizoma) 泽泻 9–12g
ju hua (Chrysanthemi Flos) 菊花 9–12g
gou qi zi (Lycii Fructus) 枸杞子 9–12g
bai shao (Paeoniae Radix alba) 白芍 12–15g

Method: Decoction or powders. **Shu di** enriches Liver and Kidney yin and blood; the large dose of **shan zhu yu** astringes sweating and nourishes Liver yin; **shan yao** strengthens the Spleen and supplements qi and yin; **ze xie**, **mu dan pi** and **fu ling** drain any heat and damp and prevent the supplements from creating stagnation; **gou qi zi** and **ju hua** nourish Liver yin and blood; **bai shao** astringes yin, nourishes blood and softens the Liver. (Source: *Yi Ji Bao Jian*)

Modifications

- With profuse or persistent sweating, add **ma huang gen** (Ephedrae Radix) 麻黄根 9–12g and **wu wei zi** (Schizandrae Fructus) 五味子 3–6g, or **duan mu li** (calcined Ostreae Concha) 煅牡蛎 18–30g and **duan long gu** (calcined Fossilia Ossis Mastodi) 煅龙骨 18–30g.
- With blood deficiency, postural dizziness, a dry pink tongue and spots in the visual field, add **dang gui** (Angelicae sinensis Radix) 当归 9–12g and **he shou wu** (Polygoni multiflori Radix) 何首乌 9–12g.

Variations and additional prescriptions

Heart yin deficiency

When Heart yin deficiency is the main factor, the main features are shen disturbance, and the sweating occurs in response to anxiety. The treatment is to nourish Heart yin and calm the shen with TIAN WANG BU XIN DAN (Emperor of Heaven's Special Pill to Supplement the Heart 天王补心丹, p.904).

Liver blood deficiency with qi constraint

An excessive amount of underarm sweating can also be seen in some patients who are under a lot of mental strain. Even though they may not be physically active, the stress and resulting qi constraint can deplete blood. The blood deficiency leads to unrestrained yang which expresses itself through the shaoyang, here the armpits. The sweat is generally inoffensive, and may be more copious prior to menstruation. The treatment is to nourish Liver blood and alleviate qi constraint with a formula such as XIAO YAO SAN (Rambling Powder 逍遥散, p.841).

Prepared medicines

Concentrated powders

Qi Ju Di Huang Wan (Lycium, Chrysanthemum & Rehamannia Formula)
Zhi Bai Di Huang Wan (Anemarrhena, Phellodendron & Rehmannia Formula)
    – with significant heat
Tian Wang Bu Xin Dan (Ginseng & Zizyphus Formula)
    – with Heart yin deficiency
Xiao Yao San (Bupleurum & Tangkuei Formula)

– Liver blood deficiency with constrained qi

Pills

Qi Ju Di Huang Wan (Lycium–Rehmannia Pills)

Zhi Bai Ba Wei Wan (Eight Flavor Rehmannia Teapills)

Tian Wang Bu Xin Dan (Emperor's Teapills, Tian Wang Pu Hsin Tan)

Xiao Yao Wan (Free and Easy Wanderer Teapills, Hsiao Yao Wan)

Acupuncture (select from)

Ht.1 (jiquan).....................local point in the axilla for sweating

GB.40 (qiuxu)..................source point of the Gallbladder, alleviates sweating from the axilla

LI.4 (hegu –).....................source point of the Large Intestine, diffuses the Lungs, clears heat and stops sweating

Ht.6 (yinxi –).....................cleft point of the Heart, clears heat and assists in constricting the pores to control sweating

Ht.7 (shenmen)..................source point of the Heart, cools the Heart, calms the shen, regulates and supplements Heart yin

Liv.3 (taichong +)...............source, transport and earth point of the Liver, supplements Liver yin and blood, regulates the channels

Liv.8 (ququan –).................sea and water point of the Liver, boosts and supplements Liver blood and yin

Bl.23 (shenshu +)...............these points boost and supplement Liver and Heart

Bl.15 (xinshu +)   yin

yintang (M–HN–3)...........calms the shen

Du.20 (baihui)..................calms the shen

• Ear points: liver, heart, sympathetic, subcortex, shenmen

Clinical notes

• Excessive underarm sweating of a Liver and Heart yin deficiency type may be diagnosed as hyperhidrosis. It is rarely considered pathological.

• A yin nourishing diet is recommended. See Clinical Handbook, Vol.2, p.876.

16.4.2 LIVER GALLBLADDER DAMP HEAT

肝
胆
湿
热

Liver and Gallbladder damp heat causing excessive or offensive underarm sweating is a chronic problem. It is often related to chronic qi constraint and the development of internal heat, compounded by consumption of damp and/or heating foods and beverages. The balance of damp and heat can vary from time to time depending on the patients diet, mood and environment, and can change the nature and location of the sweating. The more heat there is the more underarm sweating occurs, and the more offensive the sweat. When damp is predominant, more sweat appears in the lower body, especially the groin and genital region.

Clinical features

• Excessive underarm sweating with a strong or offensive odor; the clothing may be stained brown or yellow by the sweat

- irritability, restlessness, easily angered
- bitter taste in the mouth
- red complexion with greasy skin; red sore eyes
- dark, concentrated or painful urination
- sluggish bowels, constipation or loose stools; stools may be pasty or clay like

T red with a thick, greasy, yellow coat
P wiry, slippery, rapid

Treatment Principle

Clear damp heat from the Liver and Gallbladder

Prescription

LONG DAN XIE GAN TANG 龙胆泻肝汤
Gentian Decoction to Purge the Liver

long dan cao (Gentianae Radix) 龙胆草 6–9g
huang qin (Scutellariae Radix) 黄芩 6–12g
shan zhi zi (Gardeniae Fructus) 山栀子 6–12g
ze xie (Alismatis Rhizoma) 泽泻 6–12g
mu tong (Akebiae Caulis) 木通 3–6g
che qian zi (Plantaginis Semen) 车前子 9–15g
sheng di (Rehmanniae Radix) 生地 9–15g
dang gui (Angelicae sinensis Radix) 当归 6–12g
chai hu (Bupleuri Radix) 柴胡 3–9g
gan cao (Glycyrrhizae Radix) 甘草 3–6g

Method: Decoction. **Che qian zi** is cooked in a cloth bag. **Long dan cao** cools the Liver and clears heat; **shan zhi zi** clears heat from all three burners; **huang qin** clears heat from the upper body; **chai hu** clears heat, dredges the Liver and relieves qi constraint; **ze xie**, **che qian zi** and **mu tong** promote urination to provide an escape route for the heat; **sheng di** cools the blood; **dang gui** nourishes and protects blood; **gan cao** protects the Stomach. (Source: *Zhong Yi Nei Ke Xue* [*Yi Fang Ji Jie*])

Modifications

- The balance of heat and damp can vary considerably. When the heat is relatively mild and the damp pronounced, the dose of **long dan cao**, **huang qin** and **shan zhi zi** should be at the lower end of the dosage range, and damp drying and leaching herbs, such as **bai zhu** (Atractylodes macrocephalae Rhizoma) 白术 9–12g and **fu ling** (Poria) 茯苓 12–15g added. See also p.766.
- With constipation, add **da huang** (Rhei Radix et Rhizoma) 大黄 6–9g and **mang xiao** (Natrii Sulfas) 芒硝 6g [dissolved in the strained decoction].
- With difficult or sluggish stools, add **zhi ke** (Aurantii Fructus) 枳壳 9–12g and **bai zhu** (Atractylodes macrocephalae Rhizoma) 白术 30g.
- With abdominal distension, add **zhi shi** (Aurantii Fructus immaturus) 枳实 9–12g, **hou po** (Magnoliae officinalis Cortex) 厚朴 9–12g and **da fu pi** (Arecae Pericarpium) 大复皮 9–12g.
- With concentrated or painful urination, add **bai mao gen** (Imperatae Rhizoma) 白茅根 12–18g and **hua shi** (Talcum) 滑石 9–12g.

Prepared medicines
Concentrated powders
Long Dan Xie Gan Tang (Gentiana Combination)
Pills
Long Dan Xie Gan Wan (Snake and Dragon Teapills)
Li Dan Pian (Lidan Tablets)

Acupuncture (select from)
Ht.1 (jiquan).....................local point in the axilla for sweating
GB.41 (zulinqi –) ....master and couple points of daimai, clear damp
SJ.5 (waiguan –)   heat from the Liver and Gallbladder, and regulate
                                 the lateral parts of the body
SJ.6 (zhigou –) ....these points clear damp heat and promote qi
GB.34 (yanglingquan –)   movement through the lateral aspect of the body
Liv.3 (taichong –)..............source point of the Liver, clears damp heat, dredges
                                 the Liver, regulates qi
Bl.18 (ganshu)...................transport point of the Liver, dredges the Liver and
                                 regulates qi, clears damp heat
Bl.19 (danshu –) ....transport point of the Gallbladder, clears damp heat
- with fever or flushing add LI.11 (quchi –)
- with abdominal distension, add Ren.12 (zhongwan –) and St.25 (tianshu –)
- with constipation or sluggish stools, add St.25 (tianshu –)
- with nausea add PC.6 (neiguan –)
- with jaundice add Du.9 (zhiyang –)
- with gallstones, add dannangxue (M–LE–23)
- Ear points: liver, gallbladder, spleen, shenmen, sympathetic, subcortex

Clinical notes
- Excessive underarm sweating from Liver and Gallbladder damp heat is likely to be diagnosed as hyperhidrosis, and patients with this pattern diagnosed with hypertension, obesity, gall stones, cholecystitis, the effects of drug or alcohol abuse or chronic liver disease.
- An important principle to observe in the treatment of damp heat is to keep the bowels moving and urination flowing to provide an escape route for both heat and damp. An increase in both bowel frequency and urinary output should be observed following ingestion of medicine or acupuncture. If **da huang** is used to initiate or encourage bowel movement, it should be reduced in dosage or deleted once this is achieved so as to avoid iatrogenic damage to Spleen yang.
- A damp heat clearing diet is essential. See Clinical Handbook, Vol.2, p.884.

心
肝
火
旺

16.4.3 HEART AND LIVER FIRE

The sweating associated with Heart fire has a significant emotional component. It can be the result of some emotional trauma or shock which impedes the circulation and distribution of Heart qi. The stagnation of Heart and Liver qi that results creates fire, which is transmitted through the pathway of the Heart and shaoyang channels. The fire forces sweat out to appear in the axilla.

Clinical features

- Profuse underarm sweating that is continuous, is not especially offensive and is significantly increased when the patient is under pressure, anxious, or in anticipation of a stressful event. The sweating may also occur on the palms of the hands.
- insomnia, dream disturbed sleep or nightmares
- restlessness, irritability or anxiety
- palpitations, tachycardia
- thirst with a desire for cold fluids
- bitter taste in the mouth
- ulceration of the mouth and tongue, particularly the tongue tip
- red complexion; red sore eyes
- concentrated or painful urination

T red with a redder tip and a dry, yellow coat; the tongue may be ulcerated
P rapid and flooding, especially in the distal position

Treatment principle

Cool the Heart and Liver and drain fire
Cool the blood and stop sweating

Prescription

QING XIN LIAN ZI YIN 清心莲子饮
Lotus Seed Decoction to Cool the Heart

shi lian zi (Nelumbinis Semen) 石莲子	9–12g
fu ling (Poria) 茯苓	15–20g
huang qi (Astragali Radix) 黄芪	15–18g
ren shen (Ginseng Radix) 人参	9–12g
huang qin (Scutellariae Radix) 黄芩	9–12g
mai dong (Ophiopogonis Radix) 麦冬	9–12g
di gu pi (Lycii Cortex) 地骨皮	12–15g
che qian zi (Plantaginis Semen) 车前子	15–20g
gan cao (Glycyrrhizae Radix) 甘草	6–9g

Method: Decoction. **Shi lian zi** cools Heart fire, alleviates irritability and clears damp heat; **huang qin** and **di gu pi** support the heat clearing action of **shi lian zi** and clear damp heat and deficient heat respectively; **fu ling** and **che qian zi** promote urination to clear heat and drain damp through the urine; **ren shen**, **huang qi** and **gan cao** supplement and protect qi; **mai dong** cools the Heart and nourishes yin. (Source: *He Ji Ju Fang*)

Modifications

- For sweating and sleep disturbances that are brought on by stress, add **he**

huan pi (Albizziae Cortex) 合欢皮 12–15g and **suan zao ren** (Ziziphi spinosae Semen) 酸枣仁 12–15g.

- For cloudy uncomfortable urination, add **bi xie** (Dioscoreae hypoglaucae Rhizoma) 萆薢 9–12g and **shi chang pu** (Acori tatarinowii Rhizoma) 石菖蒲 6–9g.
- For chronic sore throat, add **xuan shen** (Scrophulariae Radix) 玄参 12–15g.
- With edema, add **yi mu cao** (Leonurus Herba) 益母草 12–15g.
- With fever, add **chai hu** (Bupleuri Radix) 柴胡 6–9g.
- With signs that heat has begun to damage the yin, causing dry mouth, red dry tongue and thirst, add **sheng di** (Rehmanniae Radix) 生地 15–18g and **xuan shen** (Scrophulariae Radix) 玄参 12–18g.

Prepared medicines
Concentrated powders
Qing Xin Lian Zi Yin (Lotus Seed Combination)
Pills
Dao Chi Pian (Tao Chih Pien)

Acupuncture (select from)
Ht.6 (yinxi –).....................cleft point of the Heart, clears heat and constricting the pores to control sweating

LI.4 (hegu +).....................source point of the Large Intestine, diffuses the Lungs, clears heat and stops sweating

PC.8 (laogong –)................fire point of the Pericardium, clears Heart fire

Ht.8 (shaofu –) ....fire point of the Heart, clears Heart fire, regulates Heart qi and calms the shen

Bl.15 (xinshu) ....transport point of the Heart, clears heat from the Heart

Sp.6 (sanyinjiao)................strengthens the Spleen and Kidneys to generate qi and yin and cool the blood

Kid.6 (zhaohai +) ....master point of yinqiaomai, clears heat, calms the shen and supplements the Kidneys to cool the Heart

yintang (M–HN–3) ....calms the shen and clears the mind

- Ear points: shenmen, heart, kidney, sympathetic, subcortex

Clinical notes
- Heart and Liver fire may be diagnosed as autonomic nervous system dysfunction, menopausal syndrome, stress response, nervous exhaustion, the effects of drug or alcohol abuse, chronic fatigue syndrome, anxiety disorder or Behçets disease.
- This type of sweating can respond reasonably well to treatment.
- A cooling diet is recommended. See Clinical Handbook, Vol.2, p.882.

16.4.4 SHAOYANG SYNDROME

A pathogen in the shaoyang can contribute to abnormal underarm sweating due to the relationship between the shaoyang pivot and the lateral parts of the body. The sweat may be profuse, watery and inoffensive when heat is the main pathogen, or stickier and with more intense odor when damp heat is at work. The treatment is the same as for shaoyang type night sweats, p.719.

16.4.5 INSTABILITY OF THE SHEN

Instability of the shen can contribute to profuse underarm sweating. See p.728.

16.5 SWEATING ON THE HEAD AND CHEST

1. Qi and yin deficiency
2. Yang qi deficiency (p.731)
3. Liver qi constraint with heat
4. Food stagnation (accumulation disorder)
5. Lingering pathogens
   - Lingering heat in the chest
   - Damp heat in the qi level (p.714)

16.5.1 QI AND YIN DEFICIENCY

气
阴
两
虚

Qi and yin deficiency type sweating is quite common in the convalescent phase of a febrile illness, when Lungs and Heart qi and yin have been damaged by a heat pathogen. It also occurs in those with a chronic or constitutional tendency to Lung qi deficiency. The sweating is due to the combined effects of wei qi not closing the pores completely, and the heat from deficient yin pushing fluid to the surface.

Clinical features

- Sweating on the head and chest. The sweat may occur both day and night, but the patient will usually notice it most in bed, when the pillow becomes damp and uncomfortable.
- breathlessness or wheezing
- pale face with red cheeks, malar flush
- sensation of heat in the palms and soles

T pink or slightly red with a thin or peeled coat, or with multiple surface cracks
P fine, weak, or large and weak in the distal position

Treatment Principle

Supplement qi and yin and restrain yang

Prescription

SHENG MAI SAN 生脉散
Generate the Pulse Powder, modified

ren shen (Ginseng Radix) 人参 9–15g
mai dong (Ophiopogonis Radix) 麦冬 15–24g
wu wei zi (Schizandrae Fructus) 五味子 6–9g
duan long gu (calcined Fossilia Ossis Mastodi) 煅龙骨 15–30g
duan mu li (calcined Ostreae Concha) 煅牡蛎 15–30g
bai shao (Paeoniae Radix alba) 白芍 12–18g
fu xiao mai (Tritici Fructus levis) 浮小麦 15–30g
wu mei (Mume Fructus) 乌梅 9–12g

Method: Decoction. **Ren shen** and **wu wei zi** strengthen the Spleen and Lungs, supplements qi and secure the exterior; **mai dong** nourishes Lung and Stomach yin; **duan long gu** and **duan mu li** secure the exterior to stop sweating; **bai shao** nourishes and astringes yin; **fu xiao mai** and **wu mei** stop sweating. Source: *Zhong Yi Nei Ke Lin Chuang Shou Ce* [*Nei Wai Shang Bian Huo Lun*]

Variations and additional prescriptions
With anxiety and insomnia
When qi and yin deficiency specifically affects the Heart, it can disturb the shen, in addition to causing sweating on the chest and upper back. The patient experiences both day and night time sweating. The treatment is to replenish qi and yin and calm the shen with a formula such as TIAN WANG BU XIN DAN (Emperor of Heaven's Special Pill to Supplement the Heart 天王补心丹, p.904), or ZHI GAN CAO TANG (Prepared Licorice Decoction 炙甘草汤, p.811).

Prepared medicines
Concentrated powders
Sheng Mai San (Ginseng & Ophiopogon Formula)
Tian Wang Bu Xin Dan (Ginseng & Zizyphus Formula)
Zhi Gan Cao Tang (Licorice Combination)

Pills
Sheng Mai Wan (Great Pulse Teapills)
Tian Wang Bu Xin Dan (Emperor's Teapills, Tian Wang Pu Hsin Tan)
Zhi Gan Cao Wan (Zhi Gan Cao Teapills)

Acupuncture (select from)
Ht.6 (yinxi –).....................cleft point of the Heart, supplements yin and constricts the pores to control sweating
LI.4 (hegu +).....................source point of the Large Intestine, diffuses the Lungs and regulates sweating
St.36 (zusanli +) ....sea point of the Stomach, strengthens the Spleen and Stomach and supplements qi and blood
Sp.6 (sanyinjiao +)..............supplements qi and yin
Bl.15 (xinshu +) ....transport point of the Heart, supplements Heart qi, calms the Heart and shen
Bl.20 (pishu +) ....transport point of the Spleen, fortifies the Spleen and supplements qi and blood
Bl.23 (shenshu +) ....transport point of the Kidneys, strengthens the Kidneys and source of the body's yin and yang
• Ear points: heart, spleen, lung, kidney, sympathetic, subcortex, shenmen

Clinical notes
• Patients with chronic respiratory problems such as asthma and emphysema are prone to sweating predominantly on the chest. The frequent use of bronchodilator medicines such as salbutamol and inhaled steroids forcefully disperse obstructed Lung qi and relieve tightness and wheezing, but gradually disperse Lung and Heart qi and compound the weakness that gives rise to the sweating.
• Sweating from qi and yin deficiency after febrile illness responds well and quickly to treatment. When associated with a more chronic condition such as asthma or emphysema, it can still respond, but will take longer to rebuild qi and yin.
• Lung and Heart qi strengthening exercises are strongly recommended, in particular aerobic activity like long distance walking or swimming.

阳虚

16.5.2 YANG QI DEFICIENCY

The head and posterior neck, being the most yang parts of the body, are especially vulnerable to weakness of yang and that most yang type of qi, the wei qi. In addition, weak yang can be so feeble that instead powering normal physiological activity, it simply floats away to the head. The combined effect of these mechanisms gives rise to a profuse sweat on the head and neck. In severe cases of yang deficiency, a copious or oily sweating on the head may be a sign that separation of yin and yang (i.e. death) is imminent. The treatment is the same as for yang deficiency type spontaneous sweating, p.731.

肝气郁滞

16.5.3 LIVER QI CONSTRAINT

Liver qi constraint causes sweating on the head because the constrained qi is contained within the trunk and unable to circulate to the extremities. At a certain point of pressure, however, the constrained yang qi and heat generated by the constraint, looks for an exit point, and is funneled up to the head. The extra yang qi and heat in the head are released with sweating.

Clinical features

- Sweating on the head and face. The sweat is intermittent, and increases in response to escalating stress levels. The patient feels the rising yang qi and facial flushing prior to the onset of the sweat.
- cold fingers and toes, while the trunk and head feel warm
- irritability, easily angered
- chest oppression; difficulty getting a deep and satisfying breath
- abdominal distension or colicky abdominal pain; hypochondriac ache
- belching, nausea
- tight muscles in the neck and shoulders; tension headaches; tight rectus
- alternating constipation and diarrhea

T mauve or red or with red edges and a thin yellow coat
P deep, wiry, fine

Treatment Principle

Dredge the Liver, mobilize qi and alleviate qi constraint
Harmonize the Liver and Spleen and rectifies the qi dynamic

Prescription

SI NI SAN 四逆散
Frigid Extremities Powder

chai hu (Bupleuri Radix) 柴胡 6–9g
bai shao (Paeoniae Radix alba) 白芍 6–9g
zhi shi (Aurantii Fructus immaturus) 枳实 6–9g
zhi gan cao (Glycyrrhizae Radix preparata) 炙甘草 6–9g
Method: Powder or decoction. Grind the herbs to a fine powder and take 2–3 grams as a draft with water twice daily. **Chai hu** dredges the Liver, regulates qi, resolves qi constraint, raises yang qi and clears heat; **zhi shi** breaks up stagnant qi, directs qi downwards and alleviates distension, its descending action balancing the ascending nature of **chai hu** thus driving the pivotal dynamo of the qi

dynamic; **bai shao** softens the Liver and nourishes yin and blood, thus preventing excessive dispersal of, and damage to, qi and Liver yin by **chai hu**; **zhi gan cao** harmonizes the Stomach and strengthen the Spleen, and with **bai shao** eases spasms and alleviates cramping pain of both smooth and skeletal muscles. (Source: *Shi Yong Zhong Yi Er Ke Xue* [*Zheng Zhi Zhun Sheng*])

Prepared medicine
Concentrated powders
Si Ni San (Bupleurum & Aurantium Immaturus Formula)

Pills
Si Ni San Wan (Four Pillars Teapills)

Acupuncture (select from)
Ht.6 (yinxi –).....................cleft point of the Heart, constricts the pores to stop sweating

Kid.7 (fuliu +)....................metal point of the Kidneys, clears heat and stops sweating

Liv.3 (taichong –)...............the 'four gates', these points together mobilize qi and
LI.4 (hegu –)   blood, calm the shen and hun, and ease muscle spasm; LI.4 (hegu –) also works with Ht.6 (yinxi) to control sweating

PC.6 (neiguan)...................opens up qi flow through the chest, dredges the liver and moves constrained qi, calms the Heart and shen, downbears counterflow Stomach qi

GB.34 (yanglingquan –)......sea point of the Gallbladder, regulates qi and pacifies ascendant Liver yang

Liv.2 (xingjian –)................fire point of the Liver, clears heat from the Liver and alleviates constrained qi

- Ear points: liver, spleen, zero point, subcortex, endocrine, shenmen

Clinical notes
- Liver qi constraint type sweating may be diagnosed as stress response, autonomic nervous system dysfunction or idiopathic hyperhidrosis.
- This type of sweating, while most commonly restricted to the head, can also occasionally be seen on the trunk as well, or be localized to the armpits.

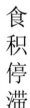

16.5.4 FOOD STAGNATION (ACCUMULATION DISORDER)
This is a pediatric condition, affecting children up to about the age of five. The sweating is due to the Spleen and Stomach (yangming) heat that is generated by the accumulated and fermenting food. The heat rises to the head through the yangming channels.

Clinical features
- Sweating on the head and back of the neck at night. This differs from a night sweat in that the child does not necessarily wake with the sweat, but is detected by the parents or seen in the damp pillow in the morning.
- distended or painful abdomen; child complains of tummy pains
- bad smelling bowel movements; smelly wind; may be constipation or diarrhea

- restlessness, irritability, fractiousness
- bad breath
- restless sleep
- bright red cheeks

T thick, greasy yellow coat
P slippery, wiry

Treatment Principle
Alleviate food stagnation, clear heat
Strengthen the Spleen and harmonize the qi dynamic

Prescription

QU MAI ZHI ZHU WAN 曲麦枳术丸
Medicated Leaven, Barley Sprout, Unripe Bitter Orange and Atractylodes Pill

jiao shen qu (scorched Massa medicata fermentata) 焦神曲 5g
chao mai ya (dry fried Hordei Fructus germinantus) 炒麦芽 5g
chao bai zhu (stir fried Atractylodes macrocephalae Rhizoma) 炒白术 ... 5g
chao zhi shi (stir fried Aurantii Fructus immaturus) 炒枳实 5g

Method: Decoction or powder. Grind the herbs to a fine powder and take 2–3 grams as a draft with water and honey twice daily. **Jiao shen qu** and **chai mai ya** dissolve accumulated food and promote digestion; **chao bai zhu** strengthens the Spleen; **chao zhi shi** directs qi downward and stimulates the qi dynamic. (Source: *Shi Yong Zhong Yi Er Ke Xue [Zheng Zhi Zhun Sheng]*)

Prepared medicine
Concentrated powders
Jin Jian Fei Er Wan (Ginseng & Poria Formula)
   – best with constipation
Xiao Er Qi Xing Cha (Children's Seven Star Tea)
Bao He Wan (Red Tangerine Peel & Crategus Formula)

Pills
Bao He Wan (Preserve Harmony Pill)
   – pills can be crushed up before being suspended in a little warm water

Acupuncture
sifeng (M–UE–9 ↓) ....the main points for accumulation disorder in infants
St.36 (zusanli) ....sea point of the Stomach, strengthens the Spleen and stimulates the qi dynamic
St.25 (tianshu)...................alarm point of the Large Intestine, promotes Intestinal function and clears stagnation
St.44 (neiting) ....water point of the Stomach, clear heat from yangming
Ear points: zero point, abdomen, sympathetic

Clinical notes
- The main treatment for accumulation disorder is dietary. The child should not be overfed, or allowed to eat too much sweet or cloying food. Snacking or constant grazing should be discouraged.

- The formulae above can be used for a few days to a week or so until the heat is cleared and digestion is working better, then dietary regulation is the best management tool.

热
郁
气
分

16.5.5 RESIDUAL HEAT IN THE CHEST

A mild and relatively common pattern in which lingering heat affects the Heart and shen, with little damage to qi or yin. This type of sweating usually follows an unresolved upper respiratory tract infection.

Clinical features
- Sweating and a sensation of stifling heat on the chest and upper back. This type of sweating can persist for some weeks after the initial cold or flu has passed.
- restlessness, irritability or depression
- tossing and turning in bed, fitful sleep
- mild but persistent feverishness
- fatigue

T red tip with a slightly yellow coat
P strong and floating in the distal position

Treatment Principle
Clear and vent heat from the qi level

Prescription

ZHI ZI CHI TANG 栀子豉汤
Gardenia and Prepared Soybean Decoction

shan zhi zi (Gardeniae Fructus) 山栀子 6–9g
dan dou chi (Sojae Semen preparatum) 淡豆豉 9–12g
Method: Decoction. **Shan zhi zi** clears heat from all three burners and alleviates irritability; **dan dou chi** vents constrained heat from the chest. (Source: *Shang Han Lun*)

Modifications
- With significant residual heat, dry mouth, bitter taste in the mouth and red tipped tongue, add **lian qiao** (Forsythiae Fructus) 连翘 9–12g and **huang qin** (Scutellariae Radix) 黄芩 6–9g.
- With any pathogen remaining on the surface, add **niu bang zi** (Arctii Fructus) 牛蒡子 9–12g and **bo he** (Mentha haplocalycis Herba) 薄荷 6–9g [added at the end of cooking].

Prepared medicines
Concentrated powders
Zhu Ye Shi Gao Tang (Bamboo Leaves & Gypsum Combination)

Acupuncture (select from)
Ht.6 (yinxi –) .... cleft point of the Heart, clears heat from the chest and constricting the pores to control sweating
LI.4 (hegu +) .... source point of the Large Intestine, diffuses the Lungs, clears heat and stops sweating

Du.14 (dazhui –)................clear heat and lingering pathogens from the chest
Du.12 (shenzhu –)
• Ear points: zero point, lung, stomach, shenmen, sympathetic

Clinical notes
• A simple condition that responds quickly to treatment.

16.5.6 DAMP HEAT IN THE QI LEVEL

湿
热
郁
蒸

The mechanism of the sweating here is damp blocking the surface of the trunk, so heat is unable to escape and is forced upwards, 'like smoke up a chimney' to emerge on the head. The treatment is the same as for damp heat in the qi level type night sweats, p.714.

16.6 SWEATING ON HALF THE BODY

1. Qi and blood deficiency
2. Cold damp

This is sweating on half the body, divided bilaterally down the midline.

气
血
虚
弱

16.6.1 QI AND BLOOD DEFICIENCY

This pattern can occur following a severe and debilitating illness, a difficult or exhausting pregnancy or delivery, sudden and catastrophic blood loss or wind stroke. It can also be a warning sign of an impending wind stroke. The sweating is due to the lack of consolidation and regulation of the pores by wei qi on the affected side.

Clinical features

- Obvious and spontaneous sweating on either the left or right half the body, with little or no sweat on the other side; numbness, coldness and weakness of the extremities on the sweating side
- pale, sallow complexion
- fatigue and lethargy
- postural dizziness
- dry skin and hair
- palpitations
- insomnia
- soft abdomen with poor tone; likes pressure; feels cool to touch

T pale and thin, with a white coat
P fine, weak

Treatment Principle

Supplement qi and blood

Prescription

SHI QUAN DA BU TANG 十全大补汤
All Inclusive Great Supplementing Decoction

shu di (Rehmanniae Radix preparata) 熟地	9–15g
dang gui (Angelicae sinensis Radix) 当归	9–12g
bai shao (Paeoniae Radix alba) 白芍	6–9g
chuan xiong (Chuanxiong Rhizoma) 川芎	3–6g
bai zhu (Atractylodes macrocephalae Rhizoma) 白术	9–12g
ren shen (Ginseng Radix) 人参	6–9g
fu ling (Poria) 茯苓	6–9g
zhi gan cao (Glycyrrhizae Radix preparata) 炙甘草	3–6g
huang qi (Astragali Radix) 黄芪	9–15g
rou gui (Cinnamomi Cortex) 肉桂	6–9g

Method: Decoction, pills or powder. **Shu di** nourishes yin and blood and supplements the Kidneys; **dang gui** and **bai shao** supplement blood and soften the Liver; **dang gui** and **chuan xiong** activate blood and move qi; **dang gui** and **huang qi** work together to build blood, and **huang qi** works with **chuan xiong** to distribute qi and blood to the extremities; **ren shen** and **huang qi** strengthen the Spleen and Stomach and supplement qi; **bai zhu** effectively strengthens the Spleen and dries damp; **fu ling** strengthen the Spleen, leaches out damp and calms the shen; **zhi gan cao** supplements qi, harmonizes the action of the other herbs, and with **bai shao** alleviates spasmodic pain; **rou gui** warms yang and promotes transformation of food into blood. (Source: *Zhong Yi Nei Ke Lin Chuang Shou Ce* [*He Ji Ju Fang*])

Modifications

- To open the channels and network vessels, add **ji xue teng** (Spatholobi Caulis) 鸡血藤 18–30g and **dan shen** (Salviae miltiorrhizae Radix) 丹参 9–12g.
- With yang deficiency, and when the pattern is more than a few months old, **zhi fu zi** (Aconiti Radix lateralis preparata) 制附子 6–9g can be added to activate the distribution of yang qi into the periphery.
- If the upper limbs are most affected, add **sang zhi** (Mori Ramulus) 桑枝 15–30g.
- If the lower limbs are most affected add **chuan niu xi** (Cyathulae Radix) 川牛膝 9–12g and **du zhong** (Eucommiae Cortex) 杜仲 9–12g.

Variations and additional prescriptions

Qi and blood deficiency with blood stasis, post wind stroke

With more loss of function on the affected side, activation of the blood and channel clearing is necessary to break through the obstructed channels and network vessels. The patient will have the features of qi and blood deficiency and the unilateral sweating, but the affected side will be partially hemiplegic, or there may be facial paralysis and slurred speech. The treatment is to supplement and move qi, activate blood and unblock the channels and network vessels with a formula such as BU YANG HUAN WU TANG (Supplement Yang to Restore Five Tenths Decoction 补阳还五汤).

huang qi (Astragali Radix) 黄芪 30–120g
dang gui wei (rootlets of Angelicae sinensis Radix) 当归尾 6–12g
chi shao (Paeoniae Radix rubra) 赤芍 6–9g
chuan xiong (Chuanxiong Rhizoma) 川芎 6–9g
tao ren (Persicae Semen) 桃仁 6–9g
hong hua (Carthami Flos) 红花 6–9g
di long (Pheretima) 地龙 6–12g

Method: Decoction. **Huang qi** supplements, and activates qi; **dang gui wei** supplements and activates the blood; **chi shao**, **chuan xiong**, **tao ren** and **hong hua** activate blood and dispel blood stasis; **di long** 'drills through' blockages in the channels and network vessels, opening them up and allowing free flow or qi and blood. (Source: *Yi Lin Gai Cuo*)

Prepared medicines

Concentrated powders

Shi Quan Da Bu Tang (Ginseng & Dang Gui Ten Combination)
Bu Yang Huan Wu Tang (Astragalus & Peony Combination)

Pills

Shi Quan Da Bu Wan (Ten Flavour Teapills)
Bu Yang Huan Wu Wan (Great Yang Restoration Teapills)

Acupuncture (select from)

SI.3 (houxi) ....These points, the master and couple points of the
Bl.62 (shenmai)   dumai and renmai help balance the distribution of
Lu.7 (lieque)   qi and blood between the two halves of the body.
Kid.6 (zhaohai)   Usually one point is used per side, with the first
                                   insertion on the affected side, e.g. if the right side
                                   is affected, SI.3 is needled on the right, followed by
                                   Bl.62 on the left, then Lu.7 on the left and Kid.6 on
                                   the right. When this treatment is used, only these
                                   points are treated. It can be alternated with treat-
                                   ment of the points below.

Ren.12 (zhongwan +▲).......alarm point of the Stomach, strengthens the Spleen
                                   and Stomach and supplements qi and blood
Ren.4 (guanyuan+▲)..........supplements yuan qi and Kidney qi
St.36 (zusanli +▲) ....sea point of the Stomach, strengthens the Spleen and
                                   Stomach and supplements qi and blood
LI.11 (quchi +)...................sea point of the Large Intestine, regulates circulation
                                   of qi and blood in the extremities
Sp.6 (sanyinjiao +▲)..........strengthens the Spleen and Kidneys and supple-
                                   ments qi and blood
Bl.15 (xinshu +) ....transport point of the Heart, supplements Heart qi
                                   and improves circulation
Bl.20 (pishu +▲) ....transport point of the Spleen, strengthens the Spleen
                                   and supplements qi and blood
Bl.25 (shenshu +▲) ....transport point of the Kidney, strengthens the
                                   Kidneys to support the Spleen and supplement qi
                                   and blood

• with hemiplegia, add points along the yangming channels of the arms and legs
• with palpitations and insomnia, add Ht.5 (tongli) and Ht.7 (shenmen +)
• with dizziness, add Du.20 (baihui ▲)
• Ear points: shenmen, heart, spleen, zero point, sympathetic, subcortex

Clinical notes
• A diet to build qi and blood is essential. See Clinical Handbook, Vol.2, p.870
  and 874.

寒
湿
痹
阻

16.6.2 COLD DAMP

This pattern is associated with a type of painful obstruction, whereby the cold
damp blocks the pores on the affected side and prevents sweat from escaping.

Clinical features
• Sweating on half the body only. The sweat is unlikely to be copious, but sufficient for the patient to notice the difference. The side without sweat is likely
  to suffer mild joint and muscle pain, stiffness, soreness, aching or heaviness.
• in the early stages there may be fever and aversion to wind
• fatigue and lethargy, worse after prolonged inactivity

T thin, greasy, white coat; maybe pale body
P soggy, floating

Treatment principle
Dispel wind, cold and damp
Mobilize qi and blood in the channels and network vessels

Prescription

CHENG SHI JUAN BI TANG 程氏蠲痹汤
Remove Painful Obstruction Decoction (from the Cheng Clan), p.651

Variations and additional prescriptions
With severe cold
When the cold is severe, the joints are quite stiff and painful, worse with cold weather and after prolonged inactivity. Treatment aims to dispels cold and activate qi and blood with a formula such as **XIAO HUO LUO DAN** (Minor Activate the Network Vessels Special Pill 小活络丹, p.656).

Prepared medicines
Concentrated powders
Juan Bi Tang (Notopterygium & Turmeric Combination)
Xiao Huo Luo Dan (Myrrh & Aconite Formula)

Pills
Juan Bi Wan (Clear Channel Teapills)
Xiao Huo Luo Dan (Xiao Huo Luo Dan Teapills)

Acupuncture (select from)
LI.11 (quchi ▲) ....together these points warms yang and dispel cold
St.36 (zusanli ▲)   and damp
Sp.6 (sanyinjiao)
Ren.4 (guanyuan ▲)
- Other points are chosen according to the location of pain. See Table 15.2, pp.647–650.

Clinical notes
- Cold damp sweating may accompany a diagnosis of chronic arthritis which has affected one side of the body more than the other, or post–stroke debilitation.

16.7 SWEATING ON THE GENITALS

1. Liver and Gallbladder damp heat
2. Kidney yang deficiency

Sweating from the genital region is rarely considered to be a problem, but can be a contributing factor to symptoms that will bring a patient into the clinic, such as itch and irritation, and secondary fungal infection.

肝
胆
湿
热

16.7.1 LIVER AND GALLBLADDER DAMP HEAT

Liver and Gallbladder damp heat is a relatively common cause of pathology of the external genitals and groin area. Excessive sweating in this area predisposes to rashes and fungal infections, and the resulting lesions, itching and irritation are what usually bring the patient into the clinic.

Clinical features

- Sweating in the genital region. The sweat is relatively copious, may smell and stain the underwear. There may be itching and irritation resulting in an embarrassing need to scratch. There may be skin lesions, frequent infections or ulceration of the skin of the genitals.
- red complexion with greasy skin; red sore eyes
- irritability, restlessness, easily angered
- bitter taste in the mouth
- dark, concentrated or painful urination
- sluggish bowels, constipation or loose stools

T red with a thick, greasy, yellow coat
P wiry, slippery, rapid

Treatment Principle

Clear damp heat from the Liver and Gallbladder

Prescription

LONG DAN XIE GAN TANG 龙胆泻肝汤
Gentian Decoction to Purge the Liver, p.746

This prescription is used when heat is greater than damp.

Modifications

- With lesions, ulceration or sores, add **pu gong ying** (Taraxaci Herba) 蒲公英 18–30g, **jin yin hua** (Lonicerae Flos) 金银花 15–30g and **lian qiao** (Forsythiae Fructus) 连翘 9–12g.
- With concentrated or painful urination, add **bai mao gen** (Imperatae Rhizoma) 白茅根 12–18g and **hua shi** (Talcum) 滑石 9–12g.
- With constipation, add **da huang** (Rhei Radix et Rhizoma) 大黄 6–9g and **mang xiao** (Natrii Sulfas) 芒硝 6g [dissolved in the strained decoction].
- With difficult or sluggish stools, add **zhi ke** (Aurantii Fructus) 枳壳 9–12g and **bai zhu** (Atractylodes macrocephalae Rhizoma) 白术 30g.

- With abdominal distension, add **zhi shi** (Aurantii Fructus immaturus) 枳实 9–12g, **hou po** (Magnoliae officinalis Cortex) 厚朴 9–12g and **da fu pi** (Arecae Pericarpium) 大复皮 9–12g.

Variations and additional prescriptions

Damp greater than heat

In cases with chronic genital sweating and irritation, over time the heat will dissipate and the damp component come to the fore. The signs of heat and inflammation are muted, and the dampness more evident in the moist genital area, a white or slightly yellow tongue coat and a soft or soggy pulse. The treatment is to dry damp and clear heat from the lower burner with BI XIE SHENG SHI TANG (Dioscorea Hypoglauca Decoction to Overcome Dampness 萆薢胜湿汤).

yi ren (Coicis Semen) 苡仁.. 24–30g
fu ling (Poria) 茯苓 12–15g
bi xie (Dioscoreae hypoglaucae Rhizoma) 萆薢 9–12g
huang bai (Phellodendri Cortex) 黄柏.. 9–12g
bai xian pi (Dictamni Cortex) 白藓皮 9–12g
ze xie (Alismatis Rhizoma) 泽泻 9–12g
cang zhu (Atractylodis Rhizoma) 苍术.. 9–12g
mu dan pi (Moutan Cortex) 牡丹皮.. 9–12g
shan zhi zi (Gardeniae Fructus) 山栀子 9–12g
tong cao (Tetrapanacis Medulla) 通草... 3–6g

Method: Decoction. **Yi ren** and **bi xie** clear damp heat from the lower burner and promote urination; **huang bai** and **shan zhi zi** clears damp heat from the lower burner; **bai xian pi** clears damp heat and stops itch; **fu ling**, **ze xie** and **tong cao** promote urination and drain damp; **cang zhu** parches damp and with **huang bai** clears damp heat from the lower body; **mu dan pi** cools and activates blood. (Source: *Yang Ke Xin De Ji*)

Topical application

- For skin lesions, ulceration or unbearable itching, a wash can be prepared by decocting 30 grams each of **ku shen** (Sophorae flavescentis Radix) 苦参, **ai ye** (Artemisiae argyi Folium) 艾叶 and **han lian cao** (Ecliptae Herba) 旱莲草. The decoction is added to a sitzbath. Soak in the sitzbath for 30 minutes once or twice daily.

Prepared medicines

Concentrated powders

Long Dan Xie Gan Tang (Gentiana Combination)

Pills

Long Dan Xie Gan Wan (Snake and Dragon Teapills)
Bi Xie Sheng Shi Wan (Subdue the Dampness Teapills)

Acupuncture (select from)

Ren.3 (zhongji) ....clears damp heat from the lower burner
Liv.5 (ligou)......................connecting point of the Liver, clears damp heat from the genitals
Liv.8 (ququan)...................sea point of the Liver, douses fire and clears damp

heat from the lower burner

Kid.7 (fuliu –).....................clears damp heat from the lower burner and regulates sweating

GB.41 (zulinqi) ....master and couple points of daimai, clear damp

SJ.5 (waiguan)   heat from the lower burner, regulate qi and drain fire
the Liver and Gallbladder

Liv.3 (taichong –)...............source point of the Liver, clears damp heat, dredges
the Liver and regulates qi

Bl.18 (ganshu)....................transport point of the Liver, dredges the Liver and
regulates qi, clears damp heat

Bl.19 (danshu –) ....transport point of the Gallbladder, clears damp heat

- with fever add LI.11 (quchi –)
- with abdominal distension, add Ren.12 (zhongwan –) and St.25 (tianshu –)
- with constipation or sluggish stools, add St.25 (tianshu –)
- with nausea add PC.6 (neiguan –)
- Ear points: liver, spleen, zero point, sympathetic, shenmen

Clinical notes

- Genital sweating from Liver and Gallbladder damp heat may be diagnosed as jock itch, tinea cruris or hyperhidrosis.
- An important principle to observe in the treatment of damp heat is to keep the bowels moving and urination flowing to provide an escape route. An increase in both should be observed following ingestion of medicine or acupuncture. If **da huang** is used to get the bowels moving, it should be reduced in dosage or deleted once this is achieved so as to avoid iatrogenic damage to Spleen yang.
- A diet aimed at clearing damp heat is essential. See Clinical Handbook, Vol.2, p.884.

肾
阳
不
足

16.7.2 KIDNEY YANG DEFICIENCY

Kidney yang deficiency sweating is due to the weakness of local lower burner yang qi that is unable to regulate local wei qi and keep the pores closed.

Clinical features

- The genital region is persistently cold and clammy, with a mild to moderate odor. There may be clamminess elsewhere on the body, especially the head.
- pale puffy complexion
- lower back and legs weak, aching and cold
- frequent urination, nocturia
- edema, worse in the lower limbs
- impotence, no libido
- patients may be overweight

T pale, swollen and scalloped with a white coat
P deep, weak, slow

Treatment Principle

Warm and supplement Kidney yang

Prescription

JIN GUI SHEN QI WAN 金匮肾气丸
Kidney Qi Pill from the Golden Cabinet, modified

shu di (Rehmanniae Radix preparata) 熟地 15–24g
shan yao (Dioscoreae Rhizoma) 山药 9–12g
shan zhu yu (Corni Fructus) 山茱萸 12–18g
mu dan pi (Moutan Cortex) 牡丹皮 6–9g
fu ling (Poria) 茯苓 6–9g
ze xie (Alismatis Rhizoma) 泽泻 6–9g
zhi fu zi (Aconiti Radix lateralis preparata) 制附子 3–6g
rou gui (Cinnamomi Cortex) 肉桂 3–6g
qian shi (Euryales Semen) 芡实 9–12g
wu wei zi (Schizandrae Fructus) 五味子 6–9g

Method: Pills or powder. May also be decocted with the doses as shown. **Shu di** nourishes yin and Blood and supplements the Kidneys; **shan zhu yu** supplements the Liver and Kidneys, while its astringency stops sweating; **shan yao** strengthens the Spleen and Kidneys and supplements qi; **ze xie** promotes urination and drains damp; **fu ling** strengthens the Spleen and leaches damp; **mu dan pi** activates and cools the Blood. **zhi fu zi** and **rou gui** warm yang and stimulate fluid metabolism. (Source: *Zhong Yi Nei Ke Xue* [*Jin Gui Yao Lüe*])

Prepared medicines
Concentrated powder
Ba Wei Di Huang Wan (Rehmannia Eight Formula) plus Jin Suo Gu Jing Wan (Lotus Stamen Formula)

Pills
Jin Kui Shen Qi Wan (Fu Gui Ba Wei Wan, Golden Book Tea)
You Gui Wan (Right Side Replenishing Teapills)

Acupuncture (select from)
Ren.4 (guanyuan +▲)........supplements source qi, warms yang and regulates qi
Kid.7 (fuliu +)...................supplements the Kidneys and regulates sweating
Kid.3 (taixi +)...................source point of the Kidneys, supplements yang
St.36 (zusanli +▲) ....sea point of the Stomach, strengthens the Spleen and supplements yang qi
Sp.6 (sanyinjiao +▲).........strengthens the Spleen and Kidneys and supplements yang qi
Bl.23 (shenshu +▲) ....transport point of the Kidneys, warms yang
Du.4 (mingmen +▲).........warms and supports Kidney yang
• Ear points: kidney, zero point, adrenal, sympathetic, subcortex

Clinical notes
• Genital sweating from Kidney yang deficiency may be diagnosed as tinea cruris, hyperhidrosis or thrush.
• A yang warming diet is recommended. See Clinical Handbook, Vol.2, p.873.

16.8 YELLOW SWEATING

Sweat that stains clothing yellow or brown.

肝
脾
湿
热

16.8.1 LIVER AND SPLEEN DAMP HEAT

The damp tends to predominant in this pattern, and it is a chronic problem. In some cases the heat may predominate (see 16.4.2, p.745), and the more heat there is the darker the sweat stains and the more intense the odor.

Clinical features

- Sweating, usually most noticeable under the arms, but can be anywhere, that stains clothing yellow or brown. There may be a strong or musty body odor.
- may be varying degrees of heat, but usually not too extreme
- heaviness in the body, lethargy
- dull hypochondriac ache
- irritability, restlessness
- bitter taste in the mouth
- red or flushed complexion with greasy skin
- abdominal distension
- poor appetite and a tendency to loose stools, or less commonly, sluggish bowels
- concentrated or turbid urination
- may be mild edema of the lower limbs

T red or slightly red with a greasy, white or yellow coat
P deep, wiry, slippery

Treatment Principle

Clear damp heat from the Liver and Spleen

Prescription

YIN CHEN WU LING SAN 茵陈五苓散
Virgate Wormwood and Five Ingredient Powder with Poria

yin chen (Artemisiae scopariae Herba) 茵陈 18–30g
fu ling (Poria) 茯苓 9–12g
zhu ling (Polyporus) 猪苓 9–12g
bai zhu (Atractylodes macrocephalae Rhizoma) 白术 9–12g
ze xie (Alismatis Rhizoma) 泽泻 12–15g
gui zhi (Cinnamomi Ramulus) 桂枝 6–9g
Method: Decoction. **Yin chen** promotes urination and drains damp; **fu ling**, **zhu ling** and **ze xie** promote urination to drain damp; **bai zhu** fortifies the Spleen and dries damp; **gui zhi** is used here to stimulate the transformation of yang qi, and the processing and elimination of fluids via the Urinary Bladder. (Source: *Shi Yong Zhong Yi Nei Ke Xue* [*Jin Gui Yao Lüe*])

Modifications

- With more heat than damp, omit **gui zhi**. See also p.745.
- With severe damp, add **cang zhu** (Atractylodis Rhizoma) 苍术 9–12g.
- With sluggish bowels, add **bing lang** (Arecae Semen) 槟榔 9–12g and **da fu**

pi (Arecae Pericarpium) 大腹皮 9–12g.
- With abdominal distension, add **zhi shi** (Aurantii Fructus immaturus) 枳实 9–12g.
- With a strong body odor, add **pu gong ying** (Taraxaci Herba) 蒲公英 18–30g.

Prepared medicines
Concentrated powders
Yin Chen Wu Ling San (Capillaris & Poria Five Formula)
Pills
Li Dan Pian (Lidan Tablets)

Acupuncture (select from)
Liv.14 (qimen –) ....alarm point of the Liver, dredges the Liver and regulates qi, activates blood and transforms blood stasis

Sp.9 (yinlingquan –)...........these points promote urination to drain damp
Sp.6 (sanyinjiao)

Liv.3 (taichong –)................source, stream and earth point of the Liver, dredges the Liver and regulates qi

Bl.18 (ganshu)....................transport point of the Liver, dredges the Liver and regulates qi, clears damp heat

Bl.19 (danshu –) ....transport point of the Gallbladder, clears damp heat
- with abdominal distension, add Ren.12 (zhongwan –) and St.25 (tianshu –)
- with constipation or sluggish stools, add St.25 (tianshu –)
- Ear points: liver, gallbladder, spleen, shenmen, sympathetic

Clinical notes
- Yellow sweating from Liver Spleen damp heat may be diagnosed as biliary stasis or hepato–biliary disease with mild jaundice, but it also may appear without any identifiable pathology.
- An important principle to observe in the treatment of damp heat is to keep the bowels moving and urination flowing to provide an escape route. An increase in both should be observed following ingestion of medicine or acupuncture.
- A diet aimed at clearing damp heat is essential. See Clinical Handbook, Vol.2, p.884.

Table 16.3 Summary of sweating patterns

Type	Pattern	Features	Prescription
Night sweats	Yin deficiency	Night sweats, afternoon fever, hot flushing, heat in the palms and soles, thirst, dryness, concentrated urine, insomnia, fatigue and restlessness, lower back ache, weight loss, amenorrhea, red, dry tongue with little or no coat, fine, rapid pulse	Dang Gui Liu Huang Wan / Da Bu Yin Wan / Zhi Bai Ba Wei Wan
	Heart blood and Spleen qi deficiency	Night sweats and spontaneous sweating, insomnia, palpitations, anxiety, breathlessness, fatigue, pale complexion, poor appetite, scanty periods, persistent uterine bleeding and easy bruising, pale tongue with a thin, white coat, weak, fine pulse	Gui Pi Tang
	Liver qi constraint	Intermittent night sweats, depression, irritability, hypochondriac ache, sense of blockage in the throat, insomnia, red complexion, red sore eyes, bitter taste, headaches, red tongue or with red edges and a thin yellow coat, wiry, rapid pulse	Jia Wei Xiao Yao San
	Lingering pathogens		
	Damp heat in the qi level	Night sweats with sticky or oily sweat, afternoon fever, muscle aches, fatigue, chest oppression, loss of appetite, nausea, diarrhea, swollen glands, thick, greasy, yellow tongue coat, slippery, wiry, rapid pulse	San Ren Tang / Huo Po Xia Ling Tang
	Heat in the qi level	Night sweats and spontaneous sweating, dryness, low grade fever, dry cough, swollen glands, fine rapid pulse	Zhu Ye Shi Gao Tang
	Shaoyang	Mild to moderate night sweats, alternating fever and chills, poor appetite, nausea, hypochondriac pain, fullness in the chest, dizziness, irritability, bitter taste, swollen glands, wiry pulse	Xiao Chai Hu Tang
	Phlegm heat	Night sweats and spontaneous sweating, insomnia and palpitations, nervousness and anxiety, productive cough, swollen glands, thick greasy yellow tongue coat, slippery pulse	Wen Dan Tang
	Heat in the ying level	Night sweats, low grade fever, disturbance of consciousness, faint maculopapular rash, dizziness, mouth ulcers, swollen glands, red or scarlet tongue with no coat, fine rapid pulse	Qing Ying Tang

Table 16.3 Summary of sweating patterns (cont.)

Type	Pattern	Features	Prescription
Spontaneous	Qi deficiency	Spontaneous daytime sweating, continuous but worse with exertion, breathlessness, weak voice, chronic cough, pale complexion, fatigue, frequent colds and flu, pale tongue with a thin white coat, fine, weak pulse	Yu Ping Feng San Bu Zhong Yi Qi Tang Fang Ji Huang Qi Tang
	Yang deficiency	Spontaneous daytime sweating, continuous but worse with exertion, cold intolerance, cold extremities, frequent urination, lower back ache, pale complexion, pale, wet and swollen tongue, weak; floating, fine pulse	Gui Zhi Jia Fu Zi Tang
	Ying and wei disharmony	Intermittent daytime sweating, aversion to wind and sudden changes of temperature, nasal congestion, muscle aches and joint stiffness, white tongue coat, floating, weak pulse	Gui Zhi Tang
	Lingering pathogens	Spontaneous sweating, red complexion, low grade fever, restlessness and insomnia, thirst, nausea, dry cough, swollen glands, red dry tongue with a patchy coat, fine, rapid pulse	Zhu Ye Shi Gao Tang
	Shaoyang	Intermittent spontaneous sweating, alternating fever and chills, poor appetite, nausea, hypochondriac pain, fullness in the chest, dizziness, irritability, bitter taste, swollen glands, wiry pulse	Xiao Chai Hu Tang
	Phlegm heat	Spontaneous sweating, insomnia and palpitations, nervousness and anxiety, productive cough, swollen glands, thick greasy yellow tongue coat, slippery pulse	Wen Dan Tang

Table 16.3 Summary of sweating patterns (cont.)

Type	Pattern		Features	Prescription
Hands and feet	Qi deficiency		Cool clammy palms, worse when the patient is anxious or nervous, insomnia, palpitations, shortness of breath, fatigue, pale complexion, poor appetite, pale tongue with a thin white coat, weak, fine or big, floating, weak pulse	Gui Pi Tang
	Yang deficiency		Cool clammy or dripping hands and feet, cold extremities, pale complexion, abdominal distension, diarrhea, pale, wet and swollen tongue, weak; floating, fine pulse	Li Zhong Wan
	Instability of the shen		Sweaty palms with stress and anxiety in an otherwise well individual	An Shen Ding Zhi Wan
	Heart fire		Warm, red, clammy palms, worse with stress, insomnia, palpitations, bitter taste, mouth ulcers, painful urination, red tipped tongue, rapid flooding pulse	Qing Xin Lian Zi Yin
	Spleen and Stomach yin deficiency		Clammy hands and feet, worse at night, dry mucous membranes, lack of saliva, muscle weakness, loose stools, easy bruising, red dry tongue, fine rapid pulse	Shen Ling Bai Zhu San
	Lingering pathogens	Heat in the qi level	Warm clammy hands and feet, low grade fever, red complexion, thirst, insomnia, restlessness and irritability, constipation, mouth ulcers, red tongue with patchy yellow coat, fine, rapid pulse	Zhu Ye Shi Gao Tang
		Damp heat in the qi level	Sweaty, smelly feet, afternoon fever or contained fever, muscle aches, thick greasy tongue coat, slippery or soggy pulse	San Ren Tang Lian Po Yin
Underarm	Heart and Liver yin deficiency		Excessive underarm sweating, inoffensive, worse towards evening, or when the patient is anxious or upset, facial flushing, heat in the palms and soles, dry mouth, red tongue with little or no coat, wiry, fine, rapid pulse	Qi Ju Di Huang Wan Tian Wang Bu Xin Dan Xiao Yao San
	Liver and Gallbladder damp heat		Excessive underarm sweating, offensive and staining, hypochondriac ache, irritability, bitter taste, red greasy complexion, concentrated urination, red tongue with a thick, greasy, yellow coat, slippery rapid pulse	Long Dan Xie Gan Tang

Table 16.3 Summary of sweating patterns (cont.)

Type	Pattern	Features	Prescription
Underarm	Heart and Liver Fire	Excessive underarm sweating, not especially offensive worse with stress and anxiety, insomnia, restlessness, anxiety, palpitations, thirst, bitter taste, mouth ulcers, red complexion, concentrated or painful urination, red tongue with a redder tip and a dry, yellow coat, rapid, flooding pulse	Qing Xin Lian Zi Yin
	Instability of the shen	Excessive underarm sweating with stress and anxiety in an otherwise well individual	An Shen Ding Zhi Wan
	Shaoyang	Excessive underarm sweating, alternating fever and chills, poor appetite, nausea, hypochondriac pain, fullness in the chest, dizziness, irritability, bitter taste, swollen glands, wiry pulse	Xiao Chai Hu Tang
Head and chest	Qi and yin deficiency	Sweating on the head and chest, breathlessness, wheezing, pale face with red cheeks, malar flush, heat in the palms and soles, pink or slightly red tongue or swollen cracked tongue, fine, weak pulse	Sheng Mai San
	Yang qi deficiency	Sweating on the head and neck, waxy pale complexion, cold intolerance, cold extremities, frequent urination, nocturia, lower back ache, weak legs, pale, wet, swollen, scalloped tongue, weak, deep pulse	Gui Zhi Jia Fu Zi Tang
	Liver qi constraint	Sweating on the head brought on by stress, irritability, cold fingers and toes, red edges on the tongue, wiry pulse	Si Ni San
	Lingering heat in the chest	Sweating on the chest and upper back, sense of heat in the chest, insomnia, restlessness, irritability, depression, low grade fever, fatigue, red tongue tip	Zhi Zi Chi Tang
	Damp heat in the qi level	Sweating on the head, worse mid afternoon, muscle aches, chest oppression, nausea, loose stools, thick greasy tongue coat, slippery or soggy pulse	San Ren Tang

Table 16.3 Summary of sweating patterns (cont.)

Type	Pattern	Features	Prescription
Half the body	Qi and blood deficiency	Sweating on half the body; numbness, coldness and weakness of the extremities on the sweating side, pallor, fatigue, dizziness, poor muscle tone, pale tongue with a white coat, fine, weak pulse	Shi Quan Da Bu Tang
	Cold damp	Sweating on half the body with stiffness, soreness, aching muscles and joints, pale or swollen tongue with a greasy, white coat, soggy, floating pulse	Juan Bi Tang
Genitals	Liver damp heat	Genital sweating with itching, irritation and odor, dark or painful urination, red tongue with a thick, greasy, yellow coat, wiry, slippery, rapid pulse	Long Dan Xie Gan Tang Bi Xie Sheng Shi Tang
	Kidney yang deficiency	Genital sweating cold and clammy, pale complexion, frequent urination, nocturia, edema, pale, swollen, scalloped tongue, deep, weak, slow pulse	Jin Gui Shen Qi Wan
Yellow	Liver and Spleen damp heat	Sweating that stains clothing yellow or brown, musty body odor, bitter taste, red complexion, greasy skin, turbid urination, edema, red or slightly red tongue with a greasy coat, deep, wiry, slippery pulse	Yin Chen Wu Ling San

THYROID DISORDERS

The main function of the thyroid gland is maintenance of basal metabolic rate. Thyroid dysfunction is one of the most common endocrine imbalances seen in clinic, with hypothyroidism and its many complications such as infertility, weight problems, depression and chronic tiredness the most frequent. It is estimated that thyroid dysfunction of some type, diagnosed by abnormal pathology results, affects as much as 10% of the population[1][2].

The two main clinical syndromes of the thyroid are over activity and under activity. The classic Chinese medical literature discusses thyroid conditions in terms of swelling of the thyroid gland, without specific reference to either hyperthyroid or hypothyroid conditions. Some of the thyroid swelling patterns noted below are clearly associated with hyperthyroidism, but a clear description of hypothyroidism is absent.

Swelling of the thyroid gland is known as *yǐng bìng* 癭病 in Chinese medicine. The term is usually translated simply as

> **BOX 17.1 PATTERNS OF THYROID DYSFUNCTION**
>
> **Goitre and nodules**
> Phlegm damp
> Liver and Kidney deficiency
> Liver qi and phlegm stagnation
> Yang deficiency with congealed phlegm
>
> **Hyperthyroid**
> Liver qi constraint with heat
> Liver qi constraint with phlegm heat
> Liver (Stomach and Heart) fire
> Wind warmth
> Heart and Kidney yin deficiency
> Heart yin and qi deficiency
> Liver and Kidney yin deficiency with heat and ascendant yang
> Liver and Heart yin deficiency
> Kidney yin and yang deficiency
> Heart blood and Spleen qi deficiency
>
> **Hypothyroid**
> Spleen and Kidney qi deficiency
> Heart and Kidney yang deficiency
> Kidney jing deficiency

goitre, but there are different types of *yǐng* that reflect a variety of thyroid problems. A typical contemporary text[3] gives the following types of *yǐng:*

- *qi yǐng* 气癭 (diffuse swelling, goitre)
- *ròu yǐng* 肉癭 (benign nodules, adenoma)
- *yǐng yōng* 癭痈 (inflammation of the thyroid, thyroiditis)
- *shí yǐng* 石癭 (malignancy)
- *yǐng qì* 癭气 (thyroid swelling with heat, overactive thyroid)

These differentiations are summarized in Appendix 5, p.930.

In clinical practice, numerous cases of thyroid dysfunction are observed without

---

1 Empson M et al. Prevalence of Thyroid disease in an older Australian Population. Intern Med J 2007 July 37(7):448–55

2 Toplis DJ, Eastmen CJ. Diagnosis and Management of hyperthyroidism and hypothyroidism. Med J Aust. 2004 Feb 16; 180(4):186–93

3 *Zhong Yi Wai Ke Xue* 中医外科学 (Traditional Chinese External Medicine 1999) Tan Xin–Hua, Lu De–Ming (eds.), Peoples Health Publishing, Beijing

swelling of the gland, so the *ying bing* analysis is of limited use. The patterns and treatments discussed in this chapter are derived from both contemporary sources and our own clinical experience. Thyroid dysfunction falls broadly into three groups:

- goitre and thyroid swellings without systemic features
- hyper–function, heat and/or yin deficiency, with or without thyroid swelling
- hypo–function, cold and yang deficiency, with or without thyroid swelling

PHYSIOLOGY OF THE THYROID

The thyroid is a master regulatory gland, controlling the growth and metabolism of many tissues in the body. It produces two hormones, thyroxine (T4) and tri–iodothyronine (T3) which control the rate of metabolism.

The production of thyroid hormone is regulated by thyroid stimulating hormone (TSH) produced in the pituitary gland. Neurons in the hypothalamus secrete thyroid releasing hormone (TRH) in response to environmental and metabolic stimuli such as cold and stress, which in turn stimulates cells in the anterior pituitary to secrete thyroid stimulating hormone (TSH).

When blood concentrations of thyroid hormones increase above a certain threshold, TRH secreting neurons in the hypothalamus are inhibited and stop secreting TRH. This is an example of negative feedback (Fig 17.1). Inhibition of TRH secretion terminates secretion of TSH, which stops manufacture and secretion of thyroid hormones. As thyroid hormone levels decay below the threshold, negative feedback is relieved, TRH is secreted and the metabolic sequence begins again.

BIOMEDICAL TREATMENT

Hyperthyroid

Antithyroid medication

Antithyroid drugs block the production of thyroxine by inhibiting enzymes involved in the production of thyroid hormone. Drugs include thionamides (Carbimazole, Methimazole) and propylthiouracil. These are usually the first line of therapy. Negative effects of drugs such as these include increase in size of the gland due to stimulation of TSH by the pituitary. This is more likely when large doses are used. More than 50% of patients relapse within 2 years of cessation.

Radiation

Radioactive iodine (^{131}I) is introduced into the body and selectively taken up by and concentrated in the thyroid. The radiation destroys a proportion of the gland. Mainly given to those beyond reproductive age as the radiation is teratogenic. The drawbacks include difficulty in calibrating a dose of ^{131}I so as to destroy enough of the gland to reduce its over activity, but not so much as to destroy it totally. Most patients end up with hypothyroidism and dependence on exogenous thyroxine.

Surgery

Partial or total removal of the thyroid, with synthetic thyroxine replacement. Surgery is usually reserved for those too young or otherwise unsuited for radiation treatment, those for whom antithyroid drug therapy has failed or who have large

Figure 17.1 Regulation of the thyroid gland – negative feedback

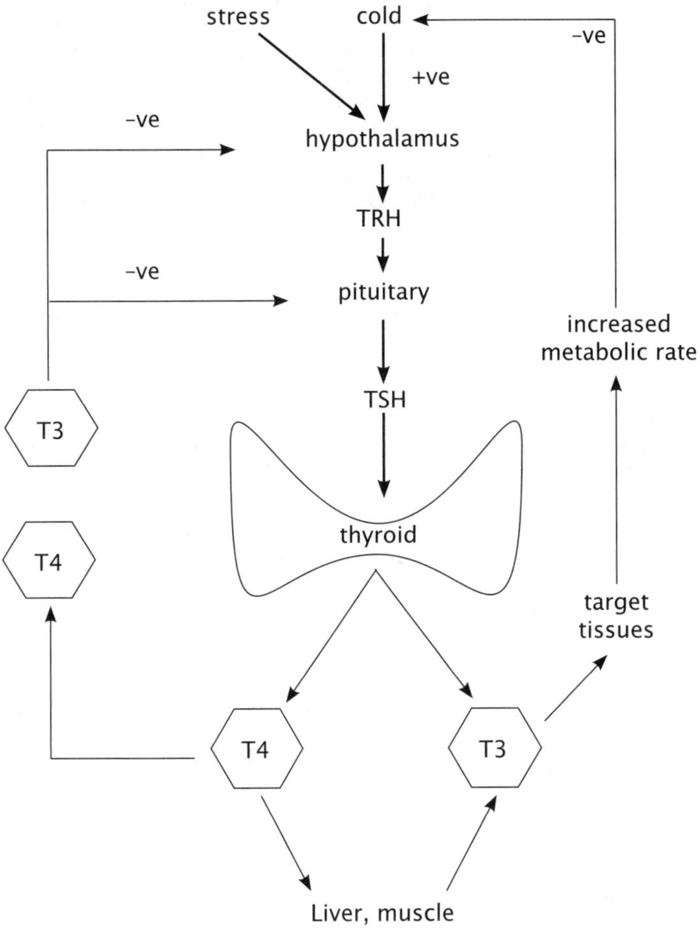

goitres. Negative effects include scarring and blood stasis, loss of thyroid tissue and damage to adjacent structures such as the parathyroid glands and laryngeal nerve.

Iodine (as potassium iodide)

Used to suppress thyroid function in acute thyroid crisis (the 'thyroid storm' or thyrotoxicosis). In pharmacological doses, iodine acts to inhibit production of T4 and T3. This effect is transitory and lasts a few days to a week, after which the iodine provides fuel for increased synthesis.

Beta blockers (such as propanolol)

Beta blockers are used symptomatically to control the adrenergic component of the condition, the tachycardia, tremor and mental symptoms. They act symptomatically and do nothing to alter the disease process.

Table 17.1 Causes of hyperthyroidism

Graves disease (thyrotoxicosis)	Accounts for about 75% of cases. Autoimmune in nature, due to stimulation of the thyroid by antibodies (TRAb, a TSH receptor antibody) which bind to TSH receptors and mimic its effects. Can occur at any age but is unusual before puberty and most commonly affects the 30–50 year old age group. Women are affected about 4 times more often than men. There is a genetic disposition and familial link. The trigger for onset of symptoms in genetically susceptible individuals may be infection, stress or emotional trauma. The course of the illness can fluctuate with periods of increase and decrease or remission, or may progress into hypothyroid.
Multinodular goitre	Most common in older women, 50+. Usually T4 and T3 are only slightly elevated, but because an older age group is affected the cardiovascular features, arrhythmia, fibrillations and palpitations predominate.
Autonomously functioning single nodule (toxic adenoma or 'hot' nodule)	Most common in women over 40. The nodule is a follicular adenoma which autonomously secretes thyroid hormone and inhibits TSH. Mild hyperthyroidism and usually only T3 is elevated.
Thyroiditis (subacute, postpartum)	May be viral (mumps, adenovirus) or postpartum. The viral type appears after an acute upper respiratory tract infection and leads to transitory hyperthyroidism due to destruction of follicle cells with release of hormone into the blood, sometime followed by hypothyroid. Postpartum thyroiditis is mild and self limiting, although 5–10% of postpartum women are affected. Treatment, if required, is usually a ß–blocker. Can recur with subsequent pregnancies with patients gradually progressing to hypothyroidism.
Iodine induced	Drugs, especially amiodarone (an anti-arrhythmic agent loaded with iodine) and radiographic contrast media can overload the gland and induce a mild hyperthyroidism.

Hypothyroid

Treatment of hypothyroidism is hormone replacement with synthetic thyroxine (trade names Synthroid, Oroxine, Eutroxsig) or a product derived from the ground up thyroid gland of various animals.

Goitre and thyroid nodules

The treatment of simple goitre is to increase iodine in the diet. Nodules can be removed surgically. Malignancy is treated surgically, with radiation or chemotherapy.

ASSESSMENT OF THYROID FUNCTION

In addition to the clinical features of thyroid dysfunction (Table 17.4, p.778), there are laboratory tests that measure the levels of various hormones involved in the thyroid chain (Table 17.5, p.779). In clinical practice, thyroid disease can be difficult to detect symptomatically and patients may exhibit few symptoms, or present with unusual symptoms that can throw the physician off the trail. For

Table 17.2 Causes of hypothyroidism

Hashimoto's thyroiditis	This is the most common cause, and is due to loss of thyroid tissue from autoimmune destruction. Antibodies are generated against thyroid follicle cells. It is initially associated with a small firm goitre which may later atrophy and become fibrotic. Often starts with a mild transitory hyperthyroid state as stored T4 and T3 are released into circulation from the ruptured cells.
Spontaneous atrophic hypothyroidism	May follow Hashimoto's thyroiditis, or Graves disease treated with anti-thyroid drugs some years earlier
Post therapeutic	Following radioactive iodine or thyroidectomy
Drug induced	Lithium carbonate for bipolar mood disorder; iodine in high doses (amiodarone, expectorants containing potassium iodide)
Iodine deficiency	Common in mountainous areas; subclinical deficiency quite common in pockets of the developed world

Table 17.3 Causes of goitre and nodules

Puberty	Diffuse enlargement, usually with no (obviously related) associated symptoms (Chinese medical analysis may find symptoms)
Pregnancy	
Iodine deficiency	Smooth soft enlargement
Thyroiditis	Painful or tender diffuse enlargement with fever, malaise; usually follows an acute upper respiratory tract infection
Hyperthyroidism	Diffuse enlargement, usually firm or rubbery
Hypothyroidism	
Cancer	Single hard or tender lump, lymphadenopathy
Cysts, adenoma	One or more rubbery well defined lumps; the more there are the less likely malignancy

example, patients with borderline or subclinical hypothyroidism may present with tiredness and unexplained weight gain (common), depression, constipation or carpal tunnel syndrome. Patients with hyperthyroidism can present with anxiety and emotional lability (common), weight loss, heat intolerance and amenorrhea (frequently mistaken for menopause) and arrhythmias. Patients may complain that their contact lenses don't fit and keep popping out, as may occur in the early stages of exopthalmos.

Laboratory results are a good way of assessing progress and in acute cases can be retested every 4–6 weeks. In more chronic cases, every few months is generally sufficient. Assessment of progress should not be wholly dependent on lab testing however. Some patients whose thyroid hormone levels do not change significantly can still get good results in terms of alleviation of acute symptoms and improvements in wellbeing and other parameters of health, as detected by Chinese medicine.

Table 17.4 Features of thyroid dysfunction

	Hyperthyroid	Hypothyroid
most common features	anxiety, nervousness, emotional lability, irritability, hyperkinesis	depression, lethargy, sluggishness
	increased sweating	coarse, dry skin
	heat intolerance, increased basal metabolic rate	cold intolerance, decreased metabolic rate
	fatigue, breathlessness with exertion	fatigue, poor memory, dementia, psychosis
	weight loss	weight gain
	increased frequency of bowel movement	constipation
	palpitations, tachycardia, arrhythmias	bradycardia
	excessive lacrimation	
other	goitre (may be absent, or nodular)	goitre (may be absent)
	increased appetite and thirst, or anorexia	decreased appetite, large, swollen tongue
	ankle edema	edema, deep or hoarse voice
	fine tremor, increased tendon reflex	slow tendon reflex
	proximal muscle weakness	general aches and pains, stiffness
	palmar erythema, warm sweaty palms, onycholysis (separation of the nail from the nail bed)	carpal tunnel syndrome
	warm clammy skin, spider nevi, pruritus	dry flaky skin and hair
	insomnia	somnolence
	alopecia	coarse dry hair; hair loss (especially lateral eyebrows)
	amenorrhea, scanty periods	menorrhagia
	infertility, loss of libido	infertility, loss of libido
	exopthalmos, lid lag, gritty eyes	puffy eyes and lids, purplish lips, malar flush
	lymphadenopathy (usually seen in Graves disease)	
		deafness
		high blood cholesterol and cardiovascular disease

Table 17.5 Thyroid function tests

	TSH	T4	T3
Hyperthyroid	undetectable	raised	raised
Subclinical hyperthyroid	undetectable	normal (usually upper end of range[2])	normal (usually upper end of range)
1# Hypothyroid[3]	raised	low	normal or low[1]
2# Hypothyroid[4]	usually undetectable	low	normal or low[1]
Subclinical hypothyroid	raised	normal (usually lower end of range)	
1. Not a sensitive indicator of hypothyroid and usually not requested 2. Reference range: T4 8.0–22.0 pmol/L; T3 2.5–6.0 pmol/L; TSH 0.30–4.0 mU/L 3. thyroid disease-Hashimoto's thyroiditis or atrophic thyroiditis 4. hypothalamic or pituitary disease-failure of TSH			
Thyroid auto-antibodies	· Anti-thyroid peroxidase in Hashimoto's thyroiditis · TSH receptor (TRAb) antibodies in Graves disease		

THE THYROID AND ITS INFLUENCES IN CHINESE MEDICINE

The anterior neck and thyroid gland are influenced primarily by the Liver, Heart, and Kidneys organ systems, and the renmai which traverses the area. The taiyin and yangming organ systems (the Lung, Spleen, Large Intestine and Stomach) can also be involved in thyroid pathology because of local influence via channel pathways, proximity of the organ itself (Lungs), and as a result of the dampness and phlegm that can be created by their weakness.

The throat and neck are also the bridge between the head and the body. The neck connects the head, the seat of the intellect, to the chest, the seat of the emotions. The throat is associated with communication and the ability to express oneself clearly. The neck is the place where emotions can get caught when their expression is repressed, inappropriate or otherwise difficult. This can manifest in disorders of the throat and vocal cords, in globus hystericus (plum pit qi) and thyroid problems.

ETIOLOGY

There are two primary pathological processes we see in patients with thyroid disorders. They manifest from disruption to two of the major energetic axes of the body, the Liver and Spleen, and the Heart and Kidney.

Disharmony between the Liver and Spleen creates some of the necessary preconditions for thyroid dysfunction, such as qi constraint, heat and phlegm, as well as weakened resistance (qi deficiency). Once these preconditions exist then any disruption to the Heart and Kidney axis by emotional trauma, persistent or increasing stress, or by pathogenic invasion such as a wind heat or a warm disease may precipitate clinical thyroid disease.

The Liver Spleen axis and the primary pathological triad

Stress is a major contributor to qi stagnation, heat, phlegm accumulation and qi deficiency. Stress, defined here as conditions leading to constrained Liver qi, includes not only classical etiological stressors such as anger, frustration and repressed emotion but any phenomena that impacts on the body's ability to adapt to change. These include activities that disrupt the body's innate clock and that run counter to the natural internal rhythms that follow the cycle of the day and seasons, such as staying up late at night processing information (i.e. watching TV or working), at a time when the body and mind should be resting. Shift workers and those who frequently cross time zones, air crew and business travellers, are particularly vulnerable.

In many cases, the physiological stress that leads to qi constraint is the accumulation of many small and seemingly trivial behaviors, which accumulate over time and alter the body's ability to adapt.

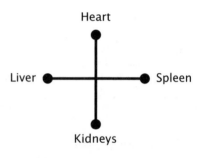

The most important ramification of prolonged or acute stress in the development of thyroid disorder is disruption to the Liver Spleen axis and development of the primary pathological triad (PPT). The primary pathological triad is three patterns of pathology that are found to occur simultaneously, are tightly interlinked and mutually engendering. The triad comprises Liver qi stagnation, Spleen yang qi deficiency, and heat of some type, typically heat from constrained qi, damp heat and/or phlegm heat. The pathology of the basic triad often leads to further complication by blood and/or yin deficiency, blood stagnation and shen disturbances. The development of the PPT is promoted by a combination of stress and worry, inappropriate or poor diet and eating habits, increasingly sedentary habits and occupations and overuse of pharmaceutical drugs.

One of the characteristic features of the PPT is its self perpetuating nature. The three main patterns of the PPT engender and reinforce each other, and if only one component is treated the condition will tend to return. Liver qi constraint impacts on the Spleen and Stomach, weakening their functions and encouraging the generation of damp. Damp is heavy in nature and tends to sink downwards to the lower body and lower gastrointestinal system. Constrained qi, and the increase in qi pressure behind an obstruction, generate heat. Heat from qi constraint, combined with pre–existing damp, creates damp heat. Qi constraint can also retard fluid movement and lead to congealing of fluids into phlegm. Damp on its own, due to its sticky obstructing nature, can also generate heat by blocking qi flow and so transform into damp heat. Once there is damp and heat, the damp can be congealed further into phlegm. The pathological relationships are summarized in Figure 17.2, p.782. The influence of the PPT is most evident in younger people, and in those whose foundation of qi, blood, yin and yang is relatively intact.

Heart Kidney axis

The Heart Kidney (shaoyin) axis is one of the fundamental relationships of the body. It connects the inherited constitution (the jing and yuan qi) with the conscious awareness and mental stability of the individual (the shen). The quality and stability of the shen is dependent on a solid base of Kidney energy and jing. When the platform of jing is weak, the shen is fragile, unstable, and easily upset. When the Heart Kidney relationship is already fragile, it doesn't take too much to cause major disruption and the onset of pathology. The Heart Kidney axis can be constitutionally weak, it can be weakened by lifestyle factors, or can suddenly be disrupted by a severe shock.

• Congenital: Thyroid disorders tend to run in families. In addition, we often see a history that suggests this axis is fragile. Weakness of the Heart Kidney axis may be reflected in a tendency to chronic anxiety or nervous disorders, chronic sleep problems, prolonged enuresis and so on.

• Acquired: This is a common effect of ageing or any of the other factors that can deplete Kidney energy, such as chronic overwork, excessive use of stimulant drugs, too much sexual activity for the individual concerned, depleting pregnancies and terminations.

• Sudden disruption: This usually occurs after a major shock or emotional trauma. A significant event is usually required, such as loss of a loved one, motor vehicle accident or major life crisis. In those with a pre–existing congenital or acquired weakness of the Heart Kidney axis, a seemingly trivial event may be sufficient to cause disruption. The effect may not be immediately apparent; anywhere between 3–12 months may lapse between the trigger event and the onset of specific features of thyroid imbalance.

• External pathogens: Pathogens can enter to the deep levels of the body when the shaoyin is weak, bypassing the surface altogether. A pathogen contacting the surface can gain direct access to the deep levels via the taiyang – shaoyin relationship. Weakness of shaoyin is often mirrored in weakness of taiyang, so little if any initial resistance is seen. This is a type of lingering pathogen (see Chapter 11).

Once the Heart Kidney axis is weak it can easily be disrupted. When it is disrupted, the pathology can develop in either a yin or yang deficient direction (Fig 17.3, p.783) depending on the initial conditions, constitutional factors, the cause of the disruption, the patients diet and the environment in which they live and work.

Heat

Heat is an important component of many thyroid disorders. The heat may be introduced by pathogenic invasion, a heating diet, be the result of the PPT or the product of yin deficiency. Xu Da–Chun, a famous physician of the early 20th century well known for trying to integrate traditional Chinese and modern Western medicine, described a clinical condition in which persistent pathogenic heat gradually merges in some way with the body's zheng qi. In such situations, the repeated attempts to eradicate the pathogen and restore homeostasis end up par-

Figure 17.2 Pathological consequences of the primary pathological triad

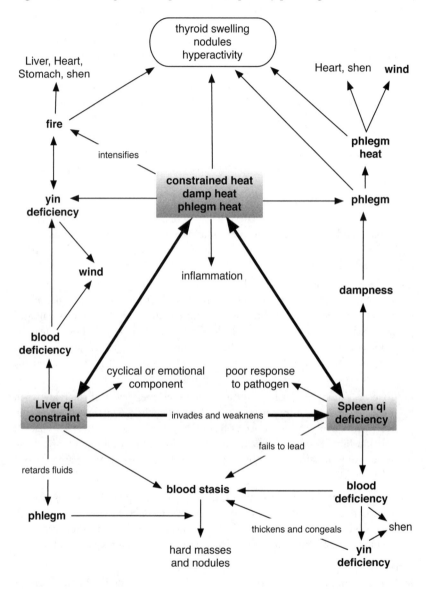

ticipating in the problem, with the misdirected defensive efforts causing collateral damage to the tissues of the body, in this case the thyroid gland. This type of heat is usually prolonged, low grade or even subclinical, and causes chronic inflammation. Persistent retention of pathological heat can also make tissues hypersensitive to other stimuli, whether infectious, neurological or environmental. In Chinese medicine, we see a strong correlation between the presence of pathological heat, and autoimmunity and allergies, at least during part of their natural history. Being a yang pathogen, heat generates systemic and local hyperactivity, but eventually burns out. This is the scenario seen in many inflammatory disorders, where the initial insult leads to over activity that is eventually replaced by loss of function. This process is clearly seen in thyroid dysfunction, where hyperthyroidism gradually gives way to hypothyroidism.

Phlegm

Phlegm is present when the thyroid gland swells, causing nodules or goitre. Phlegm can be the product of retarded fluid metabolism and weakness of the Spleen, Lungs and Kidney, yin deficiency that cooks and congeals fluids, or more commonly in the case of thyroid dysfunction, a slowing and thickening of fluids due to Liver qi constraint or failure of Lung qi descent. The phlegm congeals in response to stress or grief and emotional turmoil. Seen in this way, the phlegm that

Figure 17.3 Disruption of the Heart Kidney axis

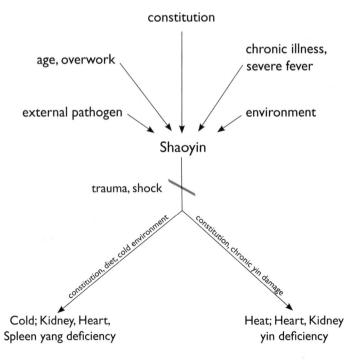

forms the substance of the thyroid swelling can be seen as a type of 'concentrated emotion' and must be gradually dispersed so as not to overwhelm the patient with difficult or painful feelings. Once phlegm has been created, it can cause further qi stagnation, generate heat or be complicated by static blood. Phlegm is carried around the body by qi, and although it may go anywhere, it tends to lodge along the pathway of the Liver channel. When there is heat, phlegm is more likely to be concentrated and elevated to the neck. With cold and yang deficiency, phlegm tends to be more diffuse and can sink into the peripheral tissues as myxedema, infiltrate the larynx (hoarse voice) or contaminate the blood (high cholesterol and triglycerides).

Constitution

A tendency to develop a thyroid disorder may be inherited. More women than men develop thyroid imbalances. Hyperthyroidism in particular, has a strong constitutional component. The pathology will develop according to weaknesses in either of the two major organ axes described above.

The most important and commonly seen factor is weakness of the Kidneys (and yuan qi) that predisposes to disruption of the Heart Kidney axis and to invasion of shaoyin by external pathogens. This weakness can influence the function of renmai and chongmai leading to pathological accumulation along their pathways, in this case the anterior and lateral neck.

The second is an inherited tendency to qi constraint and disruption of the Liver Spleen axis, which predisposes the patient to development of the primary pathological triad and phlegm.

Environment

People living in mountainous regions with iodine poor soils are more prone to goitre formation, but even soils with slightly low levels of iodine can contribute to compromised thyroid function.

Dry desiccating environments damage Kidney yin and fluids. Cold dry environments predispose people to development of yang deficiency, especially when combined with a cold, goitrogenic or otherwise inadequate diet.

Diet

Aspects of the diet can be influential in predisposing the patient to the development of thyroid problems. A low iodine diet will cause poor thyroid function and iodine deficiency is not uncommon, even with a healthy diet. A 2006 survey[4] of 1709 Australian schoolchildren found mild to moderate iodine deficiency in between 20–70% of children by region. A diet rich in goitrogenic foods (Table 17.7, p.805) can inhibit thyroid function. An excess of rich, sweet or dairy based foods, as well as simply overeating, can contribute to accumulation of phlegm. Cold raw foods that weaken the Spleen can lead to damp and phlegm, or weaken yang qi. A heating diet can contribute to an inflammatory tendency.

Selenium is an important trace element for normal thyroid functioning and is low in many soils. Selenium protects against autoimmune thyroid disease and

---

4 Medical Journal of Australia (184:165–169)

insufficient dietary selenium is correlated with thyroiditis. Supplementation with selenium in patients with Hashimoto's thyroiditis decreases autoantibodies[5].

There is also a link between gluten intolerance/celiac disease and thyroid disease in some patients. Undiagnosed or low grade celiac disease may be a part of the process that triggers autoimmunity in genetically susceptible individuals. The damage to the lining of the gut may also allow larger molecules to enter the portal circulation, possibly triggering both an immune response and inflammation. Certainly some patients diagnosed with a thyroid disorder seem to do well with a gluten free diet (Table 17.7, p.805). The link to underlying Spleen weakness is clear. Compromised Spleen function leads to both dampness and phlegm and also contributes to the qi deficiency that leads to susceptibility to infection that can trigger some thyroid disorders.

Age

The more yin deficient one is, either overt or incipient, the more vulnerable to disruption of the Heart Kidney axis, and the development of heat and inflammation. This occurs naturally in everyone with age ('by 40 half the yin is gone' is a well know aphorism of Chinese medicine), and more so in women due their unique physiology. Yin can be significantly damaged in younger people because of sleep deprivation, sexual and reproductive habits, overwork and stimulant drug use. It is also more likely in very dry or desiccating environments.

Shock and emotional trauma

It is frequently observed that the onset of hyperthyroid (most commonly) or hypothyroid states follow some weeks or months after a major trauma, such as the death of a loved one, motor vehicle accident or severe shock of some sort. Such events disrupt the Heart Kidney axis. Trauma of this magnitude is distinct from the everyday stresses and frustrations that accumulate to cause Liver qi constraint.

Infection

Invasion of shaoyin by an external pathogen which becomes a type of lingering pathogen is seen in some cases of both hyperthyroidism and hypothyroidism. It is more likely when there is pre–existing Kidney weakness. Once a pathogen is lodged in the shaoyin level, the disorder can progress in either a yin or yang deficiency direction depending on the patient. There will usually be some supporting evidence to suggest a lingering pathogen at work, such as lymphadenopathy, swollen tonsils and low grade fever.

Chemicals and drugs

A number of drugs can influence thyroid function, especially those containing large amounts of iodine (such as Amiodarone, an anti–arrhythmic agent). Iodine in large doses can cause both hyper–function and hypo–function. Lithium carbonate inhibits release of thyroxine. Dopamine, glucocorticoids and interferon can lead to decreased thyroid stimulating hormone (TSH) secretion. Beta block-

5 Gartner R et al. Selenium supplementation in patients with autoimmune thyroiditis decreases thyroid peroxidase antibody concentrations. J. Clin. Endocrinol. Metab. 2002 Apr; 87(4):1687–91

ers, amiodarone, cortisol and other glucocorticoids can inhibit the conversion of T4 to T3. Rifampicin, phenytoin, barbituates and carbamazapine can increase hepatic metabolism of T4.

A number of common industrial and environmental chemicals may interfere with the thyroid by binding to thyroid receptors and inhibiting iodine uptake. These include polychlorinated biphenyls, polybrominated biphenyls, bisphenol–A and perclorate. These are found in paints, adhesives, flame retardants and plastics.

TREATMENT

There are two broad aims of treatment. Overall Chinese medicine treatment aims to correct the constitutional imbalances that led to the disorder in the first place. When heat is extreme, however, it must be swiftly cleared to avoid damage to yin. Acupuncture is often the treatment of choice in these circumstances (particularly when Liver pathology is responsible) with its unparalleled ability to regulate qi, clear heat and calm the shen very quickly.

In cases with more deficiency, treatment of the constitutional aspects with herbal medicine is important. Basic herbal formulas can be augmented with herbs that have specific effects on the thyroid (Table 17.8, pp.806–807).

甲
状
腺
肿

17.1. GOITRE AND NODULES

These are diffuse thyroid swellings or nodules in a patient with otherwise normal (euthyroid) thyroid function. In the case of goitre from an iodine deficiency, the treatment is simply to increase intake of iodine containing foods. The swellings in this section include masses that are benign (adenomas, cysts) as well as those that may be malignant. The assessment of a mass in the neck should focus on the shape and symmetry, presence or absence of pain, irregularity of the surface, mobility of the mass and thyroid and the presence of lymphadenopathy. The harder, less mobile and more irregular the mass, the higher the index of suspicion about possible malignancy. Single irregular lumps and those that grow quickly should be regarded with particular suspicion. Regardless of the physical findings, all masses should be investigated.

Nodules and goitre are an unusual primary presentation in the Chinese medicine clinic. Most people just live with them if they are causing no problem. If they are problematic and a simple surgical option is available it is the treatment of choice for many patients, although surgery should be followed with appropriate qi regulating, phlegm resolving and supplementing treatment. For patients choosing to avoid surgery, treatment according to the guidelines below can be quite effective depending on the nature of the lesion.

痰
湿
凝
结

17.1.1 PHLEGM DAMP ACCUMULATION WITH SPLEEN DEFICIENCY

This is simple diffuse swelling of the thyroid gland in an otherwise euthyroid patient. It is associated with iodine deficiency, either from an iodine deficient diet or an excess of goitrogenic foods in the diet (Table 17.7, p.805). Some drugs can have a goitrogenic effect (p.776–777). Iodine deficiency goitre is not common in the western world.

Clinical features
• Smooth soft enlargement of the thyroid gland

Treatment principle
Transform and resolve phlegm and disperse the mass

Prescription

HAI ZAO YU HU TANG 海藻玉壶汤
Sargassum Decoction for the Jade Flask

hai zao (Sargassum) 海藻	6–9g
kun bu (Eckloniae Thallus) 昆布	6–9g
hai dai (Laminariae Thallus) 海带	9–12g
zhe bei mu (Fritillariae thunbergii Bulbus) 浙贝母	6–9g
zhi ban xia (Pinelliae Rhizoma preparatum) 制半夏	6–9g
qing pi (Citri reticulatae viride Pericarpium) 青皮	6–9g
chen pi (Citri reticulatae Pericarpium) 陈皮	6–9g
chuan xiong (Chuanxiong Rhizoma) 川芎	6–9g

dang gui (Angelicae sinensis Radix) 当归 6–9g
du huo (Angelicae Pubescentis Radix) 独活 6–9g
lian qiao (Forsythiae Fructus) 连翘 6–9g
gan cao (Glycyrrhizae Radix) 甘草 6–9g
Method: Decoction. **Hai zao**, **hai dai** and **kun bu**, soften hardness and resolve phlegm. These herbs are salty and contain significant quantities of iodine. **Zhi ban xia** and **zhe bei mu** resolve phlegm and dissipate nodules; **qing pi** and **chen pi** regulate qi, alleviate qi constraint and resolve phlegm; **dang gui** and **chuan xiong** activate blood and disperse static blood; **du huo** frees up circulation of qi through the channels and network vessels, transforms damp and dispels pathogens; **lian qiao** clears heat generated by the stagnation and dissipates nodules; **gan cao** relieves toxicity and harmonizes the actions of the other herbs in the formula. (Source: *Zhong Yi Wai Ke Xue* [*Wai Ke Zheng Zong*])

Modifications
- With hoarse voice, add **mu hu die** (Oroxyli Semen) 木蝴蝶 6–9g and **she gan** (Belamcandae Rhizoma) 射干 9–12g.
- With dysphagia, add **hou po** (Magnoliae officinalis Cortex) 厚朴 6–9g.
- With Spleen deficiency, combine with Liu Jun Zi Tang (Six Gentlemen Decoction 六君子汤, p.916).

Prepared medicines
Pills
Hai Zao Jing Wan (Sargassum Teapills, Haiodin)

Acupuncture
See Table 17.6, p.794.

Clinical notes
- This is an unusual pattern in the west, with iodine routinely added to salt and other food items.

肝
肾
不
足

17.1.2 LIVER AND KIDNEY DEFICIENCY; (chongmai and renmai deficiency)
This is diffuse thyroid swelling associated with puberty, pregnancy or menopause, without clinical or laboratory evidence of thyroid dysfunction. The etiology is thought to be associated with Kidney weakness and dysfunction of the chongmai and renmai, with subsequent accumulation of qi in regions where qi flow is more likely to be obstructed, here the neck.

Clinical features
- Diffuse goitre that is soft and regular. There may be some signs of Kidney deficiency, such as delayed onset of menstruation or irregular menses, difficulty falling pregnant, lower back ache, urinary frequency and so on. Some patients may have a history of gynecological masses such as polycystic ovaries, and fibroids.

Treatment principle
Supplement and strengthen the Liver and Kidneys
Regulate chongmai and renmai

Prescription

ER XIAN TANG 二仙汤
Two Immortal Decoction, plus
SI WU TANG 四物汤
Four Substance Decoction

xian mao (Curculiginis Rhizoma) 仙茅 9–15g
xian ling pi (Epimedii Herba) 仙灵脾 9–15g
dang gui (Angelicae sinensis Radix) 当归 9–12g
ba ji tian (Morindae officinalis Radix) 巴戟天 9–12g
huang bai (Phellodendri Cortex) 黄柏 6–9g
zhi mu (Anemarrhenae Rhizoma) 知母 6–9g
shu di (Rehmanniae Radix preparata) 熟地 9–15g
bai shao (Paeoniae Radix alba) 白芍 9–12g
chuan xiong (Chuanxiong Rhizoma) 川芎 6–9g

Method: Decoction. **Xian mao** and **xian ling pi** (also known as **yin yang huo** 淫羊藿) warm Kidney yang and support jing; **ba ji tian** warms Kidney yang and strengthens the tendons and bones; **dang gui** nourishes and protects blood and yin, softens the Liver, and combined with **xian mao** and **xian ling pi** regulates and supplements chongmai and renmai; **zhi mu** and **huang bai** nourish Kidney yin and clear heat, and balance the pungent heat of **xian mao** and **xian ling pi**; **shu di** nourishes yin and supplements blood; **bai shao** supplements blood, softens the Liver and preserves yin; **chuan xiong** ativates blood and moves qi. (Source: *Zhong Yi Wai Ke Xue* [*Shanghai Shu Guang Yi Yuan Jing Yan Fang / He Ji Ju Fang*])

Modifications

• Herbs to soften phlegm may be added, such as **zhe bei mu** (Fritillariae thunbergii Bulbus) 浙贝母 9–12g, **mu li** (Ostreae Concha) 牡蛎 15–30g, **xuan shen** (Scrophulariae Radix) 玄参 12–15g and mild qi regulators like **xiang fu** (Cyperi Rhizoma) 香附 9–12g.

Prepared medicines
Concentrated powder
Er Xian Tang (Curculigo & Epimedium Combination) plus Si Wu Tang (Tangkuei Four Combination)

Pills
Er Xian Wan (Two Immortals Teapills) plus Si Wu Wan (Four Substances for Women Teapills)

Acupuncture
See Table 17.6, p.794.

Clinical notes

• An uncommon pattern, and one for which treatment is rarely sought as the swelling is unlikely to be very large and there are no accompanying symptoms. Most swellings of this type are noticed by family and friends of the patient.
• Thyroid swelling of this type is self limiting, and the swelling usually recedes after conclusion of puberty or pregnancy.

肝
气
郁
痰
凝
滞

17.1.3 LIVER QI CONSTRAINT AND PHLEGM STAGNATION

This is the most common pattern of euthyroid swelling, usually presenting with benign thyroid nodules, either single (most common) or multiple. The basic qi and phlegm stagnation pattern can be complicated by heat, qi deficiency or blood stasis. This type of swelling has the tendency to evolve into a hyperthyroid state.

Clinical features
- Diffuse goitre, or a single (occasionally multiple) relatively soft, rubbery, regular nodule that is non tender.
- clear emotional component – the swelling comes and goes, or the perception of discomfort and fullness changes according to the emotional state of the patient
- may be a sense of some obstruction in the throat, or dysphagia
- depression, mood swings, irritability
- alternating bowel habits, loose stools or constipation
- headaches, neck and shoulder tension, tooth grinding (bruxism)
- premenstrual symptoms, irregular menses

T unremarkable tongue, or with pale or red edges
P wiry, fine pulse

Treatment principle
Regulate Liver qi, resolve phlegm and disperse the mass

Prescription

CHAI HU SHU GAN SAN 柴胡疏肝散
Bupleurum Powder to Dredge the Liver

chai hu (Bupleuri Radix) 柴胡	9–12g
bai shao (Paeoniae Radix alba) 白芍	9–15g
xiang fu (Cyperi Rhizoma) 香附	9–12g
zhi ke (Aurantii Fructus) 枳壳	6–9g
chuan xiong (Chuanxiong Rhizoma) 川芎	6–9g
chen pi (Citri reticulatae Pericarpium) 陈皮	6–6g
zhi gan cao (Glycyrrhizae Radix preparata) 炙甘草	3–6g

Method: Decoction. Pills or powder. **Chai hu** dredges the Liver and resolves qi constraint; **xiang fu** regulates Liver qi, and with **chuan xiong** activates the blood and stops pain; **bai shao** nourishes yin and blood and softens the Liver; **zhi ke** and **chen pi** regulate qi and correct the qi dynamic; **zhi ke** breaks up stagnant qi, directs qi downwards and in combination with the ascending nature of **chai hu**, kick starts the qi dynamic; **zhi gan cao** harmonizes the Stomach and strengthens the Spleen, and with **bai shao** eases spasms, thereby alleviating cramping pain of both smooth and skeletal muscles. (Source: *Zhong Yi Wai Ke Xue* [*Jing Yue Quan Shu*])

Modifications
- With a diffuse swelling, combine with **Er Chen Tang** (Two Aged [Herb] Decoction 二陈汤, p.915).
- For soft and rubbery nodules, combine with **Xiao Luo Wan** (Reduce Scrophula Pill 消瘰丸, p.921 and 806).
- For regular, but firmer nodules combine with **San Zi Yang Qin Tang** (Three Seed Decoction to Nourish One's Parents 三子养亲汤, p.918 and 806).

- With depression or mood swings, add **he huan pi** (Albizziae Cortex) 合欢皮 12–15g and **ye jiao teng** (Polygoni multiflori Caulis) 夜胶藤 15–30g.

Variations and additional prescriptions

The basic phlegm and qi stagnation pattern can be complicated by qi and blood deficiency or constrained heat. In either case the guiding formula can be replaced to suit. In the case of qi and blood deficiency, use XIAO YAO SAN (Rambling Powder 逍遥散, p.841); in the case of constrained heat use JIA WEI XIAO YAO SAN (Augmented Rambling Powder 加味逍遥散, p.713), plus the above modifications as suitable.

Prepared medicines

Concentrated powder

Chai Hu Shu Gan San (Bupleurum & Cyperus Combination)

Xiao Yao San (Bupleurum & Tangkuei Formula)
 – with blood deficiency

Jia Wei Xiao Yao San (Bupleurum & Peony Formula)
 – with heat

Ju He Wan (Citrus Seed Formula)
 – qi and phlegm masses

Pills

Chai Hu Shu Gan Wan (Bupleurum Soothe Liver Teapills)

Xiao Yao Wan (Free and Easy Wanderer Teapills, Hsiao Yao Wan)

Jia Wei Xiao Yao Wan (Free and Easy Wanderer Plus Teapills, Dan Zhi Xiao Yao Wan)

Ji Sheng Ju He Wan (Citrus Aurantium Compound Pills, Citrus Seed Pills)

Acupuncture

See Table 17.6, p.794.

Clinical notes

- This is a common cause of benign nodules and thyroid swelling, and when the nodules or swelling is uncomplicated and of recent origin, it responds well to both acupuncture and herbal treatment.

17.1.4 YANG DEFICIENCY WITH CONGEALED PHLEGM

阳
虚
痰
凝

These are chronic benign nodules and cysts.

Clinical features

- Small, usually single, non tender nodule. The overlying skin is taut and shiny, the nodule firm, rubbery and well defined. No pain with palpation and usually no abnormal thyroid activity. There may be few systemic symptoms, but some patients may display signs of yang deficiency – pale tongue, cold intolerance and urinary frequency.

Treatment principle

Warm yang qi and promote circulation of yang

Disperse and transform phlegm

Prescription

YANG HE TANG 阳和汤
Yang Heartening Decoction

shu di (Rehmanniae Radix preparata) 熟地 30g
lu jiao jiao (Cervi Cornus Colla) 鹿角胶 9g
bai jie zi (Sinapsis Semen) 白芥子 6g
rou gui (Cinnamomi Cortex) 肉桂 3g
gan cao (Glycyrrhizae Radix) 甘草 3g
pao jiang (Zingiberis Rhizoma preparatum) 炮姜 1.5g
ma huang (Ephedra Herba) 麻黄 1.5g

Method: Decoction. **Shu di** supplements yin and blood; **lu jiao jiao** nourishes blood, supports yang qi and assists **shu di** in nourishing jing and blood and strengthening the bones; **rou gui** and **pao jiang** warm yang qi, dispel cold and unblock the channels and network vessels; **ma huang** and **bai jie zi** assist **pao jiang** and **rou gui** in warming and removing blockages; **gan cao** alleviates toxicity and balances the formula. The rich and potentially congesting natures of **shu di** and **lu jiao jiao** are moderated by the dispersing and mobilizing action of the other herbs. (Source: *Zhong Yi Wai Ke Xue* [*Wai Ke Zheng Zhi Quan Sheng Ji*])

Modifications
- A few mild blood activating herbs may be added to improve access into the nodule, such as **dan shen** (Salviae miltiorrhizae Radix) 丹参 9–12g, **lu lu tong** (Liquidambaris Fructus) 路路通 12–15g and **wang bu liu xing** (Vaccariae Semen) 王不留行 6–9g.

Prepared medicines
Concentrated powder
Ba Wei Di Huang Wan (Rehmannia Eight Formula) plus Su Zi Jiang Qi Tang (Perilla Seed Combination)

Pills
Jin Kui Shen Qi Wan (Fu Gui Ba Wei Wan, Golden Book Teapills) plus Hai Zao Jing Wan (Sargassum Teapills, Haiodin)

Acupuncture
See Table 17.6, p.794.

Clinical notes
- Nodules of this type are usually benign, but are chronic and can be difficult to resolve. Persistent Chinese medical treatment can be successful, but some months will usually be required.

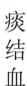

17.1.5 PHLEGM AND BLOOD STAGNATION
Masses of this type are likely to be malignant.

Clinical features
- Nodular or very firm, hard or stone like swelling of the thyroid, with skin discoloration or vascular congestion. The mass may feel irregular, tender to palpation, and is generally immobile.

- may be impingement on the larynx or trachea with hoarseness and dysphagia

Treatment principle
Activate and disperse blood and phlegm and resolve the mass

Prescription

SAN ZHONG KUI JIAN SAN 散肿溃坚散
Forsythia and Laminaria Powder

chao huang qin (stir fried Scutellariae Radix) 炒黄芩 12g
huang qin (Scutellariae Radix) 黄芩 12g
long dan cao (Gentianae Radix) 龙胆草 15g
huang bai (Phellodendri Cortex) 黄柏 15g
tian hua fen (Trichosanthes Radix) 天花粉 15g
zhi mu (Anemarrhenae Rhizoma) 知母 15g
jie geng (Platycodi Radix) 桔梗 15g
kun bu (Eckloniae Thallus) 昆布 15g
chai hu (Bupleuri Radix) 柴胡 10g
san leng (Sparganii Rhizoma) 三棱 10g
e zhu (Curcumae Rhizoma) 莪术 10g
lian qiao (Forsythiae Fructus) 连翘 10g
zhi gan cao (Glycyrrhizae Radix preparata) 炙甘草 10g
ge gen (Puerariae Radix) 葛根 6g
bai shao (Paeoniae Radix alba) 白芍 6g
dang gui wei (rootlets of Angelicae sinensis Radix) 当归尾 6g
huang lian (Coptidis Rhizoma) 黄连 6g
sheng ma (Cimicifugae Rhizoma) 升麻 1.8g

Method: Powder. **Huang qin, huang lian, huang bai** and **long dan cao** clear heat and toxic heat from the triple burner, Liver and Stomach; **tian hua fen** and **zhi mu** clear heat from the qi level, while generating fluids and protecting yin; **lian qiao** clears toxic heat and dissipates nodules; **e zhu** and **san leng** break up blood stasis masses; **kun bu** softens hardness and resolves phlegm; **chai hu, sheng ma, jie geng** and **ge gen** are used to raise yang qi and focus the action of the formula in the upper body; **jie geng** also assists in discharging pus; **dang gui wei** nourishes, protects and activates blood; **bai shao** nourishes yin and blood and softens the Liver; **zhi gan cao** harmonizes the action of the other herbs and protects the Stomach. (Source: *Zhong Yi Wai Ke Xue* [*Wan Bing Hui Chun*])

Modifications
- For malignant masses, the formula can be augmented with anticancer herbs such as **bai hua she she cao** (Hedyotidis diffusae Herba) 白花蛇舌草 30–120g, **ban zhi lian** (Scutellariae barbatae Herba) 半支莲 15–18g, **ban bian lian** (Lobeliae chinensis Herba) 半边莲 15–24g or **zhong jie feng** 肿节风 (Sarcandra glabrae Herba) 15–18g. See also Table 1.5, p.11.

Prepared medicines
Concentrated powder
San Zhong Kui Jian San (Forsythia and Laminaria Powder)
Pills
Nei Xiao Luo Li Wan (Nei Xiao Luo Li Teapills)

Acupuncture

See Table 17.6, below.

Clinical notes

- Nodules and masses of a blood and phlegm stasis type may be malignant, and should be thoroughly investigated. Chinese medicine treatment can be helpful in some cases, but should be done in conjunction with appropriate management by Western medicine.

Table 17.6 Acupuncture for thyroid goitre and nodules

The basic treatment is to mobilize qi and blood and resolve phlegm, clear heat, strengthen the Spleen and supplement yin as necessary.	
SJ.6 zhigou GB.34 yanglingquan St.40 fenglong Liv.3 taichong	Basic combination for moving qi and resolving phlegm from the neck. Used for the qi and phlegm stagnation patterns.
Lu.7 lieque Kid.6 zhaohai	Opens up the flow of qi through renmai and downbears counterflow qi; main combination for goitre during puberty, pregnancy and menopause.
Sp.4 gongsun PC.6 neiguan	Opens up flow of qi through the chongmai and downbears counterflow qi. Used when masses are firmer. The renmai and chongmai points are often used together, usually one point per side (e.g. left Lu.7 + right Kid.6; left Sp.4 + right PC.6 or visa versa, depending on palpation and tenderness).
Ren.17 shanzhong Ren. 22 tiantu Ren.12 zhongwan	Keep qi flowing through the renmai and strengthen qi
Huatuo jiaji points from C3–C5	Known as the 'ping ying 平瘿' points (literally 'alleviate goitre')
local points St.10 shuitu	Nodules can be surrounded by shallow needling obliquely towards the nodule
Liv.2 xingjian	Add with heat
Bl.17 geshu	Add with blood stasis
St.36 zusanli Sp.6 sanyinjiao	Add with Spleen qi deficiency
GB.41 zulinqi SJ.5 waiguan	Open and regulate daimai and mobilize qi to break up accumulations. Used when nodules are lateral, patients are generally robust but very tense and uptight, and there is gynecological stagnation (period pain, endometriosis, fibroids) and so on. Be careful in those with significant reproductive qi and blood stasis as this treatment can move the stagnation quickly and cause sudden discharge of pent up qi and blood.
Ear points	p.831

甲
状
腺
功
能
亢
进
证

17.2 HYPERTHYROID CONDITIONS

There are several factors that consistently emerge in the genesis of hyperthyroid disorders. These are Liver qi constraint with heat or fire, phlegm and yin deficiency. Liver qi constraint and yin deficiency tend to occur at different times of life. Liver qi constraint is more common in younger people, whereas yin deficiency tends to be seen in older people, from 40 years onwards. Liver qi constraint and its various ramifications can exist independent of yin deficiency, but may eventually contribute to it. The yin deficiency patterns may in part be due to the pathological ramifications of qi constraint, but are more associated with age, depletion of yin from various causes and susceptibility to invasion by pathogens or vulnerability to disruption of the Heart Kidney axis.

When heat is severe, the main aim of treatment is to clear away the heat as quickly as possible to further prevent damage to yin and blood. Prompt treatment with acupuncture will clear the heat, calm the shen and restore some balance (see Table 17.9, p.808). When yin or blood deficiency are prominent features, treatment with herbs is essential. Herbs with specific effects on the thyroid are listed in Table 17.8, p.806.

The patterns described below are of two types, those in which the excess is the predominant feature, and those where the deficiency is the main feature. Even though different patterns are described, in clinic we often see overlap between the various states. Because some of these patterns can appear similar, the most important differential points are highlighted in bold.

肝
郁
化
热

17.2.1 LIVER QI CONSTRAINT WITH HEAT

This is the basic pattern that often precedes other patterns of thyroid disorder. There are grades of heat, from relatively minor to extreme. The basic qi constraint pattern can be complicated in a number of ways–by qi and yin deficiency, severe heat or fire, phlegm (goitre) and blood stasis. There is an emotional component or a period of increased stress preceding the onset of symptoms.

Clinical features
- Early stage of an overactive thyroid, usually seen in younger or relatively robust patients.
- anxiety, emotional lability, mood swings, weepiness
- patient feels hot, mild to moderate heat intolerance; warm clammy skin
- excessive lacrimation; sore dry irritated eyes; exopthalmos, lid lag
- flushing on the neck and chest
- fatigue, tiredness
- premenstrual symptoms or menstrual irregularity; breast pain, dysmenorrhea, scanty periods
- ankle edema, premenstrual fluid retention
- hypochondriac aching
- may or may not be thyroid swelling or nodules

T red edges on the tongue with a thin yellow coat; paler edges with qi and blood deficiency

P wiry and rapid, or wiry and fine

Treatment principle

Soften and regulate Liver qi and clear constrained heat
Harmonize the Liver and Spleen and support qi and blood

Prescription

JIA WEI XIAO YAO SAN 加味逍遥散
Augmented Rambling Powder, modified

chai hu (Bupleuri Radix) 柴胡 6–9g
dang gui (Angelicae sinensis Radix) 当归 6–9g
bai shao (Paeoniae Radix alba) 白芍 6–9g
bai zhu (Atractylodis macrocephalae Rhizoma) 白术 6–9g
fu ling (Poria) 茯苓 9–12g
zhi gan cao (Glycyrrhizae Radix preparata) 炙甘草 3–6g
shan zhi zi (Gardeniae Fructus) 山栀子 6–9g
mu dan pi (Moutan Cortex) 牡丹皮 6–9g
sheng jiang (Zingiberis Rhizoma recens) 生姜 6–9g
bo he (Mentha haplocalycis Herba) 薄荷 2–3g
xia ku cao (Prunellae Spica) 夏枯草 18–24g
xuan shen (Scrophulariae Radix) 玄参 12–18g

Method: Decoction or powder. **Chai hu** regulates the Liver and alleviates constrained qi; **dang gui** and **bai shao** nourish Liver blood and soften the Liver; **bai zhu** and **fu ling** strengthen the Spleen and dry damp; **zhi gan cao** supplements qi and, with **bai shao**, eases muscle spasms; **sheng jiang** harmonizes the Stomach; **bo he** assists **chai hu** in moving Liver qi; **mu dan pi** activates and cools the blood; **shan zhi zi** clears heat from all three burners and promotes urination to provide an exit for the heat; **xia ku cao** cools the Liver, clears heat and dissipates masses; **xuan shen** clears heat and cools the blood, protects and nourishes yin and softens hardness. Source: *Zhong Yi Zhi Liao Yi Nan Za Bing Mi Yao* [*Nei Ke Zhai Yao*])

Modifications

• Additional herbs can be selected on the basis of the specific symptom picture from Table 17.8, p.806.
• With a diffuse goitre or nodules, combine with XIAO LUO WAN (Reduce Scrophula Pill 消瘰丸, p.921 and 806) or SAN ZI YANG QIN TANG (Three Seed Decoction to Nourish One's Parents 三子养亲汤, p.918 and 806).
• With fluid damage, add one or two of the following herbs: **mai dong** (Ophiopogonis Radix) 麦冬 9–12g, **sha shen** (Glehniae/Adenophorae Radix) 沙参 9–12g and **tian hua fen** (Trichosanthes Radix) 天花粉 12–15g.

Variations and additional prescriptions

This pattern is often complicated by varying degrees of deficiency which can diminish the expression of the heat. The most common is qi and blood deficiency (at least in the early stages) and the guiding prescription can be modified accordingly. With less heat and a paler tongue, use XIAO YAO SAN (Rambling Powder 逍遥散, p.841) as the guiding prescription, with the addition of **xia ku cao** and **xuan shen**.

Prepared medicines

Concentrated powder

Jia Wei Xiao Yao San (Bupleurum & Peony Formula)

Xiao Luo Wan (Scrophularia & Fritillaria Combination)
  – add if there are nodules

Pills

Jia Wei Xiao Yao Wan (Free and Easy Wanderer Plus Teapills, Dan Zhi Xiao Yao Wan)

Nei Xiao Luo Li Wan (Nei Xiao Luo Li Teapills)
  – add if there are nodules

Acupuncture

See Table 17.9, p.808.

Clinical notes

• Liver qi constraint with heat is a common pattern of early stage hyperthyroidism, most commonly seen in women under forty. This pattern responds reliably well to early intervention, and both symptoms and levels of thyroid hormones can usually be controlled within 4–6 weeks.

• Once an episode of hyperthyroidism has occurred, it is more likely to occur again, especially if the patient is in a stressful situation at work or home. Appropriate stress management techniques should be encouraged. Exercise is an essential component of treatment (p.103), with yoga, taijiquan very helpful in controlling stress. Relaxation techniques and meditation are also helpful.

• Hot spot therapy is helpful, p.923.

• During the acute phase, including some specific foods in the diet can assist in reducing thyroxine production. See Table 17.7, p.805. A qi regulating and cooling diet can be helpful. See Clinical Handbook, Vol.2, pp.878 and 882.

肝
郁
痰
热
阳
亢

17.2.2 LIVER QI CONSTRAINT WITH PHLEGM HEAT

The main features of this pattern are qi constraint, phlegm and heat. The phlegm component is significant, and may be substantial (thyroid swelling) or insubstantial (misting the Heart causing manic behavior and shen disturbance). The heat component is moderate to strong.

Clinical features
- **severe irritability to the point of mania, uncontrollable outbursts or psychosis**
- **anxiety, palpitations, tachycardia**
- insomnia, restlessness, agitation, nightmares or dream disturbed sleep
- heat intolerance, patient feels hot (may exude a scorched smell)
- sweating
- red complexion, facial flushing
- sore red dry eyes, exopthalmos, distension in the eyes, excessive lacrimation
- constipation or alternating constipation and diarrhea
- tremor of the hands
- bitter taste in the mouth
- soft swelling of the thyroid, may be relatively large (but not always present)

T red tongue or red edged tongue with a greasy white or yellow coat
P wiry, strong, slippery pulse

Treatment principle
Dredge the Liver and regulate qi
Transform phlegm, clear heat and calm the shen

Prescription

CHAI HU JIA LONG GU MU LI TANG 柴胡加龙骨牡蛎汤
Bupleurum plus Dragon Bone and Oyster Shell Decoction, modified

chai hu (Bupleuri Radix) 柴胡 6–12g
zhi ban xia (Pinelliae Rhizoma preparatum) 制半夏 6–9g
fu ling (Poria) 茯苓 9–12g
gui zhi (Cinnamomi Ramulus) 桂枝 3–6g
sheng jiang (Zingiberis Rhizoma recens) 生姜 6–9g
huang qin (Scutellariae Radix) 黄芩 6–9g
da huang (Rhei Radix et Rhizoma) 大黄 6–9g
ren shen (Ginseng Radix) 人参 6–9g
long gu (Fossilia Ossis Mastodi) 龙骨 15–30g
mu li (Ostreae Concha) 牡蛎 15–30g
sheng tie luo (Ferri Frusta) 生铁落 15–30g
da zao (Jujubae Fructus) 大枣 .... 4 fruit
xia ku cao (Prunellae Spica) 夏枯草 18–24g
xuan shen (Scrophulariae Radix) 玄参 12–18g

Method: Decoction or powder. When decocted, the **long gu**, **mu li** and **sheng tie luo** are cooked for 30–60 minutes prior to the other herbs, and the **da huang** is added towards the end of cooking.

Chai hu dredges the Liver and regulates qi, and with **huang qin**, clears heat and dispels pathogens from shaoyang; **huang qin** also clears heat from the upper burner; **ren shen** supplements qi and moistens dryness; **zhi ban xia** transforms phlegm; **sheng tie luo**, **long gu** and **mu li** pacify and anchor yang and calm the shen; **fu ling** strengthens the Spleen and calms the shen; **gui zhi** frees yang qi circulation in the chest and dispels pathogens from the exterior; **da huang** clears heat and open the bowels; **sheng jiang** and **da zao** harmonize the Stomach and protect it from the harsh effects of the minerals and bitter dispersing herbs; **xia ku cao** cools the Liver, clears heat and dissipates masses; **xuan shen** clears heat and cools the blood, protects and nourishes yin and dissipates masses. (Source: *Shang Han Lun*)

Modifications
- With a diffuse goitre or nodules combine with Xiao Luo Wan (Reduce Scrophula Pill 消瘰丸, p.921 and 806) or San Zi Yang Qin Tang (Three Seed Decoction to Nourish One's Parents 三子养亲汤, p.918 and 806).
- With tremors, add **shi jue ming** (Haliotidis Concha) 石决明 15–30g [cooked first] and **gou teng** (Uncariae Ramulus cum Uncis) 钩藤 12–15g [added towards the end].
- With confusion or muddled thinking, add **shi chang pu** (Acori tatarinowii Rhizoma) 石菖蒲 6–9g and **yuan zhi** (Polygalae Radix) 远志 6–9g.
- With fluid damage, add one or two of the following herbs: **mai dong** (Ophiopogonis Radix) 麦冬 9–12g, **sha shen** (Glehniae/Adenophorae Radix) 沙参 9–12g and **tian hua fen** (Trichosanthes Radix) 天花粉 12–15g.
- Without constipation, delete **da huang**.

Prepared medicines
Concentrated powder
Chai Hu Jia Long Gu Mu Li Tang (Bupleurum & Dragon Bone Combination)
Xiao Luo Wan (Scrophularia & Fritillaria Combination)
   – add if there are nodules

Acupuncture
See Table 17.9, p.808.

Clinical notes
- This is a relatively common presentation of hyperthyroidism, and one in which the mental aspects of the pattern often emerge before the physical symptoms. Patients may report that the first signs of something wrong was irrational and uncontrollable anger, and erratic behavior uncharacteristic of their usual personality. Due to the phlegm component, this pattern is also more likely to exhibit a thyroid swelling at some point.
- With frequent treatment, the phlegm and heat can be reliably cleared within 4–8 weeks, and the patient made more comfortable.
- Exercise is essential and relaxation techniques are helpful for long term management.
- Hot spot therapy is helpful, p.923.
- During the acute phase including some specific foods in the diet can assist in reducing thyroxine production. See Table 17.7, p.805. A qi regulating and cooling diet can be helpful. See Clinical Handbook, Vol.2, pp.878 and 882.

肝心胃火旺 | 17.2.3 LIVER (AND HEART, STOMACH) FIRE

This is similar to the previous pattern, 17.2.2, but the heat is more concentrated and intense. When heat is this severe the yin can be quickly damaged. The main priority of treatment is to quickly cool the heat. Once the heat is reduced, there will be more focus on regulating Liver qi.

Clinical features

- **heat intolerance, patient feels hot and unable to cool down, warm or hot clammy skin, flushing, heat intolerance**
- red, sore, dry, bloodshot eyes, exopthalmos, distension in the eyes, excessive lacrimation
- severe irritability, anger, uncontrollable temper; nervousness, restlessness
- hand tremor
- frequent bowel movements, or constipation
- pruritus
- bitter taste in the mouth
- menstrual irregularity, premenstrual syndrome, may be amenorrhea or heavy periods
- soft, maybe tender swelling of the thyroid (not always present)
- **with Stomach fire**: thirst, ravenous hunger, weight loss
- **with Heart fire**: copious sweating, severe insomnia, palpitations, mental instability

Liver, Heart, Stomach fire

↑ increasing heat

Liver qi constraint with phlegm heat

Liver qi constraint with heat

T red or red edged or red tipped tongue with a thick or dry yellow coat
P wiry strong rapid surging pulse

Treatment principle

Clear and purge fire from the Liver, Heart and Stomach

Prescription

LONG DAN XIE GAN TANG 龙胆泻肝汤
Gentian Decoction to Purge the Liver, plus
YI GUAN JIAN 一贯煎
Linking Decoction, modified

jiu long dan cao (wine fried Gentianae Radix) 酒龙胆草 3–9g
huang qin (Scutellariae Radix) 黄芩 6–12g
shan zhi zi (Gardeniae Fructus) 山栀子 6–12g
ze xie (Alismatis Rhizoma) 泽泻 6–12g
mu tong (Akebiae Caulis) 木通 3–6g
che qian zi (Plantaginis Semen) 车前子 9–15g
sheng di (Rehmanniae Radix) 生地 24–45g
dang gui (Angelicae sinensis Radix) 当归 6–12g
chai hu (Bupleuri Radix) 柴胡 3–9g
gan cao (Glycyrrhizae Radix) 甘草 3–6g

gou qi zi (Lycii Fructus) 枸杞子 9–18g
sha shen (Glehniae/Adenophorae Radix) 沙参 9–12g
mai dong (Ophiopogonis Radix) 麦冬 9–12g
chuan lian zi (Toosendan Fructus) 川楝子 3–6g
xia ku cao (Prunellae Spica) 夏枯草 18–24g
xuan shen (Scrophulariae Radix) 玄参 12–18g

Method: Decoction. **Jiu long dan cao** cools the Liver and clears heat; **shan zhi zi** clears heat from all three burners; and **huang qin** clears heat from the upper burner; **chai hu** clears heat, dredges the Liver and alleviates qi constraint; **ze xie**, **che qian zi** and **mu tong** promote urination to provide an escape route for the heat; **sheng di** cools the blood and protects yin from damage by intense heat and the bitter cold herbs; **dang gui** nourishes and protects blood; **gan cao** protects the Stomach; **gou qi zi** enriches Liver yin and blood; **sha shen** and **mai dong** protect yin; **chuan lian zi** rectifies qi and stops pain; **xia ku cao** cools the Liver, clears heat and dissipates masses; **xuan shen** clears heat and cools the blood, protects and nourishes yin and dissipates masses. (Source: *Zhong Yi Wai Ke Xue* [*Yi Fang Ji Jie* / *Xu Ming Yi Lei An*])

Modifications

- With blazing fire, a relatively high dose of the iodine containing **hai zao** (Sargassum) 海藻 30–60g and **kun bu** (Eckloniae Thallus) 昆布 30–60g can be used for a week of so to assist in quickly dampening down the heat.
- Additional herbs can be selected on the basis of the specific symptom picture from Table 17.8, p.806–807.
- With a diffuse goitre or nodules combine with Xɪᴀᴏ Lᴜᴏ Wᴀɴ (Reduce Scrophula Pill 消瘰丸, p.921 and 806) or Sᴀɴ Zɪ Yᴀɴɢ Qɪɴ Tᴀɴɢ (Three Seed Decoction to Nourish One's Parents 三子养亲汤, p.918 and 806).
- With Heart fire, add **lian zi** (Nelumbinis Semen) 莲子 6–9g and **huang lian** (Coptidis Rhizoma) 黄连 3–6g.
- With Stomach fire, add **shi gao** (Gypsum fibrosum) 石膏 15–30g [cooked first], **zhi mu** (Anemarrhenae Rhizoma) 知母 9–12g and **tian hua fen** (Trichosanthes Radix) 天花粉 12–15g.
- With tremors, add **shi jue ming** (Haliotidis Concha) 石决明 15–30g [cooked first] and **gou teng** (Uncariae Ramulus cum Uncis) 钩藤 12–15g [added towards the end].
- With phlegm heat, add **yu jin** (Curcumae Radix) 郁金 9–12g.
- To further protect fluids and yin, increase the doses of **mai dong** (Ophiopogonis Radix) 麦冬 and **sha shen** (Glehniae/Adenophorae Radix) 沙参 to 18g and add **tian hua fen** (Trichosanthes Radix) 天花粉 12–15g and **bai shao** (Paeoniae Radix alba) 白芍 9–15g.

Prepared medicines

Concentrated powder

Long Dan Xie Gan Tang (Gentiana Combination) plus Yi Guan Jian (Linking Combination)

Xiao Luo Wan (Scrophularia & Fritillaria Combination)
    – add if there are nodules

Pills

Long Dan Xie Gan Wan (Snake and Dragon Teapills) plus Yi Guan Jian Wan

(Linking Decoction Teapills)

Acupuncture

See Table 17.9, p.808.

Clinical notes

- Liver and Heart fire may be diagnosed as acute hyperthyroidism or thyrotoxicosis (also known as thyroid storm). This pattern can be more difficult than the previous two, and takes aggressive and frequent treatment to bring under control. It can be dangerous if not swiftly brought under control, and management in hospital may be necessary.
- During the acute phase including some specific foods in the diet can assist in lowering thyroxine production. See Table 17.7, p.805. When the condition is under control, a qi regulating and cooling diet can be helpful. See Clinical Handbook, Vol.2, pp.878 and 882.
- Hot spot therapy is helpful, p.923.
- The iodine rich herbs, **hai zao** (Sargassum) 海藻 and **kun bu** (Eckloniae Thallus) 昆布 can be used in the same fashion as pharmacological doses of potassium iodide (see pp.775 and 807). High doses in the order of 30–60 grams, used for a week or so, have the effect of suppressing thyroxine production and quickly dampening the heat and sparing the yin. Continued use for more than a week, however, provides more fuel to the fire, and they should be discontinued after no more than 10 days.
- Once the acute phase is under control, exercise to mobilize qi and appropriate stress management techniques to calm the shen should be encouraged. Exercise is an essential component of long term treatment (p.103), with yoga, taijiquan very helpful in controlling stress. Relaxation techniques and meditation can also be helpful in preventing reoccurrence.

风
温
瘿
痈

17.2.4 WIND HEAT OR WIND WARMTH (WARM DISEASE)

This pattern is associated with acute swelling of the thyroid due to external pathogenic invasion (either viral or bacterial) or localized heat following radiation treatment. It tends to appear in seasonal clusters, and can easily lead to yin or yang qi deficiency complications. It may also occur in postpartum women with a yin and blood deficiency predisposition.

Clinical features
- Acute tenderness and mild to moderate swelling of the thyroid with redness of the overlying skin. The swelling usually appears a couple of weeks after a wind heat invasion with sore throat, cough and fever. The main feature of this pattern is the tenderness of the thyroid, which may radiate into the jaw and throat and cause dysphagia.
- tachycardia, palpitations
- copious sweating
- tremor, shakiness
- fever
- malaise, nausea
- thirst
- restlessness
- headache

T thick, greasy, yellow tongue coat
P rapid, strong pulse

Treatment principle
Vent and resolve toxic heat and wind heat
Alleviate swelling and pain

Prescription

PU JI XIAO DU YIN 普济消毒饮
Universal Benefit Drink to Eliminate Toxin

jiu huang qin (Scutellariae Radix) 酒黄芩	6–12g
jiu huang lian (Coptidis Rhizoma) 酒黄连	3–9g
xuan shen (Scrophulariae Radix) 玄参	6–12g
niu bang zi (Arctii Fructus) 牛蒡子	9–15g
lian qiao (Forsythiae Fructus) 连翘	6–12g
ban lan gen (Isatidis/Baphicacanthis Radix) 板蓝根	9–15g
jie geng (Platycodi Radix) 桔梗	3–6g
chai hu (Bupleuri Radix) 柴胡	3–9g
gan cao (Glycyrrhizae Radix) 甘草	3–6g
chen pi (Citri reticulatae Pericarpium) 陈皮	3–6g
ma bo (Lasiosphaerae/Calvatiae) 马勃	2–3g
bai jiang can (Bombyx Batryticatus) 白僵蚕	3–9g
bo he (Mentha haplocalycis Herba) 薄荷	3–6g
sheng ma (Cimicifugae Rhizoma) 升麻	3–6g

Method: Decoction. **Jiu huang qin** and **jiu huang lian** clear heat and toxic heat from the upper burner; the wine processing focuses the action of these herbs on the upper body and head; **niu bang zi, lian qiao, bo he** and **bai jiang can** dispel wind heat from the head and upper burner; **xuan shen, ma bo, ban lan gen, jie geng** and **gan cao** clear toxic heat from the throat; **chen pi** regulates qi and assists in moving stagnant qi and alleviating pain; the ascending action of **sheng ma** and **chai hu** when used together, help the formula target the upper body, while dispersing wind heat from the face and head. (Source: *Zhong Yi Wai Ke Xue* [*Dong Yuan Shi Xiao Fang*])

Prepared medicines
Concentrated powder
Pu Ji Xiao Du Yin (Scute & Cimicifuga Combination)
Xian Fang Huo Ming Yin (Angelica & Mastic Combination)

Pills
Pu Ji Xiao Du Wan (Universal Benefit Teapills)
Huang Lian Shang Qing Pian (Huang Lien Shang Ching Pien)
Chuan Xin Lian Kang Yan Pian (Chuan Xin Lian Antiphlogistic Tablets)
 – all toxic heat patterns
Niu Huang Qing Huo Wan
 – severe cases

Acupuncture (select from)
The treatment of this condition differs from that of other patterns of hyperthyroidism.

Du.14 (dazhui –)...............meeting point of the yang channels, clears heat and drains fire

SJ.5 (waiguan)...................connecting point of the triple burner, clears heat, dispels wind heat and alleviates swelling in the neck

St.44 (neiting –)................together these points clear heat from yangming and
LI.4 (hegu –)   have a special effect on heat lesions of the jaw and neck

Lu.10 (yuji).......................fire point of the Lungs, clears heat from the Lungs and benefits the throat

LI.11 (quchi –)..................sea point of the Large Intestine, clears heat and damp from yangming, dispels wind and regulates qi and blood

Lu.11 (shaoshang ↓)...........wood point of the Lungs, clears heat from the Lungs, dispels wind heat and eases the throat

Du.10 (lingtai –)................these points have a special effect on pyogenic lesions
Du.12 (shenzhu –)
Kid.6 (zhaohai) ....protects yin from damage by the extreme heat and benefits the throat.

• with severe heat, bleed the jing points of the finger tips
• Ear points: lungs, thyroid, tonsils ↓

Clinical notes

- A wind heat or wind warmth pattern of thyroid swelling and tenderness may be diagnosed as acute or subacute thyroiditis as a result of infection or following radiation treatment for other pathology in the neck.
- This is a relatively uncommon pattern, but one which can be easily misdiagnosed. There are usually clear signs of hyperthyroid activity, but the clinching feature is the history and the degree of tenderness in the gland itself which is generally not seen in the other patterns. This is a transitory hyperthyroidism due to release of T4 and T3 from viral destruction of follicle cells.
- Because thyroid follicle cells are destroyed by the inflammatory process, patients often experience a period of hypothyroidism after resolution of the acute phase.

Table 17.7 Goitrogenic foods and a gluten free diet assist in management of hyperthyroid conditions.

These items contain substances that inhibit thyroid hormone synthesis. They can be used therapeutically in hyperthyroid cases to suppress thyroid function. When they comprise a large part of the diet they may contribute to goitre formation or hypothyroidism. They contain thiocyanates that interfere with uptake and concentration of iodine, as well as inhibiting thyroperoxidase activity. Thiocyanates are heat sensitive, so cooking can deactivate the effect to a degree.	
Brassica family	broccoli (generally considered the most effective), cabbage, cauliflower, kale, brussel sprouts, kohlrabi, mustard, mustard seed, many chinese vegetables (bok choy, choy sum, wong bok, gai lan, tatsoi, mizuna, mustard greens), canola, turnips, collard greens
Lesser known (effects for some are disputed)	cassava, millet, peanuts, cashews, almonds, areca nut (bing lang), bamboo shoots, lima beans, horseradish, maize
Gluten free diet. Especially indicated when there is known gluten intolerance or clear evidence of Spleen deficiency or damp.	
Avoid	Any product made with wheat, rye, barley and oat flours, or ingredients and by products made from those grains. As a general rule all processed foods containing wheat, gluten-derivatives, or thickeners (which is most of them). Easiest to avoid anything in a packet or can. Problematic items include ice cream, salad dressings, canned soups, dried soup mixes, processed cheeses, cream sauces, sausages, hot dogs and many others.
Include	Fresh meat, fish and poultry, corn and rice, milk, yogurt and unprocessed cheeses, dried beans, fresh or frozen fruits and vegetables

Table 17.8 Herbs with a specific effect on the thyroid

Xia Ku Cao Prunellae Spica 夏枯草		Selfheal spike; bitter, pungent, cold; Liver, Gallbladder. Cools the Liver and dissipates masses and nodules. An important herb for thyroid patterns with inflammation, swelling and nodules associated with Liver fire or phlegm fire. Added to all formulas to treat hyperthyroid conditions.
Lian Qiao Forsythiae Fructus 连翘		Forsythia fruit; pungent, cool, bitter; Heart, Lung, Gallbladder. Has the ability to penetrate deeply into dense congealed areas and assist other herbs in gaining access. For hot type thyroid nodules.
Huang Yao Zi Dioscoreaea bulbiferae Rhizoma 黄药子		Dioscorea bulbifera root; bitter, cold, toxic; Liver, Stomach, Heart, Lung. Dissipates nodules and goitre. For Liver heat and phlegm heat patterns. Also used for thyroid cancer. Can cause liver damage, and toxicity precludes its use in those with hepatic dysfunction (chronic hepatitis, cirrhosis). Usually reserved for non responsive cases.
Zhe Bei Mu Fritillaria thunbergii Bulbus 浙贝母	Xiao Luo Wan 消瘰丸	Zhejiang fritillaria tuber; bitter, cold; Heart, Lung. Dissipates nodules. An important herb for phlegm masses in the thyroid, usually in combination with **mu li** and **xuan shen**.
Mu Li Ostreae Concha 牡蛎		Oyster shell; salty, astringent, cool; Liver, Kidney. Softens hardness and dissipates masses and nodules. An important substance for a variety of masses and swellings, including goitre and thyroid nodules.
Xuan Shen Scrophulariae Radix 玄参		Scrophularia root; salty, sweet, bitter, cool; Kidney, Lung. Softens hardness, dissipates masses and nodules, cools the blood and nourishes yin. For phlegm and phlegm heat swelling and nodules in the neck and thyroid.
Bai Jie Zi Sinapsis Semen 白芥子	San Zi Yang Qin Tang 三子养亲汤	Mustard seed; pungent, warm; Lung, Stomach. Dissolves phlegm and disperses nodules. Traditionally used for cold patterns, but can inhibit thyroid hormone production (as a member of the Brassica family, see p.805) and so can be used for heat and hyperthyroid patterns, when combined with an appropriate cooling formula.
Lai Fu Zi Raphani Semen 莱菔子		Radish seed; pungent, sweet; Lung, Spleen. Dissolves phlegm and food stagnation. Member of the brassica family, p.805, so can be used for heat and hyperthyroid patterns.
Su Zi Perillae Fructus 苏子		Perilla seed; pungent, warm; Lung, Large Intestine. Dissolves phlegm and directs qi downwards. For phlegm swellings.

Table 17.8 Herbs with a specific effect on the thyroid (cont.)

Hai Zao Sargassum 海藻	Hai Zao-sargassum seaweed; bitter, salty, cold; Liver, Stomach, Kidney; Kun Bu-kelp; salty, cold; Liver, Stomach, Kidney. These herbs disperse phlegm and dissipate nodules. Used together for various types of phlegm and phlegm heat thyroid masses and nodules. Being rich in iodine they can be used in high doses (to 60 grams each) for a week or so to quickly dampen down thyroxine production in thyrotoxicosis.
Kun Bu Eckloniae Thallus 昆布	
Wa Leng Zi Arcae Concha 瓦楞子	Arc shell; sweet, salty, neutral; Liver, Spleen, Lung, Stomach. Softens hardness, activates blood, disperses phlegm and dissipates masses. Used for both phlegm and blood stasis type thyroid swelling and nodules.
Hai Fu Shi Costaziae Os 海浮石	Pumice; salty, cold; Lung. Softens hardness and dissipates nodules. For thyroid nodules from heat and phlegm heat.
Hai Ge Ke Meretricis/Cyclinae Concha 海蛤壳	Clam shell; salty, cold; Lung, Kidney. Softens hardness and dissipates masses. For thyroid nodules from heat and phlegm heat.
E Zhu Curcumae Rhizoma 莪术	E zhu-curcuma rhizome; bitter, pungent, warm. San leng-scirpus; bitter, pungent, neutral; both enter the Liver and Spleen. Together these herbs break up blood stasis and disperse masses. Used together for a variety of masses and tumors, especially when they are very firm. Used for both benign and malignant thyroid nodules and tumors.
San Leng Sparganii Rhizoma 三棱	
Symptomatic treatment	
Nodules	Xiao Luo Wan (rubbery, diffuse, euthyroid) San Zi Yang Qi Tang ('hot', firmer, smaller) e zhu + san leng (hard nodules)
Goitre	kun bu, hai zao (diffuse euthyroid), xia ku cao, huang yao zi
Tremors	shi jue ming, gou teng, shan yang jiao (山羊角 goat horn, substitute for ling yang jiao 羚羊角), bai ji li, bai shao, mu gua
Eyes (irritation, protrusion)	bai ji li, xia ku cao, jue ming zi, qing xiang zi, gou qi zi
Palpitations, tachycardia	long gu, ci shi, hu po, dan shen, yuan zhi, ye jiao teng, zhen zhu mu
Insomnia	long gu, mu li, suan zao ren, he huan pi, ye jiao teng
Thirst, ravenous hunger	shi gao, zhi mu, tian hua fen
Spider veins, peripheral numbness, left iliac fossa pressure pain (blood stasis)	dan shen, yu jin, tao ren (the latter not when there are loose or frequent bowel movements), ji xue teng, chuan niu xi

Table 17.9 Acupuncture points for the excess patterns of hyperthyroid

The basic treatment for acute patterns with marked heat, agitation and palpitations. The main aim of treatment is to quickly clear heat, regulate and move stagnant qi; secondary aims are to calm the shen, restrain ascendant yang, resolve phlegm and protect yin.	
PC.6 neiguan	Regulates the Liver, downbears counterflow qi, calms the shen and opens yinweimai. The main point for acute excess hyperthyroid patterns when the Liver is the main organ system affected. PC.6 restrains the exuberance of an overactive Liver and downbears counterflow qi from the upper body. Combined with Kid.9 zhubin to help in pulling the ascendant yang and heat away from the upper body.
Kid.9 zhubin	The cleft point of yinweimai, calms the shen and draws heat and yang downwards and away from the upper body when combined with PC.6 neiguan.
Liv.3 taichong +/– Liv.2 xingjian	Regulates the Liver and alleviates qi constraint; clears heat and fire from the Liver.
Lu.7 lieque Kid.6 zhaohai	Opens up the flow of qi through renmai and directs qi downwards; protects yin from damage by the heat.
LI.4 hegu Liv.3 taichong Du.20 baihui	This combination is a good standby when the qi stagnation, agitation and wind (tremor) components are obvious. Usually used once or twice to settle the patient down.
LI.11 quchi St.44 neiting	Clears heat and fire from yangming; used for ravenous hunger and thirst.
Liv.8 ququan	Supports Liver yin and clears heat.
St.40 fenglong	Added when there is goitre or nodules, often paired with Sp.3 taibai and PC.5 jianshi.
local points St.10 shuitu Ren.22 tiantu	Shallow needling of local points obliquely towards any swelling on the thyroid circulates qi and blood and reduces accumulation.
Ear points	p.831, plus zero point

心肾阴虚 17.2.5 HEART AND KIDNEY YIN DEFICIENCY

This is the basic pattern in chronic and persistent hyperthyroid conditions, and in older patients with hyperthyroidism. This basic yin deficiency pattern is often complicated by other pathology that alters the presentation and the treatment approach. The common variations are described below. When yin deficiency is prolonged or severe, it will usually be complicated by blood stasis. All patterns below, except the Heart and Spleen deficiency pattern, share common features although they differ in the organ primarily affected by the deficiency, and the degree of heat. In this and the patterns that follow, there is frequently a history of some significant emotional trauma or shock in the preceding 12 months.

Clinical features
- **Anxiety, panic attacks, nervousness, irritability, insomnia, dream disturbed sleep**
- palpitations, tachycardia
- tiredness and fatigue compounded by a sense of jitteriness and over stimulation (exhausted during the day, but unable to sleep or wide awake at night)
- poor concentration, forgetfulness
- heat in the hands, palmar erythema
- facial flushing
- sweating, clamminess
- may or may not present with a goitre or nodules
- may be dry, irritated eyes, excessive lacrimation, lid lag or exopthalmos
- pruritus

T dry, cracked or red tongue with little coat; may be mouth or tongue ulcers
P fine, weak pulse, maybe rapid

Treatment principle
Nourish and enrich Heart and Kidney yin, clear heat, calm the shen
Transform phlegm as necessary

Prescription

TIAN WANG BU XIN DAN 天王补心丹
Emperor of Heaven's Special Pill to Supplement the Heart

sheng di (Rehmanniae Radix) 生地	120 (24)g
xuan shen (Scrophulariae Radix) 玄参	60 (18)g
mai dong (Ophiopogonis Radix) 麦冬	30 (12)g
tian dong (Asparagi Radix) 天冬	30 (12)g
chao suan zao ren (stir fried Zizyphi spinosae Semen) 炒酸枣仁	30 (12)g
dang gui (Angelicae sinensis Radix) 当归	30 (9)g
wu wei zi (Schizandrae Fructus) 五味子	30 (9)g
bai zi ren (Platycladi Semen) 柏子仁	30 (9)g
dan shen (Salviae miltiorrhizae Radix) 丹参	15 (12)g
fu ling (Poria) 茯苓	15 (12)g
ren shen (Ginseng Radix) 人参	15 (9)g

jie geng (Platycodi Radix) 桔梗..15 (9)g
yuan zhi (Polygalae Radix) 远志...15 (6)g
Method: Pills or powder. Grind herbs to a fine powder and form into 9 gram pills with honey. The dose is one pill 2–3 times daily. Can also be decocted with the doses shown in brackets. **Sheng di** and **xuan shen** nourish and supplement Kidney yin and cool the blood; **tian dong** and **mai dong** clear heat and moisten dryness; **dan shen** and **dang gui** nourish and regulate blood and prevent the supplementing herbs from causing blood stasis; **dan shen** also clears heat; **chao suan zao ren, bai zi ren** and **yuan zhi** calm the shen; **ren shen** and **fu ling** strengthen the Spleen and supplement qi; **wu wei zi** secures Heart qi and yin, calms the shen and stops sweating; **jie geng** diffuses the Lungs and directs the action of the other herbs to the upper body; **xuan shen**, **yuan zhi** and **jie geng** transform phlegm. (Source: *Zhong Yi Zhi Liao Ning Nan Za Bing Mi Yao* [*She Sheng Mi Pou*])

Modifications
• With a diffuse goitre or nodules, combine with **Xiao Luo Wan** (Reduce Scrophula Pill 消瘰丸, p.921 and 806).

Prepared medicines
Concentrated powder
Tian Wang Bu Xin Dan (Ginseng & Zizyphus Formula)
Xiao Luo Wan (Scrophularia & Fritillaria Combination)
   – add if there are nodules

Pills
Tian Wang Bu Xin Dan (Emperor's Teapills, Tian Wang Pu Hsin Tan)
Nei Xiao Luo Li Wan (Nei Xiao Luo Li Teapills)
   – add if there are nodules

Acupuncture
See Table 17.10, p.822.

Clinical notes
• Heart and Kidney yin deficiency is a common pattern of hyperthyroidism and one that generally responds well to treatment.
• During the acute phase, including some specific foods in the diet can assist in reducing thyroxine production. See Table 17.7, p.805, otherwise a yin nourishing diet is recommended. See Clinical Handbook, Vol.2, p.876.

心
气
阴
虚

17.2.6 HEART YIN AND QI DEFICIENCY

The addition of qi deficiency in this pattern gives rise to a functional weakness in cardiac rhythm. This variation of the basic yin deficiency pattern is more common in an older age group, over 50 years.

Clinical features

- **Arrhythmia, tachycardia, palpitations.** Irregular heart beat may not be apparent to the patient and only detected during pulse examination. Irregularity may be intermittent or frequent. The more irregular the pulse and the more frequent the dropped beats the more severe the deficiency. Palpitations and tachycardia are worse at night; the patient may wake with a racing heart.
- mild anxiety, irritability, jitteriness
- insomnia, dream disturbed sleep
- tiredness, fatigue and weakness
- poor concentration, forgetfulness, poor memory
- breathlessness with exertion
- heat in the hands, palmar erythema
- facial flushing
- easy sweating, clamminess, night sweats
- pruritus
- may or may not present with a goitre or nodules; when nodules are present they are usually multiple
- dry, irritated eyes, lid lag or exopthalmos

T pink or swollen and slightly red, maybe cracked tongue with little coat

P **irregularly irregular pulse**, or fine weak pulse

Treatment principle

Nourish and supplement Heart qi and yin

Prescription

ZHI GAN CAO TANG 炙甘草汤
Prepared Licorice Decoction

zhi gan cao (Glycyrrhizae Radix preparata) 炙甘草 12–15g
sheng di (Rehmanniae Radix) 生地 24–30g
mai dong (Ophiopogonis Radix) 麦冬 15–24g
huo ma ren (Cannabis Semen) 火麻仁 9–12g
ren shen (Ginseng Radix) 人参 6–9g
sheng jiang (Zingiberis Rhizoma recens) 生姜 6–9g
gui zhi (Cinnamomi Ramulus) 桂枝 6–9g
e jiao (Asini Corii Colla) 阿胶 6–9g
da zao (Jujubae Fructus) 大枣 ....5 fruit

Method: Decoction or powder. **E jiao** is melted in the strained decoction. **Zhi gan cao** strengthens the Spleen and Stomach, supplements qi and unblocks the flow of yang qi to the Heart; **ren shen** and **da zao** strengthen the Spleen, supplement qi, nourish the Heart and support yuan qi; **sheng di**, **mai dong**, **huo ma ren** and **e jiao** nourish yin, and moisten dryness; **sheng jiang**, **gui zhi** and the rice wine promote the movement of yang qi in the chest and assist in restoring the pulse. (Source:

Zhong Yi Nei Ke Xue [Shang Han Lun])

Modifications

- With a diffuse goitre or nodules, combine with **XIAO LUO WAN** (Reduce Scrophula Pill 消瘰丸, p.921 and 806).
- With more marked anxiety, and prominent insomnia and night sweats, delete **huo ma ren** and add **bai zi ren** (Platycladi Semen) 柏子仁 9–12g and **suan zao ren** (Ziziphi spinosae Semen) 酸枣仁 12–15g.
- With marked or unsettling palpitations, add **ci shi** (Magnetitum) 磁石 15–30g or **hu po** (Succinum) 琥珀 1–3g [as powder added to strained decoction].

Prepared medicines

Concentrated powder

Zhi Gan Cao Tang (Licorice Combination)
Xiao Luo Wan (Scrophularia & Fritillaria Combination)
   – add if there are nodules

Pills

Zhi Gan Cao Wan (Zhi Gan Cao Teapills)
Nei Xiao Luo Li Wan (Nei Xiao Luo Li Teapills)
   – add if there are nodules

Acupuncture

See Table 17.10, p.822.

Clinical notes

- Heart qi and yin deficiency is a relatively common presentation of hyperthyroid in an older age group. It can respond quite well to treatment, but it usually takes some time (months) to improve and maintain a stable cardiac rhythm.
- During the acute phase, including some specific foods in the diet can assist in reducing thyroxine production. See Table 17.7, p.805, otherwise a qi and yin nourishing diet is recommended. See Clinical Handbook, Vol.2, pp.870 and 876.

17.2.7 LIVER AND KIDNEY YIN DEFICIENCY WITH HEAT, ASCENDANT YANG AND WIND

肝
肾
阴
虚
阳
亢

This variation of the basic yin deficiency pattern is characterized by more heat and more severe Kidney yin deficiency than the previous two patterns, with the addition of some wind in the form of an obvious tremor.

Clinical features
- **heat intolerance that increases in the afternoon and at night**
- **sweating, frequent drenching night sweats**
- **bone steaming fevers, tidal fever**
- **tremor usually obvious**
- **hyperkinesis**
- tiredness and fatigue, yet with a jitteriness that prevents rest
- insomnia, restlessness
- lower back ache
- weakness of the proximal muscles, especially thighs and hips
- heat in the hands and feet, palmar erythema
- urinary irritation, scanty concentrated urine
- scanty periods or amenorrhea; infertility; impotence in men; loss of libido
- alopecia
- may be lymphadenopathy

T red, dry, peeled, without coat or mirror tongue
P fine, rapid pulse

Treatment principle
Nourish and enrich Liver and Kidney yin and clear heat
Pacify ascendant yang and extinguish wind

Prescription

ZHI BAI DI HUANG WAN 知柏地黄丸
Anemarrhena, Phellodendron and Rehmannia Pill, modified

shu di (Rehmanniae Radix preparata) 熟地	18–24g
shan yao (Dioscoreae Rhizoma) 山药	12–15g
shan zhu yu (Corni Fructus) 山茱萸	12–15g
mu dan pi (Moutan Cortex) 牡丹皮	9–12g
fu ling (Poria) 茯苓	9–12g
ze xie (Alismatis Rhizoma) 泽泻	9–12g
zhi mu (Anemarrhenae Rhizoma) 知母	9–12g
huang bai (Phellodendri Cortex) 黄柏	9–12g
xia ku cao (Prunellae Spica) 夏枯草	15–24g
xuan shen (Scrophulariae Radix) 玄参	9–12g

Method: Decoction, powder or pills. Decoctions are preferred in the early stages of treatment until the heat has substantially cleared. When powdered, the herbs are ground into a fine powder and formed into 9 gram pills with honey, with one pill taken 2–3 times daily with a little salty water. **Shu di** nourishes and supplements Kidney yin and blood and augments the jing; **shan zhu yu** supplements the Liver and Kidneys; **shan yao** strengthens the Spleen and secures jing; **ze xie** clears heat and fire from the Kidneys through the urine; **mu dan pi** cools and activates the blood, and clears heat from the Liver; **fu ling** strengthens the Spleen and leaches damp out through the urine; **zhi mu** clears heat and nourishes yin; **huang bai** clears damp heat and drains fire from the Kidneys and lower burner; **xia ku cao** cools the Liver, clears heat and dissipates masses; **xuan shen** clears heat and cools the blood, protects and nourishes yin and dissipates masses. (Source: *Zhong Yi Nei Ke Shou Ce* [*Zheng Yin Mai Zhi*])

Modifications

- With a diffuse goitre or nodules, combine with **Xiao Luo Wan** (Reduce Scrophula Pill 消瘰丸, p.921 and 806).
- Additional herbs can be selected from Table 17.8, p.806–807 on the basis of the specific symptoms.
- With blazing heat, a relatively high dose, 60g each, of the iodine containing **hai zao** (Sargassum) 海藻 and **kun bu** (Eckloniae Thallus) 昆布 can be used for a week or so to assist in dampening down the heat (see p.807).
- With tremors, add **shi jue ming** (Haliotidis Concha) 石决明 15–30g [cooked first] and **gou teng** (Uncariae Ramulus cum Uncis) 钩藤 12–15g [added at the end].
- With Stomach or Heart heat (thirst, hunger and weight loss) add **shi gao** (Gypsum fibrosum) 石膏 15–30g [cooked first] and **tian hua fen** (Trichosanthes Radix) 天花粉 12–15g.

Variations and additional prescriptions

Varying degrees of heat

The degree of heat and the prominent features in this pattern can vary. The primary prescription is suitable when the heat is moderate and the Kidney yin deficiency symptoms are obvious. As the degree of heat increases, different prescriptions can be used to deal with specific aspects of the pattern, with the aim of quickly clearing the heat, stopping sweating or fever, before returning to the basic Kidney supplement for long term supplementation.

When the deficiency heat is more intense, with bone steaming or afternoon fever, **Da Bu Yin Wan** (Great Supplement the Yin Pill 大补阴丸, p.914) can be used to deeply enrich yin and cool the blood. When the night sweats are drenching and need to be quickly checked to avoid further damage to yin, select **Dang Gui Liu Huang Tang** (Tangkuei and Six Yellow Decoction 当归六黄汤, p.704). When night–time fevers without sweating are the main feature, select **Qing Hao Bie Jia Tang** (Sweet Wormwood and Soft–Shelled Turtle Shell Decoction 青蒿鳖甲汤, p.381) as guiding prescription.

Prepared medicines

Concentrated powder

Zhi Bai Di Huang Wan (Anemarrhena, Phellodendron & Rehmannia Formula)
Da Bu Yin Wan (Rehmannia & Testudinis Combination)
Dang Gui Liu Huang Tang (Tangkuei & Six Yellow Combination)
Qing Hao Bie Jia Tang (Artemesia & Turtle Shell Combination)
Xiao Luo Wan (Scrophularia & Fritillaria Combination)
    – add if there are nodules

Pills

Zhi Bai Ba Wei Wan (Zhi Bai Ba Wei Wan, Eight Flavor Rehmannia Teapills)
Da Bu Yin Wan (Da Bu Yin Wan, Abundant Yin Teapills)
Nei Xiao Luo Li Wan (Nei Xiao Luo Li Teapills)
  – add if there are nodules

Acupuncture

See Table 17.10, p.822.

Clinical notes

• Liver and Kidney yin deficiency with heat, ascendant yang and wind is a relatively severe pattern of hyperthyroidism that borders on thyrotoxicosis (thyroid storm).
• Including some specific foods in the diet can assist in reducing thyroxine production. See Table 17.7, p.805. Once the heat has cleared somewhat, a yin nourishing diet is recommended. See Clinical Handbook, Vol.2, p.876.

肝
心
阴
虚

17.2.8 LIVER AND HEART YIN DEFICIENCY

This is a minor variant of the basic yin deficiency pattern, where the Liver yin deficiency is the main feature. Pathology of the eyes, nails and upper digestive tract is prominent. The heat symptoms tend to be somewhat muted. Symptoms have an emotional component.

Clinical features
• **dry, sore, irritated eyes, lid lag, exopthalmos**
• **brittle nails, onycholysis**
• insomnia
• anxiety, depression
• acid reflux, indigestion, nagging hunger, abdominal pain
• dry mouth and throat
• muscles spasms, tremor, tics; muscle tightness, stiffness and tension
• temporal headaches
• dull hypochondriac pain
• may or may not be a goitre or nodules

T red and dry with little or no coat
P fine, wiry pulse

Treatment principle
Supplement Liver yin and regulate qi

Prescription

YI GUAN JIAN 一贯煎
Linking Decoction

sheng di (Rehmanniae Radix preparata) 生地 24–45g
gou qi zi (Lycii Fructus) 枸杞子 9–18g
sha shen (Glehniae/Adenophorae Radix) 沙参 9–12g
mai dong (Ophiopogonis Radix) 麦冬 9–12g
dang gui (Angelicae sinensis Radix) 当归 9–12g
chuan lian zi (Toosendan Fructus) 川楝子 3–6g

Method: Decoction. **Sheng di** and **gou qi zi** enrich and nourish Liver yin and blood; **sha shen** and **mai dong** nourish and supplement Stomach yin; **dang gui** supplements and activates Liver blood and softens the Liver; **chuan lian zi** regulates qi and stops pain. (Source: *Xu Ming Yi Lei An*)

Modifications
• With a diffuse goitre or nodules, combine with **XIAO LUO WAN** (Reduce Scrophula Pill 消瘰丸, p.921 and 806).
• With Heart and Stomach fire, add **jiu huang lian** (wine fried Coptidis Rhizoma) 酒黄连 1–1.5g.
• With constipation, add **huo ma ren** (Cannabis Semen) 火麻仁 9–12g or **gua lou ren** (Trichosanthis Semen) 栝楼仁 9–12g.
• With persistent hypochondriac ache, add **mei gui hua** (Rosae rugosae Flos) 玫瑰花 6–9g.
• With muscle spasms or tics, add **bai shao** (Paeoniae Radix alba) 白芍 12–18g

and **gan cao** (Glycyrrhizae Radix) 甘草 6–9g.
• With headaches, add **bai shao** (Paeoniae Radix alba) 白芍 12–18g.
• With marked acid reflux, add **hai piao xiao** (Sepiae Endoconcha) 海螵蛸 9–12g [as powder added to the strained decoction].
• With Stomach yin deficiency and a peeled or mirror tongue, add **yu zhu** (Polygonati odorati Rhizoma) 玉竹 12–15g.

Prepared medicines
Concentrated powder
Yi Guan Jian (Linking Combination)
Qi Ju Di Huang Wan (Lycium, Chrysanthemum & Rehamannia Formula)
Xiao Luo Wan (Scrophularia & Fritillaria Combination)
– add if there are nodules

Pills
Yi Guan Jian Wan (Linking Decoction Teapills)
Qi Ju Di Huang Wan (Lycium–Rehmannia Pills)
Nei Xiao Luo Li Wan (Nei Xiao Luo Li Teapills)
– add if there are nodules

Acupuncture
See Table 17.10, p.822.

Clinical notes
• Liver and Heart yin deficiency is a relatively uncommon presentation of yin deficient thyroid disorders.
• During the acute phase including some specific foods in the diet can assist in reducing thyroxine production. See Table 17.7, p.805, otherwise a yin nourishing diet is recommended. See Clinical Handbook, Vol.2, p.876.

阴阳两虚

17.2.9 KIDNEY YIN AND YANG DEFICIENCY

This is a late stage variant, where there are features of heat above and cold below. It may represent a transitional state between hyperthyroid and hypothyroid states. It is also seen in older patients and those on antithyroid medications (p.774).

Clinical features
- heat intolerance, flushing; hot and restless during the night but then cold and unable to warm up in the early hours of the morning and during the day
- sweating, night sweats
- anxiety, nervousness, depression, irritability
- insomnia, fitful sleep
- fatigue, tiredness
- fine tremor, muscle tics
- amenorrhea
- warm hands, cold legs and feet
- lower back ache and weakness; back may feel cold
- weakness of the legs and hips
- frequent urination, nocturia
- may or may not be goitre or nodules
- hypertension

T pink or reddish, swollen tongue with little or no coat
P fine, wiry pulse

Treatment principle
Strengthen and warm Kidney yang, nourish Kidney yin and clear heat

Prescription

ER XIAN TANG 二仙汤
Two Immortal Decoction

xian mao (Curculiginis Rhizoma) 仙茅	9–15g
xian ling pi (Epimedii Herba) 仙灵脾	9–15g
dang gui (Angelicae sinensis Radix) 当归	9–12g
ba ji tian (Morindae officinalis Radix) 巴戟天	9–12g
huang bai (Phellodendri Cortex) 黄柏	6–9g
zhi mu (Anemarrhenae Rhizoma) 知母	6–9g

Method: Decoction. **Xian mao** and **xian ling pi** warm Kidney yang and support jing; **ba ji tian** warms Kidney yang and strengthens the tendons and bones; **dang gui** nourishes and protects Blood and yin, softens the Liver, and combines with **xian mao** and **xian ling pi** to regulate and supplement chongmai and renmai; **zhi mu** and **huang bai** nourish Kidney yin and clear deficiency heat, and moderate the pungent heat of **xian mao** and **xian ling pi**. (Source: *Zhong Yi Wai Ke Xue* [*Shanghai Shu Guang Yi Yuan Jing Yan Fang*])

Modifications
- Even though there is obvious heat, large quantities of cooling herbs are avoided in this pattern. With goitre or nodules, combine with **ER CHEN TANG** (Two Aged [Herb] Decoction 二陈汤, p.915).

- For severe insomnia, add **wu wei zi** (Schizandrae Fructus) 五味子 6–9g, **ye jiao teng** (Polygoni multiflori Caulis) 夜交藤 18–30g and **he huan hua** (Albizziae Flos) 合欢花 9–12g.
- With copious spontaneous sweating, add **duan mu li** (calcined Ostreae Concha) 煅牡蛎 15–30g, **ma huang gen** (Ephedrae Radix) 麻黄根 9–12g, **fu xiao mai** (Tritici Fructus Levis) 浮小麦 12–15g.
- With night sweats, add **di gu pi** (Lycii Cortex) 地骨皮 12–15g and **qing hao** (Artemisiae annuae Herba) 青蒿 9–15g [added towards the end of cooking].

Prepared medicines
Concentrated powder
Er Xian Tang (Curculigo & Epimedium Combination)
Er Chen Tang (Citrus & Pinellia Combination)
   – add if there are nodules

Pills
Er Xian Wan (Two Immortals Teapills)
Er Chen Wan (Pinellia Pachyma Pills, Erh Chen Wan)
Hai Zao Jing Wan (Sargassum Teapills, Haiodin)
   – add if there are nodules

Acupuncture
See Table 17.10, p.822.

Clinical notes
- During the acute phase including some specific foods in the diet can assist in reducing thyroxine production. See Table 17.7, p.805, but moderation is necessary if the patient is at risk of becoming hypothyroid. Otherwise a balanced qi and blood supplementing diet is recommended. See Clinical Handbook, Vol.2, p.870 and 874.

心脾两虚 17.2.10 HEART BLOOD AND SPLEEN QI DEFICIENCY

In contrast to the previous deficiency patterns, in this pattern the patient is predominantly yang qi deficient. It is more common in elderly patients and postpartum women.

Clinical features

- **anxiety, nervousness, panic attacks, emotional lability, phobias**
- **fatigue, weakness, pronounced proximal muscle weakness**
- **insomnia, dream disturbed sleep**
- **breathlessness with exertion**
- **palpitations**
- pale translucent complexion
- digestive weakness: frequent loose stools, poor appetite
- postural dizziness
- visual weakness, blurred vision
- easy sweating and clamminess; may be night sweats
- edema
- poor immunity, frequent colds and superficial illnesses
- amenorrhea, scanty menses
- may be thyroid swelling or nodules (uncommon)

T pale, thin tongue with a thin white coat
P weak, fine, forceless pulse

Treatment principle

Strengthen the Spleen and Heart and supplement qi and blood

Prescription

GUI PI TANG 归脾汤
Restore the Spleen Decoction

zhi huang qi (honey fried Astragali Radix) 炙黄芪	9–12g
fu shen (Poria Sclerotium pararadicis) 茯神	9–12g
chao bai zhu (stir fried Atractylodes macrocephalae Rhizoma) 炒白术	9–12g
long yan rou (Longan Arillus) 龙眼肉	9–12g
suan zao ren (Zizyphi spinosae Semen) 酸枣仁	9–12g
ren shen (Ginseng Radix) 人参	6–9g
dang gui (Angelicae sinensis Radix) 当归	6–9g
yuan zhi (Polygalae Radix) 远志	3–6g
mu xiang (Aucklandiae Radix) 木香	3–6g
zhi gan cao (Glycyrrhizae Radix preparata) 炙甘草	3–6g

Method: Decoction. **Zhi huang qi**, **ren shen**, **chao bai zhu** and **zhi gan cao** strengthen the Spleen and supplement qi; **dang gui** and **zhi huang qi** in combination have a special effect on building blood; **suan zao ren**, **long yan rou** and **yuan zhi** nourish the Heart and calm the shen; **fu shen** strengthens the Spleen and calms the shen; **mu xiang** regulates qi and aids the Spleen in digesting the blood supplementing herbs; **zhi gan cao** supplements qi and harmonizes the Stomach. (Source: *Zhong Yi Nei Ke Xue* [*Ji Sheng Fang*])

Modifications
- With goitre or nodules, combine with ER CHEN TANG (Two Aged [Herb] Decoction 二陈汤, p.915) or **shi chang pu** (Acori tatarinowii Rhizoma) 石菖蒲 6–9g and **yuan zhi** (Polygalae Radix) 远志 6–9g. The latter combination is also good for foggy head and concentration difficulties.
- For marked anxiety, fearfulness and propensity to being easily startled, add **long chi** (Fossilia Dentis Mastodi) 龙齿 15–30g and **ci shi** (Magnetitum) 磁石 15–30g [both cooked first].
- With copious spontaneous sweating, add **duan mu li** (calcined Ostreae Concha) 煅牡蛎 15–30g [cooked first], **ma huang gen** (Ephedrae Radix) 麻黄根 9–12g, **fu xiao mai** (Tritici Fructus Levis) 浮小麦 12–15g.
- With night sweats, add **shu di** (Rehmanniae Radix preparata) 熟地 12–15g or **di gu pi** (Lycii Cortex) 地骨皮 12–15g.
- For severe insomnia, add **wu wei zi** (Schizandrae Fructus) 五味子 6–9g, **ye jiao teng** (Polygoni multiflori Caulis) 夜交藤 18–30g and **he huan hua** (Albizziae Flos) 合欢花 9–12g.
- With marked palpitations, add **ci shi** (Magnetitum) 磁石 15–30g [cooked first].
- With cold intolerance and cold extremities, add **rou gui** (Cinnamomi Cortex) 肉桂 3–6g.
- With mild heat, irritability and qi constraint, add **shan zhi zi** (Gardeniae Fructus) 山栀子 9–12g and **chai hu** (Bupleuri Radix) 柴胡 9–12g.
- With abnormal uterine bleeding, add **ai ye** (Artemisiae argyi Folium) 艾叶 6–9g, **pao jiang** (Zingiberis Rhizoma preparatum) 炮姜 6–9g and **xue yu tan** (Crinus carbonisatus) 血余炭 3–6g [as powder added to the strained decoction].

Prepared medicines
Concentrated powder
Gui Pi Tang (Ginseng & Longan Combination)
Yang Xin Tang (Astragalus & Zizyphus Combination)
Er Chen Tang (Citrus & Pinellia Combination)
– add if there are nodules

Pills
Gui Pi Wan (Kwei Be Wan, Gui Pi Teapills)
Bai Zi Yang Xin Wan (Pai Tzu Yang Hsin Wan)
Hai Zao Jing Wan (Sargassum Teapills, Haiodin)
– add if there are nodules

Acupuncture
See Table 17.10, p.822.

Clinical notes
- A qi and blood supplementing diet is recommended. See Clinical Handbook, Vol.2, pp.870 and 874.

Table 17.10 Acupuncture for deficiency patterns

Basic treatment for the yin deficiency and variant patterns. The main aim of treatment is to replenish yin, clear heat and cool the blood, and calm the shen. Secondary considerations, as necessary, are to extinguish wind, stop sweating, resolve phlegm and supplement qi	
Lu.7 lieque Kid.6 zhaohai	These points open up the flow of qi through renmai, direct rebellious qi downward, and protect yin from damage by heat.
Ren.12 zhongwan Ren.17 shanzhong Ren.4 guanyuan	Open up the flow of qi through renmai, and supplement the Kidneys (Ren.4).
Kid.3 taixi	Supplements Kidney and Liver yin.
Kid.2 rangu	Supplements yin, clears heat and cools the blood; used when the deficiency fire aspects are significant.
Liv.8 ququan	Supplements Liver yin.
Liv.3 taichong	Supplements Liver yin and extinguishes wind.
Sp.6 sanyinjiao	Supplements Liver and Kidney yin and Spleen qi.
Ht.7 shenmen	Calms the shen, supplements Heart yin.
Ht.6 yinxi	Alleviates sweating.
Ht.5 tongli	Treats arrhythmia.
Bl.15 xinshu Bl.18 ganshu Bl.23 shenshu	Transport points to supplement Heart, Liver and Kidney yin.
GB.37 guanming	Treats sore, gritty, dry and irritated eyes. Combine with Liv.8 ququan for this.
St.40 fenglong	Treats goitre or nodules, often paired with Sp.3 taibai and PC.6 jianshi.
local points St.10 shuitu Ren.22 tiantu	Shallow needling of local points obliquely towards any swelling on the thyroid circulates qi and blood and reduces accumulation.
Ear points	p.831, plus kidney and zero point

甲
状
腺
功
能
减
退
证

脾
肾
气
虚

17.3 HYPOTHYROID

Treatment of an underactive thyroid is based on supplementing and warming yang qi. Many patients who have been diagnosed as hypothyroid will have been prescribed thyroxine (trade names Synthroid, Oroxine, Eutroxsig). Exogenous thyroxine suppresses TSH and endogenous T4 and T3 production through negative feedback (Fig. 17.1, p.775). If the gland hasn't atrophied or been removed, treatment which warms yang can be attempted to stimulate better thyroid function, remembering that externally delivered thyroid hormone does not equate to yang qi.

If there is no functional thyroid tissue, the patient must always take thyroxine, but we can improve their general constitutional wellbeing and overall health. When patients are taking thyroxine but there is still functional thyroid tissue, (as may be seen in cases of recent onset and in subclinical hypothyroidism), Chinese medical treatment can restore thyroid function sufficiently so the dose requirements of any exogenous thyroxine may change.

17.3.1 SPLEEN AND KIDNEY QI DEFICIENCY

Spleen and Kidney qi deficiency is seen in subclinical hypothyroidism or the early stages of an underactive thyroid. It is frequently complicated by blood deficiency. Care must be taken in this early stage pattern, especially when there are few cold features. If strong yang warming herbs or methods are utilized too early, the yin may be damaged, or if there is a masked yin deficiency, it may be aggravated.

Clinical features
- In general the symptoms are not likely to be marked, presenting with mild digestive and genitourinary complaints. Blood tests may reveal elevated TSH but normal to low T4/T3.
- fatigue, tiredness, low exercise tolerance, increased desire to sleep
- depression
- mild sensitivity to cold
- poor appetite, early satiety, abdominal distension, food sits in the stomach for long periods
- constipation, sluggish stools, generally not dry or hard
- pale complexion with puffiness and swelling of the eyes
- weight gain, or inability to lose weight
- vague aches and pains, morning stiffness
- frequent urination, weak bladder
- low basal body temperature (close to or below 36⁰C)
- heavy or prolonged periods; irregular cycle; infertility; lower than normal temperatures in luteal phase of the menstrual cycle
- may or may not present with a goitre; when present it is relatively small, firm and rubbery

T pale, scalloped tongue
P weak, fine, deep pulse

Treatment principle
Strengthen and supplement Spleen and Kidney qi
Resolve phlegm

Prescription

SHEN LING BAI ZHU SAN 参苓白术散
Ginseng, Poria and White Atractylodes Powder, plus
ER XIAN TANG 二仙汤
Two Immortal Decoction

ren shen (Ginseng Radix) 人参 6–9g
bai zhu (Atractylodes macrocephalae Rhizoma) 白术 9–12g
fu ling (Poria) 茯苓 9–12g
shan yao (Dioscoreae Rhizoma) 山药 15–18g
zhi gan cao (Glycyrrhizae Radix preparata) 炙甘草 3–6g
bai bian dou (Dolichos Semen) 白扁豆 12–15g
chao yi ren (dry fried Coicis Semen) 炒苡仁 15–30g
lian zi (Nelumbinis Semen) 莲子 12–15g
jie geng (Platycodi Radix) 桔梗 6–9g
sha ren (Amomi Fructus) 砂仁 3–6g
xian mao (Curculiginis Rhizoma) 仙茅 9–15g
xian ling pi (Epimedii Herba) 仙灵脾 9–15g
dang gui (Angelicae sinensis Radix) 当归 9–12g
ba ji tian (Morindae officinalis Radix) 巴戟天 9–12g
huang bai (Phellodendri Cortex) 黄柏 2–3g
zhi mu (Anemarrhenae Rhizoma) 知母 2–3g

Method: Decoction. **Ren shen, bai zhu, yi ren, fu ling, bai bian dou, shan yao** and **zhi gan cao** strengthen the Spleen and supplement qi; **bai zhu** dries damp; **chao yi ren, fu ling** and **bai bian dou** leach out damp through the urine; **lian zi** astringes the Intestines and stops diarrhea; **jie geng** diffuses the Lungs and raises yang qi; **sha ren** transforms damp and elevates Spleen qi; **xian mao** and **xian ling pi** warm Kidney yang and support jing; **ba ji tian** warms Kidney yang and strengthens the tendons and bones; **dang gui** nourishes and protects Blood and yin, softens the Liver, and combines with **xian mao** and **xian ling pi** to regulate and supplement the chong and renmai; the small doses of **zhi mu** and **huang bai** balance the pungent hot dispersing nature of **xian mao** and **xian ling pi** without damaging the Spleen. (Source: *Zhong Yi Wai Ke Xue* [*He Ji Ju Fang* [*Shanghai Shu Guang Yi Yuan Jing Yan Fang*]])

Modifications
- With a goitre, combine with **ER CHEN TANG** (Two Aged [Herb] Decoction 二陈汤, p.915).
- With marked blood deficiency, add **bai shao** (Paeoniae Radix alba) 白芍 9–12g and **ji xue teng** (Spatholobi Caulis) 鸡血藤 15–30g.
- With stiffness and aching of muscles and joints, add **gui zhi** (Cinnamomi Ramulus) 桂枝 6–9g and **lu jiao jiao** (Cervi Cornus Colla) 鹿角胶 6–9g [as powder added to the strained decoction].
- With food stagnation and sluggish digestion, add **chao shan zha** (stir fried Crataegi Fructus) 炒山楂 9–12g and **chao shen qu** (stir fried Massa medicata fermentata) 炒神曲 9–12g (the latter not for those with gluten intolerance);

or **chao zhi shi** (stir fried Aurantii Fructus immaturus) 炒枳实 6–9g and **jie geng** (Platycodi Radix) 桔梗 3–6g.

- Mild elements of yin deficiency may be apparent, in which case combine with SHENG MAI SAN (Generate the Pulse Powder 生脉散, p.728).

Prepared medicines
Concentrated powder
Shen Ling Bai Zhu San (Ginseng & Atractylodes Formula) plus Er Xian Tang (Curculigo & Epimedium Combination)
Shi Quan Da Bu Tang (Ginseng & Dang Gui Ten Combination)

Pills
Shen Ling Bai Zhu Wan (Absorption and Digestion Pill, Shen Ling Bai Zhu Pian plus Er Xian Wan (Two Immortals Teapills)
Shi Quan Da Bu Wan (Ten Flavour Teapills)

Acupuncture
See Table 17.11, p.831.

Clinical notes
- Underactive thyroid of a Spleen and Kidney qi deficiency type is likely to be diagnosed as subacute hypothyroidism or Hashimoto's thyroiditis.
- Low thyroid function of a Spleen and Kidney qi deficiency type can be corrected relatively easily and the patient should feel better (more energy, improved digestive function and so on) within a few weeks. To rebuild a sustainable base of qi may take several months.
- Dietary advice should focus on warming and cooked food, and avoidance of the goitrogenic foods (Table 17.7, p.805).

脾
肾
心
阳
虚

17.3.2 SPLEEN, KIDNEY AND HEART YANG DEFICIENCY

This is the most common presentation of well developed and clinical hypothyroidism. In addition to the basic Spleen and Kidney yang deficiency aspects, cardiovascular complications are quite common, even in those already taking thyroxine.

Clinical features
- cold intolerance; cold extremities
- lethargy, somnolence; slow movement
- depression; blank or dull expression
- pale, matt, puffy complexion; puffy face and eyes
- weight gain, generalized puffiness; edema (may or may not be pitting)
- carpal tunnel syndrome
- coarse, dry skin; sparse dry hair
- thinning or loss of eyebrows (at their lateral ends)
- no sweating
- poor appetite, early satiety, food sits in the stomach for long periods
- constipation, no urge to defecate, stools generally not hard
- generalized aches, pains and stiffness, lower back ache and coldness
- frequent urination, nocturia
- loss of hearing acuity
- hoarse or husky voice; slow speech
- bradycardia; chest oppression
- low basal body temperature (close to or below 36^0C)
- heavy or prolonged periods; irregular cycle; infertility; lower than normal temperatures in luteal phase of the menstrual cycle
- may or may present with a goitre, but if there is a goitre it may be quite large and firm

T pale, swollen, scalloped tongue
P weak, slow or imperceptible pulse

Treatment principle
Warm Kidney, Spleen and Heart yang

Prescription

JIN GUI SHEN QI WAN 金匮肾气丸
Kidney Qi Pill from the Golden Cabinet

shu di (Rehmanniae Radix preparata) 熟地	240g
shan yao (Dioscoreae Rhizoma) 山药	120g
shan zhu yu (Corni Fructus) 山茱萸	120g
mu dan pi (Moutan Cortex) 牡丹皮	90g
fu ling (Poria) 茯苓	90g
ze xie (Alismatis Rhizoma) 泽泻	90g
zhi fu zi (Aconiti Radix lateralis preparata) 制附子	30g
gui zhi (Cinnamomi Ramulus) 桂枝	30g

Method: Powder or pills. Grind the herbs to a fine powder and form into 6 gram pills with honey.

The dose is one pill 2–3 times daily with warm, slightly salty water. **Shu di**, supplements the Kidneys; **shan zhu yu** supplements the Liver and Kidneys and protects yin; **shan yao** strengthens the Spleen and Kidneys and supplements qi; **zhi fu zi** and **gui zhi** support and warm Kidney yang, dispel cold and promote qi transformation and fluid metabolism; **ze xie** promotes urination and drains damp; **fu ling** strengthens the Spleen and leaches damp; **mu dan pi** activates and cools the Blood. (Source: *Jin Gui Yao Lüe*)

Variations and additional prescriptions

There are a few alternative prescriptions that warm and supplement Kidney and Spleen yang, while addressing different primary manifestations. When edema is mild to moderate, Jɪ SHENG SHEN Qɪ WAN (Kidney Qi Pill from Formulas to Aid the Living 济生肾气丸, p.248) is a better choice as primary prescription; when the edema is moderate to severe and there are cardiovascular complaints, ZHEN WU TANG (True Warrior Decoction 真武汤, p.249) is recommended.

Modifications

- With goitre or nodules, combine with ER CHEN TANG (Two Aged [Herb] Decoction 二陈汤, p.915). The goitrogenic brassicas (Table 17.7, p.805) and cooling herbs are avoided here.
- With significant Spleen deficiency and digestive difficulty, combine the selected formula with Lɪ ZHONG WAN (Regulate the Middle Pill 理中丸, p.732).
- With constipation, add **rou cong rong** (Cistanches Herba) 肉苁蓉 15–24g (or **suo yang** (Cynomorii Herba) 锁阳 12–15g) and a big dose of **bai zhu** (Atractylodis macrocephalae Rhizoma) 白术, up to 30g.
- With fullness, pain or oppression in the chest, add **gua lou** (Trichosanthis Fructus) 栝楼 12–18g, **tan xiang** (Santali albi Lignum) 檀香 9–12g and **xie bai** (Allii macrostemi Bulbus) 薤白 6–9g.
- Occasionally there are elements of yin deficiency, such as night sweats, amenorrhea and malar flush. The primary formula above has a yin supplementing action, but if the symptoms persist or get worse, which can happen with **fu zi**, some mild yin nourishing herbs can be added, **tian dong** (Asparagi Radix) 天冬 and **mai dong** (Ophiopogonis Radix) 麦冬, or **nu zhen zi** (Ligustri Fructus) 女贞子 and **han lian cao** (Ecliptae Herba) 旱莲草 may be helpful. The combination of the primary formula with ER XIAN TANG (Two Immortal Decoction 二仙汤, p.818) can be also tried.

Prepared medicines
Concentrated powder
Ba Wei Di Huang Wan (Rehmannia Eight Formula)
Ji Sheng Shen Qi Wan (Cyathula & Plantago Formula)
Zhen Wu Tang (Ginger, Aconite, Poria & Peony Combination)
You Gui Wan (Eucommia & Rehmannia Formula)

Pills
Jin Kui Shen Qi Wan (Fu Gui Ba Wei Wan, Golden Book Teapills)
You Gui Wan (Right Side Replenishing Teapills)
Zhen Wu Tang Wan (True Warrior Teapills)
Ba Ji Yin Yang Wan (Ba Ji Yin Yang Teapills)

Acupuncture

See Table 17.11, p.831.

Clinical notes

- In general, hypothyroidism of a Spleen and Kidney yang deficiency type can respond quite well to treatment, at least in terms of increased wellbeing and improved function. Depending on whether the patient has any functional thyroid tissue intact, the dose of thyroxine may be able to be gradually reduced as the thyroid is stimulated. The longer the patient has been taking thyroxine, the less the probability of being able to reduce exogenous thyroxine. For patients with a recent diagnosis of hypothyroidism, whose thyroid remains at least partially functional and who are not yet medicated, treatment may produce a good outcome.
- Diet is important, with an emphasis on warming and cooked food and avoidance of the goitrogenic foods (Table 17.7, p.805). See Clinical Handbook, Vol. 2, p.873.

肾
精
虚
损

17.3.3 KIDNEY JING DEFICIENCY

This is late stage illness where the Kidneys are severely depleted and the Marrow is being affected. Patients are usually middle aged and older.

Clinical features
- very poor memory to the point of dementia
- dull affect, expressionless or wooden face
- dizziness, headaches
- insomnia with lots of dreaming
- hearing loss, deafness, tinnitus
- lower back ache and weakness
- general weakness, weak legs and knees, difficulty walking
- dry mouth and throat
- hair loss, alopecia
- amenorrhea
- urinary frequency with scanty yellow urine

T slightly pale or pink dry tongue with no coat
P weak, fine, deep, imperceptible pulse

Treatment principle
Supplement and enrich Kidney jing

Prescription

ZUO GUI WAN 左归丸
Restore the Left [Kidney] Pill, plus
SHENG MAI SAN 生脉散
Generate the Pulse Powder

shu di (Rehmanniae Radix preparata) 熟地 240g
shan yao (Dioscoreae Rhizoma) 山药 120g
shan zhu yu (Corni Fructus) 山茱萸 120g
tu si zi (Cuscutae Semen) 菟丝子 120g
gou qi zi (Lycii Fructus) 枸杞子 120g
lu jiao jiao (Cervi Cornus Colla) 鹿角胶 120g
gui ban jiao (Testudinis Plastri Colla) 龟板胶 120g
huai niu xi (Achyranthis bidentatae Radix) 怀牛膝 90g
ren shen (Ginseng Radix) 人参 90g
mai dong (Ophiopogonis Radix) 麦冬 90g
wu wei zi (Schizandrae Fructus) 五味子 60g

Method. Pills or powder. **Shu di** nourishes and supplements Kidney yin and blood; **shan yao** strengthens the Spleen and Kidneys and supplements qi and yin; **shan zhu yu** supplements the Liver and Kidneys; **tu si zi** and **gou qi zi** benefit jing and blood and improve vision; **tu si zi** and **huai niu xi** strengthen the tendons, bones, low back and knees; **lu jiao jiao** warms and strengthens yang qi and acts to stimulate the transformation of raw materials into yin; **gui ban jiao** deeply enriches yin; **lu jiao jiao** and **gui ban jiao** have a 'meatiness' that is deeply enriching to yin, yang and jing, and supplementing to the chongmai and renmai; **ren shen** supplements yuan qi; **mai dong** nourishes yin; **wu wei zi** strengthens the Kidneys and calms the shen. (Source: *Zhong Yi Zhi Liao Ning Nan Za Bing Mi Yao* [*Jing Yue Quan Shu / Nei Wai Shang Bian Huo Lun*])

Modifications
- Add ER CHEN TANG (Two Aged [Herb] Decoction 二陈汤, p.915) if there is goitre.

Prepared medicines
Concentrated powder
Huan Shao Dan (Lycium Formula)

Pills
Huan Shao Dan (Return to Spring Teapills)
Zuo Gui Wan (Left Side Replenishing Teapills)
    – with yin deficiency
You Gui Wan (Right Side Replenishing Teapills)
    – with yang deficiency

Acupuncture
See Table 17.11, p.831.

Clinical notes
- Avoidance of the goitrogenic foods (Table 17.7, p.805), and a basic qi and blood nourishing diet is recommended. See Clinical Handbook, Vol.2, pp.870 and 874.

Table 17.11 Acupuncture for hypothyroid patterns

The main aim of treatment is to warm and supplement Kidney, Spleen and Heart yang qi, with a secondary aim of resolving phlegm when necessary. Plenty of moxa can be used, except where there are elements of both yin and yang deficiency, in which case moxa can still be used but with care.	
Ren.4 guanyuan Ren.6 qihai	Warms and stimulates Kidney yang when treated with moxa.
Ren.17 shanzhong Ren.12 zhongwan	Treated with moxa to mobilize yang qi in the upper and middle burners.
SI.3 houxi BI.62 shenmai	Opens up the dumai and allows yang qi to start to flow again. Usually used in combination with Du.14 dazhui and Du.4 mingmen.
Du.14 dazhui Du.4 mingmen	Moxa to stimulate the circulation of dumai qi.
BI.15 xinshu BI.20 pishu BI.23 shenshu	Transport points directly access and improve the function of the relevant organ systems.
St.25 tianshu Ren.8 shenque	Treated with moxa or moxa on salt (Ren.8) to warm Intestinal yang and stimulate peristalsis to relieve constipation.
Kid.3 taixi St.36 zusanli Sp.6 sanyinjiao St.40 fenglong	Additional points to warm and strengthen the Kidneys and Spleen.
Ear points	below, plus kidney, adrenal

Fig 17.4 Ear points for thyroid disorder

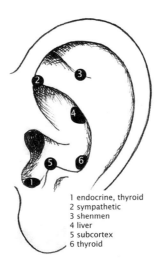

1 endocrine, thyroid
2 sympathetic
3 shenmen
4 liver
5 subcortex
6 thyroid

Table 17.12 Summary of euthyroid goitre and nodule patterns

Pattern	Features	Prescription
Phlegm damp with Spleen deficiency	Smooth soft enlargement of the thyroid	Hai Zao Yu Hu Tang
Liver and Kidney, chong-mai and renmai deficiency	Diffuse goitre that is soft and regular; signs of Kidney deficiency such as delayed onset of menstruation, infertility, irregular menses, amenorrhea or urinary frequency	Er Xian Tang + Si Wu Tang
Liver qi constraint and phlegm	Diffuse goitre or single, regular rubbery nodule; symptoms aggravated by stress, premenstrual syndrome, irritability, digestive problems	Chai Hu Shu Gan San
Phlegm and blood stasis	Nodular, firm or hard swelling of the thyroid	San Zhong Kui Jian San

Table 17.13 Summary of hypothyroid patterns

Pattern	Features	Prescription
Spleen and Kidney qi deficiency	Fatigue, lethargy, constipation, pallor, abdominal distension, pale tongue, weak pulse	Shen Ling Bai Zhu San + Er Xian Tang
Spleen, Kidney and Heart yang deficiency	Fatigue, lethargy, somnolence, cold intolerance, constipation, pallor, puffy face, abdominal distension, weight gain, pale scalloped tongue, deep, weak or imperceptible pulse	Jin Gui Shen Qi Wan
Kidney jing deficiency	Poor memory, dizziness, weakness, dull affect, hearing loss, amenorrhea, pale or pink dry tongue, deep, weak pulse	Zuo Gui Wan + Sheng Mai San

Table 17.14 Summary of hyperthyroid patterns

	Common features		Specific features	Prescription
Excess heat patterns	· heat intolerance, feels hot · warm clammy skin · hyperkinesis	Liver qi constraint with heat	early stage with mild symptoms, tongue may be relatively normal or with slightly red or pale edges depending on degree of heat and qi and blood deficiency	Jia Wei Xiao Yao San
	· irritability, anger · sore red eyes, lacrimation · red tongue or with red edges coated tongue · surging, slippery, wiry, rapid, otherwise strong pulse	Liver qi and phlegm fire	agitation, emotional lability to the point of mania, insomnia, palpitations	Chai Hu Jia Long Gu Mu Li Tang
		Liver fire	severe heat, irritability, temper outbursts, copious sweating, ravenous hunger and thirst, bloodshot eyes, photophobia	Long Dan Xie Gan Tang + Yi Guan Jian
		Wind heat (wen bing)	acute tenderness and swelling of the thyroid following an acute wind heat attack	Pu Ji Xiao Du Yin
Yin deficiency	· heat intolerance · anxiety, irritability · hyperkinesis · fatigue, weakness · muscle weakness · sweating · weight loss · thin skin · alopecia or premature greying hair · amenorrhea · often a history of emotional trauma · red tongue with no coat · fine, weak, rapid pulse	Heart yin	marked anxiety and nervousness, insomnia, red cracked, or pink, swollen, cracked tongue	Tian Wang Bu Xin Dan
		Heart qi and yin	arrhythmia, palpitations, red cracked or pink, swollen, cracked tongue, irregularly irregular pulse	Zhi Gan Cao Tang
		with fire	marked heat intolerance that increases in the afternoon and at night, drenching night sweats, bone steaming fevers, tidal fever, hyperkinesis, restlessness, tremor, hyperkinesis, tachycardia, exopthalmos, rapid pulse	Zhi Bai Ba Wei Wan Da Bu Yin Wan Dang Gui Long Hui Wan
		Liver yin	dry eyes, sore gritty eyes, visual weakness, nail disorders, onycholysis, reflux and indigestion, fine tremor, fine wiry pulse	Yi Guan Jian
		yin and yang	heat above cold below, urinary frequency and nocturia, cold legs, hot during the night then cold early in the morning and unable to warm up, hypertension	Er Xian Tang
Qi and blood deficiency	anxiety, panic attacks, insomnia, fatigue, breathlessness, digestive weakness, pale thin tongue, weak pulse			Gui Pi Tang

TIREDNESS

Tiredness is a common primary complaint in the Chinese medicine clinic, and a feature of many different disorders. Tiredness can be expressed in many ways, such as a lack of physical and mental energy, lack of motivation, excessive sleepiness, exhaustion, weariness, listlessness, feeling flat or a devastating inability to perform even the simplest of tasks. In Chinese medicine texts, tiredness falls under the heading of diseases such as 'deficiency and overwork' (*xū láo*[1] 虚痨), a category of disease resulting from overwork, exhaustion and chronic debilitating illness. Traditionally, *xū láo* describes patterns of deficiency. Clinical experience, however, reveals that many patients who complain of chronic tiredness are in fact suffering from an excess pattern of some type.

Tiredness and fatigue can be a component of almost any pattern of disharmony. However, there are some patterns in which persistent tiredness lasting weeks, months or years, is likely to be the main symptom or a major feature. These are the patterns discussed in this text.

Tiredness from a western medical point of view is often difficult to diagnose. Unless there is a demonstrable pathology, such as thyroid dysfunction, a history of infection such as Glandular fever, blood sugar problems or anemia, this symptom is left unexplored, and the patient undiagnosed, or consigned to the category of 'depression' or psychological disorder, or possibly considered a malingerer.

> **BOX 18.1 PATTERNS OF TIREDNESS**
>
> Liver qi constraint
> Damp
>   – encumbering the Spleen
>   – in the muscles
>   – damp heat
> Phlegm
>   – phlegm damp
>   – phlegm heat
>   – phlegm and qi constraint
>   – wind phlegm
> Lingering pathogens
>   – qi level
>   – shaoyang
> Blood stasis
> Qi deficiency
>   – Lung
>   – Spleen ± damp
>   – Kidney
>   – Heart
> Yang deficiency
>   – Spleen
>   – Kidney
>   – Heart
>   – Liver
> Blood deficiency
>   – Heart
>   – Liver
> Yin deficiency
>   – Lung
>   – Kidney
>   – Heart
>   – Spleen/Stomach
> Jing deficiency

Why do people feel tired?

There are two causes of tiredness according to Chinese medicine. Either patients have too little of one or more of the fundamental physiological substances–qi, blood, yin and yang, or the distribution of these substances is impaired. If the distribution of qi and blood is impaired, there must be a pathogen or a pathological

---

1 Practical Dictionary of Chinese Medicine (1998) – 'vacuity taxation'

accumulation of some sort blocking their movement. Pathogens can be external and lingering, or generated internally. The response to, and containment of, a persistent external pathogen consumes a large amount of zheng qi. In practice, a combination of insufficient qi, blood, yin or yang and some sort of pathological obstruction, such as heat, damp, phlegm, qi or blood stasis, are commonly seen.

Differentiating types of tiredness

There are certain clues that can help identify the nature of the tiredness. One of the most important is the response of the tiredness to rest. Tiredness that is worse after, or at least no better for, rest or prolonged inactivity, indicates a excess pattern. During rest, qi and blood circulation slows and yin pathogens congeal further. Their presence blocks the distribution of qi and blood. Patients with an excess type of tiredness feel better with activity, as stimulating circulation and the increasing heart rate can shift accumulations and activate qi and blood.

Tiredness that is alleviated by sleep or rest is usually of a deficient type, as rest enables the body to replenish some of the deficit. Low reserves of energy are easily spent in activity however, and patients will feel worse with exertion.

Tiredness following eating points to Spleen deficiency or damp. Tiredness with an emotional component points to Liver or Spleen qi constraint. Tiredness aggravated by cold weather indicates deficiency of the Kidneys. Other key points are noted in Box 18.2, p.836.

The clinical approach

The patient's expectations of energy should be clearly defined, and a comparison made between current and previous energy levels. Examination of sleep and work habits, diet and medications can be revealing. It is not uncommon for patients to report adequate sleep, but on questioning admit to sleep disturbances. Partners can be helpful regarding sleeping habits. Work history should include hours worked, stress levels, work relationships, deadlines and travel. The type and frequency of extracurricular activities can be influential.

Self medication with prescription, illicit and other drugs is an important and often overlooked cause of chronic tiredness. Certain pharmaceutical medications have a recognized effect on energy levels (Box 18.3, p.839). Alcohol, nicotine and stimulants are widely used and can contribute significantly to chronic tiredness.

Detailed assessment of the diet in terms of nutritional quality, balance of food groups and size and regularity of meals is essential.

Precipitating factors and history should be carefully explored. Relevant precipitating factors to be considered include pregnancy, childbirth, breast feeding and the postpartum period, lack of sleep due to disturbance by small children, recent surgery or infection, chronic pain, bereavement, trauma or change in life situation such as divorce or retirement, and travel.

PATHOLOGY

Each pattern in this chapter is discussed as a discrete entity, but reality is never as neat as a text book, and in practice patients often have multiple overlapping patterns. For example, qi and blood deficiency frequently occurs together, as does

BOX 18.2 KEY DIAGNOSTIC POINTS

Tiredness worse
- with prolonged immobility, sleeping – excess
- in the morning – excess
- in the evening, after work – deficiency
- after bowel movement – Spleen qi deficiency
- after sex – Kidney deficiency
- with emotional upset and stress – Liver qi constraint, blood stasis
- after eating – Spleen deficiency, damp
- with exposure to cold and cold weather – Kidney deficiency
- following prolonged use of the eyes or staring at a computer screen – Liver yin or blood deficiency

Tiredness improves
- with rest – deficiency patterns
- with exercise – qi constraint, phlegm damp

Worse in the morning then better during the day, then worse again in the afternoon
- Liver qi constraint, phlegm damp and Spleen deficiency

Accompanying features
- foggy head – phlegm damp, phlegm heat
- dizziness – blood deficiency, phlegm damp, shaoyang syndrome
- aching muscles – damp
- chronic pain – blood stasis
- sleep disturbance – blood or yin deficiency, lingering pathogens, Lung deficiency (with asthma or cough), Kidney deficiency (with nocturia), Liver blood deficiency (calf cramps)
- weakness in the limbs, slumping posture – qi deficiency
- minor tremor, spasms – blood or yin deficiency
- reflux and heartburn – Liver qi constraint, Spleen damp, residual pathogen in the qi level, phlegm heat
- constipation and dry stools – blood and yin deficiency
- constipation with lack of peristalsis – qi constraint

Spleen deficiency, damp and phlegm. Yin deficiency is often complicated by qi and yang deficiency, and multiple organ system pathologies are common, such as Spleen deficiency, Liver qi constraint and heat (see the Primary Pathological Triad, see p.780). The most common combined patterns are discussed in this text.

ETIOLOGY
Lingering pathogens
Persistent fatigue commonly occurs in the aftermath of a poorly managed acute febrile illness or immunization. The pathogen responsible for the initial episode may not have been completely cleared, or it may have damaged qi and/or yin, or congealed fluids into phlegm heat or damp heat. The probability of developing a persistent problem is greater among those who ignored the illness, or were treated inappropriately during the acute phase. Lingering pathogens are more likely to oc-

cur in those who neglect to rest properly during the acute phase, and thus weaken the defensive response. Improper use of purgation or emesis when the pathogen is on the surface can cause heat to be trapped in the qi level, as will diaphoresis when the pathogen is already beyond the surface. Antibiotics given for a febrile illness cool the heat but do not disperse the pathogen. Their bitter coldness can weaken the Spleen, cause diarrhea and thus act in a similar fashion to an inappropriate purge. For more on lingering pathogens, see Chapter 11, p.500.

Emotional factors

Emotional stress is an important cause of disruption to the Liver, Spleen and qi dynamic. The Liver is affected by anger, frustration and repressed emotion, while worry, obsessive thinking and prolonged concentration, in combination with a sedentary lifestyle and poor diet, weaken the Spleen. Any of these emotional factors, if prolonged or extreme, may disrupt the relationship between the Liver and Spleen. Failure of the Liver to evenly distribute qi causes tiredness that fluctuates with the emotional state and activity levels. Persistent qi constraint will eventually weaken the Spleen and disrupt qi and blood production. Spleen deficiency resulting from repeated Liver invasion can lead to damp that blocks qi and blood flow. Chronic Liver qi constraint contributes to blood stasis and phlegm that can compound tiredness. Heat generated by the constraint can damage yin.

Prolonged worry, grief and sadness can deplete Lung and Spleen qi, and diminish qi and blood production. The weakened Spleen can produce damp, further impeding the distribution of qi and blood.

A sudden or severe shock can sever the connection between the Heart and Kidneys, drain them of vitality and damage yang qi and yin.

Diet and medications

Inadequacies or irregularities in diet and digestion are important components of persistent tiredness. If the diet is lacking in essential nutrients, or if the food ingested is not being processed efficiently, qi and blood production will suffer.

Poor or erratic protein intake, restrictive or fad diets, or excessive intake of poor quality 'fast foods' lead to relative malnutrition, weaken the Spleen and reduce qi and blood production. Prolonged starvation or digestive insult, such as occurs in patients with a history of anorexia nervosa and bulimia, seriously damage Spleen yang qi. Slimming aids that suppress the appetite have a similar Spleen damaging potential. Some drugs weaken the Spleen and deplete Spleen qi and yang or create damp. These include heat clearing herbs, purgative laxatives, antibiotics and hypoglycemic agents. A wide range of common medications can cause tiredness (Box 18.3, p.839).

Excessive intake of food and alcohol in general, or a diet overly rich in heating or supplementing foods like meat and fat, can lead to dampness, heat and phlegm. Food allergy, lactose intolerance and coeliac disease are often unrecognized, especially when mild or subclinical, and can be important factors in chronic tiredness.

Overwork, exhaustion

Overwork, working excessively long hours or laboring to the point of exhaustion depletes Spleen and Kidney yang qi. Excessive energy expenditure relative to the amount of food consumed, depletes qi and jing. This is seen in athletes, who may be considered physically fit, but are often chronically tired and vulnerable to frequent pathogenic invasion.

Sleep cycle

Insufficient sleep, or a sleep cycle that is out of synchrony with the internal rhythms of the individual, are important factors contributing to tiredness. Sleeping too much or at irregular times can lead to qi stagnation, while insufficient sleep or continually 'burning the midnight oil' depletes yin and blood. This is often seen in people who do shift work and in air crew who frequently cross time zones.

Constitutional factors

A tendency to develop patterns that predispose to tiredness can be inherited. Lung, Spleen and Kidney deficiency, as well as a tendency to phlegm and qi constraint can run in families. Respiratory weakness, asthma, digestive weakness and weight problems from an early age, as well as developmental problems and persistent bed wetting may hint at weakness of yuan qi or at difficulties in acquiring or producing adequate qi.

Qi deficiency

Qi deficiency is a the result of poor production or excessive expenditure of qi. Dysfunction or weakness in either the Lungs or Spleen are major causes of qi deficiency, but weakness of other organ systems, and excessive demand for or expenditure of qi, will place a burden on the Lungs and Spleen, gradually weakening them, reducing qi production, and so on in a vicious circle. An inappropriate or poor quality diet is a significant contributor to qi deficiency.

Blood deficiency, pregnancy and childbirth

Blood deficiency is a major cause of chronic tiredness and usually derives from poor nutrition, insufficient production of blood from Spleen deficiency or inadequate replacement of blood following hemorrhage or pregnancy. This is a common pattern of chronic tiredness in mothers who return to work too soon, or who are unable to rest adequately to replenish the blood used to nurture the baby, or who breast feed for too long.

Yin deficiency

Yin is damaged by overwork, insufficient sleep, febrile disease and pathogenic heat, insufficient hydration, drug use and ageing. Drugs that are warm or dispersing in nature, such as amphetamines, cocaine and steroids, plunder the yin. Cannabis and ecstasy can damage yin when used frequently or in large quantities. Improper use of hot yang supplementing substances and herbs to increase energy levels (a common practice in these patients), such as red ginseng and deer horn, can deplete yin.

Yang deficiency

Yang deficiency is the product of a natural decline of yang by ageing, a cold na-

TIREDNESS 839

BOX 18.3 BIOMEDICAL CONDITIONS WHERE TIREDNESS IS A MAJOR COMPONENT

The subjective experience of tiredness can be a part of almost any disease process, however there are a variety of illnesses, imbalances and compulsions in which tiredness is a major complaint.

Endocrine
- thyroid dysfunction
- diabetes
- adrenal
  - Addison's disease
  - Cushing's syndrome
- hyperparathyroidism
- changing hormone levels
  - menopause
  - puberty
  - pregnancy

Cardiovascular
- cardiomyopathy
- arrhythmias
- congestive cardiac failure
- anemia

Neuromuscular
- Parkinson's disease
- multiple sclerosis

- myasthenia gravis
- post head injury

Drugs
- alcohol and nicotine
- amphetamines
- antibiotics
- anticonvulsants
- antidepressants
- antihistamines
- antihypertensives, beta blockers
- steroids
- hormones
  - oral contraceptives
  - hormone replacement therapy
- digoxin
- sedatives and hypnotics

Other
- depression, anxiety,

bereavement
- chronic fatigue synd.
- fibromyalgia
- malignancy, leukemia, lymphoma
- chronic infection
  - Glandular fever
  - HIV
  - Lyme disease
  - cryptosporidum
  - hepatitis
- malnutrition, obesity
- autoimmune disease
  - Lupus
  - Behçets disease
- sleep disorders
  - sleep apnea
  - myoclonus
  - shift work
  - sleepwalking,
  - asthma, orthopnea
  - reflux (GERD)

---

tured or insufficient diet, exhaustion of the yang through overwork, or depletion of yang by exposure to cold.

Blood stasis

Tiredness of a blood stasis type is often associated with chronic pain, poor cardiac function or depression. The blood stasis may be acute or chronic. Acute blood stasis can follow trauma, hemorrhage or surgery, while chronic patterns develop as a consequence of other prolonged pathology. Cold and yang deficiency cause blood stasis by 'freezing and constricting' the vessels and slowing circulation of qi and blood. Heat and yin deficiency cause stasis by 'evaporating' blood and increasing its viscosity and stickiness. Chronic Liver qi constraint or qi deficiency fail to lead and propel the blood.

Figure 18.1 Common patterns of tiredness

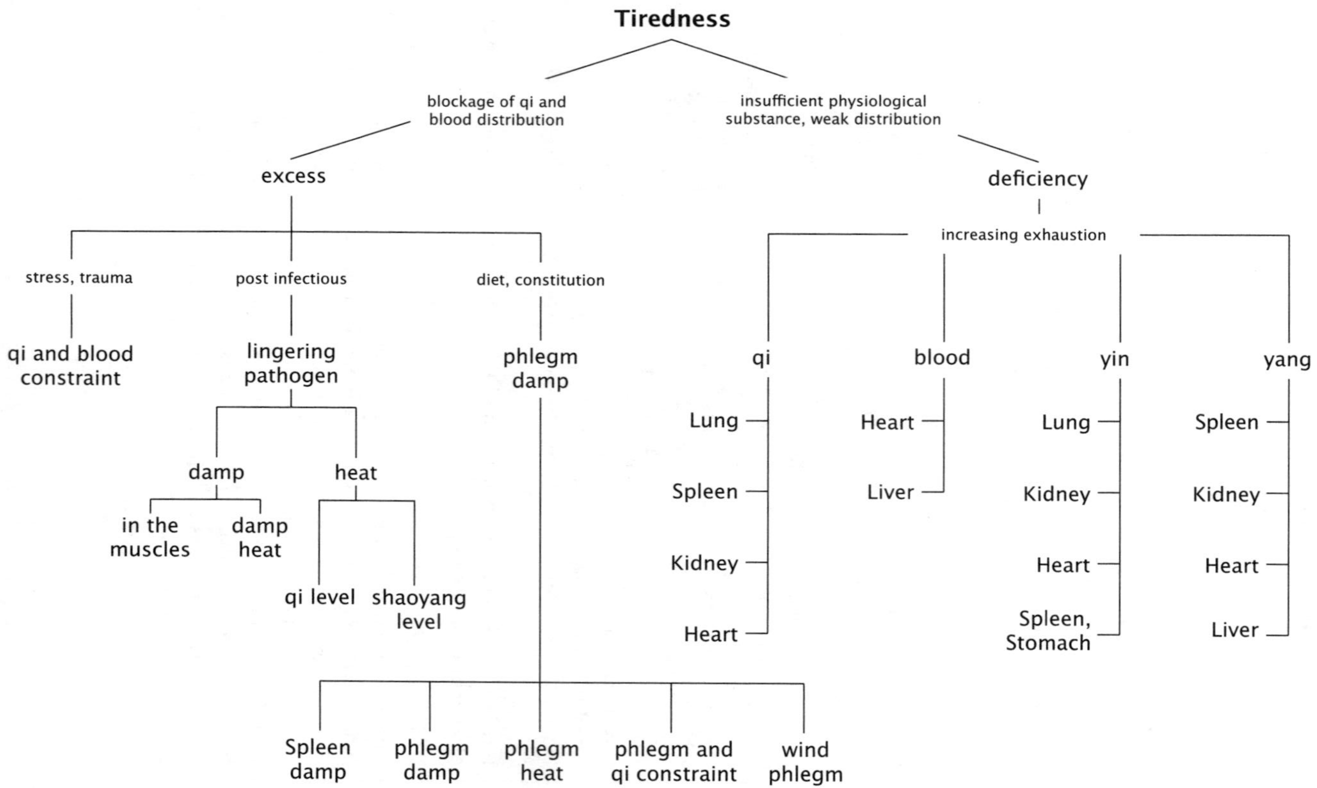

肝
气
郁
滞

18.1 LIVER QI CONSTRAINT

Liver qi constraint and its complications (see Fig. 9.1 p.411) are a common cause of tiredness and ennui. The pathology of Liver qi constraint is characterized by irregular distribution of qi and blood. The clinical features of qi constraint vary depending on the mood and activity level of the patient. Qi flows freely, with alleviation of symptoms, when the patient is emotionally relaxed or is physically moving the qi with exercise. Qi slows and gets stuck when the patient is upset or inactive.

Clinical features
- Tiredness, lack of motivation, feeling that one 'can't be bothered' or is 'flat'. Periods of feeling well are interspersed with periods of tiredness that coincide with increasing stress levels or emotional turmoil. Patients are tired, irritable and grumpy, and complain of feeling stuck and fed up. They find it hard to get started in the morning and are habitually late.
- Tiredness is worse in the morning, following periods of prolonged inactivity, before a menstrual period, and varies with the emotional state. The tiredness is alleviated as the days goes on, after exercise and when the patient is enjoying themselves or is distracted in some way.
- muscle stiffness, tightness and pain in the neck, shoulders, mid scapular and mid thoracic region; tension headaches
- constipation, or alternating constipation and diarrhea
- indigestion, heartburn, abdominal distension, belching, flatulence
- sleep disturbance; typically waking between 1–3am
- shallow breathing; frequent sighing; sense of tightness in the chest

T unremarkable or mauve, or with pale edges and a thin coat
P wiry and fine

Treatment Principle
Dredge the Liver, regulate qi and relieve qi constraint
Harmonize the middle burner and correct the qi dynamic

Prescription

XIAO YAO SAN 逍遥散
Rambling Powder

This prescription is designed for Liver qi constraint complicated by blood deficiency. The tiredness has features of both excess and deficiency. Patients are better for some activity, but too much exhausts them; fatigue levels are worse both before and after menstruation.

chai hu (Bupleuri Radix) 柴胡 9–12g
dang gui (Angelicae sinensis Radix) 当归 9–12g
bai shao (Paeoniae Radix alba) 白芍 12–18g
bai zhu (Atractylodis macrocephalae Rhizoma) 白术 9–12g
fu ling (Poria) 茯苓 12–15g
zhi gan cao (Glycyrrhizae Radix preparata) 炙甘草 3–6g

wei jiang (Zingiberis Rhizoma preparata) 煨姜 3–6g
bo he (Mentha haplocalycis Herba) 薄荷 3–6g
Method: Decoction. **Bo he** is added a few minutes before the end of cooking. **Chai hu** dredges the Liver and regulates qi; **dang gui** and **bai shao** nourish Liver blood and soften the Liver; **bai zhu** and **fu ling** strengthen the Spleen and dry damp; **zhi gan cao** supplements qi and, with **bai shao**, eases muscle spasms; **wei jiang** warms and harmonizes the Stomach; **bo he** assists **chai hu** in moving Liver qi. (Source: *He Ji Ju Fang*)

CHAI HU SHU GAN SAN 柴胡疏肝散
Bupleurum Powder to Dredge the Liver

This prescription is selected when qi constraint is uncomplicated by deficiency.
chai hu (Bupleuri Radix) 柴胡 9–12g
bai shao (Paeoniae Radix alba) 白芍 12–18g
zhi shi (Fructus Immaturus Citri Aurantii) 枳实 9–12g
xiang fu (Cyperi Rhizoma) 香附 9–12g
chuan xiong (Chuanxiong Rhizoma) 川芎 6–9g
chen pi (Citri reticulatae Pericarpium) 陈皮 6–9g
zhi gan cao (Glycyrrhizae Radix preparata) 炙甘草 3–6g
Method: Decoction. **Chai hu** dredges the Liver and regulates qi; **bai shao** softens the Liver, nourishes yin and blood and assists **chai hu** in regulating qi; **zhi shi**, **chen pi** and **xiang fu** regulate qi and correct the qi dynamic; **chuan xiong** moves qi and activates blood; **zhi gan cao** strengthens the Spleen and, with **bai shao**, alleviates cramping and spasmodic pain. (Source: *Jin Yue Quan Shu*)

Modifications (to both prescriptions, where not already included)

- With depression, add **he huan pi** (Albizziae Cortex) 合欢皮 12–15g, **yu jin** (Curcumae Radix) 郁金 9–12g and **ye jiao teng** (Polygoni multiflori Caulis) 夜交藤 18–30g.
- With tightness in the chest or difficulty getting a full breath, add **gua lou** (Trichosanthis Fructus) 栝楼 15–24g.
- With marked blood deficiency, add **shu di** (Rehmanniae Radix preparata) 熟地 9–15g.
- With heat and red edges on the tongue, add **shan zhi zi** (Gardeniae Fructus) 山栀子 6–9g and **mu dan pi** (Moutan Cortex) 牡丹皮 6–9g.
- With muscle spasm and pain, increase the dose of **bai shao** to 30g and the dose of **zhi gan cao** to 9g, or add two or three of the following herbs: **chuan lian zi** (Toosendan Fructus) 川楝子 9–12g, **yu jin** (Curcumae Radix) 郁金 9–12g, **mu xiang** (Aucklandiae Radix) 木香 6–9g and **yan hu suo** (Corydalis Rhizoma) 延胡索 9–12g or **fo shou** (Citri sarcodactylis Fructus) 佛手 9–12g.
- With constipation, add **hou po** (Magnoliae officinalis Cortex) 厚朴 9–12g, **bing lang** (Arecae Semen) 槟榔 6–9g and **zhi shi** (Aurantii Fructus immaturus) 枳实 6–9g.
- With nausea and belching, add **zhu ru** (Bambusae Caulis in taeniam) 竹茹 6–9g and **zhi ban xia** (Pinelliae Rhizoma preparatum) 制半夏 6–9g.
- With heartburn and acid reflux, add **huang lian** (Coptidis Rhizoma) 黄连 3–6g and **wu zhu yu** (Evodiae Fructus) 吴茱萸 2–3g.
- With marked abdominal distension, add **hou po** (Magnoliae officinalis Cor-

tex) 厚朴 9–12g.

- With flatulence, add **hou po** (Magnoliae officinalis Cortex) 厚朴 9–12g, **mu xiang** (Aucklandiae Radix) 木香 9–12g and **sha ren** (Amomi Fructus) 砂仁 3–6g.
- With phlegm masses or nodules in the neck, add **zhe bei mu** (Fritillariae thunbergii Bulbus) 浙贝母 9–12g and **xuan shen** (Scrophulariae Radix) 玄参 12–15g.

Variations and additional prescriptions
With phlegm
Qi constraint and phlegm frequently coexist. The constrained movement of qi leads to a slowing and congealing of fluids into phlegm, which obstruct qi flow, and so on in a vicious cycle. When qi and phlegm accumulation occur together they often get stuck in regions governed by the Liver system, such as the throat, where swelling or a sensation of obstruction may occur. The treatment is to mobilize qi and direct it downwards, and transform phlegm with BAN XIA HOU PO TANG (Pinellia and Magnolia Bark Decoction 半夏厚朴汤, p.858).

The primary pathological triad (PPT)
Qi constraint may be complicated by numerous pathologies, but a consistent theme is the triad of qi constraint, Spleen qi deficiency and heat, typically heat from constrained qi or damp heat. This is the Primary Pathological Triad (see p.780), so called due to the frequency with which it appears and its importance in many chronic patterns of illness. The PPT can be seen at work in conditions as diverse as gastrointestinal, inflammatory and autoimmune disorders, but fatigue and tiredness are common factors. There are a variety of solutions, depending on the specific balance of pathology and any other complications that may be present, however, one formula stands out in addressing equally all aspects of the triad. This is XIAO CHAI HU TANG (Minor Bupleurum Decoction 小柴胡汤, p.863).

Prepared medicines
Concentrated powder
Xiao Yao San (Bupleurum & Tangkuei Formula)
Chai Hu Shu Gan San (Bupleurum & Cyperus Combination)
Jia Wei Xiao Yao San (Bupleurum & Peony Formula)
   – with constrained heat

Pills
Xiao Yao Wan (Free and Easy Wanderer Teapills, Hsiao Yao Wan)
Chai Hu Shu Gan Wan (Bupleurum Soothe Liver Teapills)
Jia Wei Xiao Yao Wan (Free and Easy Wanderer Plus Teapills, Dan Zhi Xiao Yao Wan)

Acupuncture (select from)
Liv.13 (zhangmen –) ....alarm point of the Spleen, harmonizes the Liver and Spleen
Liv.14 (qimen –) ....alarm point of the Liver, regulates Liver qi and alleviates qi constraint

PC.6 (neiguan –)................connecting point of the Pericardium, opens up qi flow through the chest, dredges the Liver and rectifies qi

Liv.3 (taichong –)..............source point of the Liver, dredges the Liver and regulates qi and blood

LI.4 (hegu –).....................with Liv.3 (taichong), constitutes the 'four gates'; together they mobilize qi and blood, calm the shen, and relieve mental cloudiness

St.36 (zusanli +) ....sea point of the Stomach, supplements and regulates qi, and corrects the qi dynamic

SJ.5 (waiguan)...................these points stimulate qi flow and settle the hun;
GB.39 (xuanzhong)   together they alleviate qi constraint and help with the sleep disturbance that is typical of this pattern

Bl.18 (ganshu –)................transport point of the Liver, dredges the Liver and regulates qi, activates blood

• with blood deficiency, add Sp.6 (sanyinjiao +) and Bl.20 (pishu +)
• with heat, add Liv.2 (xingjian –)
• with phlegm, add St.40 (fenglong –) and PC.5 (jianshi –)
• with constipation, add St.25 (tianshu –)
• with headaches, add GB.20 (fenglong)
• Ear points: liver, zero point, sympathetic, shenmen

Clinical notes

• Liver qi constraint and its complications are common causes of tiredness, listlessness and apathy. The tiredness of qi constraint responds reliably well to treatment with herbs and acupuncture, but for long term management, changes to activity levels and contributing life habits are the best tool. In situations where qi is continually being constrained (stressful or disruptive home or work environments), exercise and stress reduction strategies are still the primary tool, but regular acupuncture over a long period can help retrain the body to respond to noxious stimuli in a more harmonious manner.
• Exercise is an essential component of treatment (see p.103).
• Hot spot therapy is helpful, p.923.
• A qi mobilizing diet can be helpful. See Clinical Handbook, Vol.2, p.878.

18.2 DAMP

1. Encumbering the Spleen/Stomach
2. In the muscles
3. Damp heat

湿
困
脾
胃

18.2.1 DAMP ENCUMBERING THE SPLEEN AND STOMACH

Damp encumbering the Spleen and Stomach is an excess pattern, most commonly the result of overconsumption of foods that introduce damp directly into the body–dairy products, sweets, rich or greasy foods, or raw uncooked food. It can also be caused by prolonged exposure to a damp environment or humid climate and poor Spleen function that produces damp as a by–product of inefficient digestion.

The damp settles over the Spleen like a thick fog, affecting digestion, the muscles and ability to concentrate. The damp also blocks the qi dynamic, impeding the distribution of qi and blood to the muscles and limbs.

Clinical features

• Fatigue, lethargy, heaviness of the body and limbs as if 'walking through treacle'; frequent desire to lie down and sleep, after which the patient feels worse. Tiredness is worse in the morning and after prolonged inactivity, and slightly better with moderate physical activity.
• poor concentration, heavy or foggy head
• abdominal distension and chest oppression
• nausea or vomiting, often in the morning
• loss of appetite, acid reflux, belching
• loose stools or diarrhea
• thrush or vaginal discharge
T thick, greasy, white coat, maybe pale, swollen or flabby tongue body
P slippery, soggy, moderate

Treatment principle

Dry and transform damp
Strengthen the Spleen and stimulate the qi dynamic

Prescription

PING WEI SAN 平胃散
Calm the Stomach Powder

cang zhu (Atractylodis Rhizoma) 苍术 12–15g
hou po (Magnoliae officinalis Cortex) 厚朴 9–12g
chen pi (Citri reticulatae Pericarpium) 陈皮 9–12g
gan cao (Glycyrrhizae Radix) 甘草 3–6g
sheng jiang (Zingiberis Rhizoma recens) 生姜 6–9g
da zao (Jujubae Fructus) 大枣 .... 4 fruit

Method: Grind the herbs into powder and take 9 grams as a draft on an empty stomach 2–3 times daily. May also be decocted. **Cang zhu** parches damp and liberates the Spleen, allowing it to function correctly; **hou po** directs qi downward, transforms damp and alleviates distension; **chen pi** transforms damp, rectifies middle burner qi and corrects the qi dynamic; **gan cao** strengthens the Spleen and harmonizes the Stomach; **sheng jiang** and **da zao** harmonize the Spleen and Stomach. (Source: *He Ji Ju Fang*)

Modifications

- With foggy head, add **shi chang pu** (Acori tatarinowii Rhizoma) 石菖蒲 6–9g and **yuan zhi** (Polygalae Radix) 远志 6–9g.
- With Spleen deficiency, reduce the dose of **cang zhu** by half, and add **chao bai zhu** (stir fried Atractylodes macrocephalae Rhizoma) 炒白术 9–12g, **chao shan yao** (stir fried Dioscoreae Rhizoma) 炒山药 12–15g and **zhi huang qi** (honey fried Astragali Radix) 炙黄芪 18–30g. See also p.870.
- With cold, add **rou gui** (Cinnamomi Cortex) 肉桂 3g and **gan jiang** (Zingiberis Rhizoma) 干姜 6–9g.

Prepared medicines

Concentrated powder

Ping Wei San (Magnolia & Ginger Formula)

Pills

Ping Wei San (Calm Stomach Teapills, Tabellae Pingwei)
Xiang Sha Yang Wei Wan (Appetite and Digestion Pill, Hsiang Sha Yang Wei Pien) – with qi stagnation

Acupuncture (select from)

Ren.12 (zhongwan –) ....alarm point of the Stomach, strengthens the Spleen and Stomach and supplements qi to transform damp

Lu.7 (lieque –)....................connecting point of the Lungs, directs Lung qi downwards to maintain the water passages and an outlet for the damp

Sp.3 (taibai).......................source and connecting points of the Spleen and
St.40 (fenglong –)   Stomach, they transform damp and supplement the Spleen, and have a special effect on heaviness and lethargy

Sp.9 (yinlingquan –)...........sea point of the Spleen, promotes urination and clears damp through the lower burner

Sp.6 (sanyinjiao –)..............strengthens the Spleen and Kidneys and transforms damp

Sp.5 (shangqiu –) ....river point of the Spleen, strengthens the Spleen and transforms damp

Bl.20 (pishu) ....transport point of the Spleen, supplements Spleen qi to promote transformation damp

- with muscle aches, add Sp.21 (dabao)
- with somnolence, add Kid.6 (zhaohai) and Bl.62 (shenmai)
- with foggy head, add St.8 (touwei), GB.20 (fengchi) and Bl.62 (shenmai)
- with Spleen deficiency, add St.36 (zusanli +)
- with edema, add St.28 (shuidao –) and Sp.6 (sanyinjiao)

- with cold, apply moxa cones to Bl.20 (pishu ▲) and Bl.21 (weishu ▲)
- Ear points: spleen, stomach, zero point, adrenal, endocrine

Clinical notes
- Damp encumbering the Spleen may be diagnosed as food allergy or intolerance, 'candida', irritable bowel syndrome, insulin resistance or the early stage of type 2 diabetes mellitus, coeliac disease or depression.
- This is a chronic pattern, and can be slow to resolve. In addition to dietary modification, damp patterns usually require substantial and persistent treatment for satisfactory results.
- A damp drying diet is essential. See Clinical Handbook, Vol.2, p.880.
- Moderate exercise is an important component of treatment.

湿 18.2.2 DAMP IN THE MUSCLES
在
肌
肉

Damp can accumulate in the muscles as a residual pathogen following an unresolved external pathogenic invasion. A lingering pathogen is more likely to occur when a patient with a pre–existing or constitutional tendency to qi deficiency is afflicted by an external pathogen, has an immunization, or they improperly use antibiotics in the course of treating an acute febrile illness.

The location of the initial pathogen is the qi level, and because the qi level is aligned with the skin, subcutaneous tissues and muscles, the viscous obstructing damp congeals in the muscle layer. This has the effect of obstructing qi and blood flow causing muscle aches, the most prominent feature of this pattern after the debilitating tiredness.

Clinical features
- Tiredness, lassitude, lethargy, heaviness in the head and limbs, foggy head, all of which are worse mid afternoon.
- muscle aches; the large proximal muscles of the limbs and buttocks are usually affected; the muscles may feel boggy or puffy when palpated
- loss of appetite; nausea
- loose stools or diarrhea
- sallow complexion
- no thirst
- chest oppression
- may be night sweats
- swollen cervical lymph nodes

T thick, greasy, white coat
P soggy, moderate or wiry

Treatment principle
Disperse and vent damp from the muscles with fragrant herbs
Promote urination to drain damp
Activate the qi dynamic

Prescription

HUO PO XIA LING TANG 藿朴夏苓汤
Agastache, Magnolia Bark, Pinellia and Poria Decoction

huo xiang (Pogostemonis/Agastaches Herba) 藿香 9–12g
zhi ban xia (Pinelliae Rhizoma preparata) 制半夏 9–12g
fu ling (Poria) 茯苓 9–12g
xing ren (Pruni Semen) 杏仁 9–12g
dan dou chi (Sojae Semen preparatum) 淡豆豉 9–12g
yi ren (Coicis Semen) 苡仁 12–15g
ze xie (Alismatis Rhizoma) 泽泻 6–9g
zhu ling (Polyporus) 猪苓 6–9g
bai dou kou (Amomi Fructus rotundus) 白豆蔻 3–6g
hou po (Magnoliae officinalis Cortex) 厚朴 3–6g
Method: Decoction. **Huo xiang** and **bai dou kou** transform and disperse damp from the muscles and qi level; **fu ling**, **ze xie** and **zhu ling** promote urination to leach out damp; **yi ren** leaches damp from the lower burner and promotes urination; **zhi ban xia** and **hou po** downbear counterflow Stomach qi and alleviate nausea and distension; **xing ren** directs Lung qi downwards, facilitating normal function of the 'upper source of water' to promote urination and provide an outlet for the damp; **dan dou chi** vents pathogens from the qi level. (Source: *Yi Yuan*)

Modifications
- With marked muscle aches and foggy head, add **shi chang pu** (Acori tatarowii Rhizoma) 石菖蒲 6–9g and **yuan zhi** (Polygalae Radix) 远志 6–9g.
- With residual exterior symptoms, add **zi su ye** (Perillae Folium) 紫苏叶 6–9g.

Prepared medicines
Concentrated powder
Xing Jun San 行军散 (Marching Powder, Five Pagodas Brand)
– a small dose (¼–½ teaspoon) several times daily will help to dry damp
Liu He Tang (Amomum Combination)

Pills
Huo Xiang Zheng Qi Pian (Huo Hsiang Cheng Chi Pien)

Acupuncture (select from)
Lu.7 (lieque –) .... connecting point of the Lungs, diffuses the Lungs and directs Lung qi downwards to vent pathogens and promote urination

SJ.6 (zhigou –) .... fire point of the triple burner, spreads the qi, disperses obstruction from the triple burner and keeps the exits open

Sp.9 (yinlingquan –) .... together these points promote urination to drain
Sp.5 (shangqiu –)   damp
Kid.7 (fuliu –) .... metal point of the Kidney, vents damp and promotes urination

Sp.21 (dabao) .... alleviates muscles aches
- with nausea, add PC.6 (neiguan)

- with diarrhea, add St.25 (tianshu) and St.37 (shangjuxu)
- Ear points: spleen, stomach, zero point, lung, shenmen, sympathetic

Clinical notes

- Damp in the muscles may be diagnosed as post viral syndrome, chronic fatigue syndrome, fibromyalgia rheumatica, glandular fever or cytomegalovirus.
- Clearing damp from the muscles can be a slow process, depending on duration of the pattern and the depth of the fatigue. It may take several weeks before any effects are noted, and treatment should continue until the myalgia has cleared. Following resolution of the myalgia, a more Spleen strengthening strategy can be adopted to prevent recurrence.
- A damp drying diet is recommended. See Clinical Handbook, Vol.2, p.880.

湿
热
疲
倦

18.2.3 DAMP HEAT

The damp heat in this pattern is usually associated with a lingering pathogen. Patients with a lingering damp heat pattern will recall an acute illness with nausea, vomiting and/or diarrhea. The sticky nature of damp heat inhibits complete clearance from the body and the pathogen lingers at a low level. The likelihood of such retention is increased by improper treatment during the acute phase, by not resting sufficiently during convalescence, or by a pre–existing Spleen deficiency.

Like the damp pattern preceding, the damp heat is in the qi level, and affects the muscles and gastrointestinal system. Damp heat also has an affinity with the Liver and Urinary Bladder, and may spill over into these systems.

Clinical features

- Tiredness, lassitude and heaviness in the head and limbs, worse mid afternoon
- muscle aches and weakness, especially large proximal muscles of the limbs and the buttocks
- low grade afternoon fever with a sticky sweat that does not break the fever; fever may alternate with chills if the Liver is involved
- night sweats
- chest oppression
- loss of appetite, nausea
- dull headache, heavy head
- foggy head, difficulty concentrating
- cloying or sticky sensation in the mouth
- dry mouth and throat with no thirst
- maybe diarrhea, painful urination or concentrated urine or yellow vaginal discharge and a tendency to thrush
- swollen lymph nodes

T thick, greasy, yellowish coat
P slippery, wiry, slightly rapid

Treatment principle

Clear and vent damp heat from the qi level
Promote urination and liberate the qi dynamic to drain damp

Prescription

SAN REN TANG 三仁汤
Three Nut Decoction

This prescription is selected when damp and heat are more or less equal, or the damp slightly more prominent than the heat.

xing ren (Pruni Semen) 杏仁...12–15g
bai dou kou (Amomi Fructus rotundus) 白豆蔻.....................................6–9g
yi ren (Coicis Semen) 苡仁..18–30g
zhi ban xia (Pinelliae Rhizoma preparata) 制半夏.................................9–12g
hou po (Magnoliae officinalis Cortex) 厚朴...6–9g
dan zhu ye (Lophatheri Herba) 淡竹叶..6–9g
hua shi (Talcum) 滑石...12–18g
tong cao (Tetrapanacis Medulla) 通草..3–6g

Method: Decoction. **Bai dou kou** is added towards the end of cooking. **Xing ren** diffuses the Lungs and directs Lung qi downwards, promotes urination and maintains an outlet for the damp heat; **bai dou kou** fragrantly transforms damp; **yi ren** promotes urination to drain damp heat; **zhi ban xia** and **hou po** downbear counterflow Stomach qi, and assist **xing ren** and **bai dou kou** in freeing up the qi dynamic; **dan zhu ye** vents pathogens from the qi level and promotes urination; **hua shi** and **tong cao** promote urination to drain damp and damp heat. (Source: *Wen Bing Tiao Bian*)

Modifications

- With marked nausea and vomiting, add **huo xiang** (Pogostemonis/Agastaches Herba) 藿香 12–15g, **pei lan** (Eupatorii Herba) 佩兰 9–12g and **shi chang pu** (Acori tatarinowii Rhizoma) 石菖蒲 6–9g.
- With alternating fever and chills, add **cao guo** (Tsaoko Fructus) 草果 6–9g and **qing hao** (Artemisiae annuae Herba) 青蒿 9–15g.
- With dysuria, add **pu gong ying** (Taraxaci Herba) 蒲公英 18–30g and **jin yin hua** (Lonicerae Flos) 金银花 15–30g.
- With a degree of yin damage (geographic tongue, dry lips, increasing thirst, delete **hou po** and **zhi ban xia**, and add **mai dong** (Ophiopogonis Radix) 麦冬 9–12g and **tian hua fen** (Trichosanthes Radix) 天花粉 30g.

Variations and additional prescriptions

With more heat

The more heat there is in a damp heat pattern, the more prominent the afternoon fever and more frequent the night sweats. Heat is also seen in concentrated urine, the yellow tongue coat and rapid slippery pulse. The treatment is to clear damp heat and correct the qi dynamic with a more cooling formula such as **LIAN PO YIN** (Coptis and Magnolia Bark Drink 连朴饮).

huang lian (Coptidis Rhizoma) 黄连 3–6g
hou po (Magnoliae officinalis Cortex) 厚朴...6–9g
shan zhi zi (Gardeniae Fructus) 山栀子 9–12g
dan dou chi (Sojae Semen preparatum) 淡豆豉 9–12g
shi chang pu (Acori tatarinowii Rhizoma) 石菖蒲 6–9g
zhi ban xia (Pinelliae Rhizoma preparatum) 制半夏 6–9g
lu gen (Phragmitis Rhizoma) 芦根 30–60g

Method: Decoction. **Huang lian** and **shan zhi zi** clear damp heat; their bitterness combines with the pungent warmth of **zhi ban xia** and the descending nature of **hou po** to correct the qi dynamic; **zhi ban xia** transforms damp, downbears counterflow Stomach qi and stops vomiting; **dan dou chi** and **shan zhi zi** clear and vent heat from the qi level and alleviate irritability; **shi chang pu** transforms damp; **lu gen** vents heat from the qi level and stops vomiting. (Source: *Huo Luan Lun*)

Prepared medicines
Concentrated powder
San Ren Tang (Triple Nut Combination)
Gan Lu Xiao Du Dan (Forsythia & Acorus Formula)
– with more heat
Xing Jun San 行军散 (Marching Powder, Five Pagodas Brand)
– a small dose (¼ – ½ teaspoon) several times daily will help to dry damp
Pills
Bi Xie Sheng Shi Wan (Subdue the Dampness Teapills)
Huo Xiang Zheng Qi Pian (Huo Hsiang Cheng Chi Pien)

Acupuncture (select from)
Lu.7 (lieque –)...................diffuses the Lungs and vents pathogens from the qi level

SJ.6 (zhigou –) ....fire point of the triple burner, rectifies qi flow through the triple burner and keeps pathways of elimination open

SI.4 (wangu –) ....source point of the Small Intestine, clears damp heat

LI.11 (quchi –)..................diffuses the Lungs and clears damp heat

Sp.9 (yinlingquan –)...........together these points promote urination to drain

Sp.5 (shangqiu –)   damp heat

Ren.5 (shimen –)...............alarm point of the triple burner, clears damp heat
* with damp heat in the Liver, add SJ.5 (waiguan –) and GB.41 (zulinqi –)
* with damp heat in the Urinary Bladder, add Ren.3 (zhongji –)
* with high fever, add Du.14 (dazhui –)
* with nausea, add PC.6 (neiguan)
* with diarrhea, add zhixie (N–CA–3) and Bl.25 (tianshu)
* with myalgia, add Sp.21 (dabao)
* Ear points: spleen, stomach, lung, zero point, shenmen, sympathetic

Clinical notes
* Damp heat tiredness may be diagnosed as a chronic infection, such as post viral syndrome, cytomegalovirus, glandular fever, cholangitis, enteric fever, pyelonephritis, hepatic or pelvic abscess or undulant fever.
* Clearing damp heat from the qi level can be a slow process, depending on duration of the pattern and the depth of the fatigue. It may take several weeks before any effects are noted, and treatment should continue until all symptoms have cleared. Following resolution of the fatigue, a more Spleen strengthening strategy can be adopted to prevent recurrence.
* A damp heat clearing diet is recommended. See Clinical Handbook, Vol.2, p.884.

18.3 PHLEGM

1. Phlegm damp
2. Phlegm heat
3. Phlegm and qi constraint
4. Wind phlegm

Phlegm is a dense pathogen, and significantly obstructs the distribution of qi and blood. Phlegm type tiredness is mostly a chronic problem, and may be constitutional, associated with the diet, or chronic Liver qi constraint. Occasionally, an acute febrile illness with a high fever can quickly congeal physiological fluids into phlegm heat, in which case the onset is more abrupt.

Prolonged phlegm will usually be complicated by Spleen qi deficiency and qi constraint.

Common features
- Phlegm tends to produce a variable tiredness. The tiredness increases as the phlegm congeals with inactivity, large volumes of food or phlegm producing foods. Tiredness improves as the phlegm is mobilized by exercise, reduced food intake, drying or pungent foods or a dry, high altitude or desert environment.
- Fatigue, lethargy, lassitude, heaviness in the body and limbs, increased desire to sleep or somnolence. After sleeping or inactivity the patient feels worse.
- Patients with phlegm patterns tend to feel 'weighed down' and may complain of heaviness of both spirit and body. They can be overweight, and often feel depressed, foggy–headed, unable to think clearly or concentrate. They may exhibit physical signs of phlegm, such as sinus congestion, productive cough, throat clearing or benign rubbery masses like subcutaneous lipomas, breast cysts or ganglia. They can suffer from relatively severe dizziness or vertigo, which is initiated or exacerbated by strong piercing odors like perfume or gasoline. Any gastrointestinal symptoms present, such as nausea or heartburn, are also aggravated by strong smells.

T swollen or flabby body, may or may not have a thick coat
P slippery

Specific features
Phlegm damp
- phlegm and damp accumulate in the middle burner and block the qi dynamic, disrupting gastrointestinal function and distribution of qi to the extremities
- anorexia or reduced appetite, loss of sense of taste
- epigastric and abdominal distension and fullness
- nausea or vomiting, often in the morning
- acid reflux, belching
- loose stools, or sluggish stools that are not dry and may have mucus
- somnolence

Phlegm heat
- In general, phlegm type tiredness is a chronic problem. It may, however, occur as a more acute condition, appearing in the aftermath of an acute febrile illness. The fever quickly congeals physiological fluids into phlegm heat. The initial illness is usually a qi level fever, affecting the Lungs, Stomach or both, but any high fever may be implicated.
- Fatigue and tiredness, but with insomnia or fitful sleep with much dreaming. Patients wake in the early hours of the morning, between 2–4am, unable to fall back to sleep.
- palpitations with anxiety and nervousness
- irritability and restlessness
- nausea, vomiting, belching, acid reflux, bitter taste in the mouth
- loss of appetite, appetite yet to return following a febrile illness
- dizziness and vertigo
- productive cough
- swollen, rubbery lymph nodes

T thick, greasy, yellow coat

Phlegm and qi constraint
- tiredness and fatigue have a clear emotional component
- sensation of a lump the throat ('plum pit qi')
- depression, sadness, obsessive thinking
- constant throat clearing, cough
- chest oppression

Wind phlegm
- Dizziness and vertigo which may be triggered by movement of the head or strong smells. The sensation is sometimes likened to being on a ship, or having the world spin around–even in bed, there may be 'bedspins'.
- headache or distending sensation in the head, also triggered by strong smells
- nausea and vomiting
- poor concentration, foggy head, 'head wrapped in a wet cloth'
- tinnitus; blurred vision

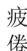
痰湿疲倦

18.3.1 PHLEGM DAMP

Treatment principle
Dry damp, transform phlegm
Strengthen the Spleen and harmonize the Stomach

Prescription

ER CHEN TANG 二陈汤
Two Aged [Herb] Decoction, modified

---

zhi ban xia (Pinelliae Rhizoma preparatum) 制半夏 9–15g
chen pi (Citri reticulatae Pericarpium) 陈皮 9–15g
fu ling (Poria) 茯苓 9–12g

zhi gan cao (Glycyrrhizae Radix preparata) 炙甘草 3–6g
sheng jiang (Zingiberis Rhizoma recens) 生姜 6–9g
chao bai zhu (stir fried Atractylodis macrocephalae Rhizoma) 炒白术 6–9g
Method: Grind the herbs into powder and take 12 grams as a draft on an empty stomach 2–3 times daily. May also be decocted. **Zhi ban xia** dries damp and transforms phlegm; **chen pi** dries damp, transforms phlegm and rectifies the qi dynamic; **fu ling** strengthens the Spleen and leaches damp out through the urine; **zhi gan cao** supplements qi and harmonizes the formula; **sheng jiang** assists the phlegm transformation of the main herbs; **chao bai zhu** strengthens the Spleen to transform phlegm damp. (Source: *He Ji Ju Fang*)

Modifications

- With cold, add **rou gui** (Cinnamomi Cortex) 肉桂 3g and **gan jiang** (Zingiberis Rhizoma) 干姜 6–9g.
- With a foggy–head, add **shi chang pu** (Acori tatarinowii Rhizoma) 石菖蒲 6–9g and **yuan zhi** (Polygalae Radix) 远志 6–9g.
- With daytime somnolence and insomnia at night, add **shi chang pu** (Acori tatarinowii Rhizoma) 石菖蒲 6–9g and **yuan zhi** (Polygalae Radix) 远志 6–9g.
- For epigastric and abdominal distension, add **cang zhu** (Atractylodis Rhizoma) 苍术 9–12g and **hou po** (Magnoliae officinalis Cortex) 厚朴 9–12g.
- With cough or nasal congestion with thin watery sputum, add **gan jiang** (Zingiberis Rhizoma) 干姜 6–9g and **xi xin** (Asari Herba) 细辛 3–6g.
- With heat, add **quan gua lou** (Trichosanthis Fructus) 全栝楼 18–24g, **zhu ru** (Bambusae Caulis in taeniam) 竹茹 6–9g and **huang qin** (Scutellariae Radix) 黄芩 6–9g.

Variations and additional prescriptions
With Spleen deficiency
Phlegm damp can be the product of Spleen qi deficiency, or its presence can disrupt Spleen function, and lead to Spleen qi deficiency. The nature of the tiredness reflects the balance between deficiency and excess. When the phlegm damp is more prominent, the patient feels worse with inactivity. When the deficiency aspects are more prominent, the patient feels worse at the end of the day. However, in patterns with both deficiency and excess aspects, activity improves energy to a certain extent, but the more activity the patient does, the more tired he or she feels. The treatment is to strengthen the Spleen and supplement qi while drying and transforming phlegm damp and moving qi with XIANG SHA LIU JUN ZI TANG (Six Gentlemen Decoction with Aucklandia and Amomum 香砂六君子汤)

ren shen (Ginseng Radix) 人参 6–9g
chao bai zhu (stir fried Atractylodis macrocephalae Rhizoma) 炒白术 12–15g
fu ling (Poria) 茯苓 12–15g
zhi ban xia (Pinelliae Rhizoma preparatum) 制半夏 9–12g
chen pi (Citri reticulatae Pericarpium) 陈皮 9–12g
sha ren (Fructus Amomi) 砂仁 6–9g
mu xiang (Aucklandiae Radix) 木香 6–9g
zhi gan cao (Glycyrrhizae Radix preparata) 炙甘草 3–6g
Method: Decoction. **Sha ren** is added towards the end of cooking time. **Ren shen** strengthens the Spleen and supplements qi; **chao bai zhu** strengthens the Spleen, supplements qi and dries damp;

fu ling strengthens the Spleen and leaches out damp through the urine; **zhi ban xia** transforms phlegm damp; **chen pi** transforms phlegm, regulates middle burner qi and corrects the qi dynamic; **zhi gan cao** strengthens the Spleen and harmonizes the Stomach; **sha ren** and **mu xiang** regulate qi and correct the qi dynamic. (Source: *Yi Fang Ji Jie*)

Prepared medicines
Concentrated powder
Er Chen Tang (Citrus & Pinellia Combination)
Xiang Sha Liu Jun Zi Tang (Vladmiria & Amomum Combination)
Pills
Er Chen Wan (Pinellia Pachyma Pills, Erh Chen Wan)
Xiang Sha Liu Jun Zi Wan (Aplotaxis–Ammomum Pills, Six Gentlemen Tea Pills)
Xiang Sha Yang Wei Wan (Appetite and Digestion Pill, Hsiang Sha Yang Wei Pien)
   – with phlegm damp and qi stagnation

Acupuncture (select from)
Ren.12 (zhongwan –) ....alarm point of the Stomach, strengthens the Spleen
                             and Stomach to transform phlegm damp
Bl.62 (shenmai) ....master points of the yangqiaomai and yinqiaomai
Kid.6 (zhaohai)   respectively, alleviate somnolence
Sp.3 (taibai).......................source and connecting points of the Spleen and
St.40 (fenglong –)   Stomach, these points transforming phlegm damp
                                 and alleviating heaviness and fatigue
St.36 (zusanli +▲) ....sea point of the Stomach, strengthens the Spleen
                                 and Stomach, supplements qi and regulates the qi
                                 dynamic
Sp.5 (shangqiu –) ....river point of the Spleen, transforms phlegm damp
PC.5 (jianshi)......................river point of the Pericardium, transforms phlegm
                                 and harmonizes the Stomach
• with foggy head, add Du.20 (baihui) and St.8 (touwei)
• with sluggish stools, add SJ.6 (zhigou –) and St.37 (shangjuxu –)
• with cold phlegm, apply moxa to Bl.20 (pishu ▲) and Bl.21 (weishu ▲)
• Ear points: spleen, stomach, zero point, shenmen, sympathetic, adrenal

Clinical notes
• Phlegm damp tiredness is chronic and can be slow to resolve. In addition to dietary modification, phlegm damp patterns usually require persistent treatment
  and dietary modification for satisfactory results. For dietary recommendations,
  see Clinical Handbook, Vol.2, p.880.
• Exercise is an important component of treatment, with moderate but sustained
  aerobic activity recommended. Walking and swimming are ideal.
• As the phlegm damp resolves, the treatment strategy should be altered to
  strengthening the Spleen and supplementing qi to prevent formation of phlegm
  and damp.

痰
热
疲
倦

18.3.2 PHLEGM HEAT

Treatment principle
Clear heat and transform phlegm
Harmonize the Stomach and calm the shen

Prescription

ZHU RU WEN DAN TANG 竹茹温胆汤
Warm Gallbladder Decoction with Bamboo

zhu ru (Bambusae Caulis in taeniam) 竹茹 12–15g
zhi shi (Aurantii Fructus immaturus) 枳实 12–15g
jie geng (Platycodi Radix) 桔梗 9–12g
chai hu (Bupleuri Radix) 柴胡 9–12g
zhi ban xia (Pinelliae Rhizoma preparatum) 制半夏 9–12g
fu ling (Poria) 茯苓 9–12g
xiang fu (Cyperi Rhizoma) 香附 6–9g
chen pi (Citri reticulatae Pericarpium) 陈皮 6–9g
ren shen (Ginseng Radix) 人参 3–6g
huang lian (Coptidis Rhizoma) 黄连 3–6g
sheng jiang (Zingiberis Rhizoma recens) 生姜 6–9g
gan cao (Glycyrrhizae Radix) 甘草 3–6g
da zao (Jujubae Fructus) 大枣 .... 3 fruit

Method: Decoction. **Zhu ru** clears phlegm heat; **zhi ban xia** dries damp and transforms phlegm; **jie geng** expels phlegm from the Lungs; **chai hu** clears heat and with **xiang fu** regulates Liver qi and resolves qi constraint; **zhi shi** breaks up qi stagnation in the abdomen and directs qi and phlegm downwards; **fu ling** strengthens the Spleen and leaches dampness out through the urine; **chen pi** dries damp, transforms phlegm and rectifies the qi dynamic; **ren shen** supplements qi; **huang lian** clears heat; **gan cao** supplements qi and harmonizes the formula; **sheng jiang** and **da zao** protect the Spleen and Stomach, while the pungent warmth of **sheng jiang** assists the phlegm transformation of the main herbs. (Source: *San Yin Ji Yi Bing Zheng Fang Lun*)

Modifications
- With marked phlegm heat, add **tian zhu huang** (Bambusae Concretio silicea) 天竺黄 9–12g, **zhu li** (Bambusae Succus) 竹沥 12–15g and **dan nan xing** (Arisaemae cum Bile) 胆南星 6–9g.
- With constipation, add **da huang** (Rhei Radix et Rhizoma) 大黄 6–9g and **gua lou ren** (Trichosanthis Semen) 栝楼仁 12–18g.

Variations and additional prescriptions
With persistent cough
Phlegm heat can persist in the Lungs after an unresolved upper respiratory tract infection. In addition to the tiredness, which can persist for weeks, the patient has a productive cough with sticky yellow sputum. The treatment is to clears phlegm heat from the Lungs and stop cough with **QING QI HUA TAN TANG** (Clear the Qi and Transform Phlegm Decoction 清气化痰汤).

dan nan xing (Arisaema cum Bile) 胆南星 45g
zhi ban xia (Pinelliae Rhizoma preparatum) 制半夏 45g
gua lou (Trichosanthis Fructus) 栝楼 30g

huang qin (Scutellariae Radix) 黄芩..30g
chen pi (Citri reticulatae Pericarpium) 陈皮..30g
zhi shi (Aurantii Fructus immaturus) 枳实..30g
xing ren (Armeniacae Semen) 杏仁..30g
fu ling (Poria) 茯苓...30g

Method: Pills or powder. **Dan nan xing** clears heat, transforms and dissipates sticky phlegm; **zhi ban xia** supports **dan nan xing** in transforming phlegm; **gua luo** transforms phlegm heat and opens up qi flow through the chest; **huang qin** clears heat from the Lungs; **chen pi** and **zhi shi** regulate qi and assist in mobilizing sticky phlegm; **xing ren** diffuses the Lungs and directs Lung qi downwards; **fu ling** strengthens the Spleen, leaches out dampness and assists **xing ren** in maintaining free flow in the water passages to enable an outlet for, and dispersal of, the phlegm. (Source: *Yi Fang Kao*)

Prepared medicines
Concentrated powder
Zhu Ru Wen Dan Tang (Bamboo & Ginseng Combination)
Qing Qi Hua Tang Wan (Pinellia & Scute Formula)

Pills
Wen Dan Wan (Rising Courage Teapills)
Qing Qi Hua Tan Wan (Clean Air Teapills, Pinellia Expectorant Pills)

Acupuncture (select from)
Ren.12 (zhongwan –).........alarm point of the Stomach, strengthens the Spleen and Stomach to transform phlegm, clears heat and harmonizes the Stomach
PC.5 (jianshi).....................river point of the Pericardium, transforms phlegm and clears heat
PC.6 (neiguan –)................connecting point of the Pericardium, calms the Heart and shen, dredges the Liver and rectifies qi
St.40 (fenglong –) ....connecting point of the Stomach, transforms phlegm and clears heat
St.36 (zusanli) ....sea point of the Stomach, strengthens the Spleen and Stomach and corrects the qi dynamic
St.43 (xianggu –)................transport and wood point of the Stomach, clears heat
• with foggy head, add Du.20 (baihui) and St.8 (touwei)
• with severe heat, add PC.8 (laogong –) and St.45 (lidui ↓)
• with epigastric pain, add St.34 (liangqiu –)
• with dizziness, add GB.43 (xiaxi –)
• with anxiety, add Du.19 (houding) and Du.24 (shenting)
• with productive cough, add Lu.5 (chize –) and Ren.17 (shanzhong –)
• Ear points: zero point, spleen, heart, liver, subcortex, sympathetic, shenmen

Clinical notes
• Tiredness of a phlegm heat type may be diagnosed as post–viral syndrome, chronic bronchitis, the convalescent phase of pneumonia or diseases with high fever, the early stages of psychosis or bipolar mood disorder.

- Phlegm heat usually responds well to treatment, although treatment needs to continue until all signs of phlegm are cleared, in particular, until the tongue coat becomes normal. Herbs are more efficient at clearing entrenched phlegm, although acupuncture often starts to improve energy levels quite quickly, especially on the day of treatment.
- A cooling, phlegm transforming diet is recommended. See Clinical Handbook, Vol.2, p.885. Avoidance of heating, rich and spicy foods, and overeating, is important.

痰气郁结 18.3.3 PHLEGM AND QI CONSTRAINT

Treatment principle
Move qi and transform phlegm
Downbear counterflow qi

Prescription

BAN XIA HOU PO TANG 半夏厚朴汤
Pinellia and Magnolia Bark Decoction

zhi ban xia (Pinelliae Rhizoma preparatum) 制半夏 9–12g
fu ling (Poria) 茯苓 9–12g
hou po (Magnoliae officinalis Cortex) 厚朴 6–9g
zi su ye (Perillae Folium) 紫苏叶 3–6g
sheng jiang (Zingiberis Rhizoma recens) 生姜 9–15g
Method: Decoction. **Zhi ban xia** transforms phlegm, promotes qi flow through areas of phlegm accumulation, and downbears counterflow qi to stop nausea and vomiting; **hou po** directs qi downwards and transforms phlegm; **sheng jiang** reinforces the phlegm transforming action of **zhi ban xia**; **fu ling** strengthens the Spleen and leaches damp; **zi su ye** opens up and diffuses qi flow from areas of constraint, while harmonizing the middle burner. (Source: *Jin Gui Yao Lue*)

Modifications
- With Liver qi constraint, add **xiang fu** (Cyperi Rhizoma) 香附 9–12g and **fo shou** (Citri sarcodacylis Fructus) 佛手 9–12g or combine with XIAO YAO SAN (Rambling Powder 逍遥散, p.841).
- With a foggy head or clouded consciousness, add **shi chang pu** (Acori tatarinowii Rhizoma) 石菖蒲 6–9g and **yuan zhi** (Polygalae Radix) 远志 6–9g.
- With somnolence, add **shi chang pu** (Acori tatarinowii Rhizoma) 石菖蒲 6–9g and **yuan zhi** (Polygalae Radix) 远志 6–9g.
- With early waking or sleep disturbance, add **mu li** (Ostreae Concha) 牡蛎 12–15g [cooked first] and **mei gui hua** (Rosae rugosae Flos) 玫瑰花 6–9g.
- With vocal cord polyps and breast lumps, add **zhe bei mu** (Fritillariae thunbergii Bulbus) 浙贝母 9–12g, **xuan shen** (Scrophulariae Radix) 玄参 12–15g and **mu li** (Ostreae Concha) 牡蛎 15–30g [cooked first].
- With hoarse voice or loss of voice, add **pang da hai** (Sterculiae lychnophorae Semen) 胖大海 2–3 pieces, and **mu hu die** (Oroxyli Semen) 木蝴蝶 1.5–3g.
- With productive cough, add **pi pa ye** (Eriobotryae Folium) 枇杷叶 9–12g, **chao xing ren** (stir fried Armeniacae Semen) 炒杏仁 9–12g and **gua lou pi** (Trichosanthis Pericarpium) 栝楼皮 9–12g.

Prepared medicines
Concentrated powder
Ban Xia Hou Po Tang (Pinellia & Magnolia Combination)
Xiao Yao San (Bupleurum & Tangkuei Formula)
Pills
Ban Xia Hou Po Wan (Pinellia and Magnolia Teapills)
Xiao Yao Wan (Free and Easy Wanderer Teapills, Hsiao Yao Wan)

Acupuncture (select from)
Ren.17 (shanzhong) ....upper 'sea of qi', diffuses the Lungs and assists descent of Lung qi, use when tender

Kid.27 (shufu) ....these points help to open the chest, aid the descent
Kid.25 (shenzang)   of Lung qi and help connect the po and zhi, use when tender

PC.5 (jianshi).....................river point of the Pericardium, transforms phlegm
PC.6 (neiguan –)................connecting point of the Pericardium, downbears counterflow qi, opens up qi flow through the chest, dredges the Liver and regulates qi

St.40 (fenglong –) ....connecting points of the Stomach and Heart, these
Ht.5 (tongli)   points transform phlegm and remove stagnation from the throat

Liv.2 (xingjian –)................these four points are the double four gates, and exert
Liv.3 (taichong –)   a powerful qi regulating and mobilizing action;
LI.3 (sanjian –)   usually needled on alternative sides (four points in
LI.4 (hegu –)   total)

- with Spleen qi deficiency, add St.36 (zusanli +) and Bl.20 (pishu +)
- with a dry or hoarse throat, add Kid.6 (zhaohai) and Lu.7 (lieque)
- with foggy head, add Du.20 (baihui)
- with dizziness, add GB.43 (xiaxi –)
- with anxiety, add Du.19 (houding) and Du.24 (shenting)
- Ear points: lung, spleen, liver, zero point, shenmen, sympathetic, adrenal

Clinical notes
- Tiredness of a phlegm and qi constraint type may be diagnosed as globus hystericus, neurosis or chronic fatigue syndrome.
- Phlegm and qi constraint is often a recurrent problem, waxing and waning according to the patient's stress levels.
- Exercise is an essential component of management in all qi and phlegm constraint patterns (p.103).
- Hot spot therapy is helpful, p.923.
- A qi mobilizing, phlegm transforming diet is recommended. See Clinical Handbook, Vol.2, pp.878–880.

风
痰
疲
倦

18.3.4 WIND PHLEGM

Treatment principle
Transform phlegm and extinguish wind
Strengthen the Spleen and harmonize the Stomach

Prescription

BAN XIA BAI ZHU TIAN MA TANG 半夏白术天麻汤
Pinellia, White Atractylodes, and Gastrodia Decoction

zhi ban xia (Pinelliae Rhizoma preparatum) 制半夏 9–12g
bai zhu (Atractylodes macrocephalae Rhizoma) 白术 12–15g
tian ma (Gastrodiae Rhizoma) 天麻 9–12g
chen pi (Citri reticulatae Pericarpium) 陈皮 6–9g
fu ling (Poria) 茯苓 9–15g
gan cao (Glycyrrhizae Radix) 甘草 3–6g
sheng jiang (Zingiberis Rhizoma recens) 生姜 9–12g
da zao (Jujubae Fructus) 大枣 .... 3 fruit

Method: Decoction. **Zhi ban xia** transforms phlegm and dries damp; **tian ma** calms the Liver and extinguishes wind; **bai zhu** and **fu ling** strengthen the Spleen, and transform phlegm; **chen pi** transforms phlegm, rectifies middle burner qi and corrects the qi dynamic; **sheng jiang** transforms phlegm and assists the other herbs in stopping nausea and vomiting; **da zao** and **gan cao** strengthen the Spleen and harmonize the Stomach. (Source: *Yi Xue Xin Wu*)

Modifications
- With frontal headache, add **bai zhi** (Angelicae dahuricae Radix) 白芷 9–12g.
- With marked qi deficiency, add **dang shen** (Codonopsis Radix) 党参 12–15g and **huang qi** (Astragali Radix) 黄芪 12–15g.
- With marked or persistent dizziness and nausea, add one or two of the following substances: **dai zhe shi** (Haematitum) 代赭石 12–18g, **xuan fu hua** (Inulae Flos) 旋复花 9–15g, **bai jiang can** (Bombyx Batryticatus) 白僵蚕 9–12g or **dan nan xing** (Arisaemae cum Bile) 胆南星 6–9g.
- With marked tinnitus, add **shi chang pu** (Acori tatarinowii Rhizoma) 石菖蒲 6–9g and **yuan zhi** (Polygalae Radix) 远志 6–9g.

Prepared medicines
Concentrated powder
Ban Xia Bai Zhu Tian Ma Tang (Pinellia & Gastrodia Combination)

Pills
Ban Xia Bai Zhu Tian Ma Wan (Head Clear Pill)

Acupuncture (select from)
St.8 (touwei) .... dispels wind phlegm from the head
GB.20 (fengchi –) .... extinguishes wind and subdues Liver yang
Liv.3 (taichong –) .... extinguishes wind and regulates qi
Bl.60 (kunlun –) .... extinguishes wind
Ren.12 (zhongwan) .... alarm point of the Stomach, strengthens Stomach
               and Spleen function to transform phlegm

St.40 (fenglong –) ....connecting point of the Stomach, transforms phlegm

St.41 (jiexi –).....................river point of the Stomach, strengthens the Spleen and Stomach, transforms phlegm

PC.5 (jianshi –)..................river point of the Pericardium, transforms phlegm

Bl.20 (pishu) ....transport point of the Spleen, strengthens the Spleen and supplements qi to transform phlegm

• with somnolence, add Kid.6 (zhaohai) and Bl.62 (shenmai)
• with foggy head, add Bl.62 (shenmai)
• with Spleen deficiency, add St.36 (zusanli +)
• with cold, apply moxa to Bl.20 (pishu ▲) and Bl.21 (weishu ▲)
• Ear points: spleen, liver, zero point, adrenal, sympathetic, shenmen

Clinical notes

• Wind phlegm tiredness may be diagnosed as Meniere's disease, benign positional vertigo, hypertension or immune weakness with chronic congestion of the middle ear.
• Patients with wind phlegm are more likely to present with vertigo and dizziness, although in some cases the vertigo episodes are quite sporadic, and tiredness, heaviness and headaches may bring them into the clinic.
• This pattern can respond well to correct treatment and dietary modification.
• Regular exercise and stress management are important components of successful treatment.
• A phlegm transforming diet is recommended. See Clinical Handbook, Vol.2, p.880.

18.4 LINGERING PATHOGENS

1. Shaoyang syndrome
2. Residual heat in the qi level (Lungs and Stomach)
3. Damp in the muscles (*see* 18.2.2 above)
4. Damp heat (*see* 18.2.3 above)
5. Phlegm heat (*see* 18.3.2 above)

Lingering pathogens are a common cause of persistent tiredness, and are often seen in the aftermath of an incompletely resolved pathogenic invasion or immunization. Certain types of pathogens are more likely to cause lingering fatigue, in particular those that are by nature cloying and heavy. Damp is especially likely to produce ongoing fatigue if not completely resolved. In addition, the qi required to fight and contain the pathogen can contribute to a continuing and gradual decline in the already weakened levels of energy.

There are many variations of lingering pathogens, all of which can cause significant fatigue. The most commonly encountered are noted in this chapter. For more on lingering pathogens, see chapter 11.

18.4.1 SHAOYANG SYNDROME

The process of containing a pathogen within the shaoyang invariably depletes qi, so one of the main features of shaoyang patterns is progressive fatigue. Although in the early to mid stages, shaoyang syndrome is predominantly an excess condition, as time passes, the deficient components become more and more prominent.

Shaoyang patterns are often diagnosed in the patient who presents days, weeks or months following a relatively trivial infection such as the flu, an upper respiratory tract or gastrointestinal infection, or immunization, saying 'I have never felt well since.......'.

Clinical features

• Persistent, continuous and progressive fatigue and tiredness in the aftermath of an unresolved infection. In some cases the initial event may have occurred long enough ago to be forgotten.
• alternating fever and chills
• reduced appetite or anorexia
• nausea, usually worse in the morning
• hypochondriac pain, distension or tenderness
• chest oppression
• dizziness
• irritability
• bitter taste in the mouth; food tastes bad

T may be unremarkable or pale depending on complicating qi deficiency, or coated only on the left side, or slightly red on the edges

P wiry

Treatment principle
Harmonize shaoyang

Prescription

XIAO CHAI HU TANG 小柴胡汤
Minor Bupleurum Decoction

chai hu (Bupleuri Radix) 柴胡 6–12g
huang qin (Scutellariae Radix) 黄芩 6–9g
zhi ban xia (Pinelliae Rhizoma preparatum) 制半夏 6–9g
ren shen (Ginseng Radix) 人参 6–9g
zhi gan cao (Glycyrrhizae Radix preparata) 炙甘草 3–6g
sheng jiang (Zingiberis Rhizoma recens) 生姜 6–9g
da zao (Jujubae Fructus) 大枣 .... 4 fruit
Method: Decoction. **Chai hu** vents pathogens from the shaoyang and rectifies qi; **huang qin** clears heat; **zhi ban xia** and **sheng jiang** harmonize the Stomach, downbear counterflow Stomach qi and stop nausea; **ren shen** and **zhi gan cao** strengthen zheng qi and prevent the pathogen from penetrating further; **sheng jiang** and **da zao** support **zhi ban xia** in harmonizing the Stomach and stopping nausea and vomiting. (Source: *Shang Han Lun*)

Modifications
• With damp in shaoyang causing marked anorexia, muscle aches, heaviness and a thick tongue coat in addition to the shaoyang symptoms, add **cang zhu** (Atractylodis Rhizoma) 苍术 12–15g, **hou po** (Magnoliae officinalis Cortex) 厚朴 9–12g and **chen pi** (Citri reticulatae Pericarpium) 陈皮 9–12g.
• To enhance the formulas ability to evict deep lying pathogens, add **qing hao** (Artemisiae annuae Herba) 青蒿 9–15g.

Variations and additional prescriptions
Damp heat in shaoyang
In humid or tropical climates the main pathogen is often damp heat. When a damp heat pathogen gains access to the shaoyang, it produces a distinct clinical picture. In addition to the fever and chill pattern with fever predominant, there is aching in the muscles, foggy head, night sweats, nausea and vomiting, thick, greasy, yellow tongue coat and a wiry, rapid and slippery pulse. The treatment is to clear damp heat from shaoyang with **HAO QIN QING DAN TANG** (Sweet Wormwood and Scutellaria Decoction to Clear the Gallbladder 蒿芩清胆汤, p.373).

Prepared medicines
Concentrated powders
Xiao Chai Hu Tang (Minor Bupleurum Combination)
Pills
Xiao Chai Hu Wan (Minor Bupleurum Teapills)

Acupuncture (select from)
SJ.5 (waiguan –) ....these points vent pathogens from shaoyang, dredge
GB.39 (xuanzhong –)   the Liver and regulate qi; they are needled on
GB.41 (zulinqi –)   alternate sides of the body (four points in total)
GB.34 (yanglingquan –)

Liv.14 (qimen –) ....alarm point of the Liver, clears heat and regulates the Liver

Bl.19 (danshu –) ....transport point of the Gallbladder, rectifies qi

- with damp heat, add Sp.9 (yinlingquan –), Liv.8 (ququan –) and Kid.7 (fuliu –)
- with qi deficiency, add Ren.12 (zhongwan +) and St.36 (zusanli +)
- Ear points: liver, spleen, zero point, shenmen, sympathetic

Clinical notes

- Shaoyang syndrome may be diagnosed as post viral syndrome, influenza, the convalescent phase of an upper respiratory tract infection, chronic fatigue syndrome, postpartum fever or cholecystitis.
- Shaoyang syndrome is one of the most commonly types of lingering pathogen, and a common presentation of chronic tiredness. Patients may harbour lurking pathogens in the shaoyang for weeks, months or even years.
- When correctly identified, shaoyang patterns respond well to treatment, indeed, patterns that have persisted for months or years can be resolved in a few weeks.

18.4.2 RESIDUAL HEAT IN THE QI LEVEL

邪
留
气
分

This pattern follows an upper respiratory or gastrointestinal tract infection associated with external heat invasion. If the heat pathogen is not completely cleared, it can linger in the qi level damaging fluids, qi and yin.

Clinical features

- persistent fatigue and tiredness in the post acute phase of an upper respiratory or gastrointestinal tract infection
- lingering low grade fever which tends to be worse in the evening and at night
- persistent dry irritating cough, or nausea and vomiting
- thirst, dry mucous membranes; may be mouth ulcers
- daytime clamminess, night sweats
- chest oppression
- irritability and restlessness
- insomnia, restlessness, fitful sleep
- dry sore throat, hoarse voice or loss of voice

T red and dry with little or no coat
P weak, fine, rapid

Treatment principle

Clear residual heat from the qi level
Generate fluids and boost qi

Prescription

ZHU YE SHI GAO TANG 竹叶石膏汤
Lophatherus and Gypsum Decoction

dan zhu ye (Lophateri Herba) 淡竹叶...9–15g
shi gao (Gypsum fibrosum) 石膏 15–30g
zhi ban xia (Pinelliae Rhizoma preparatum) 制半夏 6–9g

mai dong (Ophiopogonis Radix) 麦冬 6–15g
ren shen (Ginseng Radix) 人参 3–9g
zhi gan cao (Glycyrrhizae Radix preparata) 炙甘草 3–9g
jing mi (Oryzae Semen) 粳米 9–15g

Method: Decoction. **Shi gao** is decocted for 30 minutes prior to the other herbs. **Dan zhu ye** and **shi gao** vent heat from the qi level; **ren shen** strengthens the Spleen and supplements qi, and with **mai dong** generates fluids and protects yin; **mai dong** assists in clearing heat; **zhi ban xia** downbears counterflow Stomach qi to stop nausea and vomiting; **zhi gan cao** and **jing mi** strengthen the Spleen and protect the Stomach. (Source: *Shang Han Lun*)

Prepared medicines

Concentrated powder

Zhu Ye Shi Gao Tang (Bamboo Leaves & Gypsum Combination)

Acupuncture (select from)

Lu.7 (lieque –).....................diffuses the Lungs and vents pathogens from the qi
level

Du.14 (dazhui –Ω) ....these points clear and vent heat from the qi level

Du.12 (shenzhu –)

Du.13 (taodao –)

LI.11 (quchi –)...................these points clear heat

St.44 (neiting –)

• with cough, add Ren.17 (shanzhong) and Lu.5 (chize –)
• with nausea and vomiting, add PC.6 (neiguan)
• with dryness and thirst, add Kid.6 (zhaohai +)
• with constipation, add St.25 (tianshu –) and St.37 (shangjuxu –)
• Ear points: lung, stomach, zero point, shenmen

Clinical notes

• Qi level residual heat is a common cause of tiredness, persistent cough or nausea and low grade night time fever in the aftermath of an acute upper respiratory tract infection or gastrointestinal infection. It is especially common in children, and may persist for some time following the initial event.

• When correctly identified, a lingering in the qi level can be dispelled quite quickly, and the qi and fluids replenished quickly. Usually only a few days to a week or so of treatment are usually necessary.

血
瘀

18.5 BLOOD STASIS

Blood stasis type tiredness can be acute or chronic. When of short duration it follows a physical or emotional trauma, and many of the classic features of blood stasis may be absent. When longer term, the blood stasis intervenes in some other prolonged pathology such as qi constraint, heat and yin deficiency, cold, or yang qi deficiency. The tiredness is due to several factors. Static blood blocks the distribution of qi and blood and prevents the manufacture of new blood. It can also disrupts the function of the Liver and Heart, and compromise blood circulation. This type of fatigue is also seen in the aftermath of a wind–stroke.

Clinical features
- The tiredness of blood stasis is often associated with chronic pain or poor cardiovascular function. It may also overlap with mood disorders, and be indistinguishable from endogenous depression. Patients feel somewhat better after exercise, but not as much as with qi constraint, and will feel worse with prolonged inactivity.
- chronic pain, usually focal and sufficient to disrupt sleep and interfere with daily activity; angina; dysmenorrhea; migraine
- breathlessness or angina with exertion; palpitations
- persistent insomnia and sleep disturbances compound the fatigue
- irritability, depression, mood swings
- cold extremities with vascular congestion, varicosities and spider nevi
- skin discoloration; purplish lips, sclera, conjunctiva, nail beds
- dry, scaly skin, especially on the lower legs
- left iliac fossa pressure pain (p.925–926)
- low grade or hectic fever, worse at night
- dark rings around the eyes

T in acute cases the tongue body may be unremarkable; in chronic cases dark or red purple with brown or purple stasis spots and a thin, white coat; sublingual veins are distended and dark

P deep and choppy or wiry, or weak, intermittent and irregular

Treatment principle
Activate blood and regulate qi
Disperse static blood and promote creation of new blood

Prescription

XUE FU ZHU YU TANG 血府逐瘀汤
Drive Out Stasis in the Mansion of Blood Decoction, modified

tao ren (Persicae Semen) 桃仁	9–12g
hong hua (Carthami Flos) 红花	6–9g
sheng di (Rehmanniae Radix) 生地	9–12g
dang gui (Angelicae sinensis Radix) 当归	9–12g
chi shao (Paeoniae Radix rubra) 赤芍	9–12g
chuan xiong (Chuanxiong Rhizoma) 川芎	6–9g

chai hu (Bupleuri Radix) 柴胡 6–9g
zhi ke (Aurantii Fructus) 枳壳.. 6–9g
gan cao (Glycyrrhizae Radix) 甘草 3–6g
chuan niu xi (Cyathulae Radix) 川牛膝 9–15g
jie geng (Platycodi Radix) 桔梗 6–9g
huang qi (Astragali Radix) 黄芪 24–60g
Method: Decoction. **Tao ren, hong hua, chi shao, chuan xiong** and **chuan niu xi** activate blood and disperse stagnant blood; **sheng di, dang gui, chi shao** and **chuan xiong** nourish and regulate blood; **sheng di, dang gui, chi shao** cool the blood; **chai hu, zhi ke, chi shao** and **gan cao** dredge the Liver and rectify qi; **chai hu, chuan xiong, jie geng** and **chuan niu xi** and **zhi ke** combine ascending and descending actions to stimulate the flow of qi and blood and rectify the qi dynamic; **huang qi** supplements qi to help qi to lead the blood, and with **dang gui**, supplements blood. (Source: *Yi Lin Gai Cuo*)

Modifications
- With angina, increase the dose of **chuan xiong** to 15g and add **dan shen** (Salviae miltiorrhizae Radix) 丹参 9–12g.
- With abdominal or peripheral pain, add **yan hu suo** (Corydalis Rhizoma) 延胡索 9–12g, **zhi mo yao** (Myrrha preparata) 炙没药 6–9g and **zhi ru xiang** (Olibanum preparata) 炙乳香 6–9g.
- With headache, increase the dose of **chuan xiong** up to 30g for the duration of the headache.
- With depression and insomnia, add **he huan pi** (Albizziae Cortex) 合欢皮 12–15g and **dan shen** (Salviae miltiorrhizae Radix) 丹参 9–12g.
- With heat, add **yu jin** (Curcumae Radix) 郁金 9–12g.
- With marked qi deficiency, delete **chai hu, jie geng** and **zhi ke**, and add **dang shen** (Codonopsis Radix) 党参 18–24g and **huang jing** (Polygonati Rhizoma) 黄精 12–15g.
- With yang deficiency or cold, delete **chai hu, jie geng** and **zhi ke**, and add **zhi fu zi** (Aconiti Radix lateralis preparata) 制附子 6–9g, **rou gui** (Cinnamomi Cortex) 肉桂 3–6g, **xian ling pi** (Epimedii Herba) 仙灵脾 12–15g and **ba ji tian** (Morindae Radix) 巴戟天 9–12g.
- With yin deficiency, delete **chai hu, jie geng, chuan xiong** and **zhi ke**, and add **mai dong** (Ophiopogonis Radix) 麦冬 9–12g, **yu zhu** (Polygonati odorati Rhizoma) 玉竹 9–12g, **nu zhen zi** (Ligustri Fructus) 女贞子 9–12g and **han lian cao** (Ecliptae Herba) 旱莲草 9–12g.
- With marked blood deficiency, use **shu di** (Rehmanniae Radix preparata) 熟地 12–18g instead of **sheng di** and **bai shao** (Paeoniae Radix alba) 白芍 9–12g instead of **chi shao**.

Variations and additional prescriptions
Blood stasis and qi deficiency in the aftermath of a wind–stroke
Following wind–stroke, patients are often left with significant fatigue in addition to varying degrees of hemiplegia, facial paralysis, slurred speech or incontinence. The treatment is to supplement qi, activate blood, and unblock the channels and network vessels with **Bu Yang Huan Wu Tang** (Supplement Yang to Restore Five Tenths Decoction 补阳还五汤). This formula is also useful for loss of function,

weakness and wasting following surgery on the brain. It is quite effective but relatively slow acting, and usually requires a few months of persistent use to produce a lasting and satisfactory result. It should be given for at least two months before a judgement can be made on whether it is working for the patient. The sooner following the wind–stroke with the patient stabilized, the better the result.

huang qi (Astragali Radix) 黄芪 30–120g
dang gui wei (rootlets of Angelicae sinensis Radix) 当归尾 6–12g
chi shao (Paeoniae Radix rubra) 赤芍 6–9g
chuan xiong (Chuanxiong Rhizoma) 川芎 6–9g
tao ren (Persicae Semen) 桃仁 6–9g
hong hua (Carthami Flos) 红花 6–9g
di long (Pheretima) 地龙 6–12g

Method. Powder or decoction. **Huang qi** supplements qi and promotes circulation of qi to the extremities, and thus leads blood to the periphery; **dang gui wei** supplements and activates the blood; **chi shao, chuan xiong, tao ren** and **hong hua** activate blood and dispel stasis; **di long** 'drills through' blockages in the channels and network vessels, opening them up and allowing free flow or qi and blood. (Source: *Yi Lin Gai Cuo*)

Prepared medicines
Concentrated powder
Xue Fu Zhu Yu Tang (Persica & Carthamus Combination)
Bu Yang Huan Wu Tang (Astragalus & Peony Combination)
    – with qi deficiency
Tao Hong Si Wu Tang (Tangkuei Four, Persica & Carthamus Combination)
    – with blood deficiency

Pills
Xue Fu Zhu Yu Wan (Stasis in the Mansion of Blood Teapills)
Bu Yang Huan Wu Wan (Great Yang Restoration Teapills)
Tao Hong Si Wu Wan (Tao Hong Si Wu Tang Teapills)
Dan Shen Pian (Dan Shen Pills)
    – add to one of the above with angina
Sheng Tian Qi Pian (Raw Tian Qi Ginseng Tablets)
    – add to one of the above with angina

Acupuncture (select from)
Bl.17 (geshu –).................meeting point for blood, disperses static blood
Bl.15 (xinshu +) ....transport point of the Heart, strengthens Heart qi to activate blood
Bl.18 (ganshu –).................transport point of the Liver, dredges the Liver and regulates qi to lead blood
Sp.6 (sanyinjiao –)..............these points activate blood and disperse stagnant
Sp.10 (xuehai –)   blood
LI.4 (hegu –)
PC.6 (neiguan –).................connecting point of the Pericardium, dredges the Liver and regulates qi to lead blood
Ht.7 (shenmen).................source point of the Heart, strengthens the Heart and regulates Heart qi

- with angina, add PC.6 (ximen –) and Ren.17 (shanzhong –)
- With palpitations or tachycardia, add Ht.5 (tongli) and Ht.6 (yinxi –)
- with trauma or focal pain, add painful points (ahshi)
- with depression, add LI.4 (hegu), Liv.3 (taichong) and yintang (M–HN–3)
- Bloodletting on vascular congestion and spider nevi between the scapulae, and on congested vessels on the medial aspect of the lower leg can be helpful. See appendix 4, p.929.

Clinical notes

- Tiredness of a blood stasis type may be associated with a host of chronic conditions, a few of which should raise red flags. Chronic blood stasis patterns can involve any organ system, but have most impact on the Heart and Liver. Tiredness from blood stasis may be a sign of atherosclerotic or congestive cardiac disease, liver cirrhosis, or masses and tumors. A high incidence of suspicion is warranted in persistent tiredness of a blood stasis type and further investigations may be warranted.
- When a physical or emotional trauma is the cause, the onset of the tiredness is more abrupt and there may be few of the classic features of blood stasis. Diagnosis is based on the history, or is arrived at by a process of elimination, when other treatments have proven ineffective.
- The primary prescription above is effective at dispersing blood stasis, but can gradually deplete zheng qi and blood as well. This effect is more common after about three months or so, depending on the deficient status of the patient. If the patients qi and blood are being dispersed along with the static blood, they will start to get more fatigued again, and suffer sleep disturbances and dizziness. It is good practice to rest the patient from strong blood activating formulae every few months, changing to a more supplementing strategy for a few weeks.
- Exercise is an important component of treatment. In the early stages of treatment, and when the patient has cardiovascular complications, the gentle movement of taijiquan or yoga may be a more acceptable way to start moving.
- A qi and blood activating diet is recommended. See Clinical Handbook, Vol.2 p.878 and 886.

气
虚

18.6 QI DEFICIENCY

1. Lung
2. Spleen ± damp
3. Kidney
4. Heart

Qi is the basis of all the functional activity of the body. Insufficient qi leads to weak organ system function, poor circulation of qi and blood and insufficient energy to power the muscles and brain. Tiredness from lack of qi is often compounded by the buildup of damp, which produces a more complex type of fatigue.

The Lungs and Spleen are the organs responsible for harvesting and production of qi, so treatments to supplement qi are mainly aimed at improving their function. There are specific strategies that take the functional variations of the other systems affected by qi deficiency into account, and these are noted below.

Common features
• Lack of vitality and tiredness which is worse after activity and at the end of the day, and better after rest and a good nights sleep. The tiredness is continuous, with the patient's energy fluctuating from low to very low.
• pale, waxy complexion
• spontaneous sweating
T pale, swollen and scalloped with a thin, white coat
P deep, weak, fine

Specific features
Lung qi deficiency
• When Lung qi is weak, the tiredness takes the form of an inability to exert oneself without becoming breathless and clammy.
• weak voice, talking can be an effort and leads to increased tiredness, a hoarse voice or loss of voice, so the patient tends to speak softly or not at all
• weak immunity; easily succumbing to colds and flu
• breathlessness with exertion
• slumped shoulders, collapsed chest, shallow breathing
• wheezing, weak cough
• history of childhood asthma or chronic respiratory infections

Spleen qi deficiency
• tiredness or sleepiness, worse after eating and bowel movements, and after sustained mental activity and study; inability to concentrate
• muscles easily fatigued and tired; muscle weakness with poor muscle tone
• poor muscle tone combined with lack of energy causes a slumped posture, difficulty holding the head upright and organ prolapse
• loss of appetite, history of anorexia or bulimia
• abdominal distension
• loose stools
• menorrhagia or bruising

Kidney qi deficiency
- frequent urination or nocturia
- mild ankle edema
- dull lower back ache or weakness when tired
- tinnitus, loss of hearing acuity
- premature ejaculation
- infertility, loss of libido, impotence
- history of excessive sexual activity, multiple pregnancies or terminations

Heart qi deficiency
- palpitations and tachycardia with activity
- breathlessness with exertion
- anxiety, easily startled
- chest oppression, mild chest pain, an empty feeling in the chest
- intermittent or irregular pulse

肺
气
虚

18.6.1 LUNG QI DEFICIENCY
Treatment principle
Supplement and strengthen the Lungs and Spleen
Secure the exterior and stop sweating

Prescription

BU FEI TANG 补肺汤
Supplement the Lungs Decoction

ren shen (Ginseng Radix) 人参 6–9g
huang qi (Astragali Radix) 黄芪 18–24g
shu di (Rehmanniae Radix preparata) 熟地 15–24g
wu wei zi (Schizandrae Fructus) 五味子 6–9g
zi wan (Asteris Radix) 紫菀 6–9g
sang bai pi (Mori Cortex) 桑白皮 9–12g

Method: Decoction. **Ren shen** and **huang qi** supplement and strengthen the Lungs, fortify wei qi and secure the exterior; **sang bai pi** and **zi wan** direct Lung qi downward and stop cough; **shu di** and **wu wei zi** strengthen the Kidneys, assist them in grasping Lung qi, and enable deep respiration; **wu wei zi** also secures Lung qi and stops sweating. (Source: *Zhong Yi Nei Ke Xue* [*Yong Lei Qian Fang*])

Modifications
- Without cough, delete **sang bai pi** and **zi wan**.
- With copious spontaneous sweating, add **mu li** (Ostreae Concha) 牡蛎 15–30g, **ma huang gen** (Ephedrae Radix) 麻黄根 3–9g and **fu xiao mai** (Tritici Fructus levis) 浮小麦 12–15g.
- With frequent colds, increase the dose of **huang qi** up to 30–60 grams, and add **bai zhu** (Atractylodis macrocephalae Rhizoma) 白术 9–12g and **fang feng** (Saposhnikovae Radix) 防风 6–9g.
- With yin deficiency, a dry irritating cough and flushed cheeks, add **mai dong** (Ophiopogonis Radix) 麦冬 6–9g.
- With Spleen qi deficiency, loss of appetite and loose stools, combine with Sɪ

Jun Zi Tang (Four Gentlemen Decoction 四君子汤, p.873).
- With Kidney qi deficiency, frequent urination and lower back ache, add **bu gu zhi** (Psoraleae Fructus) 补骨脂 12–15g, **he zi** (Chebulae Fructus) 诃子 9–12g and **chen xiang** (Aquilariae Lignum resinatum) 沉香 3–6g to assist Kidneys in grasping qi.

Kidneys failing to assist inspiration of Lung qi
Chronic respiratory weakness, including asthma, often dating from childhood, will place a large demand upon not only the Spleen and Kidneys as the source of yuan qi. Tiredness is accompanied by lower back ache, weak legs and knees, urinary frequency and chronic wheezing. The treatment is to warm and supplement the Lungs and Kidneys and support yuan qi. Combine the principal prescription with a prepared medicine such as GE JIE BU SHEN WAN (Kidney Supplementing Pill with Gecko) or GE JIE DA BU WAN (Gecko Tonic Teapills).

Prepared medicines
Concentrated powder
Bu Fei Tang (Ginseng & Aster Combination)
Bu Zhong Yi Qi Tang (Ginseng & Astragalus Combination)
Si Jun Zi Tang (Four Major Herb Combination)
    – with Spleen qi deficiency
Ren Shen Ge Jie San (Ginseng & Gecko Combination)
    – Kidney failing to grasp qi

Pills
Yu Ping Feng Wan (Jade Screen Teapills)
Bu Zhong Yi Qi Wan (Central Qi Pills)
Ge Jie Bu Shen Wan (Kidney Supplementing Pill with Gecko)
Ge Jie Da Bu Wan (Gecko Tonic Teapills)

Acupuncture (select from)
Du.14 (dazhui +▲)...........meeting point of all the yang channels, strengthens the Lungs and fortifies wei qi
Bl.13 (feishu +▲)...............transport point of the Lungs, strengthens the Lungs and fortifies wei qi
Bl.20 (pishu +▲) ....transport point of the Spleen, strengthens the Spleen and supplements qi
Ren.17 (shanzhong) ....promotes correct movement of qi in the chest and assist descent of Lung qi
Ren.12 (zhongwan +▲)....... alarm point of the Stomach, strengthens the Spleen and Stomach and supplements qi
Lu.9 (taiyuan +) ....source point of the Lungs, strengthens and supplements Lung qi and yin
St.36 (zusanli +▲) ....sea point of the Stomach, strengthens the Spleen, supplements qi and stimulates the qi dynamic
- with spontaneous sweating, add LI.4 (hegu +) and Kid.7 (fuliu)
- with Kidneys not grasping qi, use Lu.7 (lieque) and Kid.6 (zhaohai) to open

renmai and strengthen the Lung Kidney axis.
- Ear points: lung, spleen, zero point, sympathetic, adrenal

Clinical notes
- Tiredness of a Lung qi deficiency type may be diagnosed as chronic asthma, weak lungs from recurrent chest infection or whooping cough, immune deficiency, unresolved grief of sadness or an excessively sedentary life with no exercise.
- Lung qi deficiency is a common cause of tiredness and lack of vitality, especially in children, and responds well to treatment.
- A qi supplementing diet is essential. See Clinical Handbook, Vol.2, see p.870.
- Moderate aerobic exercise and breathing exercises are beneficial in strengthening the Spleen and Lungs, and building qi. Swimming is especially good.

脾气虚 18.6.2 SPLEEN QI DEFICIENCY

Treatment principle
Supplement qi and strengthen the Spleen

Prescription

SI JUN ZI TANG 四君子汤
Four Gentlemen Decoction

ren shen (Ginseng Radix) 人参 6–9g
bai zhu (Atractylodis macrocephalae Rhizoma) 白术 9–12g
fu ling (Poria) 茯苓 9–12g
zhi gan cao (Glycyrrhizae Radix preparata) 炙甘草 3–6g
Method: Decoction. **Ren shen** strengthens the Spleen and supplements yuan qi; **bai zhu** strengthens Spleen and dries damp; **fu ling** strengthens the Spleen leaches out damp; **zhi gan cao** strengthens the Spleen and supplements qi. (Source: *Zhong Yi Nei Ke Xue* [*He Ji Ju Fang*])

Modifications
- With foggy head and poor concentration, add **shi chang pu** (Acori tatarinowii Rhizoma) 石菖蒲 6–9g and **yuan zhi** (Polygalae Radix) 远志 6–9g.
- With loose or watery stools, add **ge gen** (Puerariae Radix) 葛根 9–12g and **mu xiang** (Aucklandiae Radix) 木香 6–9g.
- With cold, add **gan jiang** (Zingiberis Rhizoma) 干姜 6–9g and **rou gui** (Cinnamomi Cortex) 肉桂 3–6g.
- With edema, increase the dose of **fu ling** (Poria) 茯苓 to 18g, and add **ze xie** (Alismatis Rhizoma) 泽泻 9–12g and **che qian zi** (Plantaginis Semen) 车前子 9–12g.
- With Liver qi constraint, add **chai hu** (Bupleuri Radix) 柴胡 6–9g and **bai shao** (Paeoniae Radix alba) 白芍 9–12g.
- With wei qi deficiency, add **zhi huang qi** (honey fried Astragali Radix) 炙黄芪 15–30g and **wu wei zi** (Schizandrae Fructus) 五味子 6–9g.
- With food stagnation, add **shan zha** (Crataegi Fructus) 山楂 12–15g, **chao mai ya** (stir fried Hordei Fructus germinantus) 炒麦芽 15–30g and **chao shen qu** (stir fried Massa medicata fermentata) 炒神曲 12–15g.

- With intestinal candidiasis or other parasites (*gǔ* 蠱), add **bai zhi** (Angelicae dahuricae Radix) 白芷 6–9g, **zi su ye** (Perillae Folium) 紫苏叶 6–9g and **bo he** (Mentha haplocalycis Herba) 薄荷 6–9g.

Variations and additional prescriptions
Spleen qi deficiency with damp
Spleen qi deficiency is often complicated by damp. When present, damp gives the fatigue and tiredness a slightly different quality. Patients with qi deficiency and damp, will find it hard to get started in the morning, then will improve during the morning, and feel tired again in the afternoon. Damp can settle like a mist over the consciousness, so foggy head or difficulty in concentration is more pronounced. The lack of energy and fatigue of qi deficiency are compounded by a sense of heaviness or sluggishness in the body, that makes every activity more of an effort. Patients will want to lie down and sleep a lot, but will wake feeling worse. As for all qi deficiency patterns, the tongue is pale, swollen and scalloped. The difference is in the tongue coat, the thickness and greasiness of which reflects the degree of damp. The treatment is to strengthen the Spleen, supplement qi and transform damp with a prescription such as **SHEN LING BAI ZHU SAN** (Ginseng, Poria and White Atractylodes Powder 参苓白术散).

ren shen (Ginseng Radix) 人参 100g
bai zhu (Atractylodes macrocephalae Rhizoma) 白术 100g
fu ling (Poria) 茯苓 100g
shan yao (Dioscoreae Rhizoma) 山药 100g
zhi gan cao (Glycyrrhizae Radix preparata) 炙甘草 100g
bai bian dou (Dolichos Semen) 白扁豆 75g
yi ren (Coicis Semen) 苡仁 50g
lian zi (Nelumbinis Semen) 莲子 50g
jie geng (Platycodi Radix) 桔梗 50g
sha ren (Amomi Fructus) 砂仁 50g

Method: Powder or pills. Grind the herbs to a fine powder and take in 6–9 gram doses, two or three times daily with warm water. Can also be decocted with an 80–90% reduction is dose. **Ren shen, bai zhu, yi ren, fu ling, bai bian dou, shan yao** and **zhi gan cao** strengthen the Spleen and supplement qi; **bai zhu** dries damp; **yi ren, fu ling** and **bai bian dou** leach out damp; **lian zi** astringes the Intestines and stops diarrhea; **jie geng** raises qi upwards thus alleviating the diarrhea; **sha ren** transforms damp and regulates qi. (Source: *Zhong Yi Nei Ke Xue* [*He Ji Ju Fang*])

Qi and blood deficiency
Weakness of the Spleen frequently leads to a failure of blood production or an increased tendency to bleeding disorders with subsequent blood loss and deficiency. This may manifest in heavy menstrual periods, easy bruising or rectal bleeding. Rectal bleeding is often 'occult', especially when the source of the bleeding is high in the bowel, and not easily observed in the stools. A significant amount of blood can be lost in this way. Treatment is to strengthen the Spleen and supplement qi and blood with a formula such as **GUI PI TANG** (Restore the Spleen Decoction 归脾汤, p.820). Other suitable prescriptions include **BA ZHEN TANG** (Eight Treasure Decoction 八珍汤, p.275) or **SHI QUAN DA BU TANG** (All Inclusive Great Supplementing Decoction 十全大补汤, p.758).

Qi deficiency fatigue and heat
When qi is extremely weak, it can create the illusion of heat, with the patient severely fatigued and feeling hot in the morning (see p.382 for the mechanism). The treatment is to supplement Spleen and Lung qi and elevate qi with a prescription such as **BU ZHONG YI QI TANG** (Supplement the Middle to Augment the Qi Decoction 补中益气汤 p.382).

Prepared medicines
Concentrated powders
Si Jun Zi Tang (Four Major Herb Combination)
Shen Ling Bai Zhu San (Ginseng & Atractylodes Formula)
Bu Zhong Yi Qi Tang (Ginseng & Astragalus Combination)

Pills
Si Jun Zi Wan (Four Gentlemen Teapills)
Shen Ling Bai Zhu Wan (Absorption and Digestion Pill, Shen Ling Bai Zhu Pian)
Bu Zhong Yi Qi Wan (Central Qi Pills)

Acupuncture (select from)
Ren.12 (zhongwan +▲) ....alarm point of the Stomach, strengthens the Spleen and Stomach and supplements qi

St.36 (zusanli +▲) ....sea point of the Stomach, strengthens the Spleen and Stomach, supplements qi to transforms damp

Sp.3 (taibai)........................source and connecting points of the Spleen and
St.40 (fenglong)   Stomach; these points strengthen the Spleen and have a special effect on fatigue, heaviness and lethargy from Spleen deficiency and damp

Du.20 (baihui ▲) ....clears the head and elevates qi

Bl.20 (pishu +▲) ....transport points of the Spleen and Stomach,
Bl.21 (weishu +▲)   strengthen middle burner qi

- with foggy head, add Bl.62 (shenmai)
- with edema, add Sp.9 (yinlingquan –) and Sp.6 (sanyinjiao)
- with somnolence, add Kid.6 (zhaohai) and Bl.62 (shenmai)
- with abdominal pain, add Sp.4 (gongsun)
- with diarrhea, add St.25 (tianshu ▲) and Du.20 (baihui ▲)
- with abdominal distension, add St.25 (tianshu) and Sp.15 (daheng)
- with bleeding or bruising, add Sp.1 (yinbai ▲)
- Ear points: spleen, lung, zero point, sympathetic, adrenal

Clinical notes
- Spleen qi deficiency tiredness is common, and may be diagnosed as dietary inadequacy, malnutrition, malabsorption, food intolerance or allergy, celiac disease, irritable bowel syndrome, insulin intolerance or early stage type 2 diabetes, anorexia nervosa, intestinal parasites, Vitamin B12 deficiency or anemia.
- Tiredness of a Spleen qi deficiency type usually responds reliably to treatment. In most cases, the patient should expect to see some improvement in energy within a couple of weeks, then gradual restoration and sustainability of energy

over several months.
- A qi supplementing diet is essential. See Clinical Handbook, Vol.2, see p.870.
- Moderate aerobic exercise is beneficial in strengthening the Spleen and Lungs, and building qi.

肾
气
虚

18.6.3 KIDNEY QI DEFICIENCY

Treatment principle
Supplement the Kidneys and yuan qi
Strengthen the Spleen and Lungs

Prescription

DA BU YUAN JIAN 大补元煎
Great Supplement the Basal Decoction, modified

ren shen (Ginseng Radix) 人参 3–15g
shan yao (Dioscoreae Rhizoma) 山药 6–12g
shu di (Rehmanniae Radix preparata) 熟地 6–15g
du zhong (Eucommiae Cortex) 杜仲 6–9g
dang gui (Angelicae sinensis Radix) 当归 6–9g
gou qi zi (Lycii Fructus) 枸杞子 6–9g
zhi gan cao (Glycyrrhizae Radix preparata) 炙甘草 3–6g
huang qi (Astragali Radix) 黄芪 12–18g
Method: Decoction. **Shu di** and **shan yao** supplement the Kidneys and support jing; **gou qi zi** and **du zhong** augment Kidney qi; **huang qi**, **ren shen** and **zhi gan cao** strengthen the Spleen and supplement qi; **dang gui** nourishes blood. (Source: *Zhong Yi Nei Ke Xue* [*Jing Yue Quan Shu*])

Modifications
- With frequent urination and nocturia, add **tu si zi** (Cuscutae Semen) 菟丝子 6–9g, **yi zhi ren** (Alpiniae oxyphyllae Fructus) 益智仁 6–9g and **jin ying zi** (Rosae laevigatae Fructus) 金樱子 6–9g.
- With loose stools, delete **dang gui** and **shu di** and add **bai zhu** (Atractylodis macrocephalae Rhizoma) 白术 12–15g and **fu ling** (Poria) 茯苓 12–15g.
- With premature ejaculation, add **lian xu** (Nelumbinis Stamen) 连续 3–6g, **mu li** (Ostreae Concha) 牡蛎 15–30g [cooked first] and **long gu** (Fossilia Ossis Mastodi) 龙骨 15–30g [cooked first].
- With lower abdominal pain, add **xiao hui xiang** (Foeniculi Fructus) 小茴香 9–12g.

Prepared medicines
Concentrated powder
Ba Wei Di Huang Wan (Rehmannia Eight Formula)
Liu Wei Gu Jing Wan (Rehmannia Six & Stamen Formula)
Fu Tu Dan (Poria & Cuscuta Formula)
    – the latter two for frequent urination, nocturia and leakage of fluids
Pills
Jin Kui Shen Qi Wan (Fu Gui Ba Wei Wan, Golden Book Teapills)
Ba Ji Yin Yang Wan (Ba Ji Yin Yang Teapills)

Acupuncture (select from)

Ren.4 (guanyuan +▲).......supplements Kidney qi

St.36 (zusanli +▲) ....sea point of the Stomach, strengthens the Spleen and supplements qi

Sp.6 (sanyinjiao +).............strengthens the Kidneys and Spleen

Kid.3 (taixi +)....................source point of the Kidney, supplements Kidney qi

Du.4 (ming men +▲) ....warms Kidney yang

Bl.23 (shenshu +▲) ....transport point of the Kidney, strengthens Kidney qi

Bl.52 (zhishi +▲)..............strengthens Kidney qi

- with foggy head, add Bl.62 (shenmai)
- with somnolence, add Kid.6 (zhaohai) and Bl.62 (shenmai)
- with breathlessness or asthma, add Lu.7 (lieque +)
- with urinary frequency and nocturia, add Ren.6 (qihai +▲)
- with edema, add Kid.7 (fuliu –) and Ren.9 (shuifen ▲)
- a moxa box over the lower abdomen is helpful to warm Kidney qi
- Ear points: kidney, spleen, lung, zero point, sympathetic, adrenal

Clinical notes

- Kidney qi deficiency tiredness may be diagnosed as adrenal exhaustion, Addison's disease, neurasthenia, diabetes mellitus, hypothyroidism, prostatic hypertrophy, erectile dysfunction or chronic nephritis.
- Kidney qi deficiency is usually seen in conjunction with Spleen qi deficiency. It is most common in older people, but can be seen in younger people who 'burn the candle at both ends', work all day and party all night.
- Tiredness of this type usually responds to correct treatment, but requires changes to life and work habits for full resolution. In most cases, the patient should expect to see some symptomatic improvement within a few weeks, then see gradual restoration and sustainability of energy over some months. The older and more depleted the patient, the longer rebuilding qi takes.
- A qi supplementing diet is essential. See Clinical Handbook, Vol.2, see p.870.
- Moderate aerobic exercise is beneficial in strengthening the Spleen and Lungs to supplement qi. Taijiquan and some qigong exercises are specific for building Kidney qi.

18.6.4 HEART QI DEFICIENCY

Treatment principle

Supplement qi, strengthen the Heart and calm the shen
Strengthen the Lungs and Spleen

Prescription

YANG XIN TANG 养心汤
Nourish the Heart Decoction

ren shen (Ginseng Radix) 人参 9–15g
zhi huang qi (honey fried Astragali Radix) 炙黄芪 9–18g
fu ling (Poria) 茯苓 9–12g

fu shen (Poriae Sclerotium pararadicis) 茯神 9–12g
dang gui (Angelicae sinensis Radix) 当归 9–12g
chuan xiong (Chuanxiong Rhizoma) 川芎 3–6g
zhi ban xia (Pinelliae Rhizoma preparata) 制半夏 3–6g
bai zi ren (Platycladi Semen) 柏子仁 12–15g
chao suan zao ren (stir fried Zizyphi spinosae Semen) 炒酸枣仁 12–15g
yuan zhi (Polygalae Radix) 远志 6–9g
wu wei zi (Schizandrae Fructus) 五味子 3–6g
zhi gan cao (Glycyrrhizae Radix preparata) 炙甘草 3–6g
rou gui (Cinnamomi Cortex) 肉桂 2–3g

Method: Decoction. **Ren shen**, **zhi huang qi** and **zhi gan cao** supplement qi; **dang gui** nourishes Heart blood; **fu ling**, **fu shen**, **chao suan zao ren**, **bai zi ren**, **chuan xiong** and **yuan zhi** strengthen the Heart and calm the shen; **wu wei zi** constrains Heart yin; **zhi ban xia** combined with **yuan zhi** transforms phlegm, alleviates anxiety, and harmonizes the Stomach; **rou gui** warms and supports Heart qi and promotes normal movement of blood. (Source: *Zhong Yi Nei Ke Xue* [*Zheng Zhi Zhun Sheng*])

Modifications

- In severe cases, add **huang jing** (Polygonati Rhizoma) 黄精 12–15g, and increase the dose of **zhi huang qi** to 30g.
- With loose stools, delete **bai zi ren** and **suan zao ren,** and add **bai zhu** (Atractylodis macrocephalae Rhizoma) 白术 9–12g, **ze xie** (Alismatis Rhizoma) 泽泻 6–9g and **sha ren** (Amomi Fructus) 砂仁 3–6g [added at the end of cooking].
- With phlegm, add **zhu ru** (Bambusae Caulis in taeniam) 竹茹 6–9g and **chen pi** (Citri reticulatae Pericarpium) 陈皮 6–9g.
- When anxious, easily startled and fearful, add **long chi** (Fossilia Dentis Mastodi) 龙齿 15–30g [cooked first].
- With depression, add **he huan pi** (Albizziae Cortex) 合欢皮 12–15g.
- With copious sweating, add **mu li** (Ostreae Concha) 牡蛎 15–30g [cooked first], **ma huang gen** (Ephedrae Radix) 麻黄根 9–12g and **fu xiao mai** (Tritici Fructus levis) 浮小麦 12–15g.
- With insomnia, add **ye jiao teng** (Polygoni multiflori Caulis) 夜交藤 18–30g and **long chi** (Fossilia Dentis Mastodi) 龙齿 12–18g [cooked first].
- With cold hands and feet and a deep pulse, add **zhi fu zi** (Aconiti Radix lateralis preparata) 制附子 6–9g [cooked first].
- With blood stasis and mild chest pain, add **san qi fen** (powdered Notoginseng Radix) 三七粉 3–6g [added to the strained decoction], **dan shen** (Salviae miltiorrhizae Radix) 丹参 9–12g, **tao ren** (Persicae Semen) 桃仁 6–9g and **hong hua** (Carthami Flos) 红花 6–9g.

Variations and additional prescriptions
Heart qi deficiency with arrhythmia
Heart qi deficiency is implicated in poor cardiac function. In addition to the qi deficiency symptoms noted above (p.871), the heartbeat is irregular or irregularly irregular. The more irregular the heartbeat the greater the deficiency. This is a significant contribution to poor exercise tolerance and persistent fatigue. The arrhythmias are initiated or aggravated by exertion. The treatment is to supplement

qi and blood, unblock yang qi and restore the pulse with **ZHI GAN CAO TANG** (Prepared Licorice Decoction 炙甘草汤).

zhi gan cao (Glycyrrhizae Radix preparata) 炙甘草 12–15g
sheng di (Rehmanniae Radix) 生地 24–30g
ren shen (Ginseng Radix) 人参 6–9g
sheng jiang (Zingiberis Rhizoma recens) 生姜 6–9g
gui zhi (Cinnamomi Ramulus) 桂枝 6–9g
e jiao (Asini Corii Colla) 阿胶 6–9g
mai dong (Ophiopogonis Radix) 麦冬 15–24g
huo ma ren (Cannabis Semen) 火麻仁 9–12g
da zao (Jujubae Fructus) 大枣 .... 5 fruit

Method: Decoction. **E jiao** is melted in hot water or rice wine before being added to the strained decoction. **Zhi gan cao** supplements qi, strengthens the Spleen and Stomach and unblocks the flow of yang qi to the Heart; **ren shen** and **da zao** strengthen the Spleen and supplement qi; **sheng di**, **mai dong**, **huo ma ren** and **e jiao** nourish yin and moisten dryness; **sheng jiang**, **gui zhi** and the rice wine promote the movement of yang qi in the chest and assist in restoring the pulse. (Source: *Shi Yong Zhong Yi Nei Ke Xue* [*Shang Han Lun*])

Sinking da qi

When da qi (synonymous with zong qi and thus Lung and Heart function), is significantly weak, it can collapse into the middle and lower burners. The clinical features reflect the lack of qi in the chest and accumulation of qi in the lower body. In addition to severe fatigue, the symptoms include a sense of emptiness in the chest along with fullness or bearing down in the lower abdomen, breathlessness, palpitations and a pulse that is weak or imperceptible, especially in the distal position. There may be dizziness, fainting, confusion and forgetfulness. The treatment is to strengthen and raise sinking qi with **SHENG XIAN TANG** (Raise the Sunken Decoction 升陷汤, p.273).

Prepared medicines

Concentrated powder
Yang Xin Tang (Astragalus & Zizyphus Combination)
Zhi Gan Cao Tang (Licorice Combination)
Bu Zhong Yi Qi Tang (Ginseng & Astragalus Combination)
  – to lift sinking qi

Pills
Gui Pi Wan Gui Pi Wan (Kwei Be Wan, Gui Pi Teapills)
Zhi Gan Cao Wan (Zhi Gan Cao Teapills)
Bu Zhong Yi Qi Wan (Central Chi Teapills)

Acupuncture (select from)

Bl.15 (xinshu +) ....transport point of the Heart, strengthens the Heart and supplements Heart qi, calms the Heart and shen
Ren.14 (juque +) ....alarm point of the Heart, calms the Heart and shen
Ht.7 (shenmen +)...............source point of the Heart, strengthens the Heart, supplements Heart qi and calms the shen
PC.6 (neiguan –).................connecting point of the Pericardium, opens up qi

               flow through the chest, calms the Heart and shen

Sp.6 (sanyinjiao)..................strengthens the Spleen and supplements qi

St.36 (zusanli +▲) ....sea point of the Stomach, strengthens the Spleen and supplements qi

Ren.6 (qihai +▲) ....supplements Kidney qi and supports Heart yang

yin tang (M–HN–3) ....calms the shen

- with sinking qi add Du.20 (baihui ▲)
- with spontaneous sweating, add Bl.43 (gaohuangshu) and Du.14 (dazhui ▲)
- Ear points: heart, spleen, lung, zero point, sympathetic, adrenal, shenmen

Clinical notes

- Tiredness of a Heart qi deficiency type can be quite profound, bordering on exhaustion. It may be diagnosed as anemia, congestive cardiac failure, post viral syndrome, sinus tachycardia, premature ectopic beats, anxiety, depression or sick sinus syndrome.
- This pattern is closely related to and often precedes Heart yang deficiency.
- Heart qi deficiency can respond reasonably well to treatment, but can take some months of treatment for a sustained result.
- Qi gong, taijiquan, yoga or a carefully monitored and graded exercise program can gradually build the qi and strengthen the Heart.
- A qi supplementing diet is essential. See Clinical Handbook, Vol.2, see p.870.

阳
虚
18.7 YANG DEFICIENCY

1. Spleen
2. Kidney
3. Heart
4. Liver

Yang qi is the basis of the body's warmth, vitality and drive, hence yang deficiency is characterized by profound weariness, lack of motivation and feeling cold. Yang deficiency can affect the Kidneys, Spleen, Heart and Liver, each with it own specific features. The fatigue characteristic of insufficient yang is consistent however, regardless of the organ system most affected. Because the Kidneys are at the basis of the yang of the body, warming and supplementing Kidney yang will bolster all other organ systems. Care must be taken, however, when Spleen yang is weak, as the Kidney yang supplements can be hard for some patients to digest.

Insufficient yang leads to a series of problems associated with failure of yang transformation. Processing and distribution of fluids and food requires yang input so deficiency in this area will lead to problems such as urinary frequency or edema, and weak digestion. In addition, keeping qi and blood moving requires plentiful yang, so profound circulatory and cardiovascular weaknesses can develop in yang deficiency.

Common features

- Yang deficiency produces a deep and disabling exhaustion, and an increased desire to sleep. Patients with yang deficiency have very little energy reserve and once they are at the point of exhaustion they take a long time to recover. They are better for prolonged rest. Their exhaustion is worse in winter and in cold conditions, with exertion or consumption of cold natured foods.
- cold intolerance, cold extremities; patients feel cold to the touch, especially in the lower abdomen and extremities
- depression, lack of motivation

T pale, wet, swollen and scalloped
P deep, slow

Specific features

Spleen yang deficiency

- very tired and sleepy, or unable to stay awake after meals
- energy worse after bowel movement
- muscles easily fatigued and tired; muscle weakness and poor muscle tone; organ prolapse; hard to hold head up
- poor appetite to the point of anorexia
- marked subjective abdominal distension, but abdomen feels flaccid and weak
- soft or loose stools with undigested food; urgent early morning diarrhea
- edema, especially fingers, eyelids and abdomen

Kidney yang deficiency
- lower back ache, weakness and coldness
- frequent urination, nocturia, incontinence
- edema, especially lower limb and ankles
- infertility, loss of libido, impotence

Heart yang deficiency
- icy cold extremities
- breathlessness or wheezing with exertion
- blue discoloration of the lips and around the mouth
- chest pain, chest oppression
- palpitations, bradycardia
- generalized edema
- irregular, intermittent, bound, choppy or imperceptible pulse

Liver yang deficiency
- dull persistent or vague hypochondriac ache, discomfort or fullness, worse after activity
- ashen complexion or dull yellow, dark or matt jaundice; this type of jaundice is usually mild and easy to miss in artificial lighting
- nervousness, timidity, depression, melancholy

脾
阳
虚

18.7.1 SPLEEN YANG DEFICIENCY

Treatment principle
Warm and strengthen Spleen yang
Supplement yang qi and dispel cold

Prescription

FU ZI LI ZHONG WAN 附子理中丸
Prepared Aconite Pill to Regulate the Middle

zhi fu zi (Aconiti Radix lateralis preparata) 制附子 6–15g
ren shen (Ginseng Radix) 人参 6–12g
chao bai zhu (stir fried Atractylodis macrocephalae Rhizoma) 炒白术 6–12g
gan jiang (Zingiberis Rhizoma) 干姜 3–6g
zhi gan cao (Glycyrrhizae Radix preparata) 炙甘草 3–6g
Method: Grind the herbs to a fine powder and form into small pills with honey. The dose is 6–9 grams of pills two or three times daily. **Zhi fu zi** and **gan jiang** warm yang and strengthen the Spleen; **ren shen**, **chao bai zhu** and **zhi gan cao** strengthen the Spleen and supplement qi. (Source: *Zhong Yi Nei Ke Xue* [*Shang Han Lun*])

Modifications
- With cramping abdominal pain, add **wu zhu yu** (Evodiae Fructus) 吴茱萸 3–6g and **gao liang jiang** (Alpiniae officinarum Rhizoma) 高良姜 6–9g.
- With nausea or vomiting after eating, add **sha ren** (Amomi Fructus) 砂仁 6–9g and **chen pi** (Citri reticulatae Pericarpium) 陈皮 6–9g.
- With marked abdominal distension, add **mu xiang** (Aucklandiae Radix) 木香

6–9g and **sha ren** (Amomi Fructus) 砂仁 6–9g.

- With foggy head or poor concentration, add **shi chang pu** (Acori tatarinowii Rhizoma) 石菖蒲 6–9g and **yuan zhi** (Polygalae Radix) 远志 6–9g.
- With incessant hiccough, add **ding xiang** (Caryophylli Flos) 丁香 3–6g and **xiao hui xiang** (Foeniculi Fructus) 小茴香 9–12g.
- For diarrhea with undigested food or urgent diarrhea first thing in the morning, add **rou dou kou** (Myristicae Semen) 肉豆蔻 6–9g and **bu gu zhi** (Psoraleae Fructus) 补骨脂 9–12g.

Variations and additional prescriptions

There are several variations of the Spleen yang deficiency pattern. Spleen weakness draws heavily on the Kidneys for support, so dual Spleen and Kidney yang deficiency is common. The treatment is to warm and supplement Spleen and Kidney yang by combining the primary prescription above with JIN GUI SHEN QI WAN (Kidney Qi Pill from the Golden Cabinet 金匮肾气丸, p. 826). When Spleen yang deficiency is complicated by marked edema, SHI PI YIN (Bolster the Spleen Drink 实脾饮, p.245) is recommended.

Prepared medicines

Concentrated powder

Fu Zi Li Zhong Tang (Aconite, Ginseng and Ginger Combination)

Pills

Fu Zi Li Zhong Wan (Fu Tzu Li Chung Wan, Li Chung Yuen Medical Pills)
Li Zhong Wan (Li Chung Wan)

Acupuncture (select from)

Ren.12 (zhongwan +▲) ....alarm point of the Stomach, warms and strengthens Spleen and Stomach yang qi

Ren.6 (qihai +▲) ....these points strengthen Kidney yang to support
Ren.4 (guanyuan +▲)   Spleen yang

St.36 (zusanli +▲) ....sea point of the Stomach, warms and strengthens the Spleen and Stomach and supplements yang qi

Sp.6 (sanyinjiao +▲).........strengthens the Spleen and Kidneys

Bl.20 (pishu +▲) ....transport point of the Spleen, warms Spleen yang

Bl.21 (weishu +▲) ....transport point of the Stomach, warms the middle burner

Bl.23 (shenshu +▲) ....transport point of the Kidneys, warms and supports yang

Du.4 (mingmen +▲) ....warms and supports Kidney yang

- a moxa box over the upper abdomen is helpful
- with abdominal distension, add Sp.1 (yinbai)
- with edema, add Ren.9 (shuifen ▲) and Sp.9 (yinlingquan –)
- with phlegm, add PC.5 (jianshi), St.40 (fenglong –) and Sp.3 (taibai)
- Ear points: spleen, kidney, zero point, adrenal, sympathetic

Clinical notes

- Spleen yang deficiency may be diagnosed as malnutrition, malabsorption, food intolerance or allergy, chronic gastroenteritis, celiac disease, post surgical intestinal dysfunction, anorexia nervosa, chronic peptic ulcer disease, dumping syndrome, functional weakness of the stomach, hiatus hernia or chronic colitis.
- Tiredness of a Spleen yang deficiency type generally responds well to treatment, and the patient should notice improvement in energy and digestive function within a few weeks. For lasting results however, treatment usually needs to continue for at least a few months. Depending on the duration and severity of the initial condition, 6–12 months of treatment may be required to rebuild and sustain Spleen yang.
- In the early stages of treatment, patients should be counselled to conserve their energy as it returns and use it to build more, rather than squandering it in increased activity.
- A yang warming diet is essential. See Clinical Handbook, Vol.2, p.873.

18.7.2 KIDNEY YANG DEFICIENCY

Treatment principle
Warm and supplement Kidney yang

Prescription

YOU GUI WAN 右归丸
Restore the Right [Kidney] Pill

shu di (Rehmanniae Radix preparata) 熟地 18–24g
shan yao (Dioscoreae Rhizoma) 山药 9–12g
gou qi zi (Lycii Fructus) 枸杞子 9–12g
tu si zi (Cuscutae Semen) 菟丝子 9–12g
du zhong (Eucommiae Cortex) 杜仲 9–12g
lu jiao jiao (Cervi Cornus Colla) 鹿角胶 9–12g
shan zhu yu (Corni Fructus) 山茱萸 6–9g
dang gui (Angelicae sinensis Radix) 当归 6–9g
zhi fu zi (Aconiti Radix lateralis preparata) 制附子 6–12g
rou gui (Cinnamomi Cortex) 肉桂 6–12g

Method: Pills or powder. The herbs are ground to a fine powder and formed into 9 gram pills with honey. The dose is one pill twice daily. Can also be decocted, in which case **zhi fu zi** is cooked for 30 minutes before the other herbs and **lu jiao jiao** is melted into the strained decoction. **Shu di**, **gou qi zi** and **dang gui** nourish Kidney yin and blood; **shan zhu yu** supplements the Liver; **shan yao** strengthens the Spleen and Kidneys; **tu si zi** and **du zhong** supplement Kidney yang; **zhi fu zi** and **rou gui** warm yang; **lu jiao jiao** benefits yang and jing. (Source: *Zhong Yi Nei Ke Xue* ([*Jing Yue Quan Shu*])

Modifications

- With frequent urination or nocturia, add **sang piao xiao** (Mantidis Ootheca) 桑螵蛸 6–9g, **qian shi** (Euryales Semen) 芡实 9–12g, **jin ying zi** (Rosae laevigatae Fructus) 金樱子 9–12g and **yi zhi ren** (Alpiniae oxyphyllae Fructus) 益智仁 6–9g.

- With watery diarrhea, delete **shu di** and **dang gui** and add **huang qi** (Astragali Radix) 黄芪 12–15g, **chao bai zhu** (stir fried Atractylodes macrocephalae Rhizoma) 炒白术 9–12g and **yi ren** (Coicis Semen) 苡仁 15–30g.
- With urgent early morning diarrhea, delete **shu di** and **dang gui** and add **rou dou kou** (Myristicae Semen) 肉豆蔻 3–6g and **bu gu zhi** (Psoraleae Fructus) 补骨脂 9–12g.
- With wheezing and breathing difficulty, add **bu gu zhi** (Psoraleae Fructus) 补骨脂 9–12g and **wu wei zi** (Schizandrae Fructus) 五味子 6–9g.

Variations and additional prescriptions

Kidney yang deficiency is often complicated by Spleen or Heart yang deficiency. Kidney yang supports the digestive fire of the Spleen, and dual deficiency is can be addressed with a mixture of LI ZHONG WAN (Regulate the Middle Pill 理中丸, p.732) and JIN GUI SHEN QI WAN (Kidney Qi Pill from the Golden Cabinet 金匮肾气丸, p.826).

Kidney yang supports Heart yang and the circulation, transformation and processing of fluids and blood. For Kidney and Heart yang deficiency with marked edema, breathlessness and a pale bluish cast to the face and tongue, the treatment is to support Heart and Kidney yang and mobilize fluids with ZHEN WU TANG (True Warrior Decoction 真武汤, p.249).

Prepared medicines
Concentrated powder
You Gui Wan (Eucommia & Rehmannia Formula)
Ba Wei Di Huang Wan (Rehmannia Eight Formula)
Jin Suo Gu Jing Wan (Lotus Stamen Formula)
– add when there is frequent urination and nocturia

Pills
You Gui Wan (Right Side Replenishing Teapills)
Jin Kui Shen Qi Wan (Fu Gui Ba Wei Wan, Golden Book Tea)
Ba Ji Yin Yang Wan (Ba Ji Yin Yang Teapills)

Acupuncture (select from)
Ren.6 (qihai +▲) ....these points strengthen Kidney yang
Ren.4 (guanyuan +▲)
Ren.8 (shenque ▲) ....warms Kidney yang when treated with moxa on salt; place a piece of thin cloth over the navel and fill it with salt; burn large cones of moxa on the salt. The cloth enables quick removal of the salt and prevents excessive burning.
Kid.3 (taixi +)....................source point of the Kidneys, supplements Kidney yang
St.36 (zusanli +▲) ....sea point of the Stomach, strengthens the Spleen and Stomach and supplements yang qi
Sp.6 (sanyinjiao +▲).........strengthens the Spleen and Kidneys

Bl.23 (shenshu +▲) ....transport point of the Kidneys, strengthens Kidney yang

Du.4 (mingmen +▲) ....warms and strengthens Kidney yang

- a moxa box over the lower abdomen and lower back is useful
- with abdominal distension, add Sp.1 (yinbai)
- with edema, add Kid.7 (fuliu –), Ren.9 (shuifen ▲) and Sp.9 (yinlingquan –)
- Ear points: kidney, spleen, zero point, adrenal, sympathetic

Clinical notes

- Tiredness from Kidney yang deficiency may be diagnosed as hypothyroidism, chronic nephritis, Addison's disease, prostatic hypertrophy, diabetes mellitus, menopausal syndrome or adrenal exhaustion.
- The tiredness of Kidney yang deficiency can be quite debilitating, but generally responds reasonably well to persistent treatment. For lasting results treatment usually needs to continue for at least a few months. Depending on the duration and severity of the initial condition, 6–12 months of treatment may be required to rebuild and sustain Kidney yang.
- In the early stages of treatment, patients should be counselled to conserve their energy as it returns and use it to build more, rather than squandering it in increased activity.
- A yang warming diet is essential. See Clinical Handbook, Vol.2, p.873.

心
阳
虚

18.7.3 HEART YANG DEFICIENCY

Treatment principle

Strengthen the Heart and warm and supplement Heart yang
Activate qi and blood

Prescription

GUI ZHI REN SHEN TANG 桂枝人参汤
Cinnamon Twig and Ginseng Decoction

gui zhi (Cinnamomi Ramulus) 桂枝 9–12g
ren shen (Ginseng Radix) 人参 6–9g
zhi gan cao (Glycyrrhizae Radix preparata) 炙甘草...............................9–12g
chao bai zhu (stir fried Atractylodis macrocephalae Rhizoma) 炒白术 9–12g
gan jiang (Zingiberis Rhizoma) 干姜 9–12g

Method: Grind the herbs to a fine powder and form into small pills with honey. The dose is 6–9 grams of pills two or three times daily. **Gui zhi** and **gan jiang** warm and unblock Heart yang and support the Spleen; **ren shen, chao bai zhu** and **zhi gan cao** strengthen the Spleen and supplement yang qi. (Source: *Shi Yong Zhong Yi Nei Ke Xue* [*Shang Han Lun*])

Modifications

- With intense cold, cold extremities and a bluish tint to the lips and tongue, add **zhi fu zi** (Aconiti Radix lateralis preparata) 制附子 6–12g [cooked first]. In very severe cases up to 30 grams may be used (see Clinical notes).
- With chest oppression or chest pain and a thick or greasy tongue coat from phlegm obstruction, add **gua lou** (Trichosanthis Fructus) 栝楼 15–24g, **zhi**

ban xia (Pinelliae Rhizoma preparatum) 制半夏 9–12g and **xie bai** (Allii macrostemi Bulbus) 薤白 6–9g.

- With blood stasis, add **chuan xiong** (Chuanxiong Rhizoma) 川芎 6–9g, **dan shen** (Salviae miltiorrhizae Radix) 丹参, 9–12g **san qi fen** (powdered Notoginseng Radix) 三七粉 3–6g [taken separately] and **hong hua** (Carthami Flos) 红花 6–9g.
- In critical cases the patient is cold and clammy, cyanotic, pale white and has icy extremities and a fibrillating pulse, indicating imminent collapse of Heart yang. The treatment strategy is to administer an emergency medicine such as GUAN XIN SU HE XIANG WAN (Liquid Styrax Pills for Coronary Heart Disease 冠心苏合香丸), and institute emergency acupuncture techniques (p.251) until paramedic assistance arrives.

Prepared medicines
Concentrated powder
Gui Zhi Ren Shen Tang (Cinnamon & Ginseng Combination)
Zhen Wu Tang (Ginger, Aconite, Poria & Peony Combination)

Pills
Jin Kui Shen Qi Wan (Fu Gui Ba Wei Wan, Golden Book Teapills)
Zhen Wu Tang Wan (True Warrior Teapills)
Fu Zi Li Zhong Wan (Fu Tzu Li Chung Wan, Li Chung Yuen Medical Pills)

Acupuncture (select from)
Bl.15 (xinshu +▲) ....transport point of the Heart, strengthens Heart yang
Ren.14 (juque +▲) ....alarm point of the Heart, calms the Heart and shen
Ren.4 (guanyuan +▲) ....these points strengthen Kidney yang to support
Bl.23 (shenshu +▲)   Heart yang
Du.4 (mingmen +▲)
PC.6 (neiguan –) ....connecting point of the Pericardium, regulates the Heart and opens up flow of yang qi through the chest
Ht.7 (shenmen +) ....source point of the Heart, strengthens the Heart
Ht.5 (tongli) ....connecting point of the Heart, regulates Heart qi and alleviates arrhythmia
St.36 (zusanli +▲) ....sea point of the Stomach, warms and strengthens the Spleen and Stomach and supplements yang qi
- with spontaneous sweating, add Bl.43 (gaohuangshu) and Du.14 (dazhui ▲)
- with edema or watery cough, add Ren.9 (shuifen ▲) and St.28 (shuidao ▲)
- for emergency management of collapsing Heart yang, see p.242.
- Ear points: heart, spleen, kidney, zero point, shenmen, adrenal, sympathetic

Clinical notes
- When Heart yang deficiency is critically weak, fluid can accumulate in the Lungs causing breathing difficulties and imminent collapse. Swift mobilization and elimination of fluids is imperative. In such cases, up to 30 grams of **zhi fu zi** (Aconiti Radix lateralis preparata) 制附子, boiled for an hour first, can be

used to promote strong diuresis for a few days. This may seem like an excessively high dose, but it is safe when used properly and can be life saving in the correct circumstance. Once urinary output increases, the dose of **zhi fu zi** can be reduced while phasing in a Heart and Kidney yang supplementing strategy.

- Heart yang deficiency may be diagnosed as congestive cardiac failure, cardiac arrhythmia, cor pulmonale, sick sinus syndrome, mitral valve prolapse, atherosclerosis, arteriosclerosis or cardiomyopathy.
- Heart yang deficiency can respond to treatment, as long as the initial condition is not too far advanced.
- In the early stages of treatment, patients should be counselled to conserve their energy as it returns and use it to build more, rather than squandering it in increased activity. Once energy levels are stable, gradual improvement of cardiac function is assisted by a graded and moderate exercise program.
- A yang warming diet is essential. See Clinical Handbook, Vol.2, p.873.

肝阳虚 18.7.4 LIVER YANG DEFICIENCY

Treatment principle
Warm the Liver and support yang, nourish Liver blood
Supplement qi and dispel cold

Prescription

NUAN GAN JIAN 暖肝煎
Warm the Liver Decoction, modified

dang gui (Angelicae sinensis Radix) 当归	6–9g
gou qi zi (Lycii Fructus) 枸杞子	9–12g
xiao hui xiang (Foeniculi Fructus) 小茴香	3–6g
rou gui (Cinnamomi Cortex) 肉桂	3–6g
wu yao (Linderae Radix) 乌药	6–9g
chen xiang (Aquilariae Lignum resinatum) 沉香	3–6g
fu ling (Poria) 茯苓	6–9g
sheng jiang (Zingiberis Rhizoma recens) 生姜	6–9g
huang qi (Astragali Radix) 黄芪	9–12g
ren shen (Ginseng Radix) 人参	6–9g
xi xin (Asari Herba) 细辛	2–3g

Method: Decoction. **Rou gui** is added towards the end of cooking. **Rou gui** and **xi xin** warm and supplement Liver yang, and dispel cold from the Liver channel; **xiao hui xiang**, **chen xiang** and **wu yao** warm cold and promote qi movement; **dang gui** and **gou qi zi** enrich and nourish Liver yin and blood; **ren shen**, **huang qi**, **fu ling** and **sheng jiang** strengthen the Spleen and supplement Liver qi. (Source: *Shi Yong Zhong Yi Nei Ke Xue* [*Jing Yue Quan Shu*])

Modifications
- Liver blood and/or yin will often be weak in chronic Liver illness, and need special care and preservation. If yang deficiency and cold is relatively severe, add herbs that can warm without drying or damaging yin or blood, such as **ba ji tian** (Morindae Radix) 巴戟天 12–15g, **rou cong rong** (Cistanches Herba) 肉苁蓉 18–24g, **xian ling pi** (Epimedii Herba) 仙灵脾 12–15g or **tu si zi**

(Cuscutae Semen) 菟丝子 12–15g.
- With nausea and vomiting, add **wu zhu yu** (Evodiae Fructus) 吴茱萸 2–3g and **gan jiang** (Zingiberis Rhizoma) 干姜 9–12g.
- With chronic dull jaundice, add **yin chen** (Artemisiae scopariae Herba) 茵陈 9–12g.

Variations and additional prescriptions
Liver and Spleen/Stomach yang deficiency
Liver and Spleen/Stomach yang deficiency can sometimes give rise to sporadic fatigue patterns accompanied by migraine headaches with vomiting and coldness. The headache is typically at the vertex or temples, can occur premenstrually, and is initiated when the patient is tired or stressed. The tongue is pale with a greasy, white coat. The treatment is to warm the Liver, Spleen and Stomach, downbear counterflow Stomach qi and stop vomiting with WU ZHU YU TANG (Evodia Decoction 吴茱萸汤) modified.

wu zhu yu (Evodiae Fructus) 吴茱萸 3–6g
ren shen (Ginseng Radix) 人参 9–12g
sheng jiang (Zingiberis Rhizoma recens) 生姜 15–20g
da zao (Jujubae Fructus) 大枣 .... 4 fruit
zhi fu zi (Aconiti Radix lateralis preparata) 制附子 3–6g
gan jiang (Zingiberis Rhizoma) 干姜 3–6g
Method: Decoction, best taken cool. **Wu zhu yu** warms the Stomach and Liver, downbears counterflow Stomach qi and stops vomiting; **sheng jiang** and **gan jiang** warm the middle burner and assist the **wu zhu yu** in stopping vomiting; **ren shen** strengthens the Spleen and protects Stomach qi and yin from the effects of vomiting; **da zao** moderates the dispersing and drying nature of **wu zhu yu**; **zhi fu zi** and **gan jiang** warm yang. (Source: *Shi Yong Zhong Yi Nei Ke Xue* [*Shang Han Lun*])

Prepared medicines
Concentrated powder
An Zhong San (Fennel & Galanga Formula)
Wu Zhu Yu Tang (Evodia Combination)

Pills
Tian Tai Wu Yao Wan (Lindera Combination Teapills) plus Si Wu Wan (Four Substances for Women Teapills)

Acupuncture (select from)
Du.20 (baihui ▲) ....raises yang qi, but should not be used when yang qi is ascendant
Liv.14 (qimen +▲)............alarm point of the Liver, warms the Liver and regulates qi
Liv.13 (zhangmen +▲) ......alarm point of the Spleen, strengthens the Spleen and supplements yang qi, harmonizes the Liver and Spleen
Ren.12 (zhongwan +▲) .....alarm point of the Stomach, strengthens the Spleen and Stomach and supplements qi
Ren.13 (shangwan +▲) .....warms the middle burner and dispels cold
Bl.18 (ganshu +▲)............transport point of the Liver, warms the Liver and

regulates qi

PC.6 (neiguan –) ....connecting point of the Pericardium, dredges the Liver, downbears counterflow Stomach qi and corrects the qi mechanism

St.36 (zusanli +) ....sea point of the Stomach, strengthens the Spleen and Stomach and supplements qi

Liv.3 (taichong +) ....source point of the Liver, regulates qi and activates blood, supplements Liver qi, yin and blood

• with phlegm, add PC.5 (jianshi), St.40 (fenglong –) and Sp.3 (taibai)
• with jaundice, add Du.9 (zhiyang)
• with dull hypochondriac pain, add St.21 (liangmen +) and Liv.1 (dadun ▲)
• a moxa box over the epigastrium is helpful
• Ear points: liver, spleen, zero point, adrenal, sympathetic

Clinical notes

• Tiredness of a Liver yang deficiency type may be diagnosed as chronic hepatitis, hepatic cirrhosis, chronic pancreatitis, Meniere's disease, migraine headache, menstrual migraine or chronic gastritis.
• This pattern can respond reasonably well to persistent treatment.
• Because Liver yang deficiency is frequently complicated by yin and blood deficiency, strong pungent hot herbs such as **zhi fu zi** (Aconiti Radix lateralis preparata) 制附子, **gan jiang** (Zingiberis Rhizoma) 干姜 and **rou gui** (Cinnamomi Cortex) 肉桂 must be used with caution and carefully monitored. When required, they are best started in small doses and used for relatively short periods of time, being phased out as yang warmth returns.
• A yang warming diet is essential. See Clinical Handbook, Vol.2, p.873.

血 | **18.8 BLOOD DEFICIENCY**
虚 | 1. Heart
2. Liver

Blood deficiency primarily affects the Liver and Heart, and derives from insufficient production of blood by Spleen qi deficiency, poor nutrition and inadequate replacement of blood after hemorrhage or childbirth.

Blood deficiency patterns are often complicated by other pathologies, in particular blood stasis and qi constraint. The blood stasis can be a direct result of insufficient blood or poor circulation of blood, with subsequent pooling of the remaining blood.

Common features
• The tiredness of blood deficiency is characterized by low reserve of energy, lack of vitality, feelings of apathy and increased vulnerability to the normal stresses of daily life. Patients feel drained and weak. Blood deficiency tiredness is worse with activity, at the end of the day, with prolonged use of the eyes and after a menstrual period, and is better for rest. The tiredness is compounded by difficulty in falling asleep, although once asleep patients may remain so. Exhaustion during the day is replaced by a racing mind at night and a vicious cycle can be established.
• poor concentration and memory, mental dullness
• postural dizziness or light–headedness
• dry skin and hair
• fingernails weak and brittle or ridged
• dry stools, constipation
T pale and thin, or with orangey edges
P fine

Specific features
Liver blood deficiency
• visual disturbances or spots in the visual field, dry irritated eyes
• tics, fasciculation, muscle tightness and spasm, cramps
• stiffness or creaking (crepitus) in the joints
• dull hypochondriac ache
• numbness or paresthesia in the extremities
• menstrual irregularity; scanty or long menses; amenorrhea
• dull background headaches, especially upon waking

Heart blood deficiency
• palpitations
• insomnia, dream disturbed sleep
• anxiety

肝
血
虚

18.8.1 LIVER BLOOD DEFICIENCY

Treatment principle
Supplement and nourish Liver blood
Activate blood, support the Spleen

Prescription

SI WU TANG 四物汤
Four Substance Decoction, modified

dang gui (Angelicae sinensis Radix) 当归 6–12g
shu di (Rehmanniae Radix preparata) 熟地 9–15g
bai shao (Paeoniae Radix alba) 白芍 9–12g
chuan xiong (Chuanxiong Rhizoma) 川芎 6–9g
he shou wu (Polygoni multiflori Radix) 何首乌 6–9g
e jiao (Asini Corii Colla) 阿胶 6–9g
ji xue teng (Spatholobi Caulis) 鸡血藤 12–15g
gou qi zi (Lycii Fructus) 枸杞子 9–12g

Method: Decoction. **E jiao** is melted in the strained decoction. **Shu di** nourishes yin and blood; **dang gui** and **ji xue teng** supplement and activate the blood, harmonize the Liver and regulate menstruation; **bai shao** nourishes blood and softens the Liver; **e jiao**, **he shou wu** and **gou qi zi** nourish blood and support Kidney jing to assist in generation of blood; **chuan xiong** activates blood and moves qi. (Source: *Zhong Yi Nei Ke Xue* [*He Ji Ju Fang*])

Modifications

- With blood stasis, add **tao ren** (Persicae Semen) 桃仁 9–12g, **hong hua** (Carthami Flos) 红花 6–9g and **dan shen** (Salviae miltiorrhizae Radix) 丹参 9–12g.
- With dizziness and tinnitus, add **nu zhen zi** (Ligustri Fructus) 女贞子 9–12g and **ci shi** (Magnetitum) 磁石 15–30g [cooked first].
- With marked numbness in the extremities, increase the dose of **ji xue teng** (Spatholobi Caulis) 鸡血藤 up to 30g.
- With dream disturbed sleep or nightmares, add **he huan pi** (Albizziae Cortex) 合欢皮 12–15g, **ye jiao teng** (Polygoni multiflori Caulis) 夜交藤 15–30g and **long chi** (Fossilia Dentis Mastodi) 龙齿 15–30g [cooked first].
- With Liver qi constraint, add **xiang fu** (Cyperi Rhizoma) 香附 9–12g.
- With anxiety, fearfulness and palpitations, add **long chi** (Fossilia Dentis Mastodi) 龙齿 15–30g [cooked first] and **yuan zhi** (Polygalae Radix) 远志 6–9g.
- With dull hypochondriac ache, add **chai hu** (Bupleuri Radix) 柴胡 3–6, **yu jin** (Curcumae Radix) 郁金 3–6g and **xiang fu** (Cyperi Rhizoma) 香附 6–9g.
- With visual weakness or obstruction, add **jue ming zi** (Cassiae Semen) 决明子 9–15g and **chu shi zi** (Broussonetiae Fructus) 楮实子 6–9g.
- With muscle spasms, fasciculation, tremor or numbness, add **mu gua** (Chaenomelis Fructus) 木瓜 6–9g and **tian ma** (Gastrodiae Rhizoma) 天麻 6–9g.
- With Spleen qi deficiency, diarrhea and abdominal distension, add **bai zhu** (Atractylodis macrocephalae Rhizoma) 白术 9–12g, **shan yao** (Dioscoreae Rhizoma) 山药 12–15g, **dang shen** (Codonopsis Radix) 党参 12–15g, **fu ling** (Poria) 茯苓 9–12g and **chen pi** (Citri reticulatae Pericarpium) 陈皮 6–9g.

Prepared medicines
Concentrated powder
Si Wu Tang (Tangkuei Four Combination)
Tao Hong Si Wu Tang (Tangkuei Four, Persica & Carthamus Combination)
Pills
Si Wu Wan (Four Substances for Women Teapills)
Ba Zhen Wan (Women's Precious Pills, Nu Ke Ba Zhen Wan)
Dang Gui Ji Jing (Tang Kuei Essence of Chicken)
Wu Ji Bai Feng Wan (Black Chicken White Phoenix Pill)
    – these last two have a strong blood building richness based on the medicinal
    black boned chicken, and are especially good for postpartum blood
    deficiency

Acupuncture (select from)
Ren.12 (zhongwan +▲).......alarm point of the Stomach, strengthens the Spleen
                             and Stomach and supplements qi to build blood
Ren.4 (guanyuan +▲)........boosts the Kidneys, supplements yuan qi to build
                             blood
Bl.17 (geshu +)...................meeting point for blood, regulates blood
Bl.18 (ganshu +).................transport point of the Liver, nourishes and supple-
                             ments Liver blood
Bl.20 (pishu +▲) ....transport point of the Spleen, strengthens the Spleen
                             and supplements qi and blood
Sp.6 (sanyinjiao +▲)..........strengthens the Spleen and Kidney, supplements qi
                             and blood, regulates Liver qi and menstruation
St.36 (zusanli +▲) ....sea point of the Stomach, strengthens the Spleen and
                             Stomach and supplements qi and blood
Liv.3 (taichong –)..............source point of the Liver, nourishes Liver blood
• with muscle spasm, add Liv.8 (ququan +) and Du.8 (jinsuo)
• with visual weakness or spots before the eyes, add GB.37 (guanming +)
• with dry irritated eyes, add SJ.2 (yemen +) and GB.20 (fengchi +)
• with postural dizziness, add Du.20 (baihui ▲)
• Ear points: liver, spleen, zero point, sympathetic, shenmen

18.8.2 HEART BLOOD DEFICIENCY
Treatment principle
Supplement Heart blood and Spleen qi
Strengthen the Spleen and calm the shen

Prescription

GUI PI TANG 归脾汤
Restore the Spleen Decoction, modified

zhi huang qi (honey fried Astragali Radix) 炙黄芪	9–12g
ren shen (Ginseng Radix) 人参	6–9g
fu shen (Poria Sclerotium pararadicis) 茯神	9–12g

bai zhu (Atractylodes macrocephalae Rhizoma) 白术 9–12g
dang gui (Angelicae sinensis Radix) 当归 3–6g
long yan rou (Longan Arillus) 龙眼肉 9–12g
suan zao ren (Zizyphi spinosae Semen) 酸枣仁 9–12g
yuan zhi (Polygalae Radix) 远志.. 3–6g
mu xiang (Aucklandiae Radix) 木香.. 3–6g
zhi gan cao (Glycyrrhizae Radix preparata)炙甘草.............................. 3–6g
sheng jiang (Zingiberis Rhizoma recens)生姜 3–6g
da zao (Jujubae Fructus) 大枣 .... 4 fruit
shu di (Rehmanniae Radix preparata) 熟地 9–15g
e jiao (Asini Corii Colla) 阿胶.. 6–9g
ji xue teng (Spatholobi Caulis) 鸡血藤.. 12–15g

Method: Decoction. **E jiao** is melted into the strained decoction. **Zhi huang qi**, **ren shen**, **bai zhu** and **zhi gan cao** strengthen the Spleen and supplement qi; **dang gui**, **shu di**, **ji xue teng** and **e jiao** supplement, nourish and activate blood; **dang gui** and **zhi huang qi** together have a special effect on building blood, especially following hemorrhage; **suan zao ren**, **long yan rou** and **yuan zhi** nourish the Heart and calm the shen; **fu shen** strengthens the Spleen and calms the shen; **mu xiang** regulates qi and aids the Spleen in digesting the blood supplementing herbs; **zhi gan cao** supplements qi and harmonizes the Stomach; **sheng jiang** and **da zao** assist **mu xiang** in aiding digestion of the cloying supplements. (Source: *Shi Yong Zhong Yi Nei Ke Xue* [*Ji Sheng Fang*])

Modifications
- With anxiety and sleeplessness, add **ye jiao teng** (Polygoni multiflori Caulis) 夜交藤 15–30g.
- With palpitations, add **ci shi** (Magnetitum) 磁石 15–30g.
- With diarrhea and abdominal distension, add **shan yao** (Dioscoreae Rhizoma) 山药 12–15g, **chen pi** (Citri reticulatae Pericarpium) 陈皮 6–9g and **yi ren** (Coicis Semen) 苡仁 15–30g.

Prepared medicines
Gui Pi Tang (Ginseng & Longan Combination)
Ba Zhen Tang (Tangkuei & Ginseng Eight Combination)

Pills
Gui Pi Wan (Kwei Be Wan, Gui Pi Teapills)
Shi Quan Da Bu Wan (Ten Flavour Teapills)
   – qi and blood deficiency with cold
Dang Gui Ji Jing (Tang Kuei Essence of Chicken)
Wu Ji Bai Feng Wan (Black Chicken White Phoenix Pill)
   – these last two have a strong blood building richness based on the medicinal black boned chicken, and are especially good for postpartum blood deficiency

Acupuncture (select from)
Ren.12 (zhongwan +▲).......alarm point of the Stomach, strengthens the Spleen and Stomach to supplement qi and build blood
Ren.4 (guanyuan +▲)........boosts the Kidneys, supplements yuan qi to build blood

Bl.15 (xinshu +) ....transport point of the Heart, supplements Heart blood and calms the shen

Bl.17 (geshu +)...................meeting point for blood, regulates blood

Bl.20 (pishu +▲) ....transport point of the Spleen, strengthens the Spleen and supplements qi and blood

Ht.7 (shenmen +)...............source point of the Heart, supplements Heart blood and calms the shen

Sp.6 (sanyinjiao +▲)..........strengthens the Spleen, nourishes and regulates qi and blood, calms the shen

St.36 (zusanli +▲) ....sea point of the Stomach, strengthens the Spleen and Stomach and supplements qi and blood

yintang (M–HN–3) ....calms the shen

- with dream disturbed sleep, add Bl.42 (pohu)
- with anxiety, add Du.19 (houding) and Du.24 (shenting)
- with palpitations, add Ht.5 (tongli)
- with blood stasis, add Sp.10 (xuehai –)
- Ear points: heart, spleen, zero point, sympathetic, shenmen

Clinical notes

- Herbs and appropriate dietary modification are the preferred format for blood supplementation, and are usually quicker and more reliable than acupuncture in building blood. Regardless of the modality, replenishing blood does takes time and persistence, as the well known guiding principal clearly states – 'it takes 40 parts of qi to make 1 part of blood and 40 parts of blood to make 1 part of jing (essence)'.
- A blood nourishing diet is essential. See Clinical Handbook, Vol.2, p874.
- Patients with blood and yin deficiency patterns are often hypersensitive to needles so a gentle approach with few points is recommended to begin with.

阴
虚

18.9 YIN DEFICIENCY

1. Lung
2. Kidney
3. Liver
4. Heart
5. Spleen and Stomach

The tiredness of yin deficiency is characterized by the dual elements of tiredness and exhaustion on the one hand, and a sense of jitteriness, agitation and over stimulation on the other. The tiredness arises from the deficiency, and the agitation from the deficiency heat that develops. The inability to rest satisfactorily compounds the deficiency by inhibiting the sleep that yin requires for replenishment, creating a vicious cycle.

A particular feature of yin deficiency is the anxiety that sufferers experience about their lack of energy. They feel agitated about all the things they feel they should be doing, but are unable to. This leads to a common problem that can arise early in treatment, the tendency to squander returning energy in an attempt to catch up on all they have missed out on. Patients should be firmly counselled to use the energy gains they get to build more by resting, until yin is more reliably sustained.

The basis of the body's yin is the Kidneys, and all yin nourishing prescriptions will enrich Kidney yin to one degree or another.

Common features
- Tiredness or exhaustion, compounded by a sense of jitteriness, agitation and over–stimulation that makes resting difficult. Tiredness tends to be worse in the afternoon and evening. Patients complain of being without energy or completely exhausted at the end of the day, but are unable to relax or fall sleep. If they fall asleep they may be continually woken by internal heat disturbing the shen, or by night sweats. They will often describe themselves as being on edge or feeling burned out, and will appear restless and unable to settle.
- dryness of the skin, hair, eyes, vagina, mouth and throat;
- warm, dry palms; sense of heat in the hands and feet
- dry stools or constipation
- facial flushing, night sweats, low grade fever in the evening

T red, thin and dry with little or no coat
P fine and rapid

Specific features
Lung yin deficiency
- dry, irritating cough, worse at night
- hoarse voice with frequent use
- chronic or recurrent dry or sore throat, worse in the evening
- hemoptysis
- pale face with red cheeks

Kidney yin deficiency
- tiredness and exhaustion can be profound
- lower back and legs aching and weak
- dizziness and tinnitus, worse after exertion and sex
- infertility, menstrual disorders, amenorrhea
- possibly increased sexual desire (but poor sexual response or performance)

Liver yin deficiency
- dry eyes, visual weakness
- headaches, dizziness
- irritability, easy anger
- muscle spasms, calf cramps
- numbness in the extremities
- nightmares, vivid, exhausting dreams

Heart yin deficiency
- palpitations and tachycardia with activity
- anxiety, panic attacks, easily startled
- insomnia, restless and fitful sleep with dreams or nightmares
- recurrent mouth and tongue ulcers

Spleen and Stomach yin deficiency
- poor appetite
- dry mouth and lips with little desire to drink
- constipation
- nausea, dry retching, reflux
- indeterminate gnawing hunger; mild epigastric discomfort
- oral ulceration

肺
阴
虚

18.9.1 LUNG YIN DEFICIENCY

Treatment principle
Nourish and moisten Lung yin
Clear heat and moisten dryness

Prescription

BAI HE GU JIN TANG 百合固金汤
Lily Bulb Decoction to Preserve the Metal

bai he (Lilii Bulbus) 百合	9–15g
shu di (Rehmanniae Radix preparata) 熟地	9–12g
sheng di (Rehmanniae Radix) 生地	9–12g
dang gui (Angelicae sinensis Radix) 当归	6–9g
bai shao (Paeoniae Radix alba) 白芍	6–9g
jie geng (Platycodi Radix) 桔梗	3–6g
xuan shen (Scrophulariae Radix) 玄参	6–9g
chuan bei mu (Fritillariae cirrhosae Bulbus) 川贝母	3–6g

mai dong (Ophiopogonis Radix) 麦冬 6–9g
gan cao (Glycyrrhizae Radix) 甘草 3–6g
Method: Decoction. **Bai he** nourishes yin, clears heat, moistens the Lungs and stops cough; **sheng di** and **shu di** supplement yin and blood; **sheng di** and **xuan shen** cool the blood and clear heat; **mai dong** cools and moistens the Lungs; **chuan bei mu** cools the Lungs, transforms phlegm and stops cough; **dang gui** and **bai shao** nourish and harmonize blood; **jie geng** expels phlegm, stops cough and targets the formula to the upper body; **gan cao** harmonizes the other herbs. (Source: *Shi Yong Zhong Yi Nei Ke Xue* [*Yi Fang Ji Jie*])

Modifications

- With hemoptysis, delete **dang gui** and **jie geng** and add **e jiao** (Asini Corii Colla) 阿胶 6–9g, **xing ren** (Armeniacae Semen) 杏仁 6–9g and **bai mao gen** (Imperatae Rhizoma) 白茅根 15–30g.
- With severe or frequent cough sufficient to disturb sleep, add **bai bu** (Stemonae Radix) 百部 9–12g, **zi wan** (Asteris Radix) 紫菀 9–12g and **kuan dong hua** (Farfarae Flos) 款冬花 9–12g.
- With Heart yin deficiency, irritability, palpitations, insomnia and mouth ulcers, add **dan shen** (Salviae miltiorrhizae Radix) 丹参 9–12g, **he huan hua** (Albizziae Flos) 合欢花 9–12g and **dan zhu ye** (Lophatheri Herba) 淡竹叶 3–6g.
- With qi deficiency and spontaneous sweating, add **wu wei zi** (Schizandrae Fructus) 五味子 3–6g and **ren shen** (Ginseng Radix) 人参 6–9g.
- With afternoon fever, add **yin chai hu** (Stellariae Radix) 银柴胡 9–12g and **di gu pi** (Lycii Cortex) 地骨皮 12–15g.
- With night sweats, add **mu li** (Ostreae Concha) 牡蛎 18–30g [cooked first], **fu xiao mai** (Tritici Fructus levis) 浮小麦 12–15g and **ma huang gen** (Ephedrae Radix) 麻黄根 9–12g.
- With sticky, hard to expectorate sputum, add **hai ge ke fen** (powdered Meretricis/Cyclinae) 海蛤壳粉 3g to the strained decoction.
- With constipation, add **huo ma ren** (Cannabis Semen) 火麻仁 9–12g or **hei zhi ma** (Sesame Semen nigrum) 黑芝麻 6–9g.

Variations and additional prescriptions

Lung dryness
For milder yin deficiency and more Lung dryness, as may occur in the aftermath of a febrile illness, consider SHA SHEN MAI MEN DONG TANG (Glehnia and Ophiopogonis Decoction 沙参麦门冬汤, p.918).

Lung yin deficiency and dryness following a febrile illness
Lung yin and qi can be damaged by a severe or prolonged upper respiratory tract infection. Fatigue, tiredness and cough can persist for some time after the main infection has resolved. The treatment is to clear residual heat from the Lungs and supplement qi and yin with a prescription such as ZHU YE SHI GAO TANG (Lophatherus and Gypsum Decoction 竹叶石膏汤, p.864).

Lung and Kidney yin deficiency
Chronic Lung yin deficiency will drain Kidney yin; conversely, Kidney yin deficiency can fail to support Lung yin. In either case, Lung and Kidney yin deficiency

frequently occur together, and the clinical features reflect the greater depth of the deficiency. In addition to the basic Lung deficiency symptoms there is more heat–tidal fevers, frequent night sweats, as well as concentrated urine, low back ache, tinnitus and hearing deficit. The treatment is to supplement and enrich Kidney and Lung yin with **MAI WEI DI HUANG WAN** (Ophiopogon, Schizandra and Rehmannia Pill 麦味地黄丸, p.917).

Prepared medicines
Concentrated powder
Bai He Gu Jin Tang (Lily Combination)
Sha Shen Mai Men Dong Tang (Glehnia & Ophiopogon Combination)
Pills
Bai He Gu Jin Wan (Lilium Teapills)
Mai Wei Di Huang Wan (Ba Xian Chang Shou Wan, Eight Immortals Teapills)
Yang Yin Qing Fei Wan (Pill to Nourish Yin and Cool the Lungs)

Acupuncture (select from)
Bl.13 (feishu +) ....transport point of the Lungs, nourishes Lung yin, diffuses the Lungs and directs Lung qi downwards
Bl.43 (gaohuangshu + ▲)....an important point for chronic Lung weakness patterns, can be treated with mild moxa for yin deficiency
Lu.9 (taiyuan +) ....source point of the Lungs, strengthens and nourishes Lung qi and yin
Lu.5 (chize) ....sea point of the Lungs, cools the Lungs and directs Lung qi downward
Lu.7 (lieque).......................these points open renmai, supplement Lung and
Kid.6 (zhaohai +)   Kidney yin, diffuse the Lungs and moisten dryness
Bl.23 (shenshu +) ....transport point of the Kidneys, nourishes and supplements Kidney yin
Kid.3 (taixi +)....................source point of the Kidney, supplements yin systemically
- with night sweats add Ht.6 (yinxi)
- with sore throat add Lu.10 (yuji –)
- with hemoptysis add Lu.6 (kongzui –)
- Patients with yin deficiency patterns are often hypersensitive to needles so a gentle approach with few points is recommended to begin with.
- Ear points: lung, kidney, subcortex, sympathetic, endocrine, shenmen

Clinical notes
- Tiredness of a Lung yin deficiency type may be diagnosed as pulmonary emphysema, chronic bronchitis, bronchiectasis, pulmonary tuberculosis, chronic pharyngitis or long term medicated asthma.
- When very prolonged, this type of fatigue can be difficult to alleviate and long term treatment is usually necessary. This is particularly so when Lung yin has been damaged by smoking or prolonged corticosteroid use. More recent pat-

terns due to the damaging effects of fever, can respond well and quite quickly.

- Mild activity in the form of qigong or taijiquan can be helpful in assisting Kidney yin, and therefore systemic yin. Adequate rest is essential for replenishing yin.
- A yin nourishing diet is essential. See Clinical Handbook, Vol.2, p876.

肾阴虚 18.9.2 KIDNEY YIN DEFICIENCY

Treatment principle
Nourish and supplement Kidney yin
Clear deficient heat

Prescription

ZUO GUI WAN 左归丸
Restore the Left [Kidney] Pill

shu di (Rehmanniae Radix preparata) 熟地 12–24g
shan yao (Dioscoreae Radix) 山药 12–15g
shan zhu yu (Corni Fructus) 山茱萸 12–15g
gou qi zi (Lycii Fructus) 枸杞子 9–12g
tu si zi (Cuscutae Semen) 菟丝子 9–12g
lu jiao jiao (Cervi Cornus Colla) 鹿角胶 9–12g
gui ban jiao (Testudinis Plastri Colla) 龟板胶 9–12g
huai niu xi (Achyranthis bidentatae Radix) 怀牛膝 6–9g

Method: Pills or powder. Grind the herbs to a powder and form into 9 gram pills with honey. The dose is one pill 2–3 times daily. May also be decocted with dosages as shown. When decocted **lu jiao jiao** and **gui ban jiao** are melted before being added to the strained decoction. **Shu di**, **shan yao** and **shan zhu yu** supplement Kidney yin; **gui ban jiao** and **lu jiao jiao** have a rich 'meatiness' that is especially enriching to yin, yang, blood and jing; **gou qi zi**, **tu si zi** and **huai niu xi** supplement the Kidneys and support jing. (Source: *Shi Yong Zhong Yi Nei Ke Xue* [*Jing Yue Quan Shu*])

Modifications

- With overheating and facial flushing, add **huang bai** (Phellodendri Cortex) 黄柏 6–9g and **xuan shen** (Scrophulariae Radix) 玄参 12–15g.
- With afternoon fever or bone steaming, add **qing hao** (Artemisiae annuae Herba) 青蒿 9–12g, **bie jia** (Trionycis Carapax) 鳖甲 9–15g and **yin chai hu** (Stellariae Radix) 银柴胡 9–12g.
- With marked insomnia, add **suan zao ren** (Zizyphi spinosae Semen) 酸枣仁 12–15g, **bai zi ren** (Platycladi Semen) 柏子仁 9–12g, **ye jiao teng** (Polygoni multiflori Caulis) 夜交藤 15–30g and **he huan pi** (Albizziae Cortex) 合欢皮 12–15g.

Variations and additional prescriptions

There are numerous variations of the basic Kidney yin deficiency pattern.

- With marked deficiency heat ZHI BAI DI HUANG WAN (Anemarrhena, Phellodendron and Rehmannia Pill 知柏地黄丸, p.922) or DA BU YIN WAN (Great Supplement the Yin Pill 大补阴丸, p.914) can be used.
- With Heart and Kidney yin deficiency causing severe sleeplessness, anxiety, palpitations and mouth ulcers, TIAN WANG BU XIN DAN (Emperor of Heaven's

Special Pill to Supplement the Heart 天王补心丹, p.904) can be used.

- Yin deficiency patterns usually respond quite well to prepared medicines, and it can be helpful to use different formulas at different times of the day to assist with specific aspects of the pathology. For example, LIU WEI DI HUANG WAN in the morning to nourish yin in general, and TIAN WANG BU XIN DAN when insomnia is prominent, or DA BU YIN WAN when heat is prominent, in the evening before bed.

Prepared medicines
Concentrated powder
Zuo Gui Wan (Cyathula & Rehmannia Formula)
Liu Wei Di Huang Wan (Rehmannia Six Formula)

Pills
Zuo Gui Wan (Left Side Replenishing Teapills)
Liu Wei Di Huang Wan (Six Flavor Teapills)
 – Kidney yin deficiency
Da Bu Yin Wan (Abundant Yin Teapills)
 – Kidney yin deficiency with heat
Zhi Bai Ba Wei Wan (Eight Flavor Rehmannia Teapills)
 – Kidney yin deficiency with heat
Tian Wang Bu Xin Dan (Emperor's Teapills, Tian Wang Pu Hsin Tan)

Acupuncture (select from)
Ren.4 (guanyuan +)............these points supplement Kidney yin and yuan qi
Ren.6 (qihai +)
Kid.3 (taixi +)....................source point of the Kidneys, supplements Kidney yin and clears deficiency heat
Kid.7 (fuliu –) ....connecting point of the Kidney, supplements Kidney yin and clears heat
Lu.7 (lieque).....................master and couple points of renmai, these points
Kid.6 (zhaohai)   supplement Kidney yin and moisten dryness
Sp.6 (sanyinjiao)................nourishes Kidney, Liver and Spleen yin
Bl.23 (shenshu +) ....transport point of the Kidneys, supplements Kidney yin
Bl.52 (zhishi +)..................supplements the Kidneys

- with insomnia, add Ht.7 (shenmen) and PC.6 (neiguan –)
- with night sweats, add Ht.6 (yinxi –)
- with anxiety, add yintang (M–HN–3) and Du.20 (baihui)
- with forgetfulness, add Du.20 (baihui)
- with palpitations or arrhythmias add Ht.5 (tongli)
- with dizziness, add Du.20 (baihui)
- Patients with yin deficiency patterns are often hypersensitive to needles so a gentle approach with few points is recommended to begin with.
- Ear points: kidney, liver, subcortex, sympathetic, endocrine, shenmen

Clinical notes

- Tiredness of a Kidney yin deficiency type may be diagnosed as diabetes mellitus, hyperthyroidism, Grave's disease, menopausal syndrome, neurasthenia or hypertension.
- Kidney yin deficiency can respond well to treatment.
- Mild activity in the form of qigong or taijiquan can be helpful in assisting Kidney yin. Adequate rest is essential for replenishing yin.
- Patients with yin deficiency patterns, especially Liver and Kidney, are often drawn to stimulants. Their use creates an illusory energy spike, but aggravates the deficiency. The most damaging are illicit drugs such as cocaine, speed and ice, but coffee and even tea can be overstimulating for these patients.
- A yin nourishing diet is essential. See Clinical Handbook, Vol.2, p876.

肝
阴
虚

18.9.3 LIVER YIN DEFICIENCY

Treatment principle
Nourish and enrich Liver yin
Restrain and anchor ascendant yang

Prescription

BU GAN TANG 补肝汤
Supplement the Liver Decoction

shu di (Rehmanniae Radix preparata) 熟地 15–20g
dang gui (Angelicae sinensis Radix) 当归 12–20g
bai shao (Paeoniae Radix alba) 白芍 15–20g
chuan xiong (Chuanxiong Rhizoma) 川芎 12–15g
suan zao ren (Ziziphi spinosae Semen) 酸枣仁 15–20g
mu gua (Chaenomelis Fructus) 木瓜 6–9g
zhi gan cao (Glycyrrhizae Radix preparata) 炙甘草 3–6g
Method: Decoction. **Dang gui** supplements, activates and harmonizes blood; **shu di** nourishes yin and blood and supplements the Liver and Kidneys; **bai shao** nourishes blood, softens the Liver and preserves yin; **chuan xiong** moves qi and activates blood, resolves constraint and stops pain; **suan zao ren** nourishes yin and blood and calms the shen; **mu gua** activates blood and unblocks the channels and network vessels; **zhi gan cao** augments qi and harmonizes the action of the formula. (Source: *Shi Yong Zhong Yi Nei Ke Xue* [*Yi Zong Jin Jian*])

Modifications

- With dry eyes and weak vision, add **gou qi zi** (Lycii Fructus) 枸杞子 9–12g, **sang shen** (Mori Fructus) 桑椹 6–9g, **jue ming zi** (Cassiae Semen) 决明子 9–12g and **nu zhen zi** (Ligustri Fructus) 女贞子 9–12g.
- With calf cramps or restless legs, use **bai shao** at the upper end of the dosage range and increase the dose of **zhi gan cao** to 9–12g.
- With headaches, dizziness, tinnitus or upper body muscle twitches from ascendant yang, add **shi jue ming** (Haliotidis Concha) 石决明 15–30g, **ju hua** (Chrysanthemi Flos) 菊花 9–12g, **gou teng** (Ramulus Uncariae cum Uncis) 钩藤 9–12g and **bai ji li** (Tribuli Fructus) 白蒺藜 9–12g.
- With numbness or paresthesia in the extremities, add **ji xue teng** (Spatholobi

Caulis) 鸡血藤 15–30g and **si gua luo** 丝瓜络 (Luffae Fructus) 6–12g.
- With heat in the Liver, add **shan zhi zi** (Gardeniae Fructus) 山栀子 3–6g and **huang qin** (Scutellariae Radix) 黄芩 3–6g.
- With hypochondriac pain, add **chuan lian zi** (Toosendan Fructus) 川楝子 9–12g.

Variations and additional prescriptions

There are other prescriptions that address different aspects and complications of Liver yin deficiency. For yin deficiency complicated by qi constraint, YI GUAN JIAN (Linking Decoction 一贯煎, p.816) is recommended. For Liver and Kidney yin deficiency, use QI JU DI HUANG WAN (Lycium Fruit, Chrysanthemum and Rehmannia Pill 杞菊地黄丸, p.467). For Liver yin deficiency with ascendant yang, ZHEN GAN XI FENG TANG (Sedate the Liver and Extinguish Wind Decoction 镇肝熄风汤, p.441) is selected.

Prepared medicines
Concentrated powder
Yi Guan Jian (Linking Combination)
Qi Ju Di Huang Wan (Lycium, Chrysanthemum & Rehamannia Formula)

Pills
Yi Guan Jian Wan (Linking Decoction Teapills)
Qi Ju Di Huang Wan (Lycium–Rehmannia Pills)
Ming Mu Di Huang Wan (Ming Mu Di Huang Teapills)
Suan Zao Ren Tang Pian (Tabellae Suanzaoren)
     – with insomnia

Acupuncture (select from)
Bl.18 (ganshu +)................transport points of the Liver and Kidneys, these
Bl.23 (shenshu +)   points supplement Liver and Kidney yin
Liv.13 (zhangmen +) ....alarm point of the Spleen, strengthens the Spleen, supplements qi and yin
Liv.3 (taichong +) ....source point of the Liver, supplements Liver yin and blood, alleviates spasms, pacifies ascendant yang
St.36 (zusanli +) ....sea point of the Stomach, strengthens the Spleen and Stomach, supplements qi, blood and yin
Sp.6 (sanyinjiao +)..............strengthens the Spleen and Kidneys, dredges the Liver and regulates qi, supplements qi and yin
Liv.8 (ququan –).................sea point of the Liver, supplements Liver blood and yin, relaxes the muscle channels
- Patients with yin deficiency patterns are often hypersensitive to needles so a gentle approach with few points is recommended to begin with.
- Ear points: liver, kidney, subcortex, sympathetic, endocrine, shenmen

Clinical notes
- Tiredness of a Liver yin deficiency type may be diagnosed as chronic hepatitis, menopausal syndrome, premenstrual fatigue, anemia, chronic fatigue syndrome

or hyperthyroidism.
- Liver yin deficiency can respond well to treatment.
- Mild activity in the form of qigong or taijiquan can be helpful in assisting Kidney yin, and therefore systemic yin. Adequate rest is essential for replenishing yin.
- A yin nourishing diet is essential. See Clinical Handbook, Vol.2, p876.
- Caution must be taken in this pattern, especially when complicated by qi constraint, to avoid excessive or prolonged use of qi moving herbs, as they can easily disperse qi and yin and cause aggravation of the symptoms.

心
阴
虚

18.9.4 HEART YIN DEFICIENCY

Treatment principle
Supplement Heart yin
Clear heat and calm the shen

Prescription

TIAN WANG BU XIN DAN 天王补心丹
Emperor of Heaven's Special Pill to Supplement the Heart

sheng di (Rehmanniae Radix) 熟地 ....120 (24)g
tian dong (Asparagi Radix) 天冬 ....30 (12)g
mai dong (Ophiopogonis Radix) 麦冬 ....30 (12)g
suan zao ren (Zizyphi spinosae Semen) 酸枣仁 ....30 (12)g
xuan shen (Scrophulariae Radix) 玄参 ....15 (12)g
dan shen (Salviae miltiorrhizae Radix) 丹参 ....15 (12)g
fu ling (Poria) 茯苓 ....15 (12)g
dang gui (Angelicae sinensis Radix) 当归 ....30 (9)g
wu wei zi (Schizandrae Fructus) 五味子 ....30 (9)g
bai zi ren (Platycladi Semen) 柏子仁 ....30 (9)g
ren shen (Ginseng Radix) 人参 ....15 (9)g
jie geng (Platycodi Radix) 桔梗 ....15 (9)g
yuan zhi (Polygalae Radix) 远志 ....15 (6)g

Method: Pills or powder. Grind herbs to a powder and form into 9 gram pills with honey. The dose is one pill 2–3 times daily. May also be decocted with the quantities in brackets. **Sheng di** and **xuan shen** nourish and supplement Kidney yin to restrain Heart Fire and cool the blood; **tian dong** and **mai dong** nourish yin; **dan shen** and **dang gui** nourish and activate blood and prevent the supplementing herbs from causing blood stasis; **suan zao ren**, **bai zi ren** and **yuan zhi** calm the shen; **ren shen** and **fu ling** strengthen the Spleen, supplement qi and calm the shen; **wu wei zi** secures Heart qi and yin and calms the shen; **jie geng** directs the action of the other herbs to the upper body. (Source: *Zhong Yi Nei Ke Xue* [*She Sheng Mi Pou*])

Variations and additional prescriptions
Heart yin and qi deficiency
Heart yin deficiency is often complicated by qi deficiency, with the development of various arrhythmias. Fatigue can be profound, and is aggravated by any exertion. The treatment is to boost Heart qi and yin, unblock yang qi and restore the pulse with **ZHI GAN CAO TANG** (Prepared Licorice Decoction 炙甘草汤, p.811).

After a major shock or trauma

Following a major shock or trauma there may be persistent fatigue and daytime sleepiness, night sweats, anxiety, insomnia and dream or nightmare disturbed sleep, palpitations, dizziness and depression. This is typical of interrupted communication between the Heart and Kidneys due to shock, a form of post traumatic stress. The treatment is to restore communication between the Heart and Kidneys and calm the shen with GUI ZHI JIA LONG GU MU LI TANG (Cinnamon Twig Decoction plus Dragon Bone and Oyster Shell 桂枝加龙骨牡蛎汤, p.711).

Prepared medicines

Concentrated powder

Tian Wang Bu Xin Dan (Ginseng & Zizyphus Formula)
Zhi Gan Cao Tang (Licorice Combination)
Gui Zhi Jia Long Gu Mu Li Tang (Cinnamon & Dragon Bone Combination)

Pills

Tian Wang Bu Xin Dan (Emperor's Teapills, Tian Wang Pu Hsin Tan)
Zhi Gan Cao Wan (Zhi Gan Cao Teapills)

Acupuncture (select from)

Bl.15 (xinshu +) ....transport point of the Heart, supplements Heart yin, calms the Heart and shen, clears heat

Bl.23 (shenshu +) ....transport point of the Kidneys, supplements Kidney yin to support Heart yin

Ht.6 (yinxi) ....cleft point of the Heart, clears heat, supplements Heart yin and stops sweating

Ht.7 (shenmen).................source point of the Heart, calms the shen, regulates and supplements Heart yin

Kid.3 (taixi +)....................source point of the Kidney, supplements Kidney yin and clears deficiency heat

Kid.6 (zhaohai +) ....supplements Kidney yin, clears heat and calms the shen

yintang (M–HN–3) ....calms the shen

- Patients with yin deficiency patterns are often hypersensitive to needles so a gentle approach with few points is recommended to begin with.
- Ear points: heart, kidney, subcortex, sympathetic, endocrine, shenmen

Clinical notes

- Heart yin deficiency patterns may be diagnosed as hyperthyroidism, menopausal syndrome, post traumatic stress disorder, anxiety neurosis or post febrile disease.
- Heart yin deficiency can respond well to treatment.
- Mild activity in the form of qigong or taijiquan can be helpful in assisting Kidney yin, and therefore systemic yin. Adequate rest is essential for replenishing yin.
- A yin nourishing diet is essential. See Clinical Handbook, Vol.2, p876.

脾
胃
阴
虚

18.9.5 SPLEEN AND STOMACH YIN DEFICIENCY
Treatment principle
Supplement Spleen and Stomach qi and yin
Prescription

SHEN LING BAI ZHU SAN 参苓白术散
Ginseng, Poria and White Atractylodes Powder, modified

tai zi shen (Pseudostellariae Radix) 太子参 100g
bai zhu (Atractylodes macrocephalae Rhizoma) 白术 100g
fu ling (Poria) 茯苓 100g
shan yao (Dioscoreae Rhizoma) 山药 100g
zhi gan cao (Glycyrrhizae Radix preparata) 炙甘草 100g
bai bian dou (Dolichos Semen) 白扁豆 75g
yi ren (Coicis Semen) 苡仁 50g
lian zi (Nelumbinis Semen) 莲子 50g
jie geng (Platycodi Radix) 桔梗 50g
qian shi (Euryales Semen) 芡实 50g
gu ya (Setariae Fructus germinatus) 谷芽 100g
yu zhu (Polygonati odorati Rhizoma) 玉竹 100g
Method: Pills or powder. Grind the herbs to a powder and take 9 grams, 2–3 times daily with warm water. **Tai zi shen, bai zhu, yi ren, fu ling, bai bian dou, shan yao, qian shi** and **zhi gan cao** strengthen the Spleen and Stomach and supplement yin and qi; **yi ren, fu ling** and **bai bian dou** normalize fluid metabolism; **lian zi** supplements the Spleen and alleviates diarrhea; **jie geng** and **gu ya** lightly elevate qi and alleviate diarrhea; **yu zhu** nourishes Spleen and Stomach yin. (Source: *Shi Yong Zhong Yi Nei Ke Xue* [*He Ji Ju Fang*])

Modifications
• With qi deficiency, spontaneous sweating, shortness of breath and frequent colds, add **zhi huang qi** (honey fried Radix Astragali Membranacei) 炙黄芪 15–30g and **wu wei zi** (Fructus Schizandrae Chinensis) 五味子 6–9g.
• With thirst and dryness of mucous membranes, add **mai dong** (Ophiopogonis Radix) 麦冬 6–9g, **sha shen** (Glehniae/Adenophorae Radix) 沙参 12–15g and **tian hua fen** (Trichosanthes Radix) 天花粉 12–15g.
• With heat, add **di gu pi** (Lycii Cortex) 地骨皮 12–15g and **zhi mu** (Anemarrhenae Rhizoma) 知母 9–12g.
• With abdominal distension after eating, add **shen qu** (Massa medicata fementata) 神曲 12–15g and **ji nei jin** (Gigeriae galli Endothelium corneum) 鸡内金 3–6g [powdered and taken separately].
• With constipation, add **rou cong rong** (Cistanches Herba) 肉苁蓉 15–18g and **huo ma ren** (Cannabis Semen) 火麻仁 6–9g.
• With blood deficiency, add **dang gui** (Angelicae sinensis Radix) 当归 6–12g and **ji xue teng** (Spatholobi Caulis) 鸡血藤 12–15g.

Prepared medicines
Concentrated powder
Shen Ling Bai Zhu San (Ginseng & Atractylodes Formula)
Sha Shen Mai Men Dong Tang (Glehnia & Ophiopogon Combination)

Pills

Shen Ling Bai Zhu Wan (Absorption and Digestion Pill, Shen Ling Bai Zhu Pian)

Yu Quan Wan (Jade Spring Teapills)

Acupuncture (select from)

Ren.12 (zhongwan +) ....alarm point of the Stomach, nourishes Stomach yin

Liv.13 (zhangmen +) ....alarm point of the Spleen strengthens the Spleen and Stomach, supplements qi and yin

Bl.20 (pishu +) ....transport points of the Spleen and Stomach,

Bl.21 (weishu +)   supplement yin and qi and regulate the qi dynamic

St.36 (zusanli +) ....sea point of the Stomach, strengthens the Spleen and Stomach, supplements qi and yin and stimulates the qi dynamic

Sp.6 (sanyinjiao +)..............strengthens the Spleen, benefits the Kidneys and supplements qi and yin

St.44 (neiting –) ....clears heat from the Stomach

• Ear points: spleen, zero point, subcortex, sympathetic, endocrine, shenmen

Clinical notes

• Spleen and Stomach yin deficiency type tiredness may be diagnosed as gastroesophageal reflux, chronic atrophic gastritis, chronic gastritis, peptic ulcer disease or reflux esophagitis.

• This is a relatively common cause of fatigue accompanied by chronic digestive problems. It can sometimes be difficult to treat and may take some weeks before adequate symptomatic relief is obtained with herbs and acupuncture. The underlying pattern usually requires sustained treatment for satisfactory results. Mucilaginous substances that put a lining on the esophageal and gastric walls, such as slippery elm powder, are helpful to calm irritated tissues.

• A yin nourishing diet is essential. See Clinical Handbook, Vol.2, p876.

肾
精
虚

18.10 KIDNEY JING DEFICIENCY

Kidney jing deficiency is essentially a composite of multiple organ system weakness, yin, yang, qi and blood deficiency, with all aspects profoundly depleted. Jing deficiency patterns are a common feature of the elderly, and those who have suffered a serious and debilitating illness. It can also be seen in younger people as the result of squandering jing through drug use, excessive sexual activity and 'burning the candle at both ends'.

Clinical features
- persistent and debilitating tiredness, exhaustion and weakness of mind and body
- depression, low spirits, dull eyes, flat affect
- memory problems, senility, confusion
- lower back ache, weakness; aching legs
- sleep disturbances
- emaciation
- hearing deficit, tinnitus
- urinary frequency, nocturia
- poor appetite
- loose teeth, weak gums, tooth loss
- night sweats, feverishness at night
- premature ageing

T pale, swollen
P deep, fine, weak

Treatment principle
Supplement the Liver, Spleen and Kidneys
Nourish and supplement yin, yang and jing

Prescription

HUAN SHAO DAN 还少丹
Special Pill for Rejuvenation

shan yao (Dioscoreae Rhizoma) 山药	45–60g
chuan niu xi (Cyathulae Radix) 川牛膝	45–60g
shan zhu yu (Corni Fructus) 山茱萸	30–45g
ba ji tian (Morindae officinalis Radix) 巴戟天	30–45g
du zhong (Eucommiae Cortex) 杜仲	30–45g
rou cong rong (Cistanches Herba) 肉苁蓉	30–45g
yuan zhi (Polygalae Radix) 远志	30–45g
shi chang pu (Acori tatarinowii Rhizoma) 石菖蒲	30–45g
fu ling (Poria) 茯苓	30–45g
wu wei zi (Schizandrae Fructus) 五味子	30–45g
xiao hui xiang (Foeniculi Fructus) 小茴香	30–45g
chu shi zi (Broussonetiae Fructus) 楮实子	30–45g
gou qi zi (Lycii Fructus) 枸杞子	15–30g

shu di (Rehmanniae Radix preparata) 熟地 15–30g

Method: Pills or powder. Grind the herbs to a fine powder and form in to 9 gram pills with honey. Take one pill two or three times daily with water or rice wine. Can also be decocted with a 60–70% reduction in dose. **Shan yao** and **shan zhu yu** supplement the Spleen, Liver and Kidneys; **chuan niu xi** strengthens the sinews and bones; **ba ji tian, du zhong** and **rou cong rong** warm yang and strengthen the Liver and Kidneys; **yuan zhi** and **shi chang pu** clear the mind and calm the shen; **fu ling** and **shan yao** strengthen the Spleen and supplement qi; **wu wei zi** and **shan zhu yu** fortify the exterior and stop leakage of fluids; **xiao hui xiang** dispels cold and mobilizes qi and blood; **chu shi zi, gou qi zi** and **shu di** nourish yin and supplement the Liver and Kidneys. (Source: *Hong Shi Ji Yan Fang*)

Prepared medicines

Concentrated powders

Huan Shao Dan (Lycium Formula)

Gui Lu Er Xian Jiao (Testudinis & Antler Combination)

Pills

Huan Shao Dan (Return to Spring Teapills)

Zuo Gui Wan (Left Side Replenishing Teapills)

 – tending to yin deficiency

You Gui Wan (Right Side Replenishing Teapills)

 – tending to yang deficiency

Acupuncture (select from)

Ren.4 (guanyuan +) ....these points supplement yuan qi

Ren.6 (qihai +)

St.36 (zusanli +) ....sea point of the Stomach, strengthens the Spleen and supplements yuan qi

Kid.3 (taixi +) ....source point of the Kidneys, supplements the Kidneys

Kid.7 (fuliu +) ....connecting point of the Kidneys, supplements the Kidneys

Lu.7 (lieque) ....master points of the renmai, these points open

Kid.6 (zhaohai)   up circulation of renmai qi and supplement Kidney yin; can be used with the pair below on alternate sides (left hand SI.3, right foot Bl.62, right hand Lu.7, left foot Kid.6, or visa versa) to form a circuit

SI.3 (houxi) ....master and couple points of the dumai, these points

Bl.62 (shenmai)   open up circulation of dumai qi, and strengthen Kidney yang

Sp.6 (sanyinjiao +) ....nourishes Kidney, Liver and Spleen yin

Bl.23 (shenshu +) ....transport point of the Kidneys, supplements Kidneys

Bl.52 (zhishi +) ....supplements the Kidneys

- Care must be taken with needle technique and retention times, as these patients are very depleted, and excessive sensation and treatment length can deplete them further. When in doubt, use few needles with very mild stimulation, or use moxa instead. Moxa is especially indicated if there is a tendency to cold or yang deficiency.

- with insomnia, add Ht.7 (shenmen) and PC.6 (neiguan –)
- with forgetfulness, add Du.20 (baihui) and Bl.52 (zhishi)
- with palpitations or arrhythmias add Ht.5 (tongli)
- with dizziness, add Du.20 (baihui)
- Ear points: kidney, spleen, lung, zero point, shenmen, adrenal, subcortex, endocrine

Clinical notes

- Once jing has been depleted or used up in growing old, a lot of work is required to prevent further deterioration. Jing cannot be replaced, being a fixed constitutional inheritance, but it can be conserved, and the harvesting of acquired qi can be improved to provide better daily wellbeing. The implication of this is that even though the life span may be reduced, the quality of the life remaining can be enhanced.
- A Kidney nourishing diet is essential. See Clinical Handbook, Vol.2, p876.

Table 18.1 Summary of common patterns of tiredness

Pattern	Common Features		Specific Features	Prescription
Liver qi constraint	Intermittent tiredness worse in the morning, with inactivity, premenstrually and when stressed; better with activity. Irritability, tight muscles in upper back and neck, tension headaches, a mauve tongue, or with pale edges and a thin coat, wiry fine pulse			Xiao Yao San Chai Hu Shu Gan San
Damp	Tiredness, heaviness, sleepiness, worse in the morning and with inactivity, better after activity; foggy head, thick, greasy tongue coat, slippery soggy pulse	in the Spleen	Abdominal distension, nausea, loss of appetite, belching, diarrhea, white vaginal discharge	Ping Wei San
		in the muscles	Muscle aches, night sweats, swollen cervical lymph nodes	Huo Po Xia Ling Tang
		damp heat	Muscle aches, afternoon fever, night sweats, swollen lymph nodes, urgent diarrhea, concentrated urine, yellow vaginal discharge, yellow tongue coat, slippery wiry rapid pulse	San Ren Tang Lian Po Yin
Phlegm	Tiredness and somnolence worse for inactivity and eating, better for exercise and fasting; foggy head, mucus congestion, rubbery masses, swollen or flabby tongue, slippery pulse	phlegm damp	Anorexia, loss of taste, abdominal distension nausea and vomiting, reflux, belching, diarrhea	Er Chen Tang
		phlegm heat	Insomnia, palpitations, anxiety, nausea, swollen lymph nodes, thick tongue coat	Zhu Ru Wen Dan Tang
		with qi constraint	Tiredness with an emotional component, lump in the throat, throat clearing	Ban Xia Hou Po Tang
		wind phlegm	Dizziness and vertigo, headache, tinnitus, nausea and vomiting	Ban Xia Bai Zhu Tian Ma Tang
Lingering pathogens	shaoyang		Tiredness after unresolved infection, alternating fever and chills, loss of appetite, nausea, hypochondriac pain, fullness in the chest, dizziness, irritability, bitter taste, wiry pulse	Xiao Chai Hu Tang
	qi level		Tiredness after Lung or Stomach infection, low grade fever, dry cough, nausea, thirst, sweating, irritability, insomnia, sore throat, red dry tongue with little or no coat, weak fine rapid pulse	Zhu Ye Shi Gao Tang

Table 18.1 Summary of common patterns of tiredness (cont.)

Pattern	Common Features		Specific Features	Prescription
Blood stasis	Tiredness with chronic pain and depression. Vascular congestion, skin discoloration, pressure pain in left iliac fossa, dry scaly skin, purple lips and nail, purple tongue with distended dark sublingual veins, deep choppy wiry or intermittent pulse			Xue Fu Zhu Yu Tang
Qi deficiency	Chronic tiredness worse with activity and at the end of the day, better for rest and sleep; pale complexion, daytime sweating, pale swollen scalloped tongue, weak fine pulse	Lung	breathless and clamminess with exertion, weak voice, low immunity, slumped shoulders, wheezing, weak cough	Bu Fei Tang
		Spleen	tiredness after eating, bowel movements and with mental activity, weak muscles, loss of appetite, abdominal distension, loose stools	Shen Ling Bai Zhu San Xiang Sha Liu Jun Zi Tang
		Kidney	frequent urination, nocturia, ankle edema, lower back ache, loss of hearing, premature ejaculation, impotence	Da Bu Yuan Jian
		Heart	palpitations with activity, anxiety, chest oppression, chest pain or an empty feeling in the chest, intermittent pulse	Yang Xin Tang
Yang deficiency	Exhaustion, worse during cold weather or when chilled, cold intolerance, cold to the touch, pale swollen scalloped tongue, deep slow pulse	Spleen	tiredness after meals and bowel movement, muscle weakness, anorexia, diarrhea with undigested food, bloating, edema	Fu Zi Li Zhong Wan
		Kidney	lower back ache, frequent urination, nocturia, edema, impotence, infertility	Jin Gui Shen Qi Wan You Gui Wan
		Heart	icy cold extremities, breathlessness and wheezing with exertion, chest pain, palpitations, edema, pale bluish tongue, irregular pulse	Gui Zhi Ren Shen Tang
		Liver	dull hypochondriac ache, ashen complexion or dull jaundice, anxiety, depression	Nuan Gan Jian

Table 18.1 Summary of common patterns of tiredness (cont.)

Pattern	Common Features		Specific Features	Prescription
Blood deficiency	Tiredness worse with activity, use of the eyes and blood loss. Better for rest. Insomnia, postural dizziness, poor memory, dry skin and hair, brittle nails, pale thin tongue, fine pulse	Heart	palpitations, insomnia, dream disturbed sleep, anxiety	Gui Pi Tang
		Liver	visual disturbances or spots, muscle spasm and cramps, stiff creaky, dull hypochondriac ache, numbness in the extremities, dull headaches	Si Wu Tang
Yin deficiency	Exhaustion with jitteriness, worse in the afternoon and evening. Insomnia, night sweats, dryness, constipation, low grade fever, red, thin, dry tongue with little or no coat, fine rapid pulse	Lung	dry cough, hoarse voice, recurrent sore throat, hemoptysis	Bai He Gu Jin Tang
		Kidney	lower back and legs ache, dizziness, tinnitus, infertility, menstrual disorders, amenorrhea	Liu Wei Di Huang Wan Zhi Bai Ba Wei Wan
		Liver	dry eyes, visual weakness, headaches, dizziness, irritability, muscle spasms and cramps, numbness in the extremities, nightmares	Qi Ju Di Huang Wan Yi Guan Jian
		Heart	palpitations, tachycardia, anxiety, insomnia, tongue ulcers	Tian Wang Bu Xin Dan
		Spleen, Stomach	indeterminate gnawing hunger, thirst, constipation, nausea, mouth ulcers	Yi Wei Tang Shen Ling Bai Zhu San
Jing deficiency	Debilitating exhaustion and weakness of mind and body, flat affect, memory problems, dementia, hearing deficit, loose teeth, premature ageing, pale swollen tongue, deep fine weak pulse			Huan Shao Dan

APPENDIX 1. ADDITIONAL PRESCRIPTIONS
These are the unmodified prescriptions referred to in the text.

BAN XIA XIE XIN TANG 半夏泻心汤
Pinellia Decoction to Drain the Epigastrium

---

zhi ban xia (Pinelliae Rhizoma preparata) 制半夏 9–12g
huang qin (Scutellariae Radix) 黄芩 6–9g
huang lian (Coptidis Rhizoma) 黄连 3–6g
gan jiang (Zingiberis Rhizoma) 干姜 6–9g
ren shen (Ginseng Radix) 人参 6–9g
zhi gan cao (Glycyrrhizae Radix preparata) 炙甘草 6–9g
da zao (Jujubae Fructus) 大枣 .... 4 fruit

Method: Decoction. **Zhi ban xia** transforms phlegm, dries dampness, downbears counterflow Stomach qi and stops nausea and vomiting; **gan jiang** warms the Spleen, raises yang and dispels cold; **huang qin** and **huang lian** clear heat and their bitter descending natures counterbalance the pungent ascent of **gan jiang** to correct the qi dynamic; **ren shen** and **da zao** strengthen the Spleen, supplement qi and prevent the dispersing action of the principal herbs from further injuring Spleen and Stomach qi and yin; **zhi gan cao** strengthens the Spleen and harmonizes the Stomach. (Source: *Shang Han Lun*)

DA BU YIN WAN 大补阴丸
Great Supplement the Yin Pill

---

shu di (Rehmanniae Radix preparata) 熟地 180g
gui ban (Testudinis Plastrum) 龟板 180g
yan chao huang bai (salt fried Phellodendri Cortex) 盐炒黄柏 120g
yan chao zhi mu (salt fried Anemarrhenae Rhizoma) 盐炒知母 120g

Method: Pills. Grind the herbs to a fine powder and form into 9 gram pills with a sufficient quantity of steamed pig spinal cord and honey to bind. The dose is one pill 2–3 times daily with a little salty water on an empty stomach. **Shu di** supplements Kidney yin and blood; **gui ban** and the spinal cord deeply enrich yin and jing, **gui ban** weighs down and anchors ascendant yang and fire; together these substances augment 'water to control fire'; **yan huang bai** and **yan zhi mu** are salt treated to enhance their affinity with the Kidneys; **yan huang bai** clears fire from the Kidneys, **yan zhi mu** clears heat, cools the Lungs and nourishes yin; together they clear heat from below and above–the source of the deficiency and fire, and the organ system most damaged by it, the Lungs. (Source: *Dan Xi Xin Fa*)

DA QIN JIAO TANG 大秦艽汤
Major Gentiana Qinjiao Decoction

---

qin jiao (Gentianae macrophyllae Radix) 秦艽 6–9g
qiang huo (Notopterygii Rhizoma seu Radix) 羌活 3–6g
du huo (Radix Angelicae Pubescentis) 独活 3–6g
fang feng (Saposhnikovae Radix) 防风 3–6g
bai zhi (Angelicae dahuricae Radix) 白芷 3–6g
xi xin (Asari Herba) 细辛 1–2g
dang gui (Angelicae sinensis Radix) 当归 6–9g
bai shao (Paeoniae Radix alba) 白芍 6–9g
chuan xiong (Chuanxiong Rhizoma) 川芎 3–6g
sheng di (Rehmanniae Radix) 生地 9–12g

shu di (Rehmanniae Radix preparata) 熟地 9–12g
bai zhu (Atractylodis macrocephalae Rhizoma) 白术 6–9g
fu ling (Poria) 茯苓 6–9g
huang qin (Scutellariae Radix) 黄芩 6–9g
shi gao (Gypsum fibrosum) 石膏 9–12g
gan cao (Glycyrrhizae Radix) 甘草 3–6g

Method: Decoction. **Qin jiao** dispels wind and clears heat, and opens up flow in the channels and network vessels; **qiang huo, du huo, fang feng, bai zhi** and **xi xin** dispel wind; **dang gui, bai shao, chuan xiong, sheng di** and **shu di** nourish and activate blood; **bai zhu** and **fu ling** strengthen the Spleen and dry dampness; **shi gao** and **huang qin** clear heat from the qi level; **gan cao** protects the Stomach. (Source: *Su Wen Bing Ji Qi Yi Bao Ming Ji*)

ER CHEN TANG 二陈汤
Two Aged [Herb] Decoction

zhi ban xia (Pinelliae Rhizoma preparatum) 制半夏 9–15g
chen pi (Citri reticulatae Pericarpium) 陈皮 9–15g
fu ling (Poria) 茯苓 9–12g
zhi gan cao (Glycyrrhizae Radix preparata) 炙甘草 3–6g

Method: Decoction. **Zhi ban xia** dries damp, transforms phlegm, downbears counterflow Stomach qi; **chen pi** dries damp, transforms phlegm and activates the qi dynamic; **fu ling** strengthens the Spleen and leaches out damp; **zhi gan cao** supplements qi and harmonizes the formula. (Source: *He Ji Ju Fang*)

GUI SHAO DI HUANG WAN 归芍地黄丸
Dang Gui, Peony and Rehmannia Pill

shu di (Rehmanniae Radix preparata) 熟地 24g
shan yao (Dioscoreae Rhizoma) 山药 12g
shan zhu yu (Corni Fructus) 山茱萸 12g
mu dan pi (Moutan Cortex) 牡丹皮 9g
fu ling (Poria) 茯苓 9g
ze xie (Alismatis Rhizoma) 泽泻 9g
dang gui (Angelicae sinensis Radix) 当归 9g
bai shao (Paeoniae Radix alba) 白芍 9g

Method: Pills. Grind the herbs into a fine powder and formed into 9 gram pills with honey. The dose is one pill 2–3 times daily with a little salty water. **Shu di** nourishes and supplements Kidney yin and blood and augments the jing; **shan zhu yu** supplements the Liver and Kidneys; **shan yao** strengthens the Spleen and secures jing; **ze xie** clears fire from the Kidneys through the urine; **mu dan pi** activates the blood and clears heat from the Liver; **fu ling** strengthens the Spleen and leaches damp; **dang gui** and **bai shao** nourish blood. (Source: *Tang Tou Ge Jue Zheng Xu Ji*)

HUANG LIAN WEN DAN TANG 黄连温胆汤
Warm Gallbladder Decoction with Coptis

huang lian (Coptidis Rhizoma) 黄连 3–6g
zhu ru (Bambusae Caulis in taeniam) 竹茹 12–15g
zhi shi (Aurantii Fructus immaturus) 枳实 9–12g
zhi ban xia (Pinelliae Rhizoma preparatum) 制半夏 9–12g
fu ling (Poria) 茯苓 9–12g

chen pi (Citri reticulatae Pericarpium) 陈皮 6–9g
sheng jiang (Zingiberis Rhizoma recens) 生姜 6–9g
zhi gan cao (Glycyrrhizae Radix preparata) 炙甘草 3–6g
da zao (Jujubae Fructus) 大枣 .... 3 fruit

Method: Decoction. **Huang lian** clears heat from the Heart and Stomach; **zhu ru** clears phlegm heat from the Stomach and Gallbladder, alleviates irritability and downbears counterflow qi to stop nausea; **zhi ban xia** dries dampness, transforms phlegm, downbears counterflow Stomach qi; **zhi shi** breaks up stagnation in the abdomen and directs qi downward; **fu ling** strengthens the Spleen and leaches out damp; **chen pi** dries damp, transforms phlegm and activates the qi dynamic; **zhi gan cao** supplements qi and harmonizes the formula; **sheng jiang** and **da zao** protect the Spleen and Stomach, while the pungent warmth of **sheng jiang** assists the phlegm transformation of the main herbs. (Source: *Wen Re Jing Wei*)

HUO XIANG ZHENG QI SAN 藿香正气散
Agastache Powder to Rectify the Qi

huo xiang (Pogostemonis Herba) 藿香 .... 90 (12–15)g
fu ling (Poria) 茯苓 .... 60 (12–15)g
bai zhu (Atractylodis macrocephalae Rhizoma) 白术 .... 60 (9–12)g
zi su ye (Perillae Folium) 紫苏叶 .... 60 (9–12)g
zhi ban xia (Pinelliae Rhizoma preparatum) 制半夏 .... 60 (9–12)g
da fu pi (Arecae Pericarpium) 大复皮 .... 60 (9–12)g
chen pi (Citri reticulatae Pericarpium) 陈皮 .... 60 (9–12)g
bai zhi (Angelicae dahuricae Radix) 白芷 .... 60 (9–12)g
hou po (Magnoliae officinalis Cortex) 厚朴 .... 60 (9–12)g
jie geng (Playcodi Radix) 桔梗 .... 60 (6–9)g
zhi gan cao (Glycyrrhizae Radix preparata) 炙甘草 .... 75 (3–6)g

Method: Powder. Grind the herbs to a fine powder and take in 6–9 gram drafts two or three times daily with a decoction made from 2 slices of ginger [**sheng jiang** (Zingiberis Rhizoma recens) 生姜] and one date [**da zao** (Jujubae Fructus) 大枣]. May also be decocted (no longer than 10–15 minutes) with the doses as shown in brackets. **Huo xiang** fragrantly disperses and vents damp, harmonizes the Stomach and stops vomiting; **zi su ye** and **bai zhi** dispel wind cold and transform damp; **hou po** descends qi, transforms phlegm damp and alleviates distension; **chen pi** regulates qi, corrects the qi dynamic, transforms phlegm damp and harmonizes the Stomach; **ban xia** transforms phlegm damp and stops vomiting; **da fu pi** descends qi and damp and alleviates distension; **bai zhu** and **fu ling** strengthen the Spleen, dry damp and promote urination; **jie geng** diffuses the Lungs; **gan cao**, **sheng jiang** and **da zao** harmonize the other herbs and regulate the Stomach. (Source: *He Ji Ju Fang*)

LIU JUN ZI TANG 六君子汤
Six Gentlemen Decoction

ren shen (Ginseng Radix) 人参 9–12g
bai zhu (Atractylodis macrocephalae Rhizoma) 白术 6–9g
fu ling (Poria) 茯苓 9–12g
zhi gan cao (Glycyrrhizae Radix preparata) 炙甘草 3–6g
chen pi (Citri reticulatae Pericarpium) 陈皮 6–9g
zhi ban xia (Pinelliae Rhizoma preparatum) 制半夏 6–9g

Method: Decoction. **Ren shen** strengthens the Spleen and Stomach and supplements yuan qi; **bai zhu** strengthens the Spleen and dries dampness; **fu ling** strengthens the Spleen and leaches out dampness; **zhi gan cao** strengthens the Spleen and supplements qi; **zhi ban xia** dries dampness, transforms phlegm and downbears counterflow Stomach qi; **chen pi** regulates qi, transforms phlegm and corrects the qi dynamic. (Source: *He Ji Ju Fang*)

MAI WEI DI HUANG WAN 麦味地黄丸
Ophiopogon, Schizandra and Rehmannia Pill

shu di (Rehmanniae Radix preparata) 熟地 24g
shan yao (Dioscoreae Rhizoma) 山药 12g
shan zhu yu (Corni Fructus) 山茱萸 12g
mu dan pi (Moutan Cortex) 牡丹皮 9g
fu ling (Poria) 茯苓 9g
ze xie (Alismatis Rhizoma) 泽泻 9g
mai dong (Ophiopogonis Radix) 麦冬 6g
wu wei zi (Schizandrae Fructus) 五味子 6g
Method: Pills. Grind the herbs into a fine powder and formed into 9 gram pills with honey. The dose is one pill 2–3 times daily with water. **Shu di** nourishes and supplements Kidney yin and blood and augments the jing; **shan zhu yu** supplements the Liver and Kidneys; **shan yao** strengthens the Spleen and secures jing; **ze xie** clears fire from the Kidneys through the urine; **mu dan pi** activates the blood and clears heat from the Liver; **fu ling** strengthens the Spleen and leaches damp; **mai dong** nourishes Lung yin and clears heat; **wu wei zi** astringes the Lungs and stops cough. (Source: *Yi Zong Jin Jian*)

MING MU DI HUANG WAN 明目地黄丸
Improve Vision Pill with Rehmannia

shu di (Rehmanniae Radix preparata) 熟地 24g
shan yao (Dioscoreae Rhizoma) 山药 12g
shan zhu yu (Corni Fructus) 山茱萸 12g
mu dan pi (Moutan Cortex) 牡丹皮 9g
fu ling (Poria) 茯苓 9g
ze xie (Alismatis Rhizoma) 泽泻 9g
dang gui (Angelicae sinensis Radix) 当归 9g
bai shao (Paeoniae Radix alba) 白芍 9g
bai ji li (Tribuli Fructus) 白蒺藜 9g
shi jue ming (Haliotidis Concha) 石决明 12g
Method: Pills. Grind the herbs into a fine powder and formed into 9 gram pills with honey. The dose is one pill 2–3 times daily with water. **Shu di** nourishes and supplements Kidney yin and blood and augments the jing; **shan zhu yu** supplements the Liver and Kidneys; **shan yao** strengthens the Spleen and secures jing; **ze xie** clears fire from the Kidneys through the urine; **mu dan pi** activates the blood and clears heat from the Liver; **fu ling** strengthens the Spleen and leaches out damp; **dang gui** and **bai shao** nourish blood; **bai ji li** and **shi jue ming** cool the Liver and improve vision. (Source: *Shen Shi Yao Han*)

QIAN ZHENG SAN 牵正散
Lead to Symmetry Powder

zhi bai fu zi (Typhonii Rhizoma preparatum) 制白附子 10g
bai jiang can (Bombyx Batryticatus) 白僵蚕 10g
quan xie (Scorpio) 全蝎 10
Method: Powder. Grind the herbs into a fine powder and 3 grams twice daily with water. **Zhi bai**

fu zi dispels wind, transforms phlegm and stops spasms; bai jiang can extinguishes wind phlegm and unblocks the network vessels; quan xie extinguishes wind and unblocks the network vessels. (Source: *Yang Shi Jia Zang Fang*)

SAN ZI YANG QIN TANG 三子养亲汤
Three Seed Decoction to Nourish One's Parents

su zi (Perillae Fructus) 苏子 9–12g
lai fu zi (Raphani Semen) 莱菔子 6–9g
bai jie zi (Sinapsis Semen) 白芥子 6–9g

Method: Decoction. The seeds are broken up in a mortar and pestle and placed in a cloth bag before cooking. Su zi directs qi downwards and expels phlegm; bai jie zi warms the Lungs, regulates qi and scours out phlegm; lai fu zi directs qi downward and transforms phlegm. (Source: *Han Shi Yi Tong*)

SHA SHEN MAI MEN DONG TANG 沙参麦门冬汤
Glehnia and Ophiopogonis Decoction

bei sha shen (Glehniae Radix) 北沙参 9g
mai dong (Ophiopogonis Radix) 麦冬 9g
yu zhu (Polygonati odorati Rhizoma) 玉竹 12g
sang ye (Mori Folium) 桑叶 9g
bai bian dou (Dolichos Semen) 白扁豆 9g
tian hua fen (Trichosanthes Radix) 天花粉 9g
gan cao (Glycyrrhizae Radix) 甘草 3g

Method: Decoction. Bei sha shen, mai dong, yu zhu and tian hua fen clear heat, generate fluids to moisten dryness, and thus nourish Lung and Stomach yin and fluids; bai bian dou and gan cao supplement qi and harmonize the Stomach; sang ye dredges the network vessels of the Lungs and lightly diffuses the Lungs to moisten dryness and clear heat. (Source: *Wen Bing Tiao Bian*)

SHAO YAO TANG 芍药汤
Peony Decoction

bai shao (Paeoniae Radix alba) 白芍 15–30g
huang qin (Scutellariae Radix) 黄芩 6–12g
huang lian (Coptidis Rhizoma) 黄连 3–9g
dang gui (Angelicae sinensis Radix) 当归 3–9g
bing lang (Arecae Semen) 槟榔 3–6g
da huang (Rhei Radix et Rhizoma) 大黄 3–6g
mu xiang (Aucklandiae Radix) 木香 3–6g
zhi gan cao (Glycyrrhizae Radix preparata) 炙甘草 3–6g
rou gui (Cinnamomi Cortex) 肉桂 2–3g

Method: Decoction. Bai shao and dang gui harmonize and regulate blood; bai shao and gan cao alleviate spasmodic pain; mu xiang and bing lang regulate qi, alleviate stagnation and tenesmus; huang lian and huang qin clear damp heat; da huang assists the previous two herbs in draining heat by purging according to the principle of 'promoting flow to treat excessive flow'; rou gui and gan cao prevent the bitter cold herbs from damaging yang qi. (Source: *Su Wen Bing Ji Qi Yi Bao Ming Ji*)

SHAO YAO GAN CAO TANG 芍药甘草汤
Peony and Licorice Decoction

bai shao (Paeoniae Radix alba) 白芍 30–90g
zhi gan cao (Glycyrrhizae Radix preparata) 炙甘草 10–30g
Method: Decoction. **Bai shao** softens the Liver, nourishes Liver blood and alleviates spasms; its sourness combines with the sweetness of **zhi gan cao** to create yin and harmonize the Liver and Spleen; **zhi gan cao** strengthens the Spleen and supplements qi. (Source: *Shang Han Lun*)

SHEN FU TANG 参附汤
Ginseng and Prepared Aconite Decoction

ren shen (Ginseng Radix) 人参 9–15g
zhi fu zi (Aconiti Radix lateralis preparata) 制附子 9–12g
Method: Decoction (at least 1–2 hours), or prepared as an intravenous infusion for emergency use for shock and congestive cardiac failure. **Ren shen** supplement and supports yuan qi; **zhi fu zi** warms and restores collapsing yang qi. (Source: *Fu Ren Liang Fang*)

SHENG HUA TANG 生化汤
Generation and Transformation Decoction

quan dang gui (Angelicae sinensis Radix) 全当归 12–24g
chuan xiong (Chuanxiong Rhizoma) 川芎 6–9g
tao ren (Semen Persicae) 桃仁 6–9g
pao jiang (Zingiberis Rhizoma preparatum) 炮姜 3–6g
zhi gan cao (Glycyrrhizae Radix preparata) 炙甘草 3–6g
Method: Decoction. **Quan dang gui** supplements and activates blood, and transforms blood stasis, thus allowing the generation and distribution of healthy new blood. **Quan dang gui** is the whole root, comprising both the blood supplementing body (**dang gui shen** 当归身) and the blood activating rootlets (**dang gui wei** 当归尾). **Chuan xiong** activates qi and blood; **tao ren** dispels blood stasis, and with **dang gui** lubricates the bowel and encourages healthy elimination; **pao jiang** warms the uterus, dispels cold and supports Spleen yang; **zhi gan cao** supplements zheng qi and supports the Spleen and Stomach. (Source: *Fu Qing Zhu Nü Ke*)

SHENG TIE LUO YIN 生铁落饮
Iron Filings Drink

sheng tie luo (Ferri Frusta) 生铁落 60g
dan shen (Salviae miltiorrhizae Radix) 丹参 12g
fu ling (Poria) 茯苓 12g
dan nan xing (Arisaema cum Bile) 胆南星 9g
zhe bei mu (Fritillariae thunbergii Bulbus) 浙贝母 9g
xuan shen (Scrophulariae Radix) 玄参 9g
tian dong (Asparagi Radix) 天冬 9g
mai dong (Ophiopogonis Radix) 麦冬 9g
lian qiao (Forsythiae Fructus) 连翘 9g
chen pi (Citri reticulatae Pericarpium) 陈皮 6g
shi chang pu (Acori tatarinowii Rhizoma) 石菖蒲 6g
yuan zhi (Polygalae Radix) 远志 6g
Method: Decoction. **Sheng tie luo** calms the shen; **dan shen** activates blood and calms the shen; **fu ling** strengthens the Spleen and calms the shen; **dan nan xing**, **zhe bei mu** and **xuan shen**

transform phlegm; **tian dong** and **mai dong** clear heat and nourish yin; **lian qiao** clears heat; **chen pi** regulates qi; **shi chang pu** and **yuan zhi** vaporize phlegm from the mind and calm the shen. The original prescription contained **zhu sha** (Cinnabaris) 朱砂, no longer used due to toxicity concerns. (Source: *Yi Xue Xin Wu*)

SI SHEN WAN 四神丸
Four Miracle Pill

bu gu zhi (Psoraleae Fructus) 补骨脂 120g
wu wei zi (Schizandrae Fructus) 五味子 60g
rou dou kou (Myristicae Semen) 肉豆蔻 60g
wu zhu yu (Evodiae Fructus) 吴茱萸 30g
da zao (Jujubae Fructus) 大枣 180g
sheng jiang (Zingiberis Rhizoma recens) 生姜 240g

Method: Pills. Grind the first four herbs to a fine powder, then boil the powder with the dates and ginger in sufficient water to cover until the dates are soft and well cooked, about 20–30 minutes. Remove the ginger and form the remaining paste into 9 gram pills. The dose is one pill, 2–3 times daily on an empty stomach. **Bu gu zhi** supplements Kidney yang and stops diarrhea; **rou dou kou**, **wu zhu yu** and **sheng jiang** warm Spleen and Stomach and dispel cold; **wu wei zi** astringes the Intestines and stops diarrhea; **da zao** moderates the pungent dispersing qualities of **wu zhu yu**, protect the Stomach and supplements qi. (Source: *Zheng Zhi Zhun Sheng*)

SI WU TANG 四物汤
Four Substance Decoction

dang gui (Angelicae sinensis Radix) 当归 6–12g
shu di (Rehmanniae Radix preparata) 熟地 9–15g
bai shao (Paeoniae Radix alba) 白芍 9–12g
chuan xiong (Chuanxiong Rhizoma) 川芎 6–9g

Method: Decoction. **Dang gui** supplements and gently activates blood; **shu di** nourishes yin and supplements blood; **bai shao** supplements blood, softens the Liver and preserves yin; **chuan xiong** activates qi and blood. (Source: *He Ji Ju Fang*)

TAO HE CHENG QI TANG 桃红承气汤
Peach Pit Decoction to Order the Qi

tao ren (Semen Persicae) 桃仁 9–12g
da huang (Rhei Radix et Rhizoma) 大黄 9–12g
mang xiao (Natrii Sulfas) 芒硝 6–9g
gui zhi (Cinnamomi Ramulus) 桂枝 6–9g
zhi gan cao (Glycyrrhizae Radix preparata) 炙甘草 3–6g

Method: Decoction. Boil each packet in about 300ml of water for the desired time and divide the resulting liquid into 2 or 3 doses. Dissolve the **Mang xiao** in the strained decoction, and take the dose on an empty stomach. Some diarrhea or loose bowel movements should be expected. **Tao ren** and **da huang** are the main herbs, and together break up and dispel static blood; **da huang** breaks up static blood and purges the bowels to clear stasis and Heat; **tao ren** assists in freeing the bowels by moistening the Intestines; **gui zhi** frees the channels and network vessels to clear a path for the dispersal of the static blood; the saltiness of **mang xiao** softens hardness and disperses accumulated stools and static blood; **zhi gan cao** protects the Stomach and moderates the harsh nature of the other herbs. (Source: *Shang Han Lun*)

TAO HONG SI WU TANG 桃红四物汤
Four Substance Decoction with Safflower and Peach Pit

tao ren (Persicae Semen) 桃仁 9–12g
hong hua (Carthami Flos) 红花 6–9g
dang gui (Angelicae sinensis Radix) 当归 9–12g
shu di (Rehmanniae Radix preparata) 熟地 12–15g
bai shao (Paeoniae Radix alba) 白芍 9–12g
chuan xiong (Chuanxiong Rhizoma) 川芎 6–9g

Method: Decoction. **Dang gui** supplements and activates blood; **shu di** and **bai shao** nourish and supplement blood; **bai shao** preserves yin, softens the Liver and alleviates spasmodic pain; **tao ren** and **hong hua** activate blood; **chuan xiong** activates blood, moves qi and stops pain. (Source: *Yi Zong Jin Jian*)

WU MEI WAN 乌梅丸
Mume Pill

wu mei (Mume Fructus) 乌梅 480g
gan jiang (Zingiberis Rhizoma) 干姜 300g
zhi fu zi (Aconiti Radix lateralis preparata) 制附子 180g
gui zhi (Cinnamomi Ramulus) 桂枝 180g
chuan jiao (Zanthoxyli Pericarpium) 川椒 120g
huang lian (Coptidis Rhizoma) 黄连 480g
huang bai (Phellodendri Cortex) 黄柏 180g
ren shen (Ginseng Radix) 人参 180g
xi xin (Asari Herba) 细辛 180g
dang gui (Angelicae sinensis Radix) 当归 120g

Method: Pills. Soak the **wu mei** in vinegar overnight, remove the pit and steam for 15 minutes or so until soft and cooked. Grind the other herbs to a fine powder and mix with the mashed **wu mei** and sufficient honey to form 3 gram pills. **Wu mei** astringes the Intestines and its sourness concentrates the effect of the other herbs in the jueyin; the ascending pungent heat of **gan jiang**, **zhi fu zi**, **gui zhi**, **chuan jiao** and **xi xin** warm yang and balance the descending bitter cold of **huang lian** and **huang bai** to stimulate the qi dynamic; **huang lian** and **huang bai** clear heat; **ren shen** and **dang gui** supplement and protect qi and blood. (Source: *Shang Han Lun*)

XIAO LUO WAN 消瘰丸
Reduce Scrophula Pill

duan mu li (calcined Ostreae Concha) 煅牡蛎 100g
xuan shen (Scrophulariae Radix) 玄参 100g
zhe bei mu (Fritillariae thunbergii Bulbus) 浙贝母 100g

Method: Pills or powder. Grind the herbs into a fine powder and form into 9 gram pills with water. The dose is one pill twice daily. The saltiness of **duan mu li** softens and transforms phlegm, while nourishing yin and anchoring yang; the cool, bitter, saltiness of **xuan shen** softens hardness and transforms phlegm, clears heat and nourishes yin; the pungency of **zhe bei mu** resolves constraint and dissipates phlegm nodules. (Source: *Yi Xue Xin Wu*)

YIN CHEN HAO TANG 茵陈蒿汤
Virgate Wormwood Decoction

yin chen (Artemisiae scopariae Herba) 茵陈 18–30g
shan zhi zi (Gardeniae Fructus) 山栀子 9–15g
da huang (Rhei Radix et Rhizoma) 大黄 6–9g
Method: Decoction is the preferred method as it enables alteration of the properties of the **da huang** as the jaundice resolves. The action of **da huang** varies depending on how long it is cooked; the shorter the cooking the more purgative action; when cooked for more than 20 minutes the purgative action decreases and the cholegogue action is enhanced. When the patient is constipated, **da huang** is added towards the end of cooking. When the bowels are moving, it can be deleted, the dose can be reduced, or it can be cooked for the same time as the other herbs, 20 minutes or so, depending on how much heat remains and how the Gallbladder is functioning. With the bowels moving but heat persisting, cook the **da huang** for the same time as the other herbs; with the stools loose or clay colored, add the **da huang** a few minutes before the end of cooking. One packet per day. **Yin chen** promotes urination to clear damp heat through the urine; **shan zhi zi** clears heat and damp heat from all three burners, and promotes urination to provide an escape route for the damp heat; **da huang** opens the bowels, clears heat and activates blood. (Source: *Shang Han Lun*)

ZENG YE TANG 增液汤
Increase the Fluids Decoction

xuan shen (Scrophulariae Radix) 玄参 30g
sheng di (Rehmanniae Radix) 生地 24g
mai dong (Ophiopogonis Radix) 麦冬 24g
Method: Decoction. **sheng di**, **mai dong** and **xuan shen** nourish yin and fluids and moisten dryness. (Source: *Wen Bing Tiao Bian*)

ZHI BAI DI HUANG WAN 知柏地黄丸
Anemarrhena, Phellodendron and Rehmannia Pill

shu di (Rehmanniae Radix preparata) 熟地 24g
shan yao (Dioscoreae Rhizoma) 山药 12g
shan zhu yu (Corni Fructus) 山茱萸 12g
mu dan pi (Moutan Cortex) 牡丹皮 9g
fu ling (Poria) 茯苓 9g
ze xie (Alismatis Rhizoma) 泽泻 9g
zhi mu (Anemarrhenae Rhizoma) 知母 9g
huang bai (Phellodendri Cortex) 黄柏 9g
Method: Pills. Grind the herbs into a fine powder and formed into 9 gram pills with honey. The dose is one pill 2–3 times daily with a little salty water. **Shu di** nourishes and supplements Kidney yin and blood and augments the jing; **shan zhu yu** supplements the Liver and Kidneys; **shan yao** strengthens the Spleen and secures jing; **ze xie** clears fire from the Kidneys through the urine; **mu dan pi** activates the blood and clears heat from the Liver; **fu ling** strengthens the Spleen and leaches damp; **zhi mu** clears heat and nourishes yin; **huang bai** drains fire from the Kidneys and lower burner. (Source: *Zheng Yin Mai Zhi*)

APPENDIX 2. HOT SPOT THERAPY

Hot spot therapy is a technique that utilizes sustained pressure on specific points along the Urinary Bladder channel. The technique is based on the external manifestation, through the channel pathway and associated tissues, of internal organ system dysfunction. When a particular organ system is in a pathological state the paraspinal muscles of the affected segment are usually tight or knotted. The muscle tightness constricts the vessels and nerves passing through it and further impedes the flow of qi and blood. Releasing some of this tension has a beneficial effect on qi and blood movement through the segment, and on the function of the underlying organ system. The technique is quite simple; its success relies on regularity and persistence of application. In essence it is simply sustained pressure applied to specific loci, done by the patient at home for 10 minutes or so every day. The regular pressure on the appropriate spots gradually leads to a sustained softening of the superficial tissues, better qi and blood flow and improved organ function. The technique can be applied along the length of the erector spinae muscles, from Bl.13 (feishu) to Bl.25 (dachangshu), with the main areas of interest usually the mid back, from Bl.15 (xinshu) to Bl.20 (pishu).

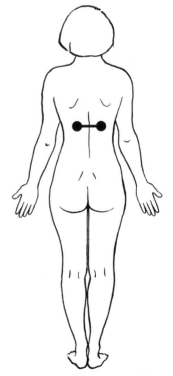

The technique involves a device made from two tennis balls placed in a sock with a knot tied between them. This enables the patient to apply pressure bilaterally with a ball sitting on both left and right Urinary Bladder channels with the knot over the spine (Fig.1). The patient lies on the bed or the floor with the tennis balls placed on either side of the spine on the Urinary Bladder channel. Using their legs to move and make fine positional adjustments they seek the sorest spots, those with the most stagnation, and once located relax into them and let their body weight provide the required pressure. The pressure should be strong and may initially hurt, but should not be so strong that the patient tenses up against it. If the pressure from the body weight is too much, a softer surface may help, in fact it is a good idea to always begin the technique on a bed and graduate to a harder surface as the stagnation resolves and firmer pressure is desired. Once the points have been located and the pressure applied, it should be maintained for a few minutes, or until the soreness clearly decreases, the tension releases and the points 'give'. Once the 'give' has occurred, move on to another point. Two or three points should

Figure 1. Placement of the hot spot device

924   APPENDIX 2 - HOT SPOT THERAPY

be treated and deactivated each session. Little by little the sore points should become harder to find, and the tissues of the segment being treated should soften and relax. For those unable to lie, the technique can also be done in a firm chair or leaning against the wall. The time is important because what is being stimulated is a neurological reflex–the pressure sends a signal to the brain, which after a certain period, usually no longer than 90–120 seconds, sends a signal back to the muscle to release, the 'give'. Pressure maintained after the release is unnecessary.

Tennis balls are selected because they have the right balance of firmness and elasticity to provide a good degree of pressure without undue discomfort. The technique is like having an acupressure massage everyday. The benefits accumulate gradually, with persistent practice providing significant and sustained result. This technique is most useful in excess patterns, especially those with a component of Liver qi constraint.

APPENDIX 3. CLINICAL FEATURES OF BLOOD STASIS

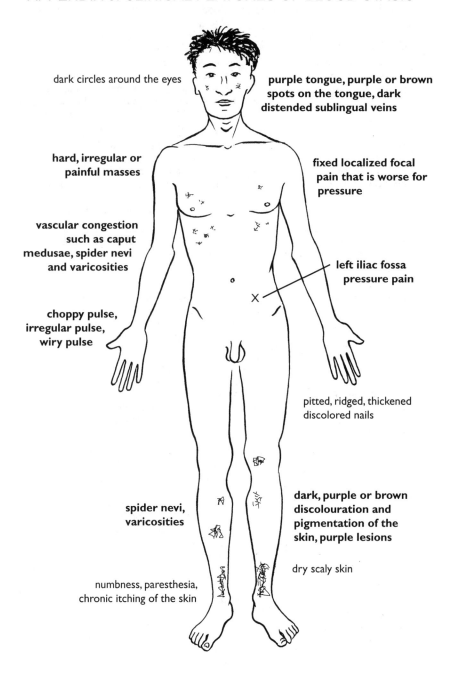

dark circles around the eyes

purple tongue, purple or brown spots on the tongue, dark distended sublingual veins

hard, irregular or painful masses

fixed localized focal pain that is worse for pressure

vascular congestion such as caput medusae, spider nevi and varicosities

left iliac fossa pressure pain

choppy pulse, irregular pulse, wiry pulse

pitted, ridged, thickened discolored nails

spider nevi, varicosities

dark, purple or brown discolouration and pigmentation of the skin, purple lesions

dry scaly skin

numbness, paresthesia, chronic itching of the skin

Table A3. Major and secondary features of blood stasis syndrome. Major features are sufficient on their own to indicate blood stasis; secondary features could be associated with other pathology and need other supporting evidence for diagnosis.

Major features	Comments
Fixed, sharp stabbing pains which are worse for pressure	The classic sign, and although common is by no means always present even in those with severe blood stasis. When present, the pain is usually focal and the patient able to point a finger at it. Although pain of this type is usually worse for pressure, this is not always the case.
Fixed, painful, irregular or hard masses and lumps, with discolored or dark overlying tissue	These are found mostly in the abdominal cavity, primarily in the Liver and pelvic basin, although they may appear anywhere. They may or may not be painful with palpation. They are not always palpable and may be detected by imaging, in which case they should be discriminated from phlegm masses.
Darkish or mottled complexion, purple lips, dark rings around the eyes, sunken eyes	Darkness appears to run right around the eye, as if the eyes have sunk into the sockets.
Purple or brown discolouration and pigmentation of the skin, including 'liver' spots	Often seen on the extremities, for example the discoloration of the lower legs seen in peripheral vascular disease and 'age' spots seen on the hands and arms of the elderly.
Vascular congestion and abnormalities such as petechiae, spider nevi, caput medusae, varicosities and angiomas which are purplish or dark, raised or flat	Spider veins and nevi are found primarily on the lower ribs, face and especially the lower limbs on the inner knee and ankle. Includes lesions such as port wine nevus. Caput medusae are large purple veins appearing on the abdomen and are a sign of severe stasis.
Left iliac fossa pressure pain	This is a specific locus of pain that can be palpated along the Stomach channel, about 2 cun below the navel. As the palpating hand moves down the channel, a small area about 1–2 centimeters in diameter is suddenly painful when pressed. As the palpation proceeds further down, the pressure pain is not felt. This is a reliable sign of blood congestion, and often one of the early indicators. The mechanism is back pressure into the rectal veins through the portal system that drains into the Liver.
A mauve or purplish tongue, or with brown or purplish stasis spots. The sublingual veins beneath the tongue are distended and dark	The tongue body is a moderately reliable indicator. Patients with gross blood stasis, such as masses, sometimes do not display the expected tongue signs. The sublingual veins seem to be more reliable, but again are sometimes inexplicably absent.

Table A3. Major and secondary features of blood stasis syndrome (cont.)

A choppy or wiry pulse, or a slow and irregular pulse, or a pulse too weak to be felt	The pulse can be quite variable depending on the complicating pathology, the location of the stasis and the main features. When the Heart is involved the pulse is often irregular or imperceptible, when there is severe pain the pulse can be wiry or choppy.
Secondary features	**Comments**
Chronic hemorrhagic disorders	Bleeding of purplish, black or clotted blood. Usually seen in menstrual bleeding, bleeding from the upper digestive tract, melena or tarry stools, vomiting of 'coffee ground' like material or subcutaneous bleeding.
Darkish, mottled palms and hands	This is more easily seen when the patient extends their fingers to stretch the palm. The hands are usually cold.
Purplish nail bed, thickened, ridged, pitted or deformed nails	The nail beds, gums and inner cheeks, and conjunctivae are a good place to assess the state of the microcirculation and network vessels, the ultimate location of much blood stasis. Either an overall purple hue, or purple or brown stasis spots can be seen.
Dark red or purple gums, receding and shrunken; gums which frequently bleed; purple or brown spots in the buccal cavity	
Purple or congested vessels in the conjunctivae	
Benign brown or purple growths on the skin	Includes moles and skin tags. Frequently seen on the neck. The number of lesions is proportional to the degree of stasis.
Recurrent hectic fever at night, not associated with sweating	This is a low grade fever that spikes at irregular intervals and is associated with very restless and fitful sleep. Also known as a tumor fever, and commonly seen in malignancy.
Dry, scaly, rough skin	Skin is nourished and moistened by blood. When blood is unable to reach the superficial layers due to local or systemic stasis it becomes rough and dry. This is most commonly seen on the lower legs.
Numbness and paraesthesia in the extremities; spasms and twitching, unusual feelings, chronic itching or cold sensations in the skin.	Numbness may be isolated in the extremities or patches of skin anywhere in the body, most commonly in the feet. Chronic itch, unusual sensations, sometimes likened to insects crawling under the skin, or coldness are due to blood unable to reach the skin.
Chronic pain or distension	Any sort of chronic pain, even when not sharp or focal will involve a degree of blood stasis.

Table A3. Major and secondary features of blood stasis syndrome (cont.)

Secondary features	Comments
Recurrent carbuncles, boils or other deep rooted sores or chronic non-healing ulcers	Seen in conditions like stasis ulcers and boils that always return to the same location and are quite painful. The upper back and buttocks are common locations.
Hemorrhoids	These are usually painful and persistent. They should be distinguished from hemorrhoids associated with qi deficiency and damp heat.
Cupping or massage draws out dark purplish marks	Cupping will usually bring out some dark or purple color, but it is the degree of darkness, almost to black, that is the feature here.
Relevant medical or family history	An important indicator of probability in subclinical blood stasis or the likelihood of developing overt blood stasis. Certain conditions should cause a high degree of suspicion, in particular a family history of connective tissue or chronic inflammatory diseases, cardiovascular disease and mental illness. Any trauma, either physical and emotional, regardless of how old or seemingly trivial should be noted, including surgery and scarring.
Age	Older people are more likely to suffer blood stasis due of declining vitality of yang qi and the increasing yin deficiency. Blood stasis should be suspected in all patients over 50.
Abnormal blood tests	Elevated erythrocyte sedimentation rate (ESR), increased erythrocyte and platelet aggregation, increased blood viscosity.
Finally, blood stagnation should be considered after excluding all other possibilities and in any condition that does not respond to other therapies.	This is the famous default position 'if all else fails, activate the blood'.

APPENDIX 4. BLOOD LETTING

Bloodletting is a excellent method of activating blood and directly eliminating blood stasis. When skillfully executed, it effectively stimulates local and upstream blood flow, and is relatively painless and hygienic. It is performed on the congested vessels, spider veins and spider nevi that are be found at various locations around the body. These congested vessels are dilating in response to an obstruction or congestion in their drainage zone. The darker and more engorged they are the greater the blood stasis. They can be due to local, distant or systemic pathology. When localized they will be found in the vicinity of the lesion, for example the congested veins seen over a chronically painful joint. In many cases they will be found at a distance from the main site of the pathology, often along the pathway of a related channel. For example, it is common to find spider veins along the pathway of the Liver, Spleen and Kidney channels around the inner knee and ankle in patients with blood stasis in the pelvic basin, manifesting as dysmenorrhea, fibroids or prostatic hypertrophy, and on the Urinary Bladder channel at the back of the knee, in patients with chronic lower back pain.

Method
Up to three or four sites can be selected per treatment. Normal precautions for the handling of body fluids apply. Surgical gloves are recommended. A surgical lancet is the best implement for sterility and ease of use. The area is cleaned with alcohol, the area squeezed between the forefinger and thumb to increase local congestion and one or two swift jabs of the lancet applied to the darkest area. The blood should run dark at first and continue until it becomes a bright red, at which time a cotton bud can be used to staunch the flow. Sometimes a lot of blood can be drawn until it becomes bright red. This is not a problem in robust patients, but it is wise to be prepared for some overflow onto the treatment surface. Cups can be applied to heavily congested areas or those that continue to run dark. Treatment can be repeated once or twice per week, usually on a different site. Some caution should be observed in those with significant deficiency, but the technique is still beneficial because blood stasis can impede supplementation of the deficient state. When deficiency is significant a milder technique can be used. Only one or two sites should be bled to extract a few drops of blood, the technique applied less frequently and cups should not be used.

APPENDIX 5. YING BING – THE TRADITIONAL ANALYSIS OF GOITRE AND NODULES

The material in this appendix is adapted from is *Zhong Yi Wai Ke Xue* 中医外科学 Traditional Chinese Medicine for Surgical Diseases (1999) Peoples Medical Publishing House, Beijing.

气
瘿

1. QI YING (diffuse goitre; literally 'qi type thyroid swelling')

These are euthyroid goiters and may be the result of iodine deficiency or iodine excess. Goitre and nodules are always associated with phlegm which may be more or less substantial. When less substantial the swelling in the neck comes and goes, when more substantial nodules and masses can always be palpated. The phlegm will usually be complicated by either qi stagnation or blood stasis.

1.1 Spleen and Stomach qi and phlegm stagnation

• This type of goitre is associated with iodine deficiency. The swelling is generally large and occurs in people who live in mountainous areas or areas otherwise deficient in iodine.

Rx: HAI ZAO SHU YU WAN (Sargassum Pills to Soothe Constraint 海藻舒郁汤), a formula rich in seaweeds and iodine containing items.

1.2 Spleen and Stomach damp heat

• This pattern corresponds to the effects of a low iodine diet that is heavy, fatty and rich. There will be digestive symptoms reflecting poor or sluggish digestion and poor absorption of nutrients.

Rx: CHU SHI WEI LING TANG (Damp Eliminating Stomach Decoction with Poria 除湿胃苓汤)

1.3 Liver and Kidney deficiency (chongmai and renmai deficiency)

• This pattern is associated with a euthyroid goitre that is congenital, or occurs during puberty, pregnancy or postpartum. There will usually be signs of Kidney deficiency such as delayed development, menstrual disorders or delayed menstruation and backache.

Rx: ER XIAN TANG (Two Immortal Decoction 二仙汤) plus SI WU TANG (Four Substance Decoction 四物汤)

1.4 Liver and Spleen disharmony with qi and phlegm stagnation

• This is a simple euthyroid goitre that is associated with stress or emotional turmoil causing constraint to the qi. It may develop over time into an overactive thyroid condition when complicated by constrained heat.

Rx: XIAO YAO SAN (Rambling Powder 逍遥散) plus ER CHEN TANG (Two Aged [Herb] Decoction 二陈汤)

2. ROU YING (literally 'flesh thyroid swelling'; benign nodules, single or multiple)

These may be simple and inactive adenomas or cysts, or 'hot' toxic nodules, that is, nodules producing excessive thyroid hormone and a hyperthyroid state. In general nodules occur in middle age and older patients. Depending on location and size they can impinge on the trachea and esophagus causing swallowing, voice and breathing difficulties.

2.1 Yang deficiency with congealed phlegm
• These are chronic benign nodules and cysts.
• Relatively small, usually single nodule. The overlying skin is taut and shiny, the nodule firm, rubbery and well defined. There is no pain with palpation and usually no abnormal thyroid activity. There may or may not be systemic signs of yang deficiency.
Rx: YANG HE TANG (Yang Heartening Decoction 阳和汤)

2.2 Liver and Spleen disharmony with congealed phlegm
• This pattern includes the most common benign thyroid nodule. May be single or multiple and appears to fluctuate with the patients emotional state.
• Relatively large, single or multiple nodules that are firm to the touch and move with swallowing; may be mild tenderness or discomfort and a sense of constriction in the throat; nodules become more obvious or uncomfortable when the patient is stressed or upset. Other qi stagnation signs and symptoms may be present, such as premenstrual syndrome, tension headaches, neck and shoulder tension, tooth grinding and wiry pulse.
Rx: XIAO YAO SAN (Rambling Powder 逍遥散) plus ER CHEN TANG (Two Aged [Herb] Decoction 二陈汤) or XIAO LUO WAN (Reduce Scrophula Pill 消瘰丸) or SAN ZI YANG QIN TANG (Three Seed Decoction to Nourish one's Parents 三子养亲汤)

2.3 Liver qi constraint with heat/fire
• This is usually associated with a 'hot' nodule, a toxic adenoma or thyroid hormone producing nodule.
• Single or multiple nodules with obvious tenderness and discomfort, weakness, weight loss, bitter taste, irritability, anger, low grade fever, red tongue with a yellow coat and a wiry rapid pulse.
Rx: KAI YU SAN (Open up Constraint Powder 开郁散)

2.4 Qi and blood stagnation
• Hard irregular mass with mottled skin overlying the lesion, hoarse voice or dysphagia, restriction of the throat.
Rx: HAI ZAO YU HU TANG (Sargassum Decoction for the Jade Flask 海藻玉壶汤)

瘿
痈

3. YING YONG (Thyroiditis; literally. 'thyroid swelling abscess')

This category includes patterns that could clearly be classed as due to heat or toxic heat, but also includes a type of chronic inflammation (equivalent to Hashimoto's thyroiditis) that would not necessarily be diagnosed as a heat pattern in Chinese medicine, and does not exhibit the classic features of a 'yong' (abscess) condition. The constitution of the patient is thought to play a major role in how these patterns present.

3.1 Wind heat or warm disease

• Associated with acute or subacute thyroiditis that may be the result of an infection (viral or bacterial) or aseptic inflammation following radiation treatment. This is a relatively uncommon pattern, but can easily lead to yin or yang qi deficiency complications. Also may occur in postpartum women, especially those with a predisposition to yin and blood deficiency.

• Redness and swelling of the thyroid and the overlying skin; the swelling is soft and tender. May be suppuration in some cases. Fever, malaise, thirst, sweating, restlessness, sore throat, headache, rapid strong pulse, thick greasy yellow tongue coat.

Rx: Niu Bang Jie Ji Tang (Burdock Seed Decoction to Release the Muscles 牛蒡解肌汤) plus Wu Wei Xiao Du Yin (Five Ingredient Drink to Eliminate Toxin 五味消毒饮); with suppuration Xian Fang Huo Ming Yin (Sublime Formula for Sustaining Life 仙方活命饮); radiation or viral thyroiditis Pu Ji Xiao Du Yin (Universal Benefit Drink to Eliminate Toxin 普济消毒饮).

3.2 Qi and yin deficiency

• Post radiation thyroiditis or subacute thyroiditis of viral origin. May follow the warm disease pattern above that damages qi and yin. Either yin or qi deficiency can be prominent.

• Swelling of the thyroid. With yang qi deficiency prominent, cold intolerance, fatigue, depression, weight gain, edema, swollen tongue. With yin deficiency, heat intolerance, palpitations, insomnia, hunger, weight loss, sweating, emotional lability.

Rx: Sheng Mai San (Generate the Pulse Powder 生脉散); Zhi Bai Di Huang Wan (Anemarrhena, Phellodendron and Rehmannia Pill 知柏地黄丸), You Gui Wan (Restore the Left [Kidney] Pill 右归丸)

3.3 Spleen and Kidney qi deficiency (with external invasion)

• Associated with chronic or autoimmune (Hashimoto's) thyroiditis. There may be an acute episode with lymphadenopathy that precedes the pattern, hence the external invasion component. This is not always apparent.

• Thyroid swelling that is firm, with or without lymphadenopathy. Gradual onset of fatigue, somnolence, diarrhea, urinary frequency, weight gain, pale swollen tongue.

Rx: Shen Ling Bai Zhu San (Ginseng, Poria and White Atractylodes Powder 参苓白术散) plus Er Xian Tang (Two Immortal Decoction 二仙汤) and Er Chen

Tang (Two Aged [Herb] Decoction 二陈汤)

3.4 Congealed phlegm

- Fibrous thyroiditis, subacute thyroiditis (remission stage), chronic autoimmune thyroiditis.
- Other than a firm mass there may be few other features, but there will be a history of some thyroid disturbance.

Rx: YANG HE TANG (Yang Heartening Decoction 阳和汤) plus ER CHEN TANG (Two Aged [Herb] Decoction 二陈汤)

石
瘿

4. SHI YING; (literally 'stone thyroid swelling; includes malignant growths)

This category includes cancer of the thyroid or hard cystic or fibrous swellings. The swelling is characteristically very firm, or hard and irregular.

4.1 Qi constraint with coagulated phlegm

- Firm irregular non tender mass without skin changes over the lesion.

Rx: HAI ZAO YU HU TANG (Sargassum Decoction for the Jade Flask 海藻玉壶汤) plus KAI YU SAN (Open up Constraint Powder 开郁散).

4.2 Qi and blood stagnation

- Slow growing hard irregular mass, with mottled, darkened skin or congested vessels overlying. May be painful. The mass doesn't move with swallowing. Dysphagia, hoarse voice, difficulty breathing. The tongue is dark or with stasis spots and swollen sublingual veins.

Rx: SAN ZHONG KUI JIAN TANG (Powder to Dissipate Swelling and Disperse Hardness 散肿溃坚散), or a modified version of DANG GUI LONG HUI WAN (Tangkuei, Gentian and Aloe Pill 当归龙会丸) if there is heat in the Liver.

4.3 Qi and blood deficiency

- Gradually increasing firm mass in a patient with weight loss, fatigue, dizziness, pale tongue and other signs of qi and blood deficiency.

Rx: HUO XUE SAN YING TANG (Activate Blood to Disperse Goitre Decoction 活血散瘿汤).

4.4 Yin deficiency with fire

- Late stage disease, seen in patients having undergone radiation, chemotherapy or surgery. Hard immobile mass. The region around the mass is stiff and hard and discolored. Emaciation, dryness, sweats, constipation and other signs of yin deficiency.

Rx: TIAO YUAN SHEN QI WAN (Regulate the Original Kidney Qi Pill 调元肾气丸), TIAN WANG BU XIN DAN (Emperor of Heaven's Special Pill to Supplement the Heart 天王补心丹)

5. YING QI (Hyperthyroid)

5.1 Liver qi constraint with fire

- This condition is triggered by stress, and presents with irritability, anger, tension, distension and pain in the hypochondrium, premenstrual syndrome, heat intolerance, copious sweating, warm skin, flushing on the chest and neck, irritated or protruding eyes, red tongue with a yellow coat, wiry rapid pulse. With Heart fire: insomnia, palpitations, sweating; with Stomach fire: ravenous hunger and thirst without weight gain.
- Mostly seen in younger patients, those that are otherwise relatively robust and in the early stages of the condition.

Rx: Long Dan Xie Gan Tang (Gentian Decoction to Purge the Liver 龙胆泻肝汤) plus Yi Guan Jian (Linking Decoction 一贯煎)

5.2 Yin deficiency with ascendant yang

- Emaciation, lower back ache, tinnitus, irritated watery eyes, amenorrhea, scanty period or irregular periods, facial flushing, heat in the palms and soles, bone steaming fever, irritability, insomnia, fine tremor, red dry tongue with little or no coat, fine rapid pulse.

Rx: Ling Yang Gou Teng Tang (Antelope Horn and Uncaria Decoction 羚羊钩藤汤)

5.3 Heart blood and Spleen qi deficiency

- Anxiety, palpitations, weakness, poor appetite, sweating, edema, frequent stools or diarrhea, breathlessness, frequent colds, pale or pink tongue with a white coat, weak, moderate pulse
- Seen in chronic cases and in those with a constitutional tendency to qi and blood deficiency or yang deficiency. Quite common in the elderly.

Rx: Gui Pi Tang (Restore the Spleen Decoction 归脾汤)

APPENDIX 6. ENDANGERED SPECIES AND POSSIBLE SUBSTITUTES

Endangered species		Substitute
The substitutes suggested here are made with the intention of reproducing a similar therapeutic effect, and thus the substitute may change depending on the problem being treated. CITES Appendix 1: all trade banned CITES Appendix 2: limited trade allowed with permits		
CITES App. 1	**hu gu** (Tigris Os)	**gou gu** (Canis Os) 狗骨, **mao gu** (Felis Os) 猫骨
	xi jiao (Rhinocerotis Cornu)	**shui niu jiao** (Bubali Cornu) 水牛角: very similar action as long as sufficiently high doses are used
	chuan shan jia (Squama Manitis)	**wang bu liu xing** (Vaccariae Semen) 王不留行: adequate substitute for blood stasis and to promote lactation **zao jiao ci** (Gleditsiae Spina) 皂角刺: for contained toxic heat lesions
	she xiang (Moschus)	**ren gong she xiang** (synthetic muscone) 人工麝香: used in prepared medicines; very similar therapeutic profile **shi chang pu** (Acori tatarinowii Rhizoma) 石菖蒲: for disturbances of consciousness **bai zhi** (Angelicae dahuricae Radix) 白芷: for headache and pain
	shi hu (Dendrobi Herba)	**yu zhu** (Polygonati odorati Rhizoma) 玉竹
CITES App. 2	**gui ban** (Testudinis Plastrum)	**mu li** (Ostreae Concha) 牡蛎: for enriching yin and anchoring yang **nu zhen zi** (Ligustri Fructus) 女贞子 plus **han lian cao** (Ecliptae Herba) 旱莲草: to nourish yin
	bie jia (Trionycis Carapax)	**san leng** (Sparganii Rhizoma) 三棱 plus **mu li** (Ostreae Concha) 牡蛎: to dissipate masses **qing hao** (Artemisiae annuae Herba) 青蒿: to clear deficient heat
	mu xiang (Aucklandiae Radix) previously known as Saussurea lappa	**tu mu xiang** (Inula Radix) 土木香: According to Bensky (2004) this was the species used as mu xiang until Saussurea Sp. was introduced from India in the 19th Cent. It has a similar therapeutic profile.
	rou cong rong (Cistanches Herba)	**suo yang** (Cynomorii Herba) 锁阳
	tian ma (Gastrodiae Rhizoma)	**gou teng** (Uncariae Ramulus cum Uncis) 钩藤
	chen xiang (Aquilariae Lignum resinatum)	**hou po** (Magnoliae officinalis Cortex) 厚朴

BIBLIOGRAPHY

The sources noted following the prescriptions are usually multiple. The first is the contemporary text from which the pattern and prescription was extracted; the second is the original text in which the prescription first appeared. When no contemporary text is cited, the prescription is drawn from the classics.

Contemporary Chinese sources

Fang Ji Xue 方剂学
  Chinese Herbal Formulae (2002). Li Fei (ed.), Peoples Medical Publishing House, Beijing

Ji Lin Di Si Lin Chuang Xue Yuan Gu Ke Jing Yan Fang 吉林第四临床学院骨科经验方 (1974) Experiential Formulas of the Jilin Fourth Clinical Teaching Hospital Orthopedic Department, Jilin

Ji Zheng Zhen Jiu 急症针灸
  Emergency Acupuncture (1988). Zhang Ren, Peoples Medical Publishing House, Beijing

Nei Fen Mi Ji Bing Bian Bing Zhuang Fang Zhi Liao 内分泌疾病辨病专方治疗
  Differentiation and Treatment of Endocrine Diseases (2000)
  Wu Xue–Gui (ed.), Peoples Medical Publishing House, Beijing

Nei Ke Chang Jian Bing Zheng Zhen Zhi Zhi Nan 内科常见病证诊治指南
  Guidebook to the Diagnosis and Treatment of Commonly Seen Internal Medicine Diseases (1997). Zhong Hong, Lou Ren (eds.) Peoples Health Publishing, Beijing

Shen Jing Ke Zhuang Bing Zhong Yi Lin Chuang Zhen Zhi 神经科专病中医临床诊治
  Chinese Medical Diagnosis and Treatment of Neurological Diseases (2000) Huang Pei–Xin, Liu Mao–Cai (eds.), Peoples Health Publishing, Beijing

Shen Zang Bing Bian Bing Zhuan Fang Zhi Liao 肾脏病辨病专方治疗
  Differentiation and Treatment of Kidney Diseases (2000). Chen Jian (ed.), Peoples Health Publishing, Beijing

Shi Yong Fang Ji Xue 实用方剂学
  Practical Chinese Herbal Formulae (1989). Zhou Feng–Wu (ed.), Shandong Science and Technology Press, Shandong

Shi Yong Zhong Yao Xue 实用中药学
  Practical Chinese Herbs (1985). Zhou Feng–Wu (ed.), Shandong Science and Technology Press, Shandong

Shi Yong Zhong Yi Er Ke Xue 实用中医儿科学
  Practical Traditional Chinese Pediatrics (1995). Jiang Yu–Ren, Zhang Qi–Wen (eds.), Shandong Science and Technology Press, Shandong

Shi Yong Zhong Yi Er Ke Xue 实用中医儿科学
Practical Traditional Chinese Pediatrics (1987). Jin Zu–Peng (ed.), Shandong Science and Technology Press, Shandong

Shi Yong Zhong Yi Fu Ke Xue 实用中医妇科学
Practical Traditional Chinese Gynaecology (1985). Zhou Feng–Wu (ed.), Shandong Science and Technology Press, Shandong

Shi Yong Zhong Yi Nei Ke Xue 实用中医内科学
Practical Traditional Chinese Internal Medicine (1984). Huang Wen–Dong (ed.), Shanghai Science and Technology Press, Shanghai

Shi Yong Zhong Yi Wai Ke Xue 实用中医外科学
Practical Traditional Chinese Medicine for Surgical Diseases (1985) Gu Bo–Hua (ed.), Shanghai Science and Technology Press, Shanghai

Shi Yong Zhong Yi Wai Ke Xue 实用中医外科学
Practical Traditional Chinese Medicine for Surgical Diseases (1986) Shang De–Jun (ed.), Shandong Science and Technology Press, Shandong

Shi Yong Zhong Yi Xue Ye Bing Xue 实用中医血液病学
Practical Traditional Chinese Hematology (1992). Wu Han–Xiang (ed.), Shanghai Science and Technology Press, Shanghai

Wai Ke Zhuang Bing Zhong Yi Lin Chuang Zhen Zhi 外科专病中医临床诊治
Chinese Medical Diagnosis and Treatment of Surgical Diseases (2000) Lin Yi, Cai Bing–Qin (eds.), Peoples Health Publishing, Beijing

Xian Zai Zhong Yi Gan Zang Bing Xue 现在中医肝脏病学
Contemporary Hepatology in Traditional Chinese Medicine (2001) Liu Ping (ed.), Peoples Medical Publishing House, Beijing

Xiao Hua Ke Zhuan Bing 消化科专病
Diseases of the Digestive Tract (2000). Luo Yun–Jian (ed.), Peoples Medical Publishing House, Beijing

Yan Ke Yu Er Bi Hou Ke Zhuan Bing 眼科与耳鼻喉科专病
TCM diagnosis and Treatment of Ear, Nose, Throat and Eye Diseases (2000) Luo Yun–Jian, Liu Mao–Cai (eds.), Peoples Medical Publishing House, Beijing

Zhen Jiu Xue 针灸学
Acupuncture (2002). Sun Guo–Jie (ed.), Peoples Medical Publishing House, Beijing

Zhen Jiu Zhi Liao Xue 针灸治疗学
Acupuncture Therapeutics (1985). Yang Zhang–Sen (ed.), Shanghai Science and Technology Press, Shanghai

Zhong Guo Zhong Yi Mi Fang Da Quan 中国中医秘方大全
A Compendium of Secret Chinese Medicine Formulas (1991). Hu Xi–Ming (ed.), Wenhui Publishing

Zhong Liu Ke Zhuan Bing 肿瘤科专病
Chinese Medical Oncology (2000). Liu Wei–Sheng (ed.), Peoples Medical Publishing House, Beijing

Zhong Xi Yi Jie He Zhi Liao Ji Fu Zheng 中西医结合治疗常见外科急腹症
Chinese and Western Medical Treatment of the Acute Abdomen (1982) Zheng Xian–Li et al., Tianjin Science and Technology Press, Shandong

Zhong Yao Xue 中药学
Chinese Herbs (1991). Yan Zheng–Hua (ed.), Peoples Medical Publishing House, Beijing

Zhong Yi Nei Ke Ji Zheng Zheng Zhi 中医内科急症政治
Proven Chinese Medical Treatments for Acute Internal Disorders (1985) Huang Xing–Yuan (ed.), Peoples Medical Publishing House, Beijing

Zhong Yi Nei Ke Lin Chuang Shou Ce 中医内科临床手册
Clinical Handbook of Traditional Chinese Internal Medicine (1984) Dang You–Lian (ed.), Henan Science and Technology Press, Henan

Zhong Yi Er Bi Hou Ke Xue 中医耳鼻喉科学
Traditional Chinese Otonasopharyngology (1985). Wang De–Jian (ed.), Peoples Medical Publishing House, Beijing

Zhong Yi Fu Chan Ke Xue 中医妇产科学
Traditional Chinese Obstetrics and Gynecology (2002) Liu Min–Ru, Tan Mo–Xin (eds.), Peoples Medical Publishing House, Beijing

Zhong Yi Tan Bing Xue 中医痰病学
Study of Phlegm Disease in Traditional Chinese Medicine (1984) Zhu Ceng–Bo, Hubei Science and Technology Press, Hubei

Zhong Yi Nei Ke Shou Ce 中医内科手册
Handbook of Traditional Chinese Medical Internal Medicine (1997) Chao En–Xiang (ed.), Fujian Science and Technology Press, Fujian

Zhong Yi Nei Ke Xue 中医内科学
Traditional Chinese Internal Medicine (1999). Wang Yong–Yan, Lu Zhao–Lin (eds.), Peoples Medical Publishing House, Beijing

Zhong Yi Wai Ke Xue 中医外科学
Traditional Chinese Medicine for Surgical Diseases (1999). Tan Xin–Hua, Lu De–Ming (eds.), Peoples Medical Publishing House, Beijing

Zhong Yi Zhi Liao Yi Nan Za Bing Mi Yao 中医治疗疑难杂病秘要
Treatment of Miscellaneous Difficult Diseases with Chinese Medicine (1993) Zhang Jing–Ren (ed.), Wenhui Publishing

Zui Xin Fang Ji Shou Ce 最新方剂手册
Handbook of the Latest Prescriptions (1998). Fan Wei–Hong (ed.), Central Plains Publishing, Henan

Classical Chinese sources of prescriptions

Ben Cao Yan Yi 本草衍义
Extension of the Materia Medica, Kou Zong–Shi 1116

Cheng Fang Bian Du 成方碥读
Convenient Reader of Established Formulas, Yu Gen–Chu 1776

Chong Ding Tong Su Shang Han Lun 重订通俗伤寒伦
Revised Popular Guide to the Discussion of Cold Induced Disorders, Zhang Bing–Cheng 1904

Chong Lou Yu Yao 重楼玉钥
Jade Key to Layered Stories, Zheng Mei–Jian 1838

Chuan Xin Shi Yong Fang 传信适用方
Transmitted Trustworthy and Suitable Formulas, Wu Yan–Kui 1180

Ci Shi Nan Zhi 此事难知
Hard Won Knowledge, Wang Hao–Gu 1308

Dan Xi Xin Fa 丹溪心法
Teachings of Zhu Dan–Xi, Zhu Dan–Xi 1481

Dan Xi Xin Fa Fu Yu 丹溪心法附馀
Additions to the Teachings of Zhu Dan–Xi, Fang Guang–Lei 1536

Dong Yuan Shi Xiao Fang 东垣试效方
Effective Formulas from Li Dong–Yuan's Practice, Li Dong–Yuan 1266

Dou Zhen Shi Yi Xin Fa 痘疹世医新法
Teachings of Generations of Physicians about Pox, Wan Quan 1568

Fu Qing Zhu Nu Ke 付青主女科
Women's Diseases According to Fu Qing–Zhu, Fu Shan (Qing–Zhu), 1827

Fu Ren Liang Fang 妇人良方
Fine Formulas for Women, Chen Zi–Ming 1237

Han Shi Yi Tong 韩氏医通
Comprehensive Medicine According to Master Han, Han Mao 1522

He Ji Ju Fang 和剂局方
Imperial Grace Formulary of the Tai Ping Era, Imperial Medical Department 1107–1110

Hong Shi Ji Yan Fang 洪氏集验方
Master Hong's Experiential Formulae, Hong Zun 1170

Huo Luan Lun 霍乱论
Discussion of Sudden Turmoil Disorders, Wan Shi–Xiong 1862

Ji Sheng Fang 济生方
Formulas to Aid the Living, Yan Yong–He 1253

Jiao Zhu Fu Ren Liang Fang 校注妇人良方
Revised Fine Formulas for Women, Chen Zi–Ming 16th C

Jin Gui Yao Lüe 金匮要略
Essentials from the Golden Cabinet, Zhang Zhong–Jing 210

Jing Yue Quan Shu 景岳全书
The Complete Works of Jing Yue, Zhang Jing–Yue 1624

Lan Shi Mi Cang 兰室秘藏
Secrets from the Orchid Chamber, Li Dong–Yuan 1336

Lei Zheng Huo Ren Shu 类证活人书
Book to Safeguard Life Arranged According to Pattern, Zhu Gong 1108

Liang Fang Ji Ye 良方集腋
Small Collection of Fine Formulas, Xie Yuan–Qing 1842

Ma Zhen Quan Shu 麻疹全书
Complete Treatise on Measles, Hua Shou (att.) Yuan dynasty

Ming Yi Zhi Zhang 明医指掌
Displays of Enlightened Physicians Huang Fu–Zhong 16th Cent.

Nan Yang Huo Ren Shu 南阳活人书
The Nanyang Book to Safeguard Life, Zhu Gong 1111

Nei Ke Zhai Yao 内科摘要
Summary of Internal Medicine, Yu Ying–Tai 19th Cent.

Nei Wai Shang Bian Huo Lun 内外伤辨惑论
Clarifying Doubts about Injury from Internal and External Causes, Li Dong–Yuan 1231

Pi Wei Lun 脾胃轮
Discussion of the Spleen and Stomach, Li Dong–Yuan 1249

Pu Ji Ben Shi Fang 普济本事方
Formulas of Universal Benefit from My Practice, Xu Shi–Wei 1132

Qi Xiao Liang Fang 奇效良方
Remarkably Effective Fine Formulas, Dong Su, Fang Xian 1470

Qian Jin Yao Fang 千金要方
Thousand Ducat Formulas, Sun Si–Miao 652

Quan Sheng Zhi Mi Fang 全生指迷方
Guiding Formulas for the Whole Life, Sun Ren–Cun, Song dynasty

Ren Zhai Zhi Zhi 仁斋直指
Straight Directions from Ren–Zhai, Yang Shi–Ying 1264

San Yin Ji Yi Bing Zheng Fang Lun 三因极一病症方论
Discussion of Illnesses, Patterns and Formulas Related to the Unification of the Three Etiologies, Chen Yan 1174

Shang Han Liu Shu 伤寒六书
Six Texts on Cold Induced Disorders, Tao Hua 1445

Shang Han Lun 伤寒论
Discussion of Cold Induced Disorders, Zhang Zhong–Jing 210

She Sheng Mi Pou 摄生秘剖
 Secret Investigations into Obtaining Health, Hong Ji 1638

She Sheng Zhong Miao Fang 摄生众妙方
 Marvelous Formulas for the Health of the Multitudes, Zhang Shi–Che 1550

Shen Shi Yao Han 审视瑶函
 Scrutiny of the Precious Jade Case, Fu Yun–Ke 1644

Shen Shi Zun Sheng Shu 沈氏尊生书
 Master Shen's Book for Revering Life, Shen Jin–Ao 1773

Shi Bing Lun 时病论
 Discussion of Seasonal Diseases, Lei Feng 1882

Shi Fang Ge Kuo 时方歌括
 Compendium of Songs on Modern Formulas, Chen Nian–Zi, 1801

Shi Re Lun 湿热论
 Discussion of Damp Heat, Jiang Sen 1989

Shi Re Tiao Bian 湿热条辨
 Systematic Differentiation of Damp Heat, Xue Sheng–Bai, Qing dynasty

Shi Yao Shen Shu 十药神书
 Miraculous Book of Ten Remedies, Ge Qian–Sun 1348

Shi Yi De Xiao Fang 世医得效方
 Effective Formulae from Generations of Physicians, Wei Yi–Lin 1345

Shi Zhai Bai Yi Yuan Fang 是斋百一选方
 Selected Formulas from the Praiseworthy Studio, Wang Qiu 1196

Su Wen Bing Ji Qi Yi Bao Ming Ji 素问病机气宜保命集
 Collection of Writings on the Mechanism of Illness, Suitability of Qi and the Safeguarding of Life as Discussed in the Basic Questions, Zhang Yuan Su 1186

Ti Ren Hui Bian 体仁汇编
 Compilation of Materials of Benevolence for the Body, Peng Yong–Guang 1549

Tong Su Shang Han Lun 通俗伤寒论
 Popular Guide to the Discussion of Cold Induced Disorders, Yu Gen–Chu 1776

Wai Ke Zheng Zhi Quan Sheng Ji 外科证治全生集
 Complete Collection of Patterns and Treatments in External Medicine, Wang Wei–De 1740

Wai Ke Zheng Zong 外科正宗
 True Lineage of External Medicine, Chen Shi–Gong 1617

Wai Tai Mi Yao 外台秘要
 Arcane Essentials from the Imperial Library, Wang Tao 752

Wan Bing Hui Chun 万病回春
 Return to Spring from the Myriad Diseases, Gong Ting–Xian 1587

Wei Sheng Bao Jian 卫生宝鉴
 Precious Mirror of Health, Luo Tian–Yi, Yuan dynasty, 13th Cent.

Wen Bing Tiao Bian 温病条辨
  Systematic Differentiation of Warm Diseases, Wu Ju–Tong, 1798

Wen Re Feng Yuan 温热逢原
  Encountering the Source of Warm–Heat Pathogen Diseases, Liu Bao–Yi, late Qing dynasty

Wen Re Jing Wei 温热经纬
  Warp and Woof of Warm Febrile Diseases, Wang Meng–Ying 1852

Wen Re Lun 温热论
  Discussion of Warm Heat Pathogen Disorders, Ye Tian–Shi 1766

Wen Yi Lun 温疫论
  Discussion of Epidemic Warm Disease, Wu You–Ke 1642

Xian Xing Zhai Yi Xue Guang Bi Ji 先醒斋医学广笔记
  Wide Ranging Medical Notes from the First Awakened Studio, Miao Xi–Hong 1613

Xiao Er Yao Zheng Zhi Jue 小儿药证直诀
  Craft of Medical Treatments for Childhood Disease Patterns, Qian Yi 1119

Xu Ming Yi Lei An 续名医类案 Continuation of Famous Physicians Cases Organized by Categories, Wei Zhi–Xiu 1770

Xuan Ming Fang Lun 宣明方论
  Clear and Open Discussion of Formulas, Liu Wan–Su 1172

Yan Fang Xin Bian 验方新编
  New Compilation of Experiential Formulas, Bao Xiang–Ao 1846

Yang Ke Xin De Ji 疡科心得集
  Collected Experience on Treating Sores, Gao Bin–Jun 1806

Yang Shi Jia Zang Fang 杨氏家藏方
  Collected Formulas of the Yang Family, Yang Tan 1178

Yang Yi Da Quan 疡医大全
  Comprehensive Treatment of Skin Sores, Gu Shi–Cheng 1760

Yi Fang Ji Jie 医方集解
  Analytic Collection of Medical Formulas, Wang Ang 1682

Yi Fang Kao 医方考
  Investigations of Medical Formulas, Wu Kun 1584

Yi Ji Bao Jian 医级宝鉴
  Precious Mirror for Advancement of Medicine, Dong Xi–Yuan 1777

Yi Lin Gai Cuo 医林改错
  Corrections of Errors among Physicians, Wang Qing–Ren 1830

Yi Men Fa Lu 医门法律
  Precepts for Physicians, Yu Chang 1658

Yi Xue Fa Ming 医学发明
  Medical Innovations, Li Dong–Yuan, 13th Cent.

Yi Xue Ru Men 医学入门
Introduction to Medicine, Li Chan 1575

Yi Xue Xin Wu 医学心悟
Medical Revelations, Cheng Guo–Peng 1732

Yi Xue Zheng Chuan 医学正传
True Lineage of Medicine, Yu Tian–Min 1515

Yi Xue Zhong Zhong Can Xi Lu 医学衷中参西录
Records of Heart Felt Experience in Medicine with Reference to the West
Zhang Xi–Chun 1918–1934

Yi Yuan 医原
Origin of Medicine, Shi Shou–Tang 1861

Yi Zhen Yi De 疫疹一得
Achievments Regarding Epidemic Rashes, Yu Shi–Yu 1794

Yi Zong Bi Du 医宗必读
Required Reading from the Masters of Medicine, Li Zhong–Zi 1637

Yi Zong Jin Jian 医宗金鉴
The Golden Mirror of Medicine, Wu Qian 1742

Yong Lei Qian Fang 永类钤方
Everlasting Categorization of Inscribed Formulas, Li Zhong–Nan 1331

Za Bing Yuan Liu Xi Zhu 杂病源流犀烛
Wondrous Lantern for Peering into the Origin and Development of Miscellaneous Diseases, Shen Jin–Ao 1773

Zheng Ti Lei Yao 正体类要
Catalogued Essentials for Correcting the Body, Bi Li–Zhai 1529

Zheng Yin Mai Zhi 症因脉治
Symptoms, Cause, Pulse and Treatment, Qin Zhi–Zhen 1706

Zheng Zhi Zhun Sheng 证治准绳
Standards of Patterns and Treatment, Wang Ken–Tang 1602

Zhong Zang Jing 中藏经
Treasury Classic, attributed to Hua Tuo, 4th Cent.

English sources and references

Abbate S (2001) The Art of Palpatory Diagnosis In Oriental Medicine, Churchill Livingstone, Edinburgh

Baldry PE (1993) Acupuncture, Trigger Points and Musculoskeletal Pain, Churchill Livingstone, Edinburgh

Bensky D and O'Connor (1985) Acupuncture: A Comprehensive Text, Eastland Press, Seattle, Washington

Bensky D, Clavey S and Stoger E (2004) Chinese Herbal Medicine: Materia Medica, (3rd ed.) Eastland Press, Seattle, Washington

Bensky D and Barolet R (1990) Chinese Herbal Medicine: Formulas and Strategies, Eastland Press, Seattle, Washington

Beers M and Berkow R, et al. (1999) The Merck Manual (17th Ed). Merck Research Laboratories, Whitehouse Station, New Jersey

Chen Ke–Ji (1994) Traditional Chinese Medicine Clinical Case Studies. Foreign Languages Press, Beijing

Chi–Shing Cho, W, et al. (2005) An outline of diabetes mellitus and its treatment by traditional Chinese medicine and acupuncture. J. Chin. Med, 78:29–36

Choate C (1998) Diabetes Mellitus 1. J. Chin. Med, 58:5–14

Choate C (1999) Diabetes Mellitus 2. J. Chin. Med, 59:5–12

Choate C (1999) Diabetes Mellitus 3. J. Chin. Med, 60:27–36

Clavey S (2003) Fluid Physiology and Pathology in Traditional Chinese Medicine 2nd ed., Churchill Livingstone, Melbourne, Australia

Clavey S (1995) Spleen and Stomach yin deficiency; differentiation and treatment. J. Chin. Med, 47:23–29

Clavey S, et al. (1998) Venting insubstantial pathogens and deep lying qi; Newsletter of the Australian Chinese Medicine Education and Research Council, Melbourne, Australia

Davis T (1992) Diabetes Mellitus: West meets East; reflections upon TCM theory. Aust. J. Acup. 19:9–19.

Deadman P, Al–Khafaji M and Baker K (1998) A Manual of Acupuncture, Journal of Chinese Medicine Publications, Hove, UK

Deadman P, Al–Khafaji M and Baker K (1998) Some acupuncture points which treat headache. J. Chin. Med, 56:5–18

Dharmananda S (2003) Treatment of diabetes with Chinese herbs and acupuncture. Internet Journal of the Institute for Traditional Medicine, Portland.

Edwards CRW et al. (1995) Davidson's Principles and Practice of Medicine (17th Ed), Churchill Livingstone, Edinburgh

Ellis A (2003) Notes from South Mountain: A Guide to Concentrated Herb Granules. Thin Moon Publishing, Berkley California.

Ellis A and Wiseman N (1994) Fundamentals of Chinese Medicine, Paradigm Publications, Brookline, Boston

Fruehauf H (1998) Gu syndrome. J. Chin. Med, 57:10–17

Gaohui Liu (2005) Warm Disease Pathogens. Eastland Press, Seattle

Gascoigne S (2001) The Clinical Medicine Guide, A Holistic Perspective, Jigme Press, Dorking, Surrey

Haines N (1993) Diabetes; Treatment by Acupuncture. J. Chin. Med. 43:5–12.

Hsu HY (1980) Commonly Used Chinese Herbal Formulas with Illustrations, Oriental Healing Arts Institute, Los Angeles, California

Jiao Shu–De (2005) Ten Lectures on the Use of Formulas from the Personal experience of Jiao Shu–De. Paradigm Publications, Taos NM

Kirschbaum B (2000) Atlas of Chinese Tongue Diagnosis. Eastland Press, Seattle

Lade H (1999) Diabetes. Pacific J. Oriental Med. 12:34–42

Legge D (2010) Close to the Bone, 2nd ed., Sydney College Press, Sydney

Leggett D (1999) Recipes for Self Healing, Meridian Press, Totnes, Devon

Leggett D (1998) Helping Ourselves: A Guide to Traditional Chinese Food Energetics, Meridian Press, Totnes, Devon

Li WL et al. (2004) Natural medicines used in the traditional Chinese medical system for therapy of diabetes mellitus. Journal of Ethnopharmacology 92:1–21

Lorenz P (1997) Differential Diagnosis (4th ed.) Social Science Press, Katoomba, NSW, Australia

Maciocia G (2004) Diagnosis in Chinese Medicine, A Comprehensive Guide, Churchill Livingstone, Edinburgh

Maciocia G (1989) The Foundations of Chinese Medicine, Churchill Livingstone, Edinburgh

Maciocia G (2007) The Practice of Chinese Medicine (2nd ed.), Churchill Livingstone, Edinburgh

Maclean W (2002) The Clinical Manual of Chinese Herbal Patent Medicines, (2nd ed.) Pangolin Press, Sydney

Maoshing Ni (1995) The Yellow Emperors Classic of Medicine; A New Translation of the Neijing Suwen with Commentary. Shambala Publications, Boston.

Matsumotos K, Birch S (1988) Hara Diagnosis: Reflections on the Sea. Paradigm Publications, Brookline, Boston

Murtagh J (2007) General Practice (4th ed.), McGraw Hill Book Company, Sydney

Neeb G (2007) Blood Stasis. Churchill Livingstone, Edinburgh

Pitchford P (1993) Healing with Whole Foods: Oriental Traditions and Modern Nutrition. North Atlantic Books, Berkeley, California

Schnyer R, Allan J (2001) Acupuncture in the Treatment of Depression. Churchill Livingstone, Edinburgh

Scott JP (1999) Acupuncture in the Treatment of Children (3rd Edition), Eastland Press, Seattle

Takako N et al (2001) A Study of Kampo Medicines in a Diabetic Nephropathy Model. J. Trad. Med 18:161–168

Travell JG and Simons DG (1983) Myofacial Pain and Dysfunction. The Trigger Point Manual, Williams and Wilkins, Baltimore

Wiseman N, Ye F (1998) A Practical Dictionary of Chinese Medicine, Paradigm Publications, Brookline, Boston

Xian L and Rodriguez J (2001) The Application of Tonifying Yang for the Treatment of Diabetes. J. Chin. Med. 67:34–36

Yin DH et al. (2009) Analysis of Chinese medicine syndrome pattern in patients with type 2 diabetes and its relationship with chronic complications. Chinese Journal of Integrated Traditional and Western Medicine 29:506–510

Yuzo Sato et al (2006) Role of Herbal Medicine in the Prevention and Treatment of Diabetes and Diabetic Complications. J. Trad. Med 23:185–195

Zhang Zhong–Jing (c. 210AD) Synopsis of Prescriptions of the Golden Chamber with 300 Cases (*Jin Gui Yao Lüe)*. Translated by Luo Xi–Wen (1995) New World Press, Beijing, China

Zhang Zhong–Jing (c. 210AD) Treatise on Febrile Diseases Caused By Cold with 500 Cases (*Shang Han Lun*). Translated by Luo Xi–Wen (1993) New World Press, Beijing, China

INDEX

Page numbers followed by *t* refer to tables; numbers followed by *f* refer to illustrations and diagrams.